UROLOGY

VOLUME ONE

Edited by

MEREDITH CAMPBELL, M.S., M.D., F.A.C.S.

EMERITUS PROFESSOR OF UROLOGY
NEW YORK UNIVERSITY

With the Collaboration of
Fifty-One Contributing Authorities

ILLUSTRATED WITH 1148 FIGURES

W. B. SAUNDERS COMPANY

Philadelphia and London

TO THOSE WHO MAY BE
HELPED BY THESE VOLUMES

CONTRIBUTING AUTHORS

CARL ABERHART, M.D., M.S. (Tor.) ....Toronto, Canada

Assistant Professor of Surgery, University of Toronto; Surgeon, Department of Urology, Toronto General Hospital; Consultant and Head of Department of Urology, Sunnybrook Hospital (D.V.A.).

EDWIN P. ALYEA, M.D., F.A.C.S. ....Durham, N.C.

Professor of Urology, Duke University Medical School; Chief, Urology Service, Duke University Hospital; Consultant, Veterans Administration Hospital, Watts Hospital, Lincoln Hospital.

J. E. ASH, M.D., Colonel (U.S.A.) Rtd. ....Washington, D.C.

Former Director, Armed Forces Institute of Pathology.

EDGAR BURNS, M.D., F.A.C.S. ....New Orleans, La.

Professor of Urology and Chairman of the Department, Tulane University School of Medicine; Head of Department of Urology, Ochsner Clinic; Director of Urologic Service, Ochsner Foundation Hospital.

MEREDITH F. CAMPBELL, M.S., M.D., F.A.C.S. ....Miami, Fla.

Emeritus Professor of Urology, New York University; Consulting Urologist, Bellevue Hospital, New York; St. Francis Hospital, Miami Beach, Fla.; Variety Children's Hospital, Miami.

ARTHUR B. CECIL, B.Sc., M.D. ....Los Angeles, Calif.

Visiting Urologist, Hospital of the Good Samaritan.

FLETCHER H. COLBY, B.S., M.D., F.A.C.S. ....Boston, Mass.

Associate Clinical Professor of Urology, Harvard Medical School; Chief of Urological Service, Massachusetts General Hospital; Consultant in Urology, Lakeville State Sanatorium.

J. A. CAMPBELL COLSTON, M.D. ....Baltimore, Md.

Associate Professor of Urology, Johns Hopkins Medical School.

EDWARD N. COOK, M.D., M.S. .... *Rochester, Minn.*

  Associate Professor of Urology, Mayo Foundation, Graduate School, University of Minnesota.

C. D. CREEVY, M.D. .... *Minneapolis, Minn.*

  Professor of Surgery and Head of Division of Urology, University of Minnesota.

ARCHIE L. DEAN, B.S., M.D. .... *New York, N.Y.*

  Professor of Urology, New York Polyclinic Medical School and Hospital; Attending Surgeon, Memorial Hospital; Attending Urologist, Polyclinic Hospital; Senior Consultant in Urology, Veterans Administration Hospital, Bronx, New York.

CLYDE L. DEMING, A.B., M.D., Sc.D., F.A.C.S. .... *New Haven, Conn.*

  Clinical Professor of Urology, Yale School of Medicine; Urologist-in-Chief, Grace-New Haven Community Hospital; Chief Consultant in Urology, Veterans Administration Hospital, West Haven, Conn.; Consulting Urologist, Norwalk, Stamford, Meriden, Willimantic and Derby, Conn. Hospitals.

AUSTIN INGRAM DODSON, M.D., F.A.C.S. .... *Richmond, Va.*

  Professor of Urology, Medical College of Virginia; Urologist, Hospital Division of Medical College of Virginia, St. Elizabeth's Hospital, St. Luke's Hospital.

JOHN L. EMMETT, M.D., M.S. .... *Rochester, Minn.*

  Professor of Urology, Mayo Foundation, Graduate School, University of Minnesota.

EARL T. ENGLE, Ph.D. .... *New York, N.Y.*

  Professor of Anatomy, College of Physicians and Surgeons, Columbia University.

P. A. FERRIER, M.D., F.A.C.S. .... *Los Angeles, Calif.*

  Department of Urology, Los Angeles General Hospital.

THOMAS E. GIBSON, A.B., M.A., M.D., F.A.C.S. ...... *San Francisco, Calif.*

  Chief, Department of Urology, Southern Pacific Hospital; Chief, Department of Urology, St. Joseph's Hospital; Visiting Urologist, St. Francis and St. Mary's Hospitals; Civilian Consultant in Urology, Letterman Army Hospital, San Francisco.

ELVIRA GOETTSCH, M.D. ....*Los Angeles, Calif.*

Formerly Associate Professor of Pediatrics, University of Southern California; Consultant, Children's Hospital.

WILLIAM GOLDRING, B.S., M.D. ....*New York, N.Y.*

Associate Professor of Medicine, New York University College of Medicine; Visiting Physician, University Hospital, Bellevue Hospital; Consulting Physician, Beth Israel Hospital, Goldwater Memorial Hospital.

BENJAMIN H. HAGER, B.S., M.S., M.D. ....*Los Angeles, Calif.*

Formerly Professor of Surgery (Urology) and Chairman of the Department of the University of Southern California.

J. HARTWELL HARRISON, M.D., F.A.C.S. ....*Boston, Mass.*

Associate Clinical Professor of Genito-Urinary Surgery, Harvard Medical School; Urologic Surgeon, Peter Bent Brigham Hospital.

S. G. HERSHEY, B.S., M.D. ....*New York, N.Y.*

Clinical Professor, Department of Anesthesiology, New York University Post Graduate Medical School; Director of Anesthesiology, Beth Israel Hospital; Assistant Visiting Anesthetist, Bellevue Hospital.

CHARLES C. HIGGINS, M.D., F.A.C.S. ....*Cleveland, Ohio*

Professor of Urology, Frank E. Bunts Educational Institute; Head, Department of Urology, Cleveland Clinic.

FRANK HINMAN, Jr., M.D., F.A.C.S. ....*San Francisco, Calif.*

Assistant Clinical Professor of Urology, University of California School of Medicine; Attending Urologist, University of California Hospital, Franklin Hospital, San Francisco Hospital.

ROBERT S. HOTCHKISS, M.D. ....*New York, N.Y.*

Professor and Chairman, Department of Urology, New York University Post-Graduate Medical School; Director of Urology, 4th Surgical Division (Urology), Bellevue Hospital; Director of Urology, University Hospital; Associate in Urology, New York Hospital; Consultant in Urology, New York Infirmary.

CHARLES B. HUGGINS, M.D., D.Sc. ....*Chicago, Ill.*

Director, Ben May Laboratory for Cancer Research, University of Chicago.

JOSEPH W. JAILER, PH.D., M.D. . . . .*New York, N.Y.*

  Associate Professor of Clinical Medicine, Columbia University; Assistant
  Attending Physician, Presbyterian Hospital.

DALTON JENKINS, M.D. . . . .*Denver, Colo.*

  Assistant Professor of Medicine, University of Colorado School of
  Medicine.

HUGH J. JEWETT, A.B., M.D. . . . .*Baltimore, Md.*

  Associate Professor of Urology, Johns Hopkins University School of
  Medicine; Urologist, Johns Hopkins Hospital.

TERENCE MILLIN, M.CH., F.R.C.S., F.R.C.S.I., F.A.C.S. . .*London, England*

  Consulting Urological Surgeon, Westminster Hospital, Royal Masonic
  Hospital; Director, Department of Urology, Queen's Gate Clinic.

CARL R. MOORE, PH.D., SC.D. . . . .*Chicago, Ill.*

  Professor of Zoology, University of Chicago.

THOMAS D. MOORE, B.A., M.D., M.S., F.A.C.S. . . . .*Memphis, Tenn.*

  Professor of Urology, University of Tennessee, College of Medicine;
  Chief, Department of Urology, John Gaston Hospital; Chief Urological
  Surgeon, Moore Clinic; Attending Urologist, Baptist Memorial Hospital.

PETER A. NARATH, M.D., DR. MED. (HEIDELBERG), F.I.C.S. .*New York, N.Y.*

  Adj. Professor of Urology, New York Polyclinic Medical School and
  Hospital; Attending Urologist, Northern Westchester Hospital, Mt.
  Kisco, New York; Associate Urologist, New York Polyclinic Medical
  School and Hospital.

REED M. NESBIT, A.B., M.D., F.A.C.S. . . . .*Ann Arbor, Mich.*

  Professor of Surgery, University of Michigan Medical School; Chief of
  Urological Service, University of Michigan Hospital.

VINCENT J. O'CONOR, B.S., M.D. . . . .*Chicago, Ill.*

  Professor and Head of the Department of Urology, Northwestern University Medical School; Chairman, Department of Urology, Wesley Memorial Hospital.

ROBERT F. PITTS, M.D., PH.D., F.A.C.P. . . . .*New York, N.Y.*

  Professor of Physiology and Biophysics, Cornell University Medical
  College.

GEORGE C. PRATHER, M.D., F.A.C.S. ....*Boston, Mass.*

Head, Department of Urology, Beth Israel Hospital; Urologist, New England Baptist Hospital; Chief, Urological Service, Newton-Wellesley Hospital; Consulting Urologist, Boston City Hospital and Boston Lying-In Hospital; Associate in Surgery, Harvard Medical School.

JAMES T. PRIESTLEY, M.D., M.S., Ph.D., F.A.C.S. ....*Rochester, Minn.*

Professor of Surgery, Mayo Foundation, Graduate School, University of Minnesota.

DALTON K. ROSE, M.D., F.A.C.S. ....*St. Louis, Mo.*

Emeritus Professor of Clinical Urology, Washington University School of Medicine; Associate Surgeon, Barnes & St. Louis Children's Hospital; Consulting Staff, St. Luke's Hospital; General Staff, Jewish Hospital; Consulting Staff, Ellis Fischel State Cancer Hospital, Columbia, Mo., and Los Alamos Medical Center, Los Alamos, N. Mex.

E. A. ROVENSTINE, A.B., M.D., Sc.D. ....*New York, N.Y.*

Professor, Department of Anesthesiology, New York Univ. Post-Graduate Medical School; Director of Anesthesia, Bellevue and University Hospitals.

CARL RUSCHE, B.Sc., M.D., F.A.C.S. ....*Los Angeles, Calif.*

Clinical Professor of Surgery, University of Southern California; Senior Attending Surgeon, Los Angeles County General Hospital, Children's Hospital, Hollywood Presbyterian Hospital, Cedars of Lebanon Hospital, St. Vincent's Hospital and Veterans Administration Hospital, Long Beach, Calif.

LUIS A. SANJURJO, M.D., F.A.C.S. ....*San Juan, Puerto Rico*

Professor of Urology and Head of Section, School of Medicine, University of Puerto Rico; Chief Urologist, San Juan City Hospital; Consulting Urologist, Veterans Administration Hospital; Attending Urologist, Mimiya Hospital.

JAMES C. SARGENT, M.D., F.A.C.S. ....*Milwaukee, Wisconsin*

Clinical Professor and Director, Department of Urology, Marquette University School of Medicine.

A. J. SCHOLL, M.D., M.S., F.A.C.S. ....*Los Angeles, Calif.*

Chief of Urology Section, St. Vincent's Hospital; Department of Urology, Cedars of Lebanon Hospital; Department of Urology, Santa Fe Hospital.

WILLIAM WALLACE SCOTT, M.D., Ph.D. ....*Baltimore, Md.*

Professor of Urology, The Johns Hopkins University School of Medicine; Urologist-in-Charge, The Johns Hopkins Hospital.

WINFIELD W. SCOTT, B.S., M.D. ....*Rochester, N.Y.*

Associate Professor of Urological Surgery, The University of Rochester School of Medicine and Dentistry; Associate Surgeon and Urologist-in-Chief, Strong Memorial and Rochester Municipal Hospitals; Consulting Urologist, Genesee Hospital.

PARKE G. SMITH, M.D., A.B., F.A.C.S. ....*Miami, Fla.*

Formerly Professor of Urology, University of Cincinnati; Director, Urologic Service, Mercy Hospital, Miami, Fla.

GERSHOM J. THOMPSON, M.D., M.S., F.A.C.S. ....*Rochester, Minn.*

Professor of Urology, Mayo Foundation, Graduate School, University of Minnesota.

IAN THOMPSON, M.D. ....*New Orleans, La.*

Assistant in Urology, Tulane University School of Medicine.

ROBERT V. THOMSON, M.D. ....*Coral Gables, Fla.*

Chief of Laboratory Service, Veterans Administration Hospital; Pathology Department, University of Miami School of Medicine, Miami.

SAMUEL A. VEST, M.D., F.A.C.S. ....*Charlottesville, Va.*

Professor and Head, Department of Urology, University of Virginia; Chief Urologist, University of Virginia Hospital.

LAWRENCE R. WHARTON, Ph.B., M.D. ....*Baltimore, Md.*

Assistant Professor of Gynecology, The Johns Hopkins University; Attending Gynecologist, The Johns Hopkins Hospital, Union Memorial Hospital, Hospital for the Women of Maryland, Sinai Hospital and Mercy Hospital.

PREFACE

A publisher's proposal to write a one-volume textbook of Urology was the nidus of this UROLOGY. I declined this proposition because today's progress and developments in this branch of medicine and its collateral fields are so amazing, rapid, and variant that it is now beyond the scope of any one person to present all phases of this subject adequately. To achieve recognized authority for UROLOGY as distinguished from mere compilation gleaned from others, outstanding collaborators were enlisted. In this corps are those nationally or internationally renowned for their intensive investigative work and unusually wide experience in the sphere of their respective topics. Many of these contributions are classic monographs.

Urology has been comprehensively brought up to date and its associated fundamental sciences such as Physiology, Biochemistry, Neurology and Endocrinology are amply considered. Yet, it is likely that here and there a lesion or condition has been slighted or even omitted. Modern key references are given in the bibliographies. Several illustrations used in my CLINICAL PEDIATRIC UROLOGY (1951) appear, but since W. B. Saunders Company published that book too, specific designation of these has not been made.

I am inexpressibly grateful to my many colleagues in this cooperative undertaking, keenly realizing that they have given to the utmost of the fruits of their own investigations, skill, and experience to make these volumes worthy and mutually creditable. I am thankful to those who have permitted use of their illustrations. Special appreciation is expressed to Miss Evelyn Northridge for her invaluable assistance in this work since its inception.

The warm cooperation of the publishers, their unusually generous latitude in these days of almost prohibitive printing costs, and their unsurpassed artistry in scientific book production have been most stimulating to our ambition that this UROLOGY be truly definitive, current, and liberally illustrated.

MEREDITH CAMPBELL

Miami, Florida

CONTENTS

VOLUME ONE

Chapter 2. INFECTIONS AND INFLAMMATIONS OF THE MALE GENITAL
            TRACT 635

Edwin P. Alyea, M.D.

Chapter 3. INFECTIONS AND DISEASES OF THE SCROTUM AND ITS
            CONTENTS 666

Samuel A. Vest, M.D.

Section VII

INFERTILITY IN THE MALE 733

Robert S. Hotchkiss, B.S., M.D.

VOLUME TWO

VOLUME THREE

Section XV

UROLOGIC SURGERY 1701

VOLUME ONE

Section I

ANATOMY AND PHYSIOLOGY

CHAPTER 1

Anatomy and Surgical Approach to the Urogenital Tract in the Male*

AUSTIN INGRAM DODSON, M.D.

THE KIDNEYS AND THEIR SUPPORTING STRUCTURES

The kidneys are two ovoid-shaped organs located in the retroperitoneal space at the level of the upper lumbar region, and lying one on each side of the spinal column. The right kidney is normally at a slightly lower level than the left. Posteriorly, they are in apposition with the diaphragm and the quadratus lumborum and psoas major muscles, and extend obliquely downward and outward from the twelfth dorsal to the upper margin of the third lumbar vertebrae (Fig. 1). The greater portion of each kidney lies within the bony thorax which affords considerable protection against injury from external trauma.

The structures in contact with the anterior and medial surfaces of each kidney vary, depending on whether the right or left organ is considered. The right kidney is in contact anteriorly with the peritoneum, liver, duodenum and ascending colon (Fig. 2). The gallbladder lies in a more anterior plane directly over the kidney. The shadows of biliary and renal calculi are at times confused. At the medial aspect of this kidney lies the vena cava. In front of the left kidney are the peritoneum, stomach, tail of the pancreas, spleen, and the descending colon. These relationships are of paramount importance in surgery of the kidney, renal pelvis or upper ureter.

Each adult kidney is from 9 to 12.3 cm. long, 4.5 to 6.5 cm. wide, and 2.5 to 3.5 cm. thick, and the average weight per kidney is in the range of 110 to 140 grams. The anterior and posterior surface of each kidney is convex, as is the external margin. The internal margin is convex at each end and concave in its central portion. This central concavity forms the hilum of the kidney and serves as the sinus through which the pelvis, blood vessels, nerves and lymphatics enter (Fig. 3).

* Special anatomic considerations in the female are discussed in Section XIII.

Each kidney is surrounded by a mass of fat and is enclosed in a fascial envelope, the renal fascia. The *renal fascia* is formed by a condensation of the retroperitoneal connective tissue and is a part of the fascia propria which reinforces the parietal peritoneum. It is composed of two layers, an anterior and a posterior. The posterior layer is a more definite structure than is the anterior. The posterior layer is also termed the fascia of Gerota

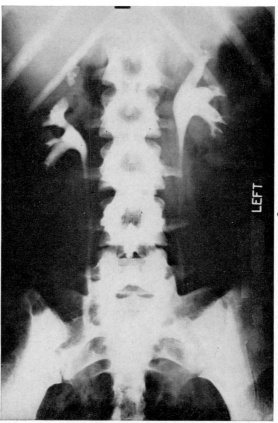

Fig. 1.   Normal position of kidneys. The right kidney is usually slightly lower than the left. Gallstones show position of gallbladder. (From Dodson, Austin I., Urological Surgery, C. V. Mosby Co., 1950.)

or Zuckerkandl. It blends loosely with the fascia overlying the psoas major and quadratus lumborum muscles (Fig. 8). Mitchell stresses this connection as providing an indirect attachment of the renal fascia to the intervertebral discs and the anterior spinal ligaments.

The anterior layer of renal fascia is a less dense structure. It is in contact with and fairly adherent to the overlying peritoneum in some areas. Where adjacent organs, i.e., the colon and duodenum, are in contact with the kidneys, the anterior fascia blends with the intervening connective tissue.

The anterior and posterior layers are firmly united above the kidney and along the lateral margin. The two halves separate above the upper pole of each kidney and after enclosing the corresponding adrenal gland unite again and become continuous with the aponeurotic covering of the diaphragm. Medially the two layers invest the pelvis and renal vessels and continue medialward to blend with the connective tissue elements surrounding the great vessels. There is no cross communication between the two sides. The fascial layers are less densely fused inferiorly and, at the inferomedial aspect, these layers blend with the periureteral fascia.

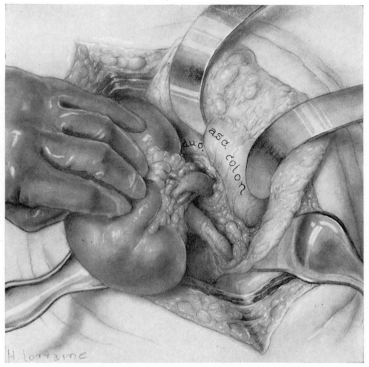

Fig. 2.   Relationship of right kidney to important viscera. (From Dodson, Austin I., Urological Surgery, C. V. Mosby Co., 1950.)

The disposition of the renal fascia is of great importance in perirenal suppuration, hematoma and urinary extravasation. The fascial compartment tends to limit the spread of these processes and serves as a protective barrier in such cases (Fig. 4).

Renal Blood Supply. The renal *arteries* are derived directly from the aorta. The right renal artery crosses behind the vena cava and is longer than its matching vessel on the left. As the renal artery reaches the kidney, it divides into anterior branches, usually two, and a posterior branch. These course between the papillae and are distributed throughout the kidney (Fig. 3). The anterior vessels are more abundant and supply slightly more than one half of the organ. The terminal branches do not anastomose.

For the most part, the ramifications of the renal arteries ultimately pass to the glomerular capillaries in the cortex. However, Trueta has shown that certain of the efferent vessels from the glomeruli lying nearest the medulla divide into straight vessels that pass toward the apices of the medullary tissue. This vascular network constitutes the Trueta shunt and on occasion is capable of transporting most, or all, of the arterial supply of the kidney, thus, in effect, shutting off the supply to the bulk of the renal cortex.

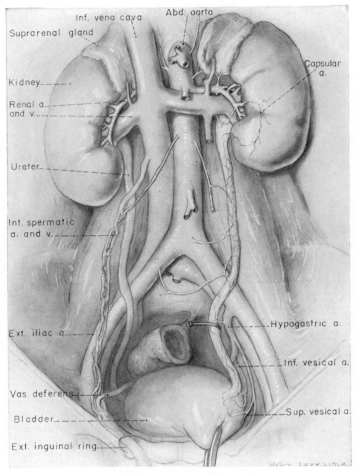

Fig. 3.   Blood supply of kidneys, ureters, bladder and adrenal glands.

Accessory renal arteries frequently arise from the aorta or from the main renal artery. Most often such vessels supply the inferior pole and anterior surface. On occasion these accessory vessels may pass in front of the ureter and interfere with drainage of the kidney. Their presence must be recognized in renal surgery. Failure to ligate these vessels when doing a nephrectomy may result in troublesome bleeding, difficult to control.

The renal *veins* drain into the vena cava and most often lie in front of and accompany the renal artery. These veins anastomose freely until they emerge at the hilum of the kidney. From this point, as a rule, the paired renal veins on each side pass directly to the vena cava, those on the left side being longer than those on the right. The vena cava is frequently in very close apposition to the renal pelvis on the right and is subject to trauma in surgical procedures (Fig. 3). This is especially true in the presence of dense peripelvic adhesions.

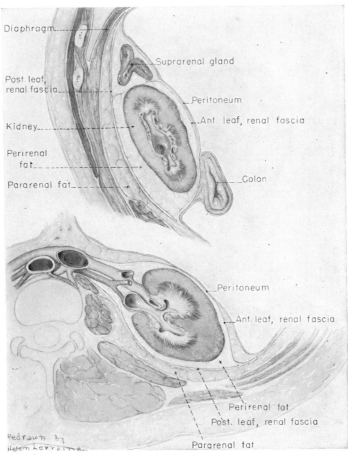

Fig. 4.   Transverse and longitudinal sections through the kidney showing relationship of the renal fascia.

Nerve Supply to the Kidneys. The nerve supply to the kidney is both sympathetic and parasympathetic in origin. The *sympathetic* fibers, derived from the sixth thoracic to the third lumbar segments, pass to the renal plexus via the splanchnic nerves and the semilunar and superior mesenteric ganglia (Fig. 5).

The *parasympathetic* branches are received in the renal plexus. Fibers of both types pass with the branching blood vessels to the arterioles, glomerular capillaries and the renal tubules. Most of the fibers accompany the renal artery to the kidney in three main groups, the superior along the upper border of the artery, the middle along the posterior aspect of the artery, and the inferior along the lower border of the artery. Some few fibers pass directly from the solar plexus and the splanchnic nerves to the kidney and its capsule. In denervation of the renal pedicle, after freeing the kidney, the pedicle must be cleaned of fat and these nerves carefully dissected from

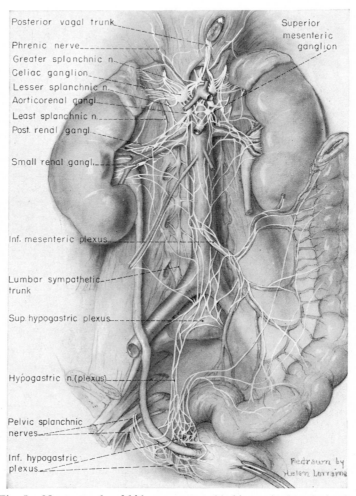

Posterior vagal trunk
Phrenic nerve
Greater splanchnic n.
Celiac ganglion
Lesser splanchnic n.
Aorticorenal gangl.
Least splanchnic n.
Post. renal gangl.

Small renal gangl.

Inf. mesenteric plexus

Lumbar sympathetic trunk

Sup. hypogastric plexus

Hypogastric n.(plexus)

Pelvic splanchnic nerves

Inf. hypogastric plexus

Superior mesenteric ganglion

Redrawn by
Helen Lorraine

Fig. 5.   Nerve supply of kidneys, ureters, bladder and adrenal glands.

the arteries. They are more densely adherent to the distal portion of the arteries (Fig. 5).

Renal Lymphatics. The smaller lymphatics, within the renal parenchyma, accompany the blood vessels and renal tubules. They communicate with the lymphatics of the renal capsule and through these with the lymphatics of the perirenal fat and fascia. The parenchymal lymphatics unite in increasingly larger trunks, emerge at the kidney hilum, and drain into the lymph nodes behind the renal pelvis. The renal lymph nodes drain into the lumbar chain of glands along the aorta and vena cava. The lymphatics of the kidney communicate with those of the periureteral sheath.

Renal Coverings. The adrenal gland lies cap fashion atop the upper pole of the kidney. The kidney itself is invested with a fairly tough, yet thin, fibrous capsule. This covering, the true capsule, is but lightly attached over

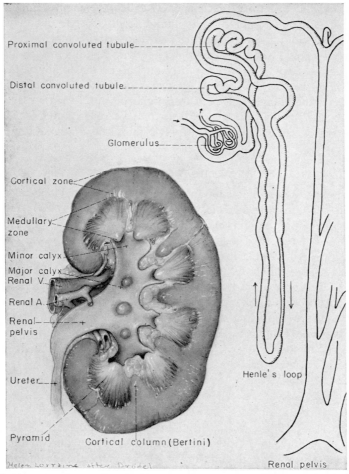

Fig. 6. Section through kidney showing structures of parenchyma. Also diagram of a nephron.

the bulk of the kidney surface. It extends into the hilum and there becomes continuous with the sheath of the renal pelvis and blood vessels. Beneath the renal capsule there is a very thin, incomplete layer of unstriped muscle fibers.

Renal Structure. The kidney parenchyma is divided into medullary and cortical portions. The *cortical* portion is the thinner, outermost layer, about 4 to 5 mm. in thickness, and dark, reddish brown in color. It is situated between the true capsule and the bases of the pyramids, and extends inward between the pyramids. These projections between the pyramids are known as the columns of Bertin. The cortex consists chiefly of the glomerular structures of the kidney (Fig. 6).

The *medullary* portion is the medial segment. It is composed of 8 to 15 reddish colored, striated, conical masses. The bases of these masses are continuous with the cortex and their apices insert into the minor calyces of the kidney pelvis. The tip of each apex is called the papilla and enters the minor calyx with three or more of its mates (Fig. 6). The openings through which these papillae present form the so-called cribriform plate.

The Pelvis of the Kidney. The renal pelvis is a funnel-shaped structure, usually situated partly within and partly outside of the hilum of the kidney. The pelvis may be entirely intrarenal or may be situated entirely outside the kidney. Its widest diameter divides into three or more major calyces. Each major calyx then further subdivides into two or more minor calyces (Fig. 6). The stem or outlet of the renal pelvis joins the ureter at the so-called ureteropelvic junction.

SURGICAL APPROACH TO THE KIDNEY

An understanding of the anatomy of the lumbar or iliocostal region is essential in the consideration of the surgical approach to the kidney. The lumbar area is quadrilateral in shape and located between the lowermost ribs above and the crest of the ilium below. It is bounded posteriorly by the vertebral column, and anteriorly by a vertical line drawn from the anterior superior iliac spine below to the costal margin above. The covering tissues of this area are the skin and two layers of superficial fascia. Lying between these two layers of fascia is a thick pad of highly vascular fat. The blood vessels and nerves supplying the superficial tissues in the lumbar area are of no surgical importance. Neglected infectious processes deep in the lumbar area may spread to the fascial and subcutaneous planes in this region and produce extensive suppuration.

Just beneath the deeper layer of the superficial fascia are found two major muscles. These are the latissimus dorsi and the external oblique muscles. The *latissimus dorsi* takes its origin from the outer edge of the iliac crest at its posterior third, from the spinous processes of the lumbar and sacral vertebrae, and from the dorsal leaf of the dorsolumbar fascia. This muscle passes upward and forward, traversing the posterior superior portion of the lumbar or iliocostal region. It is necessary to divide the anterior fibers of this muscle in order to give adequate exposure in operations upon the kidney. The *external oblique* muscle takes its origin from the ninth, tenth and eleventh ribs, then passes obliquely downward and forward, and crosses the antero-inferior portion of the iliocostal area. In the upper part of the lumbar region, the anterior fibers of the latissimus dorsi cross over the posterior fibers of the external oblique. It is frequently necessary to divide the fibers of the external oblique muscle in order to expose the kidney satisfactorily. Incisions in the lumbar area are best made parallel to the lower ribs in order to avoid division of the deeper nerves and blood vessels.

In the lower portion of the lumbar area the fibers of the latissimus dorsi and external oblique muscles diverge to form the *inferior lumbar triangle,* or Petit's triangle. The iliac crest forms the base of this triangle, the latissimus dorsi, the posterior boundary of the triangle, and the external oblique, the anterior boundary. The internal oblique muscle forms the floor of Petit's triangle. Above and somewhat medial to Petit's triangle lies the *superior*

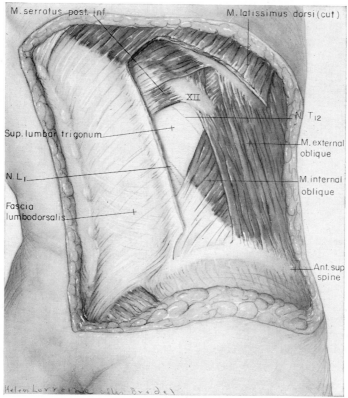

Fig. 7.   Muscles, fascia and nerves of the iliocostal region through which the kidney is usually approached surgically.

or *surgical lumbar triangle.* This triangle is bounded above by the twelfth rib, medially by the depression along the lateral margin of the sacrospinalis muscle, and below by the posterior fibers of the internal oblique muscle. It is through this triangle that the surgical approach to the kidney is most frequently made. The *internal oblique* muscle arises from the iliac crest and from the deeper layer of the lumbodorsal fascia, and passes upward and forward beneath the external oblique muscle. It is often necessary to incise the posterior fibers of this muscle during operations upon the kidney. The superior triangle lies beneath the latissimus dorsi muscle and its floor is formed by the aponeurosis of the transverse abdominis muscle (Fig. 7). The twelfth thoracic or twelfth dorsal nerve will be found running along the superior boundary of this triangle, while the ilio-inguinal and iliohypogastric divisions of the first lumbar nerve pass along the medial border and cross it at its inferior angle (Fig. 7). A knowledge of the course of these nerves is necessary in the surgical approach to the kidney, if damage to these vital structures is to be avoided.

The sacrospinalis and serratus posterior inferior are muscular structures that lie in the same plane with the internal oblique muscle. The *sacrospinalis,* or erector spinae, muscle will be found in the groove along the spinous processes of the vertebral column. This muscle is encased in a fascial sheath that is formed by the posterior and middle layers of the lumbodorsal fascia. It lies at the posterior aspect of the lumbar incisions usually made for operations on the kidney. It is rarely necessary to incise this muscle during the operation.

Crossing the upper posterior angle of the lumbar area, and lying beneath the latissimus dorsi is the *serratus posterior inferior* muscle. This is a thin, flat, quadrangular muscle that overlies the posterior lumbocostal ligament. It takes its origin from the lumbodorsal fascia, the dorsal layer, and attaches to the lower four ribs. Not infrequently this muscle, as well as the underlying lumbocostal ligament must be divided so that the lowermost rib may be displaced upward to facilitate exposure of the kidney. The pleura is in proximity with the lumbocostal ligament, and during division of this ligament may be injured. Care should be taken to protect carefully the pleura at this stage of the operation.

The deepest muscular structure in the posterior wall is the *quadratus lumborum* muscle which lies beneath and extends somewhat beyond the sacrospinalis muscle. The quadratus lumborum takes its origin from the iliac crest and the iliolumbar ligament below and courses upward to terminate in the twelfth rib. This muscle is also contained within a fascial sheath which is formed by the middle and ventral layers of the lumbodorsal fascia. As a rule, this muscle is found at the posterior margin of renal incisions, and it is unnecessary to divide its fibers. It may be retracted somewhat posteriorly, if necessary. The lumbar nerve divides into the iliohypogastric and ilioinguinal portions, which emerge beneath the quadratus lumborum near its insertion, pass along the inner surface of the muscle for a variable distance, and then pass anteriorly, the iliohypogastric branch piercing the aponeurosis of the transversalis muscle and the ilio-inguinal branch entering the transversalis muscle itself. There is a great variation in the course of these nerves, and it is important to look carefully for them during the process of making a lumbar incision and also at the time of closure of the wound.

The deepest layer of muscle and fascia in the anterior portion of the lumbar space is occupied by the aponeurosis of the *transversus abdominis* muscle. This aponeurosis is also called the lumbar fascia and developed as a result of the union of the three layers of the lumbodorsal fascia which enclose the sacrospinalis and quadratus lumborum muscles. These fascial planes pass from the spinous processes of the lumbar vertebrae, enclose the above-mentioned muscles, and then unite along the external borders of these muscles to form a single fascial sheet, the aponeurosis of the transversus abdominis. This lumbar fascia forms the floor of the surgical lumbar

triangle, and is divided in lumbar incisions made during operative procedures on the kidney. Posteriorly, the ilio-inguinal and iliohypogastric nerves
lie beneath the aponeurosis of the transversus abdominis, and as they pass
forward pierce this aponeurosis to run with the muscle fibers. Lying immediately beneath the lumbar fascia there is a layer of fat which separates
it from the perirenal fascia (Fig. 4).

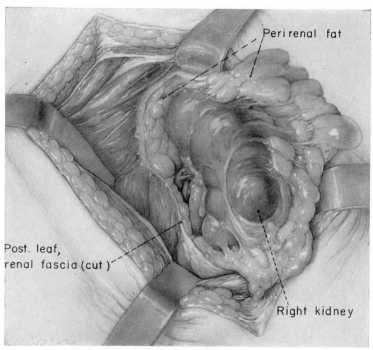

Fig. 8.   Renal fascia divided posteriorly and reflected forward exposing perirenal fat and
kidney. (From Dodson, Austin I., Urological Surgery, C. V. Mosby Co., 1950.)

The perirenal fascia previously described is a part of the fascia propria
which reinforces the peritoneum. At operation, it is divided posterior to the
kidney and reflected forward to expose the kidney (Fig. 8).

Lying below and somewhat medial to the kidney is the *psoas major*
muscle. This serves as a buffer between the kidney and the vertebral column.
The psoas major muscle takes its origin from the twelfth thoracic and all
of the lumbar vertebrae, and passes downward and laterally along the pelvic
brim, beneath the inguinal ligament, to insert into the lesser trochanter of
the femur. This muscle is not disturbed when operating upon the kidney.
Because of its insertion into the femur, there may be flexion of the thigh
when the muscle is irritated by perirenal infectious processes.

ANATOMY AND SURGICAL APPROACH TO THE URETER
ANATOMY

The ureter is a fibromuscular tube which begins at the outlet of the renal
pelvis 5 to 7 cm. below the hilum of the kidney and extends to the ureteral

orifice at one angle of the vesical trigone (Fig. 9). The ureter varies in length from 28 to 34 cm. and the left is about 1 cm. longer than the right. When the anomaly of two ureters to one kidney exists, the ureter draining the upper segment of the kidney enters the bladder below the ureter draining the lower portion. The caliber of the ureter varies in different areas and in different subjects. Three definitely constricted areas are recognized. The uppermost constriction is just below the kidney pelvis, the second where

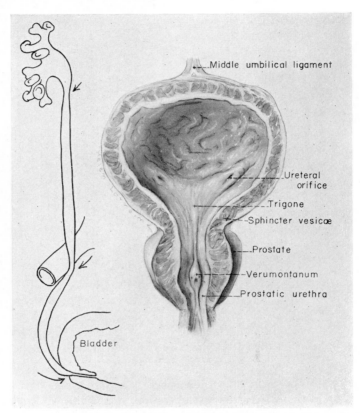

Fig. 9. Bladder and prostate sectioned to show structure of bladder wall and points of interest in base of bladder and posterior urethra. Diagram showing normal areas (arrows) of ureteral constriction.

the ureter crosses the iliac vessels at the pelvic brim, and the third within the wall of the bladder (Fig. 9). The caliber of these areas averages about 3 mm. Between the first and second constriction is the lumbar spindle which has a diameter of about 10 mm. and between the iliac vessels and the bladder is the pelvic spindle with a diameter from 4 to 6 mm. Calculi often become arrested in one of the narrow areas.

Structure of the Ureter. The ureter is composed of a fibrous, a muscular and a mucous coat. The fibrous coat is a rough elastic membrane, continuous above the fibrous covering of the kidney and blending below with the wall of the bladder. The muscular coat is continuous with the muscles of the kidney pelvis and consists of an external longitudinal and an internal circular layer. The longitudinal muscle of the ureter continues across the trigone of the bladder, a portion running along the edge of the trigone and a portion decussating with fibers from the opposite ureter to form the inter-ureteric ridge. The ureter has no sphincter. Regurgitation is prevented by a mucous membrane valve produced by the oblique course of the ureter through the bladder wall. The mucous membrane is smooth and lies in longitudinal folds when the ureter is at rest. It is composed of a stratified squamous type of epithelium.

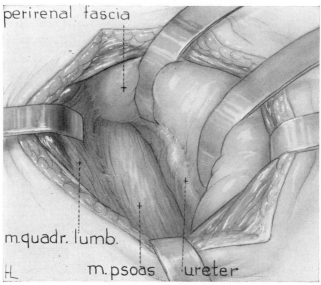

Fig. 10.   Relationship of ureter to parietal peritoneum. (From Dodson, Austin I., Urological Surgery, C. V. Mosby Co., 1950.)

Course and Relation to Other Structures. From the renal pelvis to the iliac vessels the ureter lies upon the anterior surface of the psoas major muscle and just over the tips of the transverse processes of the spinal column (Fig. 3). In front is the parietal peritoneum to which the ureter is loosely attached with the exception of the upper 4 to 5 cm. This attachment is of surgical importance. When the peritoneum is dissected up for exposure of the ureter, the ureter should be looked for on the reflected peritoneum (Fig. 10). The spermatic or ovarian vessels lie internal to the ureter for 5 to 8 cm., then cross over to continue downward as an external relation (Fig. 3). On the right side, the right colic and ileocolic vessels also pass between the ureter and the peritoneum. On the left side, the ureter is crossed by the spermatic or ovarian and by the left colic and sigmoid vessels. The genitocrural nerves cross behind the ureters. The right ureter passes behind the descending portion of the duodenum as it leaves the kidney and behind the terminal ileum and vermiform appendix just above the iliac vessels. When the appendix is retrocecal, it is in close relation with the ureter, and appendicitis may cause inflammation of the ureter with the elimination of blood and pus cells in the urine. Randall has reported constriction of the midureter resulting from inflammation of the appendix. At the pelvic brim the ureters cross the iliac vessels just at or lateral to their division into external and internal branches (Fig. 3). The ureters then follow the contour of the pelvic wall in a downward and outward direction, passing in front of all major vessels. Opposite the ischial spine the course is median-ward and downward to the base of the bladder. In the male each ureter passes under its respective vas deferens and enters the bladder in front of the upper end of the seminal vesicle (Fig. 12). Because of this relation disease of the seminal vesicles sometimes causes symptoms suggesting disease of the kidney, and periureteral inflammation may cause constriction of the ureter.

Blood Supply of the Ureter. The ureter obtains its blood supply from the renal aorta, capsular, iliacs, spermatic and superior and inferior vesicular arteries (Fig. 3). The *arteries* form a plexus of longitudinal branches in the loose fibrous outer coat of the ureter. The tributaries pierce the muscular coat at frequent intervals. A similar but more delicate plexus of arteries is formed in the submucosa of the ureter. Capillaries are given off from this plexus to the muscular coat and to the mucous membrane. The abundant blood supply and free anastomosis of the ureteral blood vessels make it possible to liberate the ureter almost completely without danger of necrosis. The *veins* form a plexus in the submucosa and drain into the veins of the adventitia. These veins drain into the spermatic or ovarian, the renal, the uterine or the vesical venous plexus.

Lymphatics. Lymph channels accompany the arteries in the submucosa and in the periureteral sheath. Those of the lower ureter drain downward. Those of the upper ureter drain toward the kidney, and those of the mid-portion medially into the pelvic and lumbar lymph glands.

Innervation of the Ureter. The nerve supply of the ureter is derived from the autonomic nervous system and is independent of the renal pelvis and bladder. The nerves supplying the ureter have been carefully dissected by Wharton who found that nerves pass to the ureter from the lowest renal ganglion at the head of the ovarian and spermatic plexus and from the aortic, hypogastric and pelvic plexuses. These ganglia are supplied by the abdominal sympathetic trunks which are derived from the solar or celiac plexus. The *celiac plexus* is formed by the greater and lesser splanchnics and the vagi, communicating branches from the upper lumbar prevertebral sympathetic ganglia, and from the sacral cord (Fig. 5). Wharton also demonstrated a connection between the ureteral innervation and the plexuses that supply the ovary, testis, and the parietal peritoneum. Complete division of the nerves to the ureter will relieve ureteral pain without disturbing ureteral peristalsis or tonus.

The neurogenic origin of motor impulses is believed to come from ganglia in the adventitia and musculature of the ureter. Peristalsis has been abolished in the ureter by complete denervation of the renal artery and vein. This does not occur when the artery alone is denervated.

THE SURGICAL APPROACH TO THE URETER

Muscles. The ureter is approached surgically through the abdominal muscles and their aponeuroses and fascial coverings. The posterior portion of the external and internal oblique muscles and the aponeurosis of the transversalis muscle have been described in discussing the surgical approach to the kidney. These structures previously described cover the lateral abdominal wall, and it is through them that incisions are made to expose the upper third of the ureter.

The lower two thirds of the ureter may be approached through a *lateral abdominal* incision somewhat similar to the McBurney incision for exposing the appendix. This incision varies in location with the portion of the ureter to be exposed. It is rarely necessary to divide muscles. The three abdominal muscles may be divided in the direction of their fibers. When more room is needed, the combined aponeuroses of the lateral abdominal muscles may be cut downward along the lateral margin of the rectus muscle. The transversalis fascia is then divided and the parietal peritoneum retracted medially. The ureter will be found attached to the peritoneum over the transverse processes of the vertebrae. Some surgeons prefer a *paramedian* incision for exposure of the lower portion of the ureter. In this case, the incision is made through the rectus abdominis muscle lateral to the midline, the rectus is divided in the direction of its fibers, after which the transversalis fascia is divided and the parietal peritoneum freed and retracted medially as in the lateral abdominal approach.

The intermediate and anterior fibers of the external oblique muscle arise from the ribs, forming the costal arch, and pass downward and inward. The intermediate fibers form the inguinal, or Poupart's ligament, and the anterior fibers, becoming aponeurotic near the linea semilunaris and below the anterior superior spine of the ilium, pass inward and downward to cross the anterior surface of the rectus abdominis muscle, and are inserted into the xiphoid, linea alba and pubic symphysis (Figs. 7 and 11).

The internal oblique muscle lies immediately beneath the external oblique. It arises from the lumbodorsal fascia, the anterior two thirds of the iliac crest, and the lateral half of the inguinal ligament. The posterior fibers are included in the iliocostal area and are inserted into the lower ribs and their cartilages. The fibers included in the anterior abdominal wall form an aponeurosis before reaching the semilunar line. Above the semicircular line, which is situated midway between the umbilicus and symphysis pubis, the aponeurosis divides into two lamellae (Fig. 11). The anterior lamella joins the aponeurosis of the external oblique to form the anterior sheath of the rectus muscle, and the posterior lamella fuses with the aponeurosis of the transversus abdominis to form the posterior rectus sheath. Below the semicircular line the aponeuroses of the external oblique, internal oblique and transversus abdominis pass in front of the rectus muscle. These anterior fibers of the internal oblique pass straight across the abdomen, those crossing the upper abdomen take a slightly upward course, and those arising from the inguinal ligament pass slightly downward. The lowermost fibers blend with corresponding fibers of the transversus abdominis to form the conjoined tendon and become attached to the pubic crest.

The transversus abdominis lies beneath the internal oblique. It arises from the lumbodorsal fascia as an aponeurosis (the transversalis fascia), the iliac crest, the lateral third of the inguinal ligament and from the inner aspects of the lower six costal cartilages. Its fibers pass directly across the

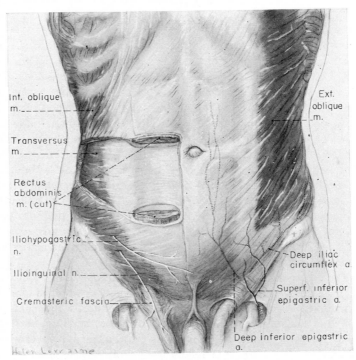

Fig. 11.   Structures of the anterior abdominal wall through which the lower two thirds of the ureter is approached surgically.

abdomen. Its aponeurosis passes behind the rectus abdominis above the semicircular line and anterior to this muscle below the semicircular line (Figs. 7 and 11).

The transversalis fascia lies beneath the muscle and lines the abdominal cavity. It is separated from the peritoneum by loose areolar tissue. Below the semicircular line it is the only fascial covering of the posterior surface of the rectus abdominis muscle.

The rectus abdominis is composed of thick, flat bands that lie on each side of the linea alba or midline of the abdomen. Each muscle arises from the anterior surface of the fifth, sixth and seventh costal cartilages and from the xiphoid process, and is inserted on the pubis between the crest and symphysis. The muscle fibers are interrupted by 3 to 5 tendinous intersections, the lineae transversae which cross the muscle, and are adherent to its anterior sheath. The anterior sheath of the rectus muscle above the semicircular line is formed by the aponeurosis of the external oblique and the anterior lamella of the internal oblique. Below the semicircular line it is composed of the aponeuroses of all three transverse muscles of the abdomen (Fig. 11). The posterior sheath, composed of the aponeurosis of the transversus abdominis and a portion of the aponeurosis of the internal oblique, terminates in a free crescentic margin, the semicircular line (semicircular fold of Douglas) midway between the umbilicus and the pubis. Below this point the transversalis fascia is the sole posterior covering of the rectus. The linea semilunaris is formed by the coalescence of the aponeuroses of the transverse abdominal muscles as they approach the margin of the rectus muscle.

Blood Vessels. The blood supply of the anterior abdominal wall is derived from the last six intercostal and the four lumbar arteries, and the superior and inferior epigastric and deep circumflex iliac arteries. These vessels anastomose freely and any of them may be divided and ligated without disturbing the nutrition of the tissues. The intercostal and lumbar arteries accompany the intercostal, iliohypogastric, and ilio-inguinal nerves between the transversus abdominis and internal oblique muscles. When it is necessary to divide these vessels, the nerve should be avoided if possible and especially should not be included in the ligature. The inferior epigastric artery arises from the external iliac and passes upward and inward, piercing the transversalis fascia to enter the rectus sheath after passing in front of the semicircular line. It is often necessary to divide this artery when exposing the lower end of the ureter. A branch of the deep circumflex iliac artery is frequently cut in muscle-splitting incisions which extend above the anterior superior spine of the ilium.

Nerves. The anterior branches of the lower six intercostal nerves pass downward and forward across the anterior abdominal wall. They run between the transversalis and internal oblique muscles. After giving off branches to supply the transverse muscles and overlying skin, their terminals pierce the rectus sheath and, after supplying the muscle, terminate in the subcutaneous tissue and skin. Oblique incisions for exposing the ureter should pass below these nerves. Division of their terminal branches is the chief objection to incisions through the semilunar line.

The ilio-inguinal and iliohypogastric nerves pass beneath the internal oblique just medial to the anterior superior spine of the ilium. They are distributed mainly to the inguinal and lower abdominal regions.

The course of these nerves varies slightly in different subjects. They are occasionally encountered when exposing the lower ureter by an oblique incision. Care should be taken to avoid including them in sutures or ligatures.

THE ANATOMY AND SURGICAL APPROACH TO THE BLADDER
ANATOMY

Situated in the pelvis is the urinary bladder. The wall of this organ is composed chiefly of muscular fibers with an inner mucosal lining. A saccular structure, it is capable of considerable distention under normal circumstances. At birth the bladder is ovoid in shape and is for the most part an abdominal organ. It is located deep to the anterior abdominal wall and its base lies behind the symphysis pubis. With growth and development the bladder descends into the true pelvis and assumes a more spherical form. In the adult, the distended bladder projects above the margin of the sym-

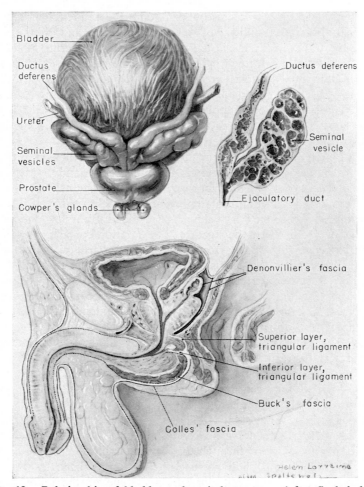

Fig. 12.   Relationship of bladder and genital structures (after Spalteholz).

physis pubis and becomes in part an abdominal organ. Its location immediately beneath the symphysis and lower abdominal wall makes it readily accessible to surgical approach (Fig. 12).

The wall of the bladder is composed of four layers, the outer fibrous, the muscular, submucosal and mucosal (Fig. 9). The fibrous layer is made up of fatty areolar tissue with considerable fibrous connective tissue interspersed throughout. This coat is thicker over the lower portion of the bladder and the areas not covered by peritoneum. It attaches in loose fashion to the underlying muscular layer and at the base of the bladder blends with the pelvic fascia.

The muscular layer is made up of three strata of unstriated muscle. The external coat consists of longitudinal fibers. Posteriorly, these fibers are blended with the deep layer of rectovesical fascia. This layer is thickest on the posterior and anterior aspects and blends over the dome of the bladder. At the lateral aspects of the bladder the longitudinal fibers are thin or absent. A thicker layer of circular fibers makes up the middle coat. These circular fibers are densely interlaced. The inner coat is longitudinal and quite thin. The external and middle coats contribute the fibers making up the internal urethral sphincter.

The trigonal muscle is a separate entity, composed of fibers derived from the longitudinal layers of the ureters (Fig. 12). These fibers intermingle in the trigone and pass downward to insert into the wall of the posterior urethra. The submucosa is a thin layer of fibrous and connective tissue, quite vascular, and serving to attach the mucosa to the underlying muscular coat. The mucosa of the bladder is a transitional type of epithelium. It is normally pale pink or salmon-colored, and in the empty bladder is thrown into folds except for the portion overlying the trigone which is smooth at all times. The mucosa of the bladder contains few glands and these are usually located over the trigone and more rarely in the area of the bladder vault.

For orientation purposes, the bladder is described as consisting of a vault or superior portion, two lateral walls, a fundus or base, and a trigone. The trigone is the triangular area lying between the ureteral orifices at its basal angles and the urethral opening at its apex.

The peritoneum is reflected from the anterior abdominal wall over the anterior surface, dome, and portions of the lateral and posterior aspects of the bladder. The urachus is covered by this peritoneal reflection. When the bladder is filled, the lower margin of this peritoneal reflection lies 1 or 2 inches above the superior margin of the symphysis pubis (Fig. 12). With the bladder empty, the peritoneal covering reaches the symphysis and may dip down behind it. Over the anterior surface of the bladder the peritoneum is attached rather loosely and may be stripped up easily. The peritoneum extends forward and downward, covering the fundus and posterior aspect, in some instances extending to the area in which the ureters reach the bladder. At this point the peritoneum reflects upward over the rectum in the male. The bladder is surrounded by a bed of loose areolar tissue that permits of considerable mobility. Anterior to the bladder and its peritoneal reflection there is a space filled with loose areolar tissue. This is the space of Retzius. Its forward boundary is formed by the posterior surface of the symphysis and superadjacent anterior abdominal wall. It is a potential area of infection in suprapubic surgery and of extravasation of blood in rupture of the extraperitoneal segment of the bladder.

The base of the bladder, the only fixed portion of the organ, is continuous with the prostate and urethra in the male (Fig. 9). The true ligaments of the bladder, fascial bands arising from the pelvic fascia, anchor this segment firmly to the pubic bones and the fascial sheaths of the levator ani muscles. Posteriorly, the rectovesical fascia, or fascia of Denonvilliers, separates the prostatovesicular structures from the anterior rectal wall, and serves to support the base of the bladder. This structure, made up of two fascial layers, is thought to be derived from the obliterated lower segment of the rectovesical peritoneal fold. The anterior layer of Denonvilliers' fascia is densely adherent to the posterior surface of the prostate and seminal vesicles. The urachus forms a portion of the middle umbilical ligament, supporting the bladder anteriorly and above (Fig. 12).

Vesical Blood Supply. The superior and inferior vesical arteries, terminal branches of the internal hypogastric artery, supply the bulk of the bladder (Fig. 3). Inconstant middle vesical arteries may arise from the superior vesical branches. Smaller arteries are derived from the middle hemorrhoidal, obturator, internal pudendal, and inferior pudic vessels.

The veins of the bladder anastomose freely and form intricate plexuses in the bladder wall. These eventually drain into the hypogastric veins via the lateral vesical plexuses.

Lymphatic Drainage of the Bladder. For the most part the lymphatics follow the veins and nerves and drain into nodes alone the external iliac and hypogastric vessels.

Nerve Supply to the Bladder. The nerve supply to the bladder is parasympathetic, sympathetic, and somatic in origin. The *parasympathetic* innervation is derived from the anterior primary divisions of the second, third and fourth sacral segments. These fibers pass through the pelvic nerves to the inferior hypogastric plexus and there are distributed to the bladder, musculature and urethra (Fig. 5). These nerve fibers mediate chiefly motor impulses to the supplied structures.

The *sympathetic* fibers arise in the spinal segments from the twelfth dorsal to the third lumbar. They pass via the presacral nerve and sacral sympathetic chains to the inferior hypogastric plexus. The presacral nerve terminates in a right and left hypogastric nerve and these latter in turn pass on to the corresponding hypogastric plexus (Fig. 5). From the plexus, the sympathetic fibers are distributed to the ureter, seminal vesicles, prostate, prostatic urethra, base of the bladder, and the blood vessels. The sympathetic is chiefly sensory, though some feel it is inhibitory to the detrusor muscles as well.

The *somatic* innervation is carried by the internal pudendal nerves. These arise from the primary divisions of the third and fourth sacral and supply motor fibers to the external sphincter and perineal muscles and sensory fibers to the perineal tissues. The pudendal nerve grouping mediates the voluntary control aspect of micturition.

Relations of the Bladder. The bladder occupies the anterior portion of the pelvic space. Anterior to the organ are the posterior surface of the pubic bone, the retropubic fat, the anterior vesical veins, and the vesicopelvic fascia (Fig. 12). Laterally, the obturator internus and levator ani muscles, the pelvic fascia, and the prostatovesical venous plexus are in apposition with the bladder. Covering a considerable portion of the upper two thirds of the bladder is the peritoneum with its contained organs. When the bladder is distended, its vault and anterior surface come in contact with the posterior aspect of the lower abdominal wall.

In the male, the base of the bladder is separated from the rectum by the seminal vesicles, terminal segments of the vasa, and the fascia of Denonvilliers (Fig. 12). The distal segments of the ureters course medial to the vasa and lie between the seminal vesicles and the bladder wall.

SURGICAL APPROACH TO THE BLADDER

The recti and pyramidalis muscles overlie the bladder. It is through these structures and their fascial and aponeurotic coverings that the bladder is exposed for surgical treatment. A median incision extending from the pubis upward is usually preferred. After dividing the skin, superficial fascia and aponeurosis, the muscles are separated in the midline, exposing a small amount of fat which overlies the transversalis fascia. When the transversalis fascia is divided, considerable fat and areolar tissue are exposed. Beneath this is the vesical layer of the pelvic fascia which is loosely attached to the surface of the bladder. The bladder is readily recognized by the large veins which course in an irregular manner over its surface. Some surgeons prefer to expose the bladder by the Pfannenstiel or the Cherney incision. These are transverse incisions. The Cherney incision is the more extensive of the two and involves transverse section of the tendinous insertions of the recti muscles.

THE MALE URETHRA AND ITS SUPPORTING STRUCTURES

Surrounding and supporting the posterior one third to one half of the male urethra are the muscular and fascial structures of the perineum. These perineal tissues are of importance because of their relation to the prostate, seminal vesicles, bladder, and rectum. Through the perineum the posterior urethra and supra-adjacent structures are approached surgically (Fig. 13).

The perineum is made up of the musculomembranous pelvic diaphragm and the soft tissues lying inferior to it and serves to close over the entire pelvic outlet. The pelvic diaphragm is composed of the triangular ligament, a dense transverse fibrous septum, and the levator ani and coccygeus muscle and their fascial investments (Figs. 12 and 13). Anterior to the anus, the perineal structures form a dense union between the anorectal junction and the apex of the prostate. This area of fusion is called the central point of the perineum. Here the bulbocavernosus, the sphincter ani, and the superficial transverse perineal muscles come together and their aponeurotic fibers fuse with the posterior margin of the triangular ligament (Figs. 12 and 13). This central tendinous ligament is an important surgical structure. Its position corresponds to a point on the perineal surface approximately midway between the anus and penoscrotal junction.

The levator ani muscles take their origin from the pelvic wall at its inner aspect, beginning at a point slightly lateral to the lower margins of the symphysis anteriorly and extending to the ischial spine posteriorly. These broad, flat muscles pass obliquely downward and inward, producing a funnel-like structure, with the walls coming together at the lower rectum and anal canal.

The more anterior fibers of the levator ani muscles, arising from the pelvic bone, pass beneath the prostate, some going to its capsule, some to the central point of the perineum, and others to the anterior and lateral walls. The

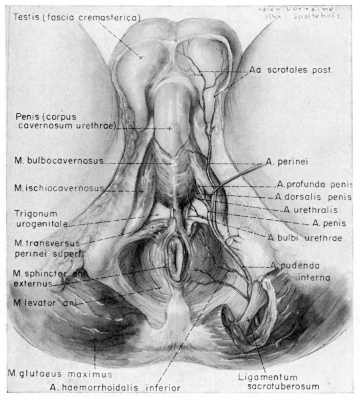

Fig. 13. Anatomy of the perineum (after Spalteholz).

more posterior fibers pass behind the rectum and insert into the sides of the coccyx and to the fibrous structures running from the coccyx to the anus.

Since the anterior portions of the levator ani muscle arise from the pelvic walls, lateral to the symphysis pubis, there is a resultant hiatus or defect in the muscular floor of the pelvic outlet at its most anterior portion. This space is partially filled by the prostate. The aponeurotic fibers bordering the medial margins of the muscle are adherent to the prostatic capsule and form the lateral puboprostatic ligaments. The superior layer of the triangular ligament helps maintain the prostate and bladder in the pelvic cavity and further seals off this hiatus (Fig. 12).

Forming the triangular ligament, or urogenital diaphragm, are two layers of fascia. These stretch across the pubic arch from one pubic ramus to the other. This ligament closes off the anterior portion of the pelvic outlet and divides the pelvis from the perineum anteriorly. The superior layer of the triangular ligament is continuous throughout the cleft between the levator muscles, with the fascia lining the pelvic wall. This particular layer is not as well defined as the inferior or superficial layer. The inferior or superficial layer, considered to arise from the obturator fascia, is deficient just behind the subpubic angle. The dense free margin is called the transverse perineal ligament. At their posterior aspect the two layers of fascia blend with each other and with Colles' fascia and the central tendon of the perineum. By this posterior fusion of the fascial components of the perineum, two partly closed areas are formed. These are designated as the superficial and deep compartments of the urogenital perineum.

The urogenital perineum includes the space between the symphysis pubis in front and the central point of the perineum behind and is limited laterally by the pubic arch. Within the confines of the urogenital perineum lie the membranous and bulbous portions of the urethra and their supporting musculomembranous structures (Fig. 12). That portion of the perineum lying posterior to the central point is referred to as the posterior perineum. These two areas at their junction contribute to the formation of the central point of the perineum. They are related in that they have a common level in the levator ani muscles and derive their innervation from the internal pudendal nerves.

Beneath the cutaneous surface of the perineum lies the superficial layer of fascia. This layer, along with the deeper layers of fascia are of primary importance from the surgical aspect. The superficial fascia consists of two layers. The outer layer is continuous with the subcutaneous fatty tissue of the body. In the region of the perineum this stratum is almost devoid of fat and presents chiefly smooth muscle fibers which are continuous anteriorly with the dartos tunic of the scrotum. Beneath this fascial plane lies Colles' fascia, a dense connective tissue membrane coating the urogenital region and attaching laterally to the periosteum of the pubic arch on each side. This layer fuses posteriorly with the margin of the triangular ligament and thus roofs the superficial perineal compartment of the urogenital diaphragm and contains the spread of infection or urinary extravasation originating in the bulbous urethra. Anteriorly, Colles' fascia is continuous over the scrotum and penis and along the spermatic cord to the anterior abdominal wall where it is in continuity with Scarpa's fascia, the deep layer of the superficial fascia (Fig. 12). Thus, infections or extravasation of urine arising in the superficial compartment will distend that area and then spread forward to the scrotum, penis, and anterior abdominal wall. Extension of the process to the thighs is prevented by the attachment of Scarpa's fascia to the fascia lata. The deep compartment of the perineum and the posterior perineum is protected by the inferior layer of the triangular ligament.

The superficial perineal compartment formed by the inferior layer of the triangular ligament and Colles' fascia is divided in two lateral spaces by a septum extending from Colles' fascia to the raphe of the bulbocavernosus muscle. The only outlet for this superficial compartment is anterior (Fig.

13). Contained within this compartment are the bulbous urethra and its surrounding cavernous body, the crura of the corpora cavernosa penis, and their overlying ischiocavernosus and bulbocavernosus muscles. The branches of the pudendal vessels and nerves pierce the inferior layer of the triangular ligament to enter this space. The corpora cavernosa of the penis have their origin near the midpoint of the ischiopubic rami and pass forward and upward, adhering to the periosteum of the pubis and the inferior surface of the triangular ligament. The bulb of the urethra originates just beyond the inferior layer of the triangular ligament, receives its corpus cavernosum and surrounding bulbocavernosus muscle, and extends forward as the central body of the penis. Abutting against the inferior surface of the triangular ligament, there is a short segment of urethra, slightly dilated in its inferior surface and free of muscular investment. This is called the cul-de-sac of the bulb (Fig. 12). This area may be involved in infection proximal to a urethral stricture and may be the point of origin of a periurethral abscess or perineal phlegmon, sometimes filling the superficial compartment and extending forward to the anterior abdominal wall. Perineal trauma, as in straddle injuries, may force the urethra up against the pubic arch or subpubic ligament and result in rupture of this area with subsequent extravasation of urine and blood.

The superficial transverse perineal muscles cross the most posterior aspect of the superficial compartment. Arising from the ischial tuberosities, these muscles pass medially and slightly forward to insert into the central point of the perineum midway between the bulb of the urethra and the anus. These muscles form an important landmark in perineal surgery. Small branches of the pudendal vessels and nerves traverse the space on each side of the bulbocavernosus muscle (Fig. 13).

The deep compartment of the urogenital diaphragm is contained between the layers of the triangular ligament. Within this space lie the membranous urethra and its enveloping sphincter. The deep transverse perineal muscle arises from the ischial ramus, traverses the deep compartment in close contact with its superior layer and fuses with its mate in a tendinous raphe behind the skeletal muscle of the sphincter urethrae (Fig. 12).

The membranous urethra extends from the apex of the prostate to the inferior layer of the triangular ligament. Its total length is about 1 cm. and it lies about 2½ cm. posterior to the subpubic ligament. It is the most fixed portion of the urethra and because of its course through the triangular ligament is subject to trauma in fracture of the pelvis and tearing of the triangular ligament. Direct blows on the perineum may force it upward against the subpubic ligament and cause its rupture. Within the deep compartment of the urogenital diaphragm lie the glands of Cowper. The draining ducts of these glands perforate the inferior layer of the triangular ligament and drain into the bulb of the urethra. The internal pudendal vessels and the dorsal nerve of the penis cross through the deep compartment (Fig. 13). The relationship of this compartment to the anterior portion of the ischiorectal fossa is of importance. This fossa runs toward the pubis between the deep layer of the compartment, the anterior portion of the levator ani muscle, and the medial surface of the obturator internus muscle. While infection and urinary extravasation in the deep compartment usually break through above and spread to the prevesical area, they can find a way into the ischiorectal fossa and eventually present in the posterior perineum at or near the anus.

The penile or pendulous portion of the urethra runs in the ventral groove between the corpora cavernosa of the penis. It is quite superficial and is covered by a thin layer of cavernous tissue, Buck's and Colles' fascia, and the skin (Fig. 12). The mobility of this segment and its protective position render it less susceptible to injury. Surgical incision in the penile portion of the urethra is avoided if possible, since the surrounding tissue is very thin and the possibility of a persistent fistula a real hazard. Urethral strictures in this area are treated by dilatation or internal urethrotomy.

The wall of the urethra is made up of mucous, submucous and muscular coats. The mucosal layer is a stratified squamous epithelium and lies in longitudinal folds. Within the mucosa are many small lacunae and mucous glands. The submucosa is a layer of highly vascular, loose connective tissue. The muscular coat has an internal longitudinal and an external circular layer of smooth muscle. Some fibers from the internal sphincter of the bladder clothe the proximal end of the urethra. The voluntary urethral sphincter, a striated muscle, surrounds the urethra as it traverses the space between the layers of the triangular ligament.

Branches of the internal pudendal and inferior vesical arteries supply the urethra. The veins drain into the pudendal or perivesical plexuses.

The lymphatic drainage is to the inguinal and hypogastric pelvic nodes (Fig. 15).

The urethra receives its innervation from the pudic and genitofemoral nerves and sympathetic fibers from the vesical plexus.

THE PENIS

The penis is an erectile organ made up of three bodies, the paired corpora cavernosa, and the corpus spongiosum. The *corpora cavernosa* originate at the midpoint of the ischiopubic rami within the superficial urogenital diaphragm. They adhere to the descending rami of the pubis and the inferior surface of the triangular ligament as they pass medially. At the subpubic angle they come in contact and are firmly united throughout the rest of their course. The corpora cavernosa are larger than the corpus spongiosum and lie in a plane above this structure (Figs. 12 and 14). The perineal portion of the corpora cavernosa is covered by the ischiocavernosus muscles (Fig. 13). These muscles arise from the ischial tuberosities and insert into the sides and under-surface of the cavernous bodies. The erectile tissue of the corpora cavernosa is a vascular sponge-like structure contained within the dense fibro-elastic tunica albuginea.

The *corpus spongiosum* is a smaller erectile body running in the ventral groove between the corpora cavernosa. It envelops the urethra from the

triangular ligament to the urinary meatus (Fig. 14). It begins at the bulb
of the urethra in the perineum where it is invested by the bulbocavernosus
muscle. This muscle arises from the central point of the perineum and
passes upward and forward to clothe the bulb. The corpus spongiosum
enters the ventral groove between the corpora cavernosa at the subpubic

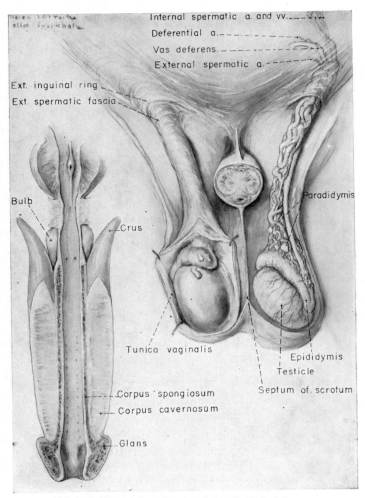

Fig. 14. Penis and testes (after Spalteholz).

angle. It then runs forward in the body of the penis to terminate as the
greatly expanded glans penis which serves to cap the rounded ends of the
corpora cavernosa (Figs. 13 and 14).

The body of the penis, or external portion, begins just below the pubic
arch and is attached to the bony structure by strong connective tissue elements (Fig. 12).

The *glans penis* is a cone-shaped structure with a prominent posterior margin called the corona glandis and a groove on the ventral surface into which the frenum inserts. At the apex of the cone there is a vertical slit, the external urethral meatus (Fig. 14). The glans is covered by a thin, semimucous membrane rich in sebaceous glands and terminal nerve fibers (Fig. 12).

The *tunica albuginea* is a dense connective tissue sheath enclosing each of the erectile bodies. The trabeculae of these sheaths surround the vascular spaces. Injury to these tunics may produce marked bleeding and swelling, and if such wounds are not carefully repaired, permanent deformity of the penis may result. Sustained erection due to disease or prolonged engorgement may cause some clotting of blood in the cavernous spaces and painful and persistent priapism. Aspiration of these blood clots may relieve the condition. While the corpora cavernosa are adherent through the body of the penis, the tunica albuginea over the contiguous portions is thicker than elsewhere and allows for separation if the bodies are carefully dissected.

All three corpora of the penis are bound together by a dense fascial coat known as *Buck's fascia* (Fig. 12). This layer is attached firmly to the base of the glans and adheres closely to the tunica albuginea covering the erectile bodies to their points of origin. It fuses with the suspensory ligament and the inferior surface of the triangular ligament.

The penis is supported by the suspensory ligament, a dense aponeurosis arising from the front of the symphysis pubis and extending downward and forward to blend with the fibrous coverings of the penis at the base of the pendulous portion (Fig. 12). Colles' fascia clothes the penis just beneath the skin and is continuous with the same layer of fascia over the scrotum and perineum.

The skin of the penis is very thin and loose and allows for considerable distention. It is devoid of fat and hair except at the base of the penis. Over the glans the skin is thrown up into a fold or hood, the prepuce, which protects this portion of the penis (Fig. 12). This structure can usually be retracted behind the glans. The internal surface of the prepuce is a delicate membrane similar to that covering the glans. The free margin of the prepuce is a somewhat narrowed area, called the preputial orifice. The foreskin is attached at the base of the glans in the coronal sulcus. A small median fold, the frenum, attaches on the ventral surface just behind the lower angle of the meatus. The frenum contains a small artery, the frenal artery, which may bleed profusely if injured.

In certain congenital or inflammatory conditions, the orifice of the prepuce may be contracted and make retraction difficult if not impossible. This condition is called phimosis and may require circumcision or dorsal slit to enlarge the opening. Unrelieved phimosis is associated with poor hygiene and may result in severe inflammation and ulceration of the glans penis and mucosal surface of the prepuce. Prophylactic circumcision at birth is an excellent means of preventing this condition and also forestalls carcinoma of the penis in later life.

The penile *blood supply* is derived chiefly from the internal pudendal artery (Fig. 13). This branch of the internal hypogastric artery after entering the base of the urogenital triangle divides into paired bulbo-urethral, dorsal, and cavernous arteries. The bulbo-urethral arteries run along with the urethra to the glans and there anastomose with branches of the dorsal

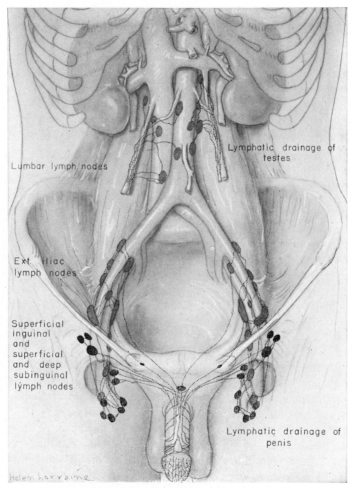

Fig. 15. Lymph nodes involved in malignancy of the genitalia.

artery. The dorsal arteries course along the dorsum of the penis beneath Buck's fascia and are accompanied by the dorsal nerves and veins. These arteries supply the glans penis and send off twigs to the penile fascia and anastomosing branches to the cavernous bodies. The cavernous arteries enter the corpora cavernosa at the point of union of these two bodies and course through the corpora somewhat eccentrically to the median side of their axis. Additional arterial supply to the penis is derived from external pudic branches of the femoral and small twigs from the superficial perineal vessels. The skin of the terminal portion of the penis is supplied chiefly by branches of the dorsal artery.

The arteries to the penis anastomose widely, and this important fact must be considered in surgery on the penis and in repair of extensive laceration of that organ. Often, very severe damage can be repaired with excellent final results.

The veins of the penis are divided into a superficial and a deep group. The superficial veins form a network beneath the skin and drain along the course of the penis, emptying into the superficial dorsal vein which courses beneath the skin over the pubis and later divides and joins the internal saphenous or femoral veins on either side, or enters the deep dorsal vein of the penis. The deep dorsal vein begins at the corona in a network encircling the base of the glans. It receives branches draining the glans and prepuce and then passes along the dorsal groove between the corpora cavernosa and beneath Buck's fascia to the base of the penis. It receives tributaries from all the cavernous bodies and at the suspensory ligament passes between the superficial and deep segments of that structure. It continues beneath the subpubic ligament and divides into three branches, a superficial branch passing upward over the bladder, and right and left lateral branches emptying into the right and left prostatovesical plexus, respectively.

The *nerves* to the penis are derived from the perineal branch of the internal pudendal nerve. They follow the course of the penile arteries. Sympathetic fibers to the blood vessels and the muscular tissue of the erectile bodies arise in the hypogastric plexus, pass through the prostatic and cavernous plexuses and join the dorsal nerves of the penis for ultimate distribution.

The penile *lymphatics,* like the veins, divide into two main groups. The superficial, beginning at the glans and prepuce and accompanying the superficial dorsal vein, drains the skin of the penis and empties into the iliac nodes (Fig. 15). The other is the deep group which begins in the glans and forms larger lymphatic channels accompanying the deep dorsal vein. This group drains the deep structures of the penis and in turn drains into the inguinal nodes and those along the iliac vessels. In some cases the lymphatic drainage of the penis is to nodes located over Scarpa's triangle. The lymphatic drainage of the penis is an important consideration in inflammation and neoplasm of that organ.

THE SCROTUM

The scrotum and the penis constitute the external male genitalia. The scrotum is a thin-skinned, contractile saccular structure containing the testes and their connecting cords and appendages. The scrotal wall consists of skin, muscle, and connective tissue. The cutaneous layer is thin and elastic and normally lies in folds. It is very deeply pigmented, covered sparsely with hair, and heavily supplied with sebaceous glands. The scrotal cavity is divided into two compartments, and this division is marked by a slight ridge or elevation on the skin, the raphe. This raphe is continuous with a similar linear projection on the ventral surface of the penis and over the perineum to the anus (Figs. 12 and 14).

Beneath the scrotal skin there are two lining tissue layers. The outermost is composed of smooth muscle and elastic fibers and is called the dartos tunic. It is attached to the ischiopubic rami laterally and at the scroto-perineal junction is continuous with Colles' fascia. In front, the dartos is continuous with the fascia of the suspensory ligament and the deep layer of the superficial fascia of the abdominal wall. These attachments explain the cleavage planes followed by infection, urinary extravasation, and hematoma formation incident to disease or injury in the perineal region.

The septum dividing the scrotum into two lateral pouches arises from the dartos layer. This division into compartments is a limiting factor in effusion processes within the scrotal cavities. The dartos layer is responsible for the contractility of the scrotal wall. These muscle fibers insert into the skin at right angles and this explains the tendency of skin edges in scrotal incisions to turn in. This point is important in the closure of such incisions.

Cowper's fascia is the deeper layer of the lining tissues of the scrotal wall. It is a loose connective tissue and permits free movement of the contained testes and their appendages within the scrotal cavity. In the surgical approach to the testis, this layer presents an easy line of cleavage. It is in this loose areolar-like layer that extravasations from the perineal regions accumulate and spread upward under the skin and superficial fascia of the abdominal wall.

The external and internal pudendal arteries and the cremasteric branch of the deep hypogastric arteries contribute the blood supply to the scrotal wall. It is well to remember that this arterial supply enters at the perineo-scrotal aspect to spread over the scrotal wall and that the vascular networks swing across the scrotal wall from the lateral aspect to the median raphe. Incisions in the region of the raphe present less trouble from bleeding than do those elsewhere in the scrotum. The veins follow the arteries.

The nerve supply to the scrotum is derived from the superficial branch of the external pudic, the inferior pudendal branch of the small sciatic, the inguinal branch of the genitocrural, and the ilio-inguinal nerves.

The scrotal lymphatics empty into the inguinal and femoral nodes.

THE SPERMATIC CORD

The spermatic cord is the suspensory element of the testicle. Originating at the internal abdominal ring, this structure courses through the inguinal canal, emerges at the external abdominal ring and extends through the scrotum to the testicle (Fig. 14). The cord is made up of the vas deferens and the blood vessels and nerves to the cord and testicle. The blood vessels are the cremasteric branch of the deep epigastric, the artery to the vas, and the spermatic artery. All of these structures are loosely connected by connective tissue elements and ensheathed by the same fascial coverings found on the testicle. The scrotal segment is readily exposed by incision through the scrotal wall at or near the median raphe. The inguinal segment is approached by an incision over the inguinal canal and carried down through the aponeurosis of the external oblique muscles.

THE TESTICLES

The testicles with their epididymides lie loosely in the scrotal cavity, suspended by the spermatic cord and their fascial investments, and attached to the floor of the scrotum by the gubernaculum testis or scrotal ligaments (Fig. 14). These ligaments must be divided before the testis can be delivered from the scrotum.

The testicles are paired oval structures, normally equal in size, consisting of closely packed seminiferous tubules enclosed by a dense fibrous sheath. The sheath of connective tissue is called the tunica albuginea and imparts to the testicle its pearly white or grayish white color. From the inner surface of the tunica albuginea, septa pass inward and divide the testicle into compartments. Within each compartment there is a mass or lobule of coiled seminiferous tubules supported by fine connective tissue stroma. These tubules exit from the lobules at their apices and unite to form the vasa recta. The vasa recta enter the mediastinum testis and combine in an irregular network, the rete testis. From this plexus a variable number of tubules, twelve to twenty, emerge. These are the vasa efferentia and they drain into the globus major of the epididymis.

The testicles are oval in shape and average 20 to 30 gm. in weight. The average length is 1½ in., width 1¼ in. anteroposteriorly, and 1 in. laterally. The epididymis caps a considerable portion of the testicle. The rest of the testicle is covered by the visceral layer of the tunica vaginalis.

THE EPIDIDYMIDES

The epididymides are compact masses of collecting tubules arranged in such fashion as to form long narrow structures. Each epididymis arises from the mediastinum of the testis at the apex of the testicle at the point where the efferent ductules pierce the tunica albuginea. They are divided into three recognizable portions: the globus major or head, the corpus or body, and the globus minor or tail (Fig. 14). The efferential ducts unite to form the coni vasculosi which make up the globus major. The body of the epididymis, which is not attached to the testicle but separated from it by the visceral layer of tunica vaginalis, contains the closely packed convoluted tubule draining the coni vasculosi. The lower portion of the epididymis is attached to the lower pole of the testicle and directly connected with the vas deferens.

THE VASA DEFERENTIA

Each vas deferens is a thick-walled, fibromuscular tubule. It is lined with ciliated epithelium and serves as a conducting channel from the epididymis to the ampulla of the vas (Fig. 14). It ascends behind the epididymis to enter the spermatic cord where it lies posterior to the vessels of that structure. At the internal abdominal ring it courses downward behind the bladder, crosses the ureter, and joins the duct of the seminal vesicle on its side to form the ejaculatory duct. Its over-all length is about 18 in.

VESTIGIAL STRUCTURES

There are several vestigial structures attached to or lying near the testicle or epididymis. The hydatid of Morgagni or appendix testis is probably the most important. It is usually found on the upper pole of the testicle in the region of the head of the epididymis. This body may be sessile or pedunculated and is occasionally of surgical interest when it undergoes torsion and gangrenous change (Fig. 14). The symptoms noted with this condition may ape those of torsion of the testicle. The hydatid of Morgagni is the remnant of the upper ends of the müllerian ducts.

An appendix epididymis or pedunculated hydatid may be found attached to the globus major of the epididymis.

The organ of Giraldès, or paradidymis, is a vestigial structure that may be found in the lower segment of the spermatic cord just above the head of the epididymis (Fig. 14). A group of rudimentary tubules, it represents the remnants of the wolffian body or progenitalis. This structure may give rise to cysts separate from the epididymis and testis. The bodies of Haller, or vasa aberrantia of Haller, may be found in the epididymis or the testicle. They are remnants of the wolffian ducts. The superior vas aberrans represents a blind ending vas efferens and in the presence of cystic dilatation forms the typical spermatocele.

THE TUNICS OF THE TESTICLES

The testicles are invested with several layers of muscle and fascia. These coverings are protective, lend active mobility to the organ, and permit a considerable passive motion of the testicles within the scrotal sac (Fig. 14). These coats are independent on the two sides and are derived from the layers of the abdominal wall during the descent of the testicle from the abdominal cavity into the scrotum. They are the tunica vaginalis from the peritoneum, the infundibuliform or internal spermatic fascia from the transversalis muscle, the cremasteric fascia from the internal oblique muscle, and the intercolumnar or external spermatic fascia from the external oblique muscle.

In its descent the testis is invested by the tunica vaginalis, an envelope-like structure derived from the tube of peritoneum which precedes and accompanies the testicle through the inguinal canal into the scrotum. The inner or visceral layer of this envelope covers the testicle and epididymis over their entire surfaces except at the points of attachment of the globus major and globus minor to the testicle proper, and posteriorly where the blood and nerve supply to the testicle enter that organ. The visceral layer dips in between the testis and epididymis to form the sinus epididymis. The outer or parietal layer of the tunica vaginalis is closely applied to the infundibuliform fascia (Fig. 14). There exists a potential space within the envelope of the tunica vaginalis, and distention of this space with fluid produces a hydrocele.

Normally, the stem or upper remnant of the peritoneal tube is obliterated and converted into a fibrous cord. Failure to obliterate in whole or in part produces a patent structure and a potential or actual indirect inguinal hernia or hydrocele of the cord.

The internal spermatic fascia is a thin layer of connective tissue elements closely adherent to the tunica vaginalis and investing the cord and testicle. The cremasteric fascia is composed of elastic tissue and striped muscle fibers. It covers the cord and testicle and attaches to the dartos at the lower angle of the scrotal cavity. The external spermatic fascia forms the outer covering of the testicle and scrotal segment of the cord (Fig. 14). Investing the cord through the inguinal canal, it blends with the arching fibers over the external inguinal ring.

THE VASCULAR SUPPLY OF THE SCROTAL CONTENTS

The main artery to the testicle is the internal spermatic artery. It arises from the aorta just below the renal arteries, passes downward, at first medial and then lateral to the ureter, distributes a branch to the ureter, then enters the inguinal canal and becomes a component of the spermatic cord (Figs. 3 and 14). It joins the testicle at the medial side of the body of the epididymis. In this area it contributes a branch to the head of the epididymis. The deferential artery is derived from the superior vesical artery, accompanies and supplies the vas deferens, and then is distributed to the lower pole of the epididymis and the testicle. The cremasteric artery springs from the deep epigastric vessel and runs in the sheath of the cord to the globus minor of the epididymis and lower pole of the testicle.

Anastomosis is known to occur between these primary arteries and hence sacrificing any one will usually retain an adequate supply to the testicle and its appendages.

The veins course with the arteries. The spermatic veins form the pampiniform plexus in the cord. This plexus is large and intricate, and the contained veins have a predisposition toward formation of varicosities. This is especially true on the left side where the spermatic vein is valvular and enters the left renal vein at a 90° angle. The condition is much less common on the right where the spermatic vein enters into the vena cava at an oblique angle.

The pampiniform plexus is composed of two networks, the outer spermatic surrounding the spermatic artery and the interior deferential accompanying the vas. The anterior group is more commonly involved in varicocele formation. In surgery for correction of varicocele, care must be taken to preserve the spermatic artery.

The Lymphatics. The lymphatics follow the arteries and veins through the cord and drain into the pre-aortic nodes. There is no direct connection with the inguinal nodes. This is explained by the intra-abdominal origin of the testicle and is an important factor in the treatment of neoplastic disease of the testicle (Fig. 15).

The Nerve Supply to the Scrotal Contents. Accompanying the spermatic artery and vas are the nerves to the testicles and epididymides. They are derived from the renal and aortic plexuses of the sympathetic system.

THE PROSTATE

The prostate is a multilobular gland, located at the base of the bladder and extending from the vesical neck to the superior aspect of the triangular ligament (Figs. 9 and 12). It is roughly conical or pyramidal, with its base contiguous with the bladder and its apex pointing toward the triangular ligament. Coursing through the gland in a vertical plane, nearer the anterior than the posterior surface, is the prostatic or first segment of the urethra. The prostate gland varies in weight from 16 to 24 gm. and is 1½ in. in its long and transverse diameter and ¾ in. thick.

The prostatic urethra presents on its lower posterior surface a rounded eminence, the verumontanum (Fig. 9). This elevation has a small depression in its lower central surface, the utricle. The ejaculatory ducts enter the prostate at the posterolateral aspects of the base on each side, traverse the gland, and open into the prostatic urethra on either side of the utricle.

The prostate is composed of 5 groups of glands or lobes, one anterior, two lateral and a median which lie in front of the ejaculatory ducts, and the posterior lobe which lies behind the ducts. Scattered profusely throughout the glandular structures are both longitudinal and circular muscle fibers. These fibers are connected with those of the bladder. The circular fibers surround the urethra. The glandular portions of the prostate are of a compound tubular type. These glands form about twenty ducts which drain into the urethra on each side of the verumontanum.

The fibromuscular stroma condenses about the periphery of the glands to form a capsule. The prostate itself is supported by the endopelvic fascia, the puboprostatic ligaments in front, the triangular ligament below, and fascia of Denonvillier behind (Fig. 12). This latter structure coats the prostate and seminal vesicles posteriorly and separates these structures from the rectum.

The *blood supply* to the prostate is derived from the inferior vesical, internal pudendal, and middle hemorrhoidal arteries. The veins form a plexus on each lateral aspect of the prostate and in common with veins from the bladder, these prostatovesical plexuses drain into the internal iliac veins.

The *nerve supply* comes from the hypogastric nerve.

THE SEMINAL VESICLES

The seminal vesicles are twin structures lying at the base of the bladder, above the prostate, and in front of the rectum. The covering of Denonvilliers' fascia over the posterior aspect of the prostate extends upward to encase the vesicles and separate them from the rectal wall (Fig. 12).

Each vesicle is made up of a single, long, thin-walled tubular structure, coiled upon itself to form a crescent-shaped pouch, about 3½ to 4 cm. long, and flattened in its anteroposterior diameter. Uncoiled, this tube reaches a length of 15 cm. or more. The wall of the vesicle is made up of a fibromuscular outer coating and a secreting type of epithelium. The vasa deferentia pass along the base of the bladder between the vesicles, and on each side the open end of the vesicle joins the vas at the base of the prostate to form the ejaculatory duct (Fig. 12).

The *blood supply* to the seminal vesicle is derived from the inferior vesicle and middle hemorrhoidal arteries. The veins accompany the arteries and drain into the prostatovesical plexuses. The *lymphatics* enter the iliac nodes, and the *nerves* are from the hypogastric plexus.

REFERENCES

CALLANDER, C. LATIMER: Surgical Anatomy. Philadelphia, W. B. Saunders Co., 1939.
DODSON, AUSTIN I.: Urological Surgery. St. Louis, C. V. Mosby Co., 1950.
MITCHELL, G. A. G.: Renal nerves. Brit. J. Urol., *22:*269–280, 1950.
MITCHELL, G. A. G.: Peri-renal fascia. Brit. J. Urol., *37:*257–266, 1950.
TRUETA, J., et al.: Studies of the Renal Circulation. Oxford, Blackwell Scientific Publications, 1947.

CHAPTER 2

The Elements of Renal Function

ROBERT F. PITTS, PH.D., M.D.

The function of the kidney in broadest terms is to regulate the composition of the internal fluid environment of the body. To consider the kidney as merely an excretory organ oversimplifies its contribution to bodily economy but, of more significance, tends to obscure the responsibility of the urologist to compensate by proper medical management for those functional deficiencies which his surgery cannot correct. True enough, the kidney excretes the wholly useless end products of protein metabolism, but it likewise excretes most of the valuable components of the body fluids when they are present in excess. Yet, if those components are present in normal or reduced amounts, the kidney jealously conserves them. Basically, the kidney regulates the osmotic pressure, the volume and the ionic structure of the blood plasma and interstitial fluid. In addition, it subserves such purely excretory functions as the elimination of urea, creatinine and uric acid. In renal disease loss of regulatory capacity is certainly of equal if not of greater import in the over-all economy of the body than is loss of excretory capacity, for the physiological disturbances characteristic of uremia are commonly better correlated with the disturbances in ionic constitution than with the waste nitrogen content of the body fluids. By properly managing diet and fluid and electrolyte balance, the urologist can compensate to a remarkable degree for deficiencies in functional capacity. An understanding of the elements of renal function is a requisite for rational management.

THE NATURE OF THE DISCRETE RENAL PROCESSES INVOLVED IN URINE FORMATION

Glomerular Filtration. The process of urine formation begins in the glomerulus with the expression of an ultrafiltrate of the blood plasma through the inert endothelial membranes of the capillary tuft. The responsible force is the hydrostatic pressure imparted to the blood by the beat of the heart. As an *ultrafiltrate,* this fluid contains all plasma constituents except those of colloidal dimensions, namely the lipids and proteins. The glomerular filtrate normally contains but trace amounts of protein, for the capillaries of the glomeruli, like those of the choroid plexuses of the brain and of the ciliary body of the eye, are essentially impermeable to colloids.

The pressure within the glomerular capillaries is thought to be about two thirds of the mean arterial pressure. Perhaps half of this pressure head, or

36

roughly 35 mm. Hg, is effective in driving fluid through the pores of the capillary membranes, for the colloid osmotic pressure exerted by the plasma proteins, amounting to some 25 mm. Hg, opposes filtration, as does a back pressure or turgor pressure of 10 mm. Hg which exists within the glomerular capsule. The glomerular capillary pores are most probably cylindrical in form with a mean radius of about 90 Angstrom units (0.000009 mm.), and a length of 0.3 microns (0.0003 mm.) or less (Pappenheimer, 1952). Because of their small size, they obstruct the movement of colloidal particles although they permit the passage of water and of substances in true solution. The proportion of the capillary surface occupied by the pores is small, probably of the order of 1 per cent or less.* The pores seem to be situated, not in the surface of the flattened endothelial cells making up the vascular tubes, but in the cement substance which holds those cells together. Damage to the cement leads first to increase in pore size, permeability to protein and proteinuria, later to capillary rupture and hematuria.

Each kidney of normal man contains about one and one-quarter million glomeruli and each glomerular tuft is composed of some 20 to 40 capillary loops. The total capillary filtering surface is variously estimated as 7,500 to 15,000 cm.²; the composite pore area, therefore, amounts to 75 to 150 cm.² (Merrill, 1952). In the average normal male 132 ml. of plasma are filtered through these glomerular pores each minute, a volume which in a day's time adds up to some 190 liters or about 50 gallons (Smith, 1951). Although this appears to be a phenomenal volume of fluid, it actually amounts to about one drop of plasma per day per glomerulus. The fact of key significance for an appreciation of the contribution of glomerular filtration to renal function is that *the entire volume of circulating blood plasma, carrying with it all waste products and valuable constituents, is filtered through the glomeruli once every 27 minutes.*

Tubular Reabsorption. The importance of tubular reabsorption in the economy of the body is immediately apparent if one considers the implications of the figures quoted above. An individual weighing 70 kg. contains in all about 40 liters of water, of which only 3.5 liters are enclosed within the vascular system as blood plasma. The filtration of 190 liters of plasma each day from an initial volume of only 3.5 liters demands the continuous cyclical return and refiltration of water. It demands no less the cyclical return and refiltration of all valuable constituents of the blood plasma with the exception of the plasma proteins, which, as we have noted, do not enter the filtrate in any significant quantity. Thus 190 liters of plasma contain 2.7 pounds of sodium chloride, 1 pound of sodium bicarbonate, 0.5 pound of glucose, 0.25 pound of amino acid and 4 gm. of vitamin C, as well as

* Per unit area of surface, glomerular capillaries filter more than 100 times the volume of fluid filtered by muscle capillaries, due first to the greater pressure head, second to the greater proportion of the capillary surface occupied by pores and third to the greater radius of the pores. Normally, muscle capillaries absorb at the venous end all fluid filtered at the arterial end. Glomerular capillaries on the other hand absorb none, for the hydrostatic pressure throughout the length of the capillary is above the sum of the colloid osmotic and turgor pressures. In other words, the glomerular capillary filters throughout its entire length, the muscle capillary does not.

appreciable quantities of many other valuable substances. In each instance the quantity filtered in a day far exceeds the total body store and even more, the quantity present in the circulating plasma. The importance of tubular reabsorption in preventing rapid and lethal depletion of water and valuable solutes is immediately apparent. There is evidence that even the traces of plasma protein which normally enter the glomerular filtrate are conserved by the renal tubules.

Cushny (1917) in his classical monograph on *The Secretion of Urine* postulated that the renal tubules, presented with a filtrate of plasma containing waste products and ions in improper proportions, reabsorb in bulk an *ideal* balanced salt solution. Waste products, unwanted ions and excess water left in the tubules after the absorption of this *ideal* fluid are eliminated as urine. This hypothesis, though attractively simple, has been shown to be untenable. Nearly all of the valuable constituents of the filtrate are absorbed independently, not in bulk as Cushny believed. Even a portion of some of the waste products (e.g., up to 60 per cent of the filtered urea) is absorbed.

The reabsorptive mechanisms fall into some four or more distinct categories.

(a) Certain substances such as urea are absorbed passively by diffusion. As the glomerular filtrate passes along the tubule, the withdrawal of water concentrates urea in the residual tubular urine. Except for water, urea is the most diffusible substance in the body. It is not surprising, therefore, to find that the lower the urine volume and the higher the urine urea concentration, the greater is the back diffusion of urea into the blood stream (Chasis and Smith, 1938). Apparently, the tubules cannot be sufficiently impermeable to exclude urea completely, and yet perform their absorptive functions adequately. The value of maintaining a volume flow of urine sufficient to limit the back diffusion of urea, especially under conditions of reduced renal function, is evident.

(b) Glucose (Shannon et al., 1941), vitamin C (Ralli et al., 1938) amino acids (Pitts and Alexander, 1944), phosphate (Pitts, 1944), and sulfate (Lotspeich, 1947) are reabsorbed by active* transport mechanisms which are capable of handling fixed and limited quantities of material per unit time. For example, the kidney of the average normal individual, filtering some 100 to 175 mg. of glucose per minute, reabsorbs all and excretes none. The tubules, however, can reabsorb as much as 375 mg. per minute before any appreciable quantity appears in the urine. If more than this quantity is filtered, either because of an increase in blood glucose level or because the rate of glomerular filtration is increased, only this limited amount is reabsorbed; all in excess of this amount is excreted. The limited capacity to reabsorb a substance when the tubules are saturated, i.e., are presented with more than they can absorb, is termed the *maximum tubular absorptive capacity* for that substance, abbreviated for glucose to read Tm_G.

---

* By active transport mechanism is meant one which operates only by the continuous expenditure of energy to move a substance from a region of low concentration to one of higher concentration.

(c) The major ions of the blood plasma and extracellular fluid, including sodium, chloride and bicarbonate, are reabsorbed by mechanisms which are no less active than those included in the category above. However, these mechanisms exhibit no true limitations of reabsorptive capacity (Pitts et al., 1949), (Wesson et al., 1948 b). Although gross renal plasma thresholds exist for each of these ion species, below which they are almost completely retained and above which they are excreted in progressively increasing amounts, the quantities filtered per unit of time are not *per se* the determinants of completeness of absorption. The concentrations of sodium, of chloride and of bicarbonate ions in the filtrate, more than the absolute quantities filtered

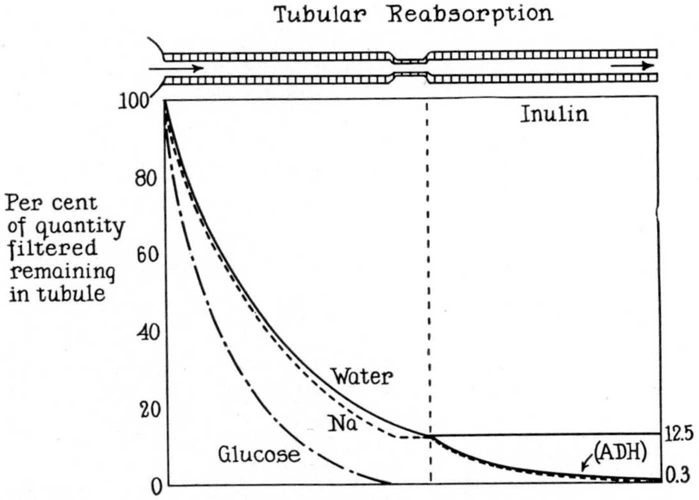

Fig. 16.   Schematic representation of the sites of reabsorption and of the amounts of several urinary constituents absorbed in the proximal and distal segments of the nephron of man.

per minute, appear to determine the relative proportions reabsorbed and excreted. Thus no Tm exists for any one of these three ion species. In fact, an increase in filtration rate is accompanied by an almost equivalent increase in the absorptive capacity for each. The situation is a fortunate one, for it protects the individual from rapid depletion of his sodium, chloride and bicarbonate reserves when his rate of filtration is moderately increased. Furthermore, a modest decrease in filtration rate and hence in quantity of salt filtered does not render him incapable of excreting that which is necessary if he is to maintain himself in salt balance. However, a sharp and significant reduction in filtration rate is one of the factors which favors salt and water retention and the accumulation of edema (*vide infra*). In addition, these ion absorptive mechanisms are regulated, at least with respect to their finer adjustments, by hormones of the adrenal cortex.

(d) The reabsorption of water is effected by no less than two distinctly different mechanisms (Wesson et al., 1948 a). The absorption of the vast bulk of the water (80 per cent or so) is dependent on the osmotic force developed by the active absorption of sodium, chloride, bicarbonate, glucose, and so forth, in the proximal segment of the renal tubule. The remainder of the filtered water (up to 20 per cent of the total) is absorbed in the distal segment of the convoluted tubule by an active process stimulated by the antidiuretic hormone, pitressin. These relationships are diagrammed in Figure 16.

Under normal conditions, salvage of water and of valuable components of the glomerular filtrate is nearly complete by the time the urine enters the renal pelvis. Only traces of glucose and amino acids escape absorption. Of the 190 liters of water filtered, only one liter or so is excreted. Of the 2.7 pounds of sodium chloride filtered, only 5 to 10 gm. are eliminated. Of the 1 pound of sodium bicarbonate filtered, essentially none appears in the urine. Energy is expended not only in forming the original filtrate, but also in performing the chemical work involved in the independent and active absorption of each of the valuable components of that filtrate. Why, in order to eliminate 20 gm. or so of urea, 5 to 10 gm. of sodium chloride, a liter of water, and perhaps 1 or 2 gm. each of creatinine, uric acid, phosphorus and sulfur, must so much useless work be performed? As Smith (1943) so aptly expresses it, "There is enough waste motion here to bankrupt any economic system other than a natural one, for nature is the only artificer who does not need to count the cost by which she achieves her ends."

Some appreciation of the foibles and contradictions of the kidney of man may be obtained from a brief consideration of its evolutionary development. Our protochordate ancestors evolved in a sea of moderate salinity and early found it advantageous to enclose a bit of this medium within their integument and to render its composition stable. The problem of maintaining constancy of the internal fluid environment was initially a simple one. These animals could drink freely of the fluid surrounding them, pump it through their vascular systems, allow it to permeate their tissues, secrete it into their body cavities and then propel it and its dissolved wastes to the outside through simple ciliated tubes. But driven by some wanderlust, the early vertebrates migrated into fresh water streams where their osmotic superiority to their environment caused them to soak up large quantities of water. The invention of a vascular glomerular tuft in association with their simple fluid conduit system enabled them to filter off this excess water from the blood stream. But filtration created the problem of conservation of those valuable solutes which found their way into the filtrate. Salt especially was at a premium in their newly adopted fresh water environment. The proximal tubule, with its capacity to absorb salts, glucose, amino acids, and so forth, was the answer to this self-created problem. Later crawling out on dry land, the problem abruptly changed from need for fluid elimination to need for fluid conservation. Instead of discarding the now unnecessary pressure filter and redesigning the kidney along the lines of an efficient secretory gland, the terrestrial vertebrates chose to add a distal segment to their tubular system to salvage the precious water. Later the mammals in their quest for independence of water developed a thin segment of the loop of Henle and a more active distal tubule capable of elaborating a highly concentrated urine from which all but a fraction of 1 per cent of the filtered water could be recovered.

In a sense the complexity and inefficiency of the kidney of man might be likened to that of our present form of federal bureaucratic government. Neither was initially created in its present form. Each developed by adding to a simple structure one new agency after another to compensate for an inadequacy of those already established in meeting new situations. Nothing, no matter how useless, has been discarded. The amazing fact about both is that they function. The normal kidney at least functions remarkably well.

Tubular Secretion. Tubular secretory mechanisms serve one or the other of two ends. First, because they favor rapid elimination, they serve to maintain the plasma concentrations of those substances which they transport at low levels. Second, they provide a means of substituting by exchange some useless substance in the plasma for a desirable one in the tubular urine. Although the number of known reabsorptive mechanisms is great, only three secretory mechanisms have so far been characterized.

The secretory mechanism which has been most completely described is that which transports phenolsulfonphthalein, penicillin, diodrast, hippuran, para-aminohippuric acid, hippuric acid, and so forth. These substances, for the most part unrelated chemically, are all carboxylic or sulfonic acids, and their transport by a single secretory system is no doubt related to their common acidic properties (Taggart, 1950). Only one, hippuric acid, is a natural excretory product and neither it nor its precursor, benzoic acid, is especially toxic. Perhaps another excretory product, more toxic but as yet unidentified, and ideally maintained at low concentration in the plasma, is the one which this mechanism was specifically devised to transport.

In a number of respects, this secretory mechanism resembles the reabsorptive mechanism for glucose (Shannon, 1939). It is, of course, polarized in the opposite direction, i.e., it transports materials from low concentration in the plasma to high concentration in the urine. Both mechanisms are active, requiring the continuous expenditure of energy. Both are limited in their transport capacity. At saturation the secretory mechanism of normal man can transport 75 mg. of para-aminohippurate, 37 mg. of phenolsulfonphthalein or 57 mg. of diodrast iodine per minute. It exhibits classically the phenomenon of competitive inhibition in that the secretory mechanism, when saturated with para-aminohippurate, is unable to transport penicillin. Certain substances, of which carinamide is an example, although not actively secreted, become tangled in the secretory machinery and prevent the transport of penicillin (Beyer et al., 1949). Clinical use is made of this secretory blocking action to obtain higher and better sustained blood levels of the antibiotic following usual therapeutic doses. It is probable that this secretory mechanism like the reabsorptive mechanism for glucose is localized in the cells of the proximal convoluted tubules.

The other secretory mechanisms are most likely localized in the distal convoluted tubule. One serves to exchange either hydrogen ions (Pitts, 1948) or potassium ions (Berliner, 1950), picked up from the peritubular blood, for sodium ions in the tubular urine. The other serves somewhat indirectly, but in like fashion, to exchange ammonium ions for sodium ions (Pitts, 1950). The net effect of the exchange of either hydrogen ions or ammonia for sodium ions is to build up the bicarbonate bound base reserves of the plasma (cf. Fig. 17). Failure of adequate operation of these mechanisms

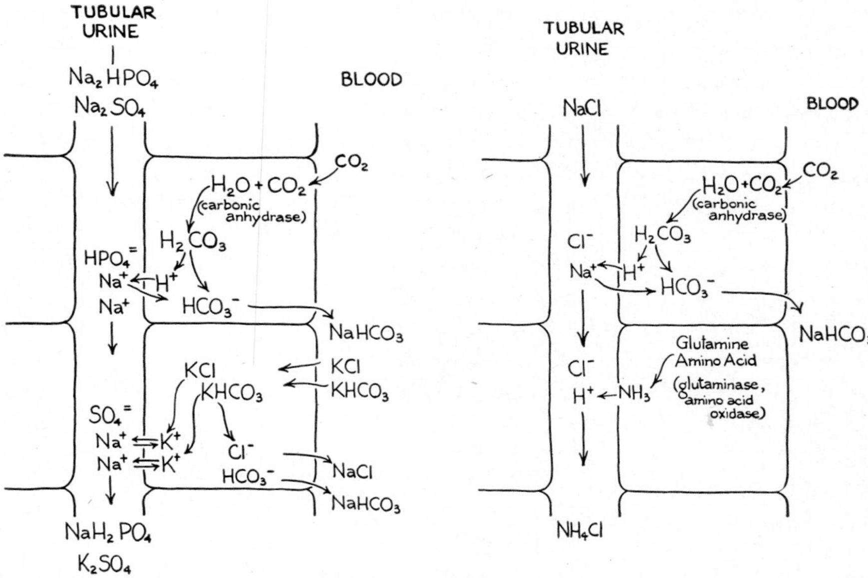

Fig. 17.   Schematic representation of the tubular secretory mechanisms concerned with the regulation of acid-base and potassium-sodium balances. Presumably all of these mechanisms are localized in cells of the distal convoluted tubules. *Left:* Hydrogen-sodium and potassium-sodium exchange mechanisms. *Left upper:* Hydration of carbon dioxide to form carbonic acid is speeded by the enzyme, carbonic anhydrase. Hydrogen ions dissociated from carbonic acid are exchanged for sodium ions in the tubular urine. Sodium and bicarbonate ions are returned to the peritubular blood stream to build up the bicarbonate bound base reserves of the body. *Left lower:* Potassium ions are likewise exchanged for sodium ions in the tubular urine, permitting excretion of potassium and conservation of sodium. Some step in this exchange mechanism appears to be common to the one concerned with hydrogen ions, for the active transfer of hydrogen ions depresses potassium exchange, and the active transfer of potassium ions depresses hydrogen exchange. *Right:* The role of ammonia in acid-base regulation. Since the tubules are incapable of elaborating urine more acid than pH 4.5, they can exchange very little hydrogen for sodium if the acid formed is a strong acid, such as hydrochloric, rather than a weak acid, such as primary phosphate, shown on the left. However, if this acid is neutralized by ammonia as rapidly as it is formed, the exchange can go on. The ammonia is formed by the hydrolysis of glutamine and amino acids and diffuses rapidly into the tubular lumen if the reaction there is an acid one.

underlies the acidosis which so frequently accompanies chronic renal disease. Recent evidence indicates that the hydrogen-sodium exchange mechanism also exchanges potassium ions for sodium ions (Berliner et al., 1951), thereby subserving the dual functions of eliminating potassium and conserving sodium.

The exchange of hydrogen ions for sodium ions is limited by the inability of the tubular cells to produce urine more acid than pH 4.5. The diffusion of ammonia from cells to urine, a process facilitated by high acidity of the urine, neutralizes the acid and permits the exchange to continue. Although ammonia is not *per se* exchanged for sodium, the net result is the same as though it were (cf. Fig. 17). Ammonia is produced in the tubular cells by the hydrolysis of glutamine and by the oxidative deamination of amino acids, not by the hydrolysis of urea as was once supposed (Van Slyke et al., 1943).

MEASURES OF RENAL FUNCTIONS

Measures Based on the Composition of the Plasma. Since regulation of the composition of the body fluids is a prime responsibility of the kidney, one would anticipate that an assessment of the degree of normalcy of concentration of the several plasma constituents would be the best indication of over-all adequacy of renal function. However, the rather broad limits of normal concentration, the dependence of concentration on dietary intake, metabolism and hydration, and the changes in concentration which occur in

Table 1. Normal Ranges of Concentration of Components of the Plasma Useful as Indicators of Adequacy of Renal Function.

Nonprotein Nitrogen	10 to 35 mg. per 100 ml.
Urea Nitrogen	5 to 20 mg. per 100 ml.
Urea	10 to 40 mg. per 100 ml.
Creatinine	0.5 to 1.5 mg. per 100 ml.
Sulfate (inorganic)	0.3 to 0.6 m.Mols per liter.
Sulfur (inorganic)	1.0 to 2.0 mg. per 100 ml.
Phosphate (inorganic)	0.5 to 1.5 m.Mols per liter.
Phosphorus (inorganic)	1.5 to 4.5 mg. per 100 ml.

circulatory insufficiency in the absence of organic renal disease, render such tests relatively unreliable as measures of the extent of renal pathology.

The constituents of the plasma commonly quantified as measures of renal function are nonprotein nitrogen, urea, creatinine, sulfate, phosphate and potassium. The upper limits of normal plasma concentration of each of these constituents are given in Table 1 (Bradley, 1945). In reality no lower limit, having any significance with respect to renal function can be given. Providing one can exclude dehydration, fever, adrenal insufficiency, absorption of blood from the gastrointestinal tract or absorption of inflammatory exudates, and either peripheral or central circulatory failure, elevation of plasma concentration of any constituent listed in this table, suggests renal pathology.

Excretion of each of the substances listed is to some degree dependent on and determined by glomerular filtration. Any reduction in the quantity of filtrate formed will result in retention of these substances and in increase in their plasma concentrations. Were this the sole factor involved, halving the rate of filtration should double the plasma concentration. However, a number of factors militate against such simple inverse proportionality. Relatively high fluid intake and urine output in patients with chronic renal insufficiency, reduces the urinary concentration of urea and hence the back diffusion of urea. Thus, even though less filtrate is formed per minute, a greater than normal proportion of the filtered urea is excreted in the urine. Furthermore, any reduction in protein intake reduces the quantity of urea presented for excretion. Creatinine is eliminated not only by filtration but an additional small moiety is secreted by the renal tubules, a fact which reduces dependence of plasma concentration on glomerular function. Some 75 per cent or so of the sulfate, phosphate and potassium delivered into the glomerular filtrate is normally absorbed by the renal tubules. Variation in completeness of absorption, rather than in quantity of filtrate formed, is the more significant determinant of plasma level. Net absorption of potassium may actually be replaced by net secretion when the plasma level increases minutely. The result of the operation of these several factors is that glomerular filtration rate must be reduced to one quarter or less of normal

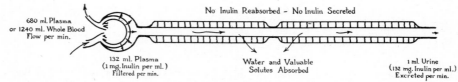

Fig. 18.   Principles involved in the use of inulin as a measure of glomerular filtration rate. The kidneys of the normal individual are represented schematically as a single large nephron rather than as some 2 million microscopic ones. The total renal whole blood flow of 1240 ml. per min. or plasma flow of 680 ml. per min. perfuses the glomeruli prior to entry into the peritubular capillary network. Roughly 20 per cent of the plasma flowing through the glomeruli (on an average 132 ml. per min.) is filtered. The inulin, entering this filtrate in the same concentration as in the original plasma, is concentrated by the reabsorption of water. No inulin is either reabsorbed or secreted. Hence all filtered inulin, no more and no less, is excreted in the urine. The rate of excretion relative to plasma concentration is therefore a measure of the rate of glomerular filtration.

before the plasma concentrations of nonprotein nitrogen and urea rise definitely above the rather overgenerous upper limit of normal. Filtration must be even more severely restricted before plasma levels of creatinine, sulfate and phosphate are significantly elevated, and only with extreme limitation of function does potassium concentration rise above the upper limit of normal.

Measures of Glomerular Filtration Rate. Only one exact measure of glomerular filtration exists, namely the *plasma clearance of inulin*. This variable is defined as the number of ml. of plasma completely cleared of inulin in one minute's time. It is expressed arithmetically in the following terms:

$$\text{Clearance of Inulin} = C_{IN} = \frac{U_{IN} \times V}{P_{IN}},$$

where U_{IN} equals the urine concentration of inulin in mg. per ml., V equals the rate of urine flow in ml. per min. and P_{IN} equals the plasma concentration of inulin in mg. per ml.

The philosophy as well as the facts upon which this test is based are illustrated in Figure 18 and in the following considerations (Smith, 1951). Inulin, though a substance of high molecular weight (approximately 5000), is a true crystalloid, not a colloid. Therefore, when injected into the blood stream, it passes through the glomerular filter with no more hindrance than does the plasma water. If 132 ml. of plasma containing 1 mg. of inulin per ml. are filtered each minute, then 132 mg. of inulin are delivered into the renal tubules each minute. Inulin is neither reabsorbed nor secreted by the renal tubular cells. Therefore, every mg. of inulin entering the filtrate is excreted in the urine, and every mg. excreted has passed through the glomerular filter.

We may, therefore, reverse our argument in the following way. If an individual excretes 1 ml. of urine per minute ($V = 1$ ml. per min.) and if that urine contains 132 mg. of inulin per ml. ($U_{IN} = 132$ mg. per ml.), then each minute he excretes 132 mg. of inulin ($U_{IN} \times V = 132$ mg. per min.). If each ml. of plasma contains 1 mg. of inulin ($P_{IN} = 1$ mg. per ml.), then 132 ml. of plasma per minute must have been filtered to account for the known rate of excretion of inulin.*

$$C_{IN} = \frac{132 \text{ mg. per ml.} \times 1 \text{ ml. per min.}}{1 \text{ mg. per ml.}} = 132 \text{ ml. per min.}$$

The following practical considerations are important if the estimation of filtration rate is to be accurate. Inulin must be injected in a priming dose in a quantity sufficient to raise the plasma level to a range adequate for accurate analysis, about 0.3 mg. per ml. In a nonedematous individual this dose in milligrams amounts to $60 \times$ body wt. in kg.** Thereafter, if inulin is infused at a rate sufficient to replace each minute the quantity filtered, the plasma level will remain constant, a condition highly desirable for accurate work. This quantity will obviously depend on the rate of glomerular filtration and it is necessary for the investigator to estimate, at least roughly, the magnitude of the variable he wishes to measure. The rate of infusion of inulin per minute to attain constancy of plasma level amounts to 40 mg. $\times$ expected fraction of normal filtration rate.† Were filtration rate normal, then 40 mg. of inulin per minute would have to be infused. If filtration rate were $\frac{1}{5}$ normal, then the quantity infused would have to be only 8 mg. per minute. Fortunately, the rate of infusion to attain adequate stability of plasma level is not especially critical.

In addition to the described priming and infusion techniques which serve to stabilize the plasma inulin concentration within the proper range, exact

---

* Using the clearance formula, $C = UV/P$, one may calculate the clearance of any substance present in the plasma. However, only inulin is freely filtered and neither secreted nor absorbed. Hence only the inulin clearance has the exact dimensions of glomerular filtration rate.

** In calculating a priming dose of any substance one must know its approximate volume of distribution. Inulin does not enter cells, but is distributed with relative rapidity through the extracellular fluid space. In the nonedematous individual extracellular volume is roughly 20 per cent of body weight. The dose in mg. therefore is equal to *desired concentration* (mg. per ml.) $\times$ body wt. (kg.) $\times 0.20 \times 1000$. In a 70 kg. individual, to attain a plasma concentration of 0.30 mg. per ml., the priming dose would be $0.30 \times 70 \times 0.2 \times 1000 = 4,200$ mg. or 4.2 gm.

† The rate of infusion must be such as to replace each minute the quantity of inulin filtered from the plasma. If the plasma inulin concentration is 0.30 mg. per ml. and the glomerular filtration rate is 132 ml. per min., then $0.30 \times 132 = 40$ mg. per min. of inulin are filtered. This quantity must be restored to the body each minute if plasma concentration is to be kept constant.

measurement of the rate of urine flow is demanded. Urine is collected over precisely measured time intervals, (usually of 15 to 20 minutes' duration) and the bladder is completely emptied of its contents through an indwelling catheter by suprapubic pressure and irrigation with sterile distilled water. To ensure accuracy of collection, it is advisable to have a flow of urine of at least 2 ml. per minute. Blood specimens are drawn at the midpoint of each urine collection period. Ultimately, of course, the validity of the measurements depends upon exact chemical analysis of plasma and urine specimens for inulin concentration.*

Two other clearance determinations may be employed as rough estimates of glomerular function, namely the endogenous creatinine clearance and the urea clearance. The procedures employed are basically the same as those described for determining the inulin clearance, except that the endogenous plasma level and rate of excretion of either creatinine or urea are measured, thus avoiding the necessity for infusing the foreign substance inulin.** The kidney of man not only filters creatinine but also secretes it. The clearance of creatinine should, therefore, be greater than the rate of glomerular filtration. However, in normal man the apparent plasma concentration of creatinine, measured by the relatively nonspecific Jaffe color reaction, is higher than the true creatinine concentration. By coincidence dividing a $U_{Cr} \times V$ term, which is too large because a secreted moiety is added to a filtered moiety, by a P_{Cr} term which is too large because of the presence of some noncreatinine chromogen, leads to a clearance having roughly the dimensions of filtration rate. The coincidence, however, is not so favorable in the presence of renal disease, and the creatinine clearance deviates considerably from the inulin clearance under such conditions.

Urea is grossly absorbed by the renal tubules. Hence the urea clearance is lower than the rate of glomerular filtration, the normal value averaging 75 ml. per minute. However, as filtration rate declines, the urea clearance drops roughly in proportion. A major difficulty with the use of the urea clearance as an index of renal function is the fact that it varies with urine flow, especially at flows below 2 ml. per minute. However, if urine flow is sustained at 2 ml. per minute or more, a reduction in urea clearance to 30 per cent of normal indicates that the rate of glomerular filtration is reduced by an approximately equivalent amount.

Measures of Renal Tubular Function. Two measures of renal tubular function in common clinical use are concentrating and diluting power and phenolsulfonphthalein (P.S.P.) excretion. The former is a measure of the ability of the kidney to regulate the osmotic pressure of the body fluids either by concentrating the urine and thus excreting solutes in preference to water, or by diluting the urine and thus excreting water in preference to solutes. The latter (P.S.P. excretion) is a rough measure of the functional capacity of the tubules to secrete the dye. As noted above on page 41, the mechanism

---

* For the analysis of inulin in plasma and urine we employ the method of Harrison, H. E.: Proc. Soc. Exp. Biol. and Med., *49:*111, 1942.

** Inulin, specially processed to be pyrogen-free, must be used. We obtain ours from U. S. Standard Products, Woodworth, Wisconsin.

which secretes P.S.P. also transports diodrast, para-aminohippurate and penicillin.

Numerous tests of concentrating and diluting power have been proposed. For the most part, concentrating power is assessed by some modification of the Addis and Shevky procedure in which the patient is instructed to take no water, milk, coffee, tea, soup, custard or junket after breakfast on the first morning. Lunch and supper are of dry toast, eggs, cheese, bacon, etc. Urine is voided at 7 P.M. and the overnight specimen is collected at 7 A.M. on the second morning. The average normal specific gravity of this overnight specimen is 1.032. Any value less than 1.026 (corrected for protein con-

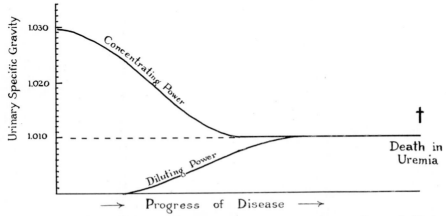

Fig. 19.   Schematic representation of progressive loss of concentrating and diluting power in the course of progressive renal disease, leading to a condition of isosthenuria or fixation of specific gravity of the urine. Once this condition is established, concentrating and diluting powers are valueless as measures of further progress of renal disease.

tent if proteinuria exists) is considered indicative of diminished renal concentrating power providing the dry regimen has been faithfully carried out and providing the patient is not in the process of losing edema. Some two thirds to three quarters of the specific gravity of the urine under such circumstances is contributed by sodium and potassium salts of chloride, sulfate and phosphate, the remainder largely by urea (Price et al., 1940). The specific gravity of a protein-free filtrate of plasma is roughly 1.010. Concentration of the urine above this value represents osmotic work performed by the renal tubules in actively absorbing water, leaving a residue of solutes. If the patient drinks a liter of water, urine flow increases and urine specific gravity falls, normally to values as low as 1.001 to 1.003.* Dilution of the urine below the specific gravity of the plasma likewise represents osmotic work performed by the renal tubules in actively absorbing salts, leaving a residue of water.

In chronic renal disease both concentrating and diluting powers are re-

* Diluting power is a rather unsatisfactory test of renal tubular function because it may be markedly altered by hepatic, adrenal cortical and cardiac disease in the absence of organic renal disease.

duced. As shown schematically in Figure 19, concentrating power is first reduced, later diluting power, and eventually there results fixation of specific gravity at a value of about 1.010, namely that of protein-free plasma. This is a precarious though not an intolerable state of affairs. It is precarious because water restriction or extrarenal loss of fluid precipitates dehydration

Table 2. Normal Values in Renal Function Tests

MEASURES OF GLOMERULAR FUNCTION
1. Inulin Clearance (male, per 1.73 sq. meters surface area)............ 132 ml. per min.
   (female, per 1.73 sq. meters surface area).......... 117 ml. per min.
2. Urea Clearance (maximal clearance at urine flows above 2 ml. per min.
   UV/P)....................................... 75 ml. per min.
   (standard clearance at urine flows less than 2 ml. per
   min. $U\sqrt{V/P}$)................................. 57 ml. per min.
3. Creatinine Clearance (endogenous), a rough approximation of inulin clearance.

MEASURES OF TUBULAR FUNCTION
1. Concentrating Power (24 hrs. on dry regimen)............. Specific Gravity > 1.026.
2. Diluting Power (after 1 liter of water)................... Specific Gravity < 1.003.
3. P.S.P. Excretion (6 mg. intramuscularly)....................... 40–60% first hour
                                                                    60–85% second hour
4. P.S.P. Excretion (6 mg. intravenously)...................... 25% first 15 minutes
5. Maximum Tubular Reabsorptive Capacity
   Glucose Tm (male, per 1.73 sq. meters surface area).............. 375 mg. per min.
   Glucose Tm (female, per 1.73 sq. meters surface area)............ 303 mg. per min.
6. Maximum Tubular Secretory Capacity
   Diodrast Tm as Iodine (male or female)....................... 57 mg. per min.
   p-Aminohippurate Tm (male or female)........................ 75 mg. per min.
   Phenolsulfonphthalein Tm (male or female).................... 37 mg. per min.

MEASURES OF RENAL VASCULAR ADEQUACY
1. Renal Plasma Flow, Clearance of PAH or Diodrast at low plasma
   levels (male or female)..................................... 680 ml. per min.
2. Renal Blood Flow, derived from above plasma flow measurements
   and hematocrit... 1,240 ml. per min.

DERIVED MEASURES OF RENAL FUNCTION
1. Adequacy of Tubular Blood Supply
   Renal Plasma Flow/Tm Glucose..................................... 1.8–2.2
   Renal Plasma Flow/Tm PAH.. 9.0–11.0
   (increased ratios, hyperemia; decreased ratios, ischemia)
2. Filtration Fraction....................................... 0.19–0.21
3. Glomerular-Tubular Balance
   Tm Glucose/Inulin Clearance...................................... 2.7–2.9
   (increased ratio, tubular preponderance; decreased ratio, glomerular
   preponderance)

and uremia. On the other hand, forcing fluids without adequate salt intake leads to depletion of body stores of sodium and chloride and the development of the low salt syndrome of lethargy, weakness and confusion.

The P.S.P. excretion test is at best only a rough indication of the extent of renal tubular dysfunction. When the dye is given intramuscularly and the one and two hour excretion rates determined, the test is sensitive only to gross impairment of function. The normal individual excretes the major fraction of the injected dose within the first half hour. Obviously the excretion of the usual normal fraction of the dye during the first hour would not rule out a 50 per cent reduction in functional capacity. However, if the excretion of P.S.P. is measured over a 15 minute interval following the intravenous administration of 6 mg. of the dye, the sensitivity of the test is considerably improved. To facilitate the collection of urine, the test is performed with the bladder full. In either instance over 90 per cent of the dye excreted is eliminated by tubular secretion. Normal values for these tests are given in Table 2.

Two exact and reproducible measures of renal tubular function are *glucose reabsorptive capacity* and *para-aminohippurate secretory capacity*. As noted on page 38, the renal tubules of normal man, when presented with an excess of glucose in the glomerular filtrate, are capable of reabsorbing, on an average, 375 mg. of glucose per minute (Smith et al., 1943). In chronic renal disease this value is reduced more or less in proportion to the reduction in tubular mass of the kidney. Glucose absorptive capacity may, therefore, be employed as a functional measure of that mass. In performing the test, glucose is infused at a rate sufficient to maintain the plasma concentration at a level of over 400 mg. per cent in order to establish frank glycuresis. Inulin is incorporated in the infusion to permit this simultaneous measurement of filtration rate. Procedures are the same as those described under the section on measurement of glomerular filtration rate, except that arterial or arterialized* venous blood specimens must be collected for analysis.

Knowing the glomerular filtration rate (C_{IN}) and plasma concentration of glucose (P_G), one may readily calculate the quantity of glucose filtered per minute in the following way:

Glucose Filtered (mg. per min.) $= C_{IN}$ (ml. per min.) $\times P_G$ (mg. per ml.)

For a normal individual having a filtration rate of 132 ml. per minute and a plasma glucose concentration of 400 mg. per cent (4 mg. per ml.),

Glucose Filtered (mg. per min.) $= 132 \times 4 = 528$ mg. per min.

Knowing the rate of urine flow (V) and the urine concentration of glucose (U_G), one may calculate the quantity of glucose excreted per minute in the following way:

Glucose Excreted (mg. per min.) $= V$ (ml. per min.) $\times U_G$ (mg. per ml.)

If the urine flow is 3 ml. per minute and the urine glucose concentration 5,100 mg. per cent (51 mg. per ml.), then

Glucose Excreted (mg. per min.) $= 3 \times 51 = 153$ mg. per min.

The quantity of glucose reabsorbed is obviously the difference between these two quantities.

Glucose Reabsorbed (mg. per min.) $=$ *Glucose Filtered* (mg. per min.)
$-$*Glucose Excreted* (mg. per min.)

In the example given, Glucose Reabsorbed (mg. per min.) $= 528 -153 =$ 375 mg. per min.

* Because a significant arteriovenous glucose difference exists under the conditions of this test, owing to utilization of glucose by the tissues of the arm, the usual venous blood specimen is unsatisfactory. However, immersing the arm for 10 minutes in water heated to 45° C. induces such marked hyperemia that the composition of the venous blood approaches that of the arterial blood.

The chief practical difficulty in performing this test lies in the estimation of the quantity of glucose which must be infused to maintain proper plasma levels, for glucose is not only excreted in the urine, it is also utilized by the body. In general, for an adult of average size (70 kg.) a priming dose of 30 to 50 gm. in 50 per cent solution should be administered rapidly to attain the desired high blood glucose level. Glucose thereafter should be infused at a rate of 1 to 2 gm. per minute to maintain this plasma level.*

Technically, the determination of maximum secretory capacity for para-aminohippurate (PAH) is a somewhat simpler measure of renal tubular function than is glucose reabsorptive capacity. As noted on page 49, the renal tubules of normal man, when presented with an excess of PAH in the peritubular capillary blood, are capable of secreting a fixed and limited quantity of PAH per min. (Chasis et al., 1945) (on an average 75 mg. per min.). However, PAH is not only secreted by the renal tubules, it also is filtered through the glomeruli. The total quantity eliminated is, therefore, the sum of the moieties filtered and secreted. The secretory capacity is determined by subtracting the quantity filtered per minute from the total quantity excreted per minute.

PAH Excreted (mg. per min.) $= V$ (ml. per min.) $\times U_{PAH}$ (mg. per ml.)

PAH Filtered (mg. per min.) $= C_{IN}$ (ml. per min.) $\times 0.83** \times P_{PAH}$ (mg. per ml.)

PAH Secreted (mg. per min.) $=$ *PAH Excreted* (mg. per min.) $-PAH$ *Filtered* (mg. per min.)

The terms U_{PAH} and P_{PAH} refer to urinary and plasma concentrations of PAH, while V refers to urine volume. The clearance of inulin (C_{IN}) must be measured simultaneously and plasma PAH must be maintained at a level of more than 30 mg. per cent.

In a normal individual in whom $P_{PAH} = 40$ mg. per cent (0.40 mg. per ml.); $C_{IN} = 132$ ml. per min.; $U_{PAH} = 2375$ mg. per cent (23.75 mg. per ml.) and $V = 5$ ml. per min.:

PAH Excreted $= 23.75 \times 5 = 118.8$ mg. per min.

PAH Filtered $= 132 \times 0.83 \times 0.40 = 43.8$ mg. per min.

PAH Secreted $= 118.8 -43.8 = 75$ mg. per min.

P.S.P. and Diodrast are secreted by this same tubular mechanism and it would be possible to measure functional tubular mass in terms of the maximal secretory capacities of either of these two substances. Normal values are given in Table 2. However, the simplicity and accuracy of the PAH determination renders this the procedure of choice.†

Measures of Renal Vascular Adequacy. About 20 per cent of the blood pumped by the heart of man at rest perfuses the kidneys. High blood flow relative to organ weight is of course related to the homeostatic functions of

* For the analysis of glucose in plasma and urine we employ the method of Shannon, J. A., Farber, S., and Troast, L.: Am. J. Physiol., *133:*752, 1941.

** The factor of 0.83 is introduced into this equation to correct for the fact that 17 per cent of the PAH is bound to the plasma proteins and hence is not filterable through the glomerular capillary membranes.

† For the analysis of PAH in plasma and urine we employ the method of Smith, H. W., Finkelstein, N., Aliminosa, L., Crawford, B., and Graber, M.: J. Clin. Investigation, *24:* 388, 1945.

the kidneys rather than to their metabolic demands. Only 1.5 ml. of oxygen are removed from each 100 ml. of blood perfusing the kidneys, in comparison with an average of 6 ml. removed by the rest of the body tissues (Cargill and Hickam, 1949). How well the kidney functions in regulating the composition of the body fluids is obviously related among other things to the adequacy of its blood perfusion.

Clinical measurement of renal blood flow depends upon the fact that certain substances such as Diodrast and para-aminohippurate, when present in very low concentration, are almost completely removed from the blood in one passage through the kidney (Chasis et al., 1945). Simultaneous measurement of the rate of excretion and plasma concentration of PAH permit calculation of the renal plasma flow, using the conventional clearance formula,

$$\text{Renal Plasma Flow (ml. per min.)} = \frac{U_{PAH} \times V}{P_{PAH}},$$

the one requisite being that P_{PAH} be maintained at levels from 0.010 to 0.040 mg. per ml. by continuous intravenous infusion. Actually the PAH clearance so determined is a measure of *effective renal plasma flow** (RPF), for the blood perfusing the capsule, perinephric fat and other nonexcretory tissues such as the pelvis does not contribute to the measured volume. *Effective renal blood flow* (RBF) may be calculated as *plasma flow* $\times$

$$\frac{1}{1 - \text{Hematocrit}}.$$

Several values derived from functional measures already described give some insight into the nature of the pathologic processes affecting the kidney in disease. Normally about 20 per cent of the plasma which flows through the kidney is filtered through the glomeruli. This datum, known as the filtration fraction (F.F.), is equal to *glomerular filtration rate divided by renal plasma flow* expressed in per cent, or $C_{IN}/C_{PAH} \times 100$. Where the pathologic process is primarily one affecting the glomeruli and reducing the rate of glomerular filtration, the filtration fraction tends to be low. On the other hand, where the pathologic process is one primarily of sclerosis of the renal arterioles, the filtration fraction is high.

The ratio of tubular mass, as measured by maximum glucose reabsorptive capacity (Tm_G) or maximum PAH secretory capacity (Tm_{PAH}), to renal plasma flow (C_{PAH}) gives an indication of the relative degree of ischemia or of hyperemia, of the renal tubules. R.P.F./$Tm_G = 2.0$ normally, an increase being indicative of hyperemia, a decrease of ischemia. Similarly RPF/$Tm_{PAH} = 10.0$ normally, with alterations in the ratio having the same connotations as above.

Application of Renal Function Tests. The actual application of certain of these function tests is illustrated by the following data.

M.F., a 30 year old colored female, was admitted for the first time on 11/14/51 to the Urological Service of the New York Hospital. She entered the hospital purely for informa-

---

* Under conditions of severe renal damage, the extraction of PAH from the blood is incomplete and the clearance of PAH no longer has the relatively exact dimensions of renal plasma flow.

tion as to her renal functional status. Some 17 years previously, following birth of her first child she suffered an acute febrile attack, followed by the development of low back pain. Three years later, following a similar acute attack, a right nephrostomy and later a right nephrectomy were performed. Roughly a month or so following operation her legs began to swell, the edema, of a brawny nonpitting type, persisting to date. About 10 years prior to admission, she developed a dull aching left flank pain which persisted until 12/50 at which time a left nephrostomy was performed. For the past year she has been symptom-free.

On examination the patient was observed to be a well-nourished, well-developed colored female in no distress. The significant physical findings were a healed right flank scar, a

Table 3. Renal Function Measurements on Left Kidney of Patient M.F.; Right Nephrectomy; Left Nephrostomy One Year Previously; Hydronephrosis, Pyelonephritis of Remaining Left Kidney.

URINE FLOW	INULIN			PARA-AMINOHIPPURATE			FILTRATION FRACTION
	Plasma Conc.	Urine Conc.	Clearance	Plasma Conc.	Urine Conc.	Clearance	
ml./min.	mg. %	mg. %	ml./min.	mg. %	mg. %	ml./min.	C_{IN}/C_{PAH}
6.37	46.2	170	23.4	2.07	15.6	48.0	0.49
5.43	42.5	166	21.2	1.87	14.1	40.2	0.53
4.95	40.7	191	23.2	1.77	13.2	36.9	0.63
			22.6			41.7	0.55
						Tm PAH	C_{PAH}
						mg./min.	Tm PAH
3.02	37.8	260	20.8	48.9	566	8.65	4.82
3.90	36.9	214	22.6	44.1	482	10.53	3.96
4.47	35.9	174	21.7	43.1	379	9.19	4.54
						9.46	4.44

large ill-defined mass in the left upper quadrant and flank extending to the umbilicus, a left nephrostomy tube, marked brawny edema of both legs and a labile hypertension varying between 170/90 and 220/150. Blood urea nitrogen on three occasions averaged 32 mg. per 100 ml.; plasma chlorides, 118 m.Eq. per liter; plasma carbon dioxide combining power, 17 m.Eq. per liter; plasma sodium, 143 m.Eq. per liter; and plasma potassium, 4.8 m.Eq. per liter. Thus, the patient exhibited moderate nitrogen retention, mild hyperchloremic acidosis and no disturbance of plasma sodium or potassium concentration.

Intravenous pyelography revealed no function by x-ray up to 3 hours. P.S.P. excretion was 10 per cent in one hour and 23 per cent in two hours. Urea clearance averaged 10 per cent of normal.

Renal function studies performed in the Department of Physiology of Cornell University Medical College are summarized in Table 3. Glomerular filtration rate averaged 22.1 ml. per minute over the 6 periods of the test, a value about 19 per cent of normal. Renal plasma flow was more seriously reduced amounting on an average to 42 ml. per minute, a value roughly 7 per cent of normal. The filtration fraction accordingly was greatly increased over the normal value of 20 per cent.* Tm_{PAH} was reduced to 13 per cent of normal. The ratio of C_{PAH}/Tm_{PAH} was very low.

One may interpret the pathology as follows. In consequence of pyelonephritis and hydronephrosis, renal tubular damage in the existing left kidney is

* It is doubtful in this patient that extraction of PAH is sufficiently complete for the clearance to have the dimensions of renal plasma flow. However, it is certain that renal plasma flow is very seriously reduced.

extensive. The glomeruli, though seriously involved, have suffered less than have the renal tubules. However, the greatest damage has occurred in the renal vascular bed with sclerosis and obliteration of small vessels, so that even the remnant of functional tissue is relatively ischemic. The hypertension is no doubt related to this ischemia of tubular tissue (Goldblatt, 1948). Tubular damage, resulting in reduction of capacity to form titratable acid and ammonia, accounts for the hyperchloremic acidosis. Despite the marked functional alterations exhibited by the kidney of this patient, its residual function is sufficient to preserve grossly the volume and composition of the body fluids.

Such function tests performed on the separately catheterized kidneys of selected patients prior to nephrectomy, should enable the urologist to gauge exactly the functional adequacy of the kidney he elects to leave. Furthermore, they should give him some insight into the nature of the pathology as well as an exact measure of the residual function of the kidney he considers removing (Chasis and Redish, 1942). The fact that the one remaining kidney of patient M.F. exhibited no function on intravenous pyelography should give the urologist some pause in his reliance on this test for determining the worth of a kidney.

NATURE OF RENAL REGULATORY MECHANISMS AND THEIR DERANGEMENTS IN DISEASE

Some appreciation of the nature of normal renal regulatory mechanisms and of their functional derangements in disease are no less significant than good surgery in the proper management of the urologic patient. Since the kidney is concerned with the regulation of osmotic pressure, volume and ionic structure of the body fluids and with the excretion of nitrogenous wastes, normal functions are complex and dysfunctions in disease are numerous. Only a few basic principles can be considered here.

Osmotic Pressure. The osmotic pressure of the body fluids is normally about 5,000 mm. Hg. Although the composition of the cell fluid is very different from that of the interstitial fluid and plasma, their osmotic pressures are essentially the same, for water is free to move across cell membranes in either direction. As a consequence, ingested water is rapidly distributed between blood plasma, interstitial fluid and cells in such a way as to maintain equality of osmotic pressure in all fluid compartments.

The osmotic pressure of the body fluids is largely determined by salts; organic solutes contribute insignificantly. Accordingly, the osmotic pressure of the extracellular fluid is dependent on the concentrations of its three most abundant ions, sodium, chloride and bicarbonate, that of the intracellular fluid, on the concentrations of potassium and phosphate complexes. The body can tolerate at most a 15 to 20 per cent increase or decrease in over-all concentration of these ionic constituents. Greater dilution leads to the convulsions of water intoxication, greater concentration to the hyperpyrexia and respiratory and circulatory failure of dehydration.

Regulation of osmotic pressure depends on the proper balance of activity of thirst mechanisms governing water intake and neuro-humoral-renal mechanisms governing water output. According to Verney (1947), small vesicles in the supraoptic nuclei of the hypothalamus are sensitive to the osmotic pressure of the circulating blood plasma. These tiny osmometers shrink as the osmotic pressure of the fluid surrounding them rises. Nerve impulses, set up in the dendrites of supraoptic neurons applied to the surfaces of these vesicles, are transmitted over the supraopticohypophyseal tracts to the pituicytes of the posterior lobe of the pituitary, causing them to liberate pitressin. This hormone in turn stimulates the distal tubules of the kidneys to conserve water and to form a concentrated hypertonic urine. Thirst, which is in part related to dryness of the mouth and in part to dehydration of body tissues, drives the individual to seek water (Adolph, 1947). The remarkable fact about the thirst experience is that it is relieved almost immediately by the ingestion of that volume of water required to satisfy the deficit, despite the fact that absorption and dilution of the body fluids may require nearly an hour to reach completion. Dilution of the body fluids and swelling of the hypothalamic osmometers inhibit the liberation of pitressin. The distal tubules of the kidney are no longer stimulated to reabsorb water actively, and a dilute, hypotonic urine is formed. In the complete absence of circulating pitressin the urine flow may rise to 20 ml. per minute, a circumstance in which some 15 per cent of the filtered water is excreted.

The severely ill patient is prone to develop dehydration, hypertonicity and oliguria, for the effort of drinking may outweigh the discomfort of thirst unless fluid is made easily available (Marriott, 1950; Newburgh, 1950). If in addition extensive renal tubular damage makes impossible the active conservation of water (isosthenuria), severe depletion of body fluid reserves may result. Vomiting, diarrhea and fever speed the processes of water depletion and may precipitate uremia. On the other hand, overenthusiastic hydration, especially with intravenous glucose, carries with it the hazard of excessive dilution of the body fluids or, under other circumstances, of dehydration despite fluid plenty. Forcing fluids above daily loss and replacement needs in an oliguric patient in an attempt to increase urine flow is especially dangerous. Oliguria on a basis other than simple dehydration is probably never favorably affected by forcing fluids. The edematous, hypotonic, water-logged patient is indeed a sorry therapeutic result. Scarcely less hazardous is the forcing of fluids without adequate attention to salt replacement in the patient who exhibits fixation of urinary specific gravity. Because a dilute urine cannot be formed, loss of salt increases *pari passu* with urine volume and reduction of extracellular fluid volume results. During the polyuric phase which occurs with the onset of recovery from acute renal shutdown, the kidney frequently exhibits a disturbing inability to regulate salt and water losses. In certain instances a very dilute urine of large volume nearly free of salt is formed, with the result that the body fluids become quite hypertonic. In others, salt is lost in excess of water and the body fluids become hypotonic.

Volume. The regulation of volume of the body fluids is by no means as well defined as is the regulation of osmotic pressure. While osmotic pressure is adjusted rapidly at the expense of volume by retention or elimination of water, volume *per se* is adjusted sluggishly by the retention or elimination of salt. Although no such mechanism has as yet been experimentally defined, an explanation of the observed stability of volume of extracellular fluid in the normal individual demands some type of volume receptor and nervous or hormonal effector system operating through the kidney (Peters, 1952). Under normal circumstances some 99 per cent or more of the filtered salt is reabsorbed by the renal tubules, the 1 per cent or less excreted being just that required to maintain constancy of salt content and hence of volume of the body fluids. This condition is defined as *glomerulotubular balance.*

In the more acute phases of renal disease a number of factors may contribute to *tubular preponderance* and thus conspire to increase the salt stores of the body and hence to expand extracellular fluid volume (Bradley, 1948). (a) A decrease in glomerular filtration rate, unaccompanied by a proportionate reduction in tubular reabsorption, leads to retention of salt and water. (b) An increase in renal venous pressure favors overabsorption of salt and water. (c) Hypersecretion of adrenal cortical hormones and pitressin, as stress responses to disease, specifically stimulate the renal tubules to greater than normal absorptive activity. (d) Finally, nerve impulses delivered to the tubules over the renal plexuses may specifically favor the absorption of salt (Pitts and Sartorius, 1950).

In the more chronic phases of renal disease, *glomerular preponderance* rather than *tubular preponderance* may dominate the functional picture. Thus, greater reduction in tubular mass than in filtration rate may lead to salt and water loss. In addition, the renal tubules may become relatively or absolutely insensitive to the actions of adrenal cortical hormones and pitressin. Hence, salt loss rather than salt retention, and dehydration rather than edema may characterize the state of chronic renal insufficiency.

In acute renal shutdown resulting from a prolonged period of hypotension, incompatible transfusion or chemical intoxication, an extreme reduction in glomerular filtration rate appears to be the major causal factor underlying the anuria or oliguria. Probably in many instances cessation of glomerular filtration results from a sharp rise in renal interstitial pressure. This may come about from leakage of plasma proteins through damaged peritubular capillaries or from liberation of protein from damaged tubular cells. In either circumstance the normal colloid osmotic force which returns the fluid absorbed by the renal tubules to the peritubular capillary network is lost and fluid collects in the interstitium. As interstitial pressure rises, blood flow is restricted and the effective filtration pressure is progressively reduced. In the anuria of instrumentation of the urinary tract, the basic factor is probably reflex vasoconstriction of afferent glomerular arterioles. If renal ischemia lasts for a sufficient time to damage capillaries or tubular cells, the factors outlined above may maintain the anuria through a rise in renal interstitial pressure.

Ionic Structure. Stabilization of total ionic concentration of the extracellular fluid is the natural consequence of stabilization of osmotic pressure, for, as pointed out above, osmotic pressure is largely determined by ionic concentration. Furthermore, since sodium is the major component of the plasma base, osmotic regulatory mechanisms effectively determine the plasma sodium level, which under normal conditions varies within the narrow limits of 138 and 145 m.Eq. per liter. However, the anion pattern and especially the relative proportions of chloride and bicarbonate are regulated independently of osmotic pressure. In general, the concentrations of these two anions are inversely related, chloride increasing as bicarbonate falls, decreasing as bicarbonate rises. Normally the plasma level of chloride is 100 to 108 m.Eq. per liter, that of bicarbonate, 25 to 27 m.Eq. per liter. One should consider the 25 to 27 m.Eq. of bicarbonate as representing an equivalent quantity of sodium, immediately available to neutralize any strong metabolic acid produced in the body. The 100 or so m.Eq. of sodium neutralized by chloride are not available for this purpose, for chloride is itself the anion of a strong acid.

The normal individual produces 30 to 50 m.Eq. of phosphoric and sulfuric acid per day in metabolizing the proteins and phospholipids of the usual mixed diet. To neutralize this acid, an amount of bicarbonate bound base equal to that contained in one to two liters of plasma is used up each day. Were this process to continue unchecked, the available base of the body would be exhausted in a little more than a week and death from acidosis would occur. The kidney in excreting phosphate and sulfate reverses the process of neutralization (see p. 42), converting the neutral sodium phosphate into free titratable acid and substituting ammonium ions for the sodium ions bound to sulfate (Pitts, 1948 and 1950). In either circumstance the sodium ions are restored to the body as bicarbonate to be re-used in neutralizing acid.

In chronic renal disease and especially in those conditions in which tubular damage is extensive, the capacity of the kidney to replenish depleted stores of available base is reduced. The ability to produce ammonia suffers first, later the capacity to form titratable acid. As a consequence acidosis is commonly associated with, and more or less proportional to, the extent of tubular damage. Even with rather marked renal pathology acidosis can be avoided or at least mitigated by restricting those foods which yield an acid ash residue in the body, and by including in the diet vegetables and fruit juices* which supply available base. The oral administration of sodium bicarbonate may accomplish the same end, but care must be exercised in the quantities given, for the damaged kidney has limited capacities to excrete this salt, and overenthusiastic therapy may lead to alkalosis and an associated further depression of renal function.

Although one might assume in renal acidosis that phosphate and sulfate would be retained and would replace bicarbonate in the body fluids, such is not the case except under conditions of severe depression of renal function. Instead, chloride replaces bicarbonate, and sulfate and phosphate are excreted. However, when glomerular filtration rate is severely reduced,

* Vegetables and fruit juices supply base mainly in the form of potassium, not sodium. If renal function is severely reduced and especially if the patient is anuric, these dietary substances should not be given because of the hazard of potassium retention and elevation of serum potassium level. Under such conditions any correction of acidosis should be accomplished by the administration of sodium bicarbonate or lactate.

phosphate and sulfate are retained. Retention of phosphate leads to depression of serum calcium, for the solubility coefficient of calcium phosphate fixes the product of the concentrations of these two ions. Neuromuscular irritability, muscle twitching and tetany are consequences of low serum calcium in uremia. Some relief of these signs may be achieved by the oral administration of colloidal aluminum hydroxide (Shorr, 1945) which increases the fecal excretion of phosphate and by the administration of calcium gluconate.

Normally, the serum concentration of *potassium* is maintained at the relatively low but constant level of 4 to 5 m.Eq. per liter. Depression below 2 m.Eq. per liter leads to weakness, paralysis and hypodynamic heart action. Elevation above 7 or 8 m.Eq. per liter leads to irregularities of heart rhythm, conduction defects, eventually to cardiac standstill and death. The capacity to regulate the plasma level of potassium is well retained until the late stages of chronic renal disease. However, restriction of dietary intake of potassium is perhaps a more valid reason for absolutely restricting protein in acute renal shutdown than is the associated reduction in nitrogen metabolism. Elevated serum potassium is an especially ominous sign in renal failure. The administration of glucose or glucose and insulin will lower the concentration of potassium temporarily, for in the process of storing glycogen, potassium is drawn from the extracellular fluid into the cells. Carbohydrate also spares the breakdown of cell protein and hence reduces loss of potassium from cells. Alkalosis, though not a common feature of renal disease, leads to excessive loss of potassium and reduction in serum concentration, and, conversely excessive loss of potassium leads to an intractable form of alkalosis (Darrow, 1950). With repeated vomiting, loss of potassium in gastric secretions may lead to reduction in serum concentration. Furthermore, the associated alkalosis may enhance the urinary loss of this ion. The hypopotassemic alkalosis may in turn be resistant to treatment with simple salt solutions and require the administration of potassium salts for correction.

PRINCIPLES OF FLUID AND ELECTROLYTE MANAGEMENT IN RENAL INSUFFICIENCY

Careful management of diet, fluid intake and electrolyte balance can often compensate to a remarkable degree for impairment of the regulatory functions of the kidney. The problem is most complex where all regulatory function is lost as in complete anuria, but where the inciting condition is self limiting, proper management of the patient is most rewarding.

The ideal approach to treatment of the anuric patient is a conservative one; all efforts being directed, not to the re-establishment of urinary flow, but to the maintenance of fluid and electrolyte balance until such time as function recovers spontaneously. (For details see Bradley, Darrow, Elkinton and Tarail, Marriott, Newburgh.) As general guiding principles, water should be given only in amounts sufficient to replace existing deficits and to cover actual daily losses. In the absence of fever and sweating, between 800 and 1000 ml. of water should be given each day to replace that vaporized from the lungs and skin. An additional 200 ml. should cover minimal sweat requirements; more is needed if obvious sweating occurs. Fecal losses of water are negligible in the absence of diarrhea, for the regimen is one of rigid restriction of all potassium, nitrogen, phosphorus and sodium containing foods, which in essence limits one to pure carbohydrates.

Ideally fluid and glucose should be given by mouth, and in the absence of vomiting small quantities of glucose solution may be taken at frequent intervals, the quantities dictated by thirst. It is difficult to administer more than 150 grams of glucose per day in this way, but even this quantity is sufficient to prevent serious ketosis and to spare to some degree breakdown of body protein. No salt should be given, for losses are negligible under these conditions. If vomiting and wound drainage are complicating factors in anuria, the total volume of fluid administered must be increased to cover these losses and some compensation must be made for sodium and chloride depletion. Wound drainage should be replaced by isotonic saline or by 3 parts of saline to 1 part of M/6 sodium lactate. Anemia should be corrected by transfusions of whole blood and hypoproteinemia by the administration of plasma. Vomitus may be replaced by one third saline, two thirds glucose in distilled water. Since gastric juice contains fair quantities of potassium, hypokalemia may result from excessive vomiting, although tissue breakdown usually liberates all that is needed. However, as renal function returns, replacement of any potassium deficit incurred is desirable, preferably by the oral administration of potassium chloride or better by orange juice as tolerated.

Frequent determinations of plasma concentration of sodium, potassium, chloride and bicarbonate are needed as guides to therapy. In fact it is impossible to control therapy in any ideal fashion without having available facilities for prompt and accurate analysis of the major ionic components of the body fluids. Practically it may be necessary to rely on chloride and bicarbonate determinations alone. Daily body weights are useful as an index of proper control of fluid intake. Under any circumstance the edema produced by too much salt or the hypotonicity of too much water is to be avoided. There is little one can do to help the anuric patient overloaded with saline, comatose, and in pulmonary edema, other than to resort to filtration-dialysis on an artificial kidney, if one is available, in an attempt to reverse the consequences of injudicious treatment. During the polyuric recovery phase following anuria attention should be directed toward anticipating either hypotonicity or hypertonicity of the body fluids, produced respectively by excessive loss of salt or by excessive loss of water.

For the patient with chronically reduced renal function but adequate urine output, management is somewhat less demanding but nevertheless rewarding. Water intake should be gauged to meet extrarenal losses and to supply an additional 2,500 to 3,000 ml. for urine formation. From the total, some 1,200 ml. may be subtracted as water contained in solid foods and derived from oxidation. The remainder should be supplied as liquids. Restriction of dietary protein must be tempered with reason. Although complete withholding of protein is an absolute *must* during the anuric phase of acute renal failure, prolonged and rigid restriction of protein in chronic renal disease is inadvisable. Certainly moderate elevation of plasma nonprotein nitrogen is no contraindication to protein intake adequate to maintain nitrogen balance. Poor appetite, malnutrition, prolonged convalescence, delayed wound healing, and certain types of edema are too high prices to pay for maintenance of pseudonormalcy of blood urea. In fact, signs and symptoms of uremia are certainly unrelated to blood urea levels per se. Nevertheless, there comes a time when judicious protein restriction will prolong life or help the patient over some self-limiting renal crisis. The matter of protein restriction requires that the physician exercise fine judgment; it cannot be decided by rule of thumb.

Salt intake adequate to meet urinary losses is necessary, with special attention to those patients who exhibit isosthenuria and hence are prone to salt depletion. Attention to exact control of daily urine volume in relation to nitrogen metabolism and salt excretion with the view of limiting renal work is superfluous, for the thermodynamically calculated work is an insignificant fraction of the actual work performed in elaborating urine. It is evident from the discussion above that the major expenditure of energy by the kidney is related to the active tubular absorption of valuable components from the glomerular filtrate, not in the excretion of the relatively much smaller quantities of waste materials. The kidneys cannot be "put at rest." However, their regulatory burdens may be lightened and compensations made for their regulatory deficiencies by proper control of diet and fluid and electrolyte intake.

REFERENCES

ADDIS, T. and SHEVKY, M. C.: A test for the capacity of the kidney to produce urine of high specific gravity. Arch. Int. Med., *30:*559, 1922.

ADOLPH, E. F.: Physiology of Man in the Desert. Interscience Publishers, New York, 1947.

BERLINER, R. W.: Renal excretion of water, sodium, chloride, potassium, calcium and magnesium. Am. J. Med., *9:*541, 1950.

BERLINER, R. W., KENNEDY, T. J. and ORLOFF, J.: Relationship between acidification of the urine and potassium metabolism. Effect of carbonic anhydrase inhibition on potassium excretion. Am. J. Med., *11:*274, 1951.

BEYER, K. H., RUSSO, H. F., TILLSON, E. K., GASS, S. R. and SCHUCHARDT, G. S.: Carinamide (4'-carboxy-phenylmethanesulfonanilide): its renal clearance and binding on plasma protein. Am. J. Physiol., *159:*181, 1949.

BRADLEY, S. E.: Laboratory findings in the blood and urine in health and disease. M. Clin. North America, *29:*1314, 1945.

BRADLEY, S. E.: The Pathologic Physiology of Uremia in Chronic Bright's Disease. American Lectures in Physiology. C. C Thomas, Springfield, Ill., 1948.

CARGILL, W. H. and HICKAM, J. B.: The oxygen consumption of the normal and the diseased human kidney. J. Clin. Investigation, *28:*526, 1949.

CHASIS, H. and REDISH, J.: Function of the separate kidneys in hypertensive subjects. Arch. Int. Med., *70:*738, 1942.

CHASIS, H., REDISH, J., GOLDRING, W., RANGES, H. A. and SMITH, H. W.: The use of sodium p-aminohippurate for the functional evaluation of the human kidney. J. Clin. Investigation, *24:*583, 1945.

CHASIS, H. and SMITH, H. W.: The excretion of urea in normal man and in subjects with glomerulo-nephritis. J. Clin. Investigation, *17:*347, 1938.

CUSHNY, A. R.: The Secretion of the Urine. Longmans, Green and Co., London, 1917.

DARROW, D. C.: Body fluid physiology: The role of potassium in clinical disturbances of body water and electrolyte. New England J. Med., *242:*978, and 1014, 1940.

ELKINTON, J. R. and TARAIL, R.: The present status of potassium therapy. Am. J. Med., *9:*200, 1950.

GOLDBLATT, H.: The Renal Origin of Hypertension. American Lectures in Pathology. C. C Thomas, Springfield, Ill., 1948.

LOTSPEICH, W. D.: Renal tubular reabsorption of inorganic sulfate in the normal dog. Am. J. Physiol., *151:*311, 1947.

MARRIOTT, H. L.: Water and Salt Depletion. American Lectures in Physiology, C. C Thomas, Springfield, Ill., 1950.

MERRILL, JOHN: The use of the artificial kidney. Chapt. 4, Renal Function, Transactions of the Third Conference, Josiah Macy, Jr., Foundation, New York, 1952.

NEWBURGH, L. H.: Significance of the Body Fluids in Clinical Medicine. American Lectures in Physiology. C. C Thomas, Springfield, Ill., 1950.

PAPPENHEIMER, JOHN: Passage of Substances Across Capillary Walls. Chapt. 1, Renal Function. Transactions of the Third Conference, Josiah Macy, Jr., Foundation, New York, 1952.

PETERS, J. P.: The problem of cardiac edema. Am. J. Med., 12:66, 1952.

PITTS, R. F.: A comparison of the renal reabsorptive processes for several amino acids. Am. J. Physiol., 140:535, 1944.

PITTS, R. F.: Renal excretion of acid. Fed. Proc., 7:418, 1948.

PITTS, R. F.: Acid-base regulation by the kidneys. Am. J. Med., 9:356, 1950.

PITTS, R. F. and ALEXANDER, R. S.: The renal reabsorptive mechanism for inorganic phosphate in normal and acidotic dogs. Am. J. Physiol., 142:648, 1944.

PITTS, R. F., AYER, J. L. and SCHIESS, W. A.: The renal regulation of acid-base balance in man. III. The reabsorption and excretion of bicarbonate. J. Clin. Investigation, 28:35, 1949.

PITTS, R. F. and SARTORIUS, O. W.: Mechanism of action and therapeutic use of diuretics. J. Pharm. and Exper. Therap., Part II, 98:161, 1950.

PRICE, J. W., MILLER, M. and HAYMAN, J. M., JR.: The relation of specific gravity to composition and total solids in normal human urine. J. Clin. Investigation, 19:537, 1940.

RALLI, E. P., FRIEDMAN, G. J. and RUBIN, S. H.: The mechanism of the execution of vitamin C by the human kidney. J. Clin. Investigation, 17:765, 1938.

SHANNON, J. A.: Renal tubular excretion. Physiol. Rev., 19:63, 1939.

SHANNON, J. A., FARBER, S. and TROAST, L.: The measurement of glucose Tm in the normal dog. Am. J. Physiol., 133:752, 1941.

SHORR, E.: The possible usefulness of estrogens and aluminum hydroxide gels in the management of renal stone. J. Urology, 53:507, 1945.

SMITH, H. W.: The Kidney. Porter Lectures. Univ. of Kansas Press, Lawrence, Kansas, 1943.

SMITH, HOMER W.: The Kidney. Structure and Function in Health and Disease. Oxford University Press, New York, 1951.

SMITH, H. W., GOLDRING, W., CHASIS, H., RANGES, H. A. and BRADLEY, S. E.: The application of saturation methods to the study of glomerular and tubular function in the human kidney. J. Mt. Sinai Hosp., 10:59, 1943.

TAGGART, J. V.: Renal Function. Transactions of the First Conference, Josiah Macy, Jr., Foundation, New York, 1950.

VERNEY, E. B.: Antidiuretic hormone and the factors which determine its release. Proc. Roy. Soc., London, B, 135:25, 1947.

VAN SLYKE, D. D., PHILLIPS, R. A., HAMILTON, P. B., ARCHIBALD, R. M., FUTCHER, P. H. and HILLER, A.: Glutamine as a source material of urinary ammonia. J. Biol. Chem., 150:481, 1943.

WESSON, L. G., JR., and ANSLOW, W. P., JR.: Excretion of sodium and water during osmotic diuresis in the dog. Am. J. Physiol., 153:465, 1948.

WESSON, L. G., JR., ANSLOW, W. P., JR. and SMITH, H. W.: The excretion of strong electrolytes. Bull. New York Acad. Med., 24:586, 1948.

CHAPTER 3

The Physiology of the Renal Pelvis and

the Ureter

PETER A. NARATH, M.D.

The physiology of the renal pelvis and ureter involves three major functions: dynamics, tonus and absorption. Interpolated between the parenchyma of the kidney and the last main reservoir, the bladder, the renal pelvis and the ureter serve essentially as a transporting system. The urine passes from the distal convoluted tubules into the collecting canaliculi (O.T., collecting tubules), i.e., the terminals of the complicated structures which derive from the ureteropelvic anlage. The transportation system begins in the canaliculus, not in the calyx. Consequently we must include the canaliculi in the upper urinary tract.

In normal physiology it is a prerequisite that the urine is transported bladderwards and does not flow back into sections of the tract which were previously passed. An ingenious muscular arrangement in the wall of the calyx, the true pelvis and the ureter provides such a one way flow.

The *dynamics of the upper urinary tract* will have our first consideration.

The amount of urine varies greatly in accordance with fluid intake and other stimulating or retarding influences. Dynamic activity, however, is not the sole factor in coping with larger or smaller amounts of urine. The lumen of the tract adjusts itself accordingly. When copious diuresis exists, the lumen of the tract will attain a wider diameter; at times of low urine production the tract can contract considerably. This adjustment is achieved by various states of tonus of the musculature, a condition similar to that found in the vascular system. There are many other causes which influence the tonicity of the tract. These questions are discussed under the heading *the tonus of the upper urinary tract*.

The wall of the canaliculi, calyx, true pelvis and ureter is lined with an epithelium of various thicknesses, which we shall call urothelium and not mucosa, since no mucous glands are present. This epithelium has absorptive capacities with areas which seem to be more capable of absorption than others. The significance of these processes is discussed under *absorption and resorption in the upper urinary tract*.

THE DYNAMICS OF THE UPPER URINARY TRACT

The complicated process of urine formation seems to be completed when the urine leaves the distal convoluted tubule and enters the adjoining canaliculus. Now the action of transportation begins.

Since the canaliculi are not equipped with muscles they have no dynamic properties of their own. They represent true canals which end in the pores of the papilla. The power which induces the urine to flow downward must come from other sources.

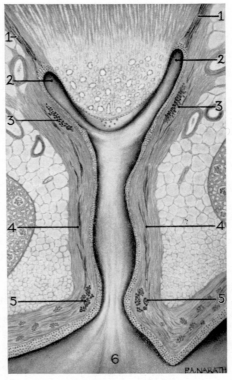

Fig. 20. Schematic drawing of a calyx and its muscular arrangement. (1) Musculus levator fornicis; (2) fornix; (3) musculus sphincter fornicis; (4) musculus longitudinalis calycis; (5) musculus sphincter calycis; (6) true pelvis. (From Narath, J. Urol., *43*, 1940.)

The wall of the calyces, true pelvis and ureter exhibits a layer of smooth muscle. A closer study of the arrangement of these delicate fibers offers a surprising explanation which enables us to understand the complicated mechanism of the various sections into which the upper urinary tract is functionally divided.

Figure 20 represents a schematic longitudinal section through the papilla, the calyx and adjoining part of the true pelvis. The wall of the calyx adheres to the papilla in an archlike formation, the fornix, which forms the rim of the goblet. Below the papilla the calyx narrows and is called the neck. Where the neck joins the true pelvis, at the calycopelvic junction, a further narrowing can be observed. The muscular structure of the calyx reveals a complicated differentiation. From the rim of the fornix longitudinal fibers extend alongside the papilla into the parenchyma, following the borderlines of the pertaining renculus. This muscle, *musculus levator fornicis* (Narath) can have only one possible action, namely, to pull the fornix upward when contracting and to let the fornix sink downward when relaxing.

At the height of the papilla, circular fibers form a sphincter, the *musculus sphincter fornicis* (Henle), first described by Henle as sphincter papillae. The function of this muscle was disputed for a long time. Henle believed that its contraction would exercise a squeezing effect (later called a milking action) on the papilla, thus facilitating the ejection of urine from the ductus papillares. This opinion proved to be incorrect for several reasons. Anatomically, there is a vast discrepancy between this delicate muscle and the rigidity and magnitude of the papilla, which it was supposed to squeeze. Moreover, in many instances, this sphincter is not ideally located in relation to the papilla; often the muscle is found below the tip of the papilla at one side and high at the other. These are cases in which the papilla dips obliquely into the calyx, so that a pressing on the papilla cannot be effected. Then there are the twin, triplet and more conjugated papillae with an utterly complicated fornix formation, most commonly in the cranial pole of the pelvis. It is quite impossible for an even stronger muscle to act as expressor on these structures. My own investigations have demonstrated that the sphincter closes below the papilla, thus shielding the pores and closing them off against the neck of the calyx during its emptying phase in order to prevent a backflow of urine into the canaliculi.

The neck of the calyx is equipped with longitudinal fibers, the *musculus longitudinalis calycis*. One must realize, however, that these fibers are not strictly longitudinal. Their course is often oblique and interwoven, though they do not form a spiral, as sometimes described. It follows that contraction of these fibers must lead to a combination of shortening and narrowing of the neck and relaxation will result in a lengthening and widening. This action is, in fact, still more differentiated, as we shall see later.

Where the neck of the calyx joins the true pelvis at the calycopelvic junction, stronger fibers of a sphincter can be seen. This is the *musculus sphincter calycis* (Disse). Its purpose is to close the calyx against the true pelvis during its own collecting phase and to prevent a backflow of pelvic contents into the calyx during the systole of the true pelvis. In Figure 20 the true pelvis and the ureter are not shown.

The arrangement of the heavy muscular layer of the true pelvis does not reveal a definite pattern. The muscular fibers are densely interwoven, and their course is longitudinal, oblique and transverse, forming a network, which in contraction must exercise a squeezing effect on the pelvis as a whole.

Physiologically, a much disputed region is the ureteropelvic junction. The closure and opening of the ureteropelvic junction can be seen roentgenologically, but histologically a sphincter cannot be demonstrated. We do not know in which way this function is achieved.

It is commonly stated that the ureter has an inner longitudinal and an outer circular muscular layer, but even though these layers exist, it seems that such statement is too simple. On serial sections it can be seen that the two layers are interwoven, sometimes to a confusing degree. These layers vary in heaviness in different parts of the ureter. No sphincter arrangement is present, although we shall find later that the ureter is usually divided into three dynamic sections. Close to the bladder an additional longitudinal outer layer, Waldeyer's sheath, extends from the bladder a few centimeters upward.

The ureterovesical junction is equipped with a complicated form of sphincter mechanism. The ureteral orifice stays closed during micturition.

From the histologic findings an important fact emerges. The presence of several sphincters in the tract proves in itself, that these sphincters cannot work synchronously since no useful action would be accomplished. These sphincters divide the tract into several sections with their own dynamic properties.

To clarify the situation, let us assume that the true pelvis is filled with urine to a degree that demands ejection into the ureter. In accordance with hydrostatic laws a contraction of the pelvis must exercise a pressure on its contents in all possible directions. This would imply that the urine is pressed not only into the ureter, but also backwards into the calyces, where it just came from. It is not plausible that nature would perform such a futile act. The urine must be transported downward, not backward. A similar process would occur in the calyx, when the calyx contracts and empties into the true pelvis, whereby the urine would be pressed against the pores of the papilla. The column of urine present in the upper part of the ureter would flow back into the true pelvis, if the closure of the ureteropelvic junction did not prevent this.

Experimental studies on the living human have corroborated the presence of single sections which work in a staggered manner.

The urine present in the canaliculi dribbles through the pores of the papilla into the calyx. The filtration pressure acts as *vis a tergo* and moves the urine through the canaliculi. But the filtration pressure is not the only force which makes the urine leave the pores.

The calyx is empty and ready to receive a new filling. In order to create the necessary room, the levator fornicis relaxes and allows the fornix to sink downward. Synchronously the sphincter fornicis relaxes and the upper part of the longitudinalis calycis contracts. Thus a goblet is formed forcefully, creating a negative pressure that sucks the urine out of the pores. As a transporting factor the negative pressure is probably just as important as the filtration pressure. During the collecting phase of the calyx the sphincter of the calycopelvic junction stays contracted to prevent any backflow of urine into the calyx in case the true pelvis starts a systole.

As soon as the calyx has been filled sufficiently to empty its contents into the true pelvis, the dynamic action of the calyx is reversed. The upper part of the musculus longitudinalis calycis relaxes, the sphincter fornicis contracts and forms a cap below the papilla, thus closing off the pores of the papilla to prevent a backflow into the canaliculi. This cap is pulled snugly to the papilla by the contraction of the levator fornicis.

At the same time or just shortly thereafter, the sphincter of the calycopelvic junction relaxes and allows the urine to flow from the calyx into the true pelvis. To facilitate this process, the lower part of the longitudinalis calycis contracts and squeezes the urinary column. This is the systole or the emptying phase of the calyx. During this time the ureteropelvic junction is closed to prevent backflow from the ureter into the pelvis. The true pelvis is now in the collecting phase, its muscles relax and a slight negative pressure which acts on the calyces is again created in the pelvis.

When the pelvis is filled to the capacity for which the existing tonus calls, the collecting phase or diastole changes to a detrusor action. The pelvis empties into the ureter. Again a synchronized action takes place. As soon as the ureteropelvic junction opens up to let the urine enter the ureter, all sphincters of the calycopelvic junctions close to prevent a backflow of urine into the calyces. The systole of the pelvis begins. Its contraction forces the urine downward into the ureter. Part of this dynamic process can be seen at time of an operation when an extrarenal pelvis is present. It is surprising how rapidly this emptying process is achieved, normally in one and one half seconds.

As soon as the pelvic contents are ejected into the ureter the ureteropelvic junction closes again. The amount of the single jet, however, is not large enough to fill the entire ureter; only the upper third will be filled. The urine remains in this section for a short time and then is shifted into the middle third, to stay there until the next jet from the pelvis takes place. During the next filling phase of the upper third, the contents of the middle section are brought into the lower third of the ureter. When the emptying of the upper third into the middle section starts, the contents of the lower third are ejected into the bladder. This can be seen during cystoscopy. The urine does not leave the ureteral orifice in a dribbling manner; it is ejected at rhythmic intervals. The intervals depend upon the amount of urine produced. Thus, under ideal conditions, the ureter is divided into three dynamic sections, of which either the upper and lower third or the middle portion is filled at one time.

When I first published this new concept of hydrodynamics of the upper urinary tract (1940), I apparently created the erroneous impression that after evacuation the single section is totally empty of urine. This is not the case. I wrote: "When the entire neck is emptied, a little urine remains between the papilla and the cap formed by the upper part of the calyx. In our investigation that means contrast medium."

The status of the various sections after their emptying phase differs considerably. The fornical space retains some urine, and only exceptionally is it totally empty. No urine will be found in the neck of the calyx during the short rest period between systole and diastole. The true pelvis, immediately after systole, is not contracted to a degree that the walls are pressed together, but its size has become much smaller. This latent retention of urine explains why in intravenous urograms the pelvis is visible throughout all exposures, save for rare exceptions. The three ureter sections contract to a degree that they appear empty, or at least the lumen is narrowed to a fine canal. The bladder is empty after micturition, unless an obstruction exists at the bladder neck.

Figure 21 summarizes in a schematic way the dynamic coordination between calyces, pelvis and ureteropelvic junction. The ureter is not shown.

The histologic concept of dynamics, already integrated with some experience gained by roentgenograms (sphincter of the ureteropelvic junction and three dynamic sections of the ureter), needs to be proved in the living human by other means.

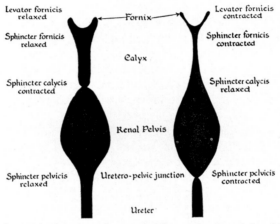

Fig. 21.   Collecting and emptying phases of calyx and true pelvis with cooperation of ureteropelvic junction. (From Narath, J. Urol., *43,* 1940.)

Roentgenocinematography would be the ideal way of studying the dynamics of the urinary tract. Machines able to take 16 exposures in one second have been constructed long ago and have yielded interesting results of the motion of various organs. However, the urinary tract, except for the action of the ureteropelvic junction and the process of micturition, did not furnish usable pictures. The exposure time for each film (of 16 exposures per one second) runs about $\frac{1}{32}$ second or less. The remainder of time is used to move the next film into position. Our equipment is improving slowly, and the day will come when $\frac{1}{50}$ of a second will suffice to take a pyelogram.

The indirect method of cinematography, namely, photographing the image on the fluoroscopic screen, is much less satisfactory even for so simple an object as a barium ball in the esophagus. Besides there is the danger of overradiation.

Fluoroscopy is inadequate, since the shadow of the renal pelvis and the calyces is not distinct enough, especially when intravenous urography is employed. Moreover, no record will be at hand for further evaluation and demonstration.

Since perfect roentgenographic pictures could not be achieved, the next thought was to take a series of exposures at short intervals. These pictures, however, are taken at random and do not present a true sequence of motion. Unfortunately, they may arrest the same dynamic phase several times and create the erroneous impression of a motionless tract.

We know today that in the calyx the switch from diastole to systole and the performance of the systole are a matter of less than a second in most instances. Consequently, an exposure time of one second cannot differentiate the action of the calyx sufficiently to give a correct impression of its motion. The configuration of the calyx will be slightly blurred and the collecting and

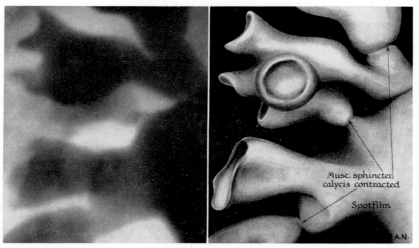

Fig. 22.   Several calyces in collecting phase. Musculus sphincter calycis contracted.
(From Narath, J. Urol., *43,* 1940.)

emptying phases appear combined on one film. Even if various stages of motion should be arrested, no dynamic sequence will be obtained.

Kymography is an excellent way of recording dynamics. As far as the urinary tract is concerned, the emptying phase of the true pelvis and the staggered motion of the ureteral sections become clearly evident. However, the dynamics of the calyces are blurred and arrested unsatisfactorily.

For the first experimental series of my own investigation I had constructed a machine which allowed a rapid change from fluoroscopic observation to film exposure, a device similar to the Berg-Kassette. But only one exposure could be taken. The advantage of this method, however, was that the exposure could be taken at an especially desired moment. A large magnifying glass was mounted over the fluoroscopic screen for better visualization of the calyces. After some experience with this procedure, the starting action of the calyx could be predicted and the picture taken. There were many failures, but the results obtained corroborated the histologic findings.

Figure 22 represents a cut out and enlargement of a retrograde pyelogram. The action of the musculus sphincter calycis is visible at three calyces, indicated by arrows. We realize that we are dealing with a disturbed physiology. The renal pelvis and the calyces are overdistended and the sphincter action of the calyces seems to be more likely a defense against further distention than the closure during the collecting phase.

Figure 23 demonstrates the emptying phase of a middle calyx. Just before the onset of the systole the diameter of this calyx was approximately that of the cranial calyx. The excess filling in this pyelogram was done purposely to

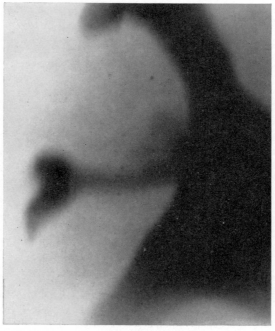

Fig. 23.   Middle calyx in emptying phase. Upper and lower calyx a little later in stage.
(From Narath, J. Urol., *43*, 1940.)

induce a more vivid dynamic activity. Hence the amount of contrast medium in the fornical space is much larger than it would appear in an intravenous urogram.

These two examples, together with a great number of other cases, were quite convincing as to the single action, but were definitely unsatisfactory for the sequence of dynamics.

Before I originated the final method of investigation, the rapid exposure of four pictures in 1.15 second, I experimented with another method, that is the triple exposure at random on one film. Most attempts were failures, but now and then various stages of dynamics could be arrested.

Figure 24 is an example of various filling degrees of one calyx with the sphincter calycis in contraction at one time. The explanatory drawing clarifies the findings. The pyelogram is enlarged for better visualization. Exposures were taken at 45 to 60 second intervals.

The results thus far obtained had shown various stages of dynamics but did not reveal a true sequence which is necessary for a clear interpretation.

Previous experience had proved the rapidity of dynamic processes and made it mandatory to take four exposures in about one second for a satisfactory sequence.

I finally succeeded in constructing a machine with which four exposures of $\frac{1}{10}$ of a second or less, at $\frac{1}{4}$ second interval, could be taken, which meant a total of 1.15 second for all four pictures. A calyx in emptying phase would be covered. The systole of the true pelvis does not extend beyond two seconds; mostly it runs for one to one and one-half second. Since the machine could be set at a speed to cover a. time up to two seconds, good pictures for the true pelvis were within reach.

There was still another difficulty. Exposures at these short intervals, taken at random, could very well fall into the collecting phase or the short rest

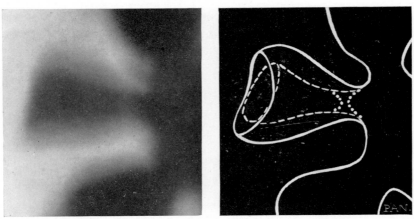

Fig. 24. Three exposures on one film at intervals of 45 to 60 seconds. Various filling degrees arrested. Sphincter calycis open and closed. (From Narath, J. Urol., *43*, 1940.)

period thereafter and thus give unsatisfactory results. Therefore the same technique of fluoroscopic observation and rapid change to exposure was used as in the first series, described above. The various parts of the pelvis were seen on the screen, a motion anticipated, and at the desired moment the cassette was moved into place to take the four exposures automatically. Notwithstanding careful evaluation in the selection of the onset of motion, there were many failures. A large number of convincing pictures, however, could be collected, of which only a few can be reproduced here.

Retrograde pyelography is the easier method for observation because of the heavier shadow on the screen, but the procedure in itself is unphysiologic and interferes with the normal dynamic function of the entire tract. Nevertheless, many interesting facts could be studied and used to substantiate the hypothesis derived at by histological examination. Intravenous urography does not disturb the physiology, but the shadows cast by the excreted contrast medium are far less intense and much more difficult to observe on the fluoroscopic screen. The conventional dose of 20 cc. of Diodrast for an adult person was increased to 30 and 40 cc. and more rapidly injected. To diminish the odds of the investigation, only very slim young girls were used as test objects. The fluoroscopic observation was thereby made easier, since the kidney came closer to the screen and less overlapping tissue was present.

For the three examples shown only intravenous urograms are selected to avoid controversial objections.

Figure 25 presents the emptying phase of a cranial calyx shown by an intravenous urogram of the left kidney. The copies are photographically enlarged. The exposure time is $\frac{1}{10}$ of a second at $\frac{1}{4}$ second interval, which means that the dynamic action shown in these four pictures extends over a period of 1.15 second.

The cranial calyx is in an emptying phase. In exposure A, the sphincter calycis is relaxed to provide for the ejection of the calycal contents into the true pelvis. In exposure B, C and D, the filling of the calyx diminishes gradually and the sphincter calycis begins to contract more and more. In D, it is nearly closed again. The emptying process is not completed. Another exposure would have shown less filling of the neck.

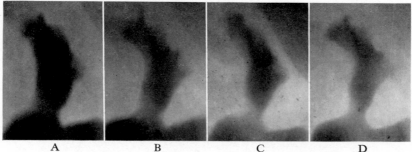

A   B   C   D

Fig. 25.   Emptying process of cranial calyx. Intravenous urogram. Exposures $\frac{1}{10}$ of a second at $\frac{1}{4}$ second interval. Total exposure time for the four pictures = 1.15 second. (From Narath, Renal Pelvis and Ureter, New York, Grune & Stratton, 1951.)

This series reveals an interesting fact, mentioned before, namely, that the expelling process does not always completely empty the calyx; this is a status, which we may call the latent filling of the calyx. It is true, however, that generally the calyx has the tendency to retain some urine only in the fornical space, as has been proved in many instances.

Figure 26 demonstrates the collecting phase of the true pelvis. A collecting phase extends over a period of time, depending upon diuresis. Usually 20 to 40 seconds elapse between the jets of the pelvis into the ureter. It is not necessary, therefore, to use a rapid succession of exposures. In the case shown the pictures were taken every 10 seconds; the total time for the four exposures required 30 seconds. The cassette was moved by hand. The emptying process was observed on the fluoroscopic screen and shortly thereafter the first film taken.

In A, the true pelvis has a crescentic form. The region of the ureteropelvic junction does not reveal any contrast medium. There is contrast medium in all fornices, but the necks of the calyces are empty and their musculus sphincter calycis is still closed, as necessary during the systole of the pelvis.

In B, the form of the pelvis has changed. The retraction near the ureteropelvic junction has subsided and a slender funnel had been formed. A larger size of the pelvis can be noted owing to increase of filling. The calyces are in various states of emptying.

In *C,* the pelvis exhibits a higher filling degree. The calyces are arrested at random.

In *D,* the true pelvis starts to perform its next jet into the ureter. The ureteropelvic junction has opened, and the contrast medium enters the ureter. The sphincters of the calyces must be arrested just before their closure.

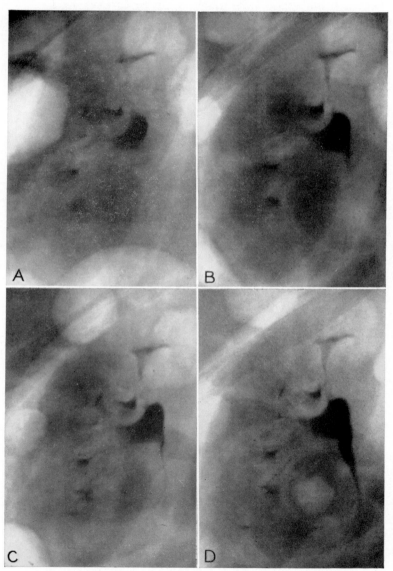

Fig. 26. Collecting phase of true pelvis in *A, B, C.* Beginning of emptying phase in *D.* Intravenous urogram. Exposures at 10 seconds interval. Total time elapsed = 30 seconds.

This series proves again that the emptying of the fornical spaces and of the pelvis is incomplete after systole; a certain amount of residual urine remains.

Figure 27 shows only two exposures of a series, number one and four.

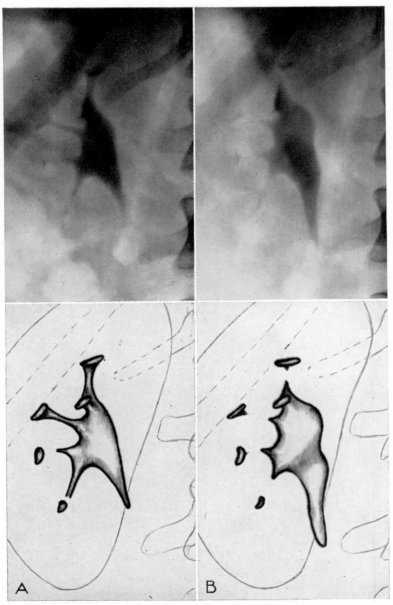

Fig. 27. Emptying phase of calyces and collecting phase of true pelvis in *A* (left). Emptying phase of true pelvis in *B* (right). Intravenous urogram. (From Narath, Renal Pelvis and Ureter, New York, Grune & Stratton, 1951.)

It is an intravenous urogram which deals with one of the rare cases in which all calyces act synchronously. In *A,* all calyces are in the process of emptying, the sphincters at the calycopelvic junction are relaxed, and in some calyces the contraction of the sphincter fornicis is visible. The ureteropelvic junction stays closed.

In *B,* all necks of the calyces are empty, the sphincters of the fornices are closed, and a small amount of urine remains in the fornical space. Now the ureteropelvic junction has opened and we see clearly the contraction wave of the true pelvis pressing the urine into the ureter.

Figure 28 demonstrates the emptying process of the true pelvis in an

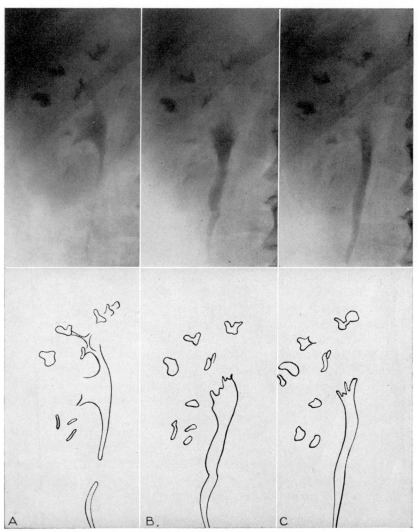

Fig. 28. Emptying phase of true pelvis. Intravenous urogram. Total exposure time 1.5 second. (From Narath, Renal Pelvis and Ureter, New York, Grune & Stratton, 1951.)

intravenous urogram. Three of the four pictures are reproduced. The machine was set at a lower speed, the total time for the four exposures being 1.5 second.

In *A,* the true pelvis, including the cranial calyx, is well filled. The calyces have closed against the pelvis. The ureteropelvic junction is located somewhat more caudally than usual and is closed.

In *B,* all calyces, including the cranial, are closed against the pelvis. The ureteropelvic junction now is wide open and the peristaltic wave running through it is plainly visible. The true pelvis is already empty except for the last extrarenal part. I wish to call the readers' attention to the upper border-line of the contrast medium column. This line is not straight, but rather notched, which means that the urothelium of the pelvis is folded together, leaving small longitudinal spaces for the contrast medium to remain.

In *C,* the extrarenal part of the pelvis seems empty, the column of the contrast medium having entered the ureter. The ureteropelvic junction is located about 2 cm. below the hilum (see explanatory drawing of *A*). When closed again some urine will remain in the last part of the extrarenal pelvis.

The urine now in the upper part of the ureter is not transported in an uninterrupted flowing motion down to the bladder. As mentioned before, the ureter is divided into dynamic sections, usually three, which have their own phases of collecting and emptying. It is a kind of a staggered process that takes place. The upper and lower thirds of the ureter are filled at the same time. The next peristaltic action transports the upper third of the column into the middle section and synchronously the lower third is ejected into the bladder. A picture obtained thereafter demonstrates that the upper and lower thirds of the ureter are empty, but the middle section is filled. With the next motion, the middle section moves into the lower third and at the same time the ureteropelvic junction opens to receive the next jet from the true pelvis into the upper third of the ureter. Figure 29 is a typical picture of this process.

In some urograms the ureter is filled with contrast medium throughout its entire length. There are differences in filling degree of the various sections. The parts with a narrower lumen are those which were emptied incompletely, as described before. Tonus variations play also an important role in the appearance of the ureter, as we shall see. Dilatations and total fillings due to obstructive processes at the ureteral orifice do not concern us here.

The question arises: which are the inducing factors for the dynamics of the upper urinary tract? Are they induced by nervous impulses, are they automatic or do they constitute a response to intrinsic pressure exercised by the volume of the accumulating urine?

The question of nervous impulses is not yet decided conclusively. Most investigators are agreed that no ganglia exist in the calyces, true pelvis and upper ureter. Only in the lowest part of the ureter near the bladder have ganglia been found. The function of these ganglia is not clearly established. We do not know how far up into the tract impulses could be transmitted from here. Denervation of the renal pedicle, as far as this is possible technically, does not influence the dynamics.

Since Engelmann's time the opinion has prevailed that an automatism of the musculature is responsible for the dynamics.

On the other hand, the amount of urine produced and transported into the urocanal definitely influences the frequency of peristalsis. When the single section is filled rapidly, it changes from collecting to emptying phase at short intervals. The theory, however, that intrinsic pressure is the sole

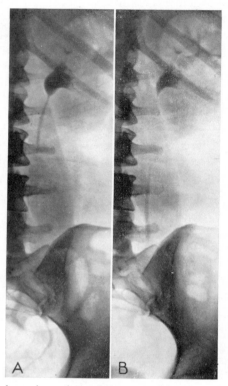

Fig. 29. The three dynamic sections of the ureter in action. In *A* (left), cranial and pelvic sections are filled. In *B* (right), cranial section shifted into middle section. Pelvic section has emptied into bladder. (From Narath, Renal Pelvis and Ureter, New York, Grune & Stratton, 1951.)

producer of dynamics can hardly be postulated. Two observations disprove this theory. (1) When during operation the blood pressure sinks below levels in which urine filtration is possible, the true pelvis, nevertheless, shows "dry action." (2) The same, even more convincingly, holds true for the stump of the ureter after nephrectomy. There is certainly no urine production, no intrinsic pressure, yet the ureteral orifice cystoscopically shows contractions.

Further histological and experimental work is necessary to decide these controversial questions.

THE TONUS OF THE UPPER URINARY TRACT

The tonic adaptations and reactions of the upper urinary tract to various conditions cannot be described and understood without including the last main reservoir, the bladder. Although this discussion deals with the renal pelvis and ureter, an exception must be granted, since the bladder is closely integrated with the upper tract.

In the discussion of *dynamics* it was shown that the renal pelvis and ureter are divided into several functional sections. The first unit consists of the canaliculi with their renculus and ends with the sphincter fornicis. The second unit comprises the calyx below the sphincter fornicis and terminates at the sphincter calycis. Between calyces and ureter is interpolated the third unit, the small reservoir of the true pelvis, which ends at the ureteropelvic junction. The ureter is usually divided into three sections; though rarely only two or four units may be found. Thus on the average there are seven functional sectors in the upper urinary tract, i.e., seven units equipped with a detrusor and sphincter mechanism. To these bilateral seven sections is added the main reservoir, the bladder.

A normal bladder is totally empty after micturition. The musculature of its wall is in a state of plastic tonus and remains in this state when the bladder fills. When the bladder has reached a filling degree which one can designate as "average individual capacity," the plastic tonus changes over to a dynamic state, the beginning of the detrusor action. The plastic tonus exercises no pressure on the urine in the bladder. With increasing filling, however, rising internal pressure can be measured. This rise is due to the intra-abdominal pressure which rests on the outside wall of the bladder and gains in magnitude, the higher up into the abdomen the filled bladder extends.

The "average individual capacity" is an acquired adjustment to the habits of the individual and to the demands of the outside world. A bladder can be trained to large capacity without the desire for micturition, or it can be emptied frequently.

When the bladder has reached a filling degree that calls for micturition, the plastic tonus changes to detrusor action. The bladder wall starts to contract, the sphincter internus opens, and an urge to urinate is manifested. If possible, the bladder will be emptied under voluntary relaxation of the sphincter externus. If, however, circumstances make a micturition impossible or undesirable, the sphincter externus can effect a stronger contraction to counteract the working detrusor. This fight between involuntary and voluntary action gives an unpleasant sensation which subsides as soon as the detrusor refrains from further contraction.

After the detrusor actions stops, a plastic tonus of a second degree is established, allowing further filling of the bladder. Such a process can repeat itself several times until the bladder capacity has finally reached an extremely high degree. The detrusor action starting from this level creates such an urge to urinate that the contracting power of the sphincter externus may yield even against the will.

The filling degree of the bladder with its various states of tonus must have repercussions on the upper urinary tract.

With the expansion and ascent of the bladder into the abdomen the pressure within the bladder rises. Against this increasing pressure the urine must be ejected from the ureteral orifice. It is necessary, therefore, that the lower third of the ureter works at a detrusor pressure somewhat higher than the pressure inside the bladder. During micturition the intravesical pressure can reach levels beyond the potential expelling power of the ureter. Therefore the ureteral orifice stays closed during micturition. If the kinetic co-operation is disturbed, which denotes that the emptying phase of the ureter is intercepted by sudden detrusor action of the bladder, a vesicoureteral reflux can occur.

The urine is ejected periodically from the ureter. There is a rest period or retention phase of varying length between the jets, depending upon the amount of diuresis. Under certain conditions the rest period may be prolonged. The staggered motion of the ureter was described previously.

How does the upper urinary tract react to increased bladder pressure and prolonged retention phases?

When the bladder is filled to capacity, but no emptying takes place,—a condition which requires a low bladder tonus,—the tonus of ureter, true pelvis and calyces is lowered reflexly. A widening of the diameter results and more urine can be harbored in each section. The detrusor action will then, though less frequently, transport a larger amount of urine with greater force, because the muscular action on the heavier column of urine is more effective. The tendency to return to a normotonus prevails and usual caliber conditions will be restored soon after the bladder has been emptied.

Figure 30 is an example of the response of the renal pelvis to extreme bladder filling.

Exposure *A* of this intravenous urogram was taken of an empty bladder. A difference of tonus is evident between the two sides. The left side exhibits a very narrow type of pelvis and calyces. The right side is well filled, except for the lower branch of the ureter fissus. The patient suffered from a bilateral parametritis, which is known to lower the tonus in the upper urinary tract. There is certainly no low tonus at the left side, a fact that cannot be explained.

In *B,* the bladder is filled to capacity and the aspect of both pelves changes considerably. The left side shows a remarkable dilatation of the small pelvis, the calyces, and the ureter. At the right side both the cranial and the caudal sections of the double pelvis are expanded, but the calyces are not truly blunted, and the fornices are well preserved.

There is one point I wish to emphasize—the ureter fissus is empty in its entire length, except for the adjacent part of the cranial pelvis. This picture confirms the previously expressed opinion, that the tonus level has nothing, or very little, to do with the dynamic activity, unless the tonus is so low that it nears the state of elastic expansion.

Tonic adjustment has its limits with no disturbance to the single units. When the force necessary to transport the urine from one section to the next becomes too great, the retention in the tract can lead to a loss of sphincter action between the sections and render the entire tract hypotonic

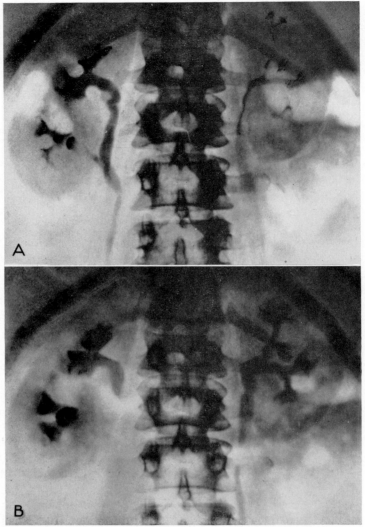

Fig. 30. Intravenous urogram exhibiting different stages of tonus of the upper urinary tract. Exposure *A* (top) is taken of an empty bladder. In exposure *B* (bottom) the bladder is filled to extreme capacity. (From Narath, Renal Pelvis and Ureter, New York, Grune & Stratton, 1951.)

to such an extent that the borderlines between the sections are lost. This is the case when a calculus in the lowest part of the ureter creates an incomplete block.

When the stagnation of urine in the tract due to a complete block gains in quantity, the detrusor action may be reduced almost to zero. Then the tract loses much of its dynamic qualities. The tonicity is reduced more and more and finally the severe hypotony ends in an elastic expansion or true atony. These conditions are reversible.

Complete obstruction depresses the renculus—the feeding section—because the urine which wants to leave the pores of the papilla is hindered by energetic contractions of the calyces, the true pelvis and the ureter in their attempt to overcome the obstacle and to press the urine into the bladder. A colic results. The pressure in the tract rises beyond the intracanalicular pressure.

Intravenous urography performed during such acute conditions does not reveal contrast medium in the affected tract. The common designation is "functionless kidney," but I do not feel that this term is correct. All one can say is, that no contrast medium is visible in the tract of the side concerned. That there is some functioning of the kidney finds its proof in the fact that the urine present in the renal pelvis of such obstructed kidneys is highly concentrated after an obstruction of longer duration. The specific gravity of such urine is much higher than the possible urine concentration within the kidney. The high concentration is due to further production of urine and water absorption in the pelvis.

In many of these cases a certain phenomenon can be observed which is called a "nephrogram," namely, an increase in density of the kidney shadow owing to storage of contrast medium in the cells of the tubules. These pictures, however, are impressive only when taken during the first hours of colic. When the obstruction subsides quickly and free passage of urine is reestablished, the stored contrast medium is excreted into the tubular lumen and transported bladderwards. If the obstruction persists, the nephrogram disappears after several hours. The constrast medium in the tubular cells is either excreted very slowly and absorbed somewhere in the tract or taken back into circulation in a different unknown way.

As an example of this situation a case is shown in which a calculus blocked the ureteral orifice for about four hours and led to severe colics. The intravenous urogram was performed within two hours after the onset of the colic and exposures were taken at intervals up to two hours. Of these films, four exposures are reproduced here (Figure 31).

Intravenous urography was started at the end of the second hour after the onset of colics in the right urinary tract. Twenty cubic centimeters of Diodrast compound solution were injected. Exposure *A* was taken 5 minutes after injection. Only the upper halves of the urograms are shown. A small calculus is visible in the intramural part of the right ureter. There is no distinct difference in shadow density of the two kidneys. The left side reveals a very narrow renal pelvis with long calyces; no true pelvis is present. The ureter splits into branches of approximately the same diameter as the ureter itself.

At the right side no contrast medium can be detected anywhere within the kidney shadow. A very faint area of increased density is visible near the hilum, suggesting the upper part of the ureter. If this is the ureter, the excretion of contrast medium is not inhibited in the right kidney, but is so slight that a pyelogram does not appear.

In *B,* after 15 minutes, the situation is not essentially changed. The only difference will be noted in a somewhat denser kidney shadow at the right side. The upper part of the ureter, which was faintly visible in the 5 minutes exposure, is better visualized and seems to be expanded.

Exposure *C*, taken after 35 minutes, shows an impressive difference in the nephrograms. The left side is unchanged. The right side, however, casts

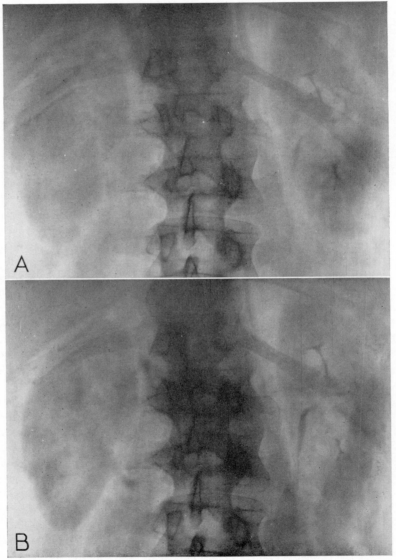

Fig. 31.   Intravenous urogram. *A,* Diodrast injection two hours after onset of colics due to calculus blocking right ureter in its intramural part. Suppression of Diodrast excretion on right side. *B,* increasing nephrogram owing to storage of Diodrast in tubular cells. Exposure *C* shows most intense nephrogram.

In exposure *D* (two hours after Diodrast injection) calculus was passed and back-pressure released. Excretion of stored Diodrast: pyelogram. Nephrogram disappears. See text.

a most intense shadow outlining the entire organ to perfection. The upper part of the ureter is no longer visible.

After the injection of the contrast medium the intermittent colics had subsided toward the end of the second hour. Exposure *D* was taken two

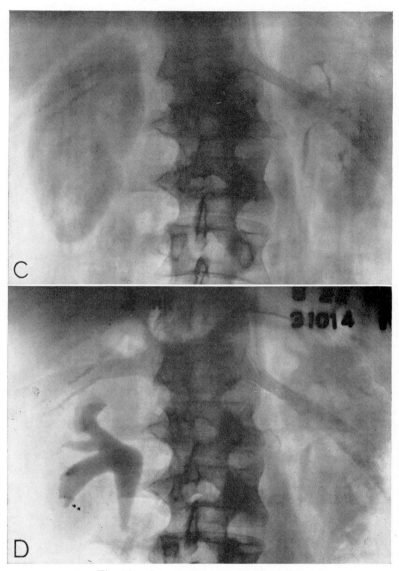

Fig. 31. *See opposite page for legend.*

hours after injection. The calculus had left the intramural part of the ureter; the passage was free.

The Diodrast, stored in the cells of the tubules, is in excretion. The dense nephrogram has disappeared, most of the contrast medium has left the tubules and is now present in the calyces, the true pelvis and the ureter. A perfect pyelogram is the result. All parts of the pelvis exhibit a very low tonus with loss of borderlines between the various sections due to the previous obstruction which lasted about four hours.

There is another interesting finding in this case. Two hours after intravenous injection of contrast medium no shadows of the medium will be visible in the renal pelves if the function of the kidneys is not impaired. The exposure in Figure 31, D was taken two hours after injection, yet the left, nonaffected kidney exhibits contrast medium in several calyces and in the upper part of the ureter. There are two possible explanations for this fact. (1) The contrast medium which is stored in the tubular cells of the right kidney, visible in the heavy nephrogram in Figure 31, C, is being slowly absorbed and returned to the general circulation. Perhaps a part of the material may be absorbed from the right renal pelvis which contains some medium. The faint excretory urogram of the left side is the result. (2) A reno-renal reflex from the right side, transmitted by the autonomous nervous system, acts on the circulation of the left kidney, constricting its arterioles and depressing filtration. Thus the contrast medium is kept in circulation for a much longer time and the delayed pyelogram is the result.

The patient did not want to submit to a second urographic study, suggested for the following week. The comparison between the two series would have been of great interest.

The tonic changes in the renal pelvis and ureter thus far presented were due either to increased bladder pressure or to obstructive conditions. Elevated pressure within the bladder is not an obstacle to urine ejection; an obstruction is. The opinion that the wider diameter of the upper tract is a result of increased intrinsic pressure must be considered. The expanding bladder does not exercise any pressure on the urine, no matter whether the bladder is filled with 50, 100 or 200 cc. It was mentioned before that the viscera of the abdomen are responsible for pressure rises. This can easily be demonstrated when pressure readings are performed in upright and extreme Trendelenburg position. In Trendelenburg position the pressure decreases. Logically, a wider diameter of the upper tract does not mean increased pressure levels *per se*, as can be proved. In a horizontal position a certain pressure level can be noted in the ureter. When the patient is placed in opposite lateral position, which means that the patient rests on the left side when pressure readings are taken in the right ureter, again a decrease of pressure will be recorded. The difference between horizontal and lateral position is due to the viscera which press on the ureter in horizontal position but slip to the other side in the lateral.

An entirely different situation arises when a block occurs in the tract. Due to further urine production the amount retained increases constantly and leads to expansion. Frequent and painful dynamics are the result. The intrapressure rises. This, however, is not a sequence of expansion and lowered tonus; the energetic action of the detrusor is responsible.

Under normal conditions both kidneys produce roughly the same amount of urine. Therefore, the same amount passes through the transporting system left and right and will exert the same intrapressure. If the intrapressure were the cause of tonus levels, no difference should be noted between the two sides. Why, then, do we find different states of tonus between left and right in many instances?

We can only illustrate the situation, record possible reasons for tonic changes and then try to find an explanation.

There is the "expanded" ureter in some cases of nephroptosis when the dislocation of the kidney produces a kink in the ureter which constitutes

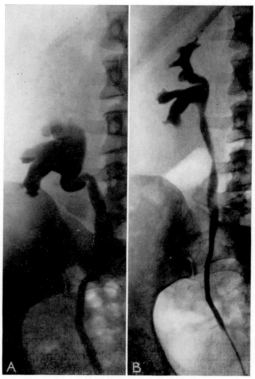

Fig. 32.   Nephroptosis. Before and after nephropexy. In *A* (before operation) severe hypotony of renal pelvis. For explanation of layer formation see text. Hypotony of unobstructed ureter below site of kinking. In *B* (38 days after operation) return to nearly normal tonus.

an obstacle to the downflow of urine. The dilatation above the kink seems plausible. Yet, also below the kink the unobstructed ureter shows a wider diameter than one would expect in a "normal" ureter or in comparison with the other side. The same lowered tonus will be found in the ureter in cases of hydronephrosis due to an aberrant vessel or a fibrous band near the ureteropelvic junction. An incompletely blocking calculus at the ureteropelvic junction produces the same picture. Figures 32 and 33 illustrate conditions of this kind. Why there are instances in which this phenomenon is not observed, cannot be explained.

Figure 32 shows a case of nephroptosis. Exposure *A* was taken in upright position after slow injection of the contrast medium. The capacity of the renal pelvis was known from the horizontal film and no attempt was made to fill the pelvis completely. The purpose of this procedure is explained in the descriptive text to Figure 35. The layer arrangement of the contrast medium does not interest us here especially, though it is very important in itself as a proof of low tonus and slackened dynamics. The kidney has descended considerably. The fornices are moderately blunted, and the necks of the calyces are very dilated, as is the true pelvis. Near the ureteropelvic junction the ureter exhibits two kinks. The tip of the ureteral catheter is visible in the second one. The upper part of the ureter is quite expanded and there may be another kinking near the linea innominata. But also below this point the ureter exhibits a distinct expansion. Since the tract is incompletely filled, it is obvious that this dilatation is not due to excess pressure within the tract. The low tonus of the ureter is due to a reflex mechanism.

Exposure B was taken 38 days after nephropexy. This early control series resulted from the fact that the patient was readmitted to the hospital because of a right pleuritis diaphragmatica. The diagnosis, however, was questionable. In order to exclude the kidney as a possible cause for the symptoms pyelography was performed. I wish to emphasize that the picture obtained does not claim to be proof of good results of a nephropexy. Two years after operation a new pyelogram will reveal the final outcome of this case.

The film was taken in upright position after the patient had jumped roughly on her heels and had coughed several times. There is an amazing difference between the pyelograms before and after operation. The size of the calyces, the true pelvis and the ureter has regressed considerably and I do not doubt that further regression will take place and will restore the kidney to normal. The tonus of the ureter is already approximately normal.

Figure 33 demonstrates the tonic response of the ureter to an intermittently blocking calculus at the ureteropelvic junction, combined with a secondary inflammatory stricture of the junction. Exposure A is shown only to visualize the calculus which escapes observation in the pyelogram in B. There is no calcified shadow in the course of the ureter. No obstruction was present in the intramural part. The pyelogram reveals a hydronephrosis of impressive size and an obstruction of the ureteropelvic junction. Below the obstruction the ureter is quite dilated in its entire length.

At operation the parenchyma was found to be heavy enough to promise a fair restoration of function. No infection was noted. Consequently, the kidney was not sacrificed; the calculus was removed by pyelotomy and a plastic procedure at the ureteropelvic junction established a good canal. The result obtained was satisfactory.

Comparative intravenous urograms taken during the first or second day of menstruation and one week after the cessation of the menstrual flow often reveal a remarkable difference in tonic aspect. The tonus is lower at times of menstruation. Tonus changes in early pregnancy must be mentioned when the uterus is not sufficiently enlarged to compress the ureter at the linea innominata. Hormonal influences have been claimed to be responsible for the lowered tonus.

There is a relationship between the urinary tract and the abdominal viscera which is most certainly effected by the autonomous nervous system. Compare the reflex response of the intestinal tract during a renal colic; vomiting, distention of the small intestines and colon. I wish to cite also the often enough erroneously interpreted digestive symptoms owing to pull on the kidney pedicle in nephroptosis, or to kinks of the ureter with resulting difficulties in urine transportation.

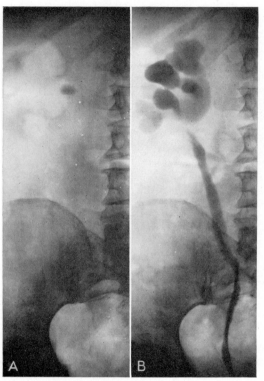

Fig. 33.   *A,* obstruction at ureteropelvic junction. *B,* unobstructed ureter below junction
shows considerable hypotony.

The autonomic apparatus is influenced by a vast reflex system of somatic nature and by cortical impulses. In the "normal" person sympathicus and vagus work in harmony. But we find quite a number of instances in which either the sympathicus or the vagus predominates. Gastroenterologists know more about these conditions than we urologists, much to our disadvantage. The previous classification of sympathicotonics and vagotonics is apparently too limited. Only certain organs may be out of autonomic balance and it is better to state that the person is stigmatized as sympathicotonic or vagotonic.

As far as the urinary tract is concerned, there is a functional spasticity as well as a hypotony. Denervations of the renal pedicle for the purpose of elimination of spastic conditions have yielded unsatisfactory results. This seems to contradict the claimed influence of nerve impulses. But

denervation of the pedicle is an unreliable procedure. A ganglionectomy
of the celiac plexus would be preferable. We do not know how far up the
ganglia at the ureter-bladder junction can send impulses. It is possible that
surgical eradication of these ganglia may produce better results.

A hypotony which persists for a longer period of time creates longer
lasting rest intervals in the sections of the tract. The dynamics are not
essentially disturbed, but the emptying process is less complete and greater
retention of urine results. This can influence absorptive processes, as discussed later.

It is not too difficult to distinguish between expansion due to back
pressure in cases of obstruction and dilatations of the tract due to lowered

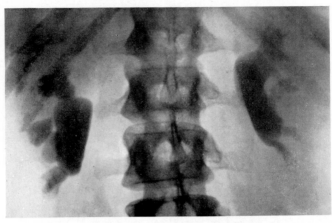

Fig. 34.   Bilateral hypotony due to parametritis. Both flabby pelves rest against psoas
edge. Hutter symptom. (From Narath, Renal Pelvis and Ureter, New York, Grune & Stratton, 1951.)

tonus. The configuration of the fornices is blunted when excess pressure is
present; the fornical arches are well maintained under hypotonic conditions.

There are other signs which are indicative of low tonus and which prove
at the same time the absence of increased intrinsic pressure. Under normotonic conditions the pelvis is not compressed by the edge of the psoas
muscle. The hypotonic pelvis is expanded and flabby and rests with its
medial side against the edge of the psoas. The psoas takes an oblique course
down to the bony pelvis and cuts off the medial side of the pelvis. A compression takes place and the ureter usually turns from the edge of the psoas
over its body in a characteristic curve. This sign is called the *Hutter
symptom,* or the psoas-edge symptom, after the urologist who described it.
Intravenous urography is used for its demonstration, since retrograde
pyelography often overdistends the pelvis and blurs the tonic aspect.

Figure 34 presents a reactive response of the urinary tract to a severe
bilateral parametritis following gonorrhea. The structure of the calyces and
fornices is normal in itself, but their diameter is widened considerably. Both
kidneys have an extrarenal type of pelvis which normally would overlap
the psoas undisturbed. Because of the lowered tonus the pelves are less

rigid, have attained a certain flabbiness, and rest with their medial side against the edge of the psoas, following its margin. On the right side, the pelvis is "cut off" in a straight line. On the left side, the situation is somewhat different, since in the upper section of the pelvis a part is filled which overlaps the psoas, indicating that the true form of this pelvis is different. The medial side is folded together owing to the protruding psoas.

I have found another sign of great loss in tonus during the course of retrograde pyelography. The ureteral catheter is introduced low and the patient placed in semi-erect position. The contrast medium is injected very slowly. In this way the heavy medium fills the pelvis gradually, carrying the

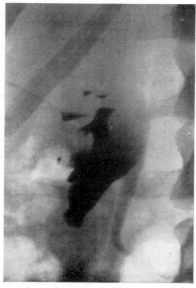

Fig. 35. Severe hypotony in ptotic kidney. Contrast medium instilled very slowly in semi-erect position. Layer formation due to slow dynamics. Narath symptom. (From Narath, Renal Pelvis and Ureter, New York, Grune & Stratton, 1951.)

lighter urine on its surface. A complete filling should not be attempted. Owing to the slow dynamics of the pelvis the contrast medium does not mix properly with the retention urine and appears in the pyelogram as if it were arranged in layers. A normotonic pelvis will never demonstrate this sign, because the rapid motion mixes urine and contrast medium readily.

Figure 35, a case of nephroptosis, not demonstrated in this single film, shows an enlarged hypotonic pelvis, but no sign of hydronephrosis, since the fornices, especially in the upper section of the kidney, are well preserved and not blunted. In the lowest part of the pelvis the borderline between urine and contrast medium is blurred. In four calyces of the cranial pole the contrast medium demarcates itself by a sharp meniscus against the invisible urine.

The influence of drugs on the tonus of the urinary tract is still a disputed topic. Though drugs are widely in use, their effect has not been satisfactorily demonstrated by intravenous urography. One must admit, however, that the investigation is much more complicated than it appears to be at first glance. Several series of urograms of the same person under varying conditions with and without stimulant and depressant drugs are necessary for comparison. The experienced reader will realize the enormous difficulties involved. No attempt, therefore, shall be made in this short resumé to discuss these questions.

The changes of tonus in the urinary tract deserve more attention than is usually offered. If properly evaluated they add valuable data for diagnosing physiologic and pathologic conditions.

ABSORPTION IN THE UPPER URINARY TRACT

The urocanal is capable of absorption as experimental work on animals and the living human has proved. Yet, it is hardly feasible that all parts of the tract perform this task equally. There may be areas of great absorptive capacity and parts which have a selective function. Absorption is accomplished by the urothelium which lines the tract. It seems necessary, therefore, to study this epithelium and its underlying structures in the various sections of the tract.

The canaliculi are joined together in the papilla to a smaller number of canals, the *ductus papillares*. The cells of their epithelium form a single layer. These cells are of cubic or prismatic form and well defined, with strictly maintained borderlines. The nuclei do not stain equally; sometimes the nucleoplasm and the nuclear body can appear to be of deeper color.

The epithelium of the papillary surface is single-layered, but there is a histological difference since a different cell type is interposed, namely, small, slender cells which extend from the base of the papilla and mostly reach the epithelial surface. It is possible that these cells constitute an intermediate stage between the single layer of the papilla and the multilayer lining of the fornix, into which the papillary layer leads. Whether they serve a definite purpose is unknown.

Experimental investigation revealed absorptive function of the epithelium of the canalicular system, but did not disclose such a faculty in the cell layer of the papilla.

The character of the papillary epithelium changes in the fornix region. A double layer is formed, evident in the state of expansion of the fornix, but folded together in a multilayer during the contracting phase. An outer margin of increased density becomes visible. This seam is not continuous, but is formed by the surface of each cell which extends into the lumen of the calyx. The borderlines of the cells are preserved. Their form varies considerably according to the filling degree of the calyx. Intermixed between the basal cells we see long cell forms with irregular nuclei and some which resemble lymphocytes. There is a distinct difference in staining quality of the fornical and upper calycal urothelium when compared with the papillary layer. The cytoplasm is lighter in color.

In the fornical region the underlying connective tissue is intensely undulated and intermixed with elastic fibers, revealing the possibility of motion and expansion. Beyond the connective fibers above the fornix and also lateral to the fornix, a venous plexus becomes visible which surrounds the upper papilla. The adventitia of the calyx begins to disperse near the fornix. Some strands are connected with the venous plexus; some penetrate higher up alongside the renculus, following the course of the musculus levator fornicis, and some are lost in the bordering fat of the sinus renalis. The entire region is amply equipped with lymph spaces and fine lymphatics.

In the neck of the calyx the transitional urothelium has essentially the same structure as in the fornix, but in the contracted state not so many layers of cells will be found. The staining quality of the epithelium gains somewhat in density the more we approach the calycopelvic junction. The nuclei seem to be unchanged.

The urothelium of the true pelvis and of the ureter does not exhibit any new features, except that it is heavier than that of the calyx.

The different staining quality of the cells and the layer arrangement distinguishes one section from the other, but the histologic appearance does not permit us to draw any conclusions as far as function is concerned.

The urine which leaves the distal convoluted tubules enters the canaliculi and is transported in rapid succession through the calyx, the true pelvis and the ureter and is ejected into the bladder. The general belief is that the urine which trickles out of the pores of the papilla is in composition the same as the urine ejected from the ureteral orifice. This is only a presumption, not proved experimentally. Theoretically there could be further changes of the urine in the transporting system, no matter how short the time may be in which resorption of water and perhaps solubles could take place.

I have expressed my doubts that calycal and low ureteral urine are identical in composition. My reluctance to accept the common concept is based on the following experiment. A ureteral catheter is introduced into the cranial pole calyx and its proper position proved roentgenologically. A second catheter is placed low into the ureter, close to the bladder. Through these two catheters urine can be collected separately. The cranial catheter will drain a urine which represents papillary urine, although this may not be entirely correct, since some fornical action cannot be excluded with certainty. The lower catheter yields a urine which has passed through the transporting system. The arrangement of the experiment has its setbacks since physiologic disturbance by foreign body reaction of the catheters is possible. But if these investigations should prove what they seem to promise, then there is a difference in composition between calycal and low ureteral urine. I wish to call the reader's attention to this very interesting problem.

In the course of this experiment a most difficult question confronts us, namely, whether the absorptive response of the upper urinary tract is different under abnormal physiologic conditions. Does a lowered tonus with widening of the diameter of the lumen of the tract and the creation of prolonged retention phases have any influence, qualitatively or quantitatively, on absorption? Does increase of intrinsic pressure due to incomplete or complete obstruction promote absorption? Does an inflammatory process of the urothelium increase or decrease absorption?

A lowered tonus stretches the urothelium and in this way increases the surface and loosens the intercellular spaces. Thus absorption should be accomplished more easily. In addition, the retention phases are prolonged, allowing the urine to remain in the calyces, pelvis and ureter for a longer period of time. The time factor, undoubtedly, is of great importance.

Increase of intrinsic pressure leads to further stretching of the urothelium, the multilayer is reduced to a lesser amount of cells, the cuticular seam is spanned and the intercellular spaces loosen more and more. Experimental work has shown that material under pressure will be absorbed more rapidly.

Whether or not inflammatory processes of the urothelium make absorption easier is difficult to say. They certainly do not inhibit it. A case of acute pyelitis (is it always a pyelonephritis?) proves the absorption of toxic substances clinically beyond doubt.

It seems nearly impossible to investigate a truly unmolested urinary tract, since all experimental work interferes with physiologic conditions. We must content ourselves for the time being with trying to gain as much knowledge as possible, aware that the results obtained come from a disturbed physiologic background.

Here are a few examples which prove absorption.

A solution of strychnine injected into the renal pelvis of a test animal does not produce any signs of poisoning. But as soon as the ureter is ligated the animal dies from strychnine poisoning very rapidly. Owing to further urine production the intrinsic pressure increases and promotes absorption. This would denote, that normally strychnine is not absorbed, but is intensely so when put under pressure.

Experimental studies in test animals proved that various chemicals injected into one side of the urinary tract could be recovered from the saliva, the blood and from the urine of the opposite side. Absorption took place sometimes under normal pressure conditions and sometimes when the intrinsic pressure of the injected side was increased. Absorption gained in direct proportion to increase of pressure. Furthermore, the higher the concentration of the material, the greater the absorption.

When a contrast medium is injected into one ureter, ligation of this ureter above the site of injection retains the material in the tract. The absorption of the medium can be followed roentgenologically. After one half to one and one half hours no contrast medium is detectable. When the injected ureter was ligated at two places above the site of injection, so that a column of contrast medium was inclosed in the ureter, a difference in time of absorption could be noted between the material in the renal pelvis and the intraureteral section. The pelvis absorbed rapidly, but the intraureteral medium was also absorbed. This proves ureteral absorption.

When in the course of retrograde pyelography both ureters are catheterized, with the catheters up into the true pelvis, but only one side injected with a 5 per cent sodium iodide solution, iodine can be recovered from the other side within 8 to 15 minutes. The objection that an injury to the injected side took place due to excess pressure must be considered. A test of this kind has convincing value only if the catheter is placed in the true pelvis and not in one calyx. Moreover, only fine catheters should be used which allow a backflow of the contrast medium, providing this is not inhibited by spastic contractions of the canal around the catheter. In order to prevent any excess pressure, small amounts of contrast medium should be used, about 3 to 4 cc.

It is difficult to follow the route of absorption of solutions. In animal experiments sodium or potassium ferrocyanate may be detected histologically, but no conclusive answer can be given whether the deposits in the cells are of absorptive nature or are transported there secondarily by the blood stream.

Small corpuscular elements may be better material for studies of absorption, provided they are absorbed at all. Many experimental studies along these lines have been published. The results are not conclusive. Ultramarine green, indigo carmine, india ink, colloid silver and bacteria have been used in these investigations. Many of these studies must be discarded for the simple reason that the material was injected with excess pressure. A rupture of the fornix, the most vulnerable place in the urinary tract, could not be excluded with certainty. Yet in some experiments, in which apparently no excess pressure was used, the injected material was found in the cells of the tubules, the canaliculi and in the urothelium, in the interstitium, the lymphatics and in the veins. The experienced reader realizes the tremendous difficulties involved in the evaluation of the findings and will accept the results with justified reluctance. Moreover, there remains the discrepancy between animal experiments and the reaction in the living human.

There is one question of great importance. Can the urocanal be ruptured by intrinsic pressure produced by continued urine production in cases of obstruction? Or can a pelvis, filled to capacity, rupture its wall somewhere owing to spastic contractions of the true pelvis? Clinically there is no evidence of such a process. The region which was suspected to be a possible site was the fornix calycis, because ruptures had been produced there experimentally with surprisingly low excess pressure. To my knowledge, no intravenous urogram has been published which proved a fornical rupture. The opinion of possible rupture was reached from retrograde pyelograms. In these cases, however, the tract was exposed to suddenly created artificial excess pressure of undetermined magnitude. Contrast medium was found beyond the borderlines of the upper calyx, similar to those deliberately produced in animals and in cadavers.

There is considerable doubt that nature should so easily sever the continuity of the urothelium and the underlying tissue, or that no better safety valve is provided to cope with such a common occurrence of excess pressure in the tract. Up to 1937 no definite proof to the contrary was at hand. Then new investigations in the living human revealed that extravasations beyond the fornical borderlines can be of different nature, namely, absorption of contrast medium by the urothelium of the fornical arch.

When during the course of retrograde pyelography contrast medium is seen in the sinus renalis, close to the fornices, no differentiation is possible between injury and absorption. The only way of proving a rupture with a high degree of certainty is to repeat the pyelogram immediately several times under the same pressure conditions. If a rupture was established, then the contrast medium will escape through the broken down tissue, time and again, and render similar pictures. In case of absorption there is undoubtedly the possibility that another exposure may show a similar extravasation at the same spot, but, peculiarly enough, it does not happen as a rule. I have seen, however, absorption at other fornices when a second and third pyelogram was taken.

There is only one form of extravasation which proves a fornical rupture with accuracy. The ingression of the contrast medium into the venous plexus around the fornix with possible filling of the vena arcuata and perhaps the interlobulares. A more or less perfect anatomical picture is visualized on the film. This means that the venous system has been ruptured by the onpressing medium and that the medium has entered the circulation. This secondary injury, which takes place in the sinus renalis or in the interstitium close to the fornix, can occur only when the fornix was ruptured primarily by excess pressure. At the end of this chapter this condition will claim our attention once more.

Consequently, routine retrograde pyelography does not seem to be the proper procedure for studying absorption since one can never exclude injuries with convincing certainty.

Based on the empirical knowledge that increase of intrinsic pressure promotes absorption, I have tried to solve the problem in the living human without creating any artificial pressure, because this would invalidate the procedure. Increase in pressure must be created by the kidney and the renal pelvis after blocking off the lowest part of the ureter by a conical and splinted catheter. No instrumentation must molest the upper tract. The situation simulates a low ureteral obstruction as seen, for instance, in cases of impacted calculus. The setup of the investigation was as follows:

A conical catheter was introduced into the ureteral orifice until an occlusion was achieved. Through this catheter 2 to 4 cc. of concentrated contrast medium were injected under fluoroscopic observation. A complete filling of the pelvis should not be attempted. Then the catheter was splinted and in this way blocked the entire tract. At this time the patient felt no sensation in his kidney region. Owing to further urine production the filling degree of the tract increased slowly but constantly. A certain discomfort resulted which finally grew into a true colic. The combined picture of overdistention and energetic, painful spastic contractions of the detrusor sections of the tract as seen in calculus occlusion was reproduced. The contrast medium was mixed with the urine due to the hypermotility of the pelvis. Starting at the time of the injection, the tract is fluoroscopically observed, using the same technique as described in the discussion on "Dynamics."

There are various kinds of reaction to an overdistended pelvis and excess pressure.

One variety was demonstrated in the discussion on "Tonus" in Figure 31. Here, after several hours of colics, the pain disappeared because further urine production was inhibited to such an extent that no more overdistention occurred. Proof is found in the storage of Diodrast in the tubular cells and the missing shadow of the contrast medium in the renal pelvis. Since in this case the blocking calculus left the ureter within four hours (two hours after the injection of Diodrast), the excess pressure in the urocanal was released and the excretion of Diodrast into the tubular lumen and ejection into the pelvis took place. Therefore the intense nephrogram faded and a perfect pyelogram was obtained after two hours. Whether or not during the time of obstruction absorptive processes were also at work in the fornical arches cannot be decided. From the results obtained by the tests in the living human this seems most likely.

This case shows clearly that urine production is suppressed (at least to a great extent) because the intrapelvic pressure supersedes the force with

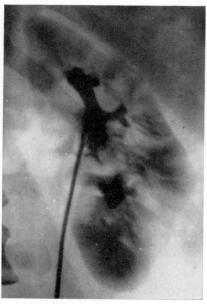

Fig. 36. Pyelocanalicular backflow. (From Narath, Renal Pelvis and Ureter, New York, Grune & Stratton, 1951.)

which the urine leaves the papillary pores. It is imaginable that the process of urine transportation could be reversed temporarily when the pressure in the pelvis rises more and more. Urine then could be pressed backwards into the canaliculi. This, indeed, would be the most natural way, the most plausible one. We observe this phenomenon now and then in retrograde pyelograms. This *"pyelocanalicular backflow"* with its brushlike formation above the calyx outlines in a most characteristic manner the anatomical structure of the canaliculi. Pyelocanalicular backflow cannot be classified as extravasation, since the material is not outside the vasae, it is inside.

There is a certain doubt whether pyelocanalicular backflow is necessarily due to excess pressure, because it is seen sometimes in, apparently, not over-distended pelves. But there may have been an overdistention shortly before the exposure was taken which is no longer evident in the pyelogram. The strongest support for the opinion of excess pressure as a prerequisite is found in the fact, that pyelocanalicular backflow has never been seen in an intravenous urogram. Occasionally faint outlines of the collecting canals in the lowest part of the papilla can be observed, but this can represent urine with high concentration of the medium in its normal flow downward into the calyx.

Figure 36 illustrates pyelocanalicular backflow throughout the entire kidney. Not one renculus has been spared. This is an exceptional case. The pyelogram was selected because it splendidly demonstrates various stages and degrees. In the upper pole and in the middle section the streaked, brush-like formations are apparent. In the lower pole the renculi seem to be imbued with contrast medium. This picture clearly delineates the renculus which

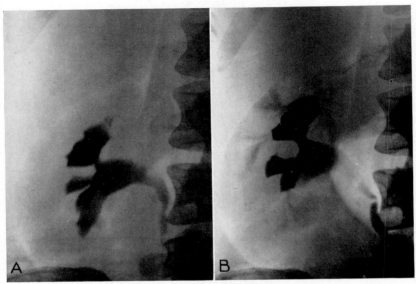

Fig. 37.   Pyelocanalicular backflow experimentally produced. See text.

belongs to one calyx. For instance, the laterally pointing calyx in the upper pole carries a twin papilla, or two renculi.

Figure 37 represents a deliberately produced excess pressure in the renal pelvis, in the hope of demonstrating absorption. Instead, extensive pyelocanalicular backflow resulted besides a small extravasation and lymphatic absorption.

In Figure 37, *A,* all calyces, the true pelvis and the region of the ureteropelvic junction are overdistended. At the cranial pole calyx an extravasation is visible, the character of which is difficult to determine. It may be an injury of the fornix, or could be due to absorption.

In the time elapsed between the two exposures the excess pressure was slowly and gently increased. In Figure 37, *B,* the calyces are still more blunted and overdistended. Compare, for instance, the neck of the cranial calyx in the two pictures. There is another interesting difference at the caudal pole. In Figure 37, *A,* a calyx major, which splits into minores, is present, but is entirely missing in *B,* notwithstanding the fact that the filling degree of the pelvis is higher in Figure 37, *B* than in Figure 37, *A*. This calyx must have succeeded in emptying against the rising intrinsic pressure. A similar action is noted at the ureteropelvic junction.

The extravasation at the cranial pole is somewhat more extensive in Figure 37, *B* and there are indications of filled venae arcuatae. If this is correct, this extravasation constitutes an injury. Pyelocanalicular backflow has occurred at most of the calyces, filling the canaliculi deep into the cortex.

In addition, lymphatic absorption takes place at the upper pole. One lymph vessel is filled with contrast medium and can be followed in its upward course toward the vertebrae.

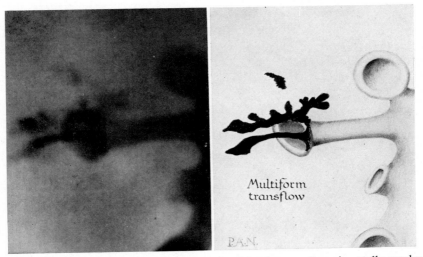

Fig. 38.   Absorption of contrast medium in the living human. Experimentally produced pyelosinous transflow. (From Narath, J. Urol., *43*, 1940.)

Pyelocanalicular backflow, peculiarly enough, cannot be produced in a cadaver kidney.

The third way in which an overdistended renal pelvis responds to increasing intrinsic pressure is by partial absorption of pelvic contents.

I have mentioned above the method employed of proving this absorption in the living human. After the injection of 2 to 4 cc. of contrast medium into the low occluding ureteral catheter, the catheter is splinted and the increase of filling degree of the tract is left to further urine production. This process is observed under the fluoroscopic screen. The renal pelvis fills more and more and the dynamics mix urine and contrast medium. At this point the patient has no sensation in his kidney region. Soon, however, a mild pressure is felt. Now starts the crucial moment of observation. A large magnifying glass over the fluoroscopic screen facilitates the recognition of changes. It is often difficult to notice the onset of absorption, and frequently enough it is overlooked. In some instances a blurring becomes evident at one or several fornices. A rapid exposure is taken instantly under vision (see technique in discussion on "Dynamics"). I have seen absorption even at a time when the patient did not complain of any unpleasant sensation. The pictures gain in clarity, however, when energetic contraction of the calyces or true pelvis produces a mild colic.

The proper term for this process would be "fornical absorption." Since the same picture as shown by absorption can be produced artificially during the course of retrograde pyelography, by rupture of the fornix using excess pressure and pressing the contrast medium into the sinus renalis, it seems better not to indicate too strongly this type of process. Therefore I suggested using a broader term, *"pyelosinous transflow,"* leaving the door open for further precision.

From the first set of experiments I want to reproduce two examples. Since in these cases no artificial injury was established, they represent true absorption.

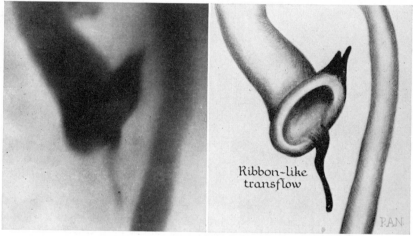

Fig. 39.   Absorption of contrast medium in the living human. Experimentally produced pyelosinous transflow. (From Narath, J. Urol., *43,* 1940.)

Figure 38 is a cut-out from a pyelogram which has been photographically enlarged for better visualization. The calyx in question is projected in semi-profile and does not give the impression of being overdistended or blunted, since the fornical rim is well maintained. From two points of the fornix an extensive extravasation arises which is distributed in an irregular pattern within the sinus renalis. In the explanatory drawing the type is designated as multiform transflow. I believe that the various forms of transflow depend on the anatomical structure of the sinus renalis around the fornix and that in themselves they have no significance. There is one form of extravasation which may be distinguished from others, however.

Figure 39 shows such a case. The caudal pole calyx of a nonrotated kidney exhibits at its fornix two types of extravasation. At the upper margin a transflow is visible which may be called "hornshaped." This is not the one which interests us just now. From the lower medial margin a ribbonlike transflow extends deep into the parenchyma beyond the borderlines of the sinus renalis. It is most likely that the absorbed contrast medium follows the course of the interstitial spaces of the musculus levator fornicis. Compare the histological drawing of Figure 20 in the discussion of "Dynamics."

In this first series the exposures were taken when absorption was expected to furnish a satisfactory picture. The next logical step was to follow the time and course of absorption more closely, using the technique of rapid serial exposures as employed in the demonstration of the dynamics.

Figure 40 gives three exposures at one second interval. In *A,* a very faint extravasation is visible on the film, but will probably not show up in the reproduction. In *B,* the absorption is more intense but does not yet allow any anatomical classification. The situation changes in *C.* Here the extravasation is very clear and must be grouped as "ribbonlike transflow,"

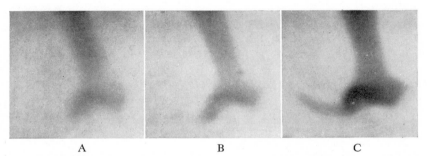

A   B   C

Fig. 40.   Absorption of contrast medium in the living human. Experimentally produced pyelosinous transflow. Exposures taken at one second interval.

following the lateral margin of the renculus in the course of the musculus levator fornicis.

Figure 41 shows in *A* a normal pyelogram of a somewhat overdistended pelvis. All fornices are sharply defined, except for the lowest one of the cranial pole which exhibits a "planelike transflow." In Figure 41, *B* the picture changes. We encounter the interesting phenomenon of a calyx of the cranial pole resisting the excess pressure and remaining closed in *A.* In *B,* it is filled (the second calyx pointing laterally). The planelike transflow of the cranial calyx has dispersed in the meantime and gives a flakier impression, a sign of further distribution and absorption from the fornices in the sinus renalis. Most interesting is the absorption from the fornices of the caudal pole. Since all three fornices are in proper projection, the site of the absorption from the rim of the fornix is clearly visible. In Figure 41, *A,* the fornix of the middle calyx in the caudal pole is not filled, probably because the sphincter fornicis managed to close. In Figure 41, *B,* the middle calyx is filled.

The entire pyelogram in Figure 41, *B* is definitely more distended. Besides the planelike transflow mentioned above, absorption can be observed at three more calyces, one at the cranial end calyx and two of the calyces of the lower pole. Arrows point to the site of absorption.

I want to add here one highly interesting case of incidental findings with immediate repetition of pyelograms which prove that no rupture of the fornix has taken place.

The case concerns a middle-aged woman. Retrograde pyelography was performed to establish a differential diagnosis between possible disease of the gallbladder or kidney. After the injection of 1.75 cc. of 40 per cent Skiodan (Abrodil) the patient suffered a sudden severe colic. The injection was interrupted and a picture taken immediately. Figure 42 shows the result in exposure *A*. The contrast medium fills the ureter to the upper end of the fourth lumbar vertebra, where it ends abruptly. No Skiodan can be detected in the true pelvis or the calyces. There are two ringlike formations which seem to represent blunted fornices. From these fornices irregular extravasations are visible which could be grouped as multiform transflow. It is not certain whether this reflects absorption or an injury to the fornix.

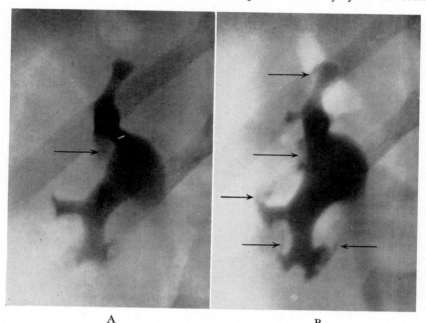

A   B

Fig. 41. Absorption of contrast medium in the living human. Experimentally produced pyelosinous transflow in stages. (From Narath, Renal Pelvis and Ureter, New York, Grune & Stratton, 1951.)

Since only 1.75 cc. of contrast medium were used, of which a part is in the ureter, it is hard to believe that this small amount should have broken through. After about 12 minutes a new film was taken which revealed that all traces of Skiodan had left the kidney. The pain had subsided in the meantime. If an injury had been done to the fornix, a second filling should show the routes of escape. Carefully the tract was reinjected, this time using 3 cc. of Skiodan. The patient had no discomfort and did not feel any pressure at all. The next exposure is shown in Figure 42, *B*. A total filling of the pelvis and calyces was achieved; no extravasation was visible.

But we could not be satisfied with the result since the objection remained that because of the small amount used no extravasation through tears in the fornix occurred. Therefore, a third injection was made this time with

9 cc. of Skiodan. This amount was tolerated without pain, but the patient indicated a feeling of pressure. The pyelogram is shown in Figure 42, *C*. There is no doubt that the renal pelvis is overdistended and the calyces are filled to capacity. Yet no extravasation occurred. The two fornices from which the absorption previously took place are totally filled, one in the upper pole, the other in the lower pole. If an injury in the fornices occurred, this pyelogram would again demonstrate an extravasation with this high degree of filling. That this is absent can be taken as definite proof that there was no rupture.

Granted that we deal here with an instance of rapid absorption, we must explain what happened at the time of the first pyelogram. Skiodan is practically

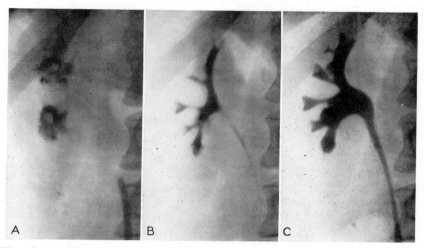

Fig. 42.   Incidental finding. Proof of absorption of contrast medium through fornix. Pyelosinous transflow in *A* with 1.75 cc. of contrast medium. In *B* pelvis filled with 3 cc. In *C* filling with 9 cc. No rupture of fornix occurred. See text. (From Narath, Renal Pelvis and Ureter, New York, Grune & Stratton, 1951.)

nonirritating; the fault, therefore, cannot be due to the contrast medium. If the patient had been sensitive to Skiodan, we would assume that the later fillings with increasing doses should have produced similar reactions. Most probably the injection coincided with the emptying phase of the pelvis, and even the small amount created a sudden excess pressure. This led to a severe, painful contraction which pressed the contrast medium backward into the two calyces and down the ureter. It seems as if the sphincter fornices had tried to close spastically and since contrast medium was in the fornical space, this material came under pressure. To release the pressure, the medium was absorbed rapidly. The importance of this case lies in the demonstration of the velocity and extensiveness of the absorption accomplished by the fornix. The fluoroscopic observation, as mentioned before, already demonstrated the surprisingly rapid absorption, which coincides with the findings in the first pyelogram of Figure 42.

The material which is absorbed by the fornices is transported into the sinus renalis or between the interrencular spaces. But we are not to infer that the medium is freely interposed between the fat and the connective tissue. Most probably it is absorbed by the capillary system and stored in the lymph spaces. X-ray follow-up can offer no conclusive proof of capillary absorption since the tiny vessels do not cast a diagnostic shadow and the flow would be too rapid to be arrested on the film.

Lymphatic absorption might offer better opportunities for roentgenologic detection, because the diameter of the lymphatics is large enough to be

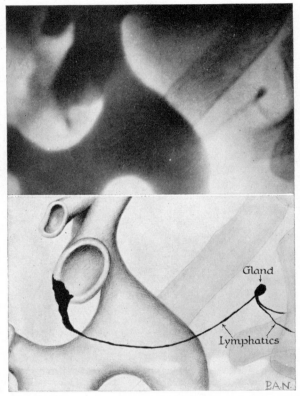

Fig. 43.   Sinolymphatic absorption. Hornshaped transflow in lymphatic absorption. Experimentally produced in the living human. (From Narath, J. Urol., *43*, 1940.)

detectable on the film and the flow of the lymph is slow enough to be arrested with a short x-ray exposure (Fig. 43).

For the following study the same technique was applied as used previously in arresting dynamic stages and pyelosinous transflow: fluoroscopic observation and rapid roentgenographic exposure under vision. The disadvantage is that one cannot observe imbued lymphatics on the fluoroscope screen. The moment to make the exposure is when the pyelosinous transflow begins to disperse. Most exposures taken at random were failures. But now and then pictures were obtained which fixed the next stage of absorption on the film. Of these pyelograms a few will be reproduced which demonstrate the phenomenon with utmost clarity. Although the flow of lymph is relatively slow, the process of further lymphatic transportation is rapid enough to eliminate a transflow in one or two minutes. Neither the pyelosinous transflow nor the lymphatics are visible anymore.

I am convinced that lymphatic absorption occurs more frequently than our ordinary pyelograms would allow us to assume. In many instances the film is not exposed at precisely the right moment or the absorption can be of minute degree and escape our observation.

Figure 43 shows a part of a pyelogram in which a transflow was observed at the lower fornix of the cranial pole. This transflow was originally broader

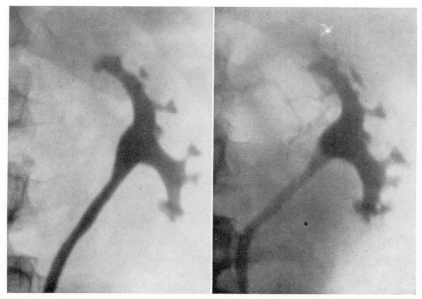

Fig. 44.   Sinolymphatic absorption of pyelosinous transflow. Experimentally produced in the living human. (From Narath, Renal Pelvis and Ureter, New York, Grune & Stratton, 1951.)

than it now appears on the film. It might have been classified as a horn-shaped transflow. As soon as the density of the shadow diminished, the next film was exposed and is the one shown here. A lymphatic crosses over the pelvis and extends toward the spine, filling a lymph gland and two smaller lymphatics which leave the gland. Neither the lymphatics nor the gland were seen under the fluoroscope. I am sure that the gland was visible, but since it is located close to the spine, no attention was paid to this region.

Figure 44 was taken with a different technique. A 4 F. ureteral catheter was introduced into the true pelvis and the pelvis was filled gently under vision. No pyelosinous transflow was noted. A picture taken at this moment, exposure *A,* reveals two doubtful areas where a pyelosinous transflow is probably beginning. First, the contour of the cranial fornix is not so sharply defined as that of the other fornices. Besides, a faint pyelocanalicular backflow is visible on the film but is lost in the reproduction. Second, a ribbonlike transflow starts at the lowest fornix.

After the first exposure the catheter was splinted and the next film taken two minutes later. Figure 44, *B* exhibits several areas of pyelosinous transflow. The cranial and caudal fornices are involved, as is one lateral fornix of the lower pole. Extensive absorption of contrast medium in the sinus renalis around the cranial fornix has taken place. Several lymph vessels are filled and reach toward the spine. One lymph gland, hardly visible in the reproduction, is faintly impregnated.

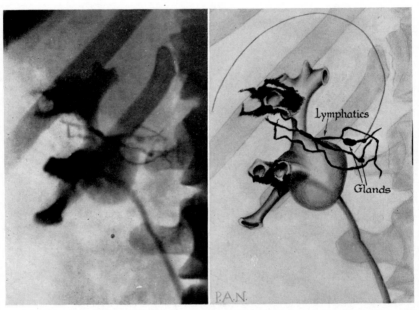

Fig. 45.   Incidental finding of sinolymphatic absorption. Several lymphatics are filled, small glands imbued with contrast medium. (From Narath, J. Urol., *43,* 1940.)

The ureteropelvic junction starts to close while the upper ureter empties and in contrast is less dense as result of the expulsion of its contents.

Figure 45 is an incidental finding, not experimentally produced. The true pelvis and calyces are overdistended. A planelike pyelosinous transflow has occurred at the upper pole and around the calyces of the lower pole. There is one point in the picture which suggests an injury at one of the lateral fornices of the upper pole with secondary rupture of a branch of the plexus venosus fornicis and ingression of the contrast medium into the venous system. The characteristics of this phenomenon will be discussed later.

Several lymphatics, arising from the cranial pole, are filled with contrast medium and are visible crossing the true pelvis toward the spine. Two small imbued lymph glands are interposed.

Figure 46 is doubly interesting. It shows two forms of deviation from the normal pyelogram. First we observe an extensive pyelocanalicular backflow which involves all calyces more or less. Furthermore, pyelosinous transflow is visible at several fornices. Several lymphatics are filled with the contrast medium. One lymphatic clearly originates from the region of the upper calyx. One (or two?) seems to derive from the region of the lowest calyx of the cranial pole. It is surprising that no lymphatic absorption was obtained

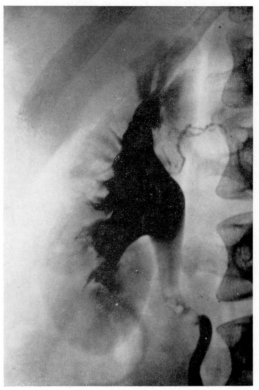

Fig. 46. Pyelocanalicular backflow, pyelosinous transflow and sinolymphatic absorption. Characteristic spindle formation of the lymphatics. (From Narath, Renal Pelvis and Ureter, New York, Grune & Stratton, 1951.)

in the caudal section of the kidney, although the extravasation here would advance such a possibility. The spindle form of the lymphatics is beautifully shown.

The reader's attention is directed to another interesting feature: the shadow of the upper part of the extrarenal pelvis and the joining ureter, the region of the ureteropelvic junction. This area is of much lesser density and shows a fine dark line in the center. This most probably constitutes a sudden contraction of the ureteropelvic junction which occurred during the exposure and was quicker than the exposure itself. The picture, therefore, seems to have arrested the ureteropelvic junction in two stages, expanded and contracted. There are air bubbles close to the filled ureter.

Attention has been called to the fact that a true injury to the fornix, a rupture, can occur as a result of excess pressure during the course of retrograde pyelography. The impossibility of discriminating in ordinary pyelograms between extravasations due to injuries and those due to absorption was mentioned, as long as these extravasations are confined to the sinus renalis. If, however, in case of injury, excess pressure is maintained, extravasating medium can expand the perifornical tissue with its venous plexus to such an extent, that a second rupture occurs. This time a branch of the plexus venosus is torn off and the way exposed for an escape of the contrast medium into the venous system.

Although extravasations due to injuries have nothing to do primarily with absorption, the material which is pressed into the sinus renalis and possibly into the interrencular spaces must be taken care of by absorption secondarily.

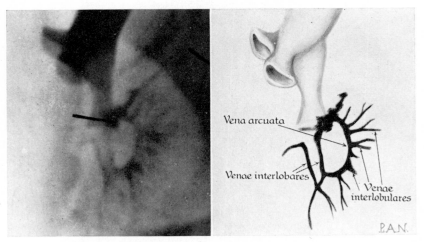

Fig. 47. Sinovenous ingression. Rupture of fornix and secondary rupture of venous plexus around fornix. Filling of venae interlobares, arcuata and venae interlobulares. (From Narath, J. Urol., *43,* 1940.)

It seems justifiable, therefore, to add to our discussion a few characteristic examples of this kind. The pictures which demonstrate what we call *"sinovenous ingression"* are most impressive because of their anatomical aspect. They are easily recognized, provided no other types of extravasation and absorption are combined in the pyelograms, which frequently is the case.

Figure 47 is an enlargement of a part of the caudal pole of a retrograde pyelogram. A rupture has taken place at the fornix (arrow) and, quite close to the fornix, there is a break in the continuity of the venous system. The contrast medium has invaded two parallel-running venae interlobares, demonstrating their anastomosis, and one arcuata which is completely filled. From this arcuata a great number of venae interlobulares are filled in their first part.

There can be no doubt of the distribution of the contrast medium. If the reader compares this picture with canalicular backflow, pyelosinous transflow or lymphatic absorption, the difference is evident.

A rupture is an established injury and the immediate repetition of the pyelogram must demonstrate the same route of escape as in the previous picture. Figure 48 splendidly illustrates the validity of this opinion. In *A* an extensive extravasation is present at the lower pole. That we are dealing with a rupture is beyond doubt, for two huge arcuatae are filled around the lateral fornix. The dense network at the medial lower calyces is difficult to distinguish. Furthermore, there is a small extravasation, possibly a small arcuata, around the lowest fornix of the cranial pole.

The next exposure, taken about five minutes after the first, disclosed an incomplete filling of the renal pelvis and no longer showed the extravasation, proving how transient those shadows are. The remnants of the first filling

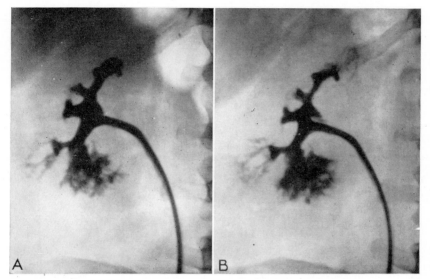

Fig. 48.   Extensive sinovenous ingression. In *A* filling of venae interlobares, arcuatae and interlobulares. After renal pelvis was drained out and ingressed contrast medium had disappeared, several refillings were performed. Each time the same picture resulted (exposure *B*) proof for the established lesion at the fornices and venous system. (From Narath, Renal Pelvis and Ureter, New York, Grune & Stratton, 1951.)

were drained out completely and a new filling begun until the patient complained of pressure in his kidney region (Fig. 48, *B*). The result resembles the first one to such an extent that one can almost superimpose these films. The filling degree of the pelvis is about the same; the extravasation is somewhat more severe. In addition, a new rupture has occurred at the cranial pole, where a new arcuata appears.

Rupture of a fornix during the course of retrograde pyelography is an accident which happens not infrequently. These accidents occur whether the gravity or the syringe method is used. I have attempted to produce sinovenous ingression at will. Of this series three cases are reproduced.

Figure 49 shows in *A* a distinctly overdistended renal pelvis and its calyces. A small extravasation of contrast medium is present at the medial fornix of the caudal pole. Were we in possession of this pyelogram alone, we should certainly not be able to state whether we are dealing with a pyelosinous transflow (absorption), or with a rupture of the fornix, though the course of the extravasation might be suspect of injury, since the beginning of an arcuata in indicated.

After sudden increased filling exposure *B* was taken. No question can exist concerning the character of these extravasations, for here a definite break is visible with a further injury to the plexus venosus. Not a single fornix has been spared from rupture. This is the more surprising, since the filling and expansion of the pelvis and calyces is not greater than in pyelogram Figure 49, *A*. This may be explained in the following manner: The degree

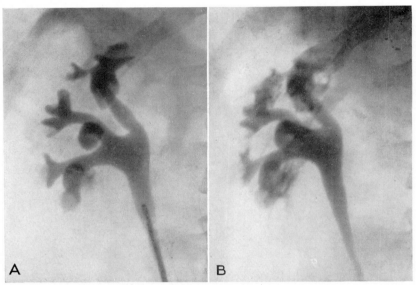

Fig. 49.   Sinovenous ingression. Experimentally produced in the living human. (From Narath, Renal Pelvis and Ureter, New York, Grune & Stratton, 1951.)

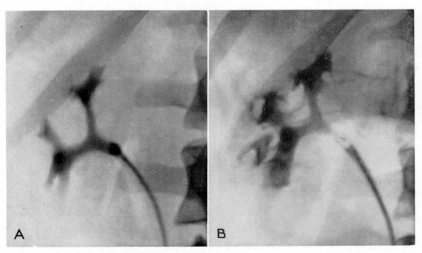

Fig. 50.   Sinovenous ingression experimentally produced in the living human. Venae interlobares, arcuatae and interlobulares are filled. Also sinolymphatic absorption takes place. (From Narath, Renal Pelvis and Ureter, New York, Grune & Stratton, 1951.)

of filling was greater before the exposure was taken and as a result of the escape of the contrast medium into the sinus renalis and venous system some excess pressure has been released. The streaks running from the caudal pole represent filled lymphatics. Their course is steeply cranial.

Figure 50 is the pyelogram of a patient who suffered from repeated colics due to a small calculus. The calculus is visible in *A*, just at the tip of the catheter at the ureteropelvic junction. The pelvis is filled to capacity, probably with slight overdistention, but no extravasation is found.

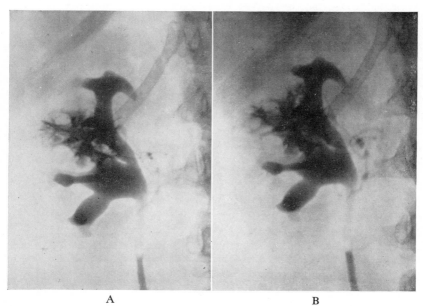

A B

Fig. 51. Sinovenous ingression experimentally produced. Technique different than in previous pictures. See text. Also sinolymphatic absorption present, which increases in exposure *B* under constant excess pressure. (From Narath, Renal Pelvis and Ureter, New York, Grune & Stratton, 1951.)

In Figure 50, *B* more contrast medium has been injected suddenly. The calculus has been pressed into the lower calyx major. Renal pelvis and calyces are overdistended. Extravasations are visible around the fornices of all calyces and at several places the venous system has been ingressed. Venae interlobares and arcuatae are filled, two of them completely, many in their basal branches. A few venae interlobulares are also demonstrated.

Simultaneously, lymphatic absorption starts from the deposit in the sinus renalis—proof of how fast this process develops. Three or four main lymphatics are carrying the contrast medium toward the spine, communicating with each other and filling a heavy branch which runs parallel to the spine toward the ductus thoracicus.

The two pyelograms in Figure 51 were obtained by a technique different from that used in Figures 49 and 50. The object was to create a sinovenous ingression at the onset, to enlarge the ingression by uninterrupted pressure and to take the second exposure after a short interval.

In *A* a huge extravasation is visible in the central section of the kidney. Whether the rupture occurred at the lowest fornix of the upper section of the pelvis or at the cranial fornix of the caudal section cannot be stated with certainty. Several arcuatae are filled, as are venae interlobulares. From the sinus renalis deposit a sinolymphatic absorption is under way. The injection was kept up slowly but constantly and about two minutes after the first, exposure film 51, *B* was taken. The pyelogram corresponds essentially with the first one, but the extravasation has gained in magnitude and the lymphatic absorption is distinctly more extensive. Not only do the lymphatics show a more complete filling, but the glands, already seen in the first exposure, appear larger in size owing to greater storage of contrast medium.

The various forms of extravasation have their anatomic characteristics and can hardly be confused as long as these pictures are not blurred by overlapping shadows or unfavorable projection. The combination of the various forms of physiologic and traumatic extravasations which lead to absorption are indicated in the accompanying diagram.

Forms of physiologic and traumatic extravasation.

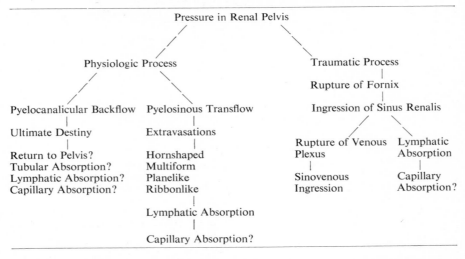

Absorption in the upper urinary tract, I believe, is of greater significance and importance than is realized today.

REFERENCES

BAKER, E. C. and LEWIS, J. S.: Comparison of the urinary tract in pregnancy and pelvic tumors. J.A.M.A., *104*:812–815, 1935.
BEAUFOND, F. H. DE and PORCHER, P.: L'exploration fonctionelle du canal excréteur du rein. Arch. mal. reins & org., genitourin., *3*:27–56, 1927.
BOEMINGHAUS, H.: Röntgenologische Untersuchungen über die Resorption schattengebender Lösungen in verschiedenen Hohlorganen, insbesondere in Niere, Nierenbecken und Ureter bei akuten Stauungszuständen. Arch. klin. Chir., *155*:451–468, 1929.
BRUNI, P.: Eccezionale reperto ottenuto con la pielographia retrograda. (Urografia da eliminazione destra con la pyelographia retrograda sinistra). La Riforma Medica, *50*: 1886–1887, 1934.

DUVERGEY, H.: Dilatations pyelo-urétérales d'origine dynamique. Bordeaux, Delma, 1937.

EHLERT, C. D.: Urologic manifestations of appendicitis. J. Urol., *43:*468–475, 1940.

ENGELMANN, TH. W.: Zur Physiologie des Ureters. Archiv. f. d. ges. Physiol., *2:*243–293, 1869.

FUMAGALLI, Z. and MARCHESI, M.: Studio anatomico dell'apparato muscolare del calice renale. Arch. Ital. Urol., *21:*1–2–3, 1944.

GIGON, C.: Recherches sur l'ischurie;—physiologie pathologique. L'Union médicale; Series 1. *10:*8–83, 85–87, 93–94, 297–299, 301–302, 1856.

GOLDSTEIN, A. E.: A scientific study of the normal human ureter by fractional ureteropyelography. J. Urol., *6:*125–133, 1921.

GRÉGOIR, W.: Les troubles moteurs de l'arbre urinaire supérieur. Congrès Belge d'Urologie, May 28, 1951.

GROEDEL, F. M.: Lehrbuch und Atlas der Röntgendiagnostik in der inneren Medizin und ihren Grenzgebieten. Lehmann, 1934, ed. 5.

HAEBLER, HANS: Zur Funktion der Nierenkelche. Z. urol. Chir., *8:*315–16, 1921.

———: Zur Funktion der Nierenkelche. Z. Urol., *16:*145–150, 1922.

———: Über die nervöse Versorgung der Nierenkelche. Z. Urol., *16:*377–384, 1922.

HINMAN, F., and LEE-BROWN, R. K.: Pyelovenous back-flow: its relation to pelvic reabsorption, to hydronephrosis and to accidents of pyelography. J.A.M.A., *82:*609–613, 1924.

HUBER: Recherches physiologiques sur la résorption rénale. Arch. Physiol., *8:*140–533, 1895.

HUTTER, KARL: Zur Röntgendarstellung der Nierenhohlräume nebst Bemerkungen über die Lagebeziehung des Nierenbeckens zum Musculus psoas. Z. urol. Chir., *30:*256–63, 1930.

JARRE, H. A. and CUMMING, R. E.: Cinex-Camera studies of the urinary tract. A new method of functional investigation. J. Urol., *24:*423–431, 1930.

JONA, J. LEON: The kidney pelvis: its normal and pathological physiology. Proc. Roy. Soc. Med., *29:*623–628, 1936.

KRETSCHMER, H. L. and KANTER, A. E.: Effect of certain gynecologic lesions on the upper urinary tract. J.A.M.A., *109:*1097–1101, 1937.

LAPIDES, J.: The physiology of the intact human ureter. J. Urol., *59:*501–537, 1948.

LEWIS, E.: The pelvic ureter in women: Effects of gynaecological lesions. Brit. J. Urol., *11:*132, 1936.

VON LICHTENBERG, A.: Kidney and ureteral lesions secondary to adnexal disease. J. Urol., *24:* 1–29, 1930.

LOMON, and COMANDON: La cinématographie radiologique. J. de radiol., *8:*433–437, 1924.

MACHT, DAVID I.: Concerning the absorption of drugs and poisons from the ureter and pelvis of the kidney. J. Urol., *2:*481–485, 1918.

MAGOUN, JAMES A. H.: Absorption from the urinary tract. J. Urol., *10:*67–80, 1923.

MARION, G.: De la dilatation de l'uretère dans les hydronephroses. Proc. Congr. Franç. d'Urol., 614, 1938.

MIRABEAU: Die Beteiligung des Harnleiters und des Nierenbeckens an den Erkrankungen der weiblichen Genitalorgane. Verhandl. deutsche Ges. Urol. 3 Kongress, Wien. 1911, pp. 158–166.

NARATH, P. A.: The hydromechanics of the calyx renalis. J. Urol., *43:*145–176, 1940.

NARATH, P. A.: Renal Pelvis and Ureter. New York, Grune & Stratton, 1951.

PASCUAL, S.: La pieloscopia. Med. ibera., *21:*328–331, 1927.

PFEIFER, W.: Grundlagen der funktionellen urologischen Röntgendiagnostik. Stuttgart, Georg Thieme, 1949.

POIRIER, M. P.: Sur quelques phénomènes consécutifs aux injections urétérales. Séance et mem. Soc. de Biologie, *3:*585–587, 1891.

SCHMIDT, W.: Pyelographische Darstellung von Harnkanälchen. Fortschr. Gebiete Röntgenstrahlen, *36:*369–371, 1927.

SHELDON, F. B.: Filling the pelvis of the kidney under direct observation with the fluoroscope. Urol. & Cutan. Rev., *28:*300–301, 1924.

STUMPF, P.: Das röntgenographische Bewegungsbild und seine Anwendung. (Flächenkymographie und Kymoskopie). Leipzig, Thieme, 1931.

SSYSGANOW, A. N.: Über das Lymphsystem der Nieren und Nierenhüllen beim Menschen. Zeitschr. f. ges. Anatomie, *91:*771–831, 1930.

THELEN, A.: Die Pathologie des Harnleiters im Röntgenbild. Stuttgart, Georg Thieme, 1949.

TUFFIER, M.: Étude clinique et expérimentale sur l'hydronephrose. Ann. mal. org. gén.-urin., *12:*14–40, 1894.
WASSINK, W. F.: Over peristaltiek van het nierbekken. Nederl. Tijdschr. v. Geneesk., *65:* 29–31, 1921.
WELD, E. H.: Renal absorption with particular reference to pyelographic mediums. M. Clin. North America, *3:*713–31, 1919.
WOOD, A. H.: Unilateral renal chyluria. J. Urol., *21:*109–117, 1929.

CHAPTER 4

Physiology of the Prostate and Seminal Vesicles

CHARLES HUGGINS, M.D.

The prostatic glands and seminal vesicles are the largest accessory sex glands of the male and their function is dependent on the presence of adequate quantities of androgenic hormones in the organism. These accessory glands are not essential to life, nor indeed to fertilization. For at least two hundred years it has been known that mashed testis tissue could in some way fertilize ova; Spallanzani obtained fertile eggs by inserting testicular cells into the oviduct of hens. While the accessory glands are in a strict sense dispensable, they are essential to fertilization by physiologic means in mammals. Since the volume of fluid emerging from the vas deferens is so small in amount (less than 5 per cent of the volume of human semen) it would doubtless be lost in the cavernous recesses of the male and female unless it were diluted, and the diluents in mammals are the secretions of the accessory glands—the semen.

The *semen* has highly remarkable properties. It contains cells, of one type only, which are not capable of division. These cells possess 3 unusual properties; they can initiate a chain reaction in an ovum (fertilization); they are highly motile; they possess a relatively small intracellular nutritional reserve. The seminal plasma provides extracellular food stuffs for the sperm.

The prostate and seminal vesicles are strictly glands of external secretion; there is no convincing evidence that they themselves produce hormones. The secretions of these glands are quite bizarre from a chemical standpoint. The semen of man contains a number of biologically unusual substances, characterized by a high concentration of fructose, citric acid, free choline and choline esters, and a number of enzymes, including acid phosphatase. All of these substances arise from the prostate or seminal vesicle. The accessory glands do nothing by halves; the secretory components are highly bizarre and apt to be either large in quantity or not present.

THE FEMALE PROSTATE

Para-urethral glands homologous to the male prostate and with identical histological appearance occur in certain female creatures. In women Virchow observed small nodules in the proximal portion of the urethra, which sometimes contained concretions similar to the prostatic calculi of men. Most of

111

the observations concerning the para-urethral glands and the effects of hormones upon them have been made in the rat. The glands are located caudal to the bladder in a position similar to the ventral prostate of the male; they are pale pink in color, contain a watery secretion, and the weight may reach 70 mg. The incidence of prostate glands in females is affected by genetic influences; in some strains of rats the incidence was 93 per cent while in other strains no vestiges or rudiments were discernible. In the gross the prostate of females is visible normally only in early life and in the last third of pregnancy, as well as in the first two weeks of subsequent lactation; however, in the multimammate mouse, Mastomys, a large prostate is present in all normal females and hypertrophies during the luteal phase of estrus. In one strain, primordia of the prostate were first observed in both males and females at $19\frac{1}{3}$ days of fetal life; ten days after delivery the ducts and lobules showed lumen formation and on the twenty-fifth day most of the acinar cells showed evidence of secretion, while between thirty and forty days evidence of involution occurred; the gland persisted for the whole lifetime of the rat but continued to show this involuted appearance.

The female prostate is stimulated by androgens and depressed by estrogens and castration. Korenchevsky and Dennison found a greater incidence of prostates with larger size in females injected with androgen than in uninjected controls, and testosterone caused the formation of the prostate in ovariectomized rats; dorsolateral prostates and coagulating glands can be induced in females with sufficiently large dosages of this hormone. In a series of normal untreated virgin rats the incidence of prostate was 9.4 per cent, in rats injected with estrone 0 per cent, and in rats injected with testosterone propionate 58.3 per cent. The glands are atrophic in spayed females. Price transplanted female prostatic tissue into other young and old, castrate and intact rats; the development was mostly good in normal males and castrate females and was poor or absent in castrate males and normal females.

The rest of this section is concerned with the prostate gland of the male.

THE MALE PROSTATE

Two Functionally Different Prostates. For many years it has been known that coagulation resulted when prostatic fluid of the rat was mixed with the secretion of the seminal vesicle. Walker observed that only secretion from a specific region of the prostate, the anterior lobes (coagulating gland) could induce clotting, the middle and posterior lobes being inactive. The coagulating gland has a slightly different cytologic appearance from the other lobes although it has the same embryologic origin. This gland occurs in rat, guinea pig and monkey; cross-coagulation is possible between the seminal vesicle of one species and the anterior prostate of another and the fluids do not induce coagulation of blood. Citrate and oxalate do not inhibit seminal clotting. The coagulation is due to the enzyme, vesiculase. A coagulating gland has not been detected as yet in man.

The evidence that human prostatic tissue consists of at least two different physiologic types derives from knowledge about the occurrence of neoplasms and also from the response of the normal human prostate to estrogen.

Geraghty and Boyd (1912) observed that prostatic cancer usually arises in the posterior lobe of the prostate and our experience supports this opinion. We believe that benign neoplasms (prostatic hypertrophy) never involve the posterior lobe and that cancer seldom arises in the anterior region of the prostate. Huggins and Webster (1948) found that there was a sharp distinction between the anterior and posterior regions of the prostate (Fig. 52). When estrogen is administered to human males for 2 to 3 months this differentiation is easily made; the epithelium of the anterior region undergoes marked atrophy, whereas the posterior lobe is much less drastically affected.

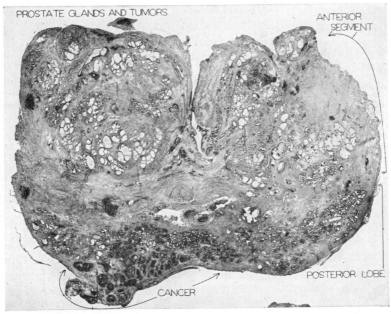

Fig. 52. Anatomical differentiation between anterior segment and posterior lobe of the human prostate. In this specimen the anterior segment is the site of spheroidal benign tumors (prostatic hypertrophy) while the posterior lobe has undergone malignant degeneration.

They concluded that these regions differ between themselves practically as much as stomach does from duodenum.

Investigative Techniques. The principal methods of investigation of prostatic function depend on determination of size of the gland, its cytology, and quantitative and qualitative studies of its secretion. The cytological evidence of secretion consists of light areas in the lumen region of the cell which appear in the rat at age 12 days and disappear in the adult within four days after castration; clearly this morphologic type of evidence is largely qualitative and inferential.

Prostatic transplants grow well in the anterior chamber of the eye and variations in size have been recorded by photography. The grafts decrease in size after orchiectomy and increase when androgen or gonadotrophic hormones are injected; continued injections of a single type of gonadotrophin (e.g., chorionic), however, do not lead to long-continued progressive increase of size, apparently because of immunity to the injected protein since later administration of another type of gonadotrophin, such as pregnant mare serum, causes an additional response.

Study of the secretion has provided quantitative data indicating more delicate changes in the prostate than the foregoing methods. The secretion may be studied directly or by indirect methods. Indirect methods concern measurement of acid phosphatase in the blood or urine; acid phosphatase values in serum are increased in certain patients with metastatic cancer of the prostate and serial study of this enzyme in clinical patients gave the first indication of the activity of hormones on disseminated human prostatic cancer. The urine of normal adult men contains 3- and 5-fold greater amounts of acid phosphatase than that of women or children and, remarkably, the daily amount of enzyme excreted in a single individual is nearly constant.

Direct studies of prostatic fluid have been made principally in man by massage of the prostate and collection of the secretion from the urethral meatus; surgical procedures have been used in the dog and the boar.

Eckhard first prepared a fistula of the prostate in the dog and discovered that stimulation of the *nervus erigens* caused abundant prostatic secretion; the dog has a well-developed prostate but no seminal vesicles. Farrell devised an operative method in 2 stages for the dog whereby many acute observations were made. At the first operation the bladder is separated from the prostate and an anastomosis is made between the bladder and penile sheath, followed later by establishing a urethral fistula in the perineum. Difficulties in the collection of fluid made chronic observations impossible in this otherwise ingenious technique. The first quantitative collections of prostatic fluid in the dog for long periods involved a new technique whereby the urine was deviated through a metallic cannula after isolation of the prostate from the bladder and a ventral slitting of the prepuce; the dogs survive for long periods in good condition and collection of prostatic fluid is easy and complete.

THE SECRETION OF PROSTATIC FLUID

The prostate excretes small amounts of fluid at frequent intervals (resting secretion) and the secretion is greatly augmented by parasympathetic stimulants (stimulated secretion); resting secretion is discharged usually from the urethra in the urine. Judging from the daily amount of acid phosphatase excreted in the urine, average 613 units per day, the amount of prostatic fluid secreted by man is in the order of 0.5 to 2 cc. per day. In the dog resting secretion is about 0.1 to 2 cc. per hour; after the urine has been deviated by the prostatic isolation operation the "tree reflex" is well preserved and dogs approach the legs of laboratory tables and void prostatic fluid at frequent intervals.

Prostatic secretion is primarily a function of androgenic activity, and secondarily of chemical and nervous stimulation; rises of acid phosphatase in the urine occur after sexual stimulation in man. In dogs frequently a steady output occurs for months while less commonly a plateau of secretory activity is interrupted by high peaks. Normal dogs may secrete as much as 4 times the weight of the prostate in one hour, but very large glands in spontaneous cystic hyperplasia do not give correspondingly large amounts of secretion, although the cysts communicate with the ducts; for example, a dog whose hypertrophied prostate weighed 102 gm. secreted from 7 to 11 cc. whereas a young normal adult of the same body weight secreted 24 to 38 cc., the prostate weighing 10.8 gm.

Pilocarpine hydrochloride, 6 mg. intramuscularly, provides a good output of secretion in normal dogs, usually without accompanying emesis and about 95 per cent of the secretion occurs in the first hour after injection. Increase of the amount of pilocarpine increases the secretion but not in a simple linear relationship and the gland does not become refractory to pilocarpine, although some signs of "prostatic fatigue" are seen after repeated stimulations in a very short time.

It was claimed that occlusion of the outflow of prostatic secretion caused atrophy of the gland but the experimental technique was defective; plugging the ducts with a transplant of muscle did not lead to prostatic atrophy in dogs injected with androgen.

Starvation of dogs injected with androgen for three weeks led to an increased secretion of prostatic fluid and definite growth of the prostate; Pazos observed further that the composition of the secretion was not disturbed by inanition.

Effect of Nerve Stimulation and Drugs on Prostatic Secretion. There is no secretion from immature or castrate dogs. The secretory pressure of the adult canine prostate has been found to be 16 to 18, and 17 to 26 mm., of mercury respectively. Stimulation of the hypogastric nerves and the *nervi erigentes* induces prostatic secretion. Faradic stimulation of the hypogastric nerves produced either large or small secretion in the dog. In man stimulation of this nerve causes ejaculation of semen.

Parasympathetic stimulating drugs greatly augment prostatic secretion. Epinephrine, nicotine and acetylcholine cause a slight increase of secretion, and pilocarpine a great increase; atropine antagonizes pilocarpine stimulation and results in cessation of secretion.

Strips of the normal prostate gland exhibit no rhythmic contractions but these occur in the prostate of castrate rats and the administration of androgen to the castrate reduced the spontaneous contractions. Epinephrine and barium chloride produced an increase of tone in prostatic strips while in most species pilocarpine added to the testing bath was without effect; in the rabbit, however, pilocarpine produced increases of tone and rhythmic activity not detected in other animals except in the prostate of castrate rats.

Pharmacodynamic Effects of Prostatic Secretion. The intravenous injection of semen is always followed by a rapid fall of blood pressure. Prostatic fluid and extracts of the prostate gland have powerful biodynamic actions. Prostatic extracts of the dog and bull when injected in the rabbit cause a pressor effect followed by a marked lowering of blood pressure, intravascular clotting and death. The pressor effect is probably due to epinephrine since this substance has been demonstrated in the prostate in considerable amounts. Euler has studied the vasodepressor substance, prostaglandin, occurring in extracts of the prostate and in prostatic fluid obtained at autopsy from man; the substance has acid properties, is dialyzable and soluble in water and alcohol; it lowers the blood pressure and increases intestinal motility in the atropinized rabbit and dilates the vessels of the hind limbs of the frog; larger quantities were found in the prostate of the adult than in children. Another highly active substance, *vesiglandin,* was found in the prostate of the monkey; this lowered the blood pressure but had no, or only a weak, effect on isolated intestine. These agents which produce vasodilatation and strong contraction of smooth muscle occur in the prostate and seminal vesicle in larger amounts than in many other organs and are assumed by Euler to function in the emptying of these glands. The prostate of the sheep contains the same amounts of vasodepressor and smooth muscle relaxing substance as human prostate; the content of organs such as liver, testis and muscle was less than 1 per cent of the prostate. The lowered blood pressure following intravenous injection is abolished by exclusion of the liver from the circulation.

The Composition of Prostatic Secretion. The chemical composition of prostatic fluid is remarkable from the standpoints of inorganic, organic and enzyme chemistry. All of the data for human prostatic fluid relate to resting secretion obtained following prostatic massage; amounts of fluid obtained are usually less than 1 cc. so that complete analyses cannot be made on a single sample and it occasionally is contaminated with fluid from the seminal vesicle or ejaculatory ducts. Quantitative data for dog prostatic fluid are more exact since technical difficulties are less. Compared with stimulated secretion, the resting secretion of dogs is more turbid, more alkaline and contains less chloride; observed values, pH 6.6, chloride 104 m. eq. per liter.

Inorganic. The prostatic secretion is more acid than plasma. Stimulated dog prostatic fluid approximates 0.16 normal $NaCl$. Human prostatic fluid contains considerably larger amounts of sodium, potassium and calcium than plasma; on the other hand, there are deficient quantities of inorganic anions with low levels of chloride, bicarbonate and phosphate. Other anions, namely, the amino acids (20 mg. per cent), proteins—peptones and proteoses, and citrate balance the cations inadequately for the observed pH of 6.45.

Organic. Most of the proteins of human prostatic fluid are derived proteins which are not coagulated by heat and pass readily through semipermeable membranes—proteoses. The content of glucose in prostatic fluid is exceedingly low. Scherstén and others found that human prostatic fluid is rich in citrate. No doubt citric acid is a factor in the accumulation of calcium, since other fluids rich in calcium salts (e.g., milk and urine) are rich in citrate, and citrate also functions in preventing the precipitation of calcium salts; however, precipitations of calcium phosphate (apatite) and cholesterol in the form of calculi often occur. Even in young men such apatite deposition occurs in the "corpora amylacea." The spermine content of human prostate is remarkably high (0.1 gm. per 100 gm. of fresh tissue) and probably most of the spermine of semen is derived from this organ; this base does not activate spermatozoa.

Enzymes. a. PHOSPHATASE. Kutscher and Wolbergs discovered that acid phosphatase is present in prostate gland and prostatic fluid in very large amount. This enzyme is a chemical secondary sex characteristic. Gutman and Gutman observed small amounts in infancy, increasing during puberty to high values in the adult. Traces in the prostate of immature monkeys became greatly augmented by androgen administration. No function for this remarkable enzyme has been discovered.

b. FIBRINOLYSIN. Proteolytic enzymes were discovered in prostatic fluid in a study of liquefaction of human semen when it was found that these fluids rapidly liquefied clotted blood and fibrin. Human semen contains fibrinolysin derived in large amount from the prostate gland. This enzyme, a physiological constituent of the prostate of man, resembles closely streptococcal fibrinolysin, and it is found that the blood of men resistant to this enzyme is easily lyzed by prostatic fibrinolysin—an immunologic difference; both streptococcal and prostatic fibrinolysins are inhibited by crystalline trypsin inhibitor.

c. FIBRINOGENASE. It was observed that the prostatic fluid of the dog destroyed fibrinogen more readily than fibrin, the activity being attributed to fibrinogenase. Both fibrinolysin and fibrinogenase are chemical activities as yet unidentified as chemical entities. Both human and dog prostatic fluids contain these activities but in different concentration. Human semen contains much fibrinolysin and little fibrinogenase; dog semen contains little fibrinolysin, much fibrinogenase. The fibrinogen of man in certain disease states is not destroyed by dog fibrinogenase. These agents may be maintained for years in refrigerated prostatic fluid.

d. MISCELLANEOUS. The prostatic secretion of normal dogs clots oxalated or heparinized rabbit and beef plasmas (these fluids are resistant to the activity of fibrinogenase) but does not clot fibrinogen alone; human prostatic fluid ranges from 0.1 to 1.1 units. Thromboplastin is present in prostatic fluid as in the juice of many other tissues.

The prostate gland and fluid of the dog have been reported to contain amylase. We have confirmed this observation but found it to be inconstant. A germicidal power in dog prostatic fluid has been described against B. coli, S. aureus and streptococci; neither complement nor lysozyme was demonstrated. Camus and Gley found that the prostatic fluid of the guinea pig contains an enzyme, *vesiculase,* which coagulates the seminal vesicle secretion but does not clot blood or milk. Diamino oxidase is present in considerable quantity but is less concentrated in prostatic tissue than in semen.

Drugs. Alcohol is excreted in dog prostatic fluid (90-594 mg. per cent) after ethyl alcohol administration; sulfonamides likewise are excreted.

Lipids of the Prostate. Thompson described the laminated corpora amylacea normally found in the prostate of adult man and monkey (and only in these species) and described yellowish refractile bodies in prostatic fluid. Fürbringer discovered that the opalescence of prostatic fluid is due to fat droplets which he named "lecithin granules"; this lipid displays double refraction in polarized light. Lipids are easily demonstrated in the epithelial cells and their presence in prostatic fluid represents a true secretion. The cholesterol content of normal prostatic tissue (0.8 gm. per cent) is lower than that of prostatic adenomas (1.10 gm.).

William W. Scott found an average total lipid content of human prostatic fluid of 286 mg. per cent, approximately half the concentration found in human plasma. Total phospholipids constituted over 60 per cent of the total lipid value. The moist-ether soluble phospholipid consisted of cephalin. Lecithin was not demonstrable indicating that the term "lecithin bodies" is not applicable to the fat bodies found in prostatic fluid. His values for total cholesterol in prostatic fluid ranged from 62 to 105 mg. per cent, considerably lower than the range of 86 to 618 mg. per cent reported by R. A. Moore. These analyses indicate that there is little if any neutral fat

Table 4. Chemical Composition of Fractions of the Ejaculate

(Fructose arises chiefly from seminal vesicle; the other components are excreted chiefly or exclusively by the prostate)

COMPONENT	FRACTION OF EJACULATE	
	First	Last
Citrate, mg. per cent (Schersténg, 1936)	770	120
Calcium, mg. per cent (Schersténg, 1936)	52	20
Acid phosphatase units, 1 cc. (Gutman and Gutman, 1941)	2760	300
Fructose, mg. per cent (MacLeod and Hotchkiss, 1942)	157	377
Fibrinolysin, minutes per test (Huggins and McDonald, 1946)	120	288

in prostatic fluid, the phospholipids and cholesterol accounting for almost all the total lipid found. Microscopic examination of prostatic fluid from normal men reveals lipids in gross aggregates while the lipids of plasma are of colloidal particulate size or are in solution. In certain prostatic inflammatory states much or all of the lipid is found in macrophages (colostrum corpuscles) in the prostatic secretion.

Time of Emptying of the Prostate During Ejaculation. In man it is known that the prostate discharges most of its secretion before the seminal vesicle in, roughly, a one-two relationship during ejaculation. The evidence is chemical in nature obtained on ejaculates fractionated according to time of delivery from the urethra (Table 4).

Relation of Hormones to Prostatic Secretion. When orchiectomy is done in dogs, a measurable decrease of secretion is observed within twenty-four hours and prostatic secretion ceases seven to twenty-three days after castration. Usually orchiectomy is followed by prompt cellular regression of the prostate, changes in the cytology of the rat being observed promptly. There is loss of the light areas within four days and then progressive reduction in epithelial height, nuclear size and acinous diameter, the epithelium becoming pseudostratified and the nuclei pycnotic. Exceptions to this rapid involution after castration were noted in benign hypertrophy in man where decreases in height of the epithelial cells were not marked at 29 days but were severe at 93 days. Also, in the guinea pig involutionary changes develop slowly after castration. Development and maintenance of well-differentiated epithelium occur in the prostate of rats and mice castrated at 1 to 3 weeks of age (the Price effect) and is apparently associated with the secretion of androgen by the X-zone in the adrenal cortex since adrenalectomy reduces the prostatic weight; the anomaly disappears spontaneously about day 40.

Testosterone propionate, 10 mg. daily in sesame oil, gives measurable prostatic secretion in immature dogs after 3 to 7 injections, and there is a steadily rising secretory curve for at least five months; in hypogonadism in the male androgens initiate and increase prostatic secretion but when administered to normal man testosterone had little effect on the seminal output. There is further evidence that androgen is less effective in intact males than in castrates; the daily administration of 0.1 to 0.5 mg. of testosterone propionate per kilogram to rabbits with intraocular prostatic transplants produced an increase of area of the graft for two weeks followed by a stillstand or regression; the same treatment in castrate rabbits produced a continuous increase for at least three months.

Burkhart studied the effects of androgen on the prostate by the colchicine technique; the male hormone effects an increase of mass of the prostatic epithelial cell followed by cell division. A single dose of testosterone propionate, 0.1 mg., in a castrate rat weighing about 170 gm. causes an increase of cell volume of the epithelium of the ventral prostate detectable 23 hours after injection followed by mitotic division at 35 hours; the effects of androgen are evident for two and one-half days after this single injection when the cells revert to a castrate condition.

Soon after the introduction of crystalline androgens it was found that the characteristic cytologic effects of androgen on the prostatic epithelium could be abolished under certain conditions by simultaneous administration of estrogenic hormones in the mouse, rat and monkey. Also with respect to the prostatic secretion estrogen is able to nullify the effect of androgen; the dosage of estrogen has been determined whereby the rising curve of prostatic secretion induced by injected androgen is converted to a plateau (neutralization), and larger doses completely vitiate the secretory effects of androgen. By this type of biological "titration" it was found that daily injections of diethylstilbestrol, 0.4 mg., neutralized testosterone propionate, 10 mg., similarly administered (a ratio of 1:25) and larger doses of this estrogen caused a cessation of secretion. When estrogen is administered to a castrate or immature dog, the acinar elements remain uninvolved while in the ducts, the lining of the posterior urethra and the utriculus, columnar epithelium is replaced by stratified squamous cells; when the acini are luminated (action of androgen) this epithelium also becomes squamous and stratified. The metaplasia is reversible by androgenic treatment. Involvement of the utriculus with squamous cells is the first cytologic sign in the dog of estrogen dominance.

The prostate gland in late fetal life and in newborn boys usually is the site of epithelial metaplasia in the utriculus and the collecting ducts; this was attributed for theoretical reasons to penetration of hormones from the mother through the placenta. The metaplasia is due to estrogen. Burrows produced these changes by injecting estrogen in adult mice and restitution to the normal state followed a cessation of estrin. Estrogen administered to infants maintained these changes for seven months—an age when the prostate in normal babies would have resumed the customary inactive appearance.

In the intact mouse, dog and monkey, administration of estrogen for long periods leads to urinary retention with uremia and death of the animal; the posterior lobe of the prostate and the utriculus become enormously distended with retained secretion. In the rat and monkey male hormone administered with estrone completely prevented the pathological changes in the prostate. Since the introduction of anti-androgenic methods of treatment of cancer of the prostate by Huggins and Hodges considerable number of men have been treated with large doses of estrogen for prolonged periods without "estrogenic urinary retention"; man is, apparently, the only mammal in which this phenomenon does not occur. Estrogen increases growth of muscle and connective tissue of the prostate.

Sharp decreases in prostatic secretion in the dog follow within one day after injection of an adequate amount of estrogen which, when maintained, leads to cessation of secretion in about ten days; desoxycorticosterone acetate causes only a slight secretory depression. The responses of the prostate to both androgenic and estrogenic stimulation appear to be unaffected by section of the hypogastric and sacral nerves.

Androgen Threshold of the Prostate. The prostate has a lower threshold to androgens than the seminal vesicle. Working with crude extracts Moore and Gallagher found that about 3 times as much androgen was required to show effects in the seminal vesicle as in the prostate. This has been confirmed with pure androgens. In the administration of estrogen to man it was found that the amount of seminal vesicle secretion in the ejaculate decreases more rapidly than the prostatic secretion; the ejaculate becomes less solid, liquefies more quickly and the concentration of glucose decreases more rapidly than fibrinolysin. There is a differential reaction of the prostatic lobes in the rat to androgen withdrawal. On the tenth day after castration involutionary changes were first detected cytologically in the anterior lobe (coagulating gland) although they had been noticed on the fifth day in the other prostatic lobes.

THE SEMINAL VESICLE

The seminal vesicle is a cul-de-sac which is strangely immune from infections despite the fact that the neighboring prostate is frequently the site of severe acute and chronic infection. An empyema of the seminal vesicle rarely is observed in clinical practise.

Spermatozoa are not found in the seminal vesicles of laboratory animals and it is believed that they rarely enter the human seminal vesicle. The most interesting components of the secretion of the seminal vesicle in man are choline esters and fructose.

Huggins and Johnson (1933) found that spermatocele fluids, although containing spermatozoa, uniformly were characterized by the absence of sugars. On the other hand, the human semen contained large amounts of reducing sugars. Vasectomy did not lower the sugar concentration. The prostate gland contained almost no sugar while the seminal vesicle fluid was rich in carbohydrate. These workers found that the sugar was fermentable by yeast and they reached the erroneous conclusion that the carbohydrate was glucose.

In 1945 the seminal sugar was purified and identified by Dr. Thaddeus Mann as D (—) fructose. This brilliant research was based on: (a) the preparation of crystalline methylphenylfructosazone, which is one of the few chemical reactions by means of which fructose can certainly be distinguished from glucose; (b) the purification of seminal fructose until it reached the same specific optical activity as pure crystalline fructose: $[\alpha] \ 20° = -92.2°$;
$$D$$
(c) the demonstration that fructose occurs in the semen in free form and that it accounts for the whole of the yeast-fermentable carbohydrate which yields the Seliwanoff reaction; (d) proof, obtained through the use of a highly specific enzyme, glucose oxidase, that in normal semen glucose is present only in traces or is entirely absent. There is no fructose in either the testes or the epididymal sperm. Thus at their site of origin the spermatozoa, still immotile, have no fructose at their disposal. At the moment of ejaculation the spermatozoa come in contact with fructose-rich secretions at a time when they become highly motile and so require a source of energy.

Human seminal plasma is distinguished by a high content of choline and also of phosphorus compounds. The concentration of inorganic phosphate ions rapidly increases after ejaculation. Dr. Frank Lundquist (1946, 1947) has investigated the nature of phosphorus compounds in semen using simple but effective techniques; the choline and phosphorus content of normal semen at room temperature was compared with semen collected in ice-cold trichloracetic acid and also by immediate freezing alone. There was 21.6 mg. per cent inorganic P in human semen frozen to $-10°C$ immediately after ejaculation but 64.2 mg. per cent after 20 minutes incubation at $+20°C$. The rise of inorganic P in semen, according to Lundquist, arises from the dephosphorylation of phosphorylcholine in human seminal plasma by the acid phosphatase of the prostatic secretion. All of the evidence suggests that phosphorylcholine arises in the human seminal vesicle. The secretion of the human seminal vesicle is rich in protein (about 9 gm. per cent).

The semen of man is delivered to the exterior in liquid form but within one minute it sets in a solid gel. Soon after coagulation the semen commences to liquefy and within ten minutes about 90 per cent of the gel has liquefied; the smaller remaining gel component requires about one hour. The mechanism of coagulation is still obscure but the events of liquefaction are understood. Huggins and Neal (1941) showed that the proteolytic enzyme concerned with liquefaction is present in the prostatic secretion. These observers mixed human semen (or prostatic secretion itself) with blood or plasma which was induced to clot and found that the blood coagulum so induced, liquefied within a matter of minutes. Because of the similarity of the proteolytic enzyme of the prostatic fluid with that discovered earlier in hemolytic streptococci by Tillett and Garner (1933) the enzyme was named fibrinolysin. It is recognized that there are both similarities to, and differences with, the streptococcal kinase.

These remarks are based on the work of many investigators and are necessarily brief. For a fuller treatment of the physiology of the prostate and seminal vesicles the reader is referred to: Mann, T. and Lutwak-Mann, C.: Secretory function of male accessory organs of reproduction mammals, Physiological Reviews, *31:*27–55, 1951, and to Huggins, C.: The prostatic secretion, The Harvey Lectures, *52:*148–193, 1946–47. Full documentation to the many references made in this paper and acknowledgment of the work of other scientists are contained in these reviews.

CHAPTER 5

Physiology of the Testis and Scrotum*

CARL R. MOORE, PH.D.

The testicle is the basic element of the male reproductive system in all vertebrates, and is closely integrated with a group of accessory reproductive organs, the size and character of which varies greatly as evolution has advanced. The scrotum, on the other hand, is an organ restricted to mammalian species; it is only temporarily apparent during the breeding season in some lower mammals but exists as a permanent structure in man and higher mammals. Whales, elephants, seals and a few others lack a scrotum, and testes remain in the abdomen as in all vertebrates below the mammals. Stages in the evolution of the scrotum involve (1) mere apposition of the testicles against a thin area on the lower abdominal wall during the breeding season (some insectivores, bats), (2) a temporary bilateral pouch into which the testicles descend during the breeding season and reascend into the abdomen during reproductive quiescence, with obliteration of an evident scrotum (wild rodents), (3) a permanent scrotum containing the testicles but with open inguinal canals that permit temporary retraction of these organs into the abdomen (rats, rabbits, guinea pigs), and (4) the permanent scrotum containing testicles incapable of being retracted into the abdomen on account of closure of the inguinal canals.

Prior to 1921 the significance of the scrotum was unknown but it is now recognized as a functional organ. It serves to regulate the environmental temperature about the testis, and in mammals spermatogenesis cannot proceed to formation of spermatozoa when testicles are subjected to the higher temperatures of the abdomen. Testicles of birds are not so sensitive to the higher body temperatures—a fact that has thus far received inadequate interpretation.

Testicular function readily falls into two principal categories, (1) germ cell production, and (2) hormone secretion. For convenience these two functions may be discussed separately.

I. SPERMATOGENESIS

The production of spermatozoa in mammals exhibits two extremes of activity—a short annual period followed by lack of spermatogenesis, and continuous activity throughout the year. Such wild rodents as the midwestern ground squirrel (Citellus tridecemlineatus) reveal active spermatogene-

* Personal researches mentioned have been greatly aided by grants from the Dr. Wallace C. and Clara A. Abbott Memorial Fund of the University of Chicago.

123

sis in January, quantities of spermatozoa by February–March, and a breeding period during April or May (Wells, 1935). In mid-June testis involution is under way; spermatozoa disappear and the testes reascend into the abdomen and remain inactive for some months. Reduction in size to a seasonal low occurs in July when testes have a fresh weight of approximately 10 per cent of the spring maximum. Spermatozoa are absent from June to February. In the bat (Courrier, 1927) early stages in spermatogenesis are present in June, and all seasonal sperm have been formed by late August. Although the testes undergo regression, the epididymis remains engorged with spermatozoa over the mating season (September) and throughout the winter. The involuted testis begins another season of spermatogenetic activity in May–June and again produces sperm for the breeding season. Similar periodicity in testicular function is characteristic of the male hedgehog, marmot, polecat, weasel, martin, deer, etc., although different species may experience their peak of spermatogenetic activity at different periods in the year.

The onset of spermatogenesis in continuous breeding mammals, such as man, cat, dog, pig, rat, mouse, rabbit, guinea pig, hamster, carry on continuous spermatogenetic activity with spermatozoa present during all months of the year. The period after birth at which mature germ cells first appear is quite variable. In general, the lower, seasonal reproducing animals become sexually mature during the first year of life, and the hamster may sire offspring prior to the fiftieth day after birth. Mature spermatozoa are produced at approximately sixty days after birth in the rat, ninety days in guinea pigs, but in man not until approximately the twelfth to fourteeth year of life. It has been stated that in cases of human *pubertas praecox* sperm may be present as early as the third or fourth year, but others hold doubts on account of the inability to advance the first appearance of spermatozoa by experimental means in continuous breeding animals such as the rat or monkey.

The onset of spermatogenesis in continuous breeding mammals introduces a continuous function of the testicle that is usually terminated only on death unless extraneous factors intervene. General health, states of nutrition, some endocrine disorders, and other unknown conditions may reduce or abolish spermatogenesis, but even in man satisfactory evidence has not been produced to show that age alone is a causative factor in spermatogenetic failure.

Thus Engle reports personal observations on the testes of 16 men past the age of 70 years in which more than one half were producing spermatozoa. He cites the report of Exner on a large series of testicles that among men of 80 to 90 years, 48 per cent were producing spermatozoa. This, naturally, does not imply that the quantity or quality of the sperm cells produced is equivalent to those produced at an earlier age. In many respects, the function of spermatogenesis appears to be a delicate one, subject to modification by many conditions, known and unknown. Sand and Okkels, by virtue of the Danish sterilization act of 1929 and 1935 and the collection of testicles immediately after sudden death from accident, suicide, or other causes not entailing long illness or obvious general pathology, were able to study histological sections on well-fixed materials from 72 individuals. Among the testicles of this group, 65 of which were obtained from men in the 30 to 40 year old group, only 17 (24 per cent) revealed a testicle of the classical textbook normal type, in which closely packed seminiferous tubules contained a full germinal epithelium, and intertubular (interstitial cell) areas were of small proportions. In approximately 50 per cent of the testicles, the intertubular areas were edematous or atypical; in 55 of the 72 organs a thickened capsule surrounded some of the seminiferous tubules; 24 of the 72 revealed grave destruction of the tubular epithelium. These findings of areas of fibrosis, hyalinization, apparent interstitial cell hyperplasia, cytolysis, edema and other atypical conditions in this 30 to 40 year old group of testes undoubtedly provided a register of previous but unknown conditions that exerted well registered influences in the absence of frank chronic illness.

The testicle is not a self-regulating organ and its function is dependent to a large extent upon general bodily conditions; it is subjected directly or indirectly to many internal physiological influences such as disordered metabolism or general deranged functions, and only within certain limits of so-called normality can its functions be carried out. One recognized influence is the activity of the organs of internal secretions, chief among which, in this respect, is the pituitary body.

The role of pituitary secretions in the function of spermatogenesis has been clearly established through the experiments of Smith when he revolutionized the operation for hypophysectomy in the rat. The removal of the pituitary gland, or its anterior lobe, from an adult breeding male is followed within a few days by loss of spermatozoa, spermatids, and some spermatocytes. Recovery of spermatogenetic function never occurs except by administration of gonadal stimulating substances. Ground, fresh, pituitary tissue repeatedly implanted in hypophysectomized males will prevent testicular degeneration, or will re-establish complete spermatogenesis after degeneration has occurred. Extracts of the gonadotrophic hormone from the anterior pituitary will effectively maintain spermatogenetic function. Removal of the pituitary from prepuberal males effectively prevents the onset of spermatogenesis, but proper treatments will induce formation of spermatozoa. Deficiencies in hypophyseal function in the intact animal, therefore, may express themselves in incomplete testicular function.

Involution of the testicle in seasonal breeding mammals is associated with a decline in pituitary secretions (Wells, 1938). Testicles which are inactive during the nonbreeding season can be stimulated to increased size and full spermatogenetic function by the introduction into the animal of fresh pituitary substance or suitable extracts. The phenomenon of a restricted annual spermatogenesis, therefore, rests upon the general physiological state of the organism, rather than upon the testicle alone, and a chief role in this regulation must be attributed to the activities of the pituitary gland.

Certain environmental influences, especially the relative length of day to night, have been shown to exert a marked control over the function of the pituitary, and thus over the spermatogenetic function. The addition of progressive short periods of artificial light, which gives a progressive increase in daily light periods, will thus lead to the establishment of full spermatogenetic function at wholly unusual periods in the annual breeding cycle. Testicles of the bird junco (Rowan, 1929), or duck (Benoit, 1936) can be caused to produce mature germ cells in mid-winter, rather than at the usual spring breeding season, and the periods of breeding in strictly seasonal reproducing mammals are subject to remarkable shifts. This influence of increased light operates through the eyes, upon the pituitary body, leading to increased secretion of gonadotrophic substances.

CRYPTORCHIDISM

Man, especially, and other mammals having closed inguinal canals occasionally experience unilateral or bilateral retention of the testicles within the abdomen. This naturally occurring cryptorchidism has long been known to involve an absence of spermatogenesis in the particular organ, and sterility in case of bilateral undescent. The cause of spermatogenetic failure revealed itself through a study of experimental cryptorchidism and other conditions to be mentioned.

When the testicle of an adult breeding guinea pig is removed from the scrotum and confined in the abdomen, with blood vessels, epididymis, and nerves intact, it reveals within five to seven days a severe derangement and dissolution of the germinal epithelium of all seminiferous tubules (Moore, 1924a). Cytolysis, cell fragmentation, and general derangement of the entire germinal epithelium are accompanied by the casting off of cells into the lumen, many being carried out into the epididymis; the formation of "giant cells," so characteristic of testicular degeneration, is prominent. Further progressive involution reduces the tubule to a basement membrane surrounding the Sertoli syncytium and a basal layer of Sertoli nuclei. The testicle becomes progressively smaller, diameters of seminiferous tubules are greatly reduced and the interstitial cells become more concentrated in the remaining intertubular spaces. No recovery in spermatogenetic function occurs as long as the testicle remains in the abdomen. The return of a testicle to the scrotum after a residence in the abdomen of three weeks, when a single layer of nuclei exists in the tubules, is followed by a resumption of spermatogenesis. Two months after scrotal placement will suffice for restoration of many normal tubules producing spermatozoa, but some tubules may fail to show recovery. Elevation of the testicles of newborn guinea pigs into the abdomen prevents the development of an active germinal epithelium and the organ remains essentially embryonic, but replacement in the scrotum three months later will be followed within a short period by development of tubules carrying on normal spermatogenesis.

Similar reactions follow the surgical removal of the normal testicle from the scrotum into the abdomen in rat, hamster, rabbit, dog, ram, and other mammals and thus is emphasized the importance of the scrotum for the process of spermatogenesis. A testicle may become so anchored in the inguinal canal that the lower portion projecting into the upper scrotum may show tubules producing spermatozoa whereas the upper part, more nearly in the abdomen, may have entirely inactive tubules.

These facts suggest the advisability of attempting to correct undescent in human cases but different opinions exist as to the most acceptable age for intervention. Delayed descent of one or both testes into the scrotum towards the approach of puberty is well known, as is the fact that not infrequently the increase of circulating male hormone encourages descent. Moderate increase of this hormone by short periods of administration of chemical androgens, or by treatments with gonadotrophic hormones to stimulate secretion by the intact testicles, while ineffectual in many cases in bringing down the testicle, has been considered advantageous in cases where surgery is required.

The results of treatment with orchidopexy are too frequently undetermined. The surgical report of Hansen may be cited, in which 30 men with bilateral cryptorchidism were treated with orchidopexy without the addition of hormones. In twenty-two cases bilateral orchidopexy was done, while eight cases were unilateral, with removal of the opposite testis or its placement in the abdomen. Age at operation ranged from 20 to 56 years. Later anatomical examination led to the characterization of 21 per cent of the 52 operated testes as normal in size and consistency. Examination of semen from 25 of the 30 operated patients revealed spermatozoa in the ejaculate in 11 cases, the oldest such patient having been operated in his fortieth year. Whereas numbers and quality of spermatozoa were not always up to a normal standard, it is to be remembered that for sperm cells to appear in the semen requires an unobstructed pathway through the rete, epididymis and ductus deferens; it is entirely probable that some cases of individuals operated upon regained spermatogenetic function without spermatozoa being delivered in a seminal discharge, and that in some testicles operated upon other pathology existed. Operation at earlier ages on uncomplicated cases of cryptorchidism would conceivably yield even better results.

TESTIS TRANSPLANTATION

It is a general biological principle that tissues of higher vertebrates can become successfully incorporated in a host only when the donor tissue comes from an animal of the same species; persistence is more probable the more closely related are host and donor, and auto-grafts provide the greatest chance for persistence. One may recall that specific types in human blood transfusions are required. During an earlier period, claims were made that higher ape testicle grafts into man were effective. Despite the alleged recovery of such grafts, six months after transplantation, that showed well-preserved testis tissue, the claim of effectiveness must still be discounted. Foreign body response to introduced strange tissues if often severe, and definite, and well circumscribed, inactive nodules may be present.

Grafts of testis tissue, transplanted from mice to rats, or the reverse, have been recovered up to a period of six months (Browman, 1937). Sections of such grafts demonstrated recognizable germinal epithelium in the tubules as well as the outlines of spermatozoa. However, such grafts were encapsulated by, and infiltrated with, calcium and phosphorus salts and upon removal could be pulverized by crushing; blood vessel invasion of the graft usually did not occur. The transplants into a host of foreign species had been so thoroughly walled off that autolysis did not occur, and visible outlines of tubules were therefore preserved. Careful tests with delicate hormone indicators in the host revealed that this type of graft was not secreting hormone. Calcification may at times be encountered in transplants of tissues between animals of the same species, and to a lesser extent when the same animal served as both donor and host (auto-transplantation). Attempts to break down this natural resistance to the implantation of foreign tissues by experimental means were not successful in the transplantation of testicular material.

Successfully incorporated testis transplants appear to be able to persist indefinitely, and under proper conditions can carry on complete testicular function; grafts of active tissue in the rat and guinea pig have been studied after persistence in the host organism for periods up to a year.

Prior to 1925, spermatozoon differentiation had never been obtained from a testis graft in a mammal. Grafts located in subcutaneous, intramuscular, or intraperitoneal positions, while showing at times well-preserved epididymis, interstitial tissue, and large areas of seminiferous tubules, most frequently did not reveal spermatogenetic activity; tubules contained for the most part a single basal layer of nuclei amid the Sertoli reticulum. Some grafts, especially in subcutaneous areas, did reveal tubules in which germinal epithelium of two or more layers contained many cells in mitosis. However, as new cells were added the more centrally placed ones escaped from the epithelium into the tubular lumen to undergo fragmentation and degeneration. When, however, the testis transplant was secured to the inside layers of the scrotum, grafts recovered six months after transplantation contained many tubules actively producing spermatozoa (Moore, 1926b). Thus, the scrotal temperature regulating mechanism was apparent. Testis grafts residing in the anterior chamber of the eye, a region of lower temperature than subcutaneous or intraperitoneal areas, is the only other locality in which transplanted testes in a mammal have produced spermatozoa (Turner, 1938).

VASOLIGATION

The closure of excurrent passageways from the testis has been held to be the cause of the degeneration of spermatogenetic tissues in this organ, in a manner analogous to degeneration of the parenchyma of salivary glands or pancreas after occlusion of their outlet ducts. In fact, since the spurious claims of the Viennese biologist, E. Steinach, that a marvelous rejuvenation occurred in senile rats when they were subjected to ductus deferens ligation, a similar operation, or one involving ligation of portions of the epididymis, has been performed on man for purposes of rejuvenation.

The theory of rejuvenation by vasoligation rested upon the claims (1) that closure of the outlet passages from the testicle led to degeneration of spermatogenetic tissues, (2) that tubular degeneration was accompanied by a compensatory hypertrophy of the interstitial tissue, (3) that such alleged compensatory hypertrophy assured an increased secretion of male hormone, and (4) that the effects of this excessive male hormone was the cause of the alleged rejuvenation. Each aspect of this hypothetical chain of events has been thoroughly discredited.

Ligation of the ductus deferens, or portions of the epididymis, has now been followed by a thorough study on the rat, guinea pig, dog, ram, and other mammalian species. In man, occlusion of the excurrent passages from the testis has been effected by operation, or by pathological causes, and testes of adult guinea pigs with congenital absence of the ductus deferens and epididymis have been studied. In all these cases seminiferous tubules have been found to be actively producing spermatozoa, in some instances several years subsequent to the occlusion (Moore, 1939; Moore and Quick, 1924). The tubules may become sufficiently engorged with accumulated cells that pressure atrophy occurs temporarily; with dissolution of accumulated products spermatogenetic activity is again renewed. In the adult guinea pig with congenital atrophy of all outlet passages, more than 50 per cent of the tubules contained spermatozoa. When the ductus deferens is ligated spermatogenesis will continue, and sperm cells will be carried out into the epididymis against pressures so great that the engorged epididymis may become triple its normal size. Compensatory hypertrophy of interstitial cells, after ductus deferens ligation, does not occur. The explanation for testis degeneration following vasoligation on laboratory rodents, reported from several European laboratories, appears to rest upon the formation of adhesions that bring the testis under the influence of abdominal temperatures.

NUTRITION AND VITAMINS

Spermatogenetic activity in the mature adult animal, although influenced by vitamin intake, is fairly resistant to low nutritive levels. Some hibernating mammals emerge from burrows in the early spring in a fairly high state of general body emaciation, but the testicles exhibit rapid increase in size or have reached their height in the production of mature germ cells. Mature breeding rats, placed upon diets adequate in all vitamin requirements but sufficiently restricted in quantity of food to cause a loss of 25 per cent in their initial body weight, may continue to carry on spermatogenesis and to possess large quantities of spermatozoa in the epididymis capable of an excellent grade of motility. A decline in body weight of slightly greater proportions, however, leads to interference with germ cell formation (Mason, 1939).

Testicles of prepuberal animals appear to suffer disproportionately from inanition, and the severity of effects appear to increase as the withholding of adequate nutrition is advanced to earlier ages. General sexual underdevelopment is noted, and delayed puberty and suppression of spermatogenesis occurs. Rats maintained upon an inanition diet from the age of 3 to

4 weeks may not produce cells above the spermatocyte stage during the first year of their lives. A change to a good maintenance diet is usually followed by the establishment of full spermatogenetic function.

Vitamin A deficiency leads to an involution of the epithelium of seminiferous tubules prior to the external appearance of deficiency symptoms. Spermatogenesis is reduced and cells of the germinal line may be sloughed into the tubular lumen to degenerate locally, or to be carried out into the epididymis. Mitosis may occur in spermatogonia but the higher elements of the germinal line are not produced. Sertoli cells and interstitial cells are little affected. The addition of sufficient quantities of vitamin A usually induces an immediate response and full spermatogenesis occurs within short periods of time.

Deficiencies in vitamins B, C and D do not usually affect spermatogenesis in mammals to any marked degree, except in those conditions in which total body weight is severely reduced. In such cases it can be shown that inanition itself, and not the absence of the specific vitamin, is the causative factor. The effect is one which pituitary activity is at a low level (Moore and Samuels, 1931).

Vitamin E deficiency has a special effect upon mammalian spermatogenesis (Mason, 1939). Rats placed upon a diet deficient in this substance may at first produce seminal discharges in which spermatozoa are apparently normal but have a low fertilizing capacity; and in turn there follows morphologically normal but immotile sperm cells, spermatozoa lacking tails, and finally complete absence of the mature germ cells.

Histologically, the degenerating seminiferous tubules reveal severe disruption of the germinal epithelium, extensive chromatolysis, formation of "giant cells," liquefaction in situ, and ultimately the tubules are reduced greatly in size and contain a single basal layer of nuclei in the Sertoli syncytium.

The special feature of disorders arising from E deficiency is the apparent inability of the testicle to recover when adequate supplements of this substance are provided. Additions of adequate supplements, upon the first appearance of histological changes, do not prevent the further degeneration of the germinal epithelium. The peculiar effects that prevent testicular repair upon the addition of more than adequate replacements of this vitamin have not been determined.

RADIATIONS

The discovery of x-rays late in the nineteenth century, and the unfortunate sterility occurring among workers using them, early emphasized that the spermatogenetic tissues were very sensitive to radiations. Subsequent studies, especially those conducted on laboratory rodents in the Manhattan Project (Heller, 1948), have made it clear that external radiations with x-rays, alpha, beta and gamma rays, and fast neutrons were all injurious and produced effects that were qualitatively alike. The internal administration of radioactive isotopes has also been shown to produce effects similar to those from external radiation.

The effects of all types of radiation, while generally similar, exhibit great variability due largely perhaps to different intensities, hence in different speeds in destruction of tissues. It is generally agreed that the larger total dosages are more destructive when given in a series of fractionated doses than in one dose. There is further agreement that the most sensitive cell, and first to be affected, is the spermatogonium. Destruction of these cells may occur while further development of the spermatocytes and spermatids may continue. However, elimination of the supply of spermatogonia ultimately leads to complete absence of the germinal line and tubules may contain only Sertoli cells. Neither Sertoli cells nor interstitial cells are particularly radiation sensitive.

It is recognized that weak dosages of radiation may produce considerable damage to the testicle and yet be followed by recovery. Heller has described the recovery process and believes that new spermatogonia may arise from outstretched spindle-shaped cells on the inner surface of the basement membrane, perhaps prespermatogonia. The source of these cells was not determined.

Some idea of testicular sensitivity can be given by noting that whole body irradiation of a rabbit with one exposure of 800 r of x-rays largely obliterates spermatogenesis within a two week period. Histological studies of testicles from treated animals reveal that after such dosages some evidence of regeneration of the spermatic tubules may be evident at about thirty-five days, and that in some cases essentially normal spermatogenesis was re-established by four months after treatment. Similar results were noted from one whole body radiation of rats with 600 r of x-rays. Four months later, in some cases, a good spermatogenetic recovery could be noted, whereas in others, recovery was only partial, and in some no recovery effects were to be noted. It has been held by some that permanent sterility is induced in cases that fail to show some evident recovery within a four month period subsequent to treatment.

The internal administration of radioactive isotopes produced effects upon the testicle similar to those following external radiation although quantitative differences were great when alpha, beta or gamma emitters were employed; this may perhaps be correlated with the deposition of substances employed in different areas of the body. Heller found that treatments with internal sources of radiation, which resulted in destruction of all spermatogenetic activity, was not followed by later recovery.

II. TEMPERATURE AND SCROTAL FUNCTION

It has already been emphasized that the position of the testicle in relation to the scrotum has great importance for the function of spermatogenesis, on account of the thermoregulatory function of the scrotum. This function became apparent gradually during the course of experiments on laboratory animals involving studies on experimental cryptorchidism, vasectomy and testis transplantation, with the crucial evidence coming from experiments on heat application, determination of temperature differences and insulation of the scrotum to mask its function (Moore, 1924a).

HEAT APPLICATION

In terms of the conception that abdominal temperature was the cause of tubular degeneration when the testicle was elevated from the scrotum into the abdomen, with recovery of spermatogenesis upon scrotal return, heat was applied to the scrotum to test the susceptibility of the spermatogenetic tissues to temperatures slightly above the normal.

A ten-minute exposure of the scrotum of an adult guinea pig to water warmed at 6° C. to 8° C. above normal body temperature resulted in great damage to the tubules. Three to six days after such a single exposure, histological study demonstrated the disorganization of the germinal epithelium, degeneration of loosened cells, cytolysis and liquefaction. Submergence of the testicle in warmed saline solution through a low abdominal incision, exposure of the unoperated scrotum to heat from an electric hot plate, electric light or diathermy, revealed the high susceptibility of the spermatogenetic tissues to temporary exposure to 5° C. above normal temperature of the body. Complete removal of all germinal epithelium to a single basal row of nuclei occurred. Recovery within some weeks followed such exposures when the treatments had not been too severe, but permanent sterility was easily induced (Moore, 1924b).

ABDOMINAL TEMPERATURES

Simultaneous measurements reveal that in unanesthetized laboratory rodents, with open inguinal canals, the temperature of the body cavity is from 2° C. to 4° C. higher than in the scrotum, with greater differences occurring as environmental temperatures became reduced (Moore and Quick, 1924). The scrotal temperature in anesthetized human patients on the operating table is lower than abdominal temperature. Single exposure of normal men to a cabinet temperature of 43° C. for 30 minutes leads to a marked drop in sperm count within three weeks after treatment (Macleod and Hotchkiss, 1941).

SCROTAL INSULATION

The clinching evidence for the scrotal temperature regulatory mechanism was provided through the utilization of adult rams whose scrotum was insulated against loss of heat by loose woolen materials and a waterproof covering (Moore and Oslund, 1924). The pendent scrotum, prevented from exercising its function, was thus unable to reduce the temperature and the testicles of rams thus treated were demonstrated to lack normal tubules within several weeks after being insulated. It was later shown that seminal discharges by rams trained to ejaculate in a receptacle exhibited a gradual and final loss of all spermatozoa a few weeks after insulation, with gradual and complete recovery subsequent to removal of the insulation. In Australia, rams in summer heat at the sea coast would be devoid of spermatozoa in ejaculates, whereas others in the same environment, but maintained inside cooled sheds, exhibited normal semen containing spermatozoa.

The function of the scrotum as a thermoregulator for the testis is made possible by virtue of its constitution. Such elements are important as (a) a thin modified and rugose skin richly provided with sweat glands, (b) lack of subcutaneous fat, and (c) a thin cremasteric muscle capable of relaxation and contraction in keeping with the environmental temperature; the rich surface blood plexus of the testicle undoubtedly plays a part.

III. EPIDIDYMAL FUNCTION AND LIFE OF THE SPERMATOZOON

Spermatozoa within the seminiferous tubules of constantly breeding mammals are continuously produced from metamorphosing spermatids. The sperm cells become loosened from the germinal epithelium and are transported through the tubuli recti, rete tubules, and vasa efferentia into the head of the epididymis. Whereas inadequate information prevails, it is probable that ciliary action, as well as smooth muscle contractions, are responsible for this transport. The older notion that spermatozoa swim through these passages is largely discounted since observations of sperm quiescence, and in many cases inability of sperm cells to show motility under suitable conditions when they are removed from the testis, rete and vasa efferentia, suggest that, although morphologically normal, the spermatozoa are physiologically immature; fertilizing capacity of spermatozoa from upper parts of the epididymis, in contrast to those from lower epididymal levels, is low or absent. Numerous experiments appear to demonstrate a physiological maturity of spermatozoa begun in the testis and continued in the epididymis; complete physiological maturity marked by high motility on dilution, and high fertilizing capacity, is followed by a natural decline and death of unvoided cells.

It has been demonstrated that sperm enter the epididymis from the testis against considerable pressures. Ligation of the ductus deferens of rabbits, rats, and sheep results in the retention of sperm in the epididymis with, often, a three-fold increase in the size of this organ; severance of the ductus above the ligation results in the immediate outflow of quantities of a milky substance containing packed masses of spermatozoa.

The length of time that spermatozoa remain in the epididymis depends to some extent upon the number of ejaculations. In normal, sexually inactive, guinea pigs Toothill and Young determined that carbon particles introduced into the head of the epididymis reached the junction of epididymis and ductus deferens in fourteen to eighteen days, which presumably represents the speed of transport of the inactive spermatozoa. Ligation of vasa efferentia, to prevent entrance of additional spermatozoa into the epididymis, subsequent to the introduction of the carbon particles, caused a doubling of time required for the passage. It has furthermore been shown that guinea pigs with vasa efferentia ligated to prevent further entrance of sperm cells, and which have mated with 20 females during the course of thirty days after operation, still had spermatozoa in the epididymis (Young, 1929). In the rabbit (Hammond and Asdell, 1926) and in the guinea pig (Moore, 1928) spermatozoa in the epididymis remain alive and reveal capacities for movement, upon proper stimulation, for a period of sixty days or longer, but the capacity for fertilization is of shorter duration. Hormones from the testis exercise an influence on the life of the spermatozoon within the epididymal passages in as much as testis removal in the guinea pig reduces the potential capacity for motility from sixty days or longer to less than thirty days. It thus appears that spermatozoa in a sexually quiescent mammal enter the epididymis in an inactive state; processes of physiological development continue until a maximum capacity for fertility and motility is acquired; and subsequently spermatozoa undergo an ageing process characterized by lowered motility and fertility, death, fragmentation and resorption in the lower ductus deferens.

The life of the spermatozoon after ejaculation varies with conditions. Motility persists in untreated semen held at room temperatures for approximately twenty-four hours, for much shorter periods as semen is held at higher temperatures, but when stored in ice chambers motility may be re-initiated for periods up to a week or longer. Spermatozoa of mammals or lower vertebrates may be subjected to rapid freezing and retain capacity for motility for days, although fertilizing capacity under such conditions is not well known.

Spermatozoon life in the female reproductive tract is ordinarily of short duration, and is affected by such conditions as vaginal acidity, bacterial action, continuous motility, and by body temperature. In the majority of mammals, including man, most observations suggest the life of the spermatozoon after insemination as less than 72 hours, and in many cases of the order of 24 to 36 hours, but fertilizing capacity is ordinarily shorter than the period of motility. Soderwall and Young (1940) demonstrated impaired fertility in guinea pig spermatozoa 17 hours after introduction into the female tract, with no fertility after a period of 30 hours. Exceptions occur, however, and Day claims that spermatozoa in the mare live and fertilize the ovum for a period of five to six days. Other extremes are known since the bat copulates in the fall months and retains spermatozoa in the uterus in a quiescent state during winter hibernation, with fertilization occurring after the spring awakening. In lower forms spermatozoa have been reported living in the female tract, and maintaining fertilizing capacity, for such extreme periods as 21 days in the bird, 10 months in some viviparous fish and up to 3 or 4 years in some reptiles.

IV. THE INTERNAL SECRETION OF THE TESTIS

Since biblical times the eunuch has provided a demonstration in man of the effects produced when the testis is removed early in life, but it remained for Berthold in 1849 to show that the effects of castration were due to loss of substances produced in the testicle and liberated in the blood stream, rather than to the interruption of nervous pathways of a special or prescribed variety. Berthold noted that the removal of the testicles from the cock led to the development of the capon, but transfer of testicular tissue into another castrated rooster, in the abdomen or in subcutaneous areas, prevented development of the characteristic castration changes (comb regression, cessation of crowing, loss of sexual interest in hens), provided that the transplant became vascularized and persisted as living tissue. It was recognized that some substance entered the blood stream from the living graft tissue, irrespective of its location, that was responsible for the masculine characters and behavior.

Investigations involving surgical manipulations of living tissues provided our principal source of knowledge of the secretion of testis hormone, and its effects within the organism, until McGee in 1927 successfully obtained extracts from fresh testicles of the bull that were capable of preventing castration changes in the rooster, or of re-establishing the typical masculine characters and behavior in capons, injected with these lipoidal extracts. Extraction of human male urine with chloroform also yielded substances that stimulated comb growth in capons; hence, two sources of masculinizing substances were available for further biochemical investigations. The development and use of biological tests for male hormone activity in laboratory mammals (spermatozoon motility; electric ejaculation; cytology of seminal vesicles, prostate, and Cowper's glands, ductus deferens, see Moore, 1939) very soon established that the androgenic activity recoverable from testis and urine extracts provided an effective substitute for the internal secretions of mammalian testes. Further extensions of these studies to lower vertebrates revealed that the androgenic activity recovered from extracts was not species specific, but that the same extract served as an effective substitute for the internal secretion of the testicles in the different species of vertebrates.

Biochemical investigations of extraction methods, purification of extracts, and quantitative studies by Koch and his students demonstrated that hormonal substances from urine and testicles were of different chemical natures. From human male urine, Butenandt (1931, 1932, 1934) obtained two androgens in crystalline form—androsterone and dehydroandrosterone— that were very soon produced in the laboratory by synthetic processes (Ruzicka et al., 1934). In 1935 the pure chemical androgen, testosterone, was obtained in crystalline form from fresh testis tissue, and the substance was prepared by synthetic procedures in the laboratory almost at once. Many different compounds of these basic substances have revealed high androgenic potency, and at the present time testosterone propionate is perhaps the androgen most frequently employed in clinical practice. It must be pointed out that, despite the high masculinizing activity of such chemical substances, it is yet unknown whether any one of them is the actual substance secreted as the testis hormone by the living tissues, or whether the same hormonal substance is secreted by different species of vertebrates.

The secretion of testis hormone, as well as the process of spermatogenesis, is characterized by two extremes, (a) a short seasonal period of activity in males of annual breeding species, and (b) continuous activity in the constantly breeding animal. Also, as with spermatogenesis, the gonadotrophic hormone of the anterior pituitary body represents the controlling influence over testis hormone secretion. Removal of the pituitary gland leads to immediate cessation of testis hormone secretion, and the introduction of gonadotrophic substances into seasonally quiescent males initiates intense secretion of testicular androgens at once. Low secretion of hormone, therefore, may be related to imperfect pituitary physiology as well as to inherent defects in the testicle. The parallel between spermatogenesis and hormone secretion does not always prevail, as it is known that cryptorchid testes, naturally occurring or artificially produced, secrete essentially normal amounts of testis hormone in the absence of spermatogenesis.

The complete effects in the organism of the internal secretion of the testes are not yet known. It is clear that some of the principal physiological actions of the hormone relate to the maintenance of function of the accessory organs of reproduction as well as of the other male secondary sex characters, including the sex drive. The latter function is quite important in most subprimate animals but in man, especially, psychological factors play such a predominant role in human relations that sex hormones appear to have a less important role in the general sex drive than is true for lower animals. Male dogs, monkeys, man, and other species may carry on copulation for many months after castration.

The internal secretion of the testes enable the epididymis, prostate gland, seminal vesicles, ductus deferens, Cowper's gland and others to produce the major portion of the semen; spermatozoa and probably small amounts of secretion are contributed from the testis proper. In the rat each gland, having its own particular type of secretory epithelium, quickly displays involution of secretory cells upon removal of the testes, or upon discontinuance of androgen injections in castrated individuals. Less distinct involutional changes occur in the accessory reproductive organs of the guinea pig, but the cessation of secretory activity is easily demonstrated for the prostate gland and seminal vesicles by loss of a coagulable ejaculate; seminal discharges are easily obtained by electric stimulation of the head. The collective secretions, discharged along with spermatozoa from the ductus deferens and lower epididymis, provide a viscous medium for the transport of spermatozoa, and serve to activate the previously inactive sperm cells. The semen also contains a high concentration of fructose and citric acid secreted by the accessory reproductive organs; the former provides an extra source of energy and is metabolized by spermatozoa (Mann, 1949) but the function of the citric acid is not yet well established.

Although the most important function of the testis hormone appears to center on the functional state of the accessory reproductive organs, including the copulatory apparatus, it exerts an influence upon other conditions. Brought into prominence, or maintained, by the testis hormone are the comb and wattles of the cock, the sex drive, crowing and combative behavior, antler or horn growth in some ruminants, and in man, voice changes, certain regional hair growth, the size of muscles, and closure of the epiphyses of the long bones. It also exercises a nitrogen sparing influence in man and frequently leads to increases in weight. Basal metabolism is not markedly influenced but some glands of the skin, and hair follicles, are influenced by it and the level of the erythrocyte count is elevated above that in the castrate.

The influence of androgens upon the testis itself is a controversial subject. Prepuberal testes of the rat, mouse, guinea pig, dog, and other mammals are definitely injured by the administration of approximately physiological dosages of androgen; testes fail to grow or to produce spermatozoa at the normal time. It is generally accepted that androgens inhibit the secretion, or the release, of effective amounts of gonadotrophic hormone by the pituitary gland, thus simulating a physiological hypophysectomy. It has been shown, however, that administration of androgens to some seasonal breeding animals, during the period of reproductive quiescence, induces testicular activity with spermatozoon production; this is true for the ground squirrel and the sparrow as well as some other species. It is further demonstrated that administration of androgens immediately following hypophysectomy effectively prevents testis degeneration, although similar dosages do not repair testis damage from hypophysectomy when given after testis involution. Testis repair, while reported effective after the use of very high dosages of the compound, is not proportional to the androgenic effects of the substance; some very weak androgens are the most effective in protecting against hypophysectomy damage, whereas some of the strongest androgenic substances may be quite ineffective in protecting the testis from hypophysectomy damage. Since some steroidal substances that lack ordinary androgenic powers protect against hypophysectomy damage, as does also progesterone and yeast extract, it is not clear that the testis secretions can be regarded as stimulants for spermatogenesis. Again, whereas pellets of some androgenic substances implanted into the testis of hypophysectomized males will show local stimulation of spermatogenesis, reports continue to reveal that the administration of androgens to normal men consistently causes a drop, or entire loss, of spermatozoa in the seminal discharge. The problem requires further study.

NUMBER OF TESTIS HORMONES

Claims have been made that, in addition to the hormone that controls the physiology of the accessory reproductive organs, generally accepted to be secreted by the interstitial cells, the germinal epithelium secretes a second hormone whose function is the control of gonadotrophic secretion by the pituitary body. On the basis of evidence thus far submitted, it would appear questionable whether more than one hormone is secreted. Since castration changes in the pituitary are prevented or repaired by the administration of compounds of testosterone, and at the same time other changes that develop as a result of the absence of testis hormone are likewise repaired, it appears that a single chemical substance can effectively substitute for the natural secretions of the male gonad. Whether this substance is testosterone or a closely related substance, or whether different species secrete the same compound as a hormone is yet to be demonstrated. The adrenal gland appears to secrete some type of androgenic substance under pathological conditions (some hyperplasias and tumors) but it is not clearly established that in the normal physiology of the adrenal, androgenic substances of an effective nature are delivered into the circulation of the male.

PERIOD OF HORMONE SECRETION

Testis hormone secretion is detectable throughout mature reproductive life in constantly breeding animals, and during the breeding period in the cyclically reproducing ones. In the former, the development of almost immediate castration changes in target organs demonstrates that the hormone is not stored within the organism but is secreted continuously. Puberal changes, developing over short periods of time as in the rat, or over longer periods in monkey and man, are hormonally conditioned. The induced changes appear to depend as well upon the differentiation of the body tissues of the organism, to a state where they effectively respond to hormones, as to the actual appearance of the hormone in the organism. Differences of opinion exist as to the time when hormones are first secreted and exert a controlling influence, but in any event the evidence suggests this onset to be a gradual rather than a precipitous one.

Studies on the free martin (Lillie, 1917) laid the foundation for the concept that the gonads secrete hormones during the early developmental stages, and that these substances exercise a controlling influence over the development and differentiation of the accessory reproductive organs. This interpretation has been questioned, however, because of observations that reveal typical differentiation of the reproductive system in both sexes subsequent to removal of the developing gonad, and at a time when the reproductive system exists as the two embryonic sex ducts that characterize development of all higher vertebrates (Moore, 1950).

The possibility exists that during embryonic development the testis may in some manner exert an influence upon the development of the accessory reproductive organs but it must be regarded as questionable, if in fact it is true, that such an influence is imparted through a steroidal secretion of the nature of the testis hormone, that is so effective in later reproductive physiology. In normal development many examples exist in which one part exercises an influence upon another without invoking hormonal actions, and it is yet to be clearly demonstrated that embryonic testes secrete hormones that play an important role in development. The exact period in which testis hormone is first secreted naturally varies with species but the appearance of puberal changes provides a clear demonstration of the action of such substances.

CLINICAL APPLICATION OF HORMONES

The application of hormones in clinical practice would appear to be indicated only in cases of frank absence, or observable deficiencies, in testicular secretions. The contention of some that administration of chemical androgens to men past the ordinary period of reproductive life is beneficial for its general "tonic" effects appears to rest upon inconclusive evidence. Whether supplements of such substances during periods of declining testis hormone secretion aid muscular action, blood vessel or heart function, digestion, sleep, and other subjective symptoms, without producing effects that may be decidedly harmful, must be determined on the basis of a large experimental group. Opinions differ with regard to the actuality of the so-called male climacteric. It is known, however, that in cases of prostatic carcinoma administration of androgens is definitely contraindicated. It is not known that testis hormone exercises any influence in the origin of this condition, but it has been stated that prostatic carcinoma does not occur in castrates.

The choice of hormones for administration differs to some extent on whether (a) testis tissue is absent due either to congenital absence, or through surgery in diseased conditions, or loss through accidental trauma or (b) when testis tissue is present but is apparently defective in secretion. In the former condition androgenic substances, representing replacement of testis hormone secretions, are indicated; in the latter case gonadotrophic hormones would be suggested in an attempt to stimulate hormone secretion by whatever testis tissue may be present.

Congenital absence or early loss of testicles produce the eunuch in which body proportions may depart conspicuously from the normal, but in any event, voice changes do not attain the male quality, and external genitalia remain relatively infantile. Androgenic treatments over sufficient periods of time can modify these obvious peculiarities with proper voice changes, growth of genitalia, development of masculine hair distribution, and the development of sexual interests beyond those that might otherwise have been present. Subsequent to definite puberal development, with establishment of a normal physique, the continuance of such treatments would appear to rest upon psychological factors.

The presence of palpable testis tissue, accompanied by obvious low androgen secretion, suggests the administration of gonadotrophic substances for the stimulation of the natural secretions, rather than the administration of androgens. Potential testis hormone secreting tissues may be inactive on account of ineffective pituitary activity, due to disorders in the latter gland; pituitary deficiency may depend upon intrinsic disorders in this body, perhaps also upon general nutritional inadequacy. The claim that obviously undersized testicles have shown improvement in some cases under androgen administration needs substantiation; it is true, however, that testes of seasonally breeding animals have shown spermatogenetic responses when treatments were given during the sexually inactive period. It has also been established that diminished androgenic effects may prevail when there exists a deficiency in thyroid hormone; animals thyroidectomized and castrated show less response to androgen administration than do castrates with intact thyroid glands. A reasonable degree of otherwise normal conditions in the organism is required for the full expression of the effects of testis hormone.

REFERENCES

BENOIT, J.: Facteurs externes et internes de l'activité sexuelle. 1. Stimulation par la lumière de l'activité sexuelle chez le Canard et la Cana domestiques. Bull. Biol. France-Belg., *70:*487, 1936.

BROWMAN, L. G.: Testicular heterotransplantation in rats and mice. J. Exp. Zool., *75:*283, 1937.

BUTENANDT, A.: Über die chemische Untersuchung der Sexualhormone. Ztschr. f. angew. Chem., *44:*905, 1931.

BUTENANDT, A.: Über die Chemie der Sexualhormone. Ztschr. f. angew. Chem., *45:*655, 1932.

BUTENANDT, A. and H. DANNENBAUM: Über Androsteron. III. Isolierung eines neuen, physiologisch unwirksamen Sterinderivatives aus Männerharn, seine Verknüpfung mit Androsteron. Ztschr. f. physiol. Chem., *229:*192, 1934.

COURRIER, R.: Étude sur le determinisme des charactères sexuels secondaires chez quelques mammifères à l'activité testiculaire periodique. Arch. de Biol., *37:*175, 1927.

DAY, F. T.: Survival of spermatozoa in the genital tract of the mare. J. Agric. Sci., *32:*108, 1941.

ENGLE, EARL T.: Male Reproductive System. Chapt. 15, Problems of Ageing, p. 441, Williams & Wilkins Co., 1939.

HAMMOND, J. and S. A. ASDELL: The vitality of the spermatozoon in the male and female reproductive tracts. Brit. J. Exp. Biol., *4:*155, 1926.

HANSEN, T. SWED: Fertiliteten ved operativt kryptorchisme jnar munksgaard. Kobenhaven. 190 pages, 1945.

HELLER, MINNIE: Histopathology of Irradiation from External and Internal Sources. Chapt. 12, The Testis. National nuclear energy series, Edited by Wm. Bloom. McGraw-Hill Pub., p. 550, 1948.

KOCH, F. C.: The Biochemistry of Androgens. Chapt. 12, Sex and Internal Secretions. Baltimore, Williams & Wilkins Co., 2nd ed. p. 807, 1939.

LILLIE, F. R.: The free martin: a study of the action of sex hormones in the foetal life of cattle. J. Exp. Zool., *23:*371, 1917.

McGEE, L. C.: The effect of the injection of a lipoid portion of bull testicle in capons. Proc. Inst. Medicine Chicago, *6:*242, 1927.

MACLEOD, J. and R. S. HOTCHKISS: The effect of hyperpyrexia upon spermatozoa count in men. Endocrinology, *28:*780, 1941.

MANN, T.: Metabolism of semen. Adv. Enzymology, *9:*329, 1949.

MASON, KARL E.: Relation of the Vitamines to the Sex Glands. Chapt. 22, Sex and Internal Secretions. Baltimore, Williams and Wilkins Co., p. 1149, 1939.

MOORE, CARL R.: Testicular reactions in experimental cryptorchidism. Am. J. Anat., *34:* 269, 1924a.

MOORE, CARL R.: Heat application and testicular degeneration; the function of the scrotum. Am. J. Anat., *34:*337, 1924b.

MOORE, CARL R.: The biology of the mammalian testis and scrotum. Quart. Rev. Biol., *1:* 4, 1926.

MOORE, CARL R.: Testis-graft reactions in different environments (rat). Am. J. Anat., *37:* 351, 1926b.

MOORE, CARL R.: Spermatozoon activity and the testis hormone. J. Exp. Zool., *50:*455, 1928.

MOORE, CARL R.: Biology of the Testis. Chapt. 7, Sex and Internal Secretions. Baltimore, Williams and Wilkins Co., p. 353, 1939.

MOORE, CARL R.: The role of the fetal endocrine glands in development. J. Clin. Endocrinol., *10:*942, 1950.

MOORE, CARL R. and R. OSLUND: Experiments on the sheep testis—cryptorchidism, vasectomy and scrotal insulation. Am. J. Physiol., *67:*595, 1924.

MOORE, CARL R. and WM. J. QUICK: Vasectomy in the rabbit. Am. J. Anat., *34:*317, 1924.

MOORE, CARL R. and WM. J. QUICK: The scrotum as a temperature regulator for the testes. Am. J. Physiol., *68:*70, 1924.

MOORE, CARL R. and L. T. SAMUELS: The action of testis hormone in correcting changes induced in the rat prostate and seminal vesicles by vitamine B deficiency or partial inanition. Am. J. Physiol., *96:*278, 1931.

ROWAN, WM.: Experiments in bird migration. I. Manipulation of the reproductive cycle; seasonal histological changes in the gonads. Proc. Boston Soc. Nat. Hist., *39:*151, 1929.

RUZICKA, L., W. M. GOLDBERG, J. MEYER, H. BRÜNGGER and E. EICHELBERGER: Über die Synthese des Testikelhormons (Androsteron) and Steriosomerer desselben durch Abbau hydrierter Sterine. Helv. Chim. Act., *17:*1395, 1934.

SAND, K. and H. OKKELS: The histological variability of the testis from normal and sexual-abnormal castrated men. Endokrin., *19:*369, 1938.

SMITH, P. E.: Hypophysectomy and a replacement therapy in the rat. Am. J. Anat., *45:* 205, 1930.

SMITH, P. E. and E .T. ENGLE: Experimental evidence regarding the role of the anterior pituitary in the development and regulation of the genital system. Am. J. Anat., *40:*159, 1927.

SODERWALL, A. L. and W. C. YOUNG: The effect of aging in the female genital tract on the fertilizing capacity of guinea pig spermatozoa. Anat. Rec., *78:*19, 1940.

STEINACH, E.: Verjüngung durch experimentelle Neubelebung der alternden Pubertätsdrüse. Arch. f. Entw.'mech., *46:*557, 1920.

TOOTHILL, M. C. and W. C. YOUNG: The time consumed by spermatozoa in passing through the ductus epididymis of the guinea pig as determined by means of India-ink injection. Anat. Rec., *50:*95, 1931.

TURNER, C. D.: Intra-ocular homotransplantation of prepuberal testes in the rat. Am. J. Anat., *63:*101, 1938.

WELLS, L. J.: Seasonal sexual rhythms and its experimental modification in the male of the thirteen-lined groundsquirrel (Citellus tridecemlineatus). Anat. Rec., *62:*409, 1935.

WELLS, L. J.: Gonadotrophic potency of the hypophysis in a wild male rodent with annual rut. Endocrinology, *22:*588, 1938.

YOUNG, W. C.: A study of the function of the epididymis. II. The importance of an aging process in sperm for the length of the period during which fertilizing capacity is retained by sperm isolated in the epididymis of the guinea pig. J. Morph. and Physiol., *48:*475, 1929.

Section II

PRINCIPLES OF DIAGNOSIS

CHAPTER 1

The Urologic Examination

GERSHOM J. THOMPSON, M.D.

The patient who seeks a physician's advice expects *thorough* consideration of his problem. He has the right to feel that in due time his problem will be solved because of the physician's training and experience, the use of his God-given senses, and his will to reason and to employ necessary diagnostic facilities. Cursory effort generally goes unrewarded and instead of obtaining good service the patient sometimes must seek the help of some other practitioner, perhaps less capable but one willing to hear the story and complete a real examination. While in rare instances the urologist can determine in but a few moments the true nature of a complaint for which relief is sought, often the situation is complex and several or many visits, a number of laboratory tests and perhaps the collaboration of other practitioners are needed to provide the solution of the problem. Campbell (1951) has aptly stated: "Yielding to investigative short cuts may lead to serious diagnostic error."

In recent years increasing numbers of people have become cognizant of the value of periodic examinations which are intended to ferret out disease in its incipiency. Large insurance companies often urge their clients to send specimens of urine for routine examination at regular intervals. These sometimes reveal positive findings which require further investigation; hence many patients seek the counsel of urologists or other specialists to determine the source of the abnormal laboratory findings. Investigation must be thorough in order to establish the importance of these laboratory data. Often relatively trivial conditions account for the presence of blood in microscopic quantities in the urine but occasionally important lesions which are asymptomatic are uncovered and their correction is possible by comparatively simple treatment. The physician and urologist must be familiar with accepted routine diagnostic procedure which will enable him to examine and advise the patient properly.

THE HISTORY

Sincere interest in the patient's story is an absolute requisite in any case.
The physician who is so busy that he cannot listen to the patient's complaint and further develop it by appropriate questions must delegate this task to some intelligent person who has the patience to hear every bit of information which is offered. It is surprising how often important leads to the diagnosis are established by only a few statements. However, these must be clarified, and sometimes prompting which leads to reiteration of various facts in the history is necessary. It is usually best to rely upon the patient's story; but now and then, especially in the very young or very old and perhaps senile individual, other members of the family can provide more reliable data.

Not infrequently one sees individuals who either willingly or not profess to have symptoms which obviously do not fit any certain pattern; in such cases the history taker must be on his guard lest he be misled and jump to the conclusion that psychosomatic disease is the predominant factor. Often, repeating the questions on another day, perhaps when additional data are available, will clarify uncertain points or establish their relative importance. The ability to properly evaluate the history comes with practice, and the directness of questions and answers many times will convince the patient that he is in the hands of an experienced physician and he will therefore be reassured.

Taking a history should not be a laborious task. It is perhaps well to follow a rough outline when questioning a patient, but certainly it is unnecessary to make many dozens of queries, and one can almost certainly say that the form sheets which are sometimes used wherein one puts check marks opposite standard items of a long list represent a waste of time. Much effort expended on these might be better spent developing firm answers to comparatively few questions.

Chief Complaint. This should be recorded in the patient's own words, along with the mode of onset of symptoms, their severity and the sequence of appearance; the time of day or night when the disturbance is at its worst and the degree of disability which results are important items. It is often well to develop a definite idea of how bad a pain becomes in comparison with its intensity at the time of the interview. Many times a patient will thus reveal that because of worry or other factors he is unwittingly magnifying comparatively trivial discomfort. The location of pain and its radiation, if any, is a point of value. Knowledge of the measure which the patient has employed to obtain relief is helpful in estimating the actual importance of the symptoms. One cannot, of course, discount such symptoms as hematuria, fever and chills but various aspects of even these, if proper questions are asked, provide data which are helpful in diagnosis.

Family History. The presence of renal or other urologic disease in other members of the family is a point of great interest. The occurrence of polycystic disease of the kidney, calculous disease, and any disorder of micturition not only in the immediate family but in other relatives should be inquired about. Congenital disorders often appear in several members of a family in the same or succeeding generations.

Past History. The recurring nature of a complaint for which advice is sought is often brought out by questions. One of the interesting aspects of urologic disease is its tendency to right itself, especially with the help of modern methods of therapy. Relief by chemotherapy from infection secondary to congenital obstruction in the urinary passages often obscures and delays recognition of the basic lesion. Its correction will be brought about by the physician who is not content to treat merely the most obvious symptom. Failure to pursue the problem may result in only temporary relief or in remission.

Present Illness. As a general rule it is best, when taking a history, to develop the facts which are uppermost in the patient's mind and in which he is at the moment chiefly interested. The order, therefore, in which any particular history is recorded will vary considerably. For instance, if it concerns an acute attack of epididymitis he will not look with particular favor on the person who asks about the cause of his grandfather's death. Seemingly irrelevant information must be sought after, if at all, at the proper time.

Occupational factors must be considered in many phases of urologic disease. The occurrence of renal brucellosis in packing-house employees and of vesical neoplasm in dye workers, for instance, is well known.

One phase of the history which should be developed thoroughly is the degree of economic disability which has resulted from the illness. A patient's tendency to exaggerate can sometimes be estimated on this basis.

There are many outlines which the novice can follow until he gains experience in history taking and soon it will become almost second nature to go through the long list of essential inquiry with minimal delay. Campbell (1951) suggests the following useful outline:

1. *Pyuria*
     Time, nature of onset and recurrences
     Duration and nature of course
     Character—initial, total (throughout), or terminal with urination
     Bacteria, present or not
     Associated pain, stone, injury, exposure or infection
     Associated gastrointestinal or neurologic disturbances
2. *Disturbances of urination*
     Frequency
         Character and time of onset and recurrences
         Duration and degree
         Periodicity—constant, intermittent, diuria, nocturia
         Nycturia (passing more urine at night than in daytime)
     Enuresis
         Duration, events preceding onset
         Night wetting
         Day wetting
         Sociologic factors—home training, neurotic mother or nurse, other children
             in family, punishments, institutional life, and so forth
         Past treatment
     Dysuria
         Duration and character of onset and recurrences
     Character of disturbance

Constant, intermittent, tenesmus, urgency, hesitancy, change in stream (small, divided, lack of force, dribbling), crying on urination

Relation to

Other urologic symptoms, instrumentation or known infections elsewhere in the body

Retention

Character of onset and recurrences

Degree, periodicity

Relation to neurologic symptoms, injury to urethra or bladder, urethral stricture, instrumentation and acute infections elsewhere in the body

3. *Pain*

Location

Character—sharp, dull, mild, severe, constant, periodic

Cry—character, duration, relation to other symptoms

Radiation

Duration of present and past attacks

Relation to urination, vomiting and so forth

Relation to urinalysis—before, during, or after pain

4. *Hematuria*

Time and duration of onset and recurrences

Character—clots, initial, during or terminal to voiding

Degree of bleeding

Relation to injury, pain, stone, exposure or known infection elsewhere in the body

5. *Fever*

Chills

Character and duration of onset and recurrences

Relation to urologic symptoms

Relation to pyuria

Associated gastrointestinal and neurologic symptoms

6. *Abdominal tumor*

Location, duration, consistency

Movable or fixed

Size—constant, variable, disappearing, factors altering, associated symptoms

7. *Injury*

Character, duration, point of impact

Urinary symptoms before and after

Pain, hematuria, fever, masses, effect of movement and position

8. *Stone passage or crystalluria*

Time and character of onset, duration

Pain—location, radiation, duration

Hematuria

Pyuria

Recurrence

9. *Genital lesions*

Malformations

Interference with normal function

Symptoms produced

Phimosis, balanitis, urethritis, vaginitis

Epididymitis, orchitis

Location, duration, character of onset

Pain, radiation, crying and so forth

Relation to infection elsewhere

Relation to other urologic disease

Relation to trauma or straining (torsion of spermatic cord)

Hydrocele

Duration, character

Relation to infection or trauma

Size—constant, increasing or variable

Varicocele

Side involved, character, rapidity of size increase

Relation to abdominal tumor and to abdominal cutaneous vascular dilatations or varices

Testicular tumor
  Side, duration, character, rapidity of enlargement
  Pain, metastasis, loss of weight
10. *Pneumaturia*
  Duration, coexistent fecaluria

History Pertaining to Nonurologic Disease. The urologist often is consulted by a patient who has concluded erroneously that his disease concerns some disorder of the genitourinary tract when in fact it is of some other bodily structure. Furthermore, it is well known that important disease which should be recognized and treated occurs coincidentally with urologic complaints. It is imperative that reasonably accurate appraisal of all the patient's symptoms be made and that the study be broad enough to uncover any and all disease which might be present. While close collaboration of the urologist and other specialists must be commended, it is possible for the urologist alone to make use of laboratory and particularly x-ray facilities to develop at least the early phases of a so-called general examination.

For instance, pain, which at first glance seems to originate in the kidney, may actually be due to skeletal disease or to a disturbance of the gallbladder or its ducts. Recurring vesical disorders in the female might be due to endometriosis. The elderly patient with prostatic disease can be suffering as well from a carcinoma of the gastrointestinal tract and the patient with recurring urinary calculi can have hyperparathyroidism. These are only a few of the many conditions which must be kept in mind and about which the urologist must have more than just a passing curiosity. Among the most appreciative patients are those whose attention has been called to some coincidental but, nevertheless, important condition of which he was totally unaware. It is, therefore, best to be on the alert and, when taking the history and while treating the patient, to be interested in his entire body and not just the urinary tract.

THE EVALUATION OF UROLOGIC SYMPTOMS

In many instances symptoms which seem to be attributable to urologic abnormality may be due to disease which neither originates in nor is confined to the urinary tract. Furthermore, the severity of the symptoms does not necessarily measure the degree of involvement or lack of involvement of the various parts of this system. Great care and the exercise of judgment in estimating the impairment of the different parts of the urinary apparatus are necessary. Experience increases with each year of practice, but one must be ever wakeful or he may overlook things which should be obvious. Indeed, errors do creep in no matter how much precaution is exercised. In this connection it must be emphasized that few symptoms may be considered singly; generally, several others enter the picture when the patient's problem is evaluated.

Pain. Anyone who has closely observed a patient suffering from renal colic has a definite idea what this must be like even though he himself has not suffered an attack. Yet it is common knowledge that a kidney can become entirely functionless owing to a "silent stone" or other obstruction and cause not the slightest discomfort.

The *location* of pain will depend upon the particular structures involved and to some extent upon the type of disease. Mechanical factors which cause obstruction in any portion of the tract, and inflammatory factors which result in swelling and distortion of the organs and disturbances in blood supply, all contribute to pain of varying degree.

Renal pain often extends to the groin, though not always. Sometimes when it is intense there will be hyperesthesia of the skin of the inner aspect of the thigh. Severe colic usually results from the passage of even a tiny calculus down the ureter but often one sees a patient who is living quite comfortably in spite of a large staghorn calculus in the kidney.

Ureteral kinks and strictures have been blamed for many of the psychosomatic complaints of middle-aged women. The worst ureteral strictures I have ever seen caused no pain whatever. The colic caused by the passage of a ureteral calculus is due to obstruction to the free flow of urine and is usually identical with that due to the presence of a stone in the kidney. Sometimes, however, when the stone is passing through the intramural portion of the ureter the patient will also note frequency and tenesmus due to swelling and edema of the wall of the bladder. That the pain caused by ureteral calculus often simulates an attack of appendicitis is attested by the fact that any series of cases of ureteral calculus reveals in the history a much higher incidence of appendectomy than does any similar-aged group in the average population. One cannot be critical of this, however, when he reflects that a large proportion of ureteral calculi will pass spontaneously, whereas a ruptured appendix may be fatal.

Vesical pain due to overdistention is familiar to all medical students. But the bladder can contain several liters of urine without causing any discomfort. There are on record any number of patients who were operated upon for an abdominal cyst which proved to be a distended bladder. Catheterization would have prevented these errors. Hunner ulcer sometimes causes pain of unusual type, producing a trigger area of sensitivity somewhere on the lower part of the abdomen—urination will relieve it. Acute cystitis most often results in pain of two types: a dull, constant discomfort, and tenesmus at the termination of voiding. Stone in the bladder causes pain which is particularly noticeable after the patient has taken a ride over a rough road or he has been on a tractor for several hours. Or he may say that short-lasting, sharp pain was noted when he stepped off a high curbstone.

Any inflammatory process of the *urethra* or neck of the *bladder* or its adnexa can cause exquisite spasms of the bladder. Acute prostatitis may cause pain which is referred principally to the rectum, although often urinary retention also results from it and there is also pain due to the distended bladder.

Pain in the *penis* and *scrotal* region, when it is real, is usually due to inflammation, though there are other causes. The psychoneurotic individual will often mislead the physician without any encouragement, and unless some real cause for pain can be elicited by careful study it is best to bend one's efforts to reassurance.

Penile pain at the time of erection is almost certainly due to Peyronie's disease, though it can also be due to extensive stricture and periurethritis.

Testicular pain which comes on at night may be due to torsion of the cord, and unless this is corrected promptly, atrophy can and usually will result. Inflammation of the testes or epididymides or their tunics always produces pain, although tuberculosis of these structures may cause very little discomfort. A calculus lodged in the ureter or in the kidney in rare instances causes pain which is noticeable only in the testicle.

In the *female,* urethral pain may result from stenosis of the meatus or from prolapse of the mucosa or from caruncle. Seldom in recent years have my colleagues and I encountered skenitis as a cause.

Pain originating in any of the structures of the external genitalia may extend to the inguinal region or even to the renal region or down the inner aspects of the thigh.

Pyuria. The appearance of pus in the urine is perhaps the most important sign of disease somewhere within or immediately adjacent to the urinary tract. The degree of pyuria is of interest especially during observations incidental to treatment. It is almost axiomatic that bacteria are found when pus is present, but these can be extremely difficult to demonstrate and even harder to identify. *The specimen for analysis must be accurately obtained.* In the female, the finding of pyuria is worthless unless the specimen is obtained by catheterization. The specimen must be fresh; it cannot stand in the laboratory for hours before it is studied. In an alkaline urine, pus cells disintegrate quickly so that only amorphous debris remains. Lack of knowledge of this often denies patients the investigation they should receive when their physician gets a negative report on the microscopic study and fails to observe that the reaction of the urine is alkaline.

The existence of *pyuria without bacteria* being found by ordinary staining methods or by ordinary culture should always arouse suspicion of tuberculosis. However, virus infections may cause pyuria without bacteria being found. Intermittent pyuria of extreme degree should arouse suspicion of pericystitis with an abscess pocket (sometimes seen in association with sigmoidal diverticulitis) which drains into the bladder only when there is a sufficient collection of pus in the cavity to force its way through the small sinus tract. A ureteral stump or a chronic prostatic abscess cavity containing stones also exhibits this intermittent ability to cloud an otherwise clear urine. Anomalies such as an ectopic ureter emptying in the urethra can also cause it. Pyuria can be localized with reasonable accuracy by using the two-glass or three-glass test in the male but there are other more reliable methods which will be discussed later on (Fig. 53).

Hematuria. The source of gross bleeding usually can be found if one has the advantage of examining the patient while it is going on. If one postpones the examination until the next day, the bleeding may cease and no obvious cause for it may be found. In such instances, all one can do is prove or attempt to prove the normality of the urinary tract or at least exclude the

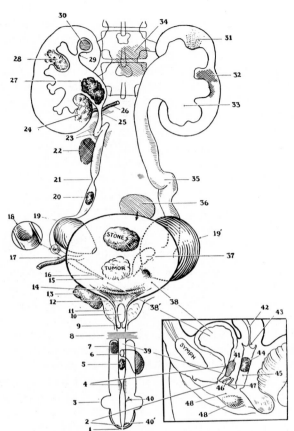

Fig. 53. Direct and indirect causes of pyuria: 1, stenosis of prepuce; 2, stenosis of urethral meatus and so forth; 3, paraphimosis; 4, urethral stricture; 5, urethral stone; 6, urethral diverticulum; 7, periurethritis, periurethral abscess; 8, cowperitis, chronic external sphincterospasm; 9, congenital valves of posterior urethra; 10, hypertrophy of verumontanum, verumontanitis, enlarged utricle or utricular diverticulum; 11, prostatitis, prostatic abscess; 12, contracted neck of bladder, median bar; 13, periprostatitis or pelvic suppuration; 14, mucosal fold at outlet of bladder, trigonal curtain; 15, stricture of ureteral meatus, ureterocele; 16, stricture of ureterovesical junction; 17, vascular obstruction of lower part of ureter; 18, congenital ureteral valves; 19, ureteral obstruction by compression from diverticulum; 19′, diverticulum; 20, ureteral stone; 21, ureteral stricture; 22, periureteritis, periureteral phlegmon or abscess; 23, ureteral kink, periureteral fibrous bands; 24, renal tumor; 25, stricture of ureteropelvic junction; 26, aberrant vessel (obstruction of upper part of ureter); 27, pelvic stone; 28, renal tuberculosis; 29, stricture of calyceal outlet; 30, calyceal stone; 31, pyelonephritis; 32, pyonephrosis; 33, "pyelitis," infected hydronephrosis; 34, perirenal suppuration invading urinary tract, spinal disease (Pott's disease and so forth); 35, hydroureter; 36, pericystic abscess rupturing into bladder; 37, seminal vesiculitis; 38, neuromuscular vesical disease; 38′, cystitis; 39, urethritis; 40, folliculitis (Littre); 40′, folliculitis (Morgagni); 41, periurethritis, periurethral abscess; 42, endometritis; 43, cervicitis; 44, foreign body in vagina; 45, vaginitis, hydrocolpos, fusion of labia minora; 46, skenitis; 47, folliculitis of introitus; 48, bartholinitis. (From Campbell, Clinical Pediatric Urology.)

presence of malignant disease. This is not as gratifying as to be able to observe a spurt of bloody urine issuing from one or the other ureteral orifice.

Some importance can be attached to the observation as to whether the bleeding is initial or terminal or total, but this information should be used only to supplement other data.

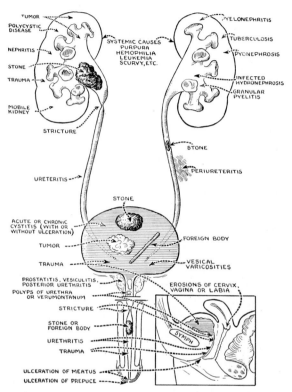

Fig. 54.   Usual causes of hematuria. Additional systemic, allergic, toxic and other unusual causes of hematuria are enumerated in the text. (Campbell, Clinical Pediatric Urology.)

There are many lesions which cause hematuria, as indicated in Figure 54. In addition there are several other causes which will be discussed in later chapters of this book.

So-called *essential hematuria* which appears intermittently in an otherwise healthy individual wherein one or the other kidney bleeds profusely for a few hours or a day or even a week is an interesting and puzzling condition. One might describe it as *renal epistaxis*. In spite of all study of the kidney, even if it is excised and sectioned serially, no abnormality may be found. Nor can one find any abnormality of the blood or its constituents or bleeding factors. If one has, after thorough pyelography, the courage to allow such kidneys to remain in the patient he is most often rewarded by a perfect recovery for many months or many years, when the patient may again be alarmed by another episode of bleeding, sometimes from the opposite kidney.

Microscopic hematuria or the presence of only a few erythrocytes in the voided specimen can be one of the most difficult conditions to localize that can be encountered in the entire practice of urology. In fact, it may be impossible to determine the source of these erythrocytes. The practice wherein patients mail specimens of urine to laboratories for analysis and receive reports directly from the laboratories has led to a great deal of worry and sometimes unnecessary expense. Interpretation of the report on a urinalysis should always be made by the patient's physician, and advice concerning the results of the tests should come from him. Nevertheless, urologists will continue to have this problem to face, and a great deal of meticulous investigation will be required in the future to try to find the cause of microscopic hematuria. Reassurance that no serious disease is present is perhaps of greatest importance in many cases.

Dysuria. Obstruction to urination or pain during the act can be classed under the broad heading of dysuria. Urinary hesitancy, decrease in the voiding distance, terminal dribbling and tenesmus or spasm of the perineal and bladder-neck musculature all signify mechanical or inflammatory disturbances of the urinary passages. Descriptive terms used by patients vary a great deal but any complaint should be carefully considered, and as a rule it is only through cystoscopic and urethroscopic study that the explanation of the symptoms becomes apparent. It is, of course, necessary for the urologist to be familiar with the normal as well as the abnormal in order to assess the condition of the patient properly and determine the need for treatment. For instance, an elderly man cannot, as a rule, expect to void as vigorously or freely as a teen-aged boy even though each can empty his bladder completely.

Oliguria or the passage of a substantially reduced amount of urine leading to anuria or complete cessation of the formation of urine is a symptom which one must be on the alert to observe as quickly as possible after it develops. Remedial measures can then be instituted early, as a rule to the patient's great advantage.

Uremia is the inevitable consequence of long-continued oliguria or anuria. It is due to retention in the blood of the nitrogenous waste products ordinarily eliminated by the kidneys. The causes of such retention will not be discussed here. The urologist should learn to recognize this condition by physical examination. There is no standard level of urea retention at which all patients exhibit certain symptoms. In most cases, however, anorexia, nausea and vomiting precede dehydration of the skin, dryness of the tongue, foul breath and mental torpor. It is only in extreme uremia, practically coma, that muscular twitchings and finally convulsions develop. Chronic renal insufficiency with moderate elevation of the level of blood urea and other nitrogenous elements results in secondary anemia. The lack of color in the patient's face and pale color of the nail beds and mucous membranes are valuable, often overlooked, signs of moderate uremia.

Fever. Elevations of temperature which accompany infections in the urogenital tract usually occur coordinately with other signs and symptoms which help in the diagnosis. But this is not always true. Sometimes fever is the earliest indication of disease, and the other signs do not appear for a number of hours or even days. Pain in one or both flanks with extension to the ureteral region justifies suspicion of pyelonephritis and, as a rule, urostasis. Frequency of urination, urgency and tenesmus develop as the bladder becomes inflamed.

Acute prostatitis, prostatic abscess and prostatic urethritis of severe extent usually cause temperature increases of several degrees. Obstruction to urination and retention of urine usually ensue. The cause of the trouble does not remain obscure very long in such acute conditions. On the other hand, recurring fever of mild degree is often caused by infections in the urinary or genital structures which result in slight or even intermittent pyuria. These cases present a more difficult diagnostic problem. Only by complete and thorough investigation, including careful roentgenographic study, are some of the problems solved. Anomalies of the kidneys and ureters must be suspected. An ectopic insertion of a supernumerary ureter may cause mild infection of the urinary tract which flares up so infrequently that it remains undiagnosed for years. Prostatic calculi contained in a small abscess cavity sometimes cause fever of so-called undetermined origin until a careful urologist notices that x-ray films have not included the prostatic region. Oddly enough, perineal discomfort usually is absent in such cases even though fever of high degree results from the condition.

Seminal vesiculitis can be responsible for low-grade fever for months before an attack of acute epididymitis directs attention to it.

Incontinence of urine in children or young adults should make one suspicious of an anomaly of the ureter with insertion of the ectopic orifice in the urethra or adjacent to the urethral orifice. In older women it is usually the result of relaxation of the perineal muscles following repeated childbirth. However, true incontinence must not be confused with urgency. In elderly men incontinence, especially nocturnal, is associated with obstruction of the vesical neck due to hypertrophy of the prostate—so-called paradoxical or overflow type. The incontinence due to disease or anomaly of the spinal cord results from faulty innervation of the urinary sphincters and as a rule is quite obvious because of other physical findings.

PHYSICAL EXAMINATION

The urologist cannot be expected to perform a general examination with the same skill as an internist. But he should be familiar with the requirements of a so-called basic examination. Not all patients who consult the urologist require thorough and complete general study. For instance, a man who appears in the office with a urethral discharge which has developed after intercourse does not need a roentgenogram of the chest or even of the bladder and renal area unless he has symptoms other than the chief complaint. It therefore behooves the urologist to collaborate with the general practitioner or the internist in most cases. The patient is best served in this way.

When the urologist finds a urologic condition which requires surgical treatment, he must insist that the patient undergo a thorough general physical survey before the operation is performed. The details of such an examination need not be discussed here. However, it seems proper to point out briefly a few things which are sometimes obvious in the course of general physical examination and which have an important bearing on urologic disease and on urologic therapy. The alert urologist often observes signs which are useful in planning his management of a condition. Obviously, one cannot discuss within the limits of this chapter much of the minutiae which clinicians through the decades have tried to get their students to observe, but if only a fraction of what is there waiting to be seen can be mentioned it may stress the fact that even modern medicine with its plethora of laboratory aids is practiced best by those physicians who keep their eyes open.

Head and Neck. The facies often tells the urologist a great deal about the patient's condition, especially as it changes from day to day during the course of therapy. Even in a primary examination the severity of a complaint may be indicated at least to some extent by the relative complacency of the visage. The sclerae and the pupils should be observed—sometimes one can practically clinch the diagnosis of tabetic bladder by recognizing an Argyll Robertson pupil. Pale conjunctivae may indicate the status of renal function. The slowness of the ocular movements and the stare of the unseeing eye mark the severely ill patient.

On many occasions one can detect an enlarged supraclavicular lymph node in a patient with malignant disease of the urinary tract. Rarely can an enlarged parathyroid gland be found in calculous disease but it is well to keep it in mind. Among other things, loss of weight may be made quite apparent by the looseness of a man's collar.

Thorax. The man with obvious enlargement of the breast may be ignorant of the fact that his home doctor has been treating him for prostatic cancer, but the evidence is usually convincing enough even though the prostate gland may now be small and soft.

The expansile power of the lungs and the percussion note, to say nothing of the breath sounds, give some knowledge of the general condition of the patient and his ability to withstand surgical procedures. A question or two as to whether any discomfort occurs in the substernal or precordial region while he is carrying on his daily tasks often proves worth while; in fact, the answers may be more significant than the electrocardiographic findings. The presence of a heart murmur may suggest the wisdom of employing antibiotic therapy if an operation on the urinary tract is contemplated. Axillary lymphadenopathy should arouse the suspicion of the urologist sufficiently to lead to special studies of the blood.

Abdomen. The general appearance of the abdomen should be studied carefully. If it is distended the examination may be unsatisfactory until another day when the bowel has emptied better. It is well not to be satisfied with palpation of the patient's abdomen on one particular day but to try again on succeeding days while he is under observation. I have often been able to feel a renal enlargement on a second or third try when the initial examination revealed nothing significant.

Tenderness over the *gallbladder,* if detected, may lead to other studies more important than urographic investigation in the patient who has related a vague story which has led one to suspect disease in the right kidney. A mass in the right upper quadrant has, on several occasions in my experience, proved to represent hydrops of the gallbladder and not a cyst in the kidney. Likewise, I have erroneously diagnosed a cyst in the left kidney which proved on operation to be a pancreatic cyst. Splenomegaly also can be falsely interpreted as a left renal mass.

Careful palpation often reveals the multiple grapelike clusters typical of congenital polycystic disease of the kidneys when pyelographic studies are equivocal.

Palpation of an *enlarged kidney* is usually not difficult if one remembers not to feel too high up in the abdomen but gently places the hand well down toward the lower quadrant while gently supporting the flank with the other hand. Having the patient breathe in and out slowly while this effort is being carried on is a useful maneuver well known to all examiners.

The distended bladder generally presents a mass that is easy to detect. It may push out more to one side, exciting a suspicion of a diverticulum. While one may be present, such an asymmetric shape more often represents a sacculation which projects well beyond the rest of the enlarged bladder. Often the patient is unaware of a distended bladder in advanced prostatic disease, although he may say that he has noticed in recent months that he has had to let out his belt repeatedly.

Many patients who consult a urologist because of urinary symptoms have lived long enough to have tumors in the colon or rectum; hence it behooves the examiner to palpate the entire abdomen carefully and to ask appropriate questions concerning bowel habits. In a fair proportion, roentgenograms of the gastrointestinal tract should supplement urologic investigation.

Rectum. It seems unnecessary to stress the need to include careful digital examination of the anus and rectum in every physical examination. But many practitioners avoid it entirely or depend upon what an associate or the intern finds. Some of this reluctance on the part of the physician is probably due to the aversion of the patient to this routine. The examination is not painful if the gloved finger is lubricated carefully in its entirety. Any patient reacts badly to forceful insertion of a rubber-covered finger lubricated on perhaps one fourth of its circumference. He tightens up and pulls away, and little useful information is obtained. One physician associate of mine insists that he has very willingly done rectal examinations on patients with whom he could not shake hands with any great enthusiasm. While the remark is rather facetious, it does stress the wisdom of not failing to include rectal examinations as routine.

The **prostate gland** should be palpated carefully, particular attention being given to feeling the extreme lateral borders and the apex. It is in this region that early malignant disease is often missed while the examiner palpates well beyond the growth. Gentle palpation sometimes permits detection of crepitation due to prostatic calculi. Tuberculosis of the genitourinary tract may be first suspected after a nodular area is felt in the prostate gland or in the seminal vesicle.

One important point that is often forgotten is that *the prostate gland should be examined when the bladder is empty.* Failure to observe this precaution may result in gross overestimation of the size of the prostate. In many cases, what seems to be a huge benign gland proves, after catheter drainage of the bladder, to be only a slightly or moderately enlarged gland. Furthermore, following catheter drainage, one frequently can detect areas of induration typical of malignant disease in what previously seemed to be a region of soft benign hypertrophy.

If blood is found on the examining finger, one must suspect a rectal neoplasm and insist on proctoscopic examination. Usually hemorrhoids are the cause.

Extremities. The general appearance of the arms and hands offers some evidence of the physical condition of the patient. Aside from this there are several things of interest to the urologist. For instance, one may find a radial artery of pipestem consistency resulting from generalized arteriosclerosis. The risk of any surgical procedure is often increased in such cases. On the contrary, when one finds thick calluses on the hands and good muscle tone, it is proof of excellent vigor, at least until a short time prior thereto.

Gouty tophi are occasionally found around the elbows of some patients, thus explaining renal colic due to nonopaque calculous disease. However, not all patients with gout form calculi.

The general appearance of the legs, the mobility of the hips, the presence of large varicose veins, and the condition of the arteries in the feet are points of interest. Contemplated surgical procedures and certainly postoperative care must often be altered in accordance with these findings. The presence of edema of the extremities not only should be noted at the time of initial examination but also should be watched for later on.

In both children and adults the arches and the toes should be examined for any deformity which may suggest myelodysplasia. This simple observation sometimes helps to explain dysfunction of the bladder. Obstructive uropathy due to congenital disease of the nervous system often does not appear until after several decades of life have passed.

URINALYSIS

The collection of urine for laboratory study should be made in such a way that the sample represents a portion of that passed during a period of twenty-four hours. This is essential because of the fact that urine passed about three hours after a meal is most likely to contain pathologic substances. Normally, about 60 gm. of solid constituents are carried off in a period of twenty-four hours, of which about 35 gm. are organic and 25 gm. inorganic substances. Urea constitutes about half of all the solids, or 30 gm. Other important organic constituents are uric acid and creatinine.

The inorganic matter consists chiefly of chlorides, phosphates, sulfates and ammonia. Sodium chloride makes up about half of the total amount of inorganic matter passed in a period of twenty-four hours.

In pathologic conditions such substances as proteins, bile, hemoglobin, carbohydrates and acetone appear.

Of chief interest to the urologist are the microscopic elements which urine contains. Normally these consist of epithelial cells, crystals of various sorts depending upon the pH of the specimen, and mucous threads. When disease is present, other things appear in the urine such as pus cells, erythrocytes, casts and bacteria of various kinds.

It is axiomatic that the specimen of urine to be examined should be a fresh one. Much time is often wasted if this fact is overlooked. An alkaline urine dissolves or disintegrates cellular elements, leaving only the débris which is sometimes mistaken for nonpathologic amorphous matter. One should make it a rule to be highly suspicious of an alkaline urine; the chances are that the patient has saved it over too long a period or has kept the specimen in some warm place where decomposition quickly sets in.

In the female the microscopic examination, if it is to be reliable, must usually be made on a catheterized specimen. In most instances the voided specimen contains pus cells which are usually present in the vaginal secretion, and in addition a flora of bacteria. This point is often overlooked by the general practitioner. Even if care is taken to collect a specimen after cleansing of the vaginal introitus, bacteria and pus cells often are found. Therefore, catheterization after sponging of the region of the urethral meatus provides a specimen upon which the best reliance can be placed.

In the male the urethra often contains mucus and secretion that harbor pus cells which contaminate the first few cubic centimeters of voided urine. For this reason the two-glass test gives a better index of the presence or absence of infection or inflammation of real urologic significance than does study of a catheterized specimen. As a general rule, it is best to rely on the analysis of the second-glass specimen.

The general aspects of urinalysis are familiar to all students of urology and will not be dealt with here. Those who are interested in the various technical details are referred to standard texts such as that of Todd, Sanford and Wells (1953).

However, there are two methods which seem worth stressing. The first is Gram's method of *differential staining of the urinary sediment.* This is very useful as an aid in classifying bacteria into the broad groups of gram-positive and gram-negative organisms. The choice of a urinary antiseptic to be used in treatment can often be made on this basis. Nevertheless, cultures of the urine and, further than that, sensitivity studies may be necessary if prompt response to treatment is lacking.

A rapid method of making a Gram's stain is as follows:

1. Make smears of a few drops of the sediment obtained by centrifuging, dry and fix by heat.

2. Cover the preparation for half a minute with a 2 per cent solution of crystal violet in methyl alcohol.

3. Wash with water.

4. Apply Gram's solution of iodine for half a minute.

5. Wash with alcohol until all the purple color ceases to come off.

6. Apply a contrast solution consisting of a 1 per cent aqueous solution of safranine.

7. Wash in water, dry thoroughly and study under the oil immersion objective.

The other staining method which will be mentioned is the *fluorescent-dye method of staining for acid-fast organisms*. Mycobacterium tuberculosis can best be found in the urine in this way. Auramine O is the dye used and the procedure involves use of the fluorescent microscope. If a careful search is made in a suspected case and several smears are studied, the organisms can often be found lying in clusters among the pus cells. A detailed description of the method is found in Todd, Sanford and Wells' textbook. Complete identification of the tubercle bacillus either by culture methods or by guinea-pig inoculation is regarded as necessary before surgical therapy can be advised.

The identification of pus cells in the fresh specimen of urine and the estimation of their number constitute one of the basic examinations upon which the practice of urology depends. The great majority of pus cells are polymorphonuclear leukocytes. These appear as granular spheric cells, about 10 to 12 microns in diameter, or somewhat larger than erythrocytes. The granules are partly the normal neutrophilic granules and partly granular products of degeneration. Each pus cell contains one irregular nucleus or several small rounded nuclei. These may be brought clearly into view by running a little dilute acetic acid under the cover glass. Thus cells in question can be differentiated from epithelial cells which have a single, rather large, round nucleus. In moderately acid urine the structure of the pus cell is well preserved. In strongly acid urine the cells may be shrunken and irregularly shaped. When the urine is strongly alkaline the cells are destroyed and converted into unrecognizable gelatinous débris.

While there is no generally accepted standard of what constitutes a normal or abnormal amount of pus in the urine specimen, I consider anything over 5 leukocytes per high power field found in the centrifuged fresh specimen as abnormal. Yet each year I see a great many patients who have several times this number but who have not the slightest symptom. Too often this lack of symptoms has been their misfortune. Moreover, persistence of a mild pyuria is of clinical importance.

Day-to-day estimation of the number of pus cells is a fairly reliable index of the degree of improvement which results from treatment. This estimation at first can sometimes be made best by the gross appearance of the specimen of urine. Of course one must often add a few drops of acetic acid to clear the haze resulting from phosphates which are present. As reduction in the degree of infection occurs, the estimation of the number of cells present in the high-power field of the microscope shows a steady fall until only a rare pus cell is present. The study of Gram's stain of the sediment likewise reveals a decrease and finally a total elimination of bacteria. Some urologists feel that this method is more reliable than cultural studies.

Erythrocytes when present in the urine always cause a positive reaction for albumin. In small quantities they impart a "smoky" color to the urine. They are usually not difficult to recognize with the microscope. However, fat, yeast and oxalate crystals may cause confusion, so that it is well to identify erythrocytes positively by examining them with the high-power dry objective.

Trichomonas vaginalis is sometimes found even in a catheterized specimen of urine. These parasites cause an intense cystitis at times and also persistent prostatitis. It is, therefore, imperative that wet smears of the centrifuged urine be studied in each case.

Extraneous structures sometimes found in the specimen of urine include yeast cells, mold fungi, and fibers of wool, cotton or silk derived from the dust in the air. Droplets of fat may be derived from unclean catheters or bottles in which the specimen is collected.

ESTIMATION OF RENAL FUNCTION

Several reliable tests of renal function are available to the urologist. The ones used most frequently are (1) estimation of nitrogen retention, (2) determination of phenolsulfonphthalein excretion and (3) determination of indigo carmine excretion. Other tests of importance include Volhard and Fahr's concentration and dilution tests, determination of the excretion of urea, and determination of the excretion of urographic media as revealed in the urogram. Most urologists depend for the most part on blood chemical studies such as estimation of the concentration of blood urea or urea nitrogen and, when indicated by elevation of these values, determination of the blood creatinine. In conjunction with these, the total volume of urine excreted in a period of twenty-four hours is usually closely followed in hospital cases, especially preoperatively and postoperatively. When the total amount of urine excreted is 1,500 cc. or more in twenty-four hours, renal function is usually adequate. However, in some cases in which the specific gravity is unusually low, several times this amount must be excreted if the kidneys are to eliminate a sufficient quantity of waste products from the blood stream.

The specific gravity of the urine often provides a rough indication of renal function; thus, if the specific gravity is 1.020 or above and there is no sugar present in the urine, one rarely finds that renal function is impaired. If Neo-iopax (sodium iodomethamate) or Diodrast (iodopyracet) or any other standard medium is visualized promptly (in the five-minute roentgenogram), it is almost a certainty that other tests of renal function will be found to give normal results. However, at least one other test for renal function should be made in any case in which an operation is contemplated.

Tests for phenolsulfonphthalein and indigo carmine excretion are used principally during cystoscopy for differential functional studies. But it is a fact that even these are seldom employed if the kidneys visualize well in the excretory urogram. When such visualization is lacking, however, the indigo carmine and the phenolsulfonphthalein excretion of each kidney should be carefully estimated. The difficulties sometimes encountered in the collection of specimens with ureteral catheters prompt the urologist to exercise good judgment in his evaluation of function in any case.

Other useful tests of renal function, especially if nephritis is suspected, are the urea clearance test and the determination of serum sulfates.

Most of the blood chemical tests which are useful to the urologist are listed in Table 5.

SPECIAL UROLOGIC INVESTIGATION

There are several methods of examination which can properly be included under this heading. This is especially true in regard to the male patient.

Table 5. Blood Chemical Tests: Normal Ranges

Calcium	9 to 11 mg. per 100 cc. of serum
Carbon dioxide combining power	25 to 29 mEq. per liter Adult: 53 to 65 volumes per 100 cc. of plasma Child: 40 to 50 volumes per 100 cc. of plasma
Chlorides	97 to 106 mEq. per liter 570 to 620 mg. of NaCl per 100 cc. of plasma
Creatinine	1 to 2 mg. per 100 cc. of blood
Nonprotein nitrogen	15 to 40 mg. per 100 cc. of serum
Phosphatase (alkaline) (acid)	5 Bodansky units or 14 King and Armstrong units or less per 100 cc. of serum (higher in children) 5 King and Armstrong units or less per 100 cc. of serum
Phosphorus (inorganic)	Adults: 1.6 to 3.0 mEq. per liter 2.5 to 4.5 mg. per 100 cc. of serum Children: 4.5 to 5.5 mg. per 100 cc. of serum Infants: 5.5 to 6.5 mg. per 100 cc. of serum
Potassium	4.0 to 5.0 mEq. per liter 15.5 to 19.5 mg. per 100 cc. of serum
Proteins (total)	15 to 19 mEq. per liter 6.4 to 7.8 gm. per 100 cc. of serum
Sodium	135 to 145 mEq. per liter 315 to 333 mg. per 100 cc. of serum
Sugar (glucose)	80 to 120 mg. per 100 cc. of blood
Sulfates (inorganic)	0.5 to 1.0 mEq. per liter 2.5 to 5.0 mg. of SO_4 per 100 cc. of serum
Urea	10 to 40 mg. per 100 cc. of blood
Urea nitrogen	9 to 17 mg. per 100 cc. of blood
Uric acid	3 to 6 mg. per 100 cc. of serum

Prostatitis and chronic nonspecific urethritis are often suspected. The symptoms which incite this suspicion need not be discussed in this chapter.

After a few questions are asked concerning urinary function, such as whether a urethral discharge has been noted (if so, smears should be made and perhaps a culture taken) and whether the patient has a specific complaint concerning the external genitals, he should be asked to void his urine into two glasses. The gross appearance of this specimen is noted. Brief questions concerning frequency of intercourse and sexual habits are then asked; any complaint of impotence should be recorded.

Thorough examination of the external genitalia should then be done even though the patient has no complaint. Palpation of each testicle, epididymis, vas deferens and spermatic cord, as well as the inguinal rings, should be done carefully in order to detect enlargement, induration, unusual tenderness or other abnormality of these structures. In order to detect pathologic conditions it is essential to be familiar with the normal. This justifies careful examination of every patient. The penis should be inspected to detect evidence of urethral discharge such as meatitis or excoriation. The penis should then be palpated, especially the corpora on the dorsal surface to note plaques which are characteristic of Peyronie's disease.

Then a careful *rectal examination* is made and the contour of the prostate gland and its immediate borders is noted. The size, shape and consistency of the prostate should be studied. If adenomatous enlargement is found, it is probably not wise to massage the gland, or if massage is given it should be gentle. In some patients the seminal vesicles can be palpated, but as a rule this is difficult in the average patient.

In order to obtain a specimen of the *prostatic secretion* for microscopic study, each lobe is massaged, using moderate pressure and directing the stroke downward toward the apex. Several strokes on each side and a final stroke through the prostatic sulcus between the lobes will, as a rule, express a few drops of fluid which can be collected on a slide, covered with a cover slip and then examined under the microscope. The normal secretion is slightly opalescent and contains numerous small granules and lecithin bodies. Corpora amylacea are sometimes found. When prostatitis exists, pus cells are present singly and in clumps. However, it is generally agreed that even the normal secretion contains a few leukocytes.

In some cases, especially when prostatitis is present, very little secretion can be obtained at the time of the first massage. Therefore, it is usually well to repeat the examination the next day when a better flow of secretion will result.

Smears of the prostatic secretion are generally difficult to stain. Therefore, if one wishes to determine whether bacteria are present, cultures should be made.

Tests for Residual Urine. This test is indicated whenever there is a history of urinary difficulty or whenever in any patient beyond the fifth decade of life there is any reason to suspect retention of urine. The patient is given plenty of time to void before the test, and as a rule it is best to ask him to hold his urine for at least thirty minutes before the test is planned. This will insure there being sufficient urine in the bladder to permit a reasonably normal urination. He should then be placed on the examining table with the legs extended where, under aseptic precautions, a small soft-rubber catheter, preferably with a Coudé tip and well lubricated, is passed. If any obstruction is encountered in the penile portion of the urethra, one can assume that it is due to stricture. Calibration with bougies may then be advisable. Normally, if the catheter passes readily, only a few drops of urine or at most a few cubic centimeters will be found. Any substantial amount suggests obstruction of the vesical neck.

In the female a substantial amount of residual urine is not infrequently found when there is a history of recurring cystitis extending through many months or years. Often these patients are not aware of urinary difficulty. The retention in most cases is caused by contracture of the vesical neck or cicatricial changes due to infection.

EXCRETORY UROGRAPHY

It is probably not an overstatement to say that no other single examination provides as much useful information for the physician as a well-made excretory urogram. While cystoscopic examination combined with retrograde pyelographic study might subsequently be necessary, there are many urologists who insist that the excretory urogram should be a part of every thorough urologic investigation, and furthermore it should in most cases precede cystoscopy for several reasons. Chief among these is the fact that enough information may be obtained with the excretory urogram to make instrumental examination entirely unnecessary. Also the excretory study may reveal anomalies of the upper part of the urinary tract which might be overlooked during the course of cystoscopy. Then, too, the method affords an excellent test of renal function in most cases. During the course of cystoscopy there is always some risk of introducing infection into the urinary tract which, if stasis exists, will result in a severe febrile reaction. If, for instance, a patient has hydronephrosis and retrograde study is not done with the utmost precaution, severe pyelitis or even cortical infection can result. This complication may cause serious delay in surgical therapy.

The main *contraindication* to the use of the excretory urogram is the idiosyncrasy to the medium that is encountered occasionally. Usually this cannot be detected until a large amount of the drug has been injected. In these days the patient usually has already suffered a reaction from a previously attempted excretory study. In such cases one should elect retrograde pyelography instead. Extremely ill patients or extremely old ones and those with obvious renal insufficiency should not be subjected to the excretory test. As a general rule in these cases the drug does not visualize well. Seldom is there any visualization whatever when the concentration of urea in the blood exceeds 70 mg. per 100 cc.

One of the chief disadvantages of excretory urography is the incomplete visualization and lack of detail of the calyces, or at least some of them, in a fair proportion of cases. This is probably due to intermittent peristaltic activity of the calyces and the renal pelvis and ureter. Methods to establish pressure on the terminal third of the ureter with corsets containing inflatable bags, sometimes with the addition of blocks of balsa wood of various shapes, usually fail to produce consistent results. In the occasional case one finds the entire length of both ureters, as well as both pelvis and all the calyces, well filled; however, in some cases this procedure results in abnormal dilatation which may be misleading. It is usually best to rely only on the pressure of the large bag placed under the canvas band that is used only to establish pressure chiefly intended to hold the abdomen firmly and restrict or deter the patient from taking a breath while the exposure is made. All other devices are usually abandoned after a period of trial.

If one pieces together the several roentgenograms obtained during the course of the urographic study he will usually have a reasonably complete picture of the entire urinary tract. However, one must avoid any tendency to read more into the urogram than is actually present. In case of doubt, retrograde pyelography should be done.

The medium employed is any one of the several standard preparations. It should be given intravenously whenever possible. About the only exception is in the case of very small infants when venipuncture is impossible. In these patients the contrast medium can be diluted with isotonic saline solution to a total volume of 100 cc. and injected subcutaneously in divided amounts of 50 cc. over the angle of each scapula. The addition of a small amount of hyaluronidase solution (Simon and Narins, 1949) will speed up the absorption of the medium.

The method of giving the medium intravenously has been debated for years. A good one that has been used for many years at the Mayo Clinic is to use a 20 cc. Luer syringe equipped with a 21-gauge needle. After careful venipuncture, 1 or 2 cc. of the solution are injected slowly. If no untoward reaction is observed within thirty seconds, the entire amount is then rapidly injected within an additional two minutes. Less arm pain will result if the medium is injected very rapidly than is experienced if it is injected slowly.

The plain roentgenogram made prior to injection and the one obtained five minutes after completion of the injection should be developed immediately and examined as soon as possible. An experienced technician will note whether or not there are any shadows in the usual course of the ureter or in the renal area. If such are found, the straight anteroposterior roentgenogram which is obtained twenty minutes after completion of the injection may be profitably supplemented with additional films obtained by slight angulation of the patient's body on the x-ray table. Such films usually throw phleboliths or other shadows lying directly over the ureter away from it. Likewise, shadows such as gallstones which sometimes lie over the renal area are similarly projected away from the kidney. As a general rule, if renal function is normal, the five-minute and twenty-minute roentgenograms suffice, but when function is reduced or delayed, films should be taken forty-five minutes after injection. In rare cases when there is considerable hydronephrosis, additional films obtained as long as eight or ten hours after injection will provide the best picture.

Excellent roentgenographic technique is an art learned by trial and error through a long period of apprenticeship. Absolute essentials are the accurate placement of the patient on the table, careful measurement of the thickness of each individual in order to calculate the exposure time correctly, use of clean cassettes, exposure while the patient holds his breath to avoid movement, and finally development of the film in solutions which are of proper strength and properly cooled. Lack of attention to any of these details produces films which are blurred or muddy in appearance or of poor texture, and they can be easily detected by the expert whose duty it is to read them. Excretory urography can quickly fall into disrepute in x-ray laboratories or hospitals where carelessness in details of roentgenographic technique is condoned. The method itself should not be criticized under these circumstances. It is the duty of the urologist to insist on better effort by the technicians.

The interpretation of the completed excretory urogram is a subject which can be considered only superficially in this chapter. A complete treatise has been written by Braasch and Emmett (1951). The variations of the normal urogram itself constitute a topic requiring extensive description. The deviations from normal caused by various pathologic changes produce a variety of patterns consisting of calyceal deformity and alterations of contour of the renal pelvis and ureter of many types.

In addition to changes in contour of the hollow structure of the kidney, the changes in position and outline of the cortical portion of the organ must be considered in making the final interpretation. If one keeps in mind the many possible lesions which alter the normal anatomic structure, the diagnosis is usually not difficult. Subsequent chapters will contain illustrations of urograms of various patterns which with other data make an accurate diagnosis probable in a high percentage of cases.

INSTRUMENTAL EXAMINATIONS

The art of urology is demonstrated best in the use of instruments for urethral, bladder and ureteral investigation. Many tools have been devised during the past 150 years by countless urologists for various purposes. The methods of using these are truly the most important part of the education of any student of the specialty. He must be familiar with the various types that are available, and the selection of the proper instrument to employ in diagnosing or treating the affliction that besets the patient is of paramount importance. Furthermore, the proper preparation for use and the care of the instruments to keep them in first-class condition and readily available when they are needed are highly essential if the diagnosis is to be established with skill and precision. Too often, ingenious manufacturers have fabricated beautiful catheters, sounds, dilators, cystoscopes of all sizes and countless other devices which cannot serve their purpose if they are abused or if they are not selected with due consideration and handled gently.

Figures 55 and 56 illustrate some of the *catheters* and *bougies* with which the student must become familiar. Practice extending through a period of years will finally result in the development of a sense of touch which is almost as important in urethral instrumentation as is good eyesight in the art of cystoscopy.

A frequently encountered example of urologic art is the ease with which a urologist catheterizes a patient with a properly selected catheter after someone else has made many unsuccessful attempts with an oversized, worn out, improperly prepared piece of rubber which resembles a coiled bedspring.

Sounds of the van Buren or LeFort filiform type are useful in calibrating the urethra or in dilating strictures. These must be passed with gentleness and caution, usually after the instillation of some suitable anesthetic agent. The filiform to which sounds or catheters may be attached is not a difficult instrument to pass if one will slowly roll it back and forth between the thumb and index finger while advancing and retracting it as it is passed through the urethra. This method will be found much more efficient than

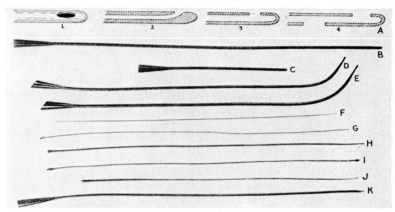

Fig. 55.   Various types of urethral instruments required for urologic investigation in the young. A, tips of soft rubber catheters; 2, "velvet eye"; 3, single eye, hollow tip; 4, double eye, Robinson type. B, Robinson catheter, male type; C, Robinson catheter, female type; D, modified natural curve silk catheter; E, natural curve silk catheter; F, whalebone filiform; G, silk urethral filiform; H, woven silk bougie; I, olivary bougie, acorn bougie; J, Phillips whip filiform; K, Phillips follower catheter. (Campbell, Clinical Pediatric Urology.)

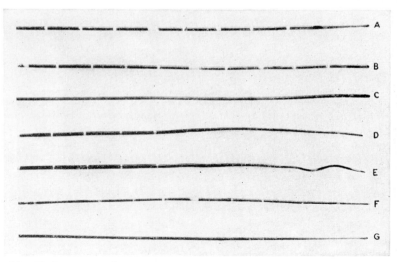

Fig. 56.   Various types of ureteral catheters. Note centimeter markings with broad band indicating 5 cm. A, olivary tip; B, round tip; C, whistle tip; D, Blasucci filiform (rat-tail); E, spiral rat-tail; F, calibrated olivary tip silk bougie; G, whalebone tip bougie. (Campbell, Clinical Pediatric Urology.)

filling the urethra with a half dozen or more filiforms in the hope that one of them will find its way through the narrow point.

Palpation of the urethra over a sound is occasionally useful in detecting areas of induration or small periurethral pockets which form in the glands of Littre.

The use of the *urethrogram* as an aid in diagnosis has been established on rather firm ground during the past decade or two. The method is described in the chapter by Emmett on neuromuscular dysfunction (Section XI) and

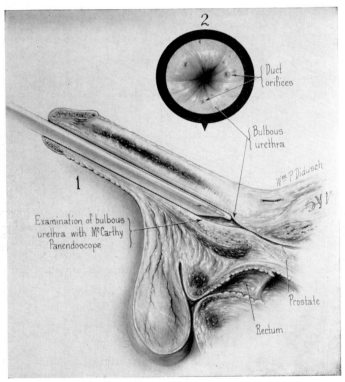

Fig. 57.   The McCarthy panendoscope permits inspection of the entire course of the urethra. (Figures 57–69 reproduced from Urological and Allied Diagnostic Instruments and High Frequency Equipment, American Cystoscope Makers, Inc., New York.)

need not be repeated here. He also describes *cystography* which, of course, is often combined with urethrography in order to portray graphically by means of the roentgenogram urethral and bladder deformities of all types.

Urethroscopy should be employed whenever it seems necessary to visualize the urethra accurately. The early urethroscopes were equipped with an attachment which allowed one to distend the urethra with air (Gordon). The best urethroscope, in my opinion, is a small-caliber beakless sheath devised by McCarthy. The foroblique lens system visualizes the entire circumference of the urethra, and with the aid of water distention the urethra can be ballooned out and accurately visualized throughout by passing the sheath slowly from the external meatus through the navicular portion, the anterior urethra, the bulb and finally the region of the external sphincter and the prostatic urethra (Fig. 57). Inflammatory conditions, strictures, papillomas, diverticula, neoplasms and so forth can be brought into clear view with this instrument. Urethral investigation is certainly not complete until this has been done; however, not all patients require it.

CYSTOSCOPY

The development of the *cystoscope* has been discussed adequately in 1933 in a publication of the American Urological Association. The invention of the electric light by Edison was the real necessity in its development. Reinhold Wappler and his associates produced lenses of superb quality and during the past decade the method of coating lenses to increase their efficacy has finally brought forth instruments which are practically perfect. The cystoscope used for examination of the adult by almost all urologists is of the Brown-Buerger type, usually 21 F. in caliber, equipped with both examining and double catheterizing telescopes. Another instrument which is very efficient is the Braasch direct-vision cystoscope. This is also equipped with an examining right-angle lens and a catheterizing sheath through which ureteral catheters can be passed.

For the examination of infants and children smaller, very efficient cystoscopes have been devised. Among these are the Meredith Campbell cystoscope, the McCarthy infant cystoscope, and the Butterfield cystoscope (see Section XIII). With any of these instruments, examination of tiny babies can be done with ease and if necessary the ureters can be catheterized with great precision. Special types of cystoscopes include those equipped with a retrograde lens telescope with which the neck of the bladder can be seen with greater clarity than is possible with any other instrument. The skilled urologist learns how to use all of these instruments, for each has certain advantages that help to increase his efficiency in diagnosis.

Anesthesia. The need for adequate anesthesia is obvious. In men one efficient type is the *local instillation* of freshly prepared 1 per cent solution of cocaine hydrochloride. Two tablets, each containing 2.28 grains of the drug, are dissolved in 1 ounce of sterile distilled water. The resulting solution is injected into the urethra with a rubber-bulb urethral syringe. In addition, a small swab of 10 per cent solution of cocaine hydrochloride is placed in the urethral meatus and with the help of a penis clamp or pressure of a rubber band the solution is kept in place for about ten minutes prior to examination. In the female one needs only to place the swab of 10 per cent solution of cocaine in the urethral meatus—no instillation of solution is necessary.

Another drug which has remarkable anesthetic action is Pyribenzamine (tripelennamine)—a 1 per cent solution injected into the urethra and retained for ten minutes seems to produce just as much anesthesia as 1 per cent solution of cocaine hydrochloride. In a series of 400 cases, cocaine and Pyribenzamine were injected alternately. Careful analysis disclosed that these drugs were equally effective.

General anesthesia is necessary in approximately 10 per cent of cases in order to perform cystoscopic examination efficiently. It must be recognized that patients differ considerably, and the very apprehensive individual suffers a great deal in spite of adequate local anesthesia. The urologist must never be satisfied with inadequate inspection of the bladder. A hurried examination is seldom satisfactory. Inhalation anesthetics have to a large extent been replaced or at least supplemented by Pentothal (thiopental) sodium or Surital (thiamylal) sodium injected intravenously. Either of these drugs injected slowly in 2.5 per cent solution produces sufficient relaxation to permit thorough cystoscopy in all but exceptional cases.

Young children who fear venipuncture and all the other unpleasantness of an operating room can be spared the ordeal by *intrarectal injection* of Pentothal sodium. The drug can be introduced into the rectum in 10 per cent solution, the effective dose being 15 to 20 mg. per pound of body weight. However, this should always be done under the careful supervision of a physician who then stays with the child if it is done in the patient's room and continues with constant observation on the trip to the operating room. Here the addition of a small amount of nitrous oxide may or may not be necessary. This method of anesthesia is particularly appropriate for those patients for whom multiple trips to the operating room become necessary. It has been used successfully in infants less than a year old, and worried parents think it is a particularly pleasing method of anesthesia.

Spinal anesthesia induced by the injection of procaine hydrochloride is unsurpassed for those cases in which thorough relaxation for an hour or more is desirable. It probably interferes less with renal function than any other anesthetic agent, and for this reason it may be desirable in those instances in which differential functional studies are needed.

Indications. The indications for cystoscopy are numerous and it is no doubt true that any list which can be made will fail to include all of them. It is a certainty that the procedure should be carried out in any case wherein one has any good reason to suspect abnormality of the urinary or genital tract. Without it any examination of the urinary tract must be considered incomplete. However, the mere fact that other examinations and tests have not disclosed significant data is not necessarily justification for cystoscopic examination, with the discomfort and minimal temporary physical disability which it may inflict. The evidence must be weighed carefully before any patient can be advised or urged to submit to the procedure. Cystoscopy seems indicated for the following purposes:

1. To determine the source of hematuria.
2. To determine the source of pyuria.
3. To determine the cause of dysuria.
4. To catheterize the ureters.
5. To take biopsy specimens from suspected intravesical lesions.
6. To treat lesions within the bladder or neck of the bladder.
7. To determine the cause of failure of medical therapy.

The contraindications to cystoscopy are few. Perhaps the most important ones are:

1. Advanced renal insufficiency which can be improved by appropriate therapy before cystoscopy is attempted.
2. Acute specific urethritis.
3. Severe prostrating illness due to acute disease of organs other than those of the urogenital tract.

EQUIPMENT FOR CYSTOSCOPIC EXAMINATION

Any good standard table with leg rests will serve the purposes of ordinary cystoscopy. For urographic study a Bucky diaphragm and tube stand must be added. A Bucky diaphragm with a 50-line grid or one of the newer reciprocating types is best, and a rotating anode x-ray tube makes very short exposures possible, thus reducing to a minimum blurring of the film due to motion. Refinements in table construction such as the electric hydraulic base increase the efficiency of the cystoscopist; they make possible rapid changes in position and save a great deal of back strain. The patients benefit by shortening of the time of cystoscopy.

Thorough preparation for cystoscopy is highly desirable. Nothing does more to insure failure than lack of equipment or lack of sufficient foresight to have it properly sterilized and ready for use.

The sterilization and proper packaging of supplies constitute a problem which varies in any office, hospital or clinic depending upon the demands. If only a few cases are listed, there may be time to assemble and sterilize all the necessary items in the half hour prior to examination. In some hospitals this seems necessary because each urologist owns his own equipment and as a rule brings it with him for the nurse to prepare while he dons his operating room uniform. This can lead to slovenly preparation and as a result infection and febrile postcystoscopic reactions. A better method would be to bring the cystoscope and any additional accessories wrapped in sterile towels ready for immediate use. Of course, this would involve preliminary preparation of them in the urologist's office or by the nurse who last assisted him with a case.

At the Mayo Clinic, cystoscopes after they are used are thoroughly washed with water and soap solution and carefully rinsed in running water. The light is then tested and the various telescopes and accessories after similar cleansing are finally immersed completely in oxycyanide of mercury solution (1:1,000) to remain for twenty minutes. They are lifted from this solution with a forceps and placed in a pan with a well-fitting cover previously autoclaved. The light cord is immersed in 70 per cent alcohol and this too is finally placed in the pan. The instrument is now ready for immediate use and will remain sterile for several days or a week if necessary. If preferred, the instrument can be wrapped in a sterile towel. Linen used to drape the patient's legs and abdomen is packaged and autoclaved separately.

Ureteral catheters, after being thoroughly washed, are sterilized by first siphoning a solution of oxycyanide of mercury through the lumen for fifteen minutes and then soaking the entire catheter in the solution. Unless the preliminary siphoning is done, no amount of soaking of the entire catheter will sterilize its interior. Ureteral catheters are sterilized in this way in lots of a dozen or more but are packaged in pairs, doubling them only once in a flat sterile towel. It is a deplorable practice to wind ureteral catheters in a circle, place them in a few layers of gauze and immerse them in an antiseptic solution or even attempt their sterilization in a formaldehyde cabinet. Even boiling ureteral catheters will fail to sterilize the interior of them if the lumen contains air. Our experience dictates that the siphon method of sterilization is the best even though it is somewhat tedious and exacting.

TECHNIQUE OF CYSTOSCOPY

After the patient has been properly anesthetized and after the cystoscope, the ureteral catheters properly threaded in the catheterizing sheath, the small

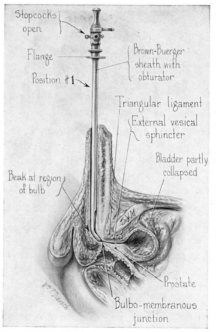

Fig. 58.   Cystoscopy. Introduction of the cystoscope in the male; initial step (see text). (American Cystoscope Makers.)

pans for specimens, and the syringes have all been laid out on a small sterile table, the urologist should first check the light to see that it is properly regulated and of sufficient intensity and that it does not flicker. A poorly fitting light cord is a great handicap. The cystoscope should be further inspected to see that the obturator fits properly and that there are no sharp or rough edges on it anywhere in its length. Thorough lubrication of the cystoscope with a water-soluble jelly will permit the passage of the instrument with much greater facility than is possible if one merely dips the tip into a small quantity of mineral oil.

During the cystoscopic examination, gentleness in every movement and the avoidance of quick jerky efforts will reassure the patient and will avoid unnecessary trauma. One should not just push the cystoscope after it is introduced into the meatus but instead should hold it steadily and try to feel with it as it is passed. In the male the instrument should at first be passed down in the direction of the table until the floor of the bulbous urethra is reached (Fig. 58); at this point the tip of the instrument should be lifted a fraction of an inch and the ocular end should then be depressed so that the beak will rise up over the sphincter and slip into the prostatic urethra (Fig. 59). At this point, if there is much enlargement of the middle

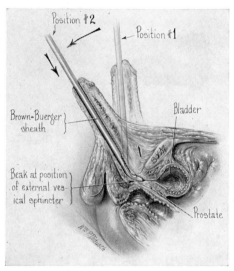

Fig. 59. Cystoscopy. Ocular end of cystoscope is depressed as the beak enters and passes through the prostatic urethra (see text). (American Cystoscope Makers.)

lobe of the prostate gland, or if there is a bar formation, further downward excursion of the ocular end may be necessary so that the beak will ride up over the obstruction and pass into the bladder. If the instrument tends to catch at any point, one should not force it through. Instead, the cystoscope should be withdrawn slightly and the direction of its passage changed to the right or left or up or down. If, on further attempts the instrument fails to pass, it should be withdrawn entirely and a curved van Buren sound or, if necessary, a LeFort filiform sound should be used to dilate the narrow point. In females, not infrequently one finds stenosis of the urethral meatus which requires meatotomy or dilatation with a Kelly tapered dilator before it is possible to introduce the cystoscope.

When the tip of the instrument has passed into the bladder the obturator is withdrawn and the urine present is collected in a sterile test tube for culture and, if there is enough of it, for microscopic examination (Fig. 60). One always finds at least the few cubic centimeters which have formed during the time the patient has been prepared for examination. The presence of a large amount, if the patient was carefully instructed to empty the bladder before getting on the table, causes one to suspect that he has obstruction of the neck of the bladder; however, it must be remembered that some of the solution used for anesthesia will find its way into the bladder, so that this amount must be deducted in computing the residual.

After the water line has been connected, care should be taken to prevent the air present in it from entering the bladder in large quantity lest the resulting air bubble obscure a large part of the dome. The wall of the bladder should be watched carefully as it distends; the flexibility of the wall is an indication of its normality. The *atonic bladder* hangs down in folds and is often sacculated. *Trabeculation* of the wall excites suspicion of obstruction of the vesical neck. *Areas of inflammation* can be easily recognized; small

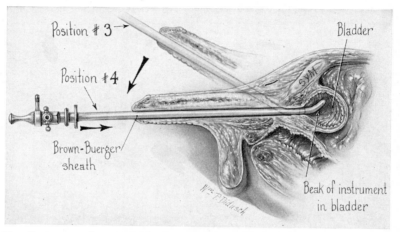

Fig. 60.   Cystoscopy. Instrument in proper position for study of the bladder interior and to catheterize the ureters (see text). (American Cystoscope Makers.)

inflammatory cysts studded in patches over the bladder, so-called *cystitis cystica,* are an indication of chronic infection of many months' or years' standing. The color of the mucosa, the way the light reflects from it, and the appearance of the small vessels in the submucosa are all important points noted by the practiced eye.

The best opportunity for examining the bladder with a patient under local anesthesia is during its first filling, and one should add water at a rate that is slow enough to permit inspection of the entire interior before the wall of the bladder is put on a stretch. Now and then one encounters a patient, usually a female, in whom the results of preliminary urinalysis have been negative and whose bladder seems unusually irritable. If careful, the cystoscopist may note a small salmon-colored patch on one of the lateral walls or dome which, as the bladder distends more, providing the patient will permit it, gradually fades away and finally blanches. This is Hunner's elusive ulcer or interstitial cystitis. Many such patients, because of the lack of positive urinary findings, have been accused of being neurotics.

The several types of cystoscopes have certain disadvantages as well as advantages. For instance, when the physician is using a Brown-Buerger cystoscope he must be sure, when looking at the posterior wall, to rock the instrument from side to side or it will be impossible to visualize an area directly posterior. This is the so-called blind spot. I have seen a number of patients in whom tumors in this area were overlooked by expert urologists. The posterior wall is best visualized with a McCarthy panendoscope or a Braasch cystoscope. However, neither of the latter instruments provides accurate visualization of the anterior wall or of the lateral walls just proximal to the vesical neck. As previously stated, only a retrograde lens will permit

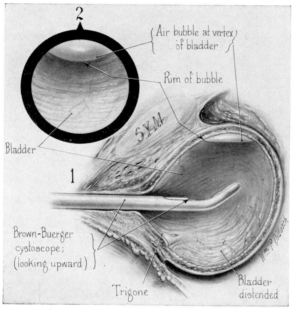

Fig. 61. Cystoscopy. The air bubble is always found at the highest point of the bladder interior and serves as a landmark for orientation (see text). (American Cystoscope Makers.)

complete visualization of the internal urethral orifice when any substantial degree of deformity in this area is present. Hence, it behooves the expert urologist to familiarize himself with all the available instruments and furthermore to make use of them when the occasion demands.

Normal bladders vary considerably in appearance, even as much as faces. In addition, the bladder changes through the decades of life so that the same bladder examined in youth will be somewhat different in appearance in middle age or in advanced age, though it must still be considered normal. Furthermore, these minor differences resulting from aging have no clinical significance.

The neck of the bladder and the prostatic urethra must be inspected carefully (Figs. 61–65). Minimal enlargement of the prostate gland may be noted as a collar or welt of tissue projecting up into the cavity of the bladder or there may be enlargement of only the middle lobe. Equal or unequal enlargements of the lateral lobes may project into the cavity of the bladder or only into the urethra. All these variations appear as differ-

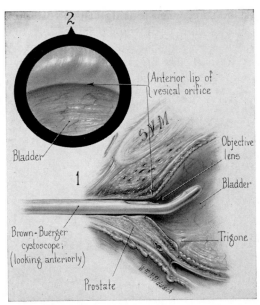

Fig. 62.   Cystoscopy. Observation of the superior segment of the bladder outlet (see text). (American Cystoscope Makers.)

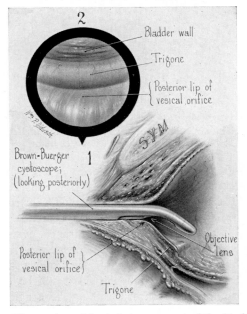

Fig. 63.   Cystoscopy. Observation of the inferior segment of the bladder outlet (see text). (American Cystoscope Makers.)

ences in the clefts or angles in the anterior commissure or in the lateral angles or in what is sometimes referred to as the 7 and 8 o'clock or the 4 and 5 o'clock positions. Further than this, the amount of approximation of the lateral lobes of the prostate gland within the urethra and their length should all be carefully noted. If there is no enlargement of the prostate gland, the prostatic portion of the urethra may be entirely normal in texture, color and contour, or if inflamed, it will be reddened and injected and may bleed easily or there may be dilated ducts which exude purulent secretion on the slightest pressure. This indicates prostatitis, or abscess of a prostatic duct.

In the female the urethra may be smooth, soft and pliable or it can be scarred and cicatricial; polypoid masses of inflammatory tissue or inflammatory cysts may be present (Fig. 65); or one may find an opening leading to a diverticulum.

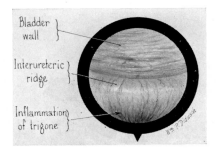

Fig. 64.   Cystoscopy. Study of the trigone (see text). (American Cystoscope Makers.)

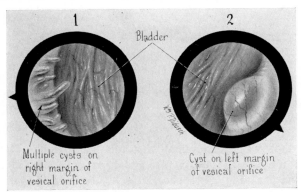

Fig. 65.   Cystoscopy. Cystic changes about the vesical outlet (see text). (American Cystoscope Makers.)

Of greatest importance in cystoscopic examination is recognition of the normal. To be able to judge what is normal the student must have the opportunity to examine many hundreds of patients. Naturally one may see in any patient a normal urethra along with a diseased bladder, or for instance, one may see one ureteral orifice that is quite normal in appearance while the other is involved in some pathologic process. The art of cystoscopy can be acquired rapidly if one has a good teacher to point out these things.

The most skilful urologist can be handicapped by various unexpected difficulties. The bladder often becomes irritable and goes into spasm before it can be thoroughly examined. Unless this subsides promptly it may be wise to stop the procedure and try again on another day, perhaps with the advantage of general anesthesia. Mistakes will creep in if one is inclined to draw final conclusions from what is actually an unsatisfactory examination. A week of treatment may soothe an inflamed bladder, and re-examination may reveal an underlying neoplasm. Nor must one be deluded into thinking that any cystoscopic examination always reveals everything that is present. As previously pointed out, if therapy fails, the wise urologist after a reasonable interval will look into the bladder again.

It is often impossible to accomplish accurate urethroscopy with a Brown-Buerger type of cystoscope. In fact, one might go so far as to say that it

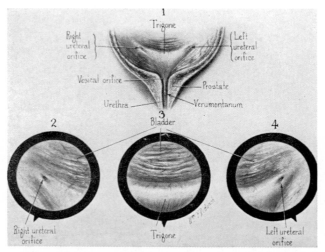

Fig. 66.   Ureteral orifices viewed cystoscopically. (Reproduced from Urological and Allied Diagnostic Instruments and High Frequency Equipment, American Cystoscope Makers, Inc., New York, p. 43.)

is seldom possible. I have seen many women suffering from a urethral diverticulum that was overlooked with this instrument. Therefore, it is often wise to use the McCarthy panendoscope or a similar instrument to examine the urethra (Fig. 57). The Braasch direct-vision cystoscope is also an excellent urethroscope. It is a good practice to examine the entire length of the urethra as the instrument is withdrawn. Wide-caliber strictures, neoplasms and diverticula may be found.

Ureteral catheterization is an integral part of cystoscopy. However, since the advent of excretory urography, it has been found necessary in far fewer cases. It is sometimes essential to supplement excretory studies with retrograde pyelography, so that the ureters must be catheterized for this reason; further, it is an absolute necessity when one wishes to determine whether pyuria is of renal origin.

The ureteral orifices can be found easily, as a rule, by searching along the ureteral ridge from the midline of the trigone laterally on each side (Fig. 66). Usually, there are only two orifices but in rare instances unilateral or bilateral duplication may be found. Normally the ureteral orifice varies from a small pinpoint type of meatus to a slit several millimeters long. Their position is usually symmetric but minor deviation may be found. As one observes the orifice the areola usually contracts and a jet of urine issues from it. Normally the urine is clear but in disease it may be cloudy or purulent, or when blood is present the jet may seem smoky or even quite red, depending on the degree of hematuria. One should watch for the spurt in any case, but if the patient has been on a restricted intake of fluid, too much time must not be lost, particularly if one intends to catheterize the ureters. If either meatus is not readily found, the region of the vesical

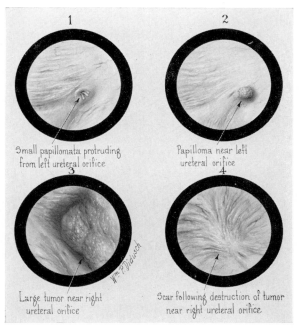

Fig. 67. Cystoscopic views of pathologic conditions. (Reproduced from Urological and Allied Diagnostic Instruments and High Frequency Equipment, American Cystoscope Makers, Inc., New York, p. 173.)

lip should be examined. Especially in the female the meatus may be found in this region, or in rare instances one may find it within the urethra.

When the orifice of the ureter is very small a ureterocele may be present and the areola may be observed to bulge into the bladder and attain the size of a grape or even a larger size. If the areola is edematous and reddened, one must suspect the presence of an intramural calculus. In cases of vesical neoplasm the meatus may be entirely obliterated by the infiltrating tumor (Figs. 67, 68, 69).

Passing the catheter when the meatus of the ureter is normal and easily found is not difficult, but of course it is a procedure which requires some practice before one becomes adept. The tip of the catheter should be advanced carefully until the meatus has been entered. Then it can be passed more rapidly up the ureter. If the tip of the catheter does not engage readily, one must not immediately suspect narrowing. Rather, the trouble is probably an anatomic variation which brings the tip up in a fold of mucosa; the catheter should be withdrawn slightly and another attempt made. If one is using a direct-vision cystoscope the catheter can be twisted slightly, thus changing the direction of the tip. As a rule, one should try No. 5 F. catheters first. If one of this size refuses to pass, a No. 4 F. catheter will usually go up without the slightest difficulty. I have seen many cases in which an erroneous diagnosis of ureteral stricture was made because some minor deviation of the lumen of the ureter prevented the immediate passage of a

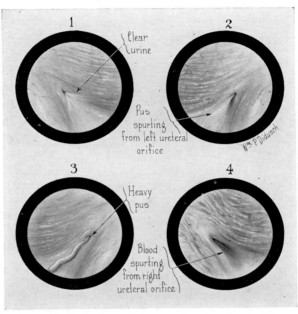

Fig. 68. Cystoscopic views of pathologic conditions (continued). (Reproduced from Urological and Allied Diagnostic Instruments and High Frequency Equipment, American Cystoscope Makers, Inc., New York, p. 173.)

catheter. It hardly seems necessary to add that one should use a catheter which is in good condition, reasonably pliable and of course with a smooth coating, uncracked and free of any blemish. Catheters which have small filiform or corkscrew ends prove very useful at times. These should be kept sterile and readily available so that no time will be lost when they are needed.

In a very small number of cases only one ureteral orifice will be found. This occurs when one kidney is congenitally absent. The ureteral ridge on that side will be missing.

A useful aid, if one anticipates difficulty in locating the ureteral orifices, is the preliminary intravenous injection of indigo-carmine solution. This is excreted normally in three or four minutes and the spurt of urine is colored light to deep blue depending upon the state of renal function. This procedure is termed "chromocystoscopy."

Ureteral spasm may prevent the passage of a catheter. When this occurs it is best to abandon one's efforts, and on another day following preliminary sedation or with the advantage of a general anesthetic, catheterization may be easily accomplished. It is much better to follow such a course than to traumatize the orifice unnecessarily. Wire stylets should seldom, if ever, be employed to stiffen the ureteral catheter; if used, great caution and judgment should be exercised.

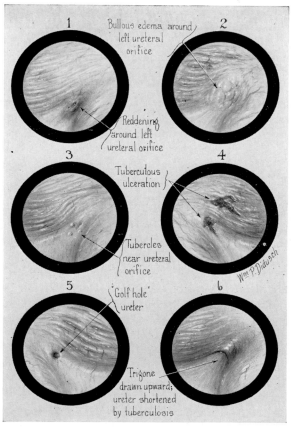

Fig. 69.   Cystoscopic views of pathologic conditions (concluded). (Reproduced from Urological and Allied Diagnostic Instruments and High Frequency Equipment, American Cystoscope Makers, Inc., New York, p. 173.)

After the catheters have been successfully passed and the pins which were used to plug the ends are removed, a steady drip of clear urine normally flows from them. If it is blood-tinged, no positive conclusions can be drawn. No matter how carefully it has been passed, the catheter may scratch the delicate normal mucous membrane which lines the ureter and renal pelvis. If considerable bleeding occurs, the catheter should be withdrawn a few centimeters and a small amount of sterile water or physiologic saline solution injected with a syringe. This maneuver often stops the bleeding and prevents plugging of the catheter. If one does not do it quickly, the entire cystoscopy may fail. Specimens of the urine are collected for microscopic examination and culture. If differential functional studies are made, either indigo carmine or phenolsulfonphthalein can be chosen. The time of appearance of the latter agent is normally three minutes after it is injected intravenously. Following this, specimens are collected from each catheter for fifteen minutes and the total excretion estimated. A normal rate from each kidney is 1 per cent per minute. Any urine which drains down the ureter alongside the catheters, rather than through them, should be recovered from the bladder with a catheter and an estimate made of the amount of the dye it contains. After collection of the specimens has been completed, retrograde pyelographic study can be made if it is indicated.

RETROGRADE PYELOGRAPHY

The injection of opaque medium into the renal pelvis and ureter preceded the excretory method by many years. Prior to the development of excretory media the most commonly used solution was 12 per cent sodium iodide. The majority of patients tolerated this very well but some experienced pronounced irritation, and in a few the iodide was retained for many hours, because of ureteral spasm, resulting in severe renal colic. Marked vesical discomfort often added to the patient's misery.

For many years at the Mayo Clinic we have used a drug called "Hippuran" (sodium ortho-iodohippurate). The most satisfactory strength is 30 per cent solution prepared as follows: Take 300 gm. of Hippuran and 100 cc. of 1:1,000 aqueous solution of merthiolate and make up to 1,000 cc. with triple distilled water. Filter several times. Put in test tubes, each containing 15 cc., and plug ends with cotton. Boil in a water bath for twenty minutes. The solution will remain sterile almost indefinitely.

The technique of making a retrograde pyelogram varies a little, depending upon the particular needs of each case. Of course, a roentgenogram should be made, prior to injection of the medium, with the patient in a horizontal position and so placed on the table as to include the entire area of the kidney, ureter and bladder. In especially tall patients this may be difficult; hence, if there is any reason to favor either the vesical area or renal area this should be done or two films should be made to insure complete visualization. The medium is then injected slowly with a 20 cc. syringe. Before the injection is started, the patient should be asked if he has any pain in the renal region; he should have none. He is asked to complain at the slightest indication of distress after the injection of medium is started. Most often, very slight discomfort will be noted when 8 or 10 cc. have been injected, but in some instances, the entire amount of 15 cc. can be injected slowly into the kidney, some of which will pass down alongside the catheter into the ureter. A roentgenogram should be made at this time after the patient has been cautioned to stop breathing and remain perfectly still. Both the film exposed before the injection (which of course will show the opaque catheters) and the film exposed after the injection should now be developed and examined. If filling is incomplete, additional medium should be injected and another film exposed. In some instances, it will be desirable to make an oblique or semi-lateral roentgenogram to rule out questionable shadows. It is not a good idea to withdraw the catheter at the time of the first injection even an inch or two, because the tip of it may lie barely within the renal pelvis and if the first attempt fails to fill the pelvis and the catheter has been pulled to a lower point during the injection the second try will almost certainly fail.

In cases in which there is any question of obstruction at the ureteropelvic juncture, a *delayed film* should be made. This is done by injecting at least

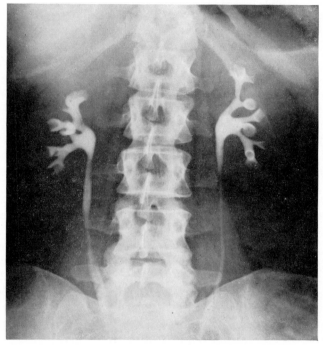

Fig. 70.   Retrograde pyelogram, bilateral. Excellent detail in visualization of pelves and calyces, which are normal. (Reproduced from Braasch, W. F. and Emmett, J. L., Clinical Urography; an Atlas and Textbook of Roentgenologic Diagnosis.)

10 cc. of medium and withdrawing the catheter. The patient is then allowed to walk around the room and remain upright for ten minutes, when another film is made in the horizontal position. If there is any important degree of ureteropelvic obstruction, medium will remain in the renal pelvis and calyces.

At times a film with the patient in the upright position is desired to delineate *renal excursion*. This is made after injection of the medium with the patient in as near an erect position as the table will permit. Normally, the kidney will descend approximately the width of one vertebra. However, in many patients in whom ptosis of several times this amount is demonstrated, one will find no evidence of pyelocaliectasis. In the absence of the latter, it is questionable whether ptosis of any degree is of clinical importance.

The ureter is often difficult to outline because of its peristaltic contractions. A good method of insuring its visualization is to pass a second catheter into the lumen a few centimeters and inject through this catheter rather than the one through which the specimen of urine was obtained. An alternate and effective method of obtaining a good ureterogram is to pass a catheter which has a bulb tip of 8 or 10 F. caliber into the intramural portion and, with the cystoscope held in place and the catheter firmly held within the ureter, to have the medium injected by an assistant while the x-ray technician exposes the film. This method practically always produces a good ureterogram although there is some possibility of overdistention, a fact which must be considered when the film is interpreted.

Bilateral pyelograms should be obtained only when strictly necessary. However, they can be made with much greater impunity since the advent of nonirritative urographic media. It must be remembered, however, that there is always a chance, even though minimal, of the introduction of infection into the kidneys by retrograde methods and that any patient can withstand a unilateral pyelonephritis better than a bilateral infection.

The interpretation of retrograde pyelograms is of course best done when all the data concerned including the microscopic urinary findings are available. The normal (Fig. 70) and variations from it due to disease are well described in textbooks on urography.

SPECIAL ROENTGENOGRAPHIC EXAMINATIONS

Several techniques of special roentgenologic investigation are occasionally found useful in examination.

Seminal vesiculography has been described by a number of investigators including McCarthy, Ritter and Klemperer (1927), and Herbst and Merricks (1939). The procedure is accomplished in most instances by catheterization of the ejaculatory ducts with the aid of a special type of panendoscope and a special sheath which directs the small catheters into the openings of the ducts which are found in the verumontanum on either side of the utriculus. After catheterization, several cubic centimeters of opaque medium are injected while the catheter is held in place. After injection, roentgenograms are made to demonstrate the seminal vesicles, the ampulla and the ductus deferens (see Fig. 568). In some cases it is impossible to outline the vas deferens in its pelvic portion. Abnormalities due to inflammation and cicatricial changes can sometimes be demonstrated. The method is difficult and the results are regarded as equivocal in the hands of all but a few investigators.

Translumbar aortography is a special roentgenographic technique which has gained considerable favor during the past decade. It is described in detail in the following chapter.

Pyeloscopy is a specialized procedure involving filling of the renal pelvis with opaque medium and observing it under the fluoroscope while the calyces and pelvis contract and force the opaque fluid down the ureter. Ureteral peristalsis can be observed and at times points of pathologic narrowing are clearly delineated. The method is difficult and has never gained great favor.

Serial pyelography is a method of recording on one film (14 by 17 inches) a number of urograms in a few minutes in the hope of outlining variations in the renal pelvis and ureter which develop during the time consumed in making the several exposures. Moore (1932) has well described the method and also the device he employs to make it possible to obtain the several pictures on one film.

Urokymography is another method which also records on an x-ray film physiologic activity of the kidney and ureter.

Laminography is an x-ray technique which provides a method of recording the appearance of the kidney in spite of the fact that it is obscured to some extent by overlying gas and feces in the intestinal tract. It has never proved to be a very practical method.

Perirenal insufflation was first advocated by Carelli in 1921; it is a method of introducing air into the perirenal fascia in order to aid in the visualization of the kidneys and the position and size of the adrenal glands. Also it sometimes helps in outlining abnormalities of other adjacent structures such as enlargement of the spleen, pancreatic cysts and other tumors which may arise in the retroperitoneal space. The method is described in Section XVIII of this book.

Presacral insufflation is another method of introducing air or, if one prefers, oxygen or helium into the retroperitoneal space. It has been described in detail by Smith and associates (1952) and by Ritter and Johnson (1953). The technique involves inserting a needle just anterior to the tip of the coccyx and injecting 1,000 to 1,200 cc. of oxygen slowly into the retroperitoneal space. After appropriate positioning of the patient to insure the passage of the gas up toward the kidney and diaphragm, roentgenograms are made in both anteroposterior and lateral positions. Normally, in the majority of cases the kidney is clearly delineated and if perirenal disease is present such as perinephritis, tumor infiltration or hematoma resulting from trauma, there is indication of it from the fact that oxygen cannot reach the perirenal region on the side where the pathologic condition exists. Simultaneous retrograde pyelography or excretory urography may be helpful in delineating pathologic processes within the kidney as well as around it.

BIOPSY AND SPECIAL CYTOLOGIC STUDY

Small specimens of tissue can be removed from lesions which are seen in the bladder or urethra or on the external genitalia. Microscopic examination of stained sections of these is often useful in establishing an early diagnosis. The positive report is of course much more valuable than a negative one for the reason that inflammation often occurs in association with tumors and tends to alter the appearance of the tissues, causing edema and swelling above and around the growth. Biopsy specimens are, as a rule, best obtained with the patient under general anesthesia. An attempt to obtain a specimen without it usually will not permit going as deep as is possible with the patient asleep. By frozen-tissue methods it is often possible to examine the small fragment of tissue removed and under the same anesthesia to proceed with treatment based on the results of the examination. But in most instances, fixed-tissue sections are desirable.

The use of biopsy in this way has been criticized by some who say that the small specimen obtained may not truly represent the larger portion of tumor underlying the surface. While this may be correct in a small number of cases, the great majority of specimens thus obtained will, in my opinion, be found to be an accurate representation of the rest of the lesion. However, as previously stated, the positive report is much more valuable than the negative. Lesions in which the biopsy gives negative results should be examined again after treatment and, if indicated, another biopsy specimen obtained.

Papanicolaou and Marshall (1945) have described a special method of cytologic study of the urine based on the theory that tumors which are present anywhere in the tract desquamate regularly so that the cells can be found in the voided specimen. They suggest the following technique: Approximately 400 cc. of urine are collected in a tube, mixed immediately with 10 to 20 cc. of 95 per cent alcohol, and centrifuged for ten minutes at 20,000 revolutions per minute. The sediment is then spread with a wire loop on glass slides which have been thinly filmed with albumin. These are fixed in a solution of equal parts of 95 per cent alcohol and ether for ten minutes. The slides are then stained and examined. The diagnosis of cancer is made on the basis of modifications and abnormalities of the nucleus such as enlargement, anisonucleosis, fragmentation, hyperchromatosis, granular arrangement of the chromatin and prominence of the nucleoli, and also on changes affecting the cytoplasm and significant deviation of cells from their normal size and form.

The foregoing method is difficult at best and certainly not reliable to any degree except in the hands of an expert pathologist. Because of the presence of epithelial cells which contain large nuclei and other changes in the cytoplasm that are perhaps the result of inflammation and metaplastic processes incidental to tissue repair, there is considerable chance of error in interpreting the results obtained by study of urinary sediment. False positive reports inevitably result and, for instance, a kidney may be sacrificed if there is a slight calyceal filling defect or other deformity which excites suspicion. Therefore it must be kept in mind at all times that the method is strictly ancillary and that the findings must not unduly influence the decision as to treatment. In case of doubt, it is best to wait until very definite pyelographic deformity can be seen rather than indulge in needless sacrifice of a kidney.

SPECIAL CHEMICAL AND HORMONAL STUDIES

Neoplasms of the testicle sometimes produce a hormone which can be detected in the urine in large quantities. This is an auxiliary aid in the diagnosis and is discussed further in the chapter on testicular tumors.

In prostatic malignancy, increased concentration of blood phosphatase is found with reasonable regularity especially when metastasis to the bone has occurred. However, some patients do not exhibit any alteration of the value for blood phosphatase even in the face of an extensive lesion.

Calculous disease of the urinary tract demands investigation to rule out hyperparathyroidism. The excess excretion of calcium in the urine can be found by making a Sulkowitch test or by quantitative studies if the twenty-four-hour excretion while the patient is eating a diet containing a known amount of calcium. Blood chemical determination reveals, when the disease is present, an elevation of the value for blood calcium and a decrease in the value for phosphate. Every patient who suffers from a calculus should be studied carefully to see whether the values for calcium and phosphate in the serum deviate from normal.

RE-EXAMINATIONS

It is important to remember that urologic examination, exact as it is in many aspects, does not always result in a complete and accurate survey in any given case. In the final analysis, the relief of symptoms and the correction of the basic lesion causing them is the object of all the detailed study. Therefore, the final proof of the various examinations is the response to the therapy employed. For instance, it may seem obvious that inflammation is the cause of vesical symptoms, but if reasonably prompt response to treatment is not obtained one must think of the possibility that an underlying neoplasm or an obstructive lesion not visualized at the time of cystoscopy is lurking in the background. Similarly, renal symptoms may be due to a nonopaque calculus which is difficult to detect, or a tuberculous infection may be obscured by other organisms which are present; likewise, a small renal neoplasm may not cause, in its incipiency, a clear-cut deformity of the calyces. Therefore, if symptoms persist in spite of treatment or if they reappear at an early date, the examiner must be quick to recognize the possibility of error in the original studies.

Experience teaches that observation over a period of weeks or even months is sometimes required to settle a diagnosis. Disease in its early phase often causes changes so minimal in degree that even the most skilful examiner overlooks them. One must be patient and sympathetic during the passage of time and yet always on the alert for other signs which are helpful in the final solution of the problem. What at first seemed so difficult and so obscure often in retrospect is amazingly obvious.

Physicians who are fully aware of the value of re-examinations succeed, while those who stubbornly or ignorantly refuse to admit the imperfections of even their best efforts, at least on some occasions, fail. In all phases of urologic examination and investigation, the wise practitioner will, when a clear-cut answer to the problem has not been obtained, be willing, and even anxious, to try again.

REFERENCES

AMERICAN UROLOGICAL ASSOCIATION: History of Urology. Baltimore, The Williams & Wilkins Company, 1933.
BRAASCH, W. F. and EMMETT, J. L.: Clinical Urography; an Atlas and Textbook of Roentgenologic Diagnosis. Philadelphia, W. B. Saunders Company, 1951.
CAMPBELL, M. F.: Pediatric Urology. New York, The Macmillan Company, 1937.
CAMPBELL, MEREDITH: Clinical Pediatric Urology. Philadelphia, W. B. Saunders Company, 1951.

CARELLI, H. H.: Sur le pneumopéritoine et sur une methode personnelle pour voir le rein sans pneumopéritoine. Bull. et mém. Soc. méd. hôp. de Paris, 2:1409–1412, 1921.

HERBST, R. H. and MERRICKS, J. W.: Visualization and treatment of seminal vesiculitis by catheterization and dilatation of the ejaculatory ducts. J. Urol., 41:733–750, 1939.

McCARTHY, J. F., RITTER, J. S. and KLEMPERER, PAUL: Anatomical and histological study of the verumontanum with especial reference to the ejaculatory ducts. J. Urol., 17:1–16, 1927.

MOORE, T. D.: The value of the serial pyelograph in diagnosis. J. Urol., 28:437–454, 1932.

PAPANICOLAOU, G. N. and MARSHALL, V. F.: Urine sediment smears as a diagnostic procedure in cancers of the urinary tract. Science, 101:519–520, 1945.

RITTER, J. S. and JOHNSON, A. A.: Perirenal oxygen insufflation. J. Internat. Coll. Surgeons, 19:732–743, 1953.

SIMON, NORMAN and NARINS, LESTER: The effect of hyaluronidase on the absorption of a subcutaneously deposited radiopaque substance. Am. J. Roentgenol., 61:91–94, 1949.

SMITH, D. R., STEINBACH, H. L., LYONS, R. P. and STRATTE, P. B.: Extraperitoneal pneumography. J. Urol., 68:953–959, 1952.

TODD, J. C., SANFORD, A. H. and WELLS, B. B.: Clinical Diagnosis by Laboratory Methods; a Working Manual of Clinical Pathology. Philadelphia, W. B. Saunders Company, 1953.

CHAPTER 2

Renal Angiography (Aortography)

PARKE G. SMITH, M.D.

The health, even the very existence, of living tissues and organs is to a great extent dependent upon the quantity as well as the quality of the arterial blood with which they are supplied. Disease of tissues or of organs may be evidenced by variations from normal of the arteries which supply these areas and, conversely, variations from normal arterial anatomy may directly affect the health of tissues. A study of the arterial circulation of a mass of living tissue commonly discloses information otherwise unobtainable about its health.

This is proved by the many techniques which have been developed for the study of the vascular anatomy of various organs and the great reliance placed upon the information obtained from these studies. Most of these techniques provide for the roentgenographic recording of the pattern of vascular structure and/or distribution revealed by a radio-opaque substance introduced into the circulating blood stream. This procedure is called *angiography,* and has reached a state of perfection that has made it universally accepted.

The value of the information to be obtained by this procedure was recognized as early as 1927, and in 1929 was discussed by the Portuguese, Dos Santos. However, his technique of injection and the contrast media he employed had inherent dangers of such magnitude that renal angiography as accomplished by the translumbar aortic puncture was, in spite of his enthusiasm, until very recently seldom employed.

In 1948, we reported our experience with a simplified technique for the production of a renal angiogram by translumbar aortic puncture. This technique varied from those previously reported by Dos Santos, A. Keller Doss, O. A. Nelson, and Vitt, in the method of injection and the quantity and character of the contrast media used. It is noteworthy for its simplicity, preciseness and the fact that excellent angiograms are obtained by using not more than 12 cc. of a nonsclerosing contrast medium. Since our original report, we have used this simplified procedure extensively and have reported a series of over 1,000 renal angiograms performed by translumbar aortic puncture with no mortality and with morbidity of only minimal degree.*

---

* Lest the reader gain the notion that lumbar aortography is a benign procedure, it should be noted that in several clinics where the method has been liberally employed, there have been many instances of grave morbidity and some deaths from its use. (Ed.)

187

TECHNIQUE

The production of a renal angiogram by means of translumbar aortic puncture, although an extremely simple procedure, is one that must be performed with precision. In the individual of average size, the puncture is accomplished by means of a 6 inch, 18 gauge, spinal puncture type of needle; in children, a 5 inch needle, and in large patients, a 7 inch or even an 8 inch needle may be advisable (Fig. 71, *B*). A needle of this gauge is recommended because it is of a size sufficiently large to allow the necessarily rapid injection of the contrast media, but is not so large that its introduction will result in excessive damage to the tissues through which it passes. A precision-made 10 cc. glass barrel syringe with a metal plunger and adequate finger and thumb rings is necessary (Fig. 71, *A*), as this type of syringe insures the

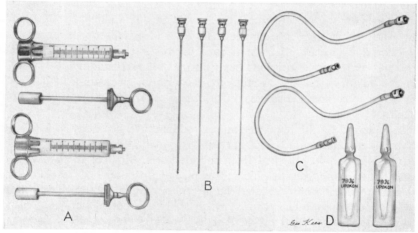

Fig. 71.   Instrument tray for translumbar aortic puncture. *A,* two syringes, *B,* two 6-inch needles. *C,* Luer tipped connecting tubes, *D,* two ampules of contrast medium. See text for description of equipment.

rapid, unimpeded stroke of the plunger essential for making a necessarily rapid injection. The syringe and needle are connected by means of plastic tubing, 12 to 15 cm. in length, 4 mm. in diameter, that has Luer adapters on either end (male and female, Fig. 71, *C*). This type of connecting tube has the flexibility necessary to prevent undue movement of the needle, offers the opportunity of inspection of the pulsations of the column of arterial blood in the tube immediately prior to the injection, will not "blow out," and is unlikely to become disconnected.

The roentgen exposure should be made at 0.1 and not more than 0.2 of a second; a high speed Potter-Bucky diaphragm and a rotary anode tube with dual control are essential parts of the equipment. Although we prefer Urokon, the contrast medium may be a 70 or 75 per cent solution of any of those now used for intravenous urography (Fig. 71, *D*). Sodium iodide in any strength is inadvisable.

The patient, who has been surgically prepared and previously tested for sensitivity to the contrast medium to be used, is placed in a prone position on the x-ray table. A scout film is made and, when inspection of this film shows that both the x-ray technique employed and the patient's position are satisfactory, the patient is anesthetized with intravenous anesthesia. The lumbar region is sterilized and draped. A point just under the edge of the twelfth rib about 7 cm. to the left of the midline is selected as the point of entrance of the needle (Fig. 72). The distance from the midline will vary slightly according to the size of the patient and the angle of the ribs with the spinal column. In cases of situs transversus the point of entrance of the needle is to the right of the midline.

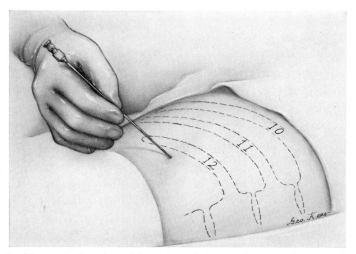

Fig. 72.   Position and direction of insertion of the needle toward the twelfth thoracic
vertebra.

The skin is punctured and the needle is directed ventrally, inward, and upward toward the body of the twelfth thoracic vertebra. When the point of the needle touches the bone in that location, the needle is withdrawn slightly, the point depressed and reintroduced. That procedure is repeated until the point of the needle passes just under the body of the vertebra (Fig. 73). The obturator of the needle is then withdrawn and the needle is advanced until resistance is suddenly overcome with a "pop" similar to that experienced when introducing a needle into the spinal canal. The flow of blood should be free but it seldom spurts. The connecting plastic tubing is attached to the needle, the rotor of the x-ray tube is started, pulsations of the blood in the connecting tube are studied and, if satisfactory, the injection is completed as rapidly as possible (1 or 2 seconds). The exposure is made as the last few cc. of the contrast medium are being injected. The needle is immediately withdrawn and a second film is made as rapidly as the cassettes can be changed. This last film is known as a *renogram* or *nephrogram*.

Local, rather than general, anesthesia may at times be advisable. Perfection of technique and cooperation between the urologist and the roentgenologist will insure excellent films, will obviate the necessity of multiple injections, multiple aortic punctures, and the use of larger than the above recommended amount of contrast media.

Multiple exposures made during the course of the injection procedure may be obtained by the use of either a rapid cassette changer or of the continuous film (Fairchild) technique. Intriguing possibilities are offered by these rapid multiple exposures and their employment may extent the usefulness of renal angiography into as yet unexplored fields of investigation.

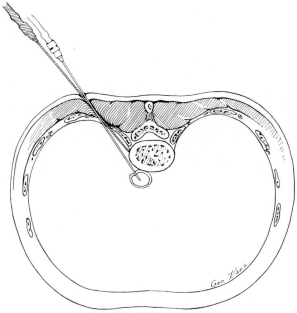

Fig. 73.   The consecutive steps in making aortic puncture at the level of the twelfth thoracic vertebra.

THE NORMAL RENAL ANGIOGRAM

The renal arteries branch from the aorta at the level of the second lumbar vertebral body and are at right angles to the aorta. The primary division which is usually into two branches occurs just within, or close to, the hilum of the kidney. From this point the branches spread throughout the kidney with diminishing caliber; most of the precortical branching is bifid and is not multiple. The interlobar and arcuate branches pass between the pyramids and spread out in graceful, minute curves in the cortex, the so-called fan-like arrangement. The small or cortical branches arise at acute angles (Fig. 74).

THE ABNORMAL RENAL ANGIOGRAM

In the clinical study of vascular and other anomalies of the upper urinary tract, accurate knowledge of the number and distribution of the renal arteries, as obtained by renal angiography, is of extreme value, particularly when the therapeutic program contemplates a surgical procedure.

Although we have had the opportunity of studying the arterial patterns in a rather large series of congenital renal anomalies of all types, we are not prepared to form any conclusion about them as a group other than that there is a great variation in their arterial patterns. This is true even in cases in which retrograde studies have shown great similarity in type. Nevertheless, there are certain facts about each of the following classes of renal anomalies that are of importance.

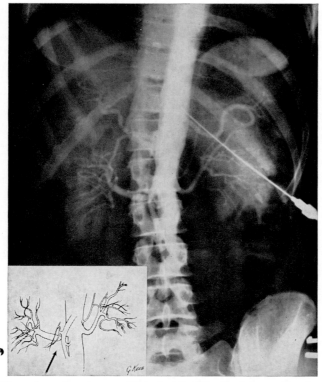

Fig. 74. Normal renal angiogram. Note that the "load" of the medium has not reached the lower portion of the aorta and that other vessels have not been filled, thus eliminating confusion resulting from visualizing other aortic branches.

Bifurcation of the Renal Pelvis. In the bifid type of renal pelvis particularly when the bifurcation extends into the ureter, it is extremely unusual to find only one renal artery. In these cases, the upper portion of the renal pelvis is seldom the one of major importance, but the contrary is true of the arteries as it is the upper artery which is always the larger and more important, supplying not only the renal parenchyma of the smaller upper segment, but also a large portion of the parenchyma draining into the larger lower segment of the renal pelvis (Fig. 75). Apparently few urologists are aware of this fact or its importance. This dominance of the upper of the two renal arteries is also a constant finding in patients whose renal pelves do not vary from normal configuration.

Congenital Renal Ectopia. The lack of complete ascent of the renal mass is usually attributed to a persistence of some of the arterial supply arising from the lower portion of the aorta or from the pelvic vessels themselves. It is not uncommon to find that some of these arteries arise from the pelvic vessels even on the opposite side. In making a renal angiogram of a patient with a known congenital ectopic kidney and one with crossed ectopia, it is important to remember that there should be a very slight delay, possibly one half second, in asking for the exposure, a time sufficient to allow the "load" to reach that portion of the aorta and iliac vessels from which the

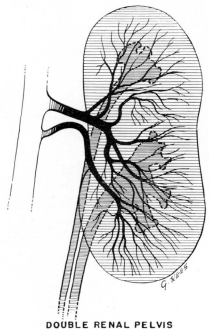

DOUBLE RENAL PELVIS

Fig. 75.   Angiogram in renal pelvic reduplication illustrating the major importance of the upper of the two renal arteries.

arterial supply of the renal mass may arise. Preoperative knowledge of the number and location of these vessels allows the urologist to locate them easily and, when necessary, to ligate them during the surgical procedure, thus reducing the danger of an accidental tear.

Hypoplastic and Aplastic Kidneys. In the study of hypertension, particularly in older children and young adults, the presence of a functionless kidney may assume great importance.

In the cases in which this unilateral lack of renal function is thought to be due to a congenital lack of adequate renal tissue, it is sometimes extremely difficult, except by translumbar aortography and renal angiography, to determine whether the condition is a simple congenital hypoplasia or a true aplasia of the renal mass.

The arterial pattern of congenital hypoplasia of the kidney is usually rather normal except that all vessels and their branches are extremely small and the terminal fan-like cortical circulation is seldom visualized (Fig. 76). In congenital renal aplasia there is complete absence of arterial pattern.

Fused Renal Masses. In fused kidneys, such as in crossed ectopia and in horseshoe formation, there is usually a multiplicity of renal arteries, some of which may arise from the iliacs (Fig. 77) or even from the hypogastrics. Some extremely unusual arterial patterns have been observed; on one oc-

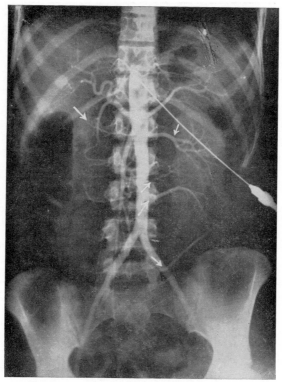

Fig. 76. Renal angiography. There is a small renal artery entering the hypoplastic right kidney. There is incomplete left renal rotation with four renal arteries but arising from the common renal artery.

casion, we demonstrated a true crossed ectopia that received its entire arterial supply from the renal artery on the side where the mass was located. We have also been informed of a horseshoe kidney that likewise was supplied by only one renal artery.

The importance of accurate preoperative knowledge of the number, distribution and areas supplied by these numerous renal arteries is obvious. This information is absolutely essential when bisection of renal masses or the resection of portions of the renal parenchyma is contemplated; an accurate surgical procedure can be planned and precisely performed.

Obstruction of the Upper Urinary Tract. Obstruction at the ureteropelvic junction may result from the pressure of an artery crossing the ureter at that point. The rapidity with which the resulting hydronephrosis develops will vary according to the source of the artery which produces this pressure. I do not believe it is generally known that when the pressure is the result of an anomalous branch of the renal artery, the obstruction is more effective, the hydronephrosis develops more rapidly, and there is an earlier tendency for the hydronephrotic sac to herniate over the artery thereby causing more complete obstruction than when the offending vessel is a true renal artery

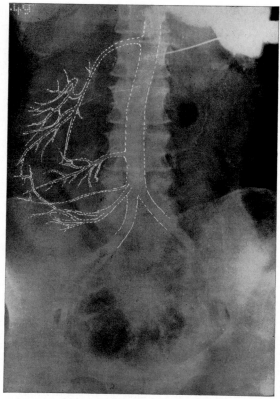

Fig. 77.   Renal angiography in crossed ectopia. The multiple renal arteries usually found in the common types of renal fusion are here demonstrated.

arising from the aorta (Figs. 78, 79). Arteries of this latter type are much less effective in producing obstruction, and the process of developing a hydrone-phrosis, consequently, may be greatly prolonged.

When these cases of hydronephrosis resulting from ureteropelvic obstruc-tion of this type are seen early, it is important for the urologist to know the source of the offending vessel that he may make a more scientific prognosis and be in a position to determine more accurately if and when reparative surgery is advisable.

Intraureteral Obstruction. When the ureter is completely occluded by a calculus, blood clot, ligature, and so forth, and intravenous urography has

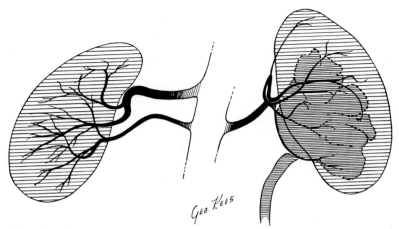

Fig. 78. Renal angiography in hydronephrosis due to vascular ureteral obstruction. The major importance of the upper renal artery, the increased effectiveness of a branch of the renal artery in producing hydronephrosis as compared with an accessory renal artery is evident in this line drawing of an actual renal angiogram and left pyelogram. The loss of blood supply in the involved organ is shown by the lack of cortical circulation and diminished caliber of all vessels.

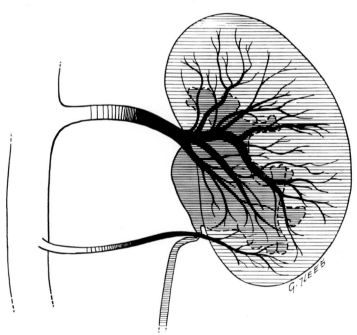

ABERRANT RENAL ARTERY

Fig. 79. Renal angiography in hydronephrosis caused by an aberrant renal artery. This line drawing made from a renal angiogram illustrates the lessened effectiveness of an accessory renal vessel in the production of hydronephrosis as compared with the condition shown in Figure 78. The persistence of cortical circulation and the normal caliber of all renal vessels demand that, if surgical therapy is indicated, it be reparative rather than nephrectomy.

demonstrated a lack of function of the kidney on the obstructed side, a renal angiogram will give accurate information about the quantity and quality of the renal parenchyma. With this information, the clinician can then plan his therapeutic program with assurance.

Renal Hypertension. It is well recognized that a pressor substance may be elaborated in the renal parenchyma as the result of the ischemia produced by partial compression of the renal artery. It has also been demonstrated that a similar pressor substance is elaborated as the result of the congestion following compression of the renal vein. In patients with an unusual amount of renal mobility and in whom there is an anomalous renal artery, the axis of rotation of the renal pedicle when movement occurs may be altered in such a manner as to twist the renal pedicle, compress the renal vein, and possibly produce this pressor substance that induces hypertension.

We believe we have recognized several such cases and are certain that in three of them the correction of the abnormal mobility and/or the ligation of the anomalous vessel has been followed by the elimination of the hypertension.

Hydronephrosis. The caliber of the renal artery and its immediate branches are factors of great importance in determining the renal arterial supply and evaluating the potential recoverability of the parenchyma of a hydronephrotic kidney. As the hydronephrosis progresses, a loss of the normal multiple branches of the cortical vessels and a diminution in the caliber of the renal artery and its branches occur (Fig. 78).

We believe that a renal angiogram is a necessary part of the preoperative examination of patients with hydronephrosis, for the quality of the renal circulation as determined by renal angiography is a more reliable indication of the salvage value of the renal parenchyma than any of the functional tests now used to determine the advisability of reparative surgery versus nephrectomy.

Renal Infarcts. Our experience with arteriography in renal infarction has been extremely illuminating. We have been unable to find any reference to renal angiographic studies in this type of kidney injury. As the result of a study of five patients with proved renal infarction, we believe we have been able to recognize an arterial pattern that is characteristic of this condition. Four of these five patients had malignant hypertension; one patient with blood pressure of 280 mm. Hg systolic and 166 mm. Hg diastolic illustrates our feeling of security about the safety of this procedure. In four of these patients, three of whom had multiple large infarcts and one of whom had a single massive infarct, the renal angiogram showed exactly what one would expect it to show, that is, a sharp termination of an otherwise unimpeded arterial branch with a wedge-shaped area of avascularity extending from that point to the parenchymal edge (Fig. 80). In one of the patients, who was found at autopsy to have innumerable small renal infarcts, the angiograms were not characteristic although on close study it was noticed that we could not identify the cortical renal branches as easily as we ordinarily do.

Renal Tumors. From the standpoint of angiographic studies renal tumors can easily be divided into two types, the clear-cell and the granular-cell. In

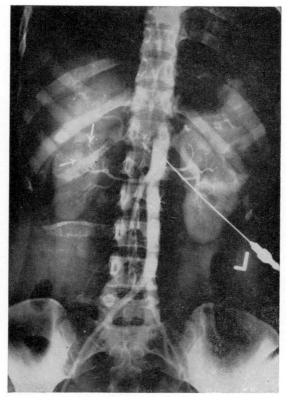

Fig. 80. Renal angiography in infarction of the kidney. The arrows point to the abrupt termination of vessels later proved to be at the apex of renal infarcts.

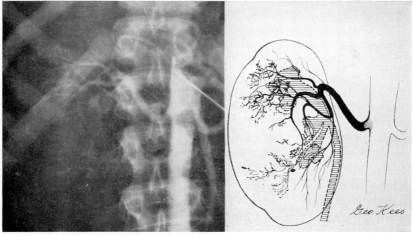

Fig. 81. Renal angiography in clear-cell tumor of the kidney. The pooling and laking of the radiopaque medium in the tumor area is diagnostically confirmative.

the former, the vascularity is sinusoid-like in character and gives a characteristic angiographic pattern with "pooling" or "puddling" of the contrast
media within the sinusoid-like areas of the neoplasm (Fig. 81, see also Figs.
430 to 433). In some of these tumors that have grown rapidly or in some
extremely old tumors, there may be little or no demonstrable vascularity

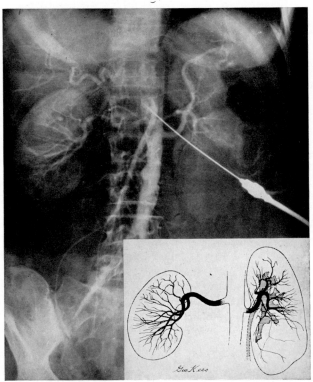

Fig. 82.   Renal angiography in solitary cyst of the kidney. In this case the cyst had
ruptured and bled into the renal pelvis. Note the comparative lack of vascularity and
absence of pooling in the involved area at the lower pole of the left kidney. (Courtesy of
Dr. Lee Elgin.)

of the central portion and, as a result, the characteristic "pooling" of the
contrast medium may be recognized only in the periphery of the tumor itself
(Fig. 81).

In the granular cell type tumor, we have been unable to recognize an
alteration in the angiographic pattern that can be regarded as characteristic
of the condition.

Solitary Renal Cysts. Solitary renal cysts are devoid of arterial supply.
They may be partially covered by a thin layer of renal parenchyma in which
some arteries may be present (Fig. 82). A renal angiogram shows a complete
avascularity of the cyst-bearing area unless the cyst is covered in part by a
thin layer of renal parenchyma. In the last event, one may see outlined small
caliber, widely dispersed arterial branches (Fig. 82).

Polycystic Renal Disease. Renal angiographic studies of polycystic kidney disease show a pattern quite similar to that of hydronephrosis; the caliber of the renal artery and its branches is definitely reduced, the entire arterial pattern is spread out, and there are no multiple or fan-like, terminal, cortical branches. There is a marked tendency for the small renal branches to assume smooth, graceful curves around the larger cysts (Fig. 83). This latter and

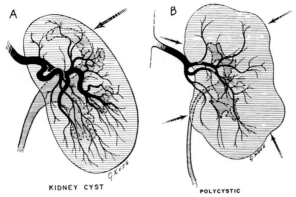

KIDNEY CYST   POLYCYSTIC

Fig. 83.   Renal angiography in *A,* solitary cystic disease and *B,* polycystic kidney disease (see text).

the widely dispersed arterial pattern are differential points between this condition and that of hydronephrosis.

REFERENCES

BISQUERTT, J. L., and CANTIN, F.: Abdominal aortography in renal affections. Urol. & Cutan. Rev., *41:*436–440, 1937.

Doss, A. K.: Translumbar aortography; its diagnostic value in urology. J. Urol., *55:*594–606, 1946.

————: Management of ureteropelvic juncture obstruction; translumbar aortography an adjunct. J. Urol., *57:*521–541, 1947.

————: Translumbar aortography; aid in management of hydronephrotic kidney. South. M. J., *40:*376–382, 1947.

Doss, A. K., THOMAS, H. C. and BOND, T. B.: Renal arteriography, its clinical value. Texas State J. Med., *38:*277–280, 1942.

DOS SANTOS, R.: L'aortographie dans les tumeurs rénales et pararénales. Arch. d. mal. d. reins, *8:*313–334, 1934.

————: Novelles applications cliniques de l'aortographie à quelques problèmes de chirurgie rénale. Bull. Soc. franc. d'urol., 1934, pp. 48–56.

DOS SANTOS, R., LAMAS, A. C. and CALDAS PEREIRA, J.: Arteriografia da aorta e dos vasos abdominais. Med. contemp., *47:*93–96, 1929.

————: Artériographie des Membres et de l'Aorte abdominale. Masson et Cie., Paris, 1931.

————: Les récents progrès dans la technique de l'artériographie de l'aorte abdominale. Presse méd., *39:*574–577, 1931.

EVANS, A. T.: Translumbar arteriography. Cincinnati J. Med., *32:*47–56, 1951.

GRAHAM, R. S.: Study of circulation in normal and pathologic kidney with roentgenographic visualization of arterial tree, including glomeruli. Am. J. Path., *4:*17–32, 1928.

HELMSWORTH, J. A., McGUIRE, J. and FELSON, B.: Arteriography of aorta and its branches by means of polyethylene catheter. Am J. Roentgenol. & Rad. Therapy, *64:*196–213, 1950.

LERICHE, R., KUNLIN, J. and BOELY, C.: Lessons of aortography. Angiology, 1, 109–132, 1950.

LINDQVIST, T.: Arterit i de fran aortabagen urgaende artarerna. Nord. med., *37:*322–324, 1948.

MELICK, W. F. and VITT, A. E.: Present status of aortography. J. Urol., *60:*321–334, 1948.
NELSON, O. A.: Arteriography of abdominal organs by aortic injection. Surg., Gynec. & Obst., *74:*655–662, 1942.
————: Arteriography in diagnosis of upper abdominal conditions. Northwest Med., *44:* 314–322, 1945.
————: Arteriography in renal and abdominal conditions. J. Urol., *53:*521–533, 1945.
SMITH, P. G.: Renal angiography; its use in 1500 cases. Trans. Am. Assn. Gen. Urin. Surgeons, 1953, in press.
SMITH, P. G., RUSH, T. W. and EVANS, A. T.: Evaluation of translumbar arteriography. J. Urol., *65:*911–921, 1951.
————: Technique of translumbar arteriography, J.A.M.A., *148:*255, 1952.
VITT, A. E. and MELICK, W. F.: Studies on translumbar aortography; simple apparatus for translumbar aortography. J. Missouri M.A., *44:*749, 1947.
WAGNER, F. B., JR.: Arteriography in renal diagnosis. J. Urol., *56:*625–635, 1946.
WAGNER, F. B., JR., PRICE, A. H. and SWENSON, P. C.: Abdominal arteriography; technique and diagnostic application. Am. J. Roentgenol. & Rad. Therapy, *58:*591–598, 1947.
WAGNER, F. B., JR. and PRICE, A. H.: Fatality after abdominal arteriography. Surgery. *27,* 621–626, 1950.

Section III

THE PATHOLOGY OF URINARY OBSTRUCTION

FRANK HINMAN, JR., M.D.

Renal function is of first importance to the urologist, and urinary obstruction his greatest foe. Renal damage is the inevitable effect of obstruction whether high or low. Further damage to the nephron comes from stasis with its sequelae of infection and calculus formation.

Let us start with hydronephrosis, the ultimate effect of obstruction, then pass down the urinary tract recording the effects of and treatment for obstructions at each level: calyx, ureteropelvic junction, ureter, ureterovesical junction and lower tract (Fig. 84). Even though we focus on a particular obstructive lesion, we cannot overlook its effect on the kidney.

THE PATHOGENESIS OF HYDRONEPHROSIS

Obstruction of the kidney differs from obstruction of other organs by one peculiar circumstance: renal function continues. The formation of urine is slowed but does not stop altogether. The urine so formed, blocked from its usual routes of excretion, is resorbed. This interplay between excretion and absorption allows the gradual dilatation of hydronephrosis. Hydronephrotic atrophy differs from primary atrophy by these dynamic changes. Obstruction of most ducts completely represses the secretion of the gland, but the kidney, as it goes on to hydronephrotic atrophy, continues as a functioning organ.

To understand the process of hydronephrosis, we must realize that the pathologic changes after partial obstruction in which urinary excretion is reduced are not essentially different from those after complete obstruction, in which the actual external excretion of urine has ceased. The same factors of formation, excretion, and resorption are common to both.

The study of hydronephrotic atrophy begins with urine formation, goes through resorption and excretion, and ends with the results of imbalance between formation and disposal.

URINE FORMATION

Urine is delivered by three distinct processes: glomerular filtration, tubular secretion, and muscular conduction.

Glomerular Filtration. Glomerular filtration is of great importance in the pathogenesis of hydronephrosis. It is a purely mechanical process not relying on cellular transport mechanisms and so could be expected to be less affected by mere compression. It is well established that the urine in the glomerular capsule is an ultrafiltrate from the pressure of blood in glomerular capillaries against the colloid osmotic pressure of the plasma and against tubular resistance. Glomerular filtration rises with increased renal blood flow and with increased blood pressure in the glomerular capillaries. Greater filtration may be brought about either by an increase in systemic blood pressure or

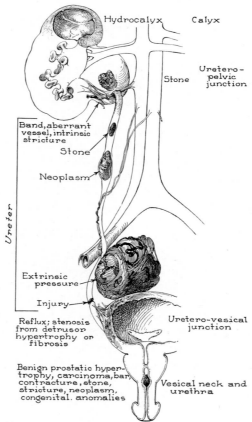

Fig. 84.   Causes of obstruction at the various levels from calyx to meatus.

by vasoconstriction of the efferent arterioles. To use actual figures, there exists on the one hand an intravascular hydrostatic pressure of about 80 mm. Hg and, opposing this, a colloid osmotic pressure of 25 mm. Hg plus a tubular resistance which approximates 25 mm. Hg. The resultant filtration pressure of the glomerulus therefore is around 30 mm. of mercury.

Obstruction anywhere along the urinary tract, while not directly affecting the intra-arterial hydrostatic pressure and having no influence on the osmotic forces, will, however, increase the pressure within Bowman's space and thereby decrease the effective filtration pressure. This consequently decreases the amount of urine secreted. (This was Ludwig's original theory, now

substantiated.) It has been estimated experimentally that in early hydronephrosis the filtration pressure falls to less than 10 mm. Hg in contrast to the
normal pressure of 30 mm.

Partial obstruction of the renal artery decreases renal blood flow and
also decreases the capillary blood pressure. This in turn causes reduction in
glomerular filtration. One would expect that since the excretion of urine from
the glomerulus was diminished, the process of hydronephrotic atrophy would
proceed more slowly. However, experiments show such is not the case (Hin-

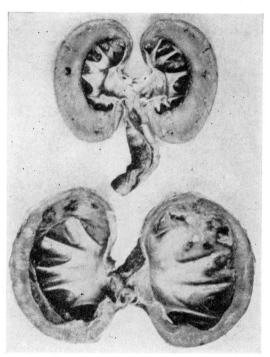

Fig. 85.   Upper renal hemisections show effect of 2 weeks' complete obstruction. Lower
kidney, in addition, had partial constriction of the renal artery. (From Hinman, F., Principles and Practice of Urology, Philadelphia, W. B. Saunders Company, 1935.)

man and Hepler, 1925), but that there is an increase in the rate and degree
of hydronephrotic atrophy as shown in Figure 85, because the changes of
hydronephrosis are closely linked with nutrition of the tissues. The limited
supply of blood causes more rapid parenchymal degeneration which in turn
speeds up the hydronephrotic dilatation in spite of the lowered rate of
glomerular filtration.

Partial obstruction of the renal vein, if not excessive, causes a temporary
increase in the secretory pressure of the nephron even though the rate of
blood flow and total urinary secretion are diminished. However, the effect
of such venous ligation is similar to that of arterial obstruction in that
hydronephrotic atrophy progresses at a more rapid rate, presumably due to
nutritional disturbance secondary to the inadequate blood supply and venous
stasis.

Tubular Secretion. Tubular secretion (in contrast to simple glomerular filtration) is a much more active physiologic process requiring actual work on the part of cells. It must be remembered that, in part, tubular function is passive, as in the proximal convoluted tubule where a large proportion of the filtrate is reabsorbed without regard for the body's requirements. Similarly, the passive diffusion and reabsorption of urea in the distal con-

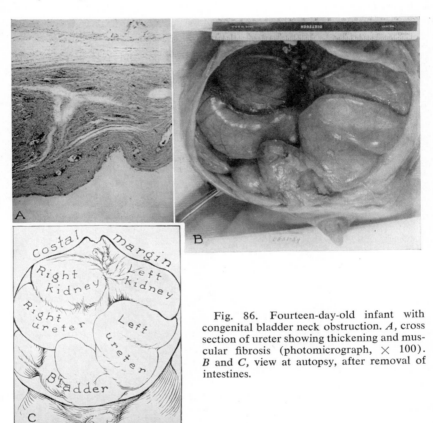

Fig. 86. Fourteen-day-old infant with congenital bladder neck obstruction. *A*, cross section of ureter showing thickening and muscular fibrosis (photomicrograph, × 100). *B* and *C*, view at autopsy, after removal of intestines.

voluted tubule and collecting tubules is well known and accounts for the error in interpretation of the urea clearance test. However, the active transport of substances by the enzyme systems of the renal tubular cells to the tubular lumen can be performed against a differential in concentration. That the tubules alone are capable of considerable secretory pressure is illustrated by two series of experiments. By obstructing the mesonephric tubule of the chick embryo in two places, Boyden (1924) was able to observe the accumulation of phenolsulfonphthalein in the lumen between and see the tubule gradually dilate. Similarly, Schmidt* demonstrated tubular dilatation after obstructing the primary excretory duct of the aglomerular

* Unpublished work.

kidney of a certain marine teleost (Midshipman). Hydronephrosis therefore is not entirely dependent on glomerular function.

Secretory pressure is roughly the result of the combined pressures of glomerular filtration and tubular secretion. If the ureter is blocked and the intrapelvic pressure measured, it will be found to be between 50 and 70 mm. Hg, and will gradually decrease as the obstruction continues.

Muscular Conduction. In addition to the forces of glomerular filtration and tubular secretion, urinary pressure is also influenced by the muscular activity of the calyces and renal pelvis and of the ureter. This activity is a smooth muscle reflex brought on by the fluid stretching the wall of the conducting tube as it enters and passes downward. The ureter alone will lift mercury 28 mm. by its peristaltic activity (Gruber, 1930) but cannot continue to do so for long, since ureteral peristalsis is incomplete at such high pressures (Trattner, 1932). Secretory pressure after approximately two weeks' obstruction is about the same as that required for maximum peristaltic activity. One would expect some correlation of the degree of muscular hypertrophy from prolonged hyperactive peristalsis with the duration and degree of obstruction, although we can find no reports of such a study. Of course, prolonged obstruction with long continued peristaltic hyperactivity of ureter, pelvis and calyx results in increasing dilatation of these structures in that order, leading to muscular decompensation, and ending in muscular atrophy and fibrosis (Fig. 86, *A*).

RESORPTION OF URINE

If glomerular filtration is a mechanical process dependent on purely physical factors and if tubular secretion can continue as well against complete obstruction, especially if muscular conduction continues up to a certain point, there must be either excretion externally of the urine so formed or resorption of it some place along the excretory pathway. Otherwise, the pressure within the conducting structures would rapidly rise until glomerular filtration and tubular secretion were stopped altogether, in which case the progressive dilatation of hydronephrosis would not occur, but rather primary atrophy would intervene.

The actual evidence for such resorption is from several sources. Study of the composition of the urine at successive stages during hydronephrotic atrophy reveals a progression from normal to markedly abnormal. At no time is the fluid in the renal pelvis stagnant. Instead, there is continuous inflow and outflow. The inflow can be demonstrated by inference: at first, the urine in the pelvis contains most of the usual urinary constituents, but as obstruction continues, there is some increase in sugar and chlorides, and only a moderate decrease in urea (Fig. 87). This is best interpreted as evidence of continued inflow. The outflow can be demonstrated by placing dye in the renal pelvis and noting its progressive disappearance in a few days. After four days, the 6 or 7 cc. of hydronephrotic fluid in the rabbit kidney (normal capacity 1½ to 3 cc.) is free of phenolsulfonphthalein.

There are several possible sites for this resorption of fluid (and dye).

It may return by way of the fornices and venous system (pyelovenous back-flow), through the tubules (tubular backflow), or by way of the interstitial tissue and lymphatics (interstitial backflow)* (Table 6).

Pyelovenous backflow is probably the most important route for the resorption of urine in hydronephrosis. In certain animals a much lower pressure is

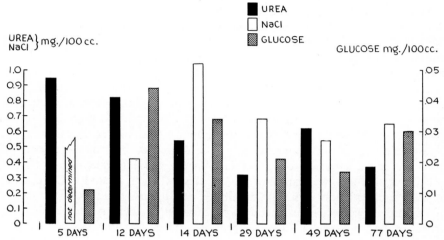

Fig. 87.   Graph showing persistence of sugar, chlorides and urea in hydronephrotic sac.

Table 6. Routes of Fluid Resorption

ROUTE OF BACKFLOW	WITHOUT OBSTRUCTION	AFTER OBSTRUCTION
via tubules...............	by transudation into pericana-licular spaces where reabsorption occurs (Narath, 1940)	a, by actual tubular rupture b, by lacerations in papillary area
and glomerular membrane...	None	by reverse flow in glomeruli with low secretory pressure (?)
via fornices...............	directly through epithelium into tissue spaces or even into vessels (polyuria, Fuchs; and antiperistalsis, Narath)	by direct rupture into tissue spaces or even into vessels
via interstitial tissue........	see above	rarely by actual rupture of pelvic membrane (see above)

required to produce backflow in the early stages of hydronephrosis than in the normal opposite kidney (Hinman and Lee-Brown, 1924). The balance between renal excretion and backflow is a fine one. It would appear that an increase in secretion raises the intrapelvic pressure which hastens the back-flow, and this, in turn, reduces the backpressure so allowing further renal secretion. Pelvic and ureteral peristalsis foster this activity by dissipating some of the pressure, as shown by the finding that high ureteral obstructions

* The reader is also referred to Narath's contribution (Section I, Chapter 3) in which he discusses in extenso these phenomena as phases of pelviocalyceal physiology.

cause a more rapid development of hydronephrosis than low obstructions. The crucial experiment compares the secretory pressure actually found after varying periods of obstruction with the pressure required to cause pyelovenous backflow at that time. The injection pressure needed for backflow in an obstructed kidney falls with the duration of obstruction and this closely parallels the fall in secretory pressure after such obstruction. These findings can be explained by assuming that a pathway is established which is then readily accessible for resorption of urine (Table 7).

Thus there is little doubt that pyelovenous backflow actually occurs and that it is of great importance in the development of hydronephrotic atrophy. We are all familiar with the picture of veins and lymphatics filled with dye during retrograde pyelography, especially if excessive pressure is used for injection or if the kidney is damaged by obstruction or infection. Histologic, roentgenographic, and experimental evidence points to the fornix of the minor calyx as the site of this resorption. The pelvic epithelium of transitional type changes suddenly at the edge of the papilla to become much more

Table 7. Intra-Ureteral Pressure Necessary to Cause Pyelovenous Backflow

	INTRAPELVIC PRESSURE in mm. Hg	PRESSURE NECESSARY FOR BACKFLOW in mm. Hg
Rabbit, 30 days' obstruction	15	10
Dog, 70 days' obstruction	21	15

endothelial. Narath (1940) and Fuchs (1930, 1944) have demonstrated with reasonable certainty that absorption of total urine may occur under certain physiologic conditions (diuresis and ? reverse peristalsis) without actual rupture at the fornix, agreeing with Winton (1937) who suggests that " . . . when flow from the ureter ceases, urine flow down the tubules still takes place, this urine leaking back into the blood at some point distal to the site of reabsorption of water." Fuchs, at the time of observing pyelovenous backflow through the fornical system, has noted the sudden fall of the secretory pressure from perhaps 70 mm. Hg to around 30 or 40. This low pressure then persists, since a pathway has been established.

During pyelovenous backflow from the fornical system, there is also pyelolymphatic backflow. Fuchs observed that simultaneously with the marked difference in the pressure gradient between the ruptured fornices and the veins, the lymphatics become highly dilated.

After the second week of obstruction with the disappearance of the fornices by pelvic dilatation and with the thickening of the pelvic and papillary epithelium the transfornical edema disappears. Pyelovenous backflow with fornical rupture ceases as the interstitial spaces become filled with new connective tissue. Tubular backflow now becomes relatively more important.

Tubular backflow is often seen in retrograde pyelography. The typical tuft formation is a not uncommon sight, especially if the kidney is inflamed. But it is difficult in the rabbit, for instance, to inject very far up the collecting duct no matter what pressure is used. In the dog and monkey and, to a lesser extent, the human kidney, dye can be forced a considerable distance up the collecting system. This tubular backflow is made easier by several days of ureteral obstruction in most experimental animals.

Of course, retrograde flow into the tubule does not explain exactly how the urine returns to the blood stream. Tubulovenous backflow would explain the more rapid, if localized, development of atrophy in the rabbit after papillary obstruction than after ureteral obstruction. Tubular backflow allows hydronephrosis to occur in animals without pelves because it permits continued excretion.* It also explains why certain other glands with a high excretory pressure go on to primary atrophy with obstruction of the duct since they have a poorer blood supply, a less advantageous arrangement of circulation, irritative secretory products, and, consequently, less opportunity for flow of the products of secretion out of their collecting system back into the circulation and so to allow the balanced process of dilatation to occur.

The work of Morison (1929) suggests a reason for the difficulty of causing immediate tubular backflow by increasing pelvic pressure early in hydronephrosis in the rabbit and explains why it may occur later as atrophy progresses. A normal papilla has a proliferative epithelium surrounding the ductal orifices. In early ureteral obstruction, hydrostatic compression of this tissue closes the papillary ducts and prevents fluid from running into the tubules. As hydronephrosis advances, the destruction and radial distention of the pelvis opens the ducts to allow tubular backflow.

Accompanying the tubulovenous, there may be tubulolymphatic backflow which has not been directly differentiated experimentally.

It seems obvious that it is not necessary for the urine actually to be discharged into the obstructed pelvis for such backflow to occur, but rather that tubulovenous or tubulolymphatic backflow can occur directly from the tubule when pressure there equals the pelvic pressure secondary to ureteral obstruction (Morison, 1939).

Glomerular back filtration has been suggested (Fuchs, 1930): " . . . Glomerular filtrate produced in some part of the parenchyma reaches the pyelon and proceeds thence into collecting tubules of a different part of the parenchyma and finally reaches glomeruli with decreased or completely eliminated filtration pressure. A sufficient difference in blood pressure in the two major groups of glomeruli causes back filtration into the low pressure glomeruli of the filtrate of the high pressure glomeruli. Thus, the flow of urine never ceases, pyelovenous and lymphatic reabsorption having been substituted by glomerular back filtration."

Interstitial absorption through the wall of the pelvis has been suggested as another route for urinary resorption with ureteral obstruction. Actually, experimental evidence suggests that this route is unimportant in hydronephrosis since it is very difficult to produce interstitial backflow in the experimental animal unless tubular or pyelovenous backflow has already occurred. If rupture into the parenchyma of the kidney does occur (true interstitial backflow), the fluid immediately enters the venous and lymphatic systems.

* Schmidt, unpublished work.

HYDRONEPHROSIS, THE RESULT OF IMBALANCE BETWEEN FORMATION AND RESORPTION-EXCRETION

The physiopathologic effects of obstruction to the outflow of urine upon the ureters and kidney can be divided roughly into three stages which are not mutually exclusive in point of time: the first is that of *trauma;* second, *hypertrophy of the conducting structures;* and the third, *atony, dilatation and parenchymal destruction.* These changes are best illustrated in acute complete obstruction.

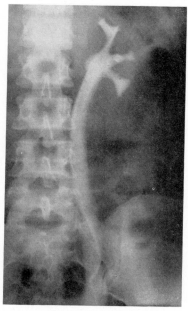

Fig. 88. Retrograde urogram showing ureteral but no pelvic or calyceal dilatation.

The Stage of Trauma. The immediate results of ligation of the ureter can be followed easily in the rabbit and similar changes have been found clinically. During the first few days, the contents of the renal pelvis increase in volume and in hemoglobin content. The source of the blood is not difficult to find, for section of the kidney shows marked vascular engorgement, especially at the corticomedullary junction. Hemorrhagic areas are seen which radiate along the tubules outward towards the capsule and inward along the collecting ducts to the pelvis. In the unipapillary kidney of the rabbit we find early degeneration of the papilla around the ducts of Bellini, so that after 8 to 14 days' obstruction the papilla is an excavated hillock with four gaping papillary ducts at the bottom of the crater. At about this same time, the renal parenchyma accommodates itself to the increased intrapelvic and intrarenal pressure to allow partial resorption of the bloody exudate and healing of the epithelial surfaces.

The Stage of Muscular Hypertrophy. The second stage blends into the first stage and in turn is continuous with the third stage. Muscular hypertrophy is much more prominent in partial obstruction than in complete obstruction. It has been incompletely studied in animals since most of the experimental work deals with complete obstruction. Muscular hypertrophy is marked above obstructions in clinical practice, which are usually partial. It begins at the most distal portion of the urinary tract, just above the obstruction; and it is here that decompensation first occurs. For this reason, isolated changes can be observed in the terminal portion of the ureter (Fig. 88). With continued muscular activity, dilatation takes place when the obstruction cannot even be overcome by the increased contractile force of ureteral peristalsis. An excellent example of the end stages of this muscular

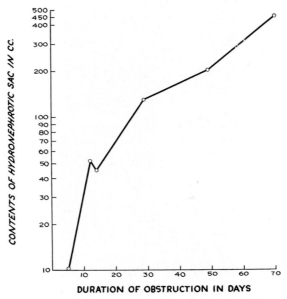

Fig. 89.   Relation of pelvic contents to duration of obstruction.

hypertrophy with progressive dilatation is seen with congenital obstruction. The ureters are left as dilated sacs with thick walls in which the hypertrophied muscle is being replaced with fibrous tissue. The dilatation occurs not only transversely, but also longitudinally, causing the characteristic tortuosity (Fig. 86, *B* and *C*).

The State of Dilatation and Parenchymal Destruction. The atony and dilatation of the third stage follows muscular decompensation since the hyperactive peristalsis and muscular hypertrophy in the second stage is no longer able to empty the ureter, pelvis or calyx. Prostatic obstruction produces analogous detrusor decompensation and atony, after initial hypertrophy.

This third stage is the most damaging in the process of hydronephrosis. Dilatation of all the obstructed segments causes parenchymal destruction by: (1) atony of the calyces, pelvis, and ureter; (2) parenchymal compression against the capsule; (3) vascular derangement; and, (4) tubular dilatation and cellular compression.

Atony of the conducting structures increases throughout the course of hydronephrosis, as reflected in dilatation with increasing volumes of fluid within them. With partial obstruction, enormous quantities of fluid may accumulate, ending in complete atony and atrophy of the pelvic and ureteral walls. In complete obstruction, on the other hand, the dilatation is usually less complete since intrapelvic pressure rises more rapidly and is held at a higher pressure than with incomplete obstruction. This results in more rapid destruction of the tubules and glomeruli, the continued secretion of which

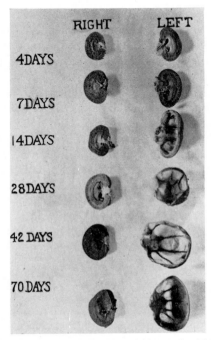

Fig. 90.   Progressive dilatation of obstructed left kidney of rabbit compared with hypertrophy of right kidney.

is necessary for further dilatation. In very late obstruction, after the secreting tissue is almost completely destroyed, the conducting structures fibrose and the small bit of remaining cortex contracts so that the total renal volume may diminish. Figure 89 shows the relation of the contents of the hydronephrotic sac of the rabbit and dog to the duration of the obstruction and Figure 90 illustrates the typical gross changes in the rat.

Parenchymal compression against the capsule had traditionally been considered the prime cause of hydronephrotic atrophy, but experimentally it has been shown to be relatively less important than derangement of the blood supply and dilatation of the tubules. Strong (1940) from his study of hydronephrosis by the maceration and microdissection technique concluded that the renal parenchyma persisting after varying periods of obstruction was related to the distortion of the kidney by the encroaching pelvis. He could not find any relation between the preservation of nephrons and their blood supply, especially since in certain specimens he was able to find zones of preserved nephrons at right angles to the course of the larger renal vessels. Certain anatomic relations to be noted in the next paragraph cast some doubt on his conclusions.

Vascular derangement during progressive hydronephrosis affects the nephron through the particular relationship of the blood vessels to the renal parenchyma. The arcuate arteries and veins swing around the calyces at the corticomedullary junction in a plane parallel to the surface of the kidney as well as parallel to the surface of the renal pelvis and of the dilating calyces. This arrangement places the vital portions of the kidney (glomeruli, and proximal and distal convoluted tubules) outside this network of major vessels. Injection studies show elongation and compression of these vessels by pelvic dilatation, such as to gradually decrease the blood supply to the cortex. (Earlier we commented on the rapid advance of hydronephrosis after partial arterial occlusion because of disturbed nutrition of the tissues.) The ischemia is not uniform throughout the kidney, but affects the lateral groups of nephrons more than the central. This patchy involvement is the basis for the formation of nodules of repair after release of the obstruction. Vascular compression affects some parts of the individual nephron selectively, the proximal convoluted tubule being most sensitive to ischemia.

The reduction of blood flow in early hydronephrosis has been found to average 41 per cent (Levy et al., 1937). Trueta's co-workers have suggested the presence of a shunt which would, by vascular reflex, make the cortex ischemic. By cineangiography, Herdman and Jaco (1950) directly observed reduction of blood flow as early as 24 hours after ureteral ligation, ascribing it to backpressure and dilatation of the tubules which in turn obstruct the capillaries. The delay in flow would indicate that under these experimental circumstances, an intrarenal shunt is not active.

Tubular dilatation with compression of tubular cells plays a major part in hydronephrotic atrophy (Strong, 1940). Increasing pressure is accompanied by dilatation of the collecting and distal convoluted tubules (the proximal tubule atrophies rather early), to a degree which varies with the topographic position of the nephron. Those with long pathways along the margin of the dilating pelvis are more compressed than dilated; those in the central portion are usually distended.

Partial obstruction in a way illustrates better than complete obstruction the interplay between urine formation and resorption-excretion. Here, instead of resorption entirely assuming the task of balancing urine formation, excretion takes over part or most of that function. But the pathologic changes in partial obstruction are the same. Because the balance is more delicate and is held at a lower pressure, which delays renal atrophy, the size of the hydronephrosis may be much greater. It should be noted here that complete ureteral obstruction, as by ligation at operation, does not result in primary renal atrophy. Rather, the kidney goes through the dilatation and final atrophy characteristic of hydronephrosis, even though this may be asymptomatic.

ADJUSTMENTS TO IMBALANCE

Compensatory hypertrophy occurs after occlusion of the ureter of the opposite kidney just as it does after unilateral nephrectomy (Arataki, 1926). Partial obstruction causes partial compensation by the other kidney. The stimulating factor is principally nitrogenous wastes. Experimentally, feeding urea will increase renal size and testosterone (Lattimer, 1932; Selye and Friedman, 1941) will cause proximal tubular hypertrophy by its effect on protein anabolism and perhaps by a direct renotrophic effect (Hinman, Jr., 1953).

Renal counterbalance is the theory that a sufficiently damaged kidney cannot compete with its mate. The normal kidney removes so much of the waste products (which are the stimulus to the nephron for compensatory hypertrophy) that the damaged kidney which requires relatively greater stimulation for hypertrophy receives less and less as the good kidney compensates. The result in the injured kidney can be considered an atrophy of disuse.

An experiment which illustrates this was done by Addis* for another reason. The upper and lower quarters of one kidney were excised from rats. If the other kidney was removed, the resected one would hypertrophy and take over total excretion. If it was not removed, the injured kidney would atrophy. Presumably, partial nephrectomy so interfered with renal blood supply that the nephrons could not compete with the normal ones in the kidney not operated upon.

Counterbalance has clinical application for the patient with rather advanced destruction of a kidney in the presence of a more normal mate. For practical purposes it has been found that if the damaged kidney has less than a fifth of the total renal function and would alone be unable to support life, it likewise is liable to atrophy in the presence of a normal kidney even if plastic procedures are effective in restoring it anatomically.

Repair of the hydronephrotic kidney after removal of the obstruction is not a generalized process. It occurs in localized areas depending on the two physical factors already mentioned: vascular derangement, and tubular compression and dilatation. In general, the central sagittal areas are more resistant and, consequently, show the most repair, while the lateral and polar areas show less. But even in these regions, the rate and degree of repair is not uniform, for patches of nephrons, presumably grouped about an intact arterial system, will hypertrophy so that they stand out on microscopic section as repair nodules. Recent work (Homburger et al., 1950) has suggested that methyl androstenediol hastens this repair in a degree greater than testosterone, but these experiments have yet to be verified adequately. It is probable that the androgens have effects favorable for repair after release of obstruction.

SECONDARY EFFECTS OF OBSTRUCTION

Stasis has two sequelae: infection and calculus formation.

Infection is common in hydronephrosis and part of the consequent renal

* Personal communication, 1948.

damage must be blamed on it. The line between infected hydronephrosis and frank pyonephrosis is poorly defined. Perhaps the only tenable division is that in pyonephrosis the pelvic contents are appreciably thicker than urine and that the pelvic contents increase at the expense of pelvic erosion. Pyonephrosis can be the end stage of infected hydronephrosis, for as the obstruction increases and function falls, the bacteria and pus accumulate to eventually fill the closed sac.

The formation of stones with stasis is common. In fact, the stone, becoming partially obstructive, may hasten its own growth. A stone that is too obstructive will grow at a less rapid rate since it will simultaneously depress renal function and hence its supply of chemicals. A discussion of the formation of stones in recumbency and in the presence of infection will be found in Section VIII, Chapter 1. Many small stones would be passed spontaneously if obstruction were not present but a calculus itself can be the primary cause of obstruction.

In summary, hydronephrosis is the result of imbalance between urine formation and its excretion or resorption. When excretion is blocked, urine formation is slowed but not stopped, and resorption from pelvis and tubules maintains the balance.

The kidney reacts to obstruction first by evidence of trauma, then by compensatory backflow with progressive dilatation in which the rate of excretion is slightly greater than that of resorption and, finally, by atrophy as the secretory ability of the parenchyma is destroyed.

Repair, after release of the obstruction, occurs in areas least damaged by pressure, fibrosis, or vascular disturbance. Waste products stimulate repair; if a good contralateral kidney efficiently removes these wastes, the injured kidney (whose damaged nephrons need even more stimulation than normal ones) atrophies, illustrating "renal counterbalance." Compensatory hypertrophy occurs in the good kidney as it is stimulated by assuming the excretory load of its mate.

The renal surgeon must take into account the possibilities of surgical injury, infection, irreversible vascular and tissue changes, as well as of renal counterbalance in weighing the chances for repair of the hydronephrotic kidney against the forces working for further atrophy.

THE CLINICAL CAUSES OF HYDRONEPHROSIS AND THEIR TREATMENT

Rationale for Therapy. Clinical evidence is accumulating that many so-called conservative plastic procedures for hydronephrosis are in reality radical, since so often secondary nephrectomy is required to remove the functionless infected kidney. Certain factors in each case will determine the choice of procedure:

Age of the patient is a prime factor. A young person deserves a more conservative procedure for three reasons: He may need the surplus renal tissue later if injury or other disease occurs; he is able to stand two operative procedures if subsequent nephrectomy should be necessary; and he will heal better, as repair is much more complete in infants and children, and even in young adults, because of intrinsic tissue reactions and better arterial supply. A patient over 55 or 60 years, on the contrary, with a shorter life expectancy, has statistically less chance of contralateral renal damage, and the operative mortality and morbidity is higher if two operations are necessary. Besides, his resistance to infection introduced during intubation and his capacity for healing are less.

The degree of destruction of the kidney, as we have noted, is of great importance. The rule-of-thumb that the kidney should have one fifth of the total function and be able to assume total excretion in the event of loss of the good kidney is workable in practice, and is based on sound experimental evidence. Infection with the obstruction can be expected later to decrease renal function by continued activity and by scarring, and the operation itself, especially if it includes nephrostomy drainage, will further damage the kidney.

Compensatory hypertrophy of the opposite kidney decreases the chances of a good functional result. Conversely, plastic procedures on the better of two kidneys are more likely to succeed. Following the same reasoning, the poor side in bilateral hydronephrosis should be repaired first: the needed stimulation for repair of that side is greater before the good side is improved by operation. Delay after repair of one of two diseased kidneys may allow the unoperated kidney to atrophy to such a degree that nephrectomy is the best treatment (renal counterbalance).

Hydronephrosis in infancy and childhood differs from that in the adult patient only in the greater ability of the young kidney to repair itself. All upper tract dilatations in childhood should be considered obstructive (Hinman, Jr., 1952), hence the basic principles of hydronephrosis which have been outlined above can be applied.

OBSTRUCTION AT THE LEVEL OF THE CALYX (HYDROCALICOSIS)

The term hydrocalyx is applied only to a cyst in the renal cortex caused by obstruction at the infundibulum, such that the entire calyx is dilated to form the wall of the cyst. It may be considered a miniature, localized hydronephrosis.

A typical case is due to retained calculus (Fig. 91). A hydrocalyx must be differentiated from (1) a parenchymal cyst with or without rupture into the pelvis; (2) a communicating pyelogenic cyst (or calyceal diverticulum); (3) localized obliterative pyelonephritis, and from (4) a communicating abscess (Fig. 92).

Treatment. If the symptoms of pain or infection warrant interference, simple transureteral catheterization may drain the area adequately (Beneventi, 1943), but more often partial or total nephrectomy is necessary.

OBSTRUCTION AT THE PELVIC LEVEL (URETEROPELVIC JUNCTION)

Pathogenesis. The most frequent finding with unilateral (as well as some cases of bilateral) hydronephrosis is obstruction at the ureteropelvic junction. A large staghorn calculus is not obstructive; a small stone is if it cannot negotiate the outlet of the renal pelvis. More often stones are secondary to renal obstruction than the cause of it.

The basic cause of obstruction at the junction of ureter with pelvis would appear to be congenitally poor design. Seldom is intrapelvic infection, stone, or tumor, or extrapelvic disease the primary cause of the obstruction, but

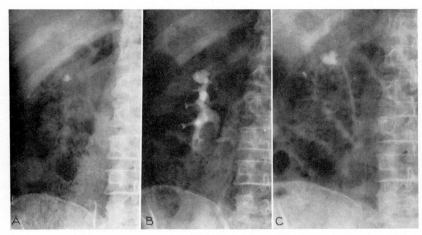

Fig. 91.   Hydrocalyx with retained calculus. *A*, plain film. *B*, retrograde pyelogram. *C*, emptying film.

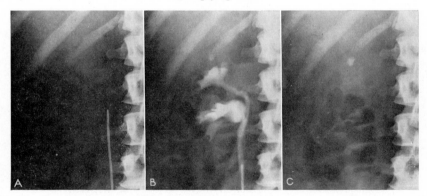

Fig. 92.   Communicating cortical abscess. *A*, plain film. *B*, retrograde film. *C*, emptying film.

more often they are factors which promote the speed of development and the degree of hydronephrosis. Most urologists no longer expect to find an aberrant vessel in every case, but look for a fibrous band or layer which pulls up and constricts the upper end of the ureter. Less common is a simple stricture at the ureteropelvic juncture which is not associated with displacement of the ureter at the pelvis as well. Consequently, plastic repair of the stricture will often be accompanied by replacement of the ureter to its normal position.

Indications for Operation. The *signs* and *symptoms* of obstruction at the ureteropelvic juncture will range from severe sharp or, more usually, aching pain in the costovertebral angle and marked tenderness to the complete absence of pain and tenderness depending whether the obstruction is acute (stone, inflammation, Dietl's crisis) or chronic. Gastrointestinal symptoms are not rare. Overhydration may be a factor. Extensive radiation of pain would not be expected, excepting testicular sensitivity because of that organ's origin from the same body segment as the kidney. A mass is less often felt, except in infants with very large sacs. Hematuria may be the only urinary finding. We have produced bleeding in rabbits from the intrarenal distention after acute obstruction. Of course, pyuria will be found if infection has supervened.

While intravenous urography may suggest the nature of the lesion (we occasionally use 50 cc. of 70 per cent Urokon injected rapidly intravenously

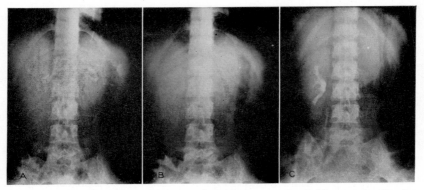

Fig. 93.   Intravenous renal angiogram and nephrogram. *A,* at 10 seconds. *B,* at one minute. *C,* at 5 minutes.

to produce a nephrogram (Fig. 93) allowing estimation of vascularity and renal cortical thickness), more often retrograde study will allow proper evaluation. One must be ready to go ahead with operative repair in some cases, for catheterization can precipitate complete obstruction as well as introduce infection which can be hard to control.

The points for study by retrograde catheterization number six: First, relative renal function is measured by phenolsulfonphthalein (PSP) test, to determine if the damaged kidney should be saved or if the interplay of renal counterbalance (q.v.) will allow its atrophy. Each normal kidney will excrete about 15 per cent PSP in fifteen minutes. Second, infection is searched for by a smear of centrifuged urine stained with methylene blue. Third, the degree of calyceal dilatation is compared with the dilatation of the pelvis, since a congenitally large pelvis may have no pathologic significance or, if acquired, may not itself require treatment, whereas calyceal dilatation usually means renal damage. At the same time, the amount of cortical thickness is estimated.

Fourth, the site and outline of the obstruction is determined. Obstruction at the ureteropelvic junction displaces the lower portion of the pelvis downward through pelvic distention. If the ureter is held up by fibers or vessels running between the lower pole and the aorta area it becomes angulated and obstructed at the point of entrance which now is on the anterior pelvic wall; such is the common picture. The surgeon will need this information in planning the plastic repair.

A fifth point is the reproduction of pain by distention of the pelvis. Since many times the patient's symptoms are vague, even gastrointestinal in character, and the visible evidence for obstruction minor, reproduction of pain may give the lie to its source.

The sixth and last point for evaluation is the time of emptying after withdrawal of the catheter. It is our observation that waiting only ten minutes may not necessarily give the normal kidney opportunity to empty; whereas significant obstruction will be picked up if there is retention on a film exposed after fifteen minutes.

Of course, all of these six factors are not present in each case, but they will form a sound basis for surgical treatment.

Contraindications to Plastic Repair. Before operating on a patient with hydronephrosis secondary to ureteropelvic juncture obstruction, one must be convinced that operation will improve the functional status of the kidney. Revision of anatomical changes alone (for example, excising a redundant dilated pelvis) will not help the patient unless at the same time renal function is improved, or infection eradicated, or perhaps pain obliterated. The surgeon must remember that plastic procedures often introduce new complications such as parenchymal scarring, resistant infection, or secondary strictures so that his patient is worse off than with the original mild hydronephrosis. This is especially true in patients older than 30 years, since obviously they have tolerated some degree of obstruction for years.

We have already reviewed the factors against plastic repair of the hydronephrotic kidney: advanced age, severe renal destruction, and marked compensatory renal hypertrophy (p. 213). These factors must be considered in each case, for nephrectomy may turn out to be the most conservative treatment.

OPERATIVE TREATMENT

Plastic procedures for relief of obstruction at the ureteropelvic junction may be grouped as follows*:
  A. Without opening into the urinary tract
        1. Pelvio-ureterolysis (with or without denervation)
        2. Nephropexy
        3. Division of aberrant vessel or band
        4. Incomplete longitudinal incisions (after Rammstedt).
  B. Ureteropelvic incision
        1. Longitudinal incision, with
              a. Intubation (Davis, 1951)
              b. Transverse closure(s) (Heinecke-Mikulicz; Fenger, 1894; Gibson, 1940)

* The technique of these procedures is given in detail in Section XV, Chapters 3 and 4.

    c. Longitudinal incision up ureter and down pelvis (Finney, von Lichtenberg, 1929; Priestley, 1939)

  2. Y-incision, with

    a. Oblique closure (Schwyzer, 1923)

    b. Inverted Y closure (Foley, 1937)

  3. W-incision (Ballenger-McDonald, 1942)

  4. With pelvic flap (Culp, personal communication, 1951)

C. Reimplantation of ureter

  1. Oblique anastomosis (Küster, 1892)

  2. Split anastomosis (Lubash, 1937)

  3. Direct anastomosis.

D. Combinations with resection of pelvis.

General Technical Details. A hydronephrotic kidney is best approached through the classical lumbar incision, with excision of the twelfth rib if that should lie over the kidney. Catgut will be used throughout since infected urine may be expected to drain from the wound. Gerota's fascia is entered posteriorly so that the perinephric fat may later be replaced to shield the repair and help support the kidney and so that the muscles of the posterior body will be left clean for later fixation of the kidney.

Exposure of the kidney must be done cautiously, since vascular anomalies are to be expected. An aberrant vessel to the upper pole, if torn, may retract and be very hard to secure. It is wise not to divide an anomalous vessel until the entire blood supply has been exposed; the vessel may be an important part of that supply. To test this the vessel may be compressed by the fingers or a rubber-shod clamp; the infarcted portion of the kidney then appears cyanotic. The injection of methylene blue into the aberrant vessel will give an outline of that vessel's area of supply. Better, because of some overlapping of arterial trees, is the injection of the dye into the main renal artery; this will leave undyed the area not supplied by the main trunk. Interrupted ureteral sutures of 4-0 chromic catgut swedged on $\frac{3}{8}$ circle cutting needles (which are better than the usual $\frac{1}{2}$ circle needle) are placed 0.5 cm. apart if plastic closure is desired. The simple incision of the stricture with intubation should not be closed.

Usually the drainage tube or ureteral splint will hold the kidney in place because of their fixation as they pass through the body wall; if not, care must be taken to fasten the kidney to the posterior body wall by several mattress sutures (more complicated techniques seem unnecessary) so that the lower pole will not fall caudally and medially and adhere to or distort the upper ureter. We seldom place heavy rubber tube drains to the peripelvic space, but find that two large-sized penrose drains provide an adequate channel for leakage of urine. Before closure, pads of fat are interposed between the ureteropelvic incisions and the posterior body wall to reduce scarring and the distorting adhesions.

Certain general rules apply to plastic operations on the ureteropelvic junction. First, an attempt should be made to restore normal anatomic relations in the hope that normal function will follow. The ureter should lie at the most dependent portion of the pelvis. The ureteropelvic junction should be funnel-shaped. Redundant portions of the pelvis may be excised so that pelvic capacity more nearly approaches normal. This is especially desirable if the pelvic wall is thick and fibrotic, without peristaltic activity. The treated area should be cleaned of all extrinsic fibrous tissue without unduly jeopardizing its blood supply and should be padded with fat after repair.

Select the plastic incision and closure which will fit the situation at the time of surgical exposure. We feel it unwise to stick to one or two plastic procedures; rather we design the operation at the table, utilizing and combining accepted procedures found useful in the past. Seldom, however, will our incision and closure look like the textbook picture since seldom is exactly the same anatomic distortion found.

A. *Operative Procedures Which Do Not Enter the Urinary Tract*. As a general rule, simple ureterolysis with or without nephropexy will not relieve symptomatic obstruction at the ureteropelvic junction. And more definitely we may state that division of an aberrant vessel or obstructing band seldom removes the obstruction, since pelvio-ureteral peristalsis acting for a long time over the obstructive bridge causes intrinsic ureteral fibrosis and stricture. This stricture must be attacked directly.

We have had little experience with longitudinal incisions in the ureter which do not incise the mucosa (as in the Rammstedt pyloroplasty); if combined with an intraluminal splint they might be of value.

B. *Ureteropelvic Incision*. The most popular procedure today is the intubated ureterostomy re-introduced by Davis (1951).

Occasionally, in simple short strictures, especially if close to the renal pelvis, we use a transverse closure of the longitudinal incision (the Heinecke-Mikulicz procedure of gastrointestinal surgery adapted to urology by Fenger, 1894 and, with a double incision, by Gibson, 1940).

If high insertion of the ureter into the pelvis is found, a U-shaped incision up the ureter and then down the pelvis behind the ureter, as in the Finney pyloroplasty (von Lichtenberg, 1929), may be applicable. Splinting is advisable.

A Y-incision may yield greater ureteral diameter than a longitudinal incision. Schwyzer's incision brings a tongue of pelvis down to widen the ureter. Foley combines this principle with the Finney operation for the case with high ureteral insertion. Culp uses a flap from the pelvis to accomplish a similar purpose.

The W-incision (Ballenger and McDonald) extends the Y-plasty of Schwyzer to allow excision of some of the redundant pelvis with the same incision.

C. *Reimplantation of the Ureters*. Many procedures have been described, ranging from division at the midportion of the pelvis with reapproximation in front of aberrant vessels to simple direct reimplantation of the divided ureter into the pelvis. An oblique anastomosis will reduce the chance of stenosis at the new opening, especially if properly splinted. Resection of redundant pelvis is done as dictated by local conditions, and the ureter obliquely reimplanted at the most dependent portion. In general, unless the pelvic wall is greatly distended and thickened, it need not be resected.

D. *Combinations with Resection of Pelvis.* We would emphasize that each case must be handled as a separate problem, hence combinations and adaptations will as often be used as the classical procedures. Occasionally, after effecting a good opening at the ureteropelvic junction, the surgeon will want to excise redundant pelvis. Simple elliptical incisions, with care to avoid blood vessels, will pare down the pelvis for a more anatomic result.

OBSTRUCTION AT THE URETERAL LEVEL

Pathogenesis. There are many causes for ureteral obstruction (the most common: stone, inflammation, injury and developmental abnormality). Their obstructive effects are similar and details of their etiology and treatment will be found in appropriate chapters. If ureteral obstruction is acute and painful, there is hyperperistalsis and local vascular spasm; if chronic, there is gradual fibrosis at the site of obstruction with progressive dilatation above. This begins just above the site of obstruction, then rises to include the remainder of the ureter, the pelvis and finally the calyces. High ureteral obstruction causes earlier caliectasis than low ureteral obstruction, since ureteral peristalsis is a buffer to carry off urine and so reduce at least temporarily the back pressure within the kidney. The symptoms are in general similar to those after higher obstruction. We have argued in a recent publication (1952) that all dilatation of the ureter is due to obstruction, intrinsic, extrinsic or in the lower tract. The hydroureter (megaloureter is a term to be avoided since it connotes a purely ureteral developmental defect) does not itself cause back pressure on the kidney; rather, the hydroureter and the hydronephrosis have a common origin in obstruction distally in the urinary tract.

OPERATIVE TREATMENT

In the last year or two interest has again been shown in plastic resection of the dilated, redundant ureter. It is my feeling that the correction of the distal obstruction (Swenson et al., 1952) rather than any local benefit to the ureter is responsible for the few successes of the procedure, since peristalsis is not regained and the valve-like folds in the redundant ureter are more apparent than real. Besides, it is usual to get reflux after reimplantation of these dilated ureters, unless the anastomosis is stenotic, which also leads to renal destruction.

Rather than be diverted by the changes secondary to obstruction, the surgeon is better advised to attack the obstructive lesion directly (as we shall discuss under lower tract obstructions). Strictures secondary to injury or operation (as after ureterolithotomy) usually require longitudinal incision and intubation, much as do those at the ureteropelvic juncture. The operative procedures are similar.

Involvement of the ureter by extrinsic processes is often seen. Most common is ureteral constriction from extension of cervical carcinoma and less common is obstruction from the fibrosis of x-ray therapy. We have recently seen such a rare etiologic agent as an aneurysm of the abdominal aorta (Fig. 94). Treatment in these cases will be influenced by the prognosis of the original lesion (for example, rapidly advancing cervical cancer would prohibit extensive procedures on the urinary tract), and by the site of the obstruction. If high, the obstruction is best treated by nephrostomy diversion.

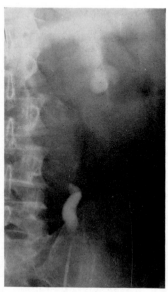

Fig. 94. Ureteral obstruction from aortic aneurysm: note calcification above dilated ureteral segment.

If low, ureteroenterostomy or ureterocutaneous anastomosis may be done. Rarely is reimplantation of the ureter practicable.

OBSTRUCTION AT THE URETEROVESICAL ORIFICE (LEVEL OF BLADDER)

Pathogenesis. Two sources for hydroureter and hydronephrosis can be found at the ureterovesical orifice: one, stenosis; and the other, the incompetent valve.

Stenosis may be caused by congenital defects, inflammatory lesions or vesical dysfunction with detrusor hypertrophy.

Often stenosis arises congenitally, commonly from ureterocele, less frequently from a malformed orifice of inadequate diameter (i.e., failure of dissolution of Chwalla's membrane). Inflammation with fibrosis of the bladder wall, after tuberculosis (Fig. 95) or after transurethral resection of prostate or bladder wall, is not rare. The hypertonic neurogenic bladder causes thickening of the detrusor, which in turn obstructs the ureteral orifices. Transurethral dilation may be tried, or reimplantation resorted to, but often transplantation of the ureters to the bowel or skin is necessary.

The incompetent ureterovesical valve may be caused by pathologic processes similar to stenosis, except that the end result differs. In children, a

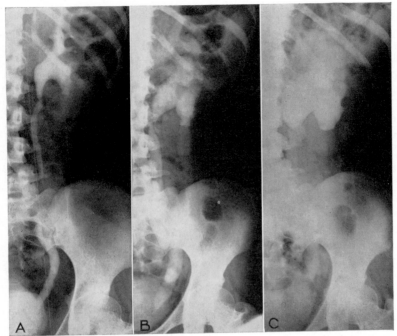

Fig. 95.   Stricture at ureterovesical junction due to tuberculous cystitis. *A*, 9-16-48. *B*, 40 months later. *C*, the following month.

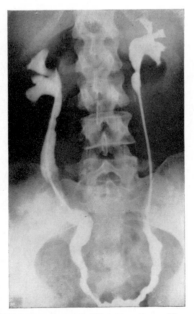

Fig. 96.   Bilateral ureteral dilatation from Hunner's ulcer.

dilated orifice means lower tract obstruction even if the other orifice is normal. Prolonged catheter drainage may be required to relieve the back pressure and allow the orifice to return to normal size. Dilated orifices may be secondary to Hunner's ulcer (Fig. 96), cord bladder, or lower tract obstruction. Reimplantation often allows reflux, although we are conducting experiments to try to prevent it.

The changes in the wall of the ureter are of interest. At first of course, there is simple hypertrophy of the muscular coats as the ureter by its peristaltic activity attempts to force the urine past the obstruction. Decompensation sets in when the size of the opening becomes too small in relation to the amount of urine presented to it. Dilatation appears first just proximal to the obstruction and moves gradually higher. Hypertrophic changes in the muscle may continue or fibrosis may intervene. In children, because of the continuation of hypertrophic processes, the ureter elongates until by urogram it appears to be angulated and obstructed at many points. Actually, this may not increase the obstruction; there is no evidence that more renal excretory pressure is required to send urine through the angulated hydroureter than through a straight, slightly dilated one.

OBSTRUCTION BELOW THE BLADDER

In other chapters (6-9; Section XV), the pathologic details and program of treatment of vesical neck obstructions and urethral lesions are discussed. In the final analysis, a higher proportion than is usually granted of hydronephrosis and ureterectasis in children is secondary to lower tract obstruction even though other lesions (incompetent or stenotic ureterovesical orifices) may appear to be primary. A systematic survey will detect meatal stenosis, urethral valves and congenital vesical neck obstruction evidenced by a small urinary stream, straining to void, residual urine, or vesical trabeculation. If these are found, and the obstructive lesion removed (by incision, simple instrumentation, progressive dilatation, or actual resection of the vesical neck), the secondary changes may regress.

After lower tract obstruction, the bladder is first involved. Intravesical pressure rises higher and higher with each voiding. Hypertrophy of the detrusor is a natural consequence, revealing itself as trabeculation. There follows cellule formation and diverticula as the mucosa and submucosa herniate between the muscle bands. In some cases, a large diverticulum may absorb the voiding force and delay damage to the upper tract, but more often the kidneys and ureters are required to push the urine into the bladder at a higher and higher pressure. So ureteral decompensation (hydroureter) may even occur before decompensation of the bladder. Or renal damage may occur without great ureteral or calyceal dilatation.

The trigone (especially the interureteric ridge) hypertrophies but probably itself does not introduce an additional obstructive factor. However, increasing attention should be paid to that portion of the detrusor lying about the neck of the bladder. Less important than the size of the benign prostatic enlargement itself may be its relation to the vesical neck, as intravesical protrusion can be more obstructive than intraurethral extension.

Sudden complete retention may temporarily reflexly suppress renal function. Chronic retention acts by the mechanisms described above (that is, by obstruction). Sudden release of pressure after chronic retention has long been considered harmful. A moment's thought, however, will show that removal of even 100 cc. will reduce intravesical pressure almost to zero, so that the usual methods of decompression cannot accomplish the desired result. In addition, most recent studies have shown less bleeding and less renal damage by rapid decompression.

SUMMARY

Obstruction to urinary outflow anywhere along the urinary tract may eventually cause renal failure through hydronephrotic atrophy. The first consideration of the urologic surgeon should be the preservation of renal function.

Hydronephrosis occurs when the rate of urine formation is greater than the rate at which it can be carried away. With any degree of obstruction, a balance is set up between the two forces of formation and reabsorption-excretion. However, enough increase in intrarenal pressure occurs to cause progressive parenchymal compression and vascular distortion, ending finally in hydronephrotic atrophy.

After release of the obstruction, repair occurs in the least damaged areas. The principal stimulus for repair is nitrogenous waste. If the good kidney on the other side removes those waste products efficiently, the injured kidney receives less stimulation and may atrophy ("renal counterbalance"). Compensatory hypertrophy, in the good kidney, occurs with the increased stimulation after loss of the other kidney.

In evaluating a patient for operation, the degree of renal damage and chance for recovery after surgical repair must be balanced against the condition of the other kidney as well as the age of the patient. Plastic operations introduce foreign bodies and infection, and may leave the kidney in poorer condition.

The choice of operative procedure will rest on the site of the obstruction. In high lesions, the exact technique for repair will often be decided after exposure of the stricture. Good technique requires diversion of the urinary stream, adequate splinting of the area of repair, and free drainage of extravasated urine.

REFERENCES

ARATAKI, M.: Experimental researches on the compensatory enlargement of the surviving kidney after unilateral nephrectomy (albino rat). Am. J. Anat., *36:*437–450, 1926.
BALLENGER, E. G. and McDONALD, H. P.: Conservation of the hydronephrotic kidney. J. Urol., *47:*203–208, 1942.
BENEVENTI, F. A.: Hydrocalyx: its relief by retrograde dilatation. Am. J. Surg., *61:*244, 1943.
BOYDEN, E. A.: Experimental obstruction of the mesonephric ducts. Proc. Soc. Exp. Biol. & Med., *24:*573, 1924.
DAVIS, DAVID M.: Intubated ureterotomy. J. Urol., *66:*77–84, 1951.
FENGER, C.: Operation for the relief of valve-formation and stricture of the ureter in hydronephrosis and pyonephrosis. J.A.M.A., *22:*335–343, 1894.
FOLEY, F. E. B.: A new plastic operation for stricture at the uretero-pelvic junction; report of 20 operations. J. Urol., *38:*643–672, 1937.

FUCHS, F.: Pyelovenous backflow in the human kidney. J. Urol., 23:181, 1930.
FUCHS, F.: The Flow of Water Through the Kidney. Manhattan Printing Co., New York, 1944.
GIBSON, T. E.: Hydronephrosis: standardization of surgical treatment. New England J. Med., 222:910–917, 1940.
GRUBER, C. M.: The function of the ureterovesical valve and the production of hydroureters without obstruction. J. Urol., 23:161, 1930.
HERDMAN, J. P. and JACO, N. T.: The renal circulation in experimental hydronephrosis. Brit. J. Urol., 22:52–55, 1950.
HINMAN, FRANK and HEPLER, A. B.: Experimental hydronephrosis. The effect of changes in blood pressure and in blood flow on its rate of development. II. Partial obstruction of the renal artery; diminished blood flow; diminished intrarenal pressure and oliguria. Arch. Surg., 11:649–659, 1925.
HINMAN, FRANK and LEE-BROWN, R. K.: Pyelovenous back-flow. J.A.M.A., 82:607–613, 1924.
HINMAN, FRANK, JR.: Congenital Ureteral and Pelvic Dilatation as Evidence of Obstruction. Monographs on Surgery, Thomas Nelson & Sons, 1952.
HINMAN, FRANK, JR.: Diseases of the kidneys: The renotrophic effects of steroid hormones. Annual Review of Medicine, 4:99–112, 1953.
HOMBURGER, F., FORBES, I. and DESJARDINS, R.: Renotropic effects of some androgens upon experimental hydronephrosis and upon the clitoris in the mouse. Endocrinol., 47: 19–25, 1950.
KUSTER, E.: Ein Fall von Resection des Ureter. Arch. f. klin. Chir., 44:850–854, 1892.
LATTIMER, J. K.: The action of testosterone propionate upon the kidneys of rats, dogs and men. J. Urol., 48:778–794, 1942.
LEVY, S. E., MASON, M. F., HARRISON, T. R. and BLALOCK, A.: The effects of ureteral occlusion on the blood flow and oxygen consumption of the kidneys of unanesthetized dogs. Surgery, 1:238–242, 1937.
VON LICHTENBERG, A.: Plastic surgery of the renal pelvis and ureter. J.A.M.A., 93:1706–1708, 1929.
LUBASH, S. and MADRID, A.: Uretero-pyeloneostomy for hydronephrosis, with case and experimental reports. J. Urol., 38:634–642, 1937.
MORISON, D. M.: Routes of absorption in hydronephrosis: experimentation with dyes in the totally obstructed ureter. Brit. J. Urol., 1:30–45, 1929.
MORISON, D. M.: Routes of absorption in total ureteral obstruction. Arch. Surg., 38:1108–1131, 1939.
NARATH, P. A.: The hydromechanics of the calyx renalis. J. Urol., 43:145, 1940.
NESBIT, R. M., BUTLER, W. J. and WHITAKER, W.: Production of epithelial lined tubes from buried strips of intact skin. J. Urol., 64:387–392, 1950.
PRIESTLEY, J. T.: The conservative surgical treatment of non-calculous hydronephrosis. Surg., Gynec. & Obst., 68:832–841, 1939.
SCHMIDT, S. S.: Ureteral obstruction in the aglomerular kidney. (Unpublished.)
SCHWYZER, A.: A new pyelo-ureteral plastic for hydronephrosis. S. Clin. North America, 3:1441–1448, 1923.
SELYE, H. and FRIEDMAN, S. M.: Beneficial action of testosterone in experimental renal atrophy caused by ligature of ureter. Endocrinology, 29:80–81, 1941.
STRONG, K. C.: Plastic studies in abnormal renal architecture; V. the parenchymal alterations in experimental hydronephrosis. Arch. Path., 29:77–119, 1940.
SWENSON, ORVAR, MACMAHON, H. E., JAQUES, W. E. and CAMPBELL, J. S.: A new concept of the etiology of megaloureters. New England J. M., 246:41–46, 1952.
TRATTNER, H. E.: Graphic registration of the function of the human ureter with the hydrophoragraph. J. Urol., 28:1, 1932.
WINTON, F. R.: Physical factors involved in the activities of the mammalian kidney. Physiol. Rev., 17:408–435, 1937 (p. 430).

Section IV

EMBRYOLOGY AND ANOMALIES OF THE UROGENITAL TRACT

MEREDITH CAMPBELL, M.D.

Embryologically and anatomically the urinary and genital tracts must be considered as a single system. The reasons for this are (1) their common origin from the mesodermal intermediate cell mass, (2) the incorporation of the primitive excretory ducts of the pronephros and mesonephros into the male genital organs, and (3) their relation with the primitive cloaca. For these reasons normal and abnormal embryology are discussed here together. Because of this intimate embryological development of the genital and urinary systems in each sex and as an important clinical corollary, it is notable that when the genitalia show malformation (vesical exstrophy, hypospadias, reduplicated uterus, uterus unicornis, etc.) the upper urinary tract is also anomalous in about a third of the cases. Conversely in upper urinary tract malformation, anomalies of the genital tract are common and in the female may occur in as high as two thirds of the cases.

Anomalous development attains its highest incidence in the urogenital tract, constituting 35 to 40 per cent of all maldevelopments. Autopsy studies have shown that more than 10 per cent of all humans are born with some urogenital tract anomaly, some observers citing this incidence as high as 14 per cent while Helmholz and Thompson (1941) put the figure at 5 per cent of all newborns which, in our experience, is a decidedly low estimate. In a postmortem study of 8905 neonatal deaths in Chicago, Bundesen et al. (1952) found malformations to be the third most common cause of death (abnormal pulmonary ventilation, 43.7 per cent; birth injury, 16.6 per cent, and malformation, 15.8 per cent), or 3.4 deaths per 1000 live births. Under one day, malformations accounted for 12 per cent of deaths; between one and twenty-nine days, 19.9 per cent, and one to eleven months, 21.6 per cent—observations copiously reflected in our autopsy studies in 19,046 infants and children. Regardless of the precise numerical incidence, the high occurrence of congenital malformations of all types as recorded in the 1948 United States* death registration rated these conditions as the second most common cause of death in infants under one year of age (4.5 per 1000 live births; no record of the etiologic incidence in stillbirths!) and as the third most common cause of death for children one to four years of age (12.6 per 100,000 population). The true incidence is, of course, much

* Vital Statistics of the United States, Part I, 1948.

higher than this despite the official recording of about 12,000 deaths per year in older children as a result of congenital malformations. These recorded lesions were in the majority of instances the readily apparent variety such as spina bifida, vesical exstrophy, or congenital hip dislocation and so forth, and in general exclude the far higher incidence discernible only by postmortem examination or by adequate urologic investigation of the urinary tract and which were performed only in a comparatively small percentage of these cases.

Urogenital maldevelopments may be single or multiple, simple and of scant clinical concern, or severe and threaten or take life. The child may be stillborn, may die immediately post partum or after a few weeks and consequent to the anomaly. On the other hand, many patients with horseshoe kidney or congenital solitary kidney, for example, live their full life span unmindful of the malformation they harbor. Urogenital malformations show a striking tendency to be multiple and only a thorough urologic examination can be expected to reveal the nature and extent of all of these anomalies in a patient. A splendid illustration of this is a ten-year-old boy initially examined because of so-called chronic pyelitis. The investigation disclosed a perineal testicle, a tight congenital urethral stricture at the penoscrotal junction, congenital hypertrophy of the verumontanum with 4 ounces of residual urine, infected hydronephrosis of the lower half of a reduplicated left kidney associated with pronounced ureterectasis and due to congenital ureterovesical junction stricture of the ureter to this renal segment, and moreover, six lumbar vertebrae, and marked spina bifida. In addition he had a curious subgrouping blood dyscrasia; crossmatching of blood from more than thirty individuals of his major blood group failed to obtain one satisfactory for transfusion. This boy's perineal testicle was properly placed in the scrotum, the urethral stricture was successfully dilated to the point of cure, the verumontanum was resected transurethrally, and left ureteroheminephrectomy was performed. A premarital examination twelve years later showed he was emptying his bladder completely, the urine was sterile, and he was otherwise functionally normal except that no spermatozoa could be found in the ejaculate, doubtless the result of fibrotic occlusion of the ejaculatory ducts following resection of the obstructing hypertrophic verumontanum. While the last finding is most regrettable, the gravity of the boy's congenital obstructive condition and infection when he was initially seen offered no course other than removal of the blockage caused by the hypertrophic verumontanum.

It is axiomatic that *an anomalous organ is more prone to disease than a normal one.* Because the majority of urinary tract anomalies are either actually or potentially obstructive and thereby engender urinary stasis which, in turn, invites infection or stone formation or may produce severe backpressure renal injury, the more important malformations are likely to manifest themselves clinically in infancy or childhood. Bigler (1934) found congenital obstructive or stasis producing lesions in half of a large series of infants and children with chronic urinary infection; in some instances there is absence or hypoplasia of one or more organs essential to the excretion or discharge of urine. Rarely a child is born with tumor. Urosurgery in this age group is predominantly concerned with the correction of anomalous development and/or the treatment of its complications.

In addition to these malformations as clinicopathologic problems, the physician is confronted by the inquiring parents of the congenitally deformed child. The questions include why did such development occur, whose fault was it, could it have been prevented, are subsequent children of theirs likely to suffer similarly and, as a corollary, should they have any more children. The information given the parents of these unfortunate children is not to be offered lightly or without the full consideration of present-day knowledge, albeit it relatively scant, of what is scientifically acceptable. These answers may have dire psychologic and domestic repercussions, particularly as concerns the prospects of having normal children subsequently.

Several explanations for the cause of anomalous development have been deduced both by observation and, more particularly, by scientific experimental study; none of these potential causes fit all cases. Our present day knowledge of these potential causes is briefly summarized in the following paragraphs.

Unfavorable Maternal Impressions Received During Pregnancy. While this ancient theory has been repeatedly advanced to explain anomalous development, it is without weight because the malformations had been embryologically established long before the impressions were received. Nevertheless, Greenfelder and Lasch (1949) experimentally observed the fetus of thirty-three days to be most susceptible to the development of factitial anomalous urogenital organs.

Vitamin deficiency has been cited by Warkany (1943, 1947) who found lack of riboflavin essential to the production of anomalous development in rats. Both Hale (1935) and Warkany and his co-workers experimentally produced malformations by vitamin A deficiency.

Chemical Substances. Chemobiologic investigations have shown that embryonic cells can be influenced by substances such as sterols and estrogens (Green et al., 1938). These and other deductions from experimental studies have been excellently summarized by Fraser and Fainstat (1951) who were able to produce cleft palate in as high as 70 per cent of the fetuses of pregnant mice by administering cortisone. A somewhat higher incidence of anomalous development in males compared with females (3:2; in greater than the birth ratio of 1055:1000) and a slightly higher incidence of left-sided over rightsided anomalous developments have been noted. Yet the carefully made studies of Murphy (1947) suggest that sex and side incidence are about equal. In Philadelphia he found the death rate from malformations in white people to be nearly twice that in Negroes (57:32 per 100,000 population).

Virus Infection. The studies of Gregg (1941) and others lend suggestive weight to the proposition that maternal virus infection particularly during the early months of pregnancy is a factor in the anomalous development in the child in many instances. He noted an unusually high incidence of congenital opacities of the eyes in children in New South Wales born of mothers who had suffered rubella (German measles) during pregnancy. Other mal-developments included deaf mutism, mental defectiveness, delayed dentition, congenital eye and heart disease, hypospadias, and talipes equinovarus. It was noted that when the maternal infection occurred after the second month of pregnancy the likelihood of malformation was greatly reduced. If the mother suffers rubella during the first two months of pregnancy, she will probably give birth to a malformed child, as will half of the mothers infected during the third month of pregnancy. These findings have been rather widely confirmed by Swan et al. (1943). Prendergast (1946) and Abel and Van Dellen (1949) found that 89 per cent of the babies born of mothers having rubella in the first three months of pregnancy were abnormal, 42 per cent when the disease occurred in the second three months, and none when it occurred in the third trimester.

Other factors which have been etiologically described in anomalous development and with suggested confirmatory evidence for each, include syphilis, x-rays (Murphy, 1947), contraceptives, alcohol, endocrine factors (infantilism, dwarfism, gigantism, cretinism), as well as hereditary and environment. Doubtless the genetic factors in heredity operate more often than do others (Mall, 1910; Gruenwald, 1949) these factors being largely gametic mutations which are recessive (92 to 95 per cent, Kemp, 1944) although some conditions such as Huntington's chorea and sickle cell anemia are hereditary dominants. Maturation of sex genes has been adduced to explain hypospadias and pseudohermaphrodism by Goldschmidt (1938), these conditions being intersex manifestations. It has long been noted that malformations or entire congenital syndromes, such as Laurence-Moon-Biedl or gargoylism, frequently occur identically in several members of the same family or there may be various combinations of anomalies with vesical exstrophy in one, spina bifida in another, or cleft palate in still another. If the child is congenitally mentally deficient, the chances of his also having structural malformation are vastly increased, a point of considerable diagnostic importance in determining whether a presenting syndrome is congenital or acquired.

Repetitive Incidence of Anomalous Development in Siblings. The most comprehensive answers to the question of the likelihood of a mother giving birth to malformed children subsequent to the birth of one anomalous child, are found in the report of Murphy who, in a masterful study of 130,132 death certificates in Philadelphia over a five-year period (January 1, 1929 to December 31, 1933), found gross congenital defects noted in 1476. In 890 of these cases the condition was recognized by postmortem examination, by external examination, or both. It is notable that 90 per cent of these defectives were stillborn or died within the year. In the 890 cases a checkback investigation was carried out with interviews with the mother in each instance and an analysis of a comprehensive questioning of her. In this manner Murphy found that the incidence of congenital defects in the first four children followed the normal proportion, but beginning with the fifth child, a sharp rise occurred in the incidence ratio of anomalies and in the seventh child was double that in any of the first four. Children born of mothers over forty years of age are three times as likely to be abnormal as in the mothers under thirty years. The mothers had their first defective child an average of five years after the birth of the preceding normal one and a long period of relative sterility preceded conception of the malformed child four times more often than when the child was normal.

In a series of 501 mothers with children dead of congenital defects in infancy, one fourth (25 per cent) of subsequent pregnancies had an unfavorable outcome, half of these being live births with one or more congenital malformations.

Defective children are born more often following a miscarriage, abortion, stillbirth, or premature birth but the month of conception is inconsequential. Dietary factors, parental age difference, illegitimacy, placenta previa, or rapid succession of pregnancy apparently played no significant part in the cases studied by Murphy, although these considerations have all been etiologically cited by others. Malformed children were found to have resulted after both the mating of a woman with two successive husbands and by a man with two successive wives. These anomalies occurred in 12.4 per cent (1:8) of families in a birth subsequent to that of a deformed child and in about half (47 per cent) of cases of malformation in two children in the same family, the anomalies will be reduplicated. In 41 per cent the same anomaly had existed in distant relatives.

Thus the information which should be given to prospective parents having one deformed child has been summarized by Murphy: *"The offspring presenting congenital malformations which are serious enough to warrant being recorded on death certificates are approximately twenty-four times as likely to occur in families possessing a congenitally deformed child as in the population at large."* Until further evidence is adduced two statements seem justified. (1) when a congenital malformation has genetic basis, there is a greatly increased chance that subsequent siblings will also be malformed; (2) when a congenital defect is due to factors which are not genetic in origin, offspring conceived subsequently should be congenitally malformed only in the same frequency as is commonly observed in the population at large.

Clinical Considerations in Anomalous Development. While many urinary tract anomalies cause death in the early months or years of life, correctly recognized in time, surgical and sometimes nonsurgical treatment will save life. This is recurrently illustrated in those patients, notably infants and children, in whom urinary infection is superimposed upon obstruction due to maldevelopment and the child commonly is optimistically and unsuccessfully treated for months or years under the diagnosis of "chronic pyelitis." Yet many of these patients with severe congenital obstructive injury of both kidneys die in uremia and without evidence of urinary infection, the diagnosis usually being chronic nephritis (cf. Campbell, 1952).

Comparably in adults, the damage caused by the urinary tract malformation may not become vitally evident until later life. Because of the gravity of many of these malformations the child does not reach adulthood and for this reason the incidence of urinary tract malformations in adults is strikingly lower than in children. Congenital abnormalities of the reproductive tract may become a matter of grave physical and psychologic, as well as reproductive, consideration. With gonadal hypoplasia there is likely to be a psychic disturbance with changes in body contour and general physical underdevelopment. Because of testicular or prostatic hypoplasia, the adult may find himself sterile. MacCallum's (1935) studies showed that 90 per cent of males bilaterally cryptorchid at puberty were sterile. In the female a pelvic kidney may seriously interfere with pregnancy and delivery. In these past few lines have been indicated but a very few of the great number of congenital malformations which greviously influence not only the pattern of life and welfare of the patient but often his assumed right to be a parent.

That the various terms employed in the designation of anomalous conditions may be properly interpreted, they are here defined.

Congenital means that the condition is present at birth.

Agenesis indicates total failure of an organ structure to develop and results from absence or lack of primordial tissue from which the structure normally arises or from failure of the particular structure growth to be initiated. Agenesis of one or both kidneys, testes, vagina and so forth are but a few of the numerous examples.

Aplasia defines incomplete development which may result from a slower than normal growth ratio, in other words, a retardation of normally progressive processes or arrest of a process already begun. Aplasia is commonly observed in the urinary tract and notably as abnormalities in renal size and position, ureteral ectopy, or imperfect descent of the testes, to cite a few examples.

Hypoplasia means defective or incomplete development and is commonly used in designating growth smaller than normal size and consequent to imperfect formation of a structure, such as a hypoplastic kidney or testis.

Paraplasia denotes the growth process with structure formation away from the normal development as observed in renal fusion, ureteral or urethral stenosis, or the growth of an homologous set of genital ducts.

To repeat, it is axiomatic that the anomalous organ is more prone to disease than a normally formed one. Urinary tract anomalies are commonly accompanied by maldevelopments elsewhere and examples involving every other system may even be found in the same patient. It is notable that anomalous upper urinary tract maldevelopment accounts for needless abdominal operation in a fifth to a fourth of the patients so afflicted. In most cases the nature and site of the anomaly can be readily determined by thorough urologic investigation; particularly is this so in the differential diagnosis of so-called chronic appendicitis, perhaps the most frequent diagnostic misadventure when unrecognized urogenital tract disease is the cause of the symptoms and notably abdominal pain.

In the subsequent discussions in this chapter and elsewhere of the various anomalies, I lean heavily upon the personal collection and study through the years of postmortem protocols totaling 51,880. These records which have been minutely abstracted and tabulated by assistants and myself were most generously made available to me at Bellevue, University, St. Vincent's, Willard Parker, Babies and New York Nursery and Childs Hospital in New York, and the Mountainside Hospital in Montclair, New Jersey by Doctors

S. L. Willens, Maurice N. Richter, A. Rottino, Laurence Smith, the late Martha Wollstein, James Wilson and John L. Work, Directors respectively of the Department of Pathology in these institutions. To these gracious colleagues, I am most deeply indebted and grateful. In 1937 the findings in 26,480 autopsies were reported in my *Pediatric Urology;* subsequent post-mortem examinations have brought the total to 51,880. Of this number 36.7 per cent (19,046) were infants and children, 63.3 per cent (32,834) were sixteen years of age and older. Of these infants and children about two thirds (68.9 per cent) were six months of age or less; slightly less than half (44.3+ per cent) were females and 55.6 per cent were males; nine tenths (90.0 per cent) were white and 9.1 per cent were black. Of the adults, nearly three fourths (71.9 per cent) were males and 28.1 per cent were females; 90.2 per cent were white, 8.6 per cent were Negroes and 1.1 per cent were of other races. It is notable that among the adults, the age group between 41 to 55 years constituted nearly a third (10,580 or 32.2 per cent).

Illustrations in this chapter are largely of private patients; where service cases or material from other sources have been shown their origin is indicated in the legends. Because anomalous development appears in greater variety in the young the illustrations here shown are largely of these conditions in infants and children. Photographs of patients and autopsy material from the New York Nursery and Childs and the Babies Hospital have been previously published by the author while associated with these institutions. Because of their higher incidence and comparably greater importance in the young, the clinical considerations of the various anomalies as they appear in this age group are purposely given special emphasis in this Section.

In order best to appreciate the origin of anomalous urogenital tract development, its clinical consideration is here sectionally preceded by a brief discussion of the normal embryologic development of this system.

EMBRYOLOGY AND ANOMALIES OF THE KIDNEY

Embryology. Three separate structures enter into the derivation and development of the kidney: the pronephros, the mesonephros (wolffian body proper) and, finally, the metanephros which becomes the permanent kidney.

The *pronephros* is an ontogenetic remnant of the excretory system in lower vertebrates, arises and develops independently cephalad on each side as six to ten pairs of tubules with a connecting duct called the wolffian or primary excretory duct which opens into the celomic cavity. The pronephros degenerates by the fourth week, leaving only the wolffian duct which rapidly grows to extend throughout the length of the nephrogenic cord and opens into the cloaca which is the dilated end of the cavity (Fig. 97, *A*).

The *mesonephros* makes its appearance just before the pronephros completely disappears and is derived from the mesoblastic intermediate cell mass. It consists of tubules at the end of the mesonephric (pronephric, wolffian) duct and appears first opposite the upper dorsal segments but when fully developed its caudad end is at the third lumbar level (Fig. 97, *B*). During its development the pronephros has functioning glomeruli and collecting tubules, but by the twelfth to the fourteenth week mesonephric degeneration occurs leaving a residuum of a small portion of collecting tubules which in the adult female reproductive tract persist as the duct of Gartner, the epoophoron and the paroophoron, and in the male as the ductuli efferentes, ductuli aberrantes, and paradidymis of the epididymis. The occasional persistence of the tubular duct of Gartner is advanced to explain ectopic ureteral opening in the vagina, cervix or uterus (see Fig. 155).

The *metanephros* or true renal secretory anlage is comprised of a secretory or glandular portion and a collecting or efferent system. This structure appears caudally (second and third sacral segment level) during mesonephric degeneration as the nephrogenic cord (renal blastema). Its vascular con-

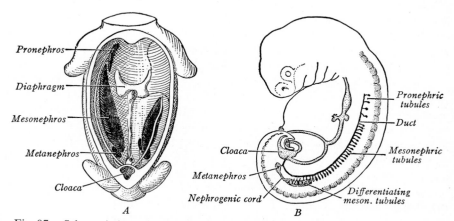

Fig. 97. Schematic indication of the location and relations of the three kidney types in mammals. *A*, note the high thoracic origin of the pronephros, the abdominal site of the mesonephros and the extremely low initial location of the metanephros. *B*, lateral schema of *A* (Arey).

nections are promptly established and simultaneously the renal collecting or drainage elements are formed by a bilateral posterior budding from the metanephric or wolffian duct which in turn enters the cloaca (Figs. 98, 99). These ureteral buds grow cephalad and form the ureters, enter and become surrounded by the metanephrogenic blastema, by division and subdivision of the upper end of the ureteral stalk form the renal pelvis, major and minor calyces, and by still further division the renal collecting tubules (Fig. 99). The primary renal collecting tubule system gives off secondary, tertiary and further branches so that by the fifth month it is estimated that as many as twelve subdivisions have formed. Up to twenty subdivisions have been described but Ludwig (1949) in extensive embryologic study could find no evidence of such dichotomous branching and believes the concept of "orders" of renal tubules should be abandoned.

The *nephrogenic cap* is carried in with, and surrounds, the tips of the newly formed collecting tubules but occasionally becomes isolated, vesiculated (nephrogenic vesicle), and encloses the capillary tuft to form the secretory glomerulus with its adjacent tubules (Fig. 100, *A-E*). It has been estimated by Traut (1923) that the human kidney contains about 4,500,000 glomeruli. This new secretory unit joins the end of the collecting tubule. Both together

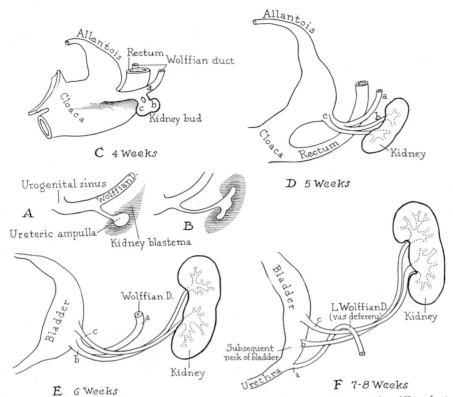

Fig. 98. Schema of origin of embryologic development of the kidney and wolffian duct. *A* and *B*, normal upper urinary tract. *C-F*, embryology of reduplicated kidney and ureter (after Kelly-Burnham).

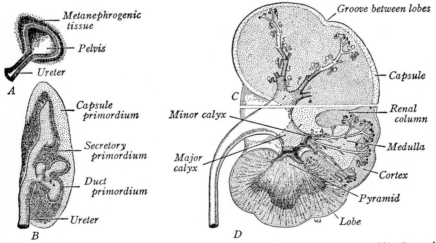

Fig. 99. Organization of the human metanephros. *A*, model at 8 mm. (× 50). *B*, model at 12 mm. (× 65). *C*, diagram of relations are nine weeks (× 40). *D*, frontal section at birth (× 15). In *D* is shown the nature of the primary and secondary renal branchings ("orders") ultimately to form the functioning kidney (Arey).

constitute the renal unit or *renculus* (Fig. 101) which is comparable to the splenic and hepatic lobule units. When these renal structures fail to join properly at this time, polycystic disease is believed to result (Fig. 100, *F, G*).

The cortex of the kidney is formed from the metanephrogenic blastema, covers the pyramid bases to impart a lobulated surface phylogenetic of lower

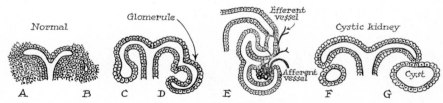

Fig. 100.   Formation of the glomerulus. *E*, ingrowth of the vascular tuft is indicated. *F, G*, schematically illustrate the prevailing theory of the etiology of renal polycystic disease, viz.: failure of union between the excretory and the collecting elements of the renal units.

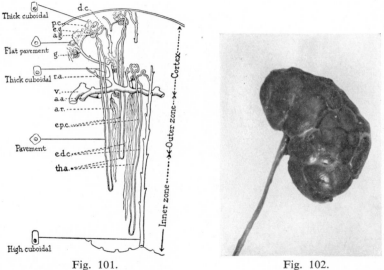

Fig. 101.   Fig. 102.

Fig. 101.   Reniculus or renal unit. Course of the renal tubules and their cellular histology at the different levels. d.c., distal convoluted tubules; p.c., proximal convoluted tubules; e.g., efferent glomerular vessel; a.g., afferent glomerular vessel; g., glomerulus; r.a., radiate artery; v., vein; a.a., arcuate artery; a.r., arteriolae rectae; e.p.c., descending loop of Henle; e.d.c., ascending loop. (Redrawn after Huber.)

Fig. 102. Fetal lobulation in an infant. This is normal until the age of four years but, according to the author's autopsy studies, in approximately 5 per cent of all individuals persists throughout life.

vertebrates and some mammals (bear, ox, bird; Fig. 102). The cortex extends centrally between the papillae of the medullary pyramids as the primary renal *columns of Bertin*. In the six-months fetus, the kidney is a lobulated organ with a small pelvis and large cortex and medulla (Fig. 101). The cortex continues to grow in thickness until some weeks after birth while the medulla thickens at a lesser rate. True cellular multiplication occurs until the fourth or fifth year after which, in renal hypertrophy, the kidney cells simply enlarge and there is no regeneration and multiplication as occurs in the liver, for example.

The kidneys at birth are disproportionately large and in a dehydrated emaciated newborn infant the comparatively huge renal masses may erroneously cause the diagnosis of polycystic disease, hydronephrosis, or tumor to be made.

The fibrous capsule of the kidney is derived from mesoderm which surrounds the fetal kidney.

Ascent of the kidney occurs between the seventh and eighth week and in rising from its initial low pelvic location, the previously forward facing

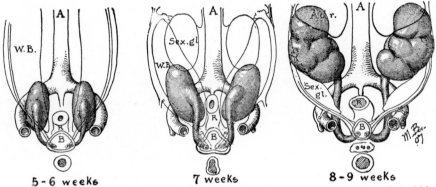

5-6 weeks   7 weeks   8-9 weeks

Fig. 103. Renal ascent and rotation during fetal life. The normal rotation of the kidney from facing forward to facing medially is shown. Fusion of either renal pole produces horseshoe kidney (compare Fig. 120). This fusion must occur by the seventh week (Kelly-Burnham).

pelvis turns medially (Fig. 103). With failure of renal rotation the clinically observed picture of malrotation results; in some instances there is overrotation and the pelvis faces posteriorly but this is most rare (Fig. 104, *A*). Rapid spinal growth caudad explains the so-called ascent of the kidney, the upper pole of which by the fifth month is at the level of the eleventh rib or the normal adult position.

The adrenal gland in early fetal life is disproportionately large, overlies and partially surrounds the kidney (see Section XVIII).

The *renal blood supply* becomes established during the eighth to ninth week from the aorta and vena cava at the second lumbar level. Prior to this, the nephrogenic blastema is supplied by vessels of more caudad origin and their persistence accounts for many cases of renal ectopy, the kidney simply being prevented from ascending by its vascular attachments which refuse to disappear. The renal vessels normally enter at the hilum but anomalous arterial polar vessels are found in a third of all individuals (Fig. 142). As shown by Anson et al. (1948) the venous renal connections are far more complex, irregular and bizarre than the arterial, particularly on the left side, and often there is no true pedicle, a matter of great importance to the surgeon.

Renal physiology is discussed in Section I, Chapter 2, and the dynamics of the pelvis and ureter in Section I, Chapter 3. The formation of urine begins by the fifth month of fetal life; Kjellberg and Rudhe (1949) injected Diodrast into the human fetus at cesarean section and showed urographically that this medium is excreted by the fourth or fifth month of intra-uterine life. Moreover, Homer W. Smith (1949, personal communication) states

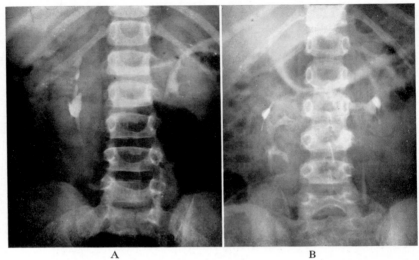

A   B

Fig. 104. Abnormal renal rotation. *A*, failure of right kidney to rotate, causing the pelvis and calyces to appear urographically in their narrowest diameter; the ureter leaves the kidney anteriorly and passes over the lower pole. Normal pelvis on the right. *B*, over-rotation (outward) of the right kidney causing the ureter to descend from the outer border of the organ. Left kidney reduplicated; urogram shows only the lower pelvis which is slightly deformed congenitally.

that in the fetal rabbit, cat, opossum and pig both the mesonephros and metanephros function in the glomerular excretion of ferrocyanide and the tubular excretion of phenol red.

CONGENITAL ANOMALIES OF THE KIDNEY

These can be conveniently classified as follows:

    I. *Anomalies of Number*
        1. Bilateral agenesis
        2. Unilateral agenesis (solitary kidney)
        3. Supernumerary kidney
   II. *Anomalies of Volume and Structure*
        1. Hypoplasia
        2. Congenital hypertrophy
        3. Solitary cystic disease
        4. Multilocular cystic disease
        5. Polycystic disease
  III. *Anomalies of Form*
        1. Short, long, round, hour-glass or lobulated kidneys
        2. Horseshoe kidney
        3. Disc or doughnut kidney
        4. Sigmoid kidney or L-shaped kidney
        5. Lump kidney

IV. *Anomalies of Location*
    1. Simple ectopia
        a. unilateral
        b. bilateral
    2. Crossed ectopia with or without fusion
    3. Movable kidney
V. *Anomalies of Rotation*
    1. Incomplete
    2. Excessive
VI. *Anomalies of the Pelvis*
    1. Double kidney
        a. unilateral
        b. bilateral
        c. complete reduplication
        d. incomplete reduplication
    2. Pseudo-spider form
    3. Congenital hydronephrosis
    4. Extrarenal pelvis
VII. *Anomalies of the Vessels*
    1. Arterial
    2. Venous

I. ANOMALIES OF NUMBER

Bilateral renal agenesis is not only extremely rare but is incompatible with life, and consequently is largely of academic interest. Its causes are those of unilateral renal agenesis (q.v.) but involving both organs. Congenital bilateral renal absence was observed seven times in 19,046 children in our necropsy series, a ratio of 1:2721. In a series of 168 cases, ninety-one were males, thirty-one were females and in forty-two the sex was not indicated (Levin); the average sex rate is about three males to one female. Of our seven cases, four were male, two were female and in one, no sex organs or genitalia were present.

Associated developmental defects in the urinary and other systems are of high incidence. These anomalies include sirenomelus, apus, monopus, undeveloped terminal lower bowel, imperforate anus, dysplasia of the genital system, wolffian and müllerian defects, hypoplastic or absent bladder and ureter, adrenal absence or malformation, acrania, hydrocephalus, meningocele, spina bifida; malformations of the upper intestinal and muscular skeletal systems have been noted. In our series of seven cases, there were foramen ovale and patent ductus arteriosus (in three each), patent interventricular septum and clubfoot, one each; the cervix and vagina were absent in a stillborn female, the uterus and tubes were malformed, and there was imperforate anus. In an anencephalic full term monster there were no kidneys, ureters, bladder nor external genitalia. In five cases the kidneys, ureters and bladder were absent, but in one, as in some cases reported in the literature, the bladder was present but there were neither ureters nor kidneys. The adrenals are often normal; they were reported as "large" in four of our seven autopsy cases but the gonads commonly are malformed.

While the substitute mechanism for renal function in bilateral total agenesis is not precisely known, this would seem to be taken over by the liver. The most striking suggestive evidence of this was reported by Moulin in a fourteen-year-old girl in whom the urine was transported by a large umbilical vein passing to the patent umbilicus. The anephric case reported by Hinman, Jr. (1940) lived ten days, which is approximately the survival period in bilateral nephrectomy in adults and suggests that neither mesonephric nor metanephric function is necessary for intra-uterine development. Seidel (1939) observed a female child who lived twenty-one days with congenital absence of the entire urinary tract. Our oldest was twenty-two hours; one lived ten minutes, another thirty minutes and the remaining four were stillborn. Most are stillborn or die within a few minutes or hours after birth.

Potter (1946) reported twenty cases observed at the Chicago Lying-In Hospital and described hypoplasia of the lungs as well as facies characteristic of the condition, as did Vaugh (1950). These children were observed to have an unusually wide interpupillary distance, inner canthus folds extending outward and downward, the appearance of advanced age or premature senility, an unusual flattened nose, receding chin from mandibular underdevelopment, and large low ears with little cartilage.

Unilateral renal agenesis (congenital solitary kidney) is caused by (1) failure of the renal bud to develop, (2) failure of the nephrogenic blastema to form, (3) both, or (4) failure of the vascular supply to form. With failure or arrest of development of the wolffian duct there is agenesis of the isolateral primitive nucleus from which the corresponding urinary tract forms, and commonly absence of the isolateral genital apparatus (cf. Boyden, 1932; Brown, 1931; Nation, 1944; Mertz and Wishard, 1950; Alexander et al., 1950; Longo and Thompson, 1952). Yet in some cases of renal agenesis a rudimentary ureter exists while in others a massive degenerated fibrolipomatous tissue has been found in the usual renal site but no ureter. Bound (1943) observed the condition in a boy whose uncle was similarly afflicted. In a three-month-old male patient of mine with a solitary cystic hydronephrotic right kidney, a brother born one year previous had no kidneys! But as a rule there is no evidence of hereditary influence as an etiologic factor in renal agenesis.

Renal agenesis is to be distinguished from renal aplasia and renal atrophy although the three conditions together with pronounced hypoplasia are of essentially equal clinical concern. Agenesis is also to be distinguished from fusion of both kidneys on one side (crossed ectopia; no kidney on the other side) but in this condition two ureters with normally located orifices in the bladder are generally demonstrable. With renal agenesis the ureter is commonly absent, as in 248 of 272 cases reported by Anders (1910), and only rudimentary in twenty-four. Renal agenesis is commonly accompanied by anomalies of the lower urinary tract or in other systems; other upper urinary tract anomalies were observed in 94 per cent of the 135 children with anomalous genitalia collected by Anders; Shumacker (1938) collected twenty-eight cases of unilateral renal agenesis accompanied by true unicornate uterus and other anomalies of the female genital tract such as isolateral absence of kidney and ovary, round ligament, broad ligament, bicornuate, septate, solid or arcuate uterus, double vagina and other malformations.

In the 51,880 autopsy cases we studied there were ninety-four cases of unilateral renal agenesis, a ratio of 1:552. In a series of 122,320 autopsies collected from the literature, the incidence was slightly lower, 1:610 cases. The isolateral adrenal is said to be absent in three fourths of the cases of solitary kidney but in the ninety-four of our series, this was so in only eight.

The vital importance of anomalous development and particularly as concerns the kidneys is splendidly illustrated in our autopsy studies showing the increased early mortality as a result of the malformations. In short, forty-five (1 in 443 or in round numbers 1 in 450) of 19,046 infants and children examined post mortem had unilateral solitary kidney, a third greater incidence than was observed (forty-nine cases; 1:662) in the 32,834 individuals over fifteen years of age.

In the ninety-four cases in this series, the anomaly occurred in sixty-four males and thirty females; autopsies were performed on approximately 10 per cent more males (55.6) than females (44.3+). In a recently reported series of eighty-seven cases, Longo and Thompson (1952) found fifty (60.6 per cent) males and thirty-seven (39.3 per cent) females, of an average thirty-seven years with age ranges from six to seventy years. The right side was recorded as involved in forty-seven and the left in forty.

Analysis of the coexisting anomalies in our ninety-four cases of renal agenesis showed the solitary kidney was hypertrophic in forty-three, reduplicated in five, ectopic in three, and polycystic in two. The ureter was absent in forty-six, strictured in six, and reduplicated in four; in three each there was idiopathic dilatation, fibrosis and partial absence; there was one case each of ureteral hypoplasia, ectopic opening in the vagina, kinking and cystic changes. There was no ureteral dimple in the bladder in eight cases, hemiatrophy of the trigone was observed in four, the bladder was exstrophic in three, and absence of the trigone, double uterus, vesical diverticulum and retrovesical fistula were found in one each. The testes were undescended in five cases with isolateral hypoplasia of the seminal vesicles. There was absence of the isolateral seminal vesicles in three each, and of the prostate in one. Gynecologic anomalies included double uterus, unicorn uterus, absent adnexa, double vagina, infantile vagina, vaginorectal fistula in one case each. The gastrointestinal tract showed six cases of imperforate anus, three of cloacal formation, three cases each of atresia of the esophagus and of esophotracheal fistula; two cases each of harelip, cleft palate, and malrotation of the cecum, and one instance each of situs inversus, pyloric stenosis, jejunal stenosis, atresia of the rectum, absence of the rectum, rectourethral fistula, hypoplastic spleen, and anomalous liver and gallbladder. Parenthetically, in a thirteen-months-old girl with a congenital solitary right kidney, there was no urethra; one was constructed (Fig. 105, *C, D*). In Peterman's case (1932) the spleen was absent.

Anomalies of the vascular tree in our series included patent ductus arteriosus in seven cases, patent foramen ovale in five, patent interventricular septum in two, and dextrocardia, patent interauricular septum, aplastic renal pedicle, anomalous left carotid artery, congenital bicuspid valve, accessory coronary arteries, and atresia of the pulmonary artery in one case each. Pulmonary anomalies found were absence of the lungs, congenital supernumerary lobes, absent lung fissures, absent diaphragm in two cases each; in one stillborn the left lung was in the abdomen. Orthopedic anomalies included clubfoot in four cases, hemivertebrae in three, and supernumerary digits, syndactylism, osteogenesis imperfecta, and absent left foot in one case each. Central nervous system anomalies were meningocele in three cases; hydrocephalus, anencephalus, and absent optic nerves in one case each. In a

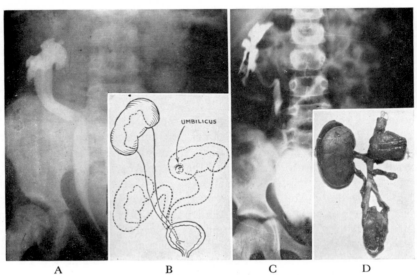

A   B   C   D

Fig. 105.   Congenital absence of one kidney (congenital solitary kidney). *A*, in a six-year-old girl admitted to Bellevue Hospital for painless "abdominal tumor." Absence of the left ureteral orifice and hemiatrophy of the trigone were observed. There is also moderate congenital narrowing of the lower ureter with ureterectasis and pyelectasis above. *B*, the freely movable solitary kidney could easily be pushed about the abdomen. *C*, in a thirteen-month-old girl with urinary incontinence from agenesis of the urethra; the last was surgically rectified with establishment of normal control. The solitary right kidney shows some malrotation with respiratory kinking of the upper ureter. (Bellevue Hospital.) *D*, autopsy specimen showing presence of left adrenal although the kidney was congenitally absent. (Babies Hospital.)

stillborn male the anterior abdominal muscular wall was absent, peritoneum and overlying skin being present but no mesenchymal derivations.

Commonly the structural volume of the solitary kidney approximates that of two normal organs and its functional capacity nearly always does. In forty-three of the ninety-four postmortem cases, the solitary kidney was hypertrophied. The pelvis of the congenitally enlarged kidney is usually large in contradistinction to the pelvis of the organ undergoing compensatory hypertrophy in later life, an observation which may be of urographic diagnostic significance (Fig. 106).

Although congenital absence of one kidney is compatible with health as long as the hypertrophied solitary kidney compensates, a single kidney is more apt to be the seat of disease than one with a normal renal mate (Campbell, 1928). One fourth of the ninety-four cases in our necropsy series died

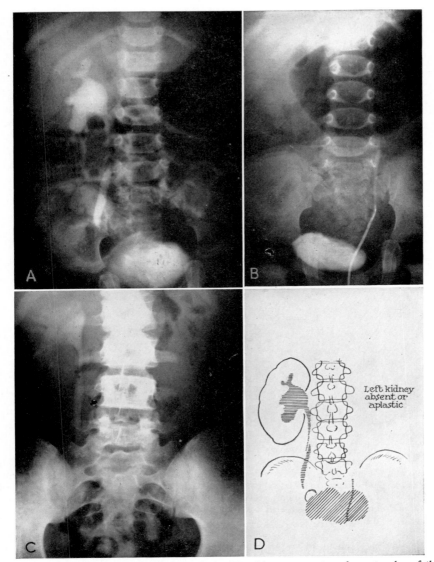

Fig. 106. Congenital left renal hypoplasia (?) with compensatory hypertrophy of the right kidney. *A*, in a boy first examined at five months of age. *B*, on the left and despite forceful injection of contrast medium, the shadow of the blind-ending ureteral stump tapers off at the level of the pelvic brim and the left kidney is believed to be congenitally absent. (Babies Hospital.) *C*, excretory urogram sixteen years later showing a normal but large pelvis of the compensatory hypertrophic right kidney. The boy's development is normal and his general physical condition excellent. *D*, schema.

of renal failure. Similar studies by others have shown that the congenital solitary kidney suffers a definitely higher incidence of disease than does the normal kidney, and in the study of children with persistent pyuria we found that one in eighty had congenital solitary kidney. In Anders' series of 170 cases of congenital solitary kidney, seventy-nine were diseased, and in 422 autopsy cases collected by Fortune, 22.6 per cent showed significant renal disease as against the general autopsy average of 15 per cent.

The solitary kidney will generally function satisfactorily unless subjected to bacterial, toxic, or obstructive assaults which will usually be manifested by pain, hematuria, pyuria, or anuria, and be clinically indistinguishable from these manifestations when two kidneys exist. In an eight-year-old boy with sulfonamide anuria reported by Malisoff (1949), sulfadiazine had been

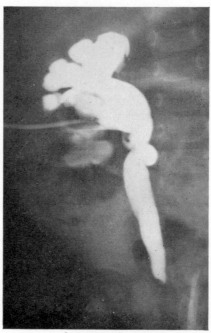

Fig. 107. Congenital ureterovesical junction stricture of a congenital solitary right kidney in a five-month-old boy examined because of persistent pyuria and recurrent severe attacks of renal infection ("recurrent hyperacute pyelitis"). No left ureteral orifice could be found and there was left hemiatrophy of the trigone. Nephrostomy drainage (above). There is irregular dilation of the ureter above the ureterovesical junction. Death by renal failure four months later.

given for the treatment of an upper respiratory tract infection; prompt establishment of urinary drainage saved the patient's life. A six-year-old girl with a freely movable, slightly tender, painful mass in the right loin was sent to Bellevue Hospital with a diagnosis of abdominal tumor which proved to be a solitary wandering kidney that could be pushed into most quarters of the abdomen (Fig. 105, *A, B*). Retroperitoneal cyst associated with renal agenesis, possibly as a mesonephric maldevelopment, has been recorded by Kornblum and Ritter (1939), and Krauss and Straus (1935).

Several surgical catastrophes following the unwitting removal of a solitary kidney have been reported, including a four-year-old boy (Morgan) and the oft-cited series of eleven cases of Ranssohof's (1911). In the last group, the kidney had been removed in seven, nephrostomy had been performed in four; in the nephrectomized cases, anuric death ensued in one to eleven days. With modern urologic methods of investigation, congenital renal absence should be identified or at least suspected, and by conservative surgery (nephrostomy, pyelostomy, ureteral transplantation) the solitary organ preserved (Fig. 107).

Diagnosis. The recognition and identification of congenital solitary kidney requires complete urologic examination in which a preliminary excretory urographic study is of suggestive value but is not conclusive. Absence of a renal pelvic urographic shadow or even of a parenchymal outline does not necessarily mean absence of the kidney. Hemiatrophy of the trigone is almost pathognomonic. Failure to find a second ureteral orifice should at once suggest unilateral renal agenesis bearing in mind that the ureter may be ectopic. Here chromocystoscopy (meatoscopy following the injection of indigo carmine intravenously) may disclose the ectopic opening in the bladder outlet, urethra, introitus, vagina, seminal vesicle or rectum. In the employment of chromocystoscopy, the ureter to the known kidney should be plugged with a large catheter to prevent ejaculation of dye from this side into the bladder. When, as in four of our cases, the solitary kidney is drained by reduplicated ureters, one of which may open normally and the other ectopic, the diagnostic problem is even more difficult. Moreover, as in three of our autopsy cases, the solitary kidney may be ectopic, forty-five such cases having been collected and reported by Berg and Kearns (1949), and in eleven Nalle et al. (1949) found vaginal aplasia.

When a blind-ending ureter exists on the side of the agenesis, a catheter can rarely be made to enter more than 2 cm.; no urinary return is obtained (Fig. 106). In a year-old male examined postmortem at Bellevue Hospital, a trilobe (clover leaf) solitary kidney was drained by a dilated ureter opening in the bladder midline, the ureteral obstruction being a congenital stricture 2.5 cm. above the ureterovesical junction. The child died of acute focal suppurative nephritis and uremia. Morris observed a similar condition in a nineteen-year-old boy dead of Bright's disease. Moreover, the ureter from the solitary kidney may cross over to open into the opposite side of the bladder as in five reported cases.

The ureter of the solitary kidney may be obstructed by stricture, aberrant blood vessel, kink, or stone, and when the blockage is complete, anuria results and demands prompt relief by ureteral catheter, ureterostomy, pyelostomy or nephrostomy (Fig. 107). Although the treatment of complicating disease in solitary congenital kidney depends upon the etiology and is fundamentally that employed when two kidneys exist, it must be far more conservative to save renal parenchyma. In short, all surgical efforts short of total nephrectomy must be exercised according to indication and this may mean the institution of permanent nephrostomy drainage which has proved the last resort in some of our patients.

Free Supernumerary Kidney. This is probably the rarest of renal anomalies; Carlson in 1950 collected forty-nine cases in one of which the ureter from the cephalic organ opened in the vaginal vestibule (Rubin, 1948), and in ónly six was the urographic diagnosis suspected or made preoperatively. To these forty-nine reported cases, three of ours are herewith added. In one of our autopsy cases, a free supernumerary kidney was found bilaterally in a child; four separate undiseased kidneys and ureters were present. In a white female there was complete reduplication of the right kidney; an extra "half kidney" was found superimposed over the lower pole of the complete kidney and each structure had its separate pelvis and ureter, the supernumerary kidney having its own arterial supply. The anomaly occurs more often in the male, and on the left side supernumerary organs up to five have been de-

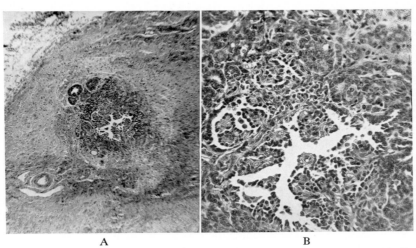

A   B

Fig. 108.   Supernumerary kidney. One of six small supernumerary kidney buds discovered at nephrectomy in a three-month-old girl whose pyelogram is shown in Fig. 109. A rouleau of these accessory structures was imbedded in a dense fibrous band passing laterally and downward from the right kidney at a point corresponding to eight on the clock face. *A,* nephrogenic tissue in the periphery of which are occasional glomeruli imbedded in fibrous tissue. Centrally there are numerous tubular structures and represent abortive attempts at glomerular formation about a central cavity (pelvis?) *B,* high magnification of the center of *A.* The tubular structures and embryonal glomeruli are readily seen.

scribed; the ureters may be completely reduplicated or bifurcated from a single stalk. In a third autopsy case, a twenty-three year old female, there were two separate kidneys on the right side, the upper being 3 inches in diameter and the lower 2½ inches, with separate ureteral openings in the bladder; the right upper urinary tract was normal. In a fourth case clinically observed in a three-month-old girl from whom a reduplicated pyonephrotic right kidney was removed, a row of six supernumerary renal buds was found in a dense fibrous bed attached to the lower outer convexity of the organ (Figs. 108, 109). At this precise point on the left kidney (heminephrectomy segment), we found an early Wilms' tumor (Fig. 109). A twenty-six-year-old woman reported by Assayer had from the age of six years suffered periodic attacks of pain in the right loin with nausea and vomiting. An elastic hard painful tumor mass, a supernumerary kidney, was felt at the level of the

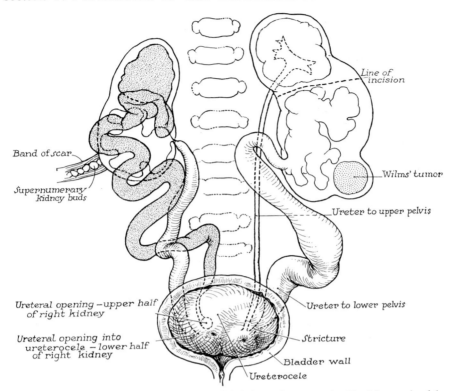

Fig. 109. Supernumerary renal buds (right) in a three-month-old girl examined be-cause of persistent severe pyuria with recurrent bouts of temperature. Her urinary tract was a veritable museum of anomalies including complete bilateral ureterorenal reduplica-tion and (1) an enormous ureterocele filling the bladder; (2) a ureterovesical junction stricture of the greatly dilated ureter draining (3) a massive infected hydronephrotic lower half of the reduplicated left kidney, and (4) a reduplicated greatly dilated right upper urinary tract, the ureter from the superior right segment opening into the uretero-cele. Only the small upper segment of the reduplicated left kidney showed a "normal" pelvis and was the sole renal tissue supporting life. Surgical treatment: removal of the entire reduplicated right urinary tract down to bladder, transvesical ureterocelectomy, left ureteroheminephrectomy, leaving only the small normally functioning segment which was the upper half of the left kidney. Right renal exposure at a point corresponding to to eight on the cock face showed a rouleau of six supernumerary renal buds imbedded in a dense band of fibrous tissue which passed laterally (Fig. 108). At a corresponding point in the left kidney (four on the clock face) was an early Wilms' tumor or renal embryoma measuring 8 mm. in diameter. Four years later the girl is well and growing normally.

umbilicus and its ureter was found joined to that of the normal right kidney. Removal of the accessory organ stopped the pain.

Supernumerary kidney develops (1) by splitting of the nephrogenic blastema, or (2) as two separate metanephric blastemas into which partially or completely reduplicated ureteral stalks enter to form two separate cap-sulated kidneys, without fusion, or at most attached to each other with only loose cellular tissue. Characteristically each supernumerary organ has its separate blood supply and ureter, points which distinguish the condition from the fused supernumerary kidney shortly to be described.

Symptoms may be absent in supernumerary kidney but when present result from complicating lesions such as obstruction, hydronephrosis, infection, calculi, tumor or, with ureteral ectopy, urinary leakage.

The diagnosis may be suspected from the excretory urographic findings and is substantiated by retrograde pyelography and particularly when the separate outlines of two kidneys are found on the one side with evidence of renal structure on the opposite. Yet it is not always this simple; in only six recorded cases has the diagnosis been made preoperatively, the condition usually being discovered at surgical exploration or post mortem.

The treatment is that of the diseased supernumerary organ, and generally requires nephrectomy, assuming adequate renal tissue will remain.

Fused Supernumerary Kidneys. These are reduplicated organs whose transverse separation is incomplete. The ureters may be incomplete, the embryologic etiology being that of renal reduplication (q.v.). The two renal divisions may be joined only by a fibrous band, as in five of our autopsy cases in children (approximately 1 to 4000). In a one-month-old boy, a normal kidney was surmounted by a loosely attached small kidney having three pyramids, the reduplicated ureters opening separately into the bladder. In a four-month-old boy, a unipyramidal kidney lay between one with two pyramids; the pelves and ureters were distinct, the two segments being joined by a fibrous band. The ureters may be completely or incompletely reduplicated. The symptoms, diagnosis and treatment are essentially those considered under free supernumerary kidney and the treatment in general is the same, heminephrectomy being the most frequent surgical indication.

II. ANOMALIES OF VOLUME AND STRUCTURE

Renal aplasia is characterized by a most meager suggestion of renal development, there being no gross evidence of true kidney, no pelvis and no true renal pedicle. The renal "parenchyma" shows most scant tubular structure. The ureter is poorly developed and has no lumen, reflecting in this immaturity an early embryonic stoppage of development and without completed nephron formation. It is agreed with Emmett et al. (1952) that if glomeruli are present, the condition should be classified as renal hypoplasia rather than aplasia. These structures, which are functionless and secrete no urine, are usually set in a fibrolipomatous mass. The condition is clinically analogous to renal agenesis, there being no true renal excretory function and usually no ureter present. The condition may also be described as an extreme variety of hypoplasia, the embryologic etiology being comparable. Occasionally the aplastic organ causes pain in the renal area by sclerotic compression of nerve endings, or it may be identified as the probable etiologic site in hypertensive vascular disease, on the basis of Goldblatt's (1940) explanation. Not infrequently symptomatic relief follows removal of the aplastic renal mass. Far more common and of greater clinical concern is renal hypoplasia, a discussion of which follows.

Renal Hypoplasia. This is characterized by subnormal growth of the kidney, the organ being small or infantile, yet with a distinct cortex and medulla recognizable as a kidney. It has excretory function although the amount of urine put out may be greatly reduced. Renal hypoplasia results from failure of (1) the metanephrogenic blastema, (2) of the metanephric duct, or (3) of the blood supply, to develop normally. It is generally unilateral although bilateral occurrence has been observed. In a male twelve hours old, both kidneys weighed only 6 grams together (normal 45–50 grams) and in a two-year-old girl both kidneys weighed 44 grams, the

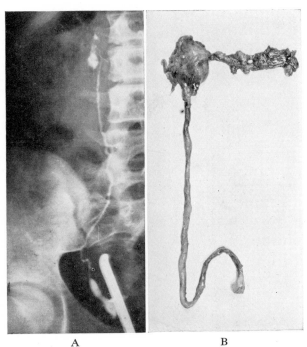

A   B

Fig. 110.   Congenital hypoplasia of the kidney and ureter. *A,* in a twelve-year-old girl examined because of recurrent hematuria proved to come from the right hypoplastic side. In the urogram is demonstrated the exceedingly small irregular renal pelvis and the hypoplastic ureter which is irregular in its course and dilated in its juxtavesical segment. Ureteronephrectomy. *B,* shows the surgical specimen; the kidney was about the size of a twenty-five cent piece.

condition causing pronounced somatic retardation and skeletal changes commonly identified as renal dwarfism or renal rickets (q.v.).

The vascular supply and notably the renal artery are correspondingly hypoplastic and commonly sclerotic (Goldblatt kidney). As a corollary, it is probable that in some instances the diminutive blood supply adversely influenced the renal development; sometimes a well developed accompanying ureter is present to suggest this (Fig. 110). Cases of hypertensive vascular disease in children with congenital unilateral renal hypoplasia have been reported in which nephrectomy markedly reduced or even cured the hypertension, as in two young patients of mine. This phase of renal hypoplasia has been well discussed by Powers and Murray (1942) and by Goldring

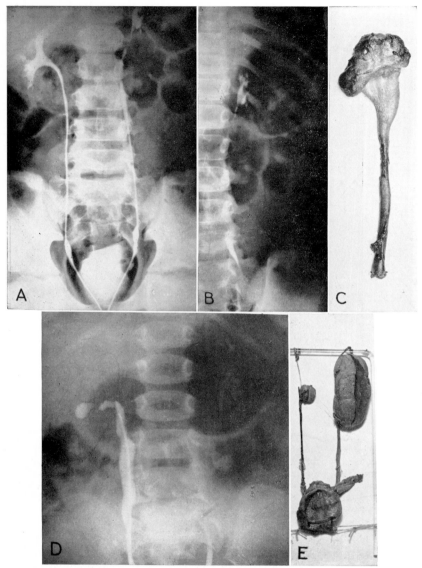

Fig. 111.   Congenital renal hypoplasia in an eight-year-old boy with recurrent pyuria and increasing blood pressure. *A*, pyelogram shows a normal right pelvis with hypoplastic left pelvis and ureter. *B*, the irregular finer markings of the hypoplastic pelvis are better shown. Ureteronephrectomy. *C*, specimen removed. Following operation the previously elevated blood pressure (135/140 mm. Hg systolic, 95/105 diastolic) returned to normal. *D*, right renal hypoplasia in a three-year-old girl examined because of persistent pyuria. Normal left renal pelvis. (University Hospital.) *E*, autopsy specimen in an infant of six months (Babies Hospital) with a condition comparable to *D*.

in Section XVII, Chapter 1, of Volume II of this book. Kruglich and Minnick (1947) found bilateral renal hypoplasia (kidneys 3 gm. each; 1.0 by 1.5 cm. in size and containing cortical cysts with dilated tubules, glomeruli, and Bowman's capsules) with occluded ureters in a ten-week-old boy dead of intracranial hemorrhage, subdural hematoma and meningitis. On the basis of this observation these authors advised that bilateral renal hypoplasia should always be considered when signs of intracranial pressure exist in infants despite normal urine.

Characteristically the hypoplastic kidney usually lies closer than normal to the spine (Figs. 110–113). The development of the parenchyma is poor, but even in young infants and without obstruction the renal substance may surround a comparatively dilated pelvis. Although glomerular and tubular development is sometimes rudimentary and may even show hyaline degeneration, many, and possibly most hypoplastic kidneys are simply normal diminutive organs whose cells are smaller than normal and the number of renal units is greatly reduced (congenitally atrophic). Although the pelvis in many of these cases appears as a "small" normal one, or longer and narrow, in some it is present as a simple bulbous dilatation of the upper end of the ureter and with few rudimentary calyces or none, or it may be of the unicalyceal (rabbit) type. Emmett et al. (1952), Gutierrez (1933), Braasch (1922), Goldblatt (1940), Lieberthal (1939) and others have drawn attention to the frequency of chronic infection and of obstruction as common etiologic factors in the production of secondarily atrophic kidneys which are too often considered to be congenitally hypoplastic, recognizing that the former condition(s) may be superimposed on the last. Cartilage is sometimes found in these kidneys as in the resected hydronephrotic upper half of a double kidney draining ectopic in a six-month-old girl (Campbell, 1937), and true bone formation with active bone marrow in the kidney was found in a twenty-five-year-old female by Tedeschi and Holtham (1952).

Compensatory hypertrophy of the sound organ usually suffices to maintain life and may function normally throughout a whole life expectancy. The hypertrophic organ is more prone to disease than is a normal organ because of its added physiologic burden and its total recipiency of nephrotoxic factors. Death was caused by renal failure in a third of our autopsy cases of unilateral hypoplasia in patients of all ages.

The *ureter* of the hypoplastic kidney is generally aplastic, especially if the kidney is nonfunctioning, or the duct may be absent. Ectopic openings into the bladder, urethra, vagina and so forth are occasionally found and, as in all other anomalies of the lower urinary tract, investigation of the upper tract may reveal the anomalous involvement.

Renal hypoplasia is of approximately the same incidence as renal agenesis having been found in thirty-three children in our autopsy series of 19,046 infants and children (1:577 bodies), and in seventy-nine cases of 32,834 adults examined post mortem, a ratio 1:462, an over-all incidence of 1 in 499 (500). Yet this autopsy finding of alleged congenital renal hypoplasia in adults bears careful scrutiny and is often inaccurate; doubtless renal degeneration or secondary sclerotic atrophy from unrecognized or unrecorded infection and/or obstruction often occurred. For this reason the cases as observed in the young are statistically more valuable (Figs. 111, 112, 113). That possible diagnostic error or confusion between renal hypoplasia and

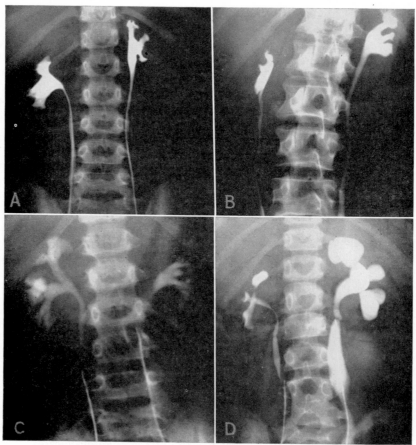

Fig. 112.   Congenital renal hypoplasia associated with vascular hypertension. *A,* involving the left kidney of a three-year-old girl. *B,* in a girl of five years, each kidney is hypoplastic, the right markedly so, the left to less degree. *C,* of the left kidney in a six-year-old boy; there is compensatory hypertrophy of the right kidney. *D,* of the right kidney in a five-year-old girl with moderate compensatory hypertrophy of the left kidney and stricture of its lower ureter with dilatation of the tract above.

renal degeneration in adults may be avoided, the following statistical data are confined to our autopsy studies in infants and children.

In the thirty-three cases of unilateral hypoplasia observed in children, the better kidney was hypoplastic in six, reduplicated in three, hypertrophic in two, ectopic in one, and together with the adrenal was absent in four. In one of the last group the adrenal on the other side was vestigial; in two cases the adrenal was aplastic. The ureter was hypoplastic in nine, showed stricture in five and was absent in three. In one instance each there was patent urachus, vesicovaginal fistula, and urethral obstruction. Double uterus and double vagina occurred in two, and atresia of the vagina and vaginorectal fistula in one each. The isolateral renal pedicle was hypoplastic in seven, patent foramen ovale existed in three, and in one each there was patent ductus arteriosus, hypoplastic aorta, cardiac hypoplasia, and "congenital heart

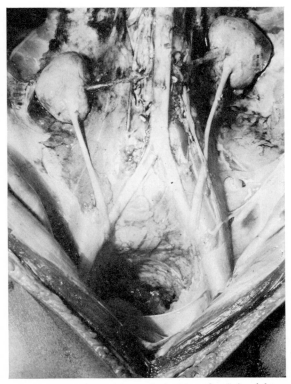

Fig. 113.   Congenital bilateral renal hypoplasia (dwarfism) in eight-year-old boy. This condition may give rise to "renal rickets" as in this case. The kidneys are about half normal size; the ureters come from the anterior renal surfaces. (Babies Hospital.)

disease." *Situs inversus* occurred in three instances, congenitally small stomach in two, and stenosis of the rectum and anomalous liver in one each. Anomalies of the lungs included dwarf lung, absent pulmonary fissure, absent diaphragm, supernumerary pulmonary fissure, anencephalus, clubfoot, supernumerary digits and absence of bones in one case each.

The chief *symptom* of renal hypoplasia is persistent pain in the loin or lumbar region and is present in about half of the cases in adults, but the only abnormal finding may be hypertension (Fig. 112) which produces its own clinical syndrome.

The *diagnosis* of renal hypoplasia is best made by urography; the renal outline is smaller than normal and the pelvis is small, undeveloped and apt to be triangular or ampullate, but may be elongated and narrowed, lacking in major calyces with the minor calyces leaving directly from the pelvis and often "squared" in outline.

While excretory urography may suggest the diagnosis, a complete urologic investigation is essential in which ureteral catheterization and divided renal function tests demonstrate an abnormally low renal function on the anomalous side. This study is particularly valuable when the total urea and phenol-sulfonphthalein output are comparatively estimated for a given time. The appearance time and concentration of the dye and the quantity of urea output per cubic centimeter from each kidney may be normal, yet a smaller total output will be obtained from the hypoplastic organ because of the greater diminished volume of secreting parenchyma. Retrograde urography commonly demonstrates an extremely small pelvis with clubbing of both minor and major calyces, or the appearance may be that of the rabbit type of

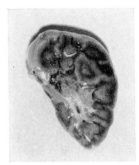

Fig. 114.   Congenital renal redundancy in a child of six months. In portions of the kidney there are two rows of pyramids, a condition thought by some to be allied with tumor formation. (Babies Hospital.)

unicalyceal kidney (Fig. 111, *D*). Occasionally the outline of the greatly thinned diminished parenchyma about the pelvis can be identified in the pyelogram. Many instances are recorded in which nephrectomy left an aplastic or hypoplastic kidney remaining to carry on the total renal secretion, a diseased organ being removed from the opposite side without knowledge of the existence of the hypoplastic organ; generally the last will not support life for many years if it is more than a third smaller than the size of a normal kidney. A uremic death from renal inadequacy occurs.

When renal hypoplasia is bilateral an early uremic death may be anticipated. These cases are exceedingly rare and while most have been recognized post mortem, the pronounced renal dysfunction may be manifested by renal dwarfism or so-called renal rickets.

The treatment of a hypoplastic kidney producing symptoms, including hypertension, is nephrectomy when the status and function of the renal mate is adequate.

Congenital renal hypertrophy is an embryologic compensatory mechanism associated with agenesis or hypoplasia of the renal mate. The organ is considerably increased both in size and functional capacity and generally its pelvis is unusually large (Fig. 106). The excretory urogram alone may suggest the diagnosis. Although solitary congenital hypertrophic kidneys often enable their bearers to reach advanced age, acute urinary infection or toxic injury associated with gastroenteritis, diphtheria, scarlet fever, measles and so forth is more likely to jeopardize life than when two kidneys of normal size and architecture exist. The hyperplastic organ may be of surgical diagnostic concern when it is mistaken for tumor and erroneously removed, as has occurred in the past; today this is inexcusable.

Redundancy of the renal parenchyma is characterized by a double row of pyramids instead of one; it is extremely rare and is to be distinguished from congenital renal hyperplasia (Fig. 114). The condition is a post mortem

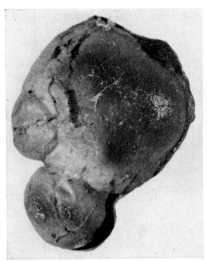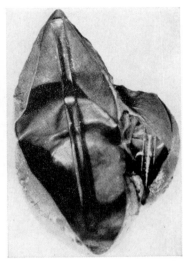

Fig. 115.   Congenital solitary cyst of the kidney in an eighteen-month-old male. The cyst measured 8 cm. in diameter and contained clear colorless fluid. A small nodule of functioning renal tissue remained at the lower pole. (Babies Hospital.)

finding; I know of two instances in the young. The cortex in each case, a stillborn boy and a five-month-old girl, was sandwiched between an outer and an inner layer of medullary pyramids. Redundancy of renal tissue was noted at autopsy in fourteen adults, twelve of whom were between forty and seventy years of age. It was present on the right in eight, on the left in four, and bilaterally in two. Parenchymal redundancy may be bilateral, is of no clinical concern, and has been thought by some to be allied to benign tumor formation (hamartoma).

Congenital solitary renal cysts are rare, are more often unilateral than bilateral and are seldom clinically important unless they produce abdominal tumor (Figs. 115, 116). Fourteen cases of solitary renal cysts have been reported in children; six of Kretschmer's (1948) cases were in patients ten years of age or less, the diagnosis being made preoperatively in two. Of 153 cases of solitary renal cyst collected by Carson, only four were children. In our autopsy studies in 19,046 infants and children, incidence was one in

1731; eight of the eleven were males. Coexisting anomalies are frequent; the kidneys showed anomalous vascularization in five cases, hydronephrosis in two, horseshoe formation in one, and in another the kidney was ectopic at the sacral level.

The *etiology* of solitary cystic renal disease is not clear; malunion or obstruction of the renal tubules is considered to be the pathogenesis as in polycystic disease (q.v.). Trauma and enlargement of one or more secretory ducts has likewise been adduced to explain the condition. The present theories regarding the etiology of renal cystic disease are discussed under congenital polycystic disease.

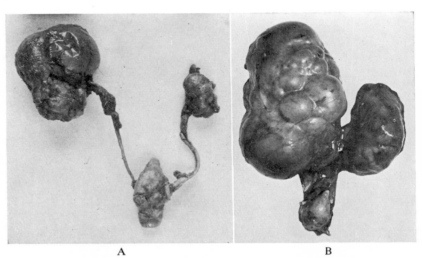

A   B

Fig. 116.   Congenital solitary renal disease. *A,* in a male infant five hours old. The lesion is unilateral and no obstructions were found. The testicle was retroperitoneal. The cyst at the right upper pole which by casual inspection appears to be a dilated pelvis, accounted for a fourth of the total renal volume. (Bellevue Hospital.) *B,* congenital muli-locular cyst of the right kidney in a boy of four years, the kidney weighing 204 gm. The upper ureter was impervious and there were neither pelvis nor calyces. The cysts developed in the cortical substance. Left kidney is normal. (Babies Hospital.)

Small solitary cortical cysts are not unusual in children (2 to 4 per cent post mortem) and generally have no significance. Several large cysts of surgical importance have been encountered; Mixter (1922) removed an enormous cyst from a thirteen-year-old girl and collected six others under ten years of age. The writer removed a large (500 cc.) solitary cyst from the left upper half of a horseshoe kidney in a seven-year-old boy (Fig. 121).

Solitary cyst must be differentiated from cystic degeneration so commonly seen in sclerotic nephritis and it is sometimes difficult in large solitary cysts encountered in the kidney of adults to determine whether the lesion was congenital or the result of postnatal factors just indicated. In adults we have encountered several solitary cysts more than 10 cm. in diameter but here, as previously indicated, it is rarely possible to be certain whether the lesion was congenital or developed as the result of inflammatory changes in the kidney with localized tubular obstruction. For this reason the data assembled by post mortem studies in infants and children are of far greater accuracy and statistical value.

In congenital solitary cyst, the lower pole is involved more often but in three of our eleven cases in children the cyst was found at the upper pole. As these cysts enlarge, they extend beyond the renal surface and laterally compress the parenchyma. The lesions vary from one to ten or more centimeters in diameter, the cyst wall being thin, its lining serosal, and its content serous, although blood clot and other debris are sometimes found. Moreover, by renal compression and damage of the renal parenchyma, hypertension may be induced as in Toulson's (1942) case, a nineteen-month-old infant. Here the blood pressure was systolic 130 and diastolic 90 mm. Hg, but a few weeks following transperitoneal nephrectomy, the systolic was 90 and the diastolic 60 mm. Hg (see also Kreutzmann, 1947).

Some of these cysts grow to enormous size and present a palpable abdominal mass which in the female is likely to be mistaken for an ovarian cyst. Compression of the bowel may produce constipation; pain is rare. In an eleven-year-old girl with right renal pain, Chalkley and Sutton (1943) found an infected solitary cyst of the lower pole of the kidney "large as a grapefruit" (12 cm. diameter). The mass had no connection with the pelvis, pushed the kidney upward, and on section was found filled with sterile pus, the pelvic walls being lined by a shaggy ivory colored material. Occasionally the solitary cyst gives rise to hematuria.

The *diagnosis* is suggested by urography when a localized and usually smoothly rounded or crescentic pelvic filling defect or pelvicalyceal distortion results from compression by the cystic mass (Figs. 117, 119). The urogram in solitary renal cyst is most often interpreted as that of malignant tumor (Figs. 117, 119). The renal axis and position are frequently changed, as is the course of the ureter, and in lateral pyelograms the cyst may be found either anterior or posterior to the kidney. Renal angiography is usually definitive in the differential diagnosis from tumor; see Section III, Chapter 2. If calcified, the cyst wall may appear as a large ring; small renal cysts rarely cause symptoms or urographic changes.

The *treatment* of solitary cyst is (1) nephrectomy when the parenchyma remaining is not worth saving and the renal mate is sound and (2) excision of the cyst or partial renal resection when the remaining parenchyma is worth saving or must be conserved. In a ten-year-old girl with complete stenosis of the pelvic outlet of the right upper reduplicated half of a horseshoe kidney, the pelvic retention cyst held more than one liter and was treated by resection through the isthmus. In a child of eighteen months the left upper kidney was replaced by a cyst 8 cm. in diameter and containing colorless clear fluid, only a small nodule of depressed renal parenchyma remained at the lower pole while the opposite kidney showed compensatory hypertrophy.

Spontaneous or traumatic rupture of these large cysts sometimes occurs and is accompanied by sharp pain and often collapse. Immediate operation, usually nephrectomy, is demanded.

Congenital multilocular cysts of the kidney are relatively rare and may be considered as an aggregation of solitary cysts and probably of the same etiology. Congenital multilocular cysts must be distinguished from congenital polycystic disease about to be described. The chief symptoms are pressure on adjacent organs, sometimes with obstruction of the bowel. Lynch and Thompson (1937) observed a female child with a left unilateral multicystic disease causing a palpable mass at four months. As it grew until its removal at fourteen months, it caused increasing dyspnea which became pronounced. A similar case was reported by Schwartz (1936; see also Kutzman and Sauer, 1950; Ravitch and Sanford, 1949).

The diagnosis conceivably may be made by urography or by pyelography but the urogram is often interpreted as that of malignant renal tumor (Fig. 119). Congenital multilocular cystic disease is to be differentiated from (1) congenital polycystic disease which characteristically involves both kidneys, and (2) from cystadenoma of the kidney (cf. Section X, Chapter 1).

The treatment is nephrectomy when (1) symptoms demand, (2) the condition of the patient warrants, and (3) the opposite kidney is able to support life.

Congenital polycystic disease is to be differentiated from cystic renal degeneration which frequently accompanies chronic nephritis. There is characteristic nodular (cystic) bilateral enlargement of the kidneys. It is said to be unilateral in less than 10 per cent of the cases (Seiber) but histologic study of the opposite kidney will almost always disclose anomalous development characteristically that of early renal changes in polycystic disease. Therefore, for practical purposes and until proved otherwise, every case of polycystic disease should be considered to be bilateral (cf. Bell, 1935), an early unrecognized disease in one kidney sometimes appearing only with advancing years. A few instances of apparently genuine unilateral cystic disease have been recorded, notably the cases of Oppenheimer and Narins (1949), and of Lich and Waud (1952); Marcel (1953) collected twelve cases from the literature and added three of his own (Fig. 117). But an incidence as high as 15 per cent as reported by some observers cannot be accepted.

Two forms of polycystic disease are recognized: (1) the group, comprising about a third of all cases, in which the condition appears in infancy, early life, or when the child is stillborn, and (2) those in whom the lesion does not appear until after puberty or in adulthood with enlarging renal masses and failing renal function.

With cystic enlargement the parenchyma shows compression atrophy and it may also be injured by infection, toxic insults, and particularly of acute febrile diseases. When the process has sufficiently damaged the kidneys, fatal renal failure occurs. Renal rickets has developed in some children with polycystic renal disease as noted by Kretschmer (1948).

Although the condition may be recognized in infancy or early childhood (Figs. 117, 119), the condition is most often discovered in mid-adult life. In a collected series of 212 cases, Seiber found twenty-eight or 15.6 per cent were between eight weeks and twenty-one years of age. The earlier the condition is discovered, the poorer is the prognosis. Sixty-nine (28.2 per cent) of 239 cases collected by Kuster (1902) did not reach the first birthday, the majority of these being born dead or dying shortly after birth. Ten died later during the first year; seven others were less than two years old. The youngest patient with this condition I have examined urologically was seven days old, and bilateral pyelography demonstrated the changes in pelvic outline characteristically produced by the disease (Fig. 119).

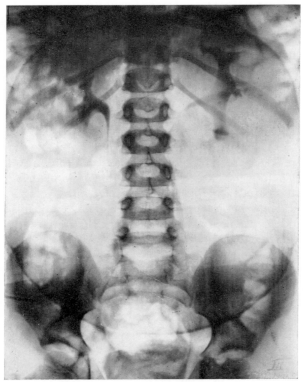

Fig. 117. Unilateral polycystic disease of left kidney in a five-year-old girl. Note the large left kidney with calyceal and pelvic deformity with ureteral displacement to the midline. Surgically confirmed. Exposure of right kidney showed it to be normal. (Courtesy of Dr. J. E. Marcel, Paris.)

Approximately one in 250 individuals is born with polycystic renal disease. In 19,046 autopsies in children studied by me, there were seventy-two cases, an incidence of 1 to 265. Of these seventy-two, there were forty-seven males and twenty-five females; allowing for the relative incidence of autopsies performed in each sex (55.6:44.3 plus), this suggests a slightly higher incidence in males. The condition was bilateral in forty-six of the seventy-two cases; in fifteen it was grossly limited to the right kidney and in eleven to the left. The medulla alone was cystic in one case, and the cortex alone in eleven, but in sixty the entire organ was involved. In eighteen the cysts were larger than 5 mm. in diameter. Polycystic kidneys were found in 114 of 32,834 adults examined post mortem, a ratio of 1 to 293. Yet it seems likely that in some of these cases at least, cystic renal degeneration from inflammatory or sclerotic disease, rather than congenital factors, engendered the cystic changes. On the other hand, minute congenital cystic lesions as they occur in early infancy may be missed by naked eye examination.

Congenital hepatic cystic disease occurs in about 5 per cent of patients with congenital polycystic renal disease, and in about 4 per cent there is also *splenic cystic disease*. Accompanying congenital cysts are also found in the bones, ovaries, epididymis, pancreas, as occurred in one case each in our autopsy series. In the 186 cases (total) here recorded, extrarenal cystic distribution was as follows: liver, 20 (2 children), lung, 4 (1 child), pancreas, 1 (child), spleen, bone and other sites 14. Large polycystic kidneys in the fetus may cause dystocia and gravely increase the maternal hazard, this being noted in two cases in one year at the Brooklyn Hospital (Denton, 1933). In the first of these cases, the kidneys each measured 10 by 6 x 5 cm. and weighed 450 gm. apiece (Fig. 118).

Coexisting anomalies in our seventy-two autopsy cases in infants and children were urologic in forty and nonurologic in eighteen. The urologic anomalies were renal reduplication in seven, aplasia in four, horseshoe fusion in one. The ureters showed idiopathic dilatation in eight, reduplication in seven, stricture in six, aplasia in three, valves and ectopia in two each. The bladder was absent in one, and diverticulum, cystic bladder, bladder atresia, ureterocele, patent urachus, permanent cloaca, urethral atresia, urethral valves, "obstruction," and hypospadias were present in one each. The testicles were undescended in eight and the right testis was absent in one. Gynecologic anomalies included double uterus, bicornate uterus, cystic uterus, cystic ovaries, atresia vulvae, and atresia of the vagina in one instance each. In the alimentary tract, stenosis of the rectum existed in four cases; harelip, cleft palate were observed in three cases each; esophageal stricture, esophagotracheal fistula, split tongue, atresia of the soft palate, atresia of the uvula, situs inversus, and Meckel's intestinal diverticulum were present in two each; accessory spleen, dwarf gallbladder, cystic gallbladder were present in one case each. The cardiovascular system showed patent foramen ovale in ten, patent ductus arteriosus in five, patent interventricular septum and dextroaortic position in one each. There were clubfoot in six, clubhand, polydactylism, hypoplasia of the mandible, hyperteleorism, vestigial tail, agenesis of skeletal muscle, spina bifida, osteogenesis imperfecta, nonfusion of the mandible, and malformed brain in one each.

Familial or hereditary tendencies appear to be more definitely pronounced in congenital polycystic renal disease than in any other anomaly. Several geneologic studies of the condition have included four or five generations, the genetic factor being recognized as a mendelian recessive (Bagg, 1925). In Crawford's (1923) study the condition existed in seventeen of forty members of one family. In history taking in this disease, it will be found that in a third to a fourth of the cases, immediate or remote family members either have known polycystic disease or, commonly, have died of "kidney" trouble. Moreover, the discovery of polycystic renal disease in a patient

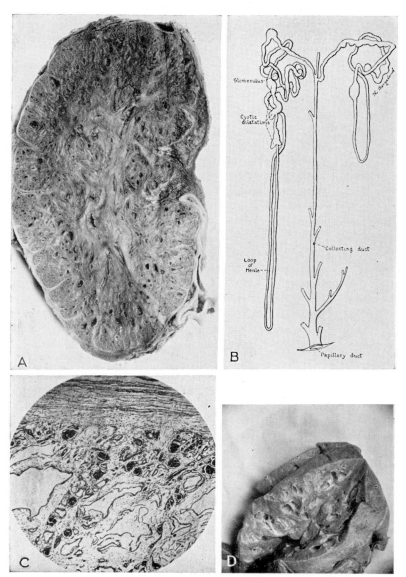

Fig. 118.   Congenital polycystic disease. *A*, congenital polycystic disease in the new-born. Each kidney weighed 450 gm. and caused dystocia. There is notable variation in size of the cysts. (Courtesy of Dr. James Denton and American Journal of Surgery.) *B*, schema showing the collecting tubule in polycystic renal disease with cystic dilatations of the duct (Greene). *C*, histology in polycystic renal disease showing pronounced dilata-tion of the tubules (Greene). *D*, congenital cystic liver disease accompanying congenital polycystic renal disease. (Bellevue Hospital.)

warrants at least a satisfactory excretory urographic study of the other members of the family and especially if more children are contemplated.

The *etiology* of polycystic renal congenital disease remains unknown, as witnessed by the many explanatory theories which have been advanced. Three of these have been outstanding but only one (Hildebrandt, 1894) has received general support. This conceives the condition to result from failure of union between the metanephroblastemic elements (glomeruli) and the collecting tubules originating in the metanephric (wolffian) duct and has been the most widely accepted theory (Fig. 100). With glomerular secretion outflow obstructed by faulty or absent union, cystic formation results. Obstruction of the papillary collecting ducts by urinary salts or inflammation (papillitis) was advanced by Virchow (1856) as an explanation theory, but this mechanism has been found to produce only tubular atrophy (Petterson, Tollens). The experimental work of Bunting, Greene (1922; see Fig. 118, *B*) and others has shown that the urinary unit is not necessarily blocked by faulty union and that retention alone is insufficient to explain cystic formation. Hepler's (1930, 1940) experimental studies indicated that interference with the parenchymal blood supply leads to cystic degeneration in the involved area and an analogous renal change is produced by the fetal type of renal circulation of the polycystic kidney which suffers compression and displacement by the cyst. Hinman and Morison (1924) found that the fetal type of renal circulation persists in the polycystic kidney and that the finer vessels of the cortex are compressed and displaced. From this, it is reasonable to assume that these vascular factors may play an etiologic role. From a histologic study of polycystic kidneys in an eight-month-old fetus, Besson (1933) concluded the condition resulted from poverty of nephrogenic tissue with resulting atypical growth of the relatively abundant tubular and vascular elements.

More recently these theories have been succeeded by those of other students of the disease. In 1923 Davis advanced the notion that polycystic renal disease results from stoppage of the development of the mesonephric tissues with subsequent degenerative changes, an observation suggested by the occurrence in lower animal life in which the adult kidney is of the mesonephric type and often shows changes similar to those observed in polycystic disease in adults. Kampmeier (1923) and McKenna and Kampmeier (1934) demonstrated that in renal development the first three or four generations or subdividings of the tubules are not permanent but become detached from the collecting tubules to persist for a time as cystic elements which normally atrophy and disappear but in polycystic disease pathologically persist (cf. Rall and Odel, 1949). Increasing in size as they persist, these cystic elements compress the adjacent tubules to increase the parenchymal tubular cyst formation.

Opposed to this notion and on the basis of studies in four cases, Norris and Herman (1941) concluded that focal cystic dilatations of tubules and collecting ducts do not develop until after differentiation of the metanephrogenic anlage and union of its elements with the collecting ducts have occurred.

Convoluted tubule segments and portions of the collecting ducts become isolated as cysts, enlarged through continuous proliferation of epithelium, and may rupture through septa and adjacent tubules to produce intercommunications and multicystic foci. These enlarging cysts cause pressure injury or even destruction of the adjacent normal tissue and thus ultimately destroy the kidney. Moreover, Norris and Herman noted similar cystogenous changes in the pancreatic and hepatic ducts. The frequent coexistence of cystic disease of the liver, spleen, pancreas and other organs is advanced to support the theory of fetal malformation as the cause of polycystic kidney (see Yarmudian and Ackerman, 1943). At present the Hildebrandt theory is probably the most generally accepted.

Pathology. Congenital polycystic kidneys are usually greatly increased in size; cystic degeneration of hypoplastic organs has been observed. The cystic renal mass often becomes five or more times normal size with totally irregular surfaces and on section is found to be composed of numerous cysts of various size between which the parenchyma is poorly developed or shows compression degeneration (Fig. 118). So extensive may the cystic development be that secreting parenchyma appears almost or totally absent and differentiation between cortex and medulla is impossible. In infancy the polycystic kidney is of normal size or only slightly enlarged, but over its surface and throughout its parenchyma are innumerable pinhead to pea size cysts (Fig. 118, *A*). In older children and adults the cystic development and renal enlargement are more pronounced. The cystic fluid is of low specific gravity (1.004–1.006), is generally watery, yellow or brown, may be colloid, mucoid, purulent, or bloody, but is never urinous. Moreover, it may contain cholesterol, leucine, cystine, uric acid, calcium oxalate, blood or pus.

Occasionally the cysts are localized to the medulla as noted by Smith and Graham (1945), Longcope, Thorn and others, or may occur only in the cortex. It is notable that there is no communication between the renal pelvis and the cysts and seldom between the cysts themselves. The existing parenchyma shows interstitial nephritis. Polycystic kidneys are particularly prone to complicating disease, both tuberculous and nontuberculous infection, hydronephrosis, calculus and other lesions which may not only jeojardize life but gravely affect the prognosis and increase the therapeutic difficulties, particularly because of the extremely narrow margin of renal reserve. When polycystic renal disease is not evident in infancy, it seldom manifests itself before puberty and generally not until the third decade or later and notably between the ages of forty and sixty.

Symptoms. The clinical picture is that of nephritis and usually with pain, hematuria, pyuria or tumor. Nephritic and/or uremic manifestations result from parenchymal irritation and destruction of the vascular tree as well as directly by compression of the tissue itself. The mass weight of the organs induces pain largely by traction on the renal pedicle. Renal colic results from acute ureteral angulation, or is induced by the passage of blood clots or complicating calculi. A fifth of all cases show hematuria, the result of nephritis or infection. Anemia in these cases is often profound and reflects the severe renal functional impairment and nitrogen retention, but is probably due especially to toxic depression of hemopoiesis rather than nitrogen retention per se (Smith and Graham, 1945; McArthur, 1942).

The enlarged kidneys can usually be palpated and when hematuria coexists, an initial diagnosis of malignant tumor is commonly made. Occasionally the nodular surface of the cystic kidneys can be detected by palpation. As the clinical course progresses there is renal insufficiency which is manifested by gastrointestinal disturbances, loss of weight, anemia, malaise, headache, increasing weakness and, generally, terminal uremia. Debilitated, these patients commonly die with intercurrent infection, chiefly pneumonia.

In adults the course is usually slow but the patient seldom lives ten years from the initial symptomatic onset. Two to four years after the onset of symptoms is the life expectancy in half of all cases, and less than two years in a fourth. When the disease is recognized in infancy or early childhood, the prognosis is unusually bad, these patients frequently dying within three months from the appearance of the initial symptoms. Simultaneous polycystic renal disease and erythroblastosis were reported in three cases by Shands (1945). In two infants under our care, the fatal course was less than six months, while a third lived for three years and a fourth for four years, yet all died in uremia.

Diagnosis. The palpation of a large nodular mass in the renal region, particularly when found bilaterally, at once suggests the diagnosis of polycystic renal disease. Thorough urologic investigation is essential and pyelographic study is generally conclusive. It is remarkable that palpation in an emaciated dehydrated newborn infant whose kidneys are three times the comparative body size ratio in adults may be misleading when two apparently enlarged organs are found. With correction of the dehydration, these seemingly enormous kidneys become no longer palpable. This possible source of diagnostic error merits serious consideration. Yet in five infant patients of ours with large bilateral palpable kidneys, polycystic disease did exist; Behr recognized it at birth on the right side in a boy; presently the left kidney became enlarged. Six weeks later at autopsy the diagnosis was confirmed.

The urinalysis shows albumin, casts, lowered specific gravity, and occasionally pus, blood and/or bacteria, but frequently it causes only the diagnosis of chronic interstitial nephritis to be made. A diminished phenolsulfonphthalein output and elevated blood nitrogen are usual but the blood pressure is not necessarily elevated.

Urography. Urographic studies are demanded in all cases of renal enlargement, especially when polycystic disease or tumor is suspected. Excretory urography may be rendered useless by a low renal function but even with moderate excretion of the radiopaque medium, the pelvic outlines may be indefinite and prohibit making a positive diagnosis. Regardless of the excretory urographic findings, retrograde pyelography should be employed. The more important pyelographic diagnostic criteria are (a) shortening, obliteration, compression, or elongation of the calyces with peculiar squared, oval or crescentic rounded outlines; (b) pelvic compression, distortion, displacement, obliteration or dilatation, and (c) with infection, the superimposed changes resulting therefrom (Section V, Chapters 1 and 2). The number and size of the cysts will largely determine the pelvic changes and by compression and distortion of the pelvic calyces suggest malignant neoplasm (Figs. 117, 119). Malignant renal tumor is seldom bilateral and part of the pelvis is likely to be normal, while in polycystic disease the entire outline is altered. An irregular but undilated pelvis with separation of the calyces is suggestive of polycystic disease. Urograms in this disease are characteristically bizarre and permit of no specifications. Sometimes the calyces

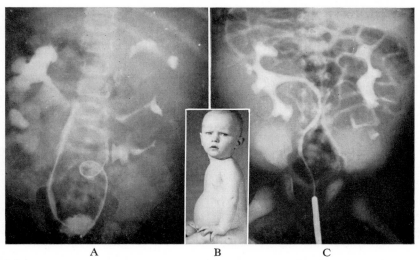

A   B   C

Fig. 119.   Congenital polycystic renal disease in a one-year-old boy. *A,* this pyelogram depicts the characteristic bizarre pelvic deformities consequent to the cystic renal changes. Patient died of renal failure three years later. *B,* patient showing abdominal enlargement caused by the polycystic kidneys. (Bellevue Hospital.) *C,* in a seven-day-old child born with comparatively enormous polycystic kidneys.

are crescentic, reflecting the cystic encroachment, but papillary cuppings may be preserved. The urographic diagnosis must usually rest on observation of some of these described pelvic changes which will usually be found and, if bilateral in part or *in toto,* will clinch the diagnosis. When these changes are unilateral, the odds favor malignant tumor.

Treatment. In uncomplicated polycystic disease, the therapy is that of chronic nephritis (Section XVII). It is axiomatic that the less surgical treatment is employed in polycystic disease, the longer the patient will live. Yet we have observed glaring exceptions to this dictum. Moreover, infection, stone, obstruction or hematuria all contribute pain, demand a complete urologic investigation, and the disclosures may call for surgical intervention in addition to chemotherapy or antibiotic therapy. Hematuria threatening life may demand nephrectomy, but lesser bleeding can sometimes be checked by liberal repeated blood transfusions, or even by the instillation of silver nitrate 1 to 5 per cent into the renal pelvis.

Cyst puncture as advocated by Rovsing (1910) has relieved pain in some cases and brought about temporary improvement in renal function. Dodson recommends surgical treatment before stricture, other obstruction, hemorrhage, infection or severe pain occurs; the superficial walls of the larger cysts are excised. Cyst puncture and marsupialization of the kidney to the wound has been advocated by Goldstein (1936); this exposure permits new formed cysts to continue to be aspirated postoperatively. Cyst aspiration and the injection of 5 per cent sodium morrhuate solution using 1 cc. for each cubic centimeter of cyst fluid withdrawn has been advocated by Young (1946); or one may inject 50 or 60 per cent dextrose solution. Following nephrectomy in polycystic disease, a half of the patients will die in the immediate postoperative period and a third will die of renal failure within the postoperative month.

III. ANOMALIES OF FORM

Fetal Lobulation. This is usual until the age of four or five years but in 3 to 4 per cent of all individuals fetal lobulation persists into later life (Fig. 102). Fetal lobulation was specifically noted at autopsy in 17.6 per cent (1408) or 7,966 children and in 3.9 per cent (671) or 18,394 adults. It has no clinical importance and is only a manifestation of comparative renal developmental immaturity.

Other frequent morphologic deviations are those in which the kidney is shorter or longer than normal with a commensurate decrease or increase in thickness or, exceptionally, is annular, hourglass or dumbbell. Sometimes one end of the kidney is unusually large or the pelvis may be entirely inter-renal or extra-renal. These changes are rarely of clinical importance but exploration of a pelvis which is entirely intrarenal is usually a difficult surgical maneuver. We have observed all of these morphologic deviations at autopsy in kidneys otherwise normal.

Renal Fusion. This may be homolateral or contralateral. Homolateral fusion is illustrated by the reduplicated or double kidney and is discussed elsewhere in this chapter (p. 285). Most reduplicated kidneys are fused, the striking exception being the isolateral supernumerary kidney.

Contralateral fusion occurs about once in 400 cases and is most often of the horseshoe variety, in which the two kidneys may be fused at the upper, lower or both poles (Fig. 120); bipolar fusion results in a disc or doughnut form (Fig. 125). The upper pole of one organ may be fused to the lower pole of its mate to produce a sigmoid or L-shaped kidney (Fig. 124, *A*), or the entire renal substance may exist as a narrowed mass, the lump kidney (Fig. 124, *B*). The weight of the combined fused renal mass averages about equal to that of two normal kidneys. Fused kidneys seldom ascend to normal level but remain in the pelvis or about the fifth lumbar vertebral level, the ascent being impeded by persistence of early fetal anomalous vascular attachments or by the size or shape of the malformed organ itself.

Horseshoe Kidney. In this frequent anomaly the two renal segments are fused across the midline by an isthmus composed of a solid mass or a thin strip of parenchyma or only a dense band of fibrous tissue (Fig. 120). Fusion occurs at the lower pole in about 90 per cent of the cases. The horseshoe kidney lies anterior to the aorta and vena cava usually, but has been found behind as well as between the vessels. In a case at Bellevue Hospital, the isthmus perforated and passed directly through the vena cava. The ureters run anterior to the isthmus, an important point in ureterotomy as for stone. Often one organ is much better developed than the other, a situation corresponding to unilateral renal hypoplasia with hypertrophy of

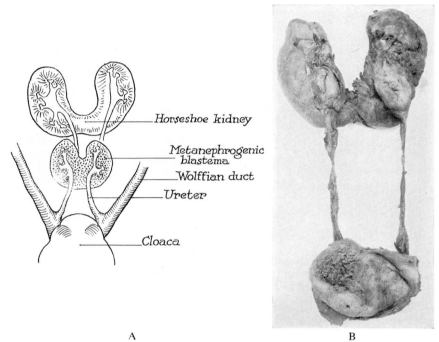

Horseshoe kidney

Metanephrogenic blastema

Wolffian duct

Ureter

Cloaca

A   B

Fig. 120.   *A,* schema indicating the embryologic etiology of horseshoe kidney formation. Lower polar fusion is here shown; superior polar fusion is most rare. *B,* horseshoe kidney resulting from fusion of the lower poles. The pelves face forward and the ureters arch over the renal isthmus.

the mate. One or both halves of the kidney may be reduplicated or be polycystic or show other congenital anomalies described in this chapter. In a seven-year-old boy with abdominal pain, a solitary cyst containing 500 cc. of clear fluid occupied the upper pole of the reduplicated left half of a horseshoe kidney and was resected (Fig. 121, *C*).

The incidence of horseshoe kidney shows reported variance from 1 in 600 to 1 in 1800 cases. Motzfeld found ninety-two cases in 73,489 collected autopsies, a ratio of 1 in 719. In our study of 51,880 autopsies there were 122, an incidence of 1 to 425. Here the anomaly occurred nearly twice as often in children (1 to 312; sixty-one in 19,046 autopsies) as in adults (1 to 538; sixty-one in 32,834), an observation which strikingly reflects the early mortality in the young with horseshoe kidney, the condition strongly predisposing to serious renal disease. A composite study of reported cases indicates horseshoe kidney occurs twice as often in males as in females. In our series of sixty-one children (postmortem study) there were forty-two males and nineteen females, and in the adults the ratio was fifty-four to seven, and in the combined autopsy study, ninety-six to twenty-six. It is notable that approximately 10 per cent more males than females were examined post mortem in this series.

Anomalies of the urogenital and other systems commonly coexist in horseshoe kidney disease and often present serious complicating clinical

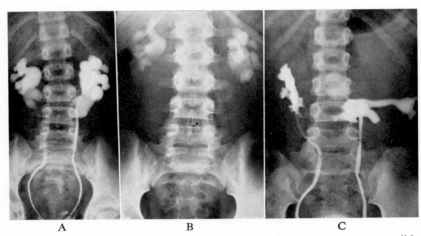

A   B   C

Fig. 121.   Horseshoe kidney disease. *A,* in a ten-year-old boy with recurrent mild abdominal pain, chronic pyuria and occasional hematuria. Bilateral ureteropelvic junction narrowing. *B,* ten-minute trap film of (*A*) showing retention of medium in each dilated pelvis, the shadow being sharply cut off at the ureteropelvic junction. Treatment: Division of the isthmus, suspension of the kidneys with tilting outward of the lower renal poles, bilateral ureteropelvioplasty. *C,* in a seven-year-old boy with large cyst (500 cc.) of the upper pole of the left half of a horseshoe kidney. The pyelogram shows pronounced transverse flattening of the left pelvis by pressure of the cyst. Treatment: Resection of the cyst.

problems. In our autopsy series of 122 cases, the fused kidneys were ectopic in twenty, polycystic in two and with absent adrenal in two. The adrenal was with the ectopic organ in five cases. The ureter showed reduplication in eleven cases, stricture in five, idiopathic dilatation in four, and aplasia in one. The bladder was aplastic in one and the urethra was obstructed in two, while the testicles were imperfectly descended in two, fused in one, and absent in one. Gastrointestinal anomalies present included Meckel's diverticulum in three, absent gallbladder, esophageal atresia, hepatic malformation and imperforate anus in two each, esophagotracheal fistula, atresia of the anus, dwarf gallbladder, incomplete rotation of the colon, rectourethral fistula in one each. Cardiovascular malformations consisted of congenital heart disease in two cases, patent ductus arteriosus in four, patent foramen ovale in five, and atresia of the right ventricle in one case. There was clubfoot in

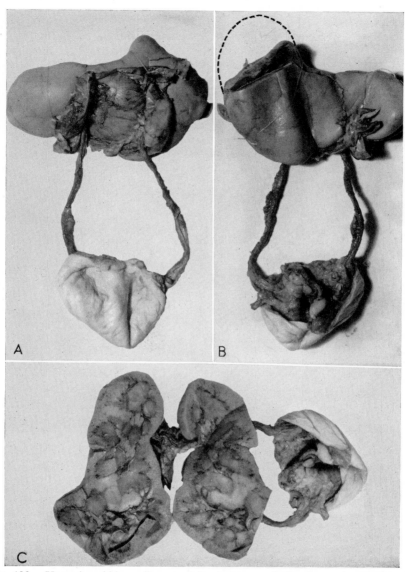

Fig. 122. Horseshoe kidney disease of the transverse fusion type. *A*, anterior view showing the ureters leaving the pelves on the anterior renal surface. *B*, posterior view. The deep sulcus in the kidney caused by the vertebral column is notable. *C*, Section of the kidney: the bizarre renal architecture indicates why renal resection in many of these anatomically unusual organs is extremely difficult or even impossible because of serious interference with the blood supply or damage of the sound segment to be left. (Mountainside Hospital, Courtesy Dr. J. L. Work.)

six, meningocele in four, mongolism and malformation of the brain in two each with optic atrophy, absent thymus, enlarged thymus, and accessory spleen in one case each.

Etiology. Horseshoe kidney results from mesial fusion of the two nephrogenic blastemas (Fig. 120). Embryologic studies suggest that fusion must take place earlier than the thirtieth day (Boyden, 1931), when the two renal masses

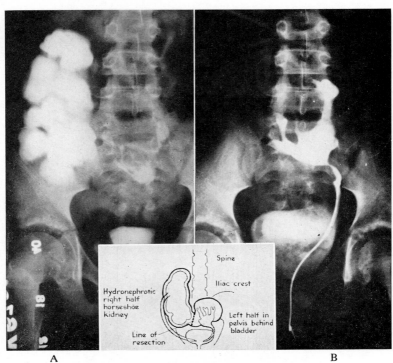

A   B

Fig. 123.   Horseshoe renal disease in pelvic ectopia in a seven-year-old boy with persistent pyuria and recurrent pain in the right lower abdomen. *A,* acute obstruction of the pelvic outlet of the enormous infected hydronephrotic right half of the horseshoe kidney caused severe pain for which the patient previously had been operated upon under the erroneous diagnosis of acute appendicitis. On opening the abdomen, the surgeon entered the distended kidney. A normal appendix was removed but a renocutaneous fistula persisted. The pyelogram of the left half of the kidney is faintly shown overlying the first sacral vertebra. *B,* remaining left renal segment six months following heminephrectomy and removal of the diseased right half of the kidney. Insert: Anatomic relations. (Bellevue Hospital.)

in the pelvis are brought into contact by the developing umbilical arteries. Yet anatomic observations indicate that fusion may occur at different periods. When fusion precedes renal rotation, the ureters will be found leaving anteriorly (eighth week) and when the pelves face medially, fusion succeeded rotation. Corresponding abnormalities in position, form and vascularization will depend therefore on the time of the fusion (Figs. 120–124). In a stillborn male, the right segment of a polycystic horseshoe kidney showed external rotation. The superior segment of the left half of the kidney contained a solitary cyst 5 cm. in diameter, the right ureter was a nonpatent threadlike structure while the urinary bladder, gallbladders and lungs were dwarfed, the thymus was absent, and there was clubfoot and hypospadias. Horseshoe kidneys are seldom found in normal position, generally being closer to the spine than separate kidneys and inclining more obliquely (Figs. 121, 123). The upper poles tilt in with superior fusion and the lower poles incline mesially with inferior fusion; for this reason calculi in horseshoe kidneys most often lie obliquely. The organs usually overlie the lower lumbar vertebrae or sacral promontory, but may be situated within the bony pelvis or, as we have seen, tucked well down behind the bladder. In a seven-year-old boy, the pyonephrotic segment of whose horseshoe kidney I resected, the fused organ was low within the bony pelvis (Fig. 123). In our 117 cases discovered at autopsy, the renal fusion occurred at the upper pole in nine, at the lower pole in ninety-eight, while there was bipolar fusion (doughnut) kidney in two and in the remainder the site of fusion was not stated. The fusion level when given was twelfth dorsal to third lumbar in eight, third to fifth lumbar in eight, and pelvic in four, and is apt to be otherwise anomalous. The kidneys are often held in low ectopia by an early established abnormally low vascular derivation from the inferior aortic or iliac vessels. The isthmus has its own blood supply in a fourth of the cases, a circumstance which together with the abnormal position of the ureters is of the utmost importance in surgery of the horseshoe kidney and usually vastly increases the technical operative difficulties. While the ureters are usually single to each pelvis and overlie the renal isthmus, they are often reduplicated or may approach the isthmus from behind. The isthmus itself may contain a pelvis, such bizarre pelvic displacement increasing both the surgical difficulties and hazards.

Symptoms. Horseshoe kidney may cause no symptoms, but the incidence of disease in these malformed organs is unusually high and is predominantly concerned with infection. More than half of the cases observed post mortem showed advanced renal disease, chiefly hydronephrosis, infection and/or stone. The abnormally ectopic renal position favors urinary stasis which favors hydronephrosis and renal stone formation, and both predispose to and perpetuate infection. The symptoms of hydronephrosis in horseshoe kidney are seldom recognized clinically until adult life, but I have encountered it in five children with persistent pyuria.

Symptoms when present are those of the complicating disease such as infection, calculus, hydronephrosis, tumor and so forth and are clinically indistinguishable from these manifestations when the kidney is unfused. Gutierrez described a so-called horseshoe kidney syndrome characterized by chronic gastrointestinal disturbances, epigastric or umbilical pain and radiating to the lumbar region. Urinary disturbances with early signs of nephritis and chronic constipation characteristically coexist. It is thought these symptoms result from renal pressure on the underlying nerve plexuses and from faulty urinary drainage. The Rovsing sign (the production of renal pain by spinal retroflexion and relief by anteflexion) is of little diagnostic significance. Pain, centered about the umbilicus, is always suggestive of horseshoe kidney, particularly when urinary infection exists, although Meckel's diverticulum and lesions of the urachus must be diagnostically excluded. Israel was able to palpate the renal isthmus in a three-year-old girl.

Diagnosis. Although pain localized about the umbilicus is always suggestive of horseshoe kidney, the precise diagnosis demands comprehensive urographic studies as part of the complete urologic investigation. A good plain urogram may indicate the normal renal outlines especially when the kidneys are tilted towards each other at the lower or upper pole and the continuity of the psoas muscle outline is broken by the shadow of the transverse renal isthmus. The urographic pelvic shadows lie closer to the midline and usually lower than normal (Figs. 121, 123), while the urogram presents a bizarre conformation dependent upon the character of the fusion and malrotation factors. Thus, by inversion, one or more calyces may point medially and downward and often overlap the pelvic shadows. Gutierrez (1934) described as pathognomonic the pyelographic horseshoe triangle in which the junction of the lines of the pelvic axes below is a minimum basic angle of twenty degrees. Computations in triangulation are seldom necessary. The curvature of the ureter conforms to the underlying renal structure over which it passes and usually arches outward first and then in towards the spine. Satisfactory preoperative urograms are most desirable for advantageous surgical approach. An operation should advisedly be withheld until reliable urographic guidance has been obtained.

Treatment. In horseshoe kidney disease therapy is predominantly that of the complicating lesions except when nonsurgical infection or nephritis is the chief consideration or problem. Surgical therapy may be extremely difficult. The horseshoe kidney is best approached by carrying the usual line of incision for renal exposure from just below the costovertebral angle downward to the midiliocostal space, then directly medially to the midline, if necessary, to obtain adequate exposure. The peritoneum is easily reflected and ample working space is afforded. When pain is the only symptom and there is no complicating disease, symphysiotomy (division of the isthmus) and suspension of the separated organs is frequently effective, chiefly by relieving the tension and drag on the renal pedicle (Campbell, 1937). When the horseshoe kidney is deep pelvic, a transperitoneal approach must usually be employed. In carrying out nephrectomy, the organ is resected through its isthmus (see Section XV, Chapter 3).

Disc, discoid, scutiform (shieldlike) or **doughnut kidney** is extremely rare, being found but three times in 51,880 autopsies (Fig. 124, *B*). The doughnut variety is formed by polar or mesial fusion of the renal anlagen before rotation begins, both kidneys being on the same level. These kidneys are usually located low over the sacral promontory or in the pelvic cavity but most of the renal mass is found on one side. The pelves and ureters emerge anteriorly while the blood vessels enter posteriorly. In a case of doughnut kidney in a seven-week-old boy examined at autopsy by the writer at Bellevue

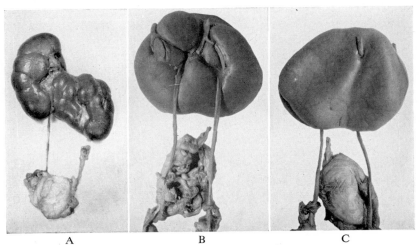

A   B   C

Fig. 124. Renal fusion. *A*, L-kidney in a one-year-old child in whom a considerable portion of the left renal segment lies across the lower lumbar spine. On each side the pelvic outlet faces anteriorly (Babies Hospital). *B*, lump kidney showing the unusual anatomy with the anterior blood supply coming from above and the ureters leaving from below. *C*, posterior view of *B*, with the blood supply entering from above and a deep grooving of the parenchyma indicating where the kidney pressed against the spine. (Courtesy of Dr. H. S. Altman.)

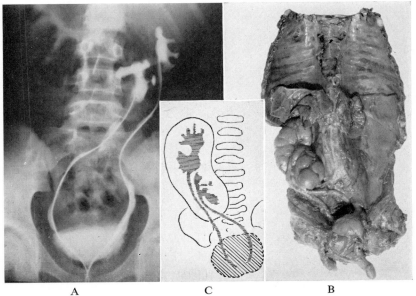

A   C   B

Fig. 125. Crossed fused renal dystopia. *A*, in an eight-year-old girl examined because of persistent pyuria and intermittent pain in the right loin (picture reversed); a normal appendix was removed during an acute attack of pain. The urogram portrays the characteristic pelvic misdirection in these cases. *B*, in a premature male in whom the kidneys show fetal lobulation, the usual course of the ureters and the normally placed left adrenal (courtesy Dr. M. J. Fein). *C*, urographic schema of *B*.

Hospital, the left renal segment was somewhat larger than the right, the ureters came from the anteromesial region, one ureter and one pelvis on each side. The left pelvis was at a higher level than the right. The cortex was circular while the medulla was somewhat irregular. In addition the child had a supernumerary left thumb as well as congenital syphilis with pneumonia alba.

Sigmoid or L-shaped Kidney. This results when the lower pole of one kidney becomes fused with the upper pole of its mate (Fig. 124, *A*). The

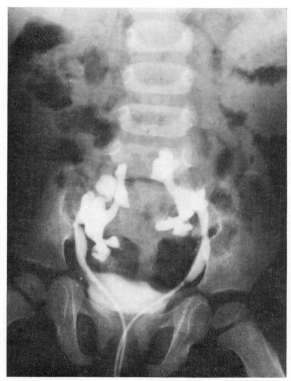

Fig. 126.   Pelvic fused kidney in a two-year-old girl examined because of the low abdominal mass thought by some to be an ovarian cyst.

pelves may be directed towards or away from each other. The condition is also designated as unilateral fused kidney or crossed renal ectopy with fusion. The malformation is believed to result from (1) growth of the ureteral stalks into a common metanephroblastema, or (2) from an excess of nephroblastema. The position of the renal components may be inverted or reversed. The condition occurred five times in our autopsy series in children (approximately 1 in 4,000) and was observed in two adults, a ratio of 1 in 16,417. The formation of these unusual kidneys is dependent upon renal dystopia plus fusion (q.v.). The ureters usually enter the bladder normally but may take a devious course in arriving. The condition was observed at autopsy in a premature male displaying the anatomic relationships shown in Figure 125.

These anomalous kidneys are more prone to disease than the normal, the symptoms being dependent on the complicating lesion(s), notably stone and infection. The diagnosis is made by urography; occasionally the fused ectopic organ can be palpated but this does not indicate its true nature. *Treatment* is that of the complicating lesion and is likely to be extremely

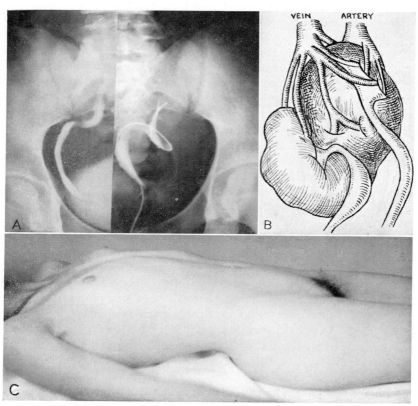

Fig. 127. Pelvic fused kidney in a twelve-year-old girl admitted to Bellevue Hospital because of "abdominal tumor." The composite pyelogram, *A,* and *B,* show the condition. *C,* suprapubic protrusion caused by the fused pelvic kidney. Not only did the ectopic organ cause lower abdominal pain but also marked pressure on the bladder dome. Treatment: Abdominal support.

difficult; forbidding surgical and technical considerations will often render the situation therapeutically hopeless.

Lump, Clump or Cake Kidney. Here both kidneys are fused into a solid irregularly lobed organ of bizarre shape, usually situated low, generally in the pelvis and toward the midline (Figs. 126, 127). The blood supply is usually derived from the lower aorta or the common iliacs although branches from the hypogastrics may exist, and generally enters the upper surface of the kidney. The blood supply may enter the fused organ between the lobules either anteriorly or posteriorly or, as we have seen, on both sides. The ureters are anterior, congenitally short, and usually enter the bladder normally. I encountered a pyonephrotic pelvic lump kidney at operation in a nineteen-year-old boy, a two-year-old girl (Fig. 126), and in a twelve-year-old girl who was referred for examination because of an asymptomatic suprapubic abdominal tumor which caused a suprapubic bulging (Fig. 127), the diagnosis being confirmed by urography in which the short ureters and closely situated bizarre renal pelves were demonstrated. The condition is extremely rare and occurred but once in our autopsy series in children—in a boy of fifteen the mass overlaid the sacral promontory.

Symptoms. The symptoms are those of the complicating infection, obstruction, calculus disease, nephritis, and so forth exactly as in horseshoe kidney disease. Dragging or pulling on the vascular pedicle by the mass weight of the ectopic kidney may cause local or lower abdominal pain which is the outstanding symptom in most cases. The paramount surgical consideration is that the solid fused organ represents the total renal tissue and may be unwittingly removed.

Diagnosis. This is established by urography which generally demonstrates the short closely approximated ureters and frequently overlying bizarre pelves (Fig. 127). Sometimes, as in the case of Kron and Meranzi (1949), the pelves intercommunicate. Unfortunately the abnormal renal mass which is usually ectopic leads to the erroneous diagnosis of tumor as in a case of a twelve-year-old girl previously cited. In the urographic diagnosis the retrograde is far more reliable than the excretory method.

Treatment. The solid fused organ represents the total renal tissue. Careful urologic examination with urography should establish the correct diagnosis; sometimes the demonstrated involvement of one portion of the fused organ gives the clue. The close and complicated relationship of the blood supply and the pelvic distribution gravely hampers surgical resection of these malformed kidneys, this procedure usually being impossible for technical and anatomic reasons. Pyelotomy or nephrostomy drainage is feasible in some cases; in a nineteen-year-old boy with a severely infected pyonephrotic pelvic lump kidney, temporary relief was afforded by pyelostomy drainage and peritoneal marsupialization, but two weeks later he died of sepsis.

IV. ANOMALIES OF LOCATION

Congenital renal ectopia may involve one or both kidneys and from the standpoint of surgical treatment it is important to know the character of the dislocation. Congenital ectopic kidneys are held in their abnormal position chiefly by anomalous vascular attachments which represent persistence of the renal blood supply of early fetal life, this attachment preventing the organ from "ascending" to its normal location. The vascular supply is characteristically abnormally multiple and is derived from adjacent large trunks—the lower aorta, iliacs, middle sacral or inferior mesenteric arteries, and the venous return follows in general the arterial supply. Ectopic kidneys are usually altered and deformed in shape, generally being smaller and more lobulated than normal and triangular, disc, round or irregularly oval.

In congenital ectopia, the length of the ureter corresponds to the situation of the kidney (Figs. 126, 128), while in acquired renal ectopia, the vascular supply is of normal origin and the ureteral length is normal but as the anatomic renal supports (perirenal fascia, perirenal fat, adjacent abdominal organs) give way, the vascular supply becomes elongated. Acquired ectopy is seen in mild form in simple renal ptosis, and is a frequently observed

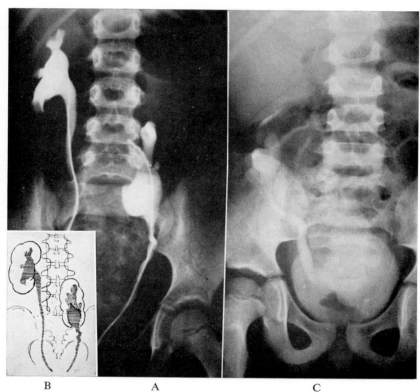

B   A   C

Fig. 128. Renal ectopia. *A,* left kidney ectopic, underrotated and infected in a five-year-old girl examined because of persistent pyuria. Normal right upper urinary tract. *B,* schema. *C,* renal malascent and malrotation in a four-year-old boy with persistent pyuria. In both cases the ureters of the ectopic organs are congenitally short and in each instance show mild obstruction in the lower segment.

condition in adults but rarely requires serious consideration in the young. In short, the renal vascular supply defines the ectopia.

The kidney may be ectopic on its own side (simple dystopia) or may be fused or unfused with its renal mate (crossed dystopia).

Simple dystopia results from early abnormal vascular fixation of the kidney which prevents it from reaching its normal position, and may be unilateral or bilateral. The ureter is shorter than normal except in high renal ectopia (Fig. 129, *B*). The incidence is about one in 1:800 persons when only one of the kidneys is involved (Campbell, 1937) and one in 2200 (Stevens, 1937) when the ectopic kidney is solitary. McCrea (1942) summarized ninety-five cases of the last variety. Simple ectopia was found by Neuman in twenty cases in 10,177 necropsies (approximately one in 500 bodies), while in 51,880 autopsies in patients of all ages, I found seventy-four cases, an incidence of approximately one in 701 individuals. Dystopia is observed three times as often on the left but a few cases of bilateral involvement have been observed. More males have the condition than females. In the twenty-two cases of congenital renal ectopy we found in a study of 15,919 autopsies in children, there were sixteen males and six females, the

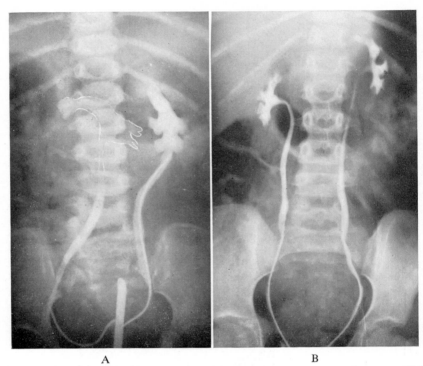

A   B

Fig. 129.   Abnormal renal position. *A*, transverse renal ectopia in a four-year-old boy with persistent pyuria. The left pelvis is malrotated. There was no evidence of fusion of the two kidneys in this instance. *B*, high ectopy of a left kidney otherwise normal. In three cases in our autopsy series the kidney was wholly or partially in the chest.

right kidney was ectopic in eight, the left in eleven, and both in three. The site of ectopy in the young was pelvic in fourteen, sacroiliac in six, and thoracic in two. In adults it was pelvic in 23, sacroiliac in four, thoracic in one, and elsewhere in four. In a white female dead at four hours, not only the kidney but the left adrenal, stomach, intestinal tract, spleen and pancreas were in the left pleural cavity. The left kidney was found ectopic in the thorax of a one-year-old boy and plugged the opening of a diaphragmatic hernia. A thoracic kidney was found also in an adult male in our autopsy group. A left, totally intrathoracic kidney was urologically demonstrated by Spillane and Prather (1949) and eight other cases have been reported not including the three additional instances noted in our autopsy series. In the cases of high renal ectopy and in which the ureter was noted to be longer than normal (Fig. 129, *B*), the blood supply originated higher than normal.

Associated urologic anomalies occurred in 15 of these seventy-four cases and nonurologic anomalies in nine. In the 22 children these include reduplicated kidney in four, ectopic adrenal in three, aplastic ureter, ureter stricture, patent foramen ovale in two each; undescended testicle, pseudo-hermaphroditism, esophageal atresia, esophagotracheal fistula, atresia of the rectum, syndactylism, diaphragmatic hernia and patent ductus arteriosus in one each.

Ectopic kidneys commonly show malrotation in which the pelvis usually faces forward and the adrenal is in its normal position, but the kidney may be overrotated and faces posteriorly or laterally. The ectopic organ may considerably displace the bowel and notably in pelvic ectopy when the sigmoid flexure may be absent because the ascending colon is forced to encroach upon the rectum from the right side. In one instance a low right kidney displaced the cecum to the midline. With this interference the function of the lower bowel is disturbed and severe constipation may result. Moreover during parturition the ectopic organ may cause dystocia or by renal impingement on the bladder, produce vesical disturbances. In one child the kidney was firmly tucked between the bladder and the rectum, in another behind the rectum, and in two adults the ectopic organ was part of the contents of a scrotal hernia.

Renal ectopia is clinically important because the involved organ (1) is often the site of surgical disease, especially infection and stone; (2) technically their surgical treatment may be extremely difficult, nephrectomy usually being the best procedure; (3) by producing pressure on nerves, blood vessels or neighboring organs the misplaced kidney may cause lower abdominal symptoms (e.g., pelvic neuralgia) and, palpated, may lead to the incorrect diagnosis of neoplasm or other disease of another organ, such as cystic ovary. Thus diseased pelvic or low kidneys have been diagnosed as appendicitis, iliocecal tumor, iliocecal tuberculosis, sigmoidal tumor and mesenteric cyst. Palpation of an ectopic kidney may be followed by albuminuria or even hematuria.

The *diagnosis* of renal ectopy is made by urography which demonstrates the displaced kidney pelvis and abnormally short (or long) ureter (Figs. 126, 128). In making the diagnosis, retrograde is far more reliable than excretory pyelography. Demonstration of a short ureter at once precludes surgical elevation of the kidney.

Crossed ectopia is characterized by fusion of one organ across the midline with its renal mate. The normal initial bilateral embryologic development occurs, but early in renal ascent one organ crosses the midline and fuses with its mate or lies adjacent. The cause of this crossing over is unknown; some believe that because of early fusion with the more normal organ, the dystopic kidney is actually drawn over. The vascular derivation shows great variety; if the dystopia has occurred late the blood supply will be from the original site of the kidney, but when the transposition has occurred early, the vessels are normally derived from the side to which the organ has crossed. The vascular supply is thoroughly anomalous, arising from the most adjacent vessel such as lower aorta, iliac or hypogastric arteries and so forth. In crossed ectopia both ureters may be expected to open normally into the bladder.

Crossed ectopia with fusion may be considered a transition form of horseshoe kidney but the mass usually extends beyond the spinal midline (Fig. 124). The position and configuration of the normal kidney are usual but the ectopic organ is situated below, is abnormal in size and form, and usually is improperly rotated. Thus the organs may be fused end to end, side to side, or in S- or L-shaped formation.

Crossed renal ectopia is said to occur about once in 2000 autopsies but it was observed in four of our 51,880 cases. Abeshouse collected 337 cases from the literature (1947); in thirty cases reported by Lee (1948) there was adenocarcinoma in two. The symptoms in crossed ectopia are those caused by the same disease in a normal organ but the site of pain in particular will be predominantly at the site of the ectopic organ. The diagnosis is made by pyelography, preferably retrograde (Figs. 125, 129). Preoperative urography is of vital consideration since in crossed dystopia with fusion the entire renal mass of the individual may unwittingly be removed, a tragedy preventable by preoperative urographic study.

The *treatment* of renal ectopia without fusion is that of the complicating disease in a kidney normally placed. The extraperitoneal exposure is preferred but in pelvic ectopy the transperitoneal approach with nephrectomy should be employed. When nephrectomy is contraindicated by solitary or ectopic fused kidney, marsupialization of the organ to the abdominal wall will generally be better than resection unless anatomic conditions and technical considerations for resection are unusually favorable. Marsupialization may eliminate postoperative peritonitis; the short ureter and blood supply make nephropexy impossible. When a surgical lesion of half of a fused crossed dystopic kidney exists, renal resection may be practicable. The inaccessibility and bizarre vascular supply in most low pelvic kidneys mitigates against conservative surgical treatment, making it extremely difficult technically and sometimes not only unwarranted but impossible. Pyelocystostomy (anastomosis of the dilated pelvis of the juxtavesical hydronephrotic ectopic kidney to the bladder) to bypass an obstructed ureter has been successfully performed by Hess (1929) in a boy of nine years and by Hess and Wright (1945) in a man of forty-two years, and by Way et al. (1946) in a boy of four months.

Abnormal renal mobility may result from an anomalous development of the blood supply and overlying peritoneum. The vascular supply is unusually long, often with engulfment of the organ by the peritoneum; the malformation of the pedicle and/or mesentery makes the kidney freely and widely movable within the peritoneal cavity (Fig. 105). The condition is essentially one of adult life, being rare before the age of twenty, although Dupoux reported thirty-seven cases in infants, seven of whom were boys. Yet it is a condition seen predominantly in long lean neurotic adults and particularly females. The perirenal vascular attachments and the perirenal capsule are abnormal while the ureter is of normal length; with changing renal positions the ureter twists, kinks, hangs over, or otherwise becomes obstructed by anomalous blood vessels or periureteral bands to produce renal pain or even acute renal colic. Because of the urinary stasis commonly present as a result of positional interference with pelvic drainage, renal infection is frequent which too often leads to the diagnosis of chronic pyelitis, pyuria and pain in the loin being the chief presenting symptoms. Constant or periodic renal pain is frequent with hydronephrosis secondary to renal ptosis; this may be manifested also by generalized abdominal pain or by reflex visceral gastrointestinal disturbances and sometimes even with vomiting. Most abnormally mobile kidneys can be freely pushed about the isolateral quadrant and sometimes even to the opposite side (Fig. 105, *A*); in a twelve-day-old boy the freely movable right kidney could be turned over to touch the normal left organ.

A persistence of renal pain with or without complicating urinary infection demands complete urologic examination during the course of which urographic study will be made both in the Trendelenburg and upright positions. Not infrequently in adults the renal excursion as demonstrated by this procedure may be as much as 6 inches. Yet here the condition is seldom congenital but rather an acquired one. Stereoscopic pyelograms will indicate the character, severity and obstructive complications of the anomaly. Surgical elevation (nephropexy) is preferable to temporizing with abdominal belts once the diagnosis has been firmly established and obstruction demonstrated, and is performed to eradicate urinary stasis and not for the relief of pain alone.

Nephroptosis is commonly observed in older patients with faulty nutrition, visceroptosis and neurasthenia and is to be differentiated from congenital abnormal renal mobility. Nephroptosis is exceedingly rare in children, yet in the older literature Comby collected eighteen cases, only two of whom were boys. In eight the condition was recognized before the tenth year, and in two before the fourth month. In a girl of thirty-three days, bilateral floating kidneys were proved at autopsy. Chicoli observed eight cases in children in thirty-six years. In some cases, as in adults, the ptosis apparently followed a fall. I have seen but one case of nephroptosis in a child of sufficient gravity to recommend renal support and have advised a belt but once. In the last case low vascular fixation of the ectopic kidney in the pelvis permitted no other therapeutic course. Irrespective of the patient's age, child or adult, and if there is pain and if coexisting urinary obstruction and stasis are demonstrated, nonsurgical or surgical correction is indicated. Belts to give renal support seldom do the trick, so nephropexy is needed.

V. ANOMALIES OF ROTATION

Faulty Rotation. At the end of the first month of embryonic life the renal pelvis faces anteriorly but with renal ascent to the upper lumbar region there is mesial rotation which is complete by the eighth week. Rotation is

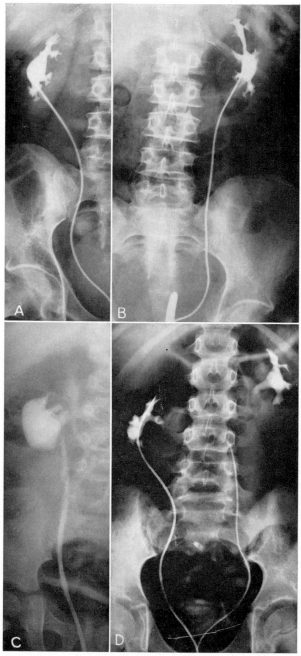

Fig. 130.   Congenital renal malrotation. *A*, complete; the pelvis faces median. *B*, pelvis faces posteriorly. *C*, complete renal rotation in a twenty-month-old girl with abnormally high insertion of the ureter into the pelvis. *D*, diminutive malrotated pelvis in a five-year-old girl. Chronic pyuria was the indication for urologic examination in cases *A–D* and in each instance the major involvement was of the malrotated organ.

interfered with chiefly by renal fusion as in horseshoe, sigmoid, discoid or lump kidney; normally placed unfused kidneys are sometimes overrotated or underrotated (Figs. 103, 104, 130). The degrees of rotation are: (1) failure of, (2) incomplete, (3) reverse, and (4) excessive rotation. In underrotation the pelvis faces forward and in overrotation it faces posteriorly. Knowledge of this rotation process assists in the interpretation of some unusual urograms. The symptoms of renal malrotation are those of disease in a normal organ, but as in other anomalous structures, the disease incidence is considerably increased. In our autopsy studies there were seven cases of malrotation in children, six of which were on the left side, and there was underrotation in six cases. At autopsy in adults we found seventeen cases (11 male, 6 female), on the right in nine, on the left in seven, and bilaterally in one. There was underrotation in thirteen, overrotation in two, and a "tipover" rotation in two. In half of these cases the malrotated organ was incompletely ascended. A boy of one month and a girl of ten months each showed left renal overrotation, the pelves leaving posteriorly. In a ten-month-old girl the ureter was compressed as it passed over the lower edge of the kidney. While malrotation is of no clinical concern except as complicating disease develops, it is essential to know preoperatively whether the location of the pelvis is normal and whether the direction of the pelvis is normal, anterior, posterior or lateral, since the surgical approach may have to be altered and needless trauma and bleeding thus avoided.

The *diagnosis* is readily made by urography. The excretory method may give the initial clue but had best be followed by satisfactory retrograde pyelographic demonstration, and this should always be done prior to surgical attack upon these kidneys. Stereoscopic urograms are preferred to indicate precisely the character and details of the malrotation. In underrotation the pelvis faces forward and in the usual anteroposterior urographic exposure the pelvic shadow is recorded in its narrow diameter (Figs. 104, 130). Here the calyceal shadows and papillary cuppings are not seen or are poorly defined and the narrowness of the pelvis may suggest pelvic compression by new growth (Fig. 104). Many horseshoe kidneys show abnormal lateral renal rotation which causes the pelvis to face laterally (Fig. 123). In faulty rotation the ureter generally proceeds to the bladder at greater than normal distance from the spine, and the course of the blood vessels may bear an abnormal relation to the pelvis and ureter to cause obstruction with massive hydronephrosis or at least to cause urinary stasis predisposing to renal infection which is the commonest complicating condition in this anomaly.

There is no corrective *treatment* of congenital renal malrotation. Urinary stasis, infection, calculi, and other complicating diseases must be treated according to indications.

VI. ANOMALIES OF THE PELVIS

Normally the pelvis is of the ampullatory type (85 per cent) with branching of the ureteral stalk ampulla into superior, medial and inferior major calyces which, in turn, subdivide into the minor calyces. The median branch may be absent. Bizarre pelvic formations are sometimes found in kidneys which are otherwise normal (Figs. 104, 130, 131). Ten per cent of normal pelves are bifid, the pelvis dividing first at or just within its entrance to the kidney to form two major calyces. Trifurcation is extremely rare. In a four-year-old girl with bilateral ureteral ectopia at the urethral meatus on each side, the left upper ureter divided into three distinct pelves (Fig. 132),

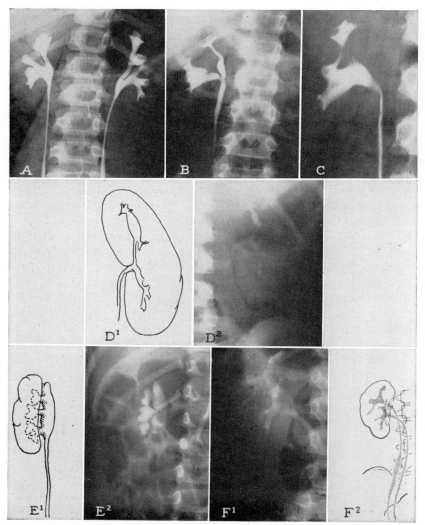

Fig. 131.   Unusual normal pyelograms in young children exhibiting attempts at pelvic reduplication. *A*, reduplicated left pelvis with localized dilatation of right upper calyx and the calyceal neck. *B*, reduplicated pelves uniting at a common ureteropelvic junction. *C*, the right superior calyx is a branch of the middle calyx. D^1, D^2, pelvic reduplication with elongated superior calyceal neck. E^1, E^2, extrarenal sausage type of pelvis. F^1, F^2, reduplicated overlying normal pelves in a six-year-old boy; here they appear to lie almost one behind the other, a rare formation. (Bellevue Hospital.)

and there was an attempt at three separate pelves on the right. As observed at autopsy in an adult at Bellevue Hospital, as many as six ureteropelvic branchings on each side may be found. In a sixty-year-old male examined because of right renal colic, a stone was found in one of three right reduplicated ureters; two ureters were present on the left side. In a patient examined post mortem there were six separate pelves, and in another patient similarly observed there were six separate branching ureteral stalks and pelves. As a rule there are as many renal pelves as there are branching stalks, but in

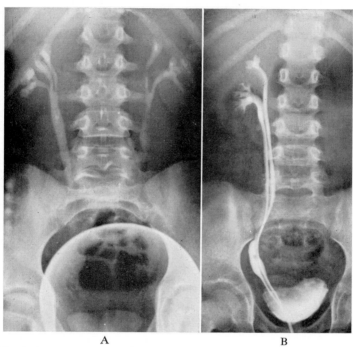

A   B

Fig. 132.   Pelvic reduplication in kidneys otherwise normal. *A,* triplication on the right and bifurcation on the left in a four-year-old female with congenital contracted bladder neck and chronic pyuria; excretory urography using ball compression. *B,* complete reduplication of pelvis and ureter in a six-year-old girl. There is mild inflammatory dilatation of the lower third of the ureters.

four cases observed post mortem, the ureteral stalks were found draining two intercommunicating renal pelves. Ureteral bifurcation may occur at any point from the bladder wall to the pelvis (Figs. 98, 131, 132, 133; cf. Kelly and Burnham, 1914). In one case the reduplicated ureters opened above into a common pelvis and fused below at the bladder wall.

Double or **reduplicated kidney** results from reduplication of the ureteral bud before it enters the nephrogenic blastema and is to be distinguished anatomically from the rare duplications in which two kidneys are formed on one side from separate blastemas. The reduplicated pelves are usually situated one above the other, but may be one behind the other. The last variety has been reported by Bumpus, and Potter and Sexton, and I ob-

served it in a ten-year-old boy with cleft palate, harelip, congenital urethrorectal fistula, rectal stricture, and other defects (Fig. 131, *F*). Occasionally
the pelvis shows only an attempt at reduplication, a condition rarely of
clinical concern and one which should readily be recognized by pyelography
(Fig. 131, *A–D*).

Reduplicated or double kidney is a relatively common condition which
apparently occurs twice as often in females as in males and more often on
the left side. It was found in 342 of our 51,880 autopsy cases, an overall
incidence of 1 to 152. In 19,046 children, there were sixty-one cases, a
ratio of 1 to 278, while in 32,834 adults there were 281 cases, an incidence of
1 to 117. This striking numerical discrepancy can be charged only to
faulty observation in recording by the pathologist, it being recognized that
the ureters in infants are often exceedingly small and when reduplicated and
passing from the kidney to the bladder in the same sheath, may appear as a
single duct. The pelvis should give a clue. Yet all of these adults were born
with their double ureters and statistical observation on the older group is more
accurate and valuable, and more in keeping with the incidence ratio as
clinically observed.

Double kidney and ureteral reduplication commonly have associated
anomalies; in 342 autopsy cases there were 129 other urologic malformations
and 63 nonurologic anomalies. The other kidney was anomalous in 22 instances, being absent and hyperplastic in two each, aplastic in one, and hypoplastic in four cases. The reduplication was part of horseshoe formation in
nine, polycystic kidney disease in five, solitary cystic kidney in two, ectopic
kidney in four, and the adrenal was ectopic in one. The ureters were aplastic
in eleven, strictured in five, showed idiopathic dilatation in three, valves and
ectopia in two each, and ureterocele formation in three. There was vesical
diverticulum in four cases, and patent urachus in one. Urethral obstruction
and undescended testicle were observed in two instances; hypospadias, persistent Gartner's duct, cystic ovaries in one each. In the gastrointestinal tract
there were two instances of pyloric stenosis and of Meckel's diverticulum.
Diverticulum of the bowel was found in four other cases, an accessory spleen
in three, imperforate anus, atresia of the rectum in one each. Cardiac anomalies included patent foramen ovale in five, patent ductus arteriosus in four,
absent pulmonary fissure in two, supernumerary pulmonary lobes, accessory
azygos lobe, "an anomalous right lung," spina bifida in two each, and
meningocele in one. Malformed bones were present in three bodies. Congenital
ureteral stricture is one of the most common coexisting anomalies in renal
reduplication and may involve one or both of the reduplicated ureters and,
as previously indicated, often at the site of bifurcation.

The *symptoms* and *clinical findings* in renal reduplication are those
of complicating obstruction, infection, calculus, and so forth. The *diagnosis*
is readily made by complete urologic examination in which the urographic
demonstration of the reduplicated pelves is made. As previously noted, the
anomalous organ is more prone to disease than a normal one and in a study
of 101 cases of hydronephrosis in children, Kretschmer (1937) found

ureterorenal anomalies in twenty-four (23.7 per cent), and in more than half of these there was pelvic reduplication. In a study of 1,102 children with persistent pyuria personally examined by me, there were 307 uretero-pelvic anomalies, chiefly reduplication (26.9 per cent). In some instances there is one ureteral orifice in the bladder and one ectopic orifice on the same side, unilaterally or bilaterally, or all ureters may open ectopic. With ureteral bifurcation above the bladder, the urographic injection of one renal

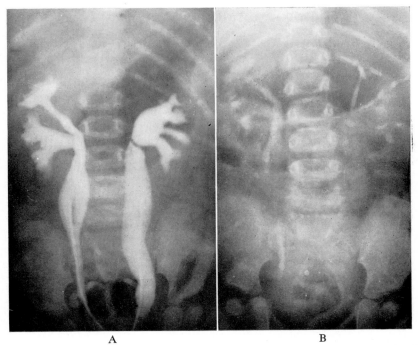

A   B

Fig. 133.   Bilateral ureteral reduplication; complete on the left, incomplete on the right in a seven-month-old girl. *A,* severely infected hydro-ureteronephrosis of the lower half of the left kidney (ureterovesical junction stricture). Preoperatively the orifice of the ureter from the left upper pelvis was not visualized but the pelvis and the course of its ureter were demonstrated by excretory urography (*B*). The bifurcation of the right ureter in its midportion is well shown. Left ureteroheminephrectomy. Cured.

segment will usually be accompanied by reflux of sufficient medium in the reduplicated ureteral segment to outline it and the pelvis it drains (Fig. 133). Excretory urography demonstrates a relatively large number of cases of this anomaly where it was wholly unsuspected. With involvement of only half of the kidney by ureteral obstruction, hemipyonephrosis or infected hydrone-phrosis commonly develops. The diagnosis here is readily made by adequate urologic examination and as a rule heminephrectomy will conserve the sound half of the reduplication as we have succeeded in doing in more than fifty infants and children (Figs. 132, 133, 134). Occasionally secondary in-volvement of the unobstructed renal segment may demand nephrectomy as it does when this segment is independently diseased.

Pseudospider pelvis identifies the congenitally small, long, thin pelvis with calyces which urographically simulate the so-called spider-leg pyelogram of renal tumor (Figs. 135, 136). The chief importance of this anomaly is the diagnostic confusion it may afford, especially when it urographically suggests renal tumor, as it did in a seven-year-old boy, which misled me as well as several other urologists. The kidney, thought to be tumor bearing, was removed but was found to be normal except for the congenital "pseudospider" pelvis. This observation is not to be confused with that often seen in renal mal-

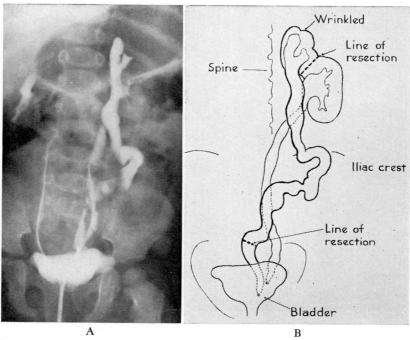

A   B

Fig. 134. *A,* complete left ureteral reduplication with a curious type of superior renal pelvis; the lower pelvis is small. The ureter to the superior pelvis is strictured at the ureterovesical junction, dilated and secondarily kinked. Ureteroheminephrectomy. *B,* schema of *A.*

rotation in which the vertical plane of the pelvis is altered so that it is morphologically recorded in its narrowest diameter (Figs. 103, 104, 135, 136).

Congenital hydronephrosis may result from a large number of obstructive lesions operating *in utero.* As in all varieties of hydronephrosis, the nearer the obstruction is to the kidney, the greater is the pelvic dilatation. In most cases in the young, in whom the condition is encountered most often by far, there is obstruction at the ureteropelvic junction and generally as congenital stricture. The next most common site of congenital ureteral obstruction is at the ureterovesical junction, and chiefly by stricture. In our autopsy series many other obstructing lesions have been demonstrated *in utero,* including

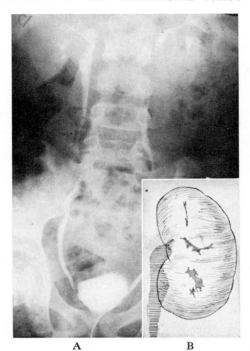

A   B

Fig. 135. Congenital left (picture reversed) "spider leg" pelvis in a seven-year-old boy admitted to Bellevue Hospital for hematuria. There was no indigo carmine excretion from this kidney on three tests. The three separate urologic examinations resulted in the same curious pyelogram suggestive of tumor but no mass could be felt in the loin. Several urologic consultants advised nephrectomy; a normal kidney with a congenitally narrowed ("spider leg") pelvis was removed.

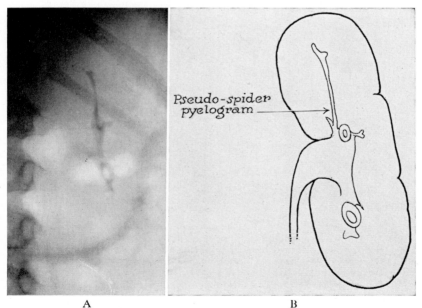

Pseudo-spider pyelogram

A   B

Fig. 136. Pseudospider-leg pyelogram in a malrotated but otherwise normal kidney in a child.

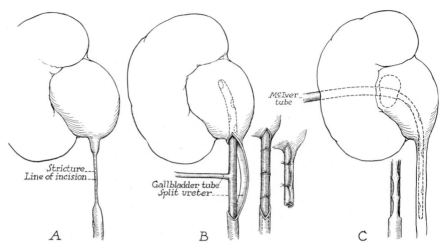

Fig. 137.   Treatment of an elongated tight lineal ureteral stricture by longitudinal incision and T-tube splinting according to the method of Davis. This is an excellent procedure for employment in children.

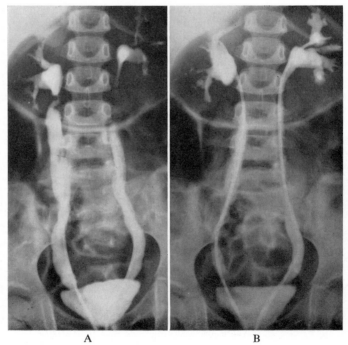

A   B

Fig. 138.   Employment of the procedure shown in Figure 137 in the treatment of a four-year-old girl with persistent pyuria since early infancy. Bilateral inflammatory ureterectasis with relatively normal renal pelves. *A, B,* there is mild pyelectasis above a constricted ureteropelvic junction and proximal ureter. Lineal slitting and inlying T-tube splinting was employed at the right ureteropelvic junction and adjacent ureter. The unobstructed left ureter shows inflammatory ureterectasis (see Fig. 139).

some cases of ureteral stone. Congenital hydronephrosis also may result on a nonobstructive basis from faulty development of the pelvic musculature and innervation; possibly in some instances pelvic inflammatory changes are overlooked.

Most hydronephrosis in children is congenital. Congenital unilateral hydronephrosis is compatible with life if the function of the opposite kidney is adequate. In advanced bilateral congenital hydronephrosis or in hydro-

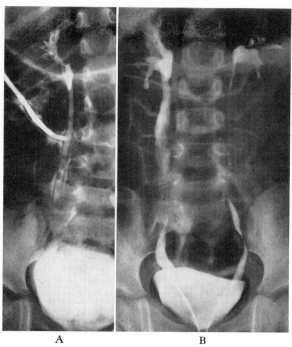

A   B

Fig. 139. *A*, indwelling T-tube intubation following longitudinal incision of the upper ureteral and juxtapelvic stricture shown in Figure 138. *B*, pyelogram four months postoperatively shows a widely patent pelvic outlet and upper ureter. There was striking improvement in anatomic appearance, functional renal improvement, and in the child's general physical condition.

nephrosis of a solitary kidney the outlook is uniformly bad, some of these victims dying *in utero* or in neonatal life because of far advanced parenchymal destruction. Yet by prompt recognition of the condition, even though bilateral, many of these kidneys can be revived and sometimes the patient restored to normal health. The diagnosis, symptoms and treatment are those common to obstruction and all types of hydronephrosis and have been splendidly discussed by Doctor Hinman in Section III. In Section XIII I have statistically indicated the outstanding features in 828 cases of hydronephrosis in infants and children; 512 of these were studied at autopsy while the remainder were personally examined and treated by me. It is notable that in nearly every case the cause was congenital obstruction. In short, permanent

nephrostomy drainage offers the only hope for life when the hydronephrosis
is unilateral and relief of obstruction by plastic operation is technically
impossible or has been unsuccessful. In two young patients of mine, ureteropelvioplasty on the only kidney was successful but too commonly the procedure is contraindicated by advanced renal injury, infection and/or insur-

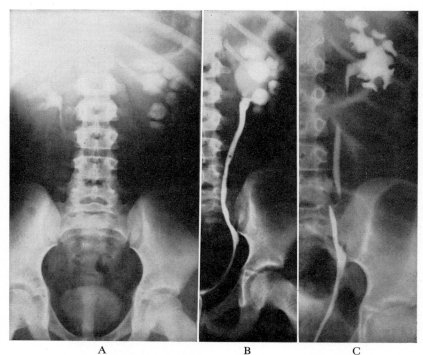

                    A   B   C

Fig. 140. Employment of the procedure shown in Figure 864 in a five-year-old girl
with severe left hydronephrosis and renal injury above a tight ureteropelvic junction stricture with secondary vascular obstruction. *A,* excretory urogram demonstrating a dilated
left pelvis and a normal right kidney. *B,* retrograde pyelography showing the severe degree
of left renal dilatation and injury. *C,* following employment of the procedure shown in
Figure 141 a most satisfactory functional and anatomic result was achieved. In this pyelogram made six months postoperative, the restitution of the renal calyces to a more normal
appearance and considerable reduction in the size of the pelvic sac (by extensive resection) is notable. Following the operative procedure and the establishment of free drainage,
the urine was readily sterilized, the child having previously suffered recurrent bouts of
fever and pyuria since birth.

mountable technical difficulties or, when employed, fails as it did in a third
child with a single kidney. In some of these patients with ureteropelvic
junction stricture, the simple longitudinal incision and intubation technique
of Davis (1948; Figs. 137–139) may offer hope; see also Figs. 140 and 141.

In **complete renal reduplication** there are two ureters and two ureteral
orifices, but one or both of these openings may be ectopic (q.v.) (Figs.
152 and 158). Regardless of how many times the completely reduplicated
ureters may cross in their downward curve, according to the Weigert-Meyer

law, the ureter from the upper pelvis almost invariably opens lowermost in the bladder (Figs. 98, 132, see ureteral anomalies).

Often the double kidney shows a circular demarcation differentiating the two segments, it sometimes being a groove, or the two portions are strikingly at variance in size or contour, the smaller segment more often showing persistence of fetal lobulation. The lower segment is generally the larger, but one segment may be rudimentary and even functionless. Such demarcation indicates the embryologic division of the two renal segments and together with proper urographic demonstration for guidance makes renal resection a relatively simple procedure. In double kidney the upper border of the lower

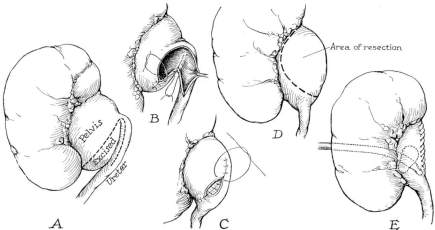

Fig. 141.   Ureteropelvic junction obstruction. Treatment by pyelo-ureteroplasty with excision of the redundant pelvis to reduce urinary stagnation. *E,* balloon catheter nephrostomy counterdrainage postoperatively.

pelvis is commonly urographically demonstrated to be flattened, squared or sheared off, an observation which at once suggests the presence of another pelvis above (Fig. 131). When the upper pelvis is small or is not in the same plane as the lower, the latter is likely to look like the pelvis of a normal kidney (Fig. 155).

Yet surface demarcations may be absent and here renal resection is guided by the essential preoperative pyelogram. The pyelogram may clearly indicate two pelves, but not infrequently the lower pelvis appears normal while associated congenital stricture is often found in one or both of the reduplicated ureters or at the point of ureteral bifurcation, whether this be at the ureterovesical junction or elsewhere. In a three-year-old girl with persistent pyuria, its source was the infected dilated upper half of a reduplicated left kidney, the ureter bifurcating 5 cm. below the kidney, at which point the dilated segment of the duct to the upper half was congenitally strictured. The strictured area was longitudinally incised on the medial surface for 3 cm., a 10-F. T-tube was left inlying for two weeks and an excellent result was obtained, normal drainage from the upper segment into the main lower ureteral segment below the bifurcation being established and the urine subsequently sterilized. Thus important disease of the obstructed half of the kidney is not uncommon although it frequently passes unrecognized. In at least half of the cases of renal reduplication the arterial blood supply is dual to the separate segments with two or more vessels passing to the kidney from the aorta or as subdivisions of a renal arterial trunk. By renal arteriography, Smith (Section II, Chapter 2) observed that the superior renal artery was consistently the largest of the reduplicated arteries. Successful heminephrectomy demands a clear identification of the renal blood supply, especially the arteries, as well as of the embryologic demarcation. When there is a sound renal mate, the hydronephrotic kidney must usually be removed because of the ravages of back pressure, injury or infection. When the obstructive damage is mild and infection is minimum, the patient should be given the benefit of ureteropelvioplasty, an unsuccessful result demanding subsequent nephrectomy.

Congenital Hydrocalycosis. This is a dilatation of a single calyx, is most rare, generally almost always results from congenital stricture or abnormal narrowing of a single calyx, and is usually a postmortem finding. Clinically it is usually associated with persistent renal infection, the etiologic factors of which also predispose to calculus formation in the dilated calyx. The condition in infancy has been splendidly discussed by Weyrauch and Fleming (1950), and in adults by Prather.

The symptoms produced are those common to all forms of hydronephrosis but there may be none. Resection of the kidney with removal of the diseased segment is the preferred treatment when technically possible.

Extrarenal Pelves. These are generally associated with anomalous kidneys whether fused, ectopic, solitary, improperly rotated or otherwise deformed. The anomalous development predisposes to poor urinary drainage with the development of urinary stasis eventually to invite acute or chronic urinary infection (Figs. 140, 141). Secondary calculous deposit is a frequent complication. Vascular obstruction of the upper ureter or ureteropelvic junction may produce hydronephrosis with pronounced extrarenal enlargement but here the readily dilating extrarenal pelvis functions as a buffer to spare the renal parenchyma, which may show a minimum of back pressure damage, the finer markings of the calyces often remaining urographically sharply defined.

Extrarenal pelves are of clinical concern only when they do not drain normally, retention being the important consideration rather than the anatomic conformation. The symptoms are those common to hydronephrosis of all varieties. The diagnosis is readily made by urography, preferably retrograde. Relief of the obstruction is the treatment when the kidney is worth saving and, in many instances, we have employed wide resection of the redundant pelvis, particularly in children, to reduce it to nearly normal size and to minimize pelvic sacculation and urinary stagnation (Figs. 140, 141).

Occasionally a portion of *the adrenal* is embryologically incorporated in the cortex of the superior renal pole, sometimes without capsular demarcation. Variable incorporation of the adrenal in the kidney was seen seven times in our autopsy series. As a rule, this anomaly is of no importance except when the kidney must be operated upon at which time serious injury of the adrenal may be unavoidable. In an eight-week-old boy at Bellevue Hospital, a spleen 2 cm. in diameter was buried in the upper half of a left kidney and adjacent to the kidney were six accessory spleens.

VII. ANOMALIES OF THE VESSELS

Aberrant renal blood vessels are of double importance: (1) to their bearer as a cause of urinary obstruction and as complicating diseases, and (2) to

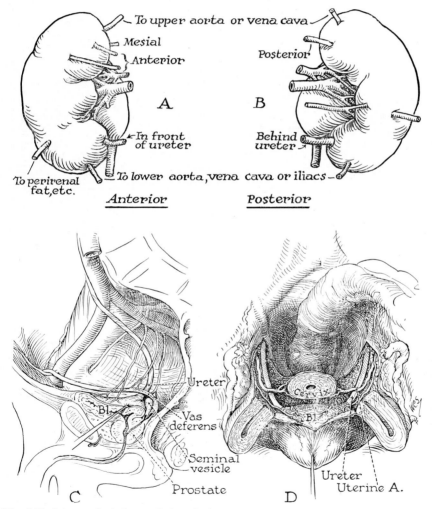

Fig. 142. Schema depicting varieties of aberrant renal vessels. *A, B,* those which cross the ureter are potential causes of hydronephrosis but all are subject to laceration during mobilization of the kidney. *C, D,* vessels of the deep pelvic organs showing the possibilities for vascular obstruction of the lower ureter analogous to conditions in *A, B.*

the surgeon who inadvertently may lacerate the structure with resulting profuse hemorrhage. Yet reduplicated and anomalous vessels are seldom of concern to the careful surgeon who cleans off well the renal pedicle and identifies its component structures before applying clamps. He also is careful in the dissection of dense fibrous structures, especially those high under the diaphragm, to be sure no anomalous aberrant vessels are accidentally cut or torn. Vessels may be given off from the pedicle, aorta or vena cava

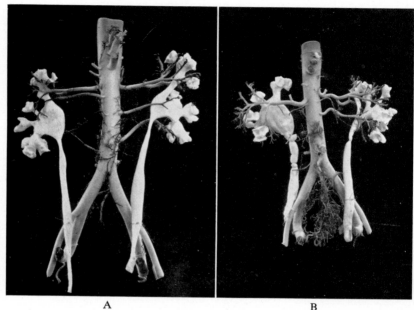

A   B

Fig. 143. Accessory renal vessels demonstrated by celluloid corrosion preparation. *A,* in a full-term fetus. The renal pelves and ureters are shown in relationship to the main arterial distribution. On each side there are two accessory renal vessels above and one below, the lower one on the left being in proximity to the ureterovesical junction. *B,* in an eight-month-old fetus in which the kidney on the right had one renal artery but the organ on the left had an accessory branch to the lower renal pole. Yet the location of the lower accessory vessel on the left does not suggest that it might cause ureteral obstruction. On the right there is early hydronephrosis, secondary kinking and narrowing at the ureterovesical junction. (Courtesy of Dr. Duncan Morison.)

to pass to the perinephric fat, diaphragm, adrenal, pancreas or liver, as well as to the renal poles; veins are even more numerous in wandering (Fig. 142). In the digital mobilization of the kidney, these vessels may be accidentally lacerated. Unfortunately the arteries in particular retract rapidly and are located and clamped with extreme difficulty. As a corollary, all dense bands encountered about the kidney may wisely be clamped before they are cut, as they frequently and unexpectedly contain fair sized vessels. In a ten-year-old girl with horseshoe kidney, with a reduplicated left half and the upper pelvis hydronephrotic (1 liter), a large upper polar artery originating high under the diaphragm was accidentally lacerated close to the aorta during mobilization of the organ. The resulting hemorrhage was a contributory cause of death (shock).

Most aberrant vessels pass to one or the other renal pole and are known as polar vessels; they originate in or communicate with comparatively distant points in the aorta, vena cava or adjacent branches of the great vessels (Fig. 143). Lower polar vessels springing from the aorta or renal arteries exist in about 6 per cent of all kidneys; they may primarily or secondarily cause ureteral compression and urinary obstruction. In a thousand autopsies in children under twelve years of age at the Boston Childrens Hospital, White and Wyatt (1942) found thirty-eight cases of lower polar aberrant renal vessels. Clinical manifestations recognize no age and have been found even in the neonatal period. The diagnosis is too often delayed until adult life by which time the kidney is frequently hopelessly damaged.

In a study of 26,060 autopsies (7,966 infants and children; 18,394 adults) renal arterial anomalies were recorded in 247 cases; 16 in the young (1:498 [500]) and 231 (1:80) in those over 15 years. This is an over-all incidence of 1 in 105 persons, which is much lower incidence than specific studies in some smaller groups have shown (cf. Anson et al., 1948). There were 169 males and 78 females. It also points up the importance of precise study of the renal blood supply, a study rarely made or recorded in most routine autopsies. There is every reason to believe the actual incidence in infants is greater than in adults. To our knowledge, fatal renal injury resulted in some infants from congenital vascular ureteral obstruction. In the young the left and right sides were each involved in six and bilaterally in four. Anomalous vessels occur unilaterally three times as often as bilaterally and are more frequent on the left side and in females. We observed the condition bilaterally in three children. In the adults the anomalies were on the left in 103, on the right in 91, and bilateral in 35. Lower polar vessels were found in 8 children and 50 adults, upper polar vessels in 4 children and 45 adults, in 68 there were other locations such as adrenal, perirenal fat, diaphragm, lower aorta and so forth, and in 84 the distribution of the anomalous vessels was not recorded. There were coexisting urologic anomalies in 76 and nonurologic in 38.

The embryologic etiology of renal vascular anomalies is concerned with the derivation of the original renal blood supply from the lower part of the aorta before the kidney ascends. These early vascular attachments are normally lost as the organ migrates upward finally to become supplied by the renal artery. Abnormally these early vascular attachments are retained and thus the renal arterial and/or venous supply may derive from the external and internal iliac, the inferior mesentery, the sacral branches, or directly from the aorta or vena cava, from the main renal vessels, adrenal, subphrenic or other adjacent branches. The lower vascular attachments are likely to produce renal ptosis by preventing ascent of the kidney.

Aside from the accidental laceration of unsuspected aberrant renal vessels at operation, we are chiefly concerned with lower polar vessels which transverse the ureter to cause obstruction. The etiologic relationship of these anomalous lower polar vessels to ureteral obstruction has divided urologists into two groups: (1) those who believe the vessel primarily traverses the ureter to cause obstruction (Quinby, Mayo, Hagedorn, Borelius), and (2) a far greater number including Hinman, Legueu, Kuster, Pannatt, Geraghty and others who believe that obstruction results because renal ptosis first causes the ureter to ride across the vessels (Figs. 143, 144). Peirson and Barney (1929), Quinby (1930), and Walters (1930) believe the arterial pulsation inhibits ureteral peristalsis at the point the vessel crosses the ureter. Yet

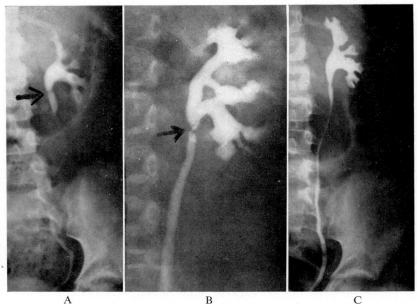

A   B   C

Fig. 144.   Early vascular obstruction of the left kidney in a seven-year-old girl examined because of left renal pain and persistent pyuria. *A, B,* a provisional urographic diagnosis of vascular obstruction was made and was confirmed by surgical exploration. Vessel resection. *C,* postoperative ureterogram which shows mild persisting ureteral narrowing at the point formerly compressed by the low aberrant vessel. Yet the symptoms were relieved and the urinary infection was cured.

clinical studies suggest that both of these etiologic factors can operate, though not simultaneously in the same patient.

A vicious cycle is thus established and the greater the hydronephrosis the more acute and pronounced the obstruction becomes. With increasing hydronephrosis there is a greater ptosis and increasing obstruction. Renal ptosis is predisposed to by a shallow lumbar gutter, scant perirenal fat, lax perirenal fascial and peritoneal attachment, generalized visceroptosis and repeated renal trauma as by jumping and jarring. Peripheral ureteral obstruction, notably congenital ureterovesical junction stricture, may be the initiating factor in the genesis of the early hydronephrosis; the variably dilated ureter is compressed against or sags over the anomalous vessel; this augments the dilatation above this point, a variety of secondary obstruction (Figs. 144–146). Secondary peripelvioureteral adhesions frequently cause ureteral fixation, add greatly to the total obstruction and it is believed by many that the initial renal ptosis results from mild hydronephrosis caused by inflammatory scarring at the ureteropelvic junction. The antecedent inflammatory process may have been a mild renal infection.

Pathology. Hydronephrosis is the most important immediate result of vascular ureteral obstruction, the kidney sometimes being enlarged fifteen to twenty times normal size. The pathologic changes in hydronephrosis have been discussed in Section III. These greatly distended organs in which the thinned out cortex and medulla can scarcely be differentiated are particularly liable to rupture even with mild trauma. Infection can always be anticipated in these cases and its advent usually leads to the diagnosis of "pyelitis." As the vicious cycle continues, local or generalized areas of suppurative nephritis appear.

Symptoms. The symptoms of ureteral blockage by an aberrant vessel are those of hydronephrosis, with or without infection and are generally intermittent. Pain in the loin is the commonest symptom and is usually a dull ache, similar to the pain caused by firmly pressing the skin against the bone. The dull ache is sometimes punctuated by sharp attacks of renal colic induced by complete ureteral obstruction (edema or sudden acute angulation). Such pain in the side and frequently referred to the thigh, and especially during an acute attack of colic with fever and vomiting, usually leads needlessly to appendectomy as it did in four young patients of mine with vascular obstruction of the ureter. Frequency of urination is commonly reflex but may result from infection. When caused by the last, dysuria, burning on urination and hematuria are often outstanding symptoms although the pyuria resulting from the infection almost always causes the diagnosis of pyelitis to be made.

Because of the attendant urinary stasis, the infection resists treatment and the diagnosis ultimately becomes "chronic pyelitis." With the onset of acute obstruction in these cases and exacerbation of the renal infection, the diagnosis is regularly changed to "acute pyelitis," even though the underlying pathology may now be acute pyonephrosis. Hematuria in these cases may be due to acute congestion of the hydronephrotic kidney or to secondary infection. When infection exists, an intermittent low-grade fever is frequently present and in more than half of the cases there are gastrointestinal disturbances which frequently overshadow the urinary symptoms. Outstanding among these gastrointestinal disturbances are malaise, anemia, dyspepsia, biliousness, constipation, chronic gastritis, anorexia, nausea, occasional vomiting, diarrhea, failure to gain or actual loss of weight. In adults the diagnosis of cholecystitis, gastric or duodenal ulcer is commonly and erroneously made in these cases as in infected hydronephrosis of any cause.

Toxemia due to diminished renal function or to the absorption from urinary infection explains the systemic symptoms of headache, irritability, malaise and gastrointestinal disturbances, these being the usual uremic manifestations, often dominating the picture. The sound kidney will gen-

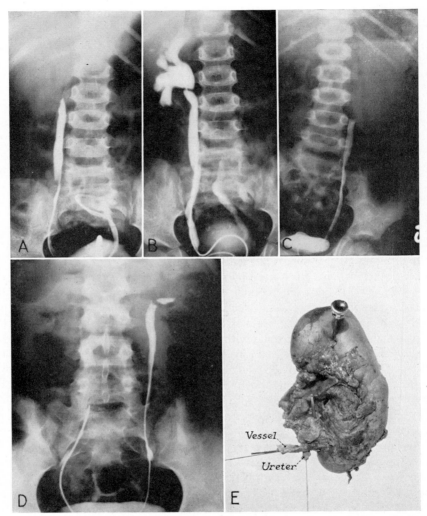

Fig. 145. *A,* vascular obstruction at the ureteropelvic junction producing pain in the right loin and accompanied by persistent pyuria in a three-year-old girl. Ureterographic injection does not extend beyond the point of vascular compression. The left kidney is ectopic over the sacrum. *B,* upon filling the renal pelvis the sharp transverse filling defect at the ureteropelvic junction is readily visualized and at this point exploration disclosed a compressing vein which was divided. There is also right ureterovesical junction stricture to which the ureteral dilatation is doubtless secondary. Were it not that the dilated ureter was pushed against the aberrant vein to produce obstruction, the vascular anomaly probably would have been of no importance. *C,* massive left hydronephrosis in a two-year-old boy. The ureterogram shows the ureter sharply cut off transversely at the site of vascular obstruction. Nephrectomy. *D,* vascular obstruction of the left ureter in an eleven-year-old boy who presented the clinical picture of chronic interstitial nephritis. The left kidney was destroyed and secondary toxic injury of the good kidney which caused a considerable depression of the total function led to the diagnosis of interstitial nephritis. Following removal of the diseased left organ, the total renal function and the urinalysis became normal. *E,* Specimen in *D.* (*D, E,* Courtesy American Journal of Surgery; author's article.)

erally care adequately for the total renal function, but when the obstruction is bilateral or in unilateral vascular obstruction, the renal mate is hypoplastic, injured by toxemia, or is surgically or congenitally absent, the symptoms of azotemia appear and will vary directly according to the degree of total renal damage. Sometimes this toxic nephritis of the good kidney causes the diagnosis of chronic interstitial nephritis with hematuria to be made because of the symptoms and laboratory findings. Yet following the removal of its diseased mate, the better kidney is usually restored to normal.

Terminally stupor appears when the renal destruction is total or nearly so. These symptoms generally date from early childhood and their significance passes unrecognized until an acute renal flare-up or complication demands surgical intervention in adulthood. Occasionally these patients learn to relieve themselves of the pain of pelvic distention by compressing the loin with the fist or against such an object as the piano or a door. As the sac refills, the intrapelvic pressure is again increased and pain results. These pains are apt to be even more pronounced when the presumably good kidney is hypoplastic, injured by toxemia, is surgically or congenitally absent, under which conditions fatal uremia and a stuporous ending occur.

Diagnosis. The history of chronic renal infection with periodic pains in the loin and remissions of acute renal symptoms suggest ureteral obstruction which, among other causes, may be the result of aberrant vascular blockage. As urinary stasis prolongs the infection despite the usual attempts at medical therapy, the diagnosis "pyelitis" becomes changed to "chronic pyelitis" while the disease progresses. The condition is generally discovered in patients of all ages by thorough urologic examination and performed most often because of persistent pyuria ("chronic pyelitis"), pain in the loin or upper abdomen, or a palpable hydronephrotic mass. In the urologic investigation there may be demonstrated a transverse urographic filling defect at the point where the vessel crosses the ureter and squeezes out the pyelographic medium leaving a nonradiopaque area (Figs. 144–148). More often one finds an enormous hydronephrosis sharply demarcated at the point of vascular obstruction; the ureter contains no opaque medium or only that which leaks out following overfilling of the pelvis (Figs. 148, 149). Conversely, by ureterography this point of filling defect may also be demonstrated, that is, the shadow of the distended ureter promptly stops at the point of vascular obstruction (Figs. 145, *A;* 149). This observation is frequent in cases in which the ureteral catheter cannot be made to pass through the obstruction to the pelvis.

Slow emptying of the pelvis of contrast medium (ten minutes or more) is also noted following removal of the ureteral catheter after pyelographic injection. When hydronephrosis is suggested by a steady ureteral drip, the urographic medium should be withdrawn to prevent subsequent renal reaction induced by edematous obstruction; these reactions, when severe, demand immediate nephrostomy or even nephrectomy. This occurred in a ten-year-old girl in whom retrograde pyelography was performed using 20 per

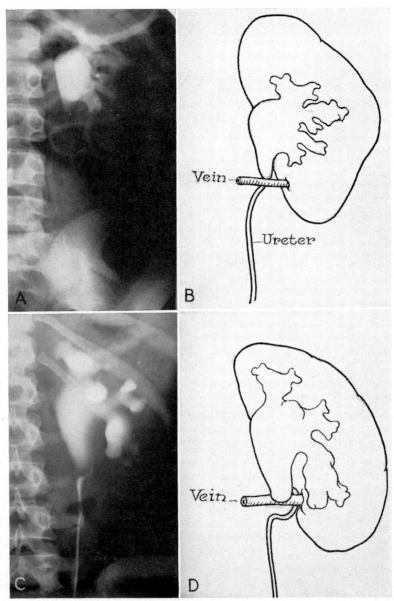

Fig. 146.   Aberrant vascular obstruction. *A, B,* in a five-year-old girl examined because of persistent pyuria. The left pelvic infundibulum is sharply blocked off by the lower polar vein. Treatment: division of the vein. *C, D,* in a six-year-old boy with pain in the left renal area and chronic pyuria. The upper ureter hooks over the vein. Treatment: division of the aberrant vein, ureteropelvioplasty for stricture at the point of venous compression, and nephropexy.

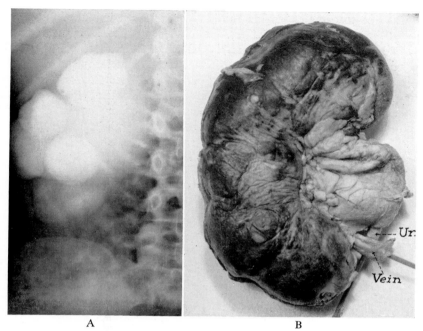

Fig. 147. Aberrant vascular obstruction of the right kidney in a ten-year-old girl examined because of chronic pyuria and pain in the right renal area. In this retrograde pyelogram, the advanced destruction of the organ is indicated. The pyelographic medium is retained in the pelvis by the obstruction and there is no medium in the ureter. Nephrectomy was performed at which time a lower polar vein 8 mm. in diameter was found to pass to the vena cava and cause the obstruction which destroyed the kidney (*B*). *B*, the surgical specimen. (Bellevue Hospital.)

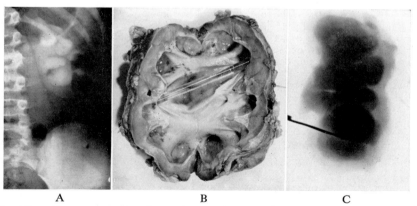

Fig. 148. Aberrant vascular obstruction causing total destruction of the left kidney in a seven-year-old boy with pain in this region. *A*, excretory urogram. Advanced hydronephrosis. *B*, surgical specimen. *C*, postoperative pyelogram of removed specimen (*B*). There is extreme hydronephrotic injury with pronounced thinning of the renal cortex.

cent Diodrast solution. Edematous closure at the point of vascular compression was due to catheter trauma rather than chemical irritation but the severity of the reaction demanded prompt removal of the kidney which previously had been shown to be irreparably damaged. For this reason and under these conditions, many urologists insist that the patient be in the hospital at the time of retrograde pyelography in order that nephrectomy or other emergency procedure can be promptly carried out should undesirable reaction or sequelae occur. Moreover and by the same logic, many urologists employ excretory pyelography only, to demonstrate not only the relative degree of

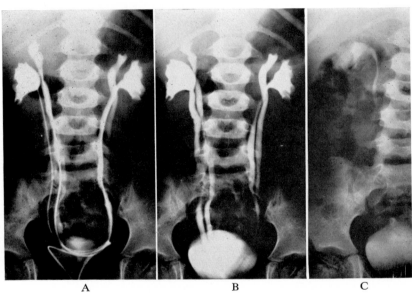

A   B   C

Fig. 149.   Aberrant vascular obstruction of the lower pelvis of a reduplicated right kidney in a three-year-old girl with persistent pyuria. There is complete bilateral ureteral reduplication. The pelvic outlet of the reduplicated lower right renal segment is sharply cut off with no downflow of medium from the injected pelvis. *B*, ureteropyelogram showing a small transverse filling defect at the outlet of the pelvis of the lower half of the right reduplicated kidney. Treatment: Resection of the aberrant vessel. *C*, postoperative trap film in *B* indicates the kidney is now draining freely.

renal function in these cases but also for suggestive diagnostic aid as to the probable initial cause of the condition. While the excretory method has the virtue of demonstrating both pelves for comparison, it is usually valueless when the renal function is low. In any event, I prefer preoperative retrograde demonstration of these lesions. Periureteral compression by a band of scar may produce a urographic filling defect indistinguishable from that caused by an anomalous vessel. The same pyelographic demonstration may also be achieved in some cases of hydronephrosis secondary to (a) ureteropelvic junction stricture, (b) high insertion of the ureter, (c) ureteropelvic spur-valve formation associated with renal sagging and rotation, the urograms being sharply cut off at the pelvic outlet. Nevertheless, all of these conditions demand renal exploration at which time the precise diagnosis will be made.

The *prognosis* in vascular obstruction of the ureter depends upon (1) the gravity of the renal damage already reflected when the diagnosis is made, (2) the presence of infection and its severity, (3) the success of treatment. When the obstructing lesion is recognized early and renal infection is unimportant, it is likely that conservative surgical treatment will save the kidney; when the renal mate is sound, surgical treatment of the diseased organ should entail a low morbidity and low mortality. In about half of the more than fifty children I have seen with vascular obstruction of the ureter, the kidney was sufficiently damaged to demand nephrectomy. In the others obstructing vessels have been ligated, pelvioplastic procedures have been carried out to permit reinstating free pelvic drainage, and with this achieved sterilization of the urine by chemotherapy completes the cure.

Treatment. This is necessarily surgical; the final decision of what to do had best be made only when the kidney has been exposed. Kidney belts, ureteral dilation and pelvic lavage, and strictly medical therapy serve only to emphasize the necessity of surgical attack. Adequate surgical exposure of these kidneys includes the clean exposure by careful dissection of the blood supply at and about the pelvic outlet with demonstration of ureteral stricture, periureteric fibrosis, stone, kinks, or other local obstruction. If exposure of the kidney reveals a substantial amount of sound parenchyma, a conservative operation is usually indicated even though infection may exist; certainly conservative renal surgery is possible in over half of the cases, and is demanded when the renal mate is absent or hopelessly diseased. Here only nephrostomy may be warranted. Occasionally the institution of nephrostomy drainage for a few days or weeks will revive the renal function and diminish infection sufficiently to justify conservative treatment. Nephrostomy should always be employed in such cases when emergency operation is necessary and the function of the other kidney is unknown.

When aberrant veins cause the ureteral blockage, they can be cut freely because of a generous collateral venous circulation in the kidney. But if an anomalous artery obstructs, the problem is more vital and difficult because the renal circulation is terminal. This means that section of the artery causes atrophy and loss of function of the segment of parenchyma it supplies. Furthermore, necrotic suppuration of the ischemic segment may occur, particularly when the area supplied by the severed artery is large. When this renal segment is small, and is determined at the operating table by noting the extent of cortical color change following compression of the artery, vascular resection is justifiable. But if this area comprises more than 25 per cent of the kidney substance, the artery should not be divided but rather plastic procedure should be carried out to circumvent the obstruction (ureteropyeloneostomy, some modification of pelvioplasty or pelvioureteroplasty). Occasionally free mobilization of the ureteropelvic junction and high nephropexy will suffice. When ureteropelvic junction stricture is an associated obstructing lesion, ureteroplasty by the Foley or Davis procedure may be employed.

(See Figs. 137–141 and Chapters 3 and 4, Section XV.) Nephropexy should be performed only when there is undue renal sagging, removal of the obstruction being the prime consideration. To date I have encountered no case in which treatment by nephropexy alone seemed indicated or warranted.

When the pyelogram or surgical exploration suggests the presence of stone, polyps, spur valve or folds, the pelvis should be explored to be sure that no intrinsic obstruction fails to be eradicated.

When the obstruction has been completely removed, urinary stagnation or stasis will disappear. Yet periodic postoperative examinations are essential to determine the degree not only of renal functional restoration but also of anatomic restoration. While we are interested primarily in functional rehabilitation, when the extrarenal hydronephrosis is large, resection of the redundant pelvis will greatly reduce urinary stasis consequent to pyelitic atony (Figs. 137, 140, 141). In turn, stronger and more active peristalsis usually follows as does restitution of the calyces to a more normal outline. While the analogy has been frequently drawn between these chronically overdistended dilated renal pelves and the comparable condition in the bladder in advanced vesical neck obstruction and the remarkable restitution to normal capacity the bladder commonly undergoes following the establishment of free drainage, this does not regularly apply to the kidney pelvis.

Failure of conservative renal surgical therapy in these cases demands nephrectomy when the renal mate permits. Nephrectomy must be performed when the hydronephrotic renal damage, complicating infection or calculus disease are too advanced to warrant employment of the conservative method just described. The infected hydronephrosis has generally been diagnosed as chronic pyelitis and permitted to terminate in hydronephrotic or pyonephrotic renal destruction. This represents the fruits of medical neglect, nearly always having its incipiency in childhood. With recognition of the indications for urologic investigation and its adequate performance, the correct diagnosis can be made and the necessity for surgical intervention revealed which, in turn, is not only life-saving but frequently means saving the kidney. In many instances in which the diagnosis has not been made, unfortunately cure or control of the renal infection is achieved by present day chemotherapy or antibiotic therapy. This false success commonly causes the nature of the underlying pathology to remain unrecognized so that when the ultimate exacerbation occurs, only nephrectomy can be employed. Moreover, these cases splendidly exemplify the dictum that even though persistent pyuria is eradicated by the improved antiseptic therapy of the present day, no patient with such a history should be discharged until at least a satisfactory excretory study has been made which may suggest the nature of the obstructive disease. Because of the consequent delay in making the diagnosis, nephrectomy will necessarily be the treatment in fully half of all children with vascular ureteral blockage and when the condition is discovered in adults the proportion requiring nephrectomy is even higher.

Vascular compression of the lower ureter is discussed on page 367.

Aneurysm of the renal artery was apparently congenital in some of the 115 reported cases analyzed by Abeshouse (1951). I found three instances of its occurrence in a child recorded, one by Reeves (1884) in a nine month old, one by Conroy (1923) in a nine-year-old boy with abdominal pain, and one by Howard et al. (1940) in a five-year-old boy with hypertension in whom this symptom promptly disappeared following isolateral nephrectomy. Lowsley and Cannon (1943) suggested a parallelism between congenital renal and cerebral aneurysm, noting their usual appearance at the angle of main artery bifurcation or at the point of branching. Yet renal aneurysms are most rare in the young, appear chiefly at branches rather than in the main artery, and their formation implies a highly selective congenital defect of particular parts of the renal artery. In older patients these lesions most commonly result from trauma or from vasculitis which is frequently syphilitic. Symptomatically they cause pain in the side in half of the cases, hematuria in a third, a palpable mass in a fourth, tenderness and hypertension in about a fifth each, and occasionally the aneurysm may produce urographic pelvic compression or filling defect and it often may be splendidly demonstrated positively by renal arteriography (Section II, Chapter 2), and negatively by pyelography.

Treatment. Nephrostomy has given the best results with the lowest mortality (about 5 per cent). Excision of the sac has been possible and successful in a few cases but too often this and other conservative procedures such as evacuation of clots, denervation of the pedicle and aneurysmolysis have required secondary nephrectomy or the patient bled to death. For large aneurysms a transperitoneal approach is advised.

EMBRYOLOGY OF THE URETER

The nature of embryonic ureteral formation as a wolffian duct derivative has been briefly indicated in embryology of the kidney. In a 6 mm. embryo (four weeks), the cloaca is present as a dilated caudal segment from whose upper portion passes the allantois and into whose lower lateral portions the wolffian ducts open (Figs. 97, 98, 150). The anterior cloacal wall is thin, is composed only of ectoderm and mesoderm, and is known as the cloacal membrane (Figs. 202–204). Between the fifth and sixth weeks a frontal fold, the urorectal septum, passes downward to divide the cloaca into a dorsal rectal and a ventral urogenital segment (Fig. 150). From the latter spring the ureteral buds which ultimately form the urinary collecting system and thus the ureter and wolffian duct come to be the vesico-urethral anlage. Ultimately the ureteral orifice is carried upward to open into the lateral angle of the trigone (Figs. 150, 208). The wolffian duct forms the posterior urethra, vas deferens, epididymis and, as a budding offshoot, the seminal vesicle (Fig. 208). This early intimate relationship of the ureteral buds and the wolffian derivatives explains the unusual types of ectopy of the ureteral orifice as, for example, when it opens into the seminal vesicles in the male or when in the female there is ectopic ureteral opening into the vagina, cervix or uterus as it occurs through persistence of a remnant of Gartner's duct, which is an early wolffian derivative.

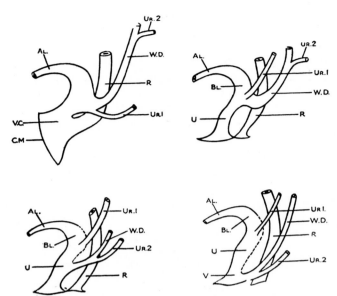

Fig. 150. Embryologic explanation of the development of ectopic ureteral opening. *A, A.L.,* allantois; *C.M.,* cloacal membrane; *V.C.,* cloaca; *R.,* rectum; *W.D.,* wolffian duct; *U.R. 1,* first reduplicated ureter; *U.R. 2,* second reduplicated ureter. Normally between the fifth and sixth week of fetal life the urorectal septum (dotted line) passes downward to separate the primitive cloaca into a dorsal rectal and a ventral urogenital segment. The ureteral buds, *U.R. 1, U.R. 2,* which ultimately form the urinary collecting system, arise from the ventral division. The wolffian ducts also open into this vesico-urethral anlage. Normally the ureteral orifices subsequently shift upward on each side to open into the lateral angle of the trigone but anomalously they may fail to do so and the result is ureteral ectopy (after Wesson).

URETERAL ANOMALIES

These may be classified as:

I. *Anomalies of Number*
    1. Agenesis
    2. Duplication
    3. Triplication and so forth

II. *Anomalies of Origin and Termination*
    1. Ectopia
    2. Ureterocele
    3. Blind ending
    4. Ureteropelvic
    5. Postcaval ureter
    6. Herniation of ureter

III. *Anomalies of Form, Caliber and Structure*
    1. Aplasia
    2. Congenital stricture
    3. Congenital valves or folds
    4. Congenital dilatation without obstruction
    5. Congenital diverticula

6. Spiral twists (torsion)
7. Kinks
8. Vascular blockage

The incidence of anomalies of the upper urinary tract is highest in the ureter. Discussion of these malformations constitutes one of the most important phases in the exposition of infection of the urinary tract and notably in the young in whom they are commonly associated etiologically with persistent pyuria which is usually erroneously designed as chronic pyelitis.

Many of these anomalies are asymptomatic and it is axiomatic that the anomalous organ is more prone to disease than is the normal one. This was exemplified in our autopsy studies in which the incidence of ureterorenal reduplication was one to 152 individuals. Yet we found it in 26.9 per cent of 1,102 children clinically examined because of persistent pyuria and in 307 of whom there were ureteropelvic anomalies, chiefly reduplication. Most of these ureteral anomalies are predominantly obstructive, supravesical obstruction being of higher incidence than intravesical. Because most ureteral anomalies are dependent upon maldevelopment of the ureteral bud, they are in genesis by the third month of fetal life.

I. ANOMALIES OF NUMBER

Bilateral ureteral agenesis is a phase of nonviable monster development associated with bilateral renal agenesis and is of no clinical concern. Instances of the condition in association with bilateral renal agenesis are cited on page 239.

Unilateral ureteral agenesis. This is due to failure of the ureteral bud to develop and is always accompanied by renal agenesis, renal aplasia or hypoplasia. Occasionally in renal agenesis the ureter is aplastic and persists as a fine fibrous thread or as a ureteral stump, indicating that there has been ureteral budding but the pelvis and metanephros have failed to develop. The clinical importance of ureteral agenesis is that of ureterorenal agenesis but a normally located and appearing ureteral dimple in the bladder may cause the upper tract anomaly to be overlooked. More commonly, the isolateral trigone shows hypoplasia, the ureteral orifice being a tiny blind dimple, or absent. In rare instances the aplastic ureter has become the site of large cyst formation to simulate tumor of abdominal organs. In a five-month-old boy with a palpable right kidney and persistent pyuria, the excretory urogram showed no renal shadow on the left, and the left ureteral catheter was stopped 4.5 cm. up the ureter (Fig. 106). With moderately forceful retrograde injection on the left, the ureter was shown to taper off to a thread just above the catheter tip. The right kidney was approximately twice normal size and showed a large pelvis such as is commonly found in congenital solitary organs. The diagnosis of renal agenesis with ureteral aplasia was made; similar urographic studies made seventeen years later showed fundamentally the same picture as that observed in early infancy (Fig. 106).

Ureteral reduplication (double ureter). In this common malformation, the reduplication may be complete or incomplete. Considerable personal data on the incidence of ureteral reduplication in its relation to renal reduplication have been given earlier in this chapter. A total of 342 instances (281 adults; 61 infants and children) of ureteral reduplication was found at autopsy in 51,880 cases, an over-all incidence of 1:161. The reduplication was complete in 101 (24 children; 77 adults), but was bilaterally complete in only four (2 children; 2 adults).

In the 342 cases the reduplication was on the right side in 144, on the left in 145, and 53, or approximately 1 in 6, were bilateral. In the incomplete ureteral reduplications, the fusion occurred in the lower third of the ureter in 69, in the middle third in 55, and in the upper third in 70. Further data on ureteral and pelvic reduplication are given under consideration of this subject on page 285. In short, unilateral reduplication occurs about once in 160 individuals, in about a third of whom it is incomplete. Double ureter is found unilaterally six times as often as bilaterally, and in one in five cases bilateral involvement is mixed with complete reduplication on one side and incomplete on the other (Fig. 132). Clinically twice as many males show the anomaly as females, but the relative incidence at autopsy is about equal. Although both segments of the reduplicated ureter are usually involved when isolateral upper tract disease exists, when only half of the organ is diseased, it is most commonly the lower segment, except when associated with ureteral ectopy. In the last, the upper segment is the one involved in nine out of ten cases.

Obstructions, congenital and otherwise, are not uncommon in reduplicated ureters. In 19,046 autopsies in infants and children, the reduplicated ureter showed obstruction in 14 of the 61 cases, there being stricture in 10, ureteral valve in 3, and stone in 1. The strictures were at the ureterovesical junction in 3, in the body of the duct in 2, and at the ureteropelvic junction in 5. In 281 autopsies in adults with ureteral reduplication, obstruction was found in 14, stone was present in 8, stricture in 4, and in two others an undesignated blockage.

In the examination of 4,774 urograms (1942 to 1946), Nordmark (1948) found 201 (4.2 per cent) cases of double pelvis; sixty-four were bilateral, 155 were unilateral (right 62; left 93), ninety-eight were men and 103 were women. There were 138 cases of double ureter (19 bilateral; 119 unilateral), and of the unilateral variety sixty (1.3 per cent) showed incomplete and 59 (1.3 per cent) complete reduplication. Eleven (0.2 per cent; 1:50) showed complete bilateral reduplication of the ureter and five (1.0 per cent) were incomplete. These figures are understandably six times higher than our autopsy findings because the examinations were made on patients with urologic disease, in whom upper urinary tract anomalies frequently play an important etiologic role.

Two embryologic explanations for ureteral reduplication have been offered: (1) the development of two ureteral buds with fusion of the nephrogenic anlagen (double kidney), or without fusion (supernumerary kidney); (2) fission or splitting of a single ureteral bud. While the first theory appears the correct one to explain such unusual findings as emptying of one ureter into the seminal vesicles, vas deferens, or ejaculatory duct when the reduplicated ureter opens normally in the bladder, and explains the exceedingly rare type in which two stalks leave the ureter but unite above, it does not explain the common incomplete reduplication usually observed. The second theory involving fission of the ureteral bud accounts for the usual types of reduplication, the splitting occurring from above downward and of any degree. Yet it does not explain the inverted Y ureter as seen in one of our cases and in which the reduplicated ureters join to open through a single duct into a single renal pelvis (Fig. 151). In short, at present no embryologic theory explains all cases.

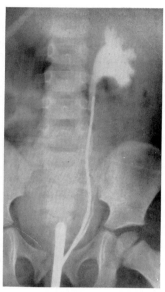

Fig. 151.   Inverted "Y" ureteral reduplication, one of the rarest anomalies of this duct. A size 6 F. catheter has been passed up the larger of the two left ureteral orifices which is superior and lateral. The size 4 F. catheter has been passed up the smaller and more mesial orifice to about 4 cm. The pyeloureterogram was obtained by injection of the smaller size 4 F. catheter only. (Courtesy Dr. W. Boyce.)

There are generally as many separate pelves as ureteral stalks, the pelves usually being situated one above the other, but rarely they are side by side or one pelvis directly behind the other (Fig. 130). Intercommunication has been noted between reduplicated pelves but is excessively rare, having been encountered in only four of our autopsy cases in the young and in no adults. Surgically, when the calyces of the two pelves are urographically distinctly separate, renal resection is usually not difficult, but when the two pelves interdigitate, this operation may be extremely arduous or even impracticable.

With complete reduplication and except when extravesical ureteral ectopy exists, both ureters pass downward side by side from the two renal pelves and just before reaching the bladder, according to the so-called Weigert-Meyer law, the ureter from the lower pelvis crosses the ureter from the upper pelvis to enter the bladder, its orifice nearly always being found situated above that of the ureter from the upper pelvis (Fig. 150). Generally the orifices lie adjacent on the ridge of the trigone one above the other, but they may be situated side by side or separated from each other. Obstruction of one or both ureters may be engendered at the point of crossing or the duct may be otherwise anomalous, congenital stricture being a frequent finding.

The inversion relation of the ureteral orifices and their corresponding pelves is explained as follows (Johnson*): "The ureter has its origin from the lower portion of the wolffian duct (Fig. 150). With continued development, the terminal portion of the wolffian duct is absorbed into the vesico-urethral anlagen so that both the wolffian duct and ureter acquire separate openings (B). By a peculiar process of growth the ureteral orifice is shifted cranially and laterally. When two ureters are present on one side, the one from the inferior half of the kidney is placed lower in the wolffian duct than that from the upper half (B). With the absorption of the wolffian duct, the inferior ureteral orifice reaches the vesico-urethral anlagen first and begins its upward and lateral shifting, while the ureter from the superior segment of the kidney is still attached to the wolffian duct (C). The latter in turn reaches the vesico-urethral anlagen and begins its upward and lateral shifting but never reaches as high a level as the first. The ureter from the inferior segment crosses in front of that from the superior segment and implants itself at a higher level. Occasionally the ureter from the superior segment does not reach the bladder, but remains attached to the wolffian duct or urethra."

This explanation defines the characteristic inversion of the ureters, the so-called *Weigert-Meyer law*. Yet rarely this so-called law is violated, the position of the ureteral orifices being that of the renal relation, the ureter from the upper pelvis opening into the bladder above that of the lower pelvis (cf. Lund, 1949). The embryologic mechanism of the inversion relation of the ureteral orifices and their corresponding pelves is indicated in Figures 98 and 150 (see also Hawthorne, 1936).

In incomplete reduplication, the ureteral branches from the reduplicated pelves join at some point so that only one orifice is present. This junction may be near the pelvis or even within the bladder wall. In about half of the cases the bifurcation occurs in the lower third of the ureter, and in the middle and upper third in about a fourth each (Fig. 149). In a girl, five years old, in whom the bifurcation occurred within the bladder wall, tilting of the ureteral catheter 3 mm. within the ureteral orifice determined which ureteral branch would be entered. The abortive or incomplete second ureter is a rare form of incomplete reduplication in which one duct is complete. Its reduplicated mate usually presents a normal appearing ureteral orifice but terminates a centimeter or so above the bladder. An abortive or incomplete ureter may develop to be a ureteral cyst or if the renal pelvis to which it is connected is infected, ureteropyonephrosis may result. In the absence of connection of this diseased segment with the bladder, the urine may remain normal and

* In Young, H. H. and Davis, D. M.: Practice of Urology. Philadelphia, W. B. Saunders Co., 1926, I, p. 39.

the condition be identified only on renal exploration or at autopsy. In short, the condition is analogous to blind ending or solitary ureter as previously described (Fig. 106). In a six-week-old boy in our autopsy series, dead of pneumonia, there was incomplete ureteral reduplication in which a second greatly dilated ureter passed downward from the kidney but ended blindly near the bladder, having no connection either with it or with its ureteral mate.

Inverse (inverted Y) ureteral reduplication has been reported in four cases and is doubtless the rarest of all anomalous ureteral branchings. Here the ureters leave the bladder as separate ducts but fuse above and as a single ureter enter the single renal pelvis (Fig. 151). This occurred in an eighteen-month-old girl in whom a stone 9 mm. in diameter was found in the lower branch of the ureter, caused persistent pyuria, and required ureteronephrectomy for cure (Burstein, 1938). In one of our autopsy cases, a three-month-old boy, the "inverted" reduplication occurred just above the bladder, one branch passing to the normal ureteral site, the other to the posterior bladder wall, In another of our autopsy cases fusion of the two ureters occurred at the bladder wall and again at the renal pelvis, the channels being separated in between.

Associated anomalies are found in at least a fourth of the cases of ureteral reduplication and include renal agenesis, hypoplasia, ectopy, polycystic disease, malrotation, ectopic ureteral orifice, and malformation of the lower urinary tract or genital system. In our 342 autopsy cases there were 105 associated urologic anomalies (75 adults; 30 children) and 42 nonurologic malformations (28 adults; 14 children).

Ureteral triplication. Ten cases of this rare condition have been reported. I have seen two others, and in a third, the condition was bilateral and found at autopsy. The difficult clinical problem this may present was illustrated by the case of a sixty-year-old man with a stone in one of three right ureters. On the left, there was complete ureteral reduplication. The reader is also referred to the paragraph covering renal reduplication.

Sometimes the pelvis is composed of several uniting extrarenal infundibula which drain separate calyces (Fig. 131, *A*). In a patient examined post mortem at Bellevue Hospital in New York, six separate stalks on each side thus joined the ureters. All of these ureteral anomalies may be splendidly demonstrated urographically (Fig. 131). The only suggestive external sign of ureteral reduplication, but not pathognomonic, is the finding of an ectopic ureteral orifice in the introitus, vagina or cervix (Figs. 152, 156).

In most cases ureteral reduplication is asymptomatic and accidentally discovered. The symptoms are those of disease of a normally formed kidney, it being an anomaly that is particularly prone to complicating infection or obstruction.

The *diagnosis* is made by urography, at operation, or at autopsy. The preliminary and initial excretory urogram will usually suggest the presence of the anomaly; an elongated renal shadow in the plain x-ray is always suggestive of a double kidney. When double orifices are found on one side, both should be catheterized and double pyelograms made. In our clinical cases of ureteral reduplication, the majority were identified at the time of complete urologic examination because of persistent pyuria. Diagnostic and therapeutic difficulties may arise since stricture, stone or other conditions involve one of the reduplicated ureters, particularly when the nature of the anomaly is undetected. It is not difficult to catheterize three or even four ureters through the ordinary operating cystoscopes in children or in adults but in infants and children whose urethra is too small to accommodate the Campbell 17 F. cystourethroscope (Section XIII), which will accommodate up to five 4 F. catheters, the miniature instrument must be withdrawn after catheterizing two ureters, rethreaded with catheters and re-introduced or, as we more often do in male infants, withdraw the catheters from one side after having completed its pyelographic demonstration and insert them on the opposite side so that the entire urinary tract may be urographically demonstrated at one sitting. In incomplete ureteral reduplication, the urographic reflux from one injected branch of the ureter will usually outline the other ureteral segment and pelvis, especially if the injection is made as the catheter is being withdrawn (Fig. 132).

Treatment in ureteral reduplication is that of the surgical or other complicating disease, and when only half of the kidney is involved ureterohemi-nephrectomy is the usual procedure to be employed. With this a renal segment, usually adequate to support life, remains.

II. ANOMALIES OF ORIGIN AND TERMINATION

Ectopy. Anomalously one or more ureteral orifices may open at some point other than the lateral angle of the vesical trigone but most cases pass unrecognized. The occurrence of ureteral ectopia in females is three to four times higher than in males; in over forty of these cases I have surgically

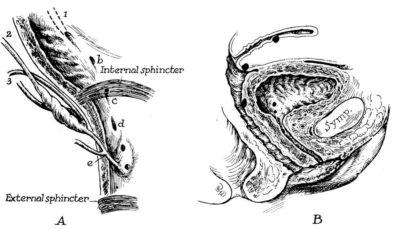

Fig. 152.   Sites of ectopic ureteral orifices; *A,* male; 1, normal; b, midtrigonal; c, vesical outlet; d, in prostate, urethra; e, ejaculatory ducts; 2, ureter joins tip of seminal vesicle; 3, ureter joins ampulla of vas. *B,* female; not only may the ureter open ectopic in the urethra and introitus, but also in the vagina and cervix. The explanation of the last is schematically indicated in Fig. 208.

treated, all were females. The condition was observed in ten of 19,046 autopsies in children (1 to 1900) but unquestionably some instances failed to be recognzied.

Embryologic Etiology. As outlined under embryology of the ureter, the ureter buds spring from the ventral urogenital cloacal segment into which the wolffian ducts also open. The ureteral orifices subsequently shift upward on each side to open into the lateral angle of the trigone (Fig. 150), but anomalously may fail to do so; this causes ureteral ectopy. In males the

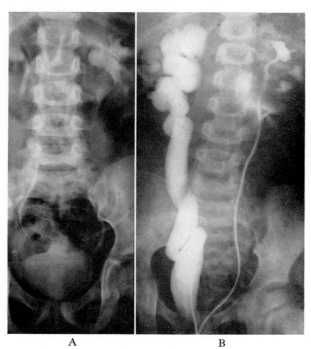

A   B

Fig. 153. *A,* left ectopic ureteral opening in the deep urethra but without causing damage to the urinary tract above in a two-year-old girl. The ectopic ureter courses lateral to the left bladder wall. *B,* ectopic ureteral opening through a strictured ureteral meatus in the posterior third of the urethra of a four-year-old girl with urinary leakage and chronic pyuria. Pronounced back-pressure damage and infection of the upper urinary tract. Ureteronephrectomy.

ectopic orifice always lies within the external sphincteric control so that no incontinence results, while in females in half of the cases the opening is beyond sphincteric control and incontinence results (Figs. 152–156).

The ectopic orifice is usually one of reduplicated ureters, by "inversion" the reduplicated ureter from the upper pelvis opens lowermost in the urinary tract, and in more than three fourths of the cases is the segment likely to be involved most seriously (Figs. 152–156). The ureter from the lower renal pelvis almost always opens in the bladder, yet both reduplicated ureters may be ectopic and even bilateral ureteral ectopia may occur. The last was observed in a four-year-old girl continually wet. Because of its wolffian duct

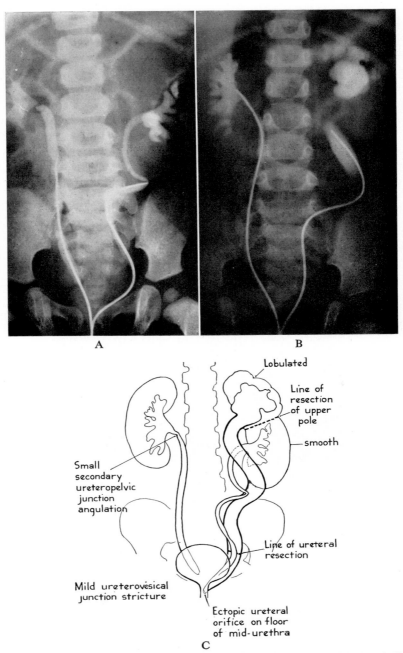

Fig. 154.   Ectopic ureteral orifice draining an infected hydronephrotic upper half of a reduplicated left kidney. *A*, the lower segment of the reduplicated organ is demonstrated; the right kidney is normal. *B*, pyelographic demonstration of the dilated infected upper half of the left kidney. In this instance the amount of urographic medium injected was wholly inadequate. Treatment: *C*, ureteroheminephrectomy removing the diseased upper half of the kidney and its ureter nearly to the bladder as shown in schema. Cure of infection.

derivation, the ureter may open into the posterior urethra, vas deferens, epididymis or seminal vesicles of the male. In a five-year-old boy with congenital solitary kidney, an attenuated ureteral stump on the opposite side opened into the seminal vesicle (cf. Engel, 1948). Pasquier and Womack (1953) collected seven cases of ectopic ureteral opening into the seminal vesicle, adding a ninth in a twenty-six-year-old male patient of theirs, and noted that thirty-two autopsy cases were also reported in the literature. By catheterization of the right seminal vesicle, and with vesiculography, they demonstrated the communication between the vesicle and right ureter. A right seminal vesicle, ureter and what was believed to be an extremely small hypoplastic right kidney were excised with successful results. In Thom's collected series of sixty-one males with ureteral ectopia, the orifice was found in the prostatic urethra in thirty-three, in the seminal vesicle in seventeen, in the vas deferens in six, and in the ejaculatory duct in five (Fig. 152). In females the anomalous orifice is generally in the urethra or just adjacent to the external urethral meatus in the introitus. In four females the ectopic ureter opened into a urethral diverticulum (cf. Willmarth, 1948), and rare instances of vaginal, cervical, or uterine openings have been reported (Wesson, 1934; Abeshouse, 1943; Hepler, 1946). Here the embryologic explanation lies in the persistence of wolffian connection through Gartner's duct which is a wolffian derivative but normally becomes atrophic or disappears in the female (Fig. 155). Perforation of unknown cause, spontaneous or traumatic rupture of a cyst of Gartner's duct explains this unusual variety of ureteral ectopy in the vagina, cervix or uterus. No instance of persistence of Gartner's duct was identified at autopsy in our series of children but was twice found (at 43 and 50 years of age) in 8,884 autopsies in adult females. In 117 cases collected by Thom (1928) the anomalous orifices were situated in the vestibule in forty-five, in the urethra in thirty-nine, in the vagina in thirty-two and in the uterus in three. In the older literature conjunction of the wolffian and müllerian systems was believed to explain ectopic ureteral opening in the fallopian tube, uterus, cervix or vagina, but analysis of these cases shows that in most the opening was really in the vestibule. We have found no authentic record of ectopic opening into a fallopian tube. In a girl at nine months and another at ten months (Babies Hospital, New York) the right ureter opened into the posterior urethra. In a ten-month-old a bicornate uterus and double vagina existed while the upper urinary tract was widely dilated, this being attributed to faulty development of the sympathetic innervation of the ureters and possibly of the musculature as well. In a three-year-old girl examined post mortem the ureter opened into the rectum, an anomaly difficult to explain on any grounds except faulty division of the cloaca by the urorectal septum. In this case the bladder was exstrophic and rectovaginal fistula existed. The right ureter opened into the rectum while the left ureter ended blindly in the tissues on the side of the bladder. When the ectopic orifice is proximal to a competent sphincter there will be no urinary leakage and for this reason in males, symptoms when present are those of infection rather than of leakage. On the other hand, in the female

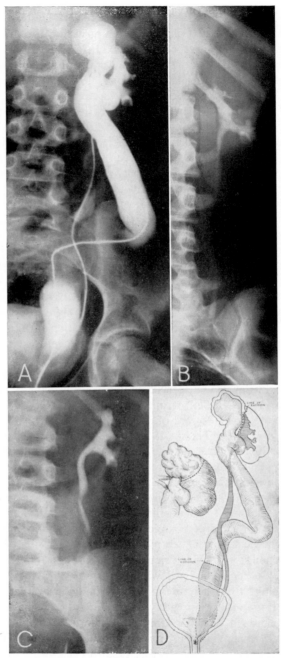

Fig. 155.   Ectopic ureteral orifice in a five-year-old girl. *A*, reduplicated left ureters have been injected which disclosed a morphologically normal lower pelvis with a greatly dilated upper pelvis and ureter. Four weeks after ureteronephrectomy it was necessary to excise the remaining pyo-ureteral stump. (Bellevue Hospital.) *B*, urographic demonstration of the remaining left upper renal segment two months and *C*, sixteen years postoperatively. Shortly before the last pyelographic examination, the girl went through pregnacy uneventfully. *D*, schema of the surgical anatomy showing the resected ureterorenal segment.

318

incontinence usually exists and the diagnosis in children is likely to be enuresis until the lower ectopic opening is recognized, or the condition in adults is thought to be bladder paralysis. In some cases the urinary leakage does not occur until after fifteen years of age (Wesson, 1934; Honke, 1946).

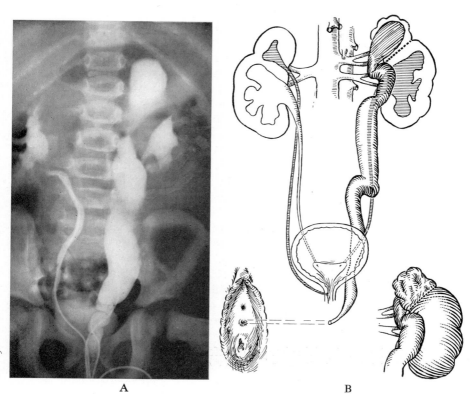

A   B

Fig. 156.   *A*, ectopic ureteral opening in a three-year-old girl examined because of persistent pyuria and "enuresis." The clinical picture and findings were similar to those indicated in Fig. 155. Ureteronephrectomy with removal of structures as indicated in schema *B*. (Bellevue Hospital.) *B*, complete bilateral ureteral reduplication in a thirteen-month-old girl with persistent pyuria. The ureter from each upper reduplicated renal segment opens ectopic, the right into the deep urethra, the left in the introitus midway between the external urethral meatus and the vaginal orifice. With squeezing of the upper portion of the left kidney, thick purulent toothpastelike material emerged from the introital ureteral opening. Left ureteroheminephrectomy. (Babies Hospital.)

Pathology. Varieties of ureteral ectopy may be classified as follows:
a. Single ureter with ectopic opening (Fig. 153).
b. Both ureters having ectopic orifices (Fig. 156).
c. Complete unilateral reduplication of the pelvis and ureter with an ectopic opening of the supernumerary ureter (Fig. 155).
d. Complete unilateral reduplication of the pelvis and ureter with ectopic opening of both ureters.
e. Supernumerary kidney, pelves and ureters, with one ectopic opening only.

    f. Bilateral reduplication of pelves and ureters, with one ectopic opening only.

    g. Bilateral reduplication of pelves and ureters, with bilateral ectopic openings.

The ureteral orifices are usually dilated so that generally urinary obstruction and back pressure are not factors in producing the dilatation which characterizes the urinary tract proximal to the anomalous orifice. While writers have described the stricturization of the ectopic orifice, in our experience this condition has been extremely rare, having been encountered in a twenty-five-year-old girl, the orifice accommodating a catheter no larger than a 3 F., and in a three-year-old girl where the stenosis was impassable. In the last case the ureter was dilated above but in the young woman with the strictured orifice, the dilatation involved only the lower 3 inches of the ureter. In the usually observed case, with widely dilated orifice and ureter, it is probable that infection plays some part in causing this change but as I believe and although it is not readily susceptible of proof, the explanation of the ureteral and pelvic dilatation lies in faulty neuromuscular development of the anomalous duct. The musculature of the ectopic ureter is usually thin and frequently shows inflammatory cellular infiltration and variable sclerosis. The pelvis it drains is frequently hydronephrotic and in several children we have seen, the pelvis of the ectopic ureter (practically always the upper) was of the small unipyramidal or rabbit type.

The microscopic picture of the renal segment drained by the ectopic ureter is that of late hydronephrotic injury with tubular dilatation, atrophy, scar, and so forth, much of the symptomatic picture resulting from complicating urinary infection, occurring as it does in about 90 per cent of these cases. The renal parenchyma shows a chronic interstitial suppurative nephritis in addition to the usual pelvic changes of infected hydronephrosis. In a thirteen-month-old girl several areas of cartilage formation were observed. She was examined because of persistent pyuria; there was bilateral ureteral reduplication, the ureters from the lower pelves opened normally in the bladder while the ureter from the right upper pelvis opened into the posterior urethra, and the ureter from the pyonephrotic left upper pelvis opened into the vestibule (Fig. 155). Left ureteroheminephrectomy was performed and examination of the removed segment showed embryonic cartilage and an embryonal formation of the glomeruli and renal tubules. A similar observation was made by Spooner and Lindsay in a newborn child, the ureter to the kidney being obstructed by a ureterocele. The greatly dilated ureter from each kidney opened into the posterior urethra of a ten-week-old girl examined post mortem. The trigone was absent, the gallbladder was lobulated and a large Meckel's diverticulum was present. Helmholz reported a nine-year-old girl with vaginal ectopia of one of reduplicated right ureters while the other opened into the bladder.

Symptoms. Urinary disturbances and infection account for the clinical picture. In females normal day and night voiding is usually accompanied by constant urinary dribbling which in turn prompts the examination that reveals the ectopic orifice. The lack of urinary control means that the external sphincter is incompetent or the ectopic orifice is peripheral to the sphincter. On the other hand, in many women we have examined with this condition incontinence existed even though the orifice was in the geographic confines of the so-called internal sphincter. When the ectopic orifice is peripheral to the sphincter, the patient is usually continually wet, although this wetness may show considerable diurnal and nocturnal variation, sometimes being related to posture with more leakage when the woman is on her feet. Children with urinary leakage from ectopic ureteral opening are commonly treated years for enuresis as adults may be also. In female patients with normal urinary control the orifice opens behind a competent "external sphincter." About half of female patients with ureteral ectopia have normal urinary control and the picture of chronic urinary infection is dominant. Sometimes the urinary leakage assumes a bizarre pattern of day incontinence with nocturnal dryness, or nocturnal incontinence beginning only in recent years, as in a twenty-one-year-old girl reported by Judd. In other cases the incontinence does not appear until after childhood while in still others incontinence of early life disappears in adulthood. Some patients will leak only when asleep while others will leak only when upright, and in vaginal ectopia with moderate ureteral drainage, the diagnosis of vaginitis erroneously may be made.

For embryologic reasons, ureteral ectopia in the male is always proximal to the external sphincter and incontinence is not a symptom. In short, males stay dry. When the ectopic segment is infected, the commonly observed "chronic pyelitis" is usually allowed to progress with only sporadic attempts at chemotherapy. With ureteral obstruction or severe complicating renal infection in these cases; isolateral renal ureteral pain is frequent.

Urinary Infection. This is generally manifested by pyuria which independently or together with urinary incontinence leads to the urologic examination which discloses the ectopic ureteral orifice. My youngest patient with this condition was six months old and was examined because of chronic pyuria (Fig. 154). Occasionally two normal ureters will be found in the bladder with one on each side and with an ectopic reduplicated ureteral mate on one or both sides. Moreover, the finding of only one ureteral orifice when the excretory urography has demonstrated ureteral reduplication isolaterally usually means ectopic ureteral orifice unless incomplete reduplication of the two channels near the bladder is shown to exist. Often the advanced hydronephrosis and infection or hypoplasia of the reduplicated superior segment draining ectopic will fail to be demonstrated by excretory urography. In these cases the presence of a second reduplicated pelvis above is suggested by a squared off or sheared off flattened urographic outline of the superior margin of the lower pelvic segment. Yet the lower pelvis may appear as that of a normal kidney. Excretory urography will yield a suggestive clue when ureteral reduplication is revealed but two isolateral orifices are not found; here retrograde pyelography may show that an incomplete ureteral reduplication does not exist.

Following injection of indigo carmine, the *diagnosis* is comparatively simple if one will carefully inspect the urethra, vagina and rectum for blue urinous discharge and particularly when the ureteral orifices which have been found are plugged by large catheters. In two of our young patients squeezing of the upper half of the involved kidney caused the ejaculation of a ribbon of toothpaste-like, purulent, urinary debris from the ectopic orifice in the vestibule just below the external urethral meatus. It is most important that a forward vision lens system be used—the foroblique type—because instruments of the Brown-Buerger type with right angled prismatic vision are of no use in the study of the urethral canal. Such ectopic ureters as can be identified should be catheterized and pyelographically injected. If the bladder is filled with a solution of methylene blue, pads will not be stained even though an ectopic ureteral orifice (plugged with a large catheter) exists but will be stained if there is true vesical incontinence.

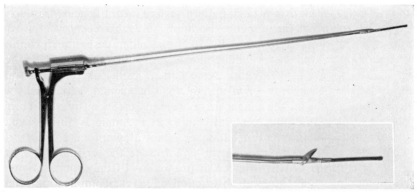

Fig. 157. Campbell's miniature (7 F.) ureteral meatome with a flexible 3 F. filiform tip employed for the division of a ureterocele, ureterovesical junction stricture, tight meatal orifice, or for slitting upward into the bladder the roof of a ureter opening ectopic in the urethra (cf. Figs. 158, 159). (Courtesy American Cystoscope Makers, Inc.)

Sometimes the identification of the ectopic ureteral orifice is exceedingly difficult. In a twenty-five-year-old girl with incontinence since infancy, the ectopic orifice of the right ureter draining the reduplicated superior renal segment was identified readily enough although it was extremely small and the ureterorenal segment hypoplastic. Ureteronephrectomy was curative, with a sharp reduction of incontinence. Yet, the patient still found it necessary to wear one or two pads a day to remain dry; on the left urography demonstrated what appeared to be a normal left upper urinary tract. Even employing chromocystoscopy and searching long and carefully it was not until the fifth examination of this patient that an extremely minute ureteral orifice was located in the left anterior urethral wall. It was successfully treated conservatively by cystoscopic electroincision of the roof of the ectopic ureter orifice and adjacent duct high up into the bladder permitting the urine to drain into the bladder rather than into the urethra, thereby curing the incontinence (Figs. 158, 159). This procedure which I have employed was suggested by Nesbit and is described in greater detail in the third succeeding paragraph.

Treatment. When the ectopic ureter is the only one for the kidney, transplantation to the bladder (ureteroneocystostomy) is commonly employed in the absence of marked renal infection and when the renal segment draining ectopic is worth conserving. When the kidney is seriously diseased by infection and the likelihood of successful conservative surgical treatment is scant, ureteronephrectomy is the indication, removing the ureter as close to the bladder as technically possible.

In reduplicated kidney with one sound segment, the upper pole is usually the one to be removed by ureteroheminephrectomy (renal resection, Figs. 154–156; see Section XV, Chapter 3). We have found the lower pole required

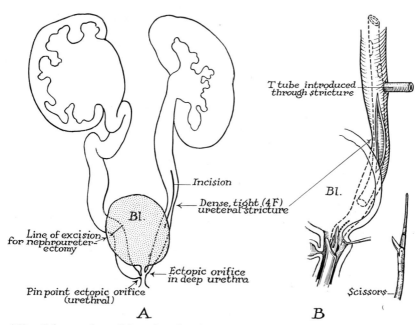

T tube introduced
through stricture

Incision

Dense, tight (4 F)
ureteral stricture

Bl.

Bl.

Line of excision
for nephroureter-
ectomy

Ectopic orifice
in deep urethra

Pin point ectopic orifice
(urethral)

Scissors

A   B

Fig. 158.   Schema of conditions found and treatment employed in the three-year-old girl whose case is discussed and pyelograms shown in Figure 182.

removal in only three out of more than fifty such resections. When both renal segments are diseased, ureteronephrectomy is the indication and particularly should the entire ureter be removed to the bladder level if it is widely dilated and/or gravely infected.

A simple transurethral procedure suggested by Nesbit (1946) has been successfully employed by me in six cases and unsuccessfully in one case of ureteral ectopia in the urethra with a salvageable renal segment above (Figs. 157–159). Using a small panendoscopic instrument and a ureteral electromeatome or scissors, the lower end of the ectopic ureter is widely cut on the roof beginning at its ureteral orifice and carrying the incision at least 1 cm. and preferably 2 to 3 cm. into the bladder, thereby causing the organ to drain normally into this viscus (Figs. 158, 159). This cures the incontinence. Ligation of the ectopic ureter should not be employed and especially when urinary infection exists. The enforced subsequent treatment of these cases thus ligated is usually ureteronephrectomy.

Ureterocele, known also as intravesical cyst of the ureter, ureterovesical cyst, or cystic dilatation of the lower end of the ureter, is an intracystic ballooning of the lower end of the ureter with involvement of all the com-

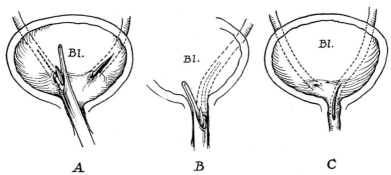

A   *B*   *C*

Fig. 159.   Methods of employment of author's miniature meatome. *A,* incision of tight ureteral meatus or ureterovesical junction stricture. *B,* incision of roof of a ureter opening ectopic in the deep urethra (Nesbit's suggestion). *C,* by carrying the incision well up into the bladder, the ureter will drain into this viscus and existing urinary leakage due to the ectopic ureteral opening stops.

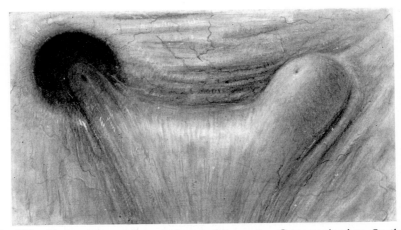

Fig. 160.   Ureterocele or intravesical cyst of the ureter. Cystoscopic view. On the top of the ureterocele is seen the extremely small ureteral meatus which causes the upper tract obstruction and is the important consideration in the genesis of ureterocele as shown in Fig. 161. On the right is shown eversion of the ureterocele in diverticulum formation with vesical overdistention.

ponent layers of the ureteral wall. Thus the cyst is covered externally by vesical mucosa, is lined internally by ureteral mucosa, and between are found diffusely scattered muscle fibers and connective tissues (Fig. 160). The condition as clinically observed is not uncommon being noted in 1 to 2 per cent of patients of all ages subjected to cystoscopic examination, but was found in one in twenty-five (4 per cent) of infants and children urologically examined by me because of chronic pyuria (1951). In our autopsy series it was observed in children but four times (1:4000). Yet this is not surprising in view of the extreme difficulty of identifying the smaller lesions after death when the ureterocele collapses. The surgeon is often unable to recognize the lesion in the opened bladder when the cystic dilatation has collapsed and looks like normal bladder wall except for unusual mucosal redundancies. This observation is cited to stress both the great importance of establishing the diagnosis of ureterocele by cystoscopy and the extreme difficulty in casually identifying a collapsed one at the operating table or post mortem, and particularly when it is small or only moderately large. A collapsed ureterocele may also be overlooked cystoscopically.

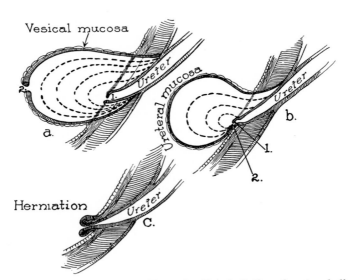

Fig. 161. Genesis of ureterocele. 1. Normal orifice. 2. Orifice of cyst. *a*, ballooning out of the vesical mucosa. *b*, asymmetrical ballooning with the orifice on the under side of the ureterocele; in the author's experience these hidden orifices are more often on the posterior surface. *C*, ureterovesical herniation (Hinman, after Petillo).

The condition is common in children, may be bilateral, and there may even be two ureteroceles on the same side as occurred in a seven-year-old boy; each drained a massive infected megaloureter and pyonephrotic pelvis of the destroyed kidney. Moreover, a congenital stricture of the lower third of the right ureter and congenital contracture of the bladder neck coexisted. In a personally examined and treated series of 100 ureteroceles in eighty-six infants and children, I found that twenty-two of these patients were males and sixty-four were females (Campbell, 1951); the lesion was on the right in thirty-three, on the left in thirty-nine, and was bilateral in fourteen. The ureterocele was observed in twenty-seven children less than one year of age, forty-one were between one and six years, and fifteen between seven and ten years, three being over eleven years.

Etiology. With one remotely possible exception, all of the 101 ureteroceles of our series to this writing were considered congenital, this conclusion being justified by their extremely high incidence in infants and young children, their frequent bilaterality (about 15 per cent as recorded in the literature and 16.3 per cent in eighty-six young patients in this series). In one case, a four-year-old girl with an enormous ureterocele, the congenital etiology was questioned because the orifice gaped slightly. Yet this meatal change may well have been the result of complicating infection. The coexistence of ureterocele and other anomalies of the urinary and other systems is of high incidence, notably with ureteral reduplication, ectopic ureteral orifice, or congenital stricture elsewhere in the ureters. When ureteral reduplication exists, the involved ureter and pelvic segment is the upper in two thirds of the cases (Fig. 164).

A congenitally small and often pinpoint ureteral meatus induces the development of a ureterocele and in this respect the condition is a phase of congenital ureteral stricture (Figs. 160, 161). Ureteroceles must be considered congenital until proved otherwise. Chwalla adduced the theory of incomplete absorption of the membrane bearing his name and this explanation is as acceptable as any thus far advanced. He noted that in embryos 12 to 30 mm. in length, epithelial downgrowth or spur-membrane formation separates the ureter from the primary excretory duct and produces a physiologic stenosis of the ureteral orifice. At a later date this membrane bursts or is absorbed and the ureteral orifice opens. He believes that failure of this process to proceed normally explains the various degrees of ureteral meatal narrowing or stenosis encountered so frequently both clinically and post mortem, and in some cases there even may be ureteral occlusion here. Others have stated that in some instances stenosis of the ureteral meatus results from local stricturization consequent to bacterial, congestive, or traumatic inflammation of the vesical wall or perimeatal area, or is secondary to pelvic inflammation, pericystitis, peripheral obstruction, infection, the passage of ureteral calculi or instrumental injury. Other alleged causes are ureteral meatitis, scarring and stricture formation subsequent to inflammation of the adjacent seminal vesicle or broad ligament, and with anatomic dilatation and intravesical protrusion of the paralyzed intramural ureteral segment (Petillo, 1925; Figs. 160, 161). Others believe an abnormal intramural course of the ureter is responsible, it being unduly oblique (Bostroem, 1884), or long and winding (Blumer, 1896). Were cystitis alone the factor, the incidence of ureterocele should be far higher in the middle-aged and the elderly than in infants and children—a situation widely contrary to the facts.

A congenital thinning or weakness of Waldeyer's sheath (the fibrous envelope of the lower end of the ureter) has been hypothecated to coexist with the meatal obstruction but convincing proof of this is lacking. Yet this assumption is not essential to the genesis of ureterocele; dilatation changes in the sheath may well result from the ensuing back pressure. The urine coming down the ureter encounters the impeding meatal stenosis and back pressure is built up, the sum of which is the renal excretory pressure and the hydrostatic pressure of the urine minus the relative drainage coefficient of the abnormally small meatal opening. Striking the meatal obstruction, the contiguous ureterovesical mucosa is dilated and ballooned outward, this process proceeding to clinical ureterocele formation as shown in Figure 161.

Pathology. Ureterocele may be classified as (1) simple (usual): (*a*) unilateral, (*b*) bilateral, (*c*) reduplicated on same side, without fusion; with fusion, (*d*) with compression of an adjacent reduplicated ureter, (*e*) with compression of a contralateral ureter; (2) prolapsed: (*a*) in female (to urethra or externally), (*b*) in male (to prostatic urethra); (3) ectopic opening: (*a*) in urethra, (*b*) in vesical diverticulum; (4) blind-ending intra-

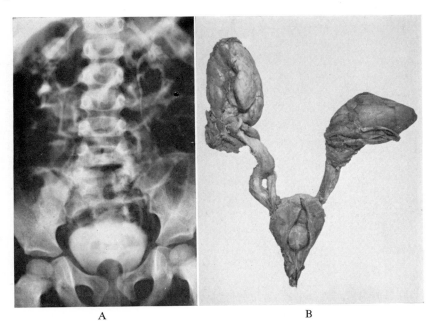

A   B

Fig. 162. Ureterocele at the vesical outlet. *A,* ureterocele blocking the vesical outlet and causing a large cystographic filling defect in a twenty-month-old girl examined because of persistent pyuria. The major condition was an advanced infected hydronephrosis of the upper half of the reduplicated right kidney, this hydronephrosis being drained through the dilated ureter which opened into the ureterocele. Right ureteroheminephrectomy; extraurethral ureterocelectomy. The ureterocele was grasped blindly with forceps, drawn out through the urethra, and cut off as shown in Fig. 907. *B,* in a thirteen-month-old girl admitted to the Babies Hospital in uremia. Reduplicated right upper urinary tract, the ureter from the upper renal segment opening into the ureterocele, the orifice of the latter being in the posterior urethra. Cystoscopically the ureterocele was so large that at first it was thought to be an accessory bladder or, when flattened, a large mucosal shelf over the trigone. Bilateral ureterostomy was performed; a third ureter (the one draining into the ureterocele) was overlooked. The ureterocele terminated essentially as a urethra within a urethra; the orifice for ureteral urinary discharge was a small slit on the roof of the ureterocele in the deep urethra. Ureterovesical junction stricture of the ureter to the left kidney and of the ureter to the lower half of the right kidney. Fatal urinary sepsis.

vesical cyst. Ureteroceles may be round, globular, oval, elongated, or broad and flat. In the pyriform variety the meatal opening is often ectopic in the urethra. They vary greatly in size, even during the filling and emptying cycle as described under diagnosis, and also as to their maximal capacity. They may vary from 1 cm. in diameter to a size completely filling the bladder as occurred in seven of our cases (Fig. 165). Prolapse of the ureterocele through the urethra occurred in seven females in this series and simulated eversion of the bladder from which it must be differentiated. The ureterocele protruded into the deep urethra in three other cases and in sixteen effectively obstructed the vesical outlet. Orr and Glanton (1953) collected forty-six cases of prolapse of a ureterocele, adding one of their own. Yet I have four cases not included in their tabulation. Their patient was an eleven-month-old white female subjected to extraurethral excision of the ureterocele and ureteronephrectomy.

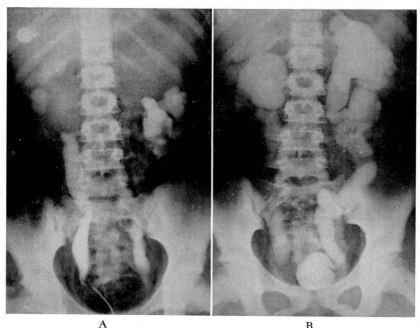

A   B

Fig. 163. Urographic demonstration of a ureterocele in a six-year-old girl examined because of persistent pyuria and recurrent fever. *A*, investigation disclosed a ureterovesical junction stricture of the right ureter and also of the left ureter which drained the lower infected hydronephrotic half of a reduplicated kidney. The upper half of the left kidney showed a massive hydronephrosis which drained through the greatly dilated angulated ureter which in turn entered the massive ureterocele which in *B* is shown as a bladderlike structure, the presence of which is faintly suggested by the negative vesical filling defect shadow in *A*.

With persistence of the ureteromeatal obstruction, the ureterocele enlarges and proximally there is progressive dilatation of the ureter and renal pelvis often with the production of megaloureter, massive hydronephrosis and even total renal destruction (Fig. 163). This renal injury caused by back pressure and commonly complicated by infection, is the factor of greatest clinical importance in ureterocele. Only rarely is the upper tract urographically normal or the changes relatively minimal, but this has been observed with a fair sized ureterocele and reflects comparatively mild meatal obstruction.

Infection may be anticipated in every case. Grossly evident chronic pyuria was the principal manifestation for urologic examination in fifty-six of the eighty-six children in this series. The urinary stasis and/or infection also favor the formation of stone which was found in six of these patients. In a twenty-five-year-old woman, a forty-year-old man, a five-year-old boy and a three-year-old girl, ureteral calculi localized in the cystic dilatation, their expulsion being prevented by the tight meatus of the ureterocele. A large branching dendritic stone filled the pelvis of a dilated pyonephrotic left kidney of a two-year-old girl with isolateral ureterocele; ureteronephrectomy was performed. Similarly in a two-year-old boy with the same clinical picture on the right side, the excised acutely infected kidney was found to be full of stones which x-ray had failed to show. In four children operated upon by suprapubic excision, we demonstrated the intraureterocele hydraulic tension to be so great as to compress firmly and completely the intramural segment of the accompanying reduplicated ureter in two cases and the adjacent contralateral ureter in the other two children, this compression causing advanced secondary hydronephrosis and hydroureter in these "innocent" structures. With incision of these tense ureteroceles and release of pressure, the secondarily compressed ureters emptied themselves with an enormous gush of dammed back urine. In a twelve-month-old boy this urine was mahogany color from old blood; the child had been referred for urologic examination because of hematuria which was thus proved to originate in the intensely congested contralateral upper tract secondarily obstructed by compression by a ureterocele of the reduplicated renal mate.

When the ureterocele is small the diminutive meatus will usually be readily found cystoscopically on the anterior or antero-superior surface (Fig. 160). As the cyst grows the meatus comes to be located on the under, lateral, median or posterior surface and not infrequently, because of technical cystoscopic difficulties and even with chromocystoscopy, the orifice cannot be found. In some instances there is no meatus; pathologically this entitles the condition to be designated as congenital intravesical dilatation of a blind-ending ureter.

Anomalies of the urogenital and other systems frequently accompany ureterocele. In our series this included isolateral complete ureteral reduplication (30), unilateral complete reduplication (16), contralateral reduplication which was complete in 10 cases and incomplete in 1. The opposite kidney was congenitally malascended, hypoplastic, or showed aberrant vascular obstruction in two cases each; renal anomalies included supernumerary buds, agenesis, multilocular cystic disease, aplasia, and vascular abnormality in one each; there was hydronephrotic atrophy in four cases, and renal sclerosis (renal rickets), renal embryoma, ureteropelvic fibrosis, stone, cortical abscesses, sclerotic nephritis and massive suppuration in one case each.

Anomalies of other body systems included spina bifida in four cases, fused labia minora in three, and one case each of clubfoot, absent anus, diaphragmatic hernia, umbilical hernia, retarded mental growth, pyloric stenosis, convergent strabismus, patent foramen ovale, accessory spleen, and ependymal rest; one child had congenital syphilis.

Symptoms. The symptoms of ureterocele reflect both the urinary obstruction and vesical irritation caused by the lesion together with complicating infection. Continuous or recurrent macroscopic pyuria and fever, frequency of urination, hematuria, dysuria, urgency and/or vesical distress are usual manifestations. Vesical irritation or even incontinence may be caused by irritation of the ureterocele mass itself in the bladder, especially when it is near the vesical outlet; here congestive inflammation, infection or both are common factors. In seven of our cases vesical retention was recurrent and in three cases acute because of ball valve obstruction of the vesical outlet by the cyst. In three cases chronic complete retention with paradoxical or overflow incontinence had existed, and three children had been clinically designated as enuretic. Pain reflects either the urinary back pressure or infection, and commonly both are present; occasionally the pain is that of chronic vesical overdistention. Moreover, complicating anomalies or diseases of the contralateral upper urinary tract may induce a symptomatology of their own. Complete retention consequent to prolapse of the ureterocele through the female urethra occurred acutely in seven of our patients but is immediately relieved by replacement of the protruding mass into the bladder. In two children cystotomy drainage had been established by other surgeons through failure to appreciate the cause of the vesical distention.

The toxemia of long-standing infection and/or obstruction is reflected in gastrointestinal disturbances with vomiting, anorexia, malaise, headache, indigestion, constipation, diarrhea, loss of weight, failure to gain and/or progressive anemia. In half the cases the complaint was that of chronic illness. With advanced bilateral renal injury by back pressure and infection the patient may die in uremia or urinary sepsis unless the obstruction, infection, and the patient's poor general condition are actively combated.

Diagnosis. Physical examination may disclose a distended bladder, renal tenderness, abdominal tenderness or rigidity, a urethral mass, prolapsed ureterocele (Fig. 167), excoriation of the genitalia, labial fusion or other findings suggestive of urinary tract disease. Malnutrition and anemia commonly reflect the long-standing infection and there even may be renal dwarfism. Examination of the catheterized urine specimen will disclose the nature of the infection. A complete urologic examination is essential in these cases, in many of whom a preliminary excretory urographic study will suggest the diagnosis, particularly when a vesical filling defect caused by the ureterocele is disclosed (Figs. 162, 164, 166) or the dilated lower end of the ureter presents the bulbous "cobra head" or "spring onion" filling outline of the intravesical cyst itself (Fig. 163, *B*). A large ureterocele may cause the cystographic shadow to appear only as a halo around the ballooned ureterocele, the medium finding only the space between the cyst and bladder wall (Fig. 165). Sometimes the ureter will be urographically seen sharply cut off at the vesical wall and without filling of the intravesical cystic portion.

While a collapsed small ureterocele may be missed, a competent cystoscopist is unlikely to overlook a ureterocele, particularly if it is distended. The classic cystoscopic picture of ureterocele is that of rhythmic filling of the cyst with urine under peristaltic projection, expanding into an easily indentable, semitranslucent balloon-like mass, which collapses as the urine slowly empties through the small meatus into the bladder. The vesical mucosa covering the cyst may be inflamed. Sometimes the stream of urine ejaculated from the meatus appears hairlike in thickness. When the meatus is extremely small, the ureterocele remains constantly distended as a large soft mass reflecting the ureteral peristaltic contractions. This factor often makes discovery of the ureteral orifice difficult or impossible, and especially when it is beneath or far on the posterior aspect of the cyst and even though indigo carmine has been given intravenously for meatal chromocystoscopy.

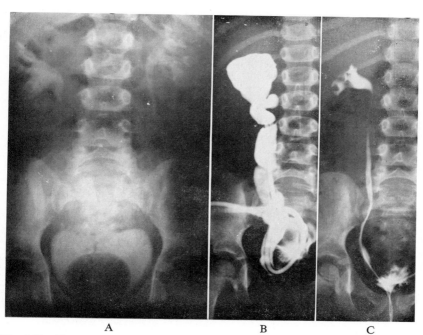

A B C

Fig. 164. Ureterocele in a twenty-two-month-old girl examined because of persistent urinary infection. *A*, excretory urography showing a normal left upper urinary tract with a mildly dilated lower segment of a reduplicated right kidney. Negative shadow filling defect in the bladder outlines the ureterocele in contrast to the demonstration of urographic filling of the ureterocele in Fig. 163 *B*. *B*, urographic demonstration of the reduplicated upper half of the right kidney. This greatly dilated ureter opened into the ureterocele. Treatment: right ureteroheminephrectomy; transvesical ureterocelectomy. *C*, remaining lower right renal segment following ureteroheminephrectomy. Cure of infection.

In some of these cases, the proper diagnosis is congenital blind ending ureteral orifice with cystic dilatation. The ureterocele should not be confused with fibroma or carcinoma. If the meatus cannot be found or catheterized and excretory urography is of no aid because of inadequate renal function, inject the upper tract through a hypodermic needle fastened to the tip of a ureteral catheter cystoscopically introduced through the wall of the cyst (Mertz, Hendricks and Garrett, 1949). I have found it easier to incise the cyst wall with miniature cystoscopic scissors and introduce a ureteral catheter through the new opening to perform the retrograde pyelographic injection in the usual manner.

It must be borne in mind that with cystoscopic overdistention of the bladder it is not unusual for a ureterocele to evaginate in diverticulum formation as was noted in thirteen of our cases (Fig. 160). Unfortunately this faulty interpretation has often led to an initial erroneous diagnosis of diverticulum. Sometimes the meatus not previously found will be identified in the cavity wall of the everted ureterocele sac. Prolapse or simple eversion of the ureteral mucosa is usually induced by the passage of stone and appears as a simple mucosal extrusion through the orifice; the outer layers of the

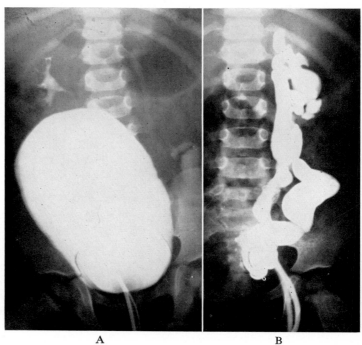

A   B

Fig. 165.   Massive ureterocele obstructing the vesical outlet and associated with persistent pyuria in a thirteen-month-old girl. *A*, the right upper urinary tract is normal. There is mild vesico-ureteral reflux into the ureter to the upper segment of the reduplicated left kidney. *B*, urographic demonstration of the diseased left upper urinary tract in which the upper reduplicated left renal segment drains into the ureterocele which in turn secondarily compresses and obstructs the intramural portion of the ureter to the lower renal pelvis. The entire left upper tract was excised. Transvesical ureterocelectomy.

ureteral wall do not participate in the process. Moreover, the prolapsed tissue is covered by ureteral mucosa while the ureterocele is covered by vesical mucosa.

A ureterocele *prolapsed through the female urethra* appears as a congested fiery red mucosal mass ballooning from the meatus (Fig. 168). When the prolapse has existed for several hours, its surface may be dull red and still later may be suggestive of severe interference with the blood supply of the mass. This condition is to be distinguished from urethral prolapse (cf.) which appears as an eversion rather than as a ballooning and lacks the fine vascularity of the bladder mucosa which covers the ureterocele. The thickness of the vesical walls in contrast to the thinness of the ureterocele walls distinguishes ureterocele prolapse from vesical prolapse in which the entire trigone and the ureteral orifices may be identified.

Treatment. The various methods for treatment of ureterocele are shown in Figure 906 (Section XV, Chapter 5). Cystoscopic dilation of the stenosed ureterocele orifice is rarely effective and is not recommended as sole therapy. Cystoscopic division of the ureterocele or wide meatotomy will usually remove the obstructive factor and can be achieved in children with a 16 F. resectoscope or by employing the Campbell 17 F. operating cysto-urethro-

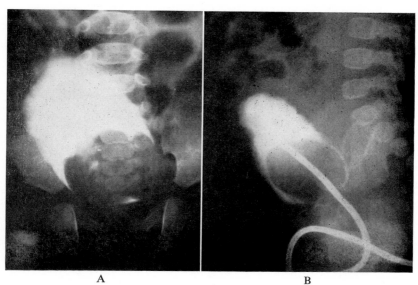

A   B

Fig. 166.   Massive ureterocele blocking the vesical outlet in an eleven-month-old boy with persistent pyuria, fever and pronounced urinary distress. Because the ureterocele blocked the vesical outlet completely by ball-valve formation, this infant instinctively learned to urinate in the knee-chest position which caused the ureterocele to fall away from the bladder orifice. *A,* anterior posterior view showing massive filling defect. *B,* lateral view showing extent of the ureterocele.

scope with miniature ureteral scissors or ureterotome. By extension of the resection, transurethral excision of the ureterocele can be carried out, progressively whittling the ureterocele tissue away. In adults these procedures are carried out with correspondingly larger instruments. Transurethral excision was employed in thirteen of our young patients with ureterocele. Electrocoagulation of bleeding points is employed for hemostasis; a small balloon catheter is left in the bladder for forty-eight hours following operation. In a thirty-five-year-old male with recurrent urinary difficulty and frequency due to a large left ureterocele, excision of the lesion with a Stern-McCarthy resectoscope was followed in three days by profuse postoperative hemorrhage which fortunately responded promptly to electrocoagulation and indwelling catheterization.

In two girls—two and four years of age—a small Kelly clamp was introduced through the urethra into the bladder to grasp the ureterocele and pull it through where it was cut off with scissors. Probably electrocautery cutting for its coagulating effect would have been better. A small balloon catheter was left indwelling in the bladder for two days; convalescence was uneventful and a satisfactory result was obtained.

The safest and most satisfactory procedure when the lesion is large and especially in children, is *ureterocelectomy* through the open bladder. A ureterocele large enough to protrude through the urethra is usually best excised suprapubically, particularly in the young or if the prolapsed segment has been strangulated. In performing hemostasis through the open bladder, topical ligation of individual bleeding vessels is generally preferred to a running hemostatic suture.

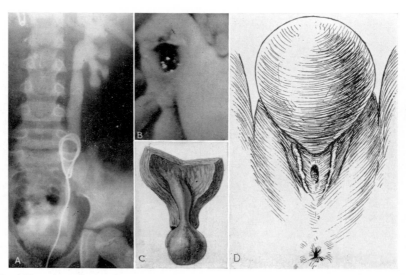

Fig. 167.   *A*, prolapse of a ureterocele in a six-year-old girl with persistent pyuria. With each voiding, the cherry red ureterocele mass ballooned through the urethra (*B, C, D*). There is marked dilatation of the ureter above. Treatment: resection of the ureterocele. *B, D*, indicate the appearance of the large prolapsed ureterocele separating the labia. (Courtesy of Dr. R. S. Cantini with whom the patient was seen.)

Coexisting stone in the ureterocele cavity is removed at the same time the cyst is excised or divided. Following resection or division of the ureterocele vesicoureteral reflux usually ensues but is seldom of clinical concern, and unquestionably injures the kidney less than did the previous obstruction.

When the upper tract is hopelessly injured, employ *ureteronephrectomy* removing the ureter down to the bladder wall or as near to it as technically possible. Less than total ureterectomy may leave a variable pyoureter—an infected diverticulum—which will continually pour infected urine into the bladder to maintain infection and to jeopardize the sound kidney and ureter. In five of our cases it was necessary to perform secondary removal of the remaining pyoureteral stump. Coexisting anomalies or other lesions of the bladder or vesical outlet are treated appropriately. Yet even though a satisfactory surgical result is achieved, no patient should be considered as cured

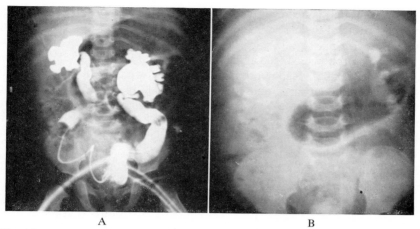

A   B

Fig. 168.   *A,* massive ureterocele draining the upper half of the infected reduplicated right kidney. The ureterocele mass was so firmly distended as effectively to compress the ureteral orifices of the lower half of the right reduplicated kidney and of the left kidney. *B,* there was pronounced secondary ureteral kinking with additional obstruction at the left ureteropelvic junction. Complicating this condition there was congenital contracture of the vesical outlet. The history was that of chronic urinary infection with recurrent bouts of fever. Treatment: right ureteroh024eminephrectomy, transurethral ureterocelectomy and transurethral resection of the contracted bladder neck. Resection of the sharply angulated left ureteropelvic junction (see Fig. 169).

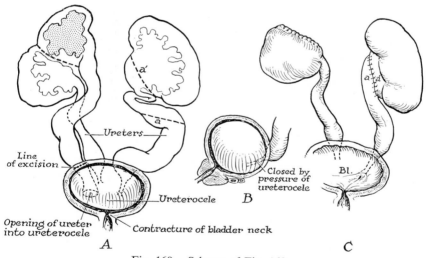

Fig. 169.   Schema of Fig. 168.

whose urine has not been sterilized by chemotherapy and/or antibiotic therapy, and according to precise bacteriologic indication.

Some of the potential complicating surgical conditions and problems in ureterocele as encountered in an eight-month-old boy are schematically suggested in Figure 169. In this case, a large tense ureterocele inadequately drained the upper half of the reduplicated right kidney. Enlarging into the bladder the cystic mass drew with it the lower segment of both the reduplicated right ureteral mate as well as the left ureter. Compression by the large tense ureterocele mass gravely obstructed both of the secondarily compressed ureters with pronounced secondary back pressure damage above. When the ureterocele was divided suprapubically the secondarily obstructed ureters gushed urine freely in large amounts, it being bloody on the left and cloudy on the right. The ureterocele was removed; the left ureteropelvic junction was resected with removal of the obstruction and 3 inches of redundant ureter with oblique side-to-side anastomosis. Later right ureteroheminephrectomy was performed (Fig. 169).

Blind Ending Ureters. The ureteral orifice may be normal in this condition but the opening is generally tiny, the ureter usually being hypoplastic throughout its course. Its lumen may be small, intermittently constricted, or completely absent. The condition must be differentiated from congenital stricture of the ureter in which the duct otherwise remains amply patent. Clinical interest derives chiefly as the blind-ending duct may become the site of a large cyst suggesting a tumor of abdominal viscera. In ten of fifty-six cases collected by Chwalla (1927), the condition was bilateral and in eleven instances a reduplicated ureter terminated blindly. Occasionally the ureter is a fibrous cord from the pelvis of an aplastic or markedly hypoplastic kidney down to the bladder where some patency may be present. Such a case is shown in Figure 106. The diagnosis will rarely be made except by surgical exploration; a patent lower segment of an otherwise congenital blind-ending ureter may be demonstrated ureterographically. Ureterectomy or ureteronephrectomy according to surgical indication should be employed.

Congenital high insertion of the ureter is a rare malformation, and is sometimes observed in an otherwise normal kidney (Fig. 170). Usually the urinary stasis and blockage coincident to the high ureteropelvic angulation produces variable hydronephrosis in which, with sagging of the distended organ, the ureteropelvic obstruction is increased, the kidney is rotated counterclockwise on the right side and clockwise on the left to cause increased angulation at the ureteropelvic junction, and sometimes a spur-valve formation. A factitial high or pseudohigh insertion of the ureter is sometimes produced with simple ureteropelvic obstruction by this rotation mechanism and is to be distinguished from the true congenital variety of high insertion in which the kidney is otherwise normal. Pelvic retention and complicating infection are the usual important considerations in congenital high insertion; pain in the side and/or chronic pyuria dominate the symptomatic picture.

The local renal pathology is progressive, for with the development of renal changes just noted, there is increased ureteropelvic angulation, and periureteral inflammation and sclerotic periureteritis. A single urogram may not demonstrate the true condition but by stereoscopic pyelography the course and nature of the angulation are immediately evident. With delayed or trap urographic exposures, the pronounced delayed emptying time and pelvic retention are demonstrated. As a result of the vicious cycle of hydronephrosis,

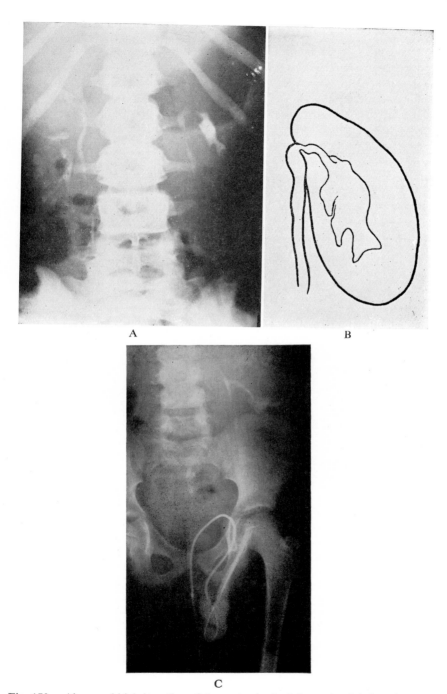

A   B

C

Fig. 170.   Abnormal high insertion of the ureter in the left renal pelvis in a four-year-old girl. As can be traced in the urogram, this ureter enters the pelvis from above. Pelvic reduplication exists on the right side. *C*, herniation of the left ureter in a nine-year-old boy with advanced hydronephrosis of the surgically solitary kidney above. There was no hernial sac; the ureter descended to the scrotum through the internal inguinal ring. A total of 26 cm. of redundant ureter was excised with oblique end-to-end anastomosis and 16 F. T-tube drainage. (Courtesy Dr. Hugh J. Jewett and Journal of Urology.)

renal sagging with increased ureteropelvic angulation and obstruction and increased hydronephrosis, total renal destruction is the usual end result.

Treatment demands relief of the obstruction and if carried out early enough, the kidney may be salvaged by ureteropelvioplastic procedures, particularly of the Y-plasty variety or, if long lineal ureterojuxtapelvioureteral stricture has developed, by the elongated incisional method of Davis with T-intubation (see Section XV, Chapters 3 and 4). Moreover, ureteropyelo-

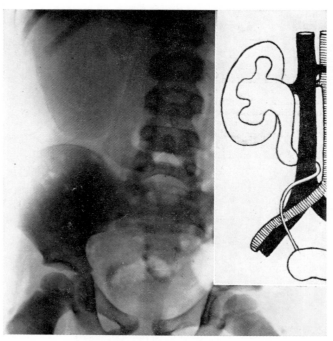

Fig. 171.   Right retrocaval ureter in a four-and-a-half-year-old boy. In the excretory urogram the greatly dilated upper third of the ureter is seen to terminate near the abdominal midline and at which point it passed behind and was compressed by the vena cava. Nephrectomy. (Courtesy of Dr. J. E. Marcel, Paris.)

neostomy may be employed with severance of the ureter from the kidney and its reimplantation into the lowermost pelvis to encourage free drainage. In carrying out plastic procedures of all varieties in these cases, postoperative infection, fibrosis and stricture commonly defeat the objective and later the kidney must be removed as it should be initially when the renal damage is hopelessly advanced and the condition of the renal mate permits. When nephrectomy is contraindicated and conservative ureteropelvioplastic procedures fail, employ permanent nephrostomy.

Congenital Postcaval or Retrocaval Ureter. This right-sided anomaly results from persistence of the early lateral fetal cardinal veins which branch around but largely lie anterior to the ureter. The mesial cardinal vein normally comes to form the inferior vena cava, yet fails to develop properly leaving the ureter encircling the anomalous vena cava from behind (Fig. 171). The clinical importance of postcaval ureter is concerned with its vascular compression by the vena cava, hydronephrotic renal injury, the common advent of severe infection and the resulting systemic symptoms. The vascular compression is brought about by squeezing of the ureter against the anterior spinal tissues by the vena cava in front. These changes and the symptoms produced define the urologic importance of the anomaly. Thirty-eight cases have been reported in which the urographic diagnosis was made preoperatively in five; operation was carried out in ten, the youngest of whom, Marcel's (1953) patient, was four and a half years of age (Shearer, 1949; Olson and Austen, 1950). Jacobson reported two cases, one of which was a child of one year, and Hofstetter also described a case in an infant one year old.

The *symptoms* are those of ureteral obstruction with or without infection. Midabdominal pain may be distressing; persistent urinary infection may be treated for long periods as "chronic pyelitis." Yet the diagnosis will rest upon complete urologic examination in which the correct identification is suggested by (1) a mesial displacement of the ureter over the spine, (2) demonstration of an S or sickle-shape ureterographic shadow at the point of obstruction with dilatation above and, as Randall (1935) noted "in the oblique films the ureter normally tends to fall away from the spine but when it passes behind the vena cava, it is observed to impinge against the lower lumbar spine." These findings were present in a three-year-old girl with abdominal pain but as yet without demonstrable ureteral obstruction and hydronephrosis.

Unless advanced renal damage by hydronephrosis and/or infection demands nephrectomy, the preferred *treatment* consists of disjoining the upper ureter well up in the pelvis so that after subsequent anastomosis, a large ostium will remain. The mobilized upper ureter is removed from behind the vena cava, and is placed in its normal position and course. Ureteropelvic anastomosis is performed making sure the mucosa-to-mucosa suture line is oblique rather than transverse in order to avoid postoperative stricture. Anderson and Hynes (1949) did this successfully. The mucosa-to-mucosa principle should guide the technical procedure. In some of the reported cases the ureter has been released by its division in the middle or at the lower end with positional correction, resection of redundancy and re-anastomosis, but this is likely to be followed by stricture. Disjoining the ureter from the bladder and restoration of the duct to the normal course may fail because of grave interruption of the blood supply of the lowermost ureteral segment. This complication or stricture has usually demanded secondary nephrectomy. More radical and questionable is section of the inferior vena cava for postcaval ureter as described and performed in one case by Cathro (1952).

Herniation of the Ureter. This rare variety of abnormal course of the duct has largely escaped urologic attention. Dourmashkin (1937) reported seventy-three collected cases of which twenty-seven were inguinal, thirty-five were femoral, and eleven were scrotal; of the last group six were associated with a hernial sac containing other structures. In four of the scrotal variety, the condition resembled that in Jewett's patient (1951), a nine-year-old boy (Fig. 170, C). The symptoms are predominantly those of ureteral obstruction which is frequently complicated by infection. Pain in the renal region and/or chronic pyuria may be the only manifestations. The diagnosis is made by urography in which the unusual looping course of the ureter into the scrotum or other hernial outlet is noted. Unless knowledge of the possibility of the anomaly exists the urogram may fail of correct interpretation, particularly when there is incomplete ureteral filling. When the condition of the kidney justifies its salvage, employ resection of the redundant ureter with oblique ureterorrhaphy; otherwise perform ureteronephrectomy.

III. ANOMALIES OF FORM, CALIBER AND STRUCTURE

Ureteral aplasia is associated with renal anomalies, notably agenesis (q.v.), but is common with hypoplasia of an entire kidney or of half of a double kidney (Fig. 106). The poorly developed ureter may have a small lumen or exist only as a fibrous cord. The orifice is smaller than normal and often cannot be catheterized or no orifice may be present. The condition is of no clinical importance except as a cyst may develop in occluded ureteral segments.

Congenital ureteral stricture is found at autopsy in about 0.6 per cent of children and is one of the most frequent discoveries at urologic examination in patients of all ages with "chronic pyelitis" or with persistent abdominal pain of ureteral origin (Campbell, 1939). We found 123 cases in 19,046 children examined post mortem, a ratio of one to 155. In adults so much upper urinary tract disease, notably infection and back pressure damage, occurs as the result of ureteral stricture that the identification of congenital ureteral stricture in this age group is statistically inaccurate because of frequent inability to distinguish between the congenital and acquired varieties.

The ureterovesical junction was involved most frequently in this series of 123 cases in infancy and childhood (51 per cent; Figs. 175–177), the ureteropelvic area in 34 per cent (Figs. 179, 180), and 15 per cent occurred in the body of the ureter (Fig. 181). The obstruction may be bilateral and multiple but we have never encountered more than three congenital strictures in the same ureter. In Bottomly's series of fifty-six cases, thirty-six were in the lower end of the ureter and eight were in the ureteropelvic area, and in eleven of his cases the ureters were reduplicated. In our series of 123 autopsy cases, the condition was on the right in thirty-one, on the left in forty-four, and bilateral in forty-eight. It is notable that three fourths of the children in whom we have demonstrated the lesion were under six months of age. This suggests its congenital nature; it has also been found in the fetus as in one of our cases at seven months. Apparently more boys than girls suffer this congenital lesion and in ratio of about two to one.

The *etiology* of congenital ureteral stricture is unknown.

Pathologically and histologically the condition is simply an abnormal narrowing of the duct comparable to similar narrowings so often observed in the lower urinary, gastrointestinal, pulmonary, vascular and biliary tracts.

Östling (1942) in an unusually fine study of autopsy material showed that many so-called ureteral strictures actually are only mucosal redundancies without adventitial changes and produce intraureteral folds and narrowings which may function as strictures (Fig. 172). Yet generally when the ureteral adventitial sheath is divided and the mucosa is drawn out longitudinally, the fold is found to represent a true narrowing. These strictures may be

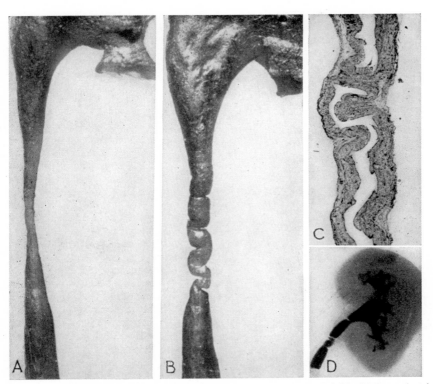

Fig. 172. Embryologic considerations in the genesis of ureteral folds, kinks and strictures. *A*, a cast of the ureter and the renal pelvis in a newborn. There is physiologic narrowing of the upper ureter below which is the normal main spindle of the ureter. No ureteral folds are present. *B*, cast of the ureter and the renal pelvis in the newborn. The ureteral folds proceed alternately from the opposite sides. *C*, ureteral kinks which appear as muscular folds with axial off-shoots of the loose adventitia. *D*, urogram of the ureter and renal pelvis in the newborn showing pronounced ureteral folds comparable to those shown in *B*, *C*. (Courtesy Dr. Karl Östling.)

sharply localized, extend over 1 to 3 cm. or more, and may be broad caliber or impassable. The usual site of elongated stricture is the ureteropelvic junction with marked hydronephrosis above. The stricture may involve one or both of reduplicated ureters. Structurally these congenital strictures show only an exaggeration of the normal ureteral narrowing although some fibrosis may be present, particularly in the mucosa (Fig. 173). Inflammatory changes are seldom observed except when secondary infection has developed; some observers have attributed the lesion to inflammatory ureteritis *in utero*.

With failure to identify stricture in reduplicated ureters, and this is

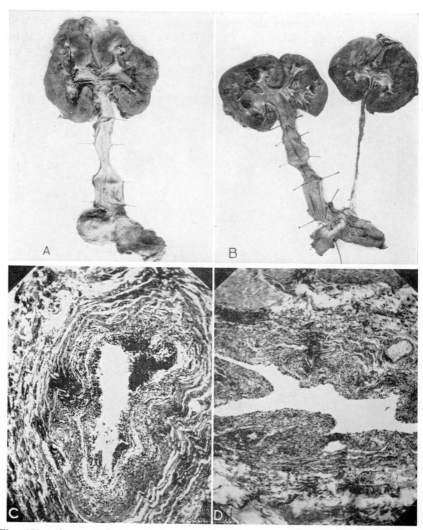

Fig. 173.   Congenital ureteral stricture as observed at autopsy. *A*, stricture at the ureteropelvic and ureterovesical junctions with marked dilatation between, in a six-month-old male. There is slight midureteral narrowing with moderate hydronephrosis above. Clinical manifestation: persistent pyuria. Histologically these obstructions showed sclerosis. *B*, pronounced dilatation and infection of the ureter and renal pelvis in a six-month-old girl with pyuria and fever. Three strictures are indicated in the right ureter: at the ureterovesical junction, at the junction of the lower and middle third, and of the middle and upper third. A probe is in the vesical outlet; the opposite kidney and ureter are normal. Histology in ureteral stricture in the young. *C*, there is moderate local mucosal inflammatory reaction because of urinary infection but there is little or no sclerotic stricture present. *D*, with prolonged infection and obstruction, scar is regularly deposited in the area of constriction. (Bellevue Hospital.)

usually due to failure to recognize that ureteral reduplication may exist, undue delay in instituting therapy is the likely result and this is of particular vital importance in infancy and early childhood. In one of our infant patients with stricture of one of reduplicated ureters, failure initially to identify the orifice of the normal ureter of the reduplicated pair greatly delayed uretero-heminephrectomy which was successfully performed when the child was

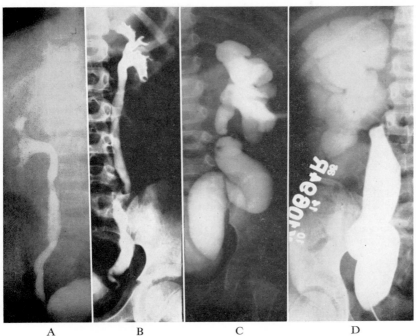

A   B   C   D

Fig. 174. Ureterovesical junction stricture. *A,* in a twelve-month-old girl with right renal infection and persistent pyuria. *B,* elongated and tortuous juxtavesical area stricture with ureterectasis and mild pyelectasis above. Chief complaint: recurrent pyuria. Treatment: ureteral resection, ureteroneocystostomy. *C,* left ureterovesical junction stricture in a twelve-month-old boy with marked urinary back-pressure injury above. Ureteronephrectomy. *D,* megalo-ureter and extreme right hydronephrosis consequent to right ureterovesical junction stricture.

twenty-eight months old; a badly infected ureter and pyonephrotic lower half of the kidney drained by the strictured ureter were excised.

Urinary tract back pressure above the stricture is manifested by ureteral dilatation, often with pronounced tortuosity or kinking, and hydronephrosis (Figs. 174–177). Extensive ureteral dilatation above a tight stricture may result in cyst formation and clinically simulate abdominal tumor while early massive hydronephrosis may even cause dystocia. Most massive hydronephrosis as discovered in late fetal life, neonatal, or early infancy results from congenital stricture of the ureteropelvic junction. The atrophic renal changes produced by compression and infection are pronounced and the end result is frequently a large fluid-filled thin walled parenchymal shell. Secondary

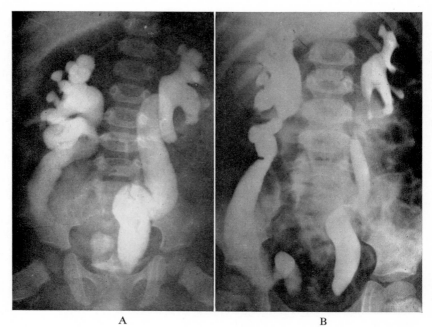

A   B

Fig. 175. Congenital bilateral ureterovesical junction stricture in a three-month-old boy with advanced upper urinary tract dilatation, infection and renal damage; examined because of persistent pyuria. Treatment: incision and plastic correction of obstruction. *B*, follow-up urogram four years later showing considerable anatomic improvement which was accompanied by striking functional improvement.

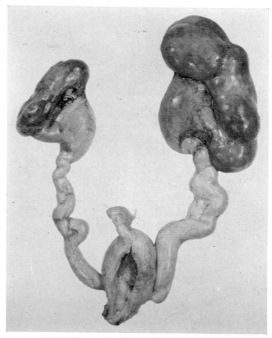

Fig. 176. Advanced bilateral ureterovesical junction stricture. Autopsy specimen in a six months old child whose condition was similar to that shown in Fig. 175 *A*. (Babies Hospital.)

344

hydronephrotic atrophy and fibrolipomatous degeneration of the kidney is a common late result, and anatomically simulates, and is to be differentiated from, congenital renal hypoplasia. Stricture at the ureterovesical junction frequently leads to massive dilatation of the ureter and a condition too frequently erroneously designated as megaloureter; here the duct may be dilated to the size of the colon and, rarely, may even be palpated trans-

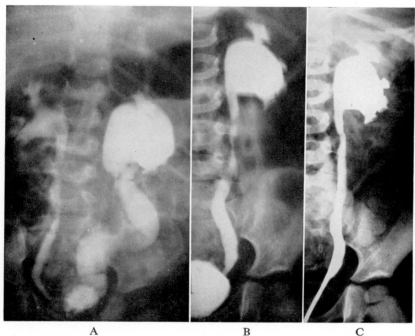

A   B   C

Fig. 177.   Congenital left ureterovesical junction stricture in an eight-week-old girl examined because of persistent pyuria since birth. There is extreme dilatation of the left upper urinary tract; the right upper tract is normal. Treatment: Periodic progressive ureteral dilatation. *B,* pyelogram after six months showing marked anatomic improvement. *C,* pyelogram two years later indicates unusual anatomic restitution; there was also striking functional improvement and the kidney was saved. This conservative therapeutic course was carried out with full knowledge that grave acute exacerbation of left renal infection would doubtless demand ureteronephrectomy. (Bellevue Hospital.)

abdominally. Properly, megaloureter must be considered a manifestation of neuromuscular dysfunction rather than as an organic obstructive disease.

Symptoms. The distressing symptoms of ureteral stricture are produced by the obstruction and reflex vesical irritation. There is commonly pain or tenderness along the course of the ureter, in the renal or general abdominal area, with backache, gastrointestinal disturbances (constipation and distention in particular); frequency and urgency of urination are the most usual vesical manifestations. In the absence of infection, bilateral ureteral stricture may give the clinical and laboratory picture of chronic interstitial nephritis as we have observed in six cases, in four of them by postmortem examination, and in two through surgical therapy. The urologic examination disclosed bilateral hydronephrosis, while the urinalysis and blood chemistry findings were those commonly considered diagnostic of advanced chronic interstitial nephritis. The renal injury and urinary toxemia causes these children to be poorly developed, pale and pasty. Although ureteral obstruction is almost never considered in the diagnosis and treatment of sclerotic nephritis, its etiologic possibilities should be more in mind. Occasionally with pronounced unilateral renal obstruction, the abnormal secretion and

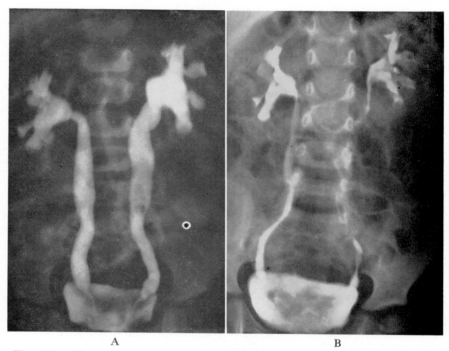

A   B

Fig. 178.   Bilateral ureterovesical junction stricture in a two-month-old female examined because of persistent pyuria. *A*, the intramural narrowing of the ureters is splendidly shown as is the dilatation of the upper ureters. Ureteral dilation. *B*, the same patient two years later; the urographic outlines of the upper urinary tract are essentially normal.

cellular content elaborated by this kidney may also cause the urinalysis to be thought indicative of nephritis as I have observed in several children and adults. This is but another indication for excretory urography which should be included as part of the diagnostic study when the clinical picture suggests nephritis. When excretory urography shows the need for further urologic examination, a complete cystoscopic study should be made.

Infection can be anticipated in all cases of ureteral stricture and the other symptoms of pyelonephritis or infected hydronephrosis are added to those of obstruction. Urinary tract infection was grossly evident at autopsy in twenty-eight of 123 cases of congenital ureteral stricture; nineteen of these were less than seven months of age. Moreover, the pyuria may be indefinitely perpetuated by the urinary stasis produced by the stricture; the usual diagnosis is "chronic pyelitis." Yet as in a twelve-month-old boy with congenital ureteropelvic junction stricture and a massive infected hydronephrosis, the diagnosis of renal neoplasm had erroneously been made.

Abdominal pain as a manifestation of ureteral stricture has not received

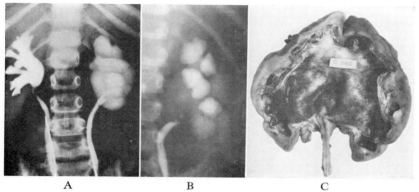

A   B   C

Fig. 179.   Ureteropelvic junction stricture; infected hydronephrosis. *A*, of the left kidney in a three-year-old boy. *B*, in a four-year-old girl examined because of "persistent pyelitis." Nephrectomy. *C*, removed kidney showing ureteropelvic junction obstruction.

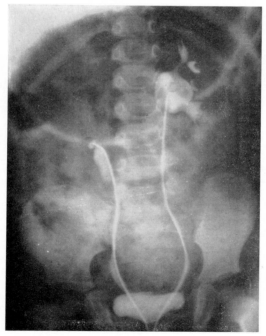

Fig. 180.   Bilateral ureteropelvic junction stricture in an eight-month-old girl examined because of persistent pyuria. The right kidney was completely destroyed by hydronephrosis; the ureterogram is sharply obstructed at the ureteropelvic junction. Nephrectomy. The left kidney was similarly obstructed but to less degree. Subsequently a Y-ureteropelvioplasty was successfully performed on the remaining kidney.

the important attention that it deserves and notably as a possible urologic symptom in young patients. The importance of this symptom in adults has been stressed but we have examined several children whose complaint was abdominal pain, particularly in the right or left lower abdominal quadrant. In practically every one of those who had right lower quadrant pain, the appendix had been previously and fruitlessly removed. Some of those with

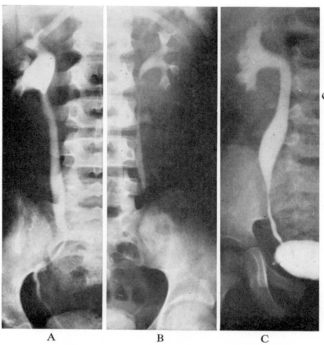

A   B   C

Fig. 181.   Stricture of the body of the ureter. *A*, in a two-year-old boy causing pain in the right lower quadrant for which the appendix had been needlessly removed. Symptomatic cure by progressive ureteral dilation. *B*, stricture of the left mid ureter in an eleven-year-old girl with continuous pain in the left lower quadrant and who had been thought to have "left-sided appendicitis." Symptomatic relief by therapeutic ureteral dilation. *C*, tight stricture at the junction of the middle and lower thirds of the right ureter in a twelve-month-old boy with balanitic hypospadias. An initial excretory urographic study was carried out because in one in three cases of genital deformity, the upper urinary tract is also anomalous. The excretory study prompted retrograde urography. Cystoscopic ureteral dilation.

left lower quadrant pain had been surgically explored on the theory that they might have inflammation of an appendix inversus or an appendicitis of a malrotated organ. Yet eradication of the urinary obstruction by periodic progressive conservative ureteral dilation regularly relieved these children of the abdominal pain. Occasionally added or more radical steps were necessary but in all instances it was observed that with the establishment of free drainage the abdominal symptoms disappeared (Fig. 181).

Diagnosis. Pyuria and pain persisting in one or both loins suggests ureteral obstruction. The diagnosis of ureteral stricture demands complete urologic examination in which satisfactory excretory urography will usually give the cue except when renal function is low. In any event, a complete urologic examination is required. Instrumentation of the ureter by the passage of catheters which are grasped by the stricture complements the urographic demonstration. A 3 F. catheter can readily be passed up the ureter of the newborn and in a child of one year a 4 F. instrument; grasping of a catheter of this size by the ureter of these respective ages or grasping of a 6 F. catheter by the ureter of an adult is presumptive of stricture. We have relied upon the grasping of ureteral catheters and the urographic demonstration of ureteral dilatation above the point of narrowing to make the diagnosis of stricture (Figs. 174–182).

These diagnostic criteria may be too conservative but they are likely to spare many patients needless ureteral instrumentation. Keyes stated that to be considered a ureteral stricture, the lesion must cause symptoms which are relieved by dilatation. We have not extensively employed in adults the diagnostic bulbs advocated by Hunner. His clinical studies on the ureter have perhaps done most to stimulate widespread interest in its lesions; Hunner relies upon the "hang" of the wax bulb for the diagnosis of stricture. A ureteral catheter tipped with an olivary wax bulb is passed to the kidney pelvis and gently withdrawn down the ureter. If the bulb is withheld at any point, and this is known as the "hang," a stricture here is inferred. His diagnoses on this criterion have been unfavorably regarded by many urologists since the hang may be caused by localized ureteral spasm or may be obtained at a point of physiologic narrowing such as the ureteroiliac crossing or at the ureterovesical junction. Yet a hang produced by ureterospasm is not repeatedly found at the same place unless a provocative local lesion exists.

Having passed the catheter, the diagnosis is confirmed by ureterography; the pelvis is usually variably dilated and the ureter above the stricture always shows ureterectasis (Figs. 174–183). Still the diagnosis of stricture should not be made on urographic findings alone; localized ureteral spasm may urographically simulate ureteral stenosis although the spasm rarely produces the identical pyelogram on all films in the same series or in films taken on different days unless there is a local pathologic basis, the nature of which should be determined.

Treatment. The conservative treatment of ureteral stricture is instrumental ureteral dilation which should be employed unless (1) the condition fails to respond promptly, (2) it is patently a surgical problem which requires ureteroplasty, or (3) when advanced renal disease demands ureteronephrectomy.

In the adult most therapeutic ureteral dilations are carried out through the McCarthy panendoscope as this instrument permits the passage of bougies up to 15 or 16 F. if so desired; it has always seemed to me that ureteral dilation to 14 F. is adequate in an adult.

In the young the problem is technically a little more difficult because of limitations occasioned by the small caliber of the urethra. In 90 per cent of children subjected to ureteral dilation by me, the Campbell 17 F. ureteral dilating cystourethroscope should be used (Section XIII); the 17 F. sheath permits the passage of Garceau or other types of ureteral dilating instruments up to 10 F. and the 19 F. sheath allows passage of ureteral instruments up to 13 F., the last caliber being considered beyond the requisites of this therapy in the young. When the urethral caliber does not permit ready

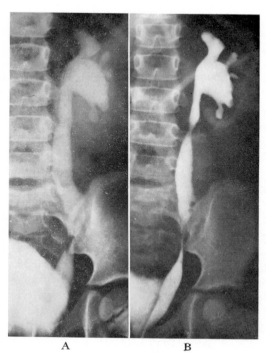

A   B

Fig. 182.   Congenital filiform stricture of the lower third of the left ureter (only kidney) in a three-year-old girl with recurrent pyuria and hematuria since birth (see Fig. 158). The right upper urinary tract was removed because of total destruction of the kidney and the massively dilated ureter which opened ectopic through a pinhole size orifice in the deep urethra. In the examination of the left upper urinary tract (A), the orifice of the ureter was found to be wide and slitlike in the posterior urethra near the bladder outlet and this caused periodic incontinence. The roof of the ectopic ureter was divided transurethrally high into the bladder to cause the urine to discharge into this viscus; this corrected the incontinence (see Fig. 158). The stricture indicated in the ureterogram was so tight that a "small" 4 F. catheter was tightly grasped. There were ureterectasis and hydronephrosis above the stricture as well as atonic (inflammatory?) dilatation below. The procedure indicated in Figure 137 was employed with longitudinal incision for 4 cm. through the stricture-bearing area with T-tube intubation for one month. B, postoperative pyelogram showing some anatomic improvement in the upper urinary tract. Although the ureterogram still suggests tight stricture at the operative site, one year postoperative a 12 F. bulb catheter could readily be passed to the kidney pelvis. Sterilization of the urine was promptly achieved.

atraumatic passage of the 17 F. cystourethroscope, it is introduced through a perineal urethrostomy opening.

In infants dilatation of stricture to 5 or 6 F. is usually adequate; for anatomic reasons a 17 F. dilating cystoscope should not be used in boys of less than four or five years old except as it is introduced through a perineal urethrostomy opening. It can usually be successfully employed in females from infancy. In many of these young patients the gravity of the ureteral obstruction, and notably at the ureterovesical junction, demands open surgical relief.

The success of ureteral dilation by catheters or bougies is proportional to the proximity of the stricture to the bladder, other factors being equal. While stricture of the body of the ureter frequently responds splendidly to ureteral dilation, instrumental dilation of stricture at the ureteropelvic junction is regularly ineffective, and here surgical therapy is indicated. As in urethral stricture, the condition is cured only when the stricture remains dilated. Sometimes, as in three children with tight ureteropelvic junction stricture of a solitary kidney, permanent nephrostomy drainage offers the only hope of relief, notably when infection deters ureteropelvioplastic procedures or, these having been done, incites fresh stricture formation. Sometimes temporary nephrostomy will spare the kidney, enabling its function to improve and its infection to be controlled.

Having achieved adequate dilatation of the ureteral stricture, the interval between subsequent dilations will vary with the individual patient, the criterion being the rapidity and degree of recurrence of the obstruction. It is unwise to repeat ureteral dilations oftener than once in ten days, particularly if general anesthesia is required. In some patients, dilation once in eight to ten weeks has been necessary while in others once in six months suffices. The fundamentals of dilatation are those observed in the conservative treatment of urethral stricture: (1) gentleness is imperative and (2) the lesion is adequately treated only when it remains dilated. Once free drainage is established, ureteral re-examination and dilatation should not be neglected. Having achieved improvement following adequate dilatation, both as to renal function and diminution of urinary infection, the patient should not be considered cured until the urine has been sterilized and free urinary drainage is maintained. As previously noted, chronic urinary infection frequently prompts the urologic examination which discloses the stricture. In some cases of chronic renal infection perpetuated by ureteral stricture, bacteriologic cure is achieved by dilatation plus chemotherapy, the last generally proving ineffective until the urinary stasis is eradicated. Occasionally cure results.

It should be borne in mind that all ureteral manipulations are traumatic despite utmost gentleness. The ureteral tissues should be given ample opportunity to regain physiologic stabilization by resorption of inflammatory indurate and postinstrumental edema, and to achieve local repair before being subjected to another instrumental assault, no matter how delicately performed. With conservative dilatation, periodic urographic check-up examination is essential and in this we are interested chiefly in the elimination of pelvic and ureteral retention, rather than the achievement of anatomic restoration. Occasionally the last is also noted (Fig. 181).

Radical surgical treatment of ureteral stricture is demanded when dilatation with bougies fails or is impossible. Several ureteroplastic procedures have been advocated for the cure of stricture but are of variable permanent value.

Strictures at the ureteropelvic junction may be treated by (1) Y-plasty of the Foley-Schwyzer type, (2) ureteropyeloneostomy with mucosa-to-mucosa suture, and (3) longitudinal incision with T-tube implantation for four weeks postoperative according to the method of Davis (Figs. 137–139). Occasionally mobilization of the ureteropelvic junction and retrograde dilation of the stricture have been successful but today are seldom employed; infection and subsequent localized scarring of the ureter frequently defeat a technically splendid operation. The advent of acute renal suppuration or hydronephrotic renal destruction demands nephrectomy. When an only

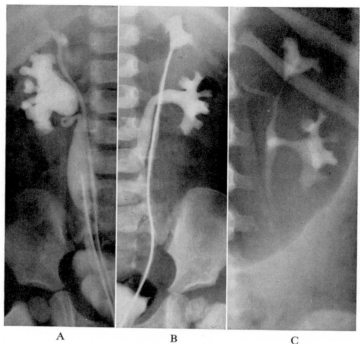

A   B   C

Fig. 183. Bilateral ureteral reduplication in a two-year-old girl examined because of persistent pyuria. There was found severe infected ureterohydronephrosis of the lower segment of the right kidney and a tight stricture of the dilated lower segment of the incompletely reduplicated left ureter at the point of bifurcation. B, preoperative composite urogram. C, postoperative urogram showing satisfactory anatomic restoration.

kidney is involved it is often necessary to establish permanent nephrostomy drainage.

If local conditions prohibit ureteropelvioplasty and especially when a ureter not sufficiently long for ureteroneopyelostomy will be left after excising the stricture bearing area at the pelvic outlet, employ longitudinal incision through the strictured area and an inlying ureteral nephrostomy tube (Cummings or McIver type) splint for two to four weeks. This has several times succeeded (Keyes, 1915; Davis, 1936, 1947) as it did in four of six children in whom I have employed it. These various procedures are described by ˙Moore in Section XV, Chapter 4; see also Figures 137 and 184.

When the only kidney is involved it is usually wiser to establish permanent nephrostomy drainage, although in two children I successfully employed the Foley-Schwyzer posterior Y-plasty on the only kidney; in two others it failed, largely because of infection and secondary sclerosis.

Stricture in the body of the ureter in our hands has responded best to longitudinal incision and postoperative intubation after the manner of Davis (see Section XV, Chapter 4). A two-year-old girl had but one kidney; a lineal ureteral stricture was situated at the level of the first sacral vertebra, and the duct opened ectopic at the bladder neck and adjoining deep urethra. Preoperatively the stricture firmly grasped a 4 F. catheter although it permitted the passage of a 3 F. instrument. Longitudinal incision of the elongated stricture was done and T-intubation was employed for one month. Twelve months postoperatively, a 14 F. bulb could be passed without difficulty through the previously constricted area (Figs. 139, 182–184). Resection of the midportion of the ureter and other varieties of ureteror-rhaphy usually fail unless the ureter is at least moderately dilated; the surgical stricture becomes as dense as that present preoperative. When ureterorrhaphy is employed with excision of the stricture-bearing area, the duct should be united by an oblique anastomosis in order that resulting scarring at the operative site will be elliptical with the maintenance of a relatively patent lumen rather than transverse and followed by a tight circular scar.

In a two-year-old girl with persistent pyuria, examination disclosed incomplete duplication of the upper third of the left ureter. At its junction with the ureteral branch to the uninvolved upper pelvis, there was a tight stricture of the dilated ureteral segment draining the lower pelvis which also was dilated. On the right, there was complete ureteral reduplication with tight ureterovesical junction stricture of the greatly dilated duct to the comparably dilated infected lower pelvis. The upper right pelvis and its ureter were small but normal (Fig. 183). Right ureteroheminephrectomy and left longitudinal incision and intubation of the strictured area was the treatment (Fig. 133, *A*).

Stricture at the ureterovesical junction not responding to dilation should be operated upon if the kidney is worth saving. Yet not all patients with congenital ureterovesical stricture require radical treatment. In an eight-week-old girl with left ureterovesical junction stricture and massive uretero-hydronephrosis and examined because of persistent pyuria, the initial findings would appear to be an indication for ureteronephrectomy (Fig. 181). Yet the mother was extremely cooperative, and conservative periodic progressive ureteral dilation was undertaken and proved strikingly successful, the procedure being carried out with full appreciation that the advent of acute exacerbation of infection might demand immediate ureteronephrectomy.

In performing the periodic progressive instrumental ureteral dilation in patients of all ages a word of caution is given against overtreatment—too many dilations, too energetic, too rapid or too frequent. Once the diagnosis is made, the first dilation usually is not carried out for ten to fourteen days, the next after an interval of three to four weeks, the next after six or eight weeks. As improvement is evidenced by increased facility of instrumentation, improved renal function, control or eradication of infection, and urographic

demonstration of favorable anatomic change, the periods between instrumental dilations is increased to three, four and six months or more. Although it is essential to have these patients under observation for what to
them may seem an unduly long time, the actual number of treatments is
relatively few. These recommendations are made to forestall treatment of
patients and notably of children according to the practice of some urologists
who carry out the same ureteral dilation every week, week in and week out.

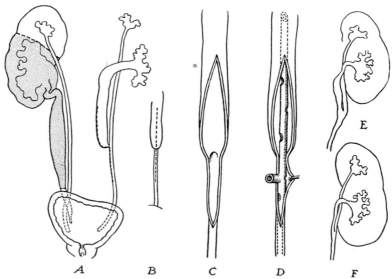

Fig. 184.   Schema of conditions in child whose urograms are shown in Figure 183. *A*,
shaded area indicates ureterorenal segment removed by a right ureteroheminephrectomy.
The major portion of the persistent pyuria originated in this segment. The condition and
function of the upper remaining part of the right kidney were good. The dotted line in the
left ureter indicates the incision made for intubation and correction of the stricture at the
junction of the moderately dilated ureter to the lower pelvis and the normal ureter to the
upper pelvis; *B*, line of incision in left ureter from mesial aspect; *C*, ureter open after *B*
indicating junction with branch to the upper left renal pelvis; *D*, T-tube intubation of *C*;
E and *F*, tracings of urograms made several months postoperative and indicating satisfactory eradication of the stricture. *F* is tracing of Figure 183, *C*.

The repetitious trauma of such therapy alone may well be expected to induce
fibrotic ureteral stricture.

Cystoscopic ureteromeatotomy employing the Campbell or other type of
ureteral meatotome (Fig. 157) is frequently successful provided adequate
follow-up ureteral dilation is employed.

When employing the ureteral meatotome, the meatus and contiguous stricture are incised upward for at least 1 cm., this to be followed by periodic
cystoscopic dilation with bougies 8 to 12 F. according to the age and size
of the patient (Fig. 159). This dilatation is employed at progressively
lengthening intervals of one to twelve months as the character of the stricture
and success of therapy demand. With the establishment of free drainage,
both functional and anatomic improvement in the injured tract above the
stricture will be observed (Fig. 181).

When ureterovesical junction stricture fails to respond to cystoscopic incision and periodic progressive dilatation, open operation should be performed if the kidney warrants saving. Transvesical ureteral meatotomy with periodic follow-up dilation is the procedure of choice (Fig. 890). When the stricture is tight and upper tract dilatation and injury are pronounced, the blockage is widely incised upward, often 1.5 to 2 cm., and oversized intubation (10 to 20 F. two-eye or four-eye catheter, according to the caliber of the dilated ureter, and preferably with whistle tip) is left indwelling for two to four weeks. It is most important that this indwelling tube fit loosely because variable contractions of the duct will occur with the relief of urinary backpressure. Suture of the incised ureteral mucosa to the bladder mucosa can be done but is not necessary. The indwelling tube in the ureter is brought out suprapubically together with the suprapubic drainage tube. When the lesion is bilateral, the procedure is carried out on both sides at the same sitting. Postoperative recontraction of the incised ureteral stricture may be anticipated unless prophylactic cystoscopic overdilation is continued at progressively lengthening intervals.

In extremely dense congenital ureterovesical junction stricture, severance of the ureter from the bladder with reimplantation (ureteroneocystostomy) has been widely advocated in recent years and in preference to wide ureteral meatotomy which generally is my choice (Fig. 903). Because of the anatomic limitations in many patients and particularly in the very young, ureteroneocystostomy may become an extensive and often traumatic operation; the blood supply and innervation of the low ureter are seriously disturbed or may be severed. The danger of postoperative surgical stricture is essentially as great as that due to recontraction of the widely incised ureterovesical junction stricture itself. Following ureteroneocystostomy, ureteral reflux practically always occurs in the absence of a tight ureteral postoperative restricturization, and on this score the procedure has little merit over cystoscopic or transvesical wide ureteromeatotomy. Yet the damage from vesical ureteral reflux is less than that caused by the initial obstruction itself.

In advanced ureterovesical junction stricture, the ureters are frequently dilated to the size of the bowel and by longitudinal dilatation may become at least twice normal length with consequent angulation and multiple kinkings, most of which become firmly fixed and frequently increase the obstructive factors. In some of these cases, the longitudinal redundancy is so great that, completely mobilized, the ureter reaches to the patient's knee.

In several cases of extreme ureterectasis and elongation, I have employed the procedure outlined in the next two paragraphs.

When the condition of the patient warrants, both as to general physical improvement and increased renal function, the bladder is opened and the ureterovesical junction is widely incised either unilaterally or bilaterally according to indication. In some cases we have mobilized one ureter from the bladder and straightened it out throughout its course to the kidney at this initial sitting. During this ureterolysis, numerous dense fibrous adhesions will be eliminated and secondary kinks released. Extreme ureteral

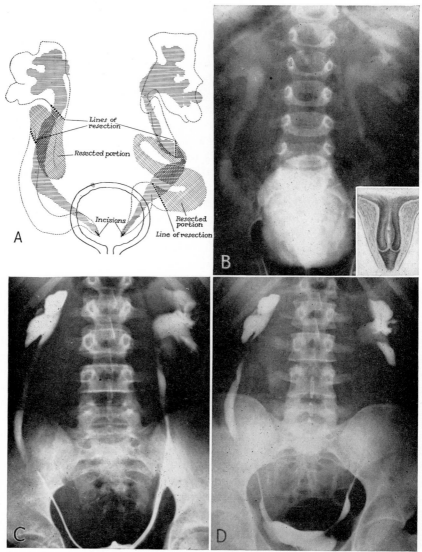

Fig. 185. Advanced bilateral ureterovesical junction stricture surgically treated. The patient, a seven-month-old boy, was examined urologically because of persistent fever for eight weeks. The initial pyelographic findings are indicated in schema *A*, being shown in dotted line; the condition is relatively similar to that shown in the urogram in Fig. 175, *A*. The boy was also found to have congenital valvular obstruction of the prostatic urethra (insert *B*). By progressive stages there was performed left nephrostomy, right ureterostomy, bilateral transvesical ureteral meatotomy, bilateral ureteral resection, transurethral resection of the urethral valves; ureterorrhaphy with resection of 5 inches of redundant ureter from the left side and 4 from the right with oblique end-to-end anastomosis. *B,* urography one year postoperative shadowing marked anatomic restitution. There is still moderate ureterectasis and ureteral irregularity. The outlines of this pyelogram are shown by transverse shading in *A. C,* pyelogram made twelve years postoperatively. The ureters are now essentially straight. The right kidney has largely undergone secondary hydronephrotic atrophy, the left kidney having taken over practically the full excretory load (phenolphthalein excretion 55 per cent in two hours). *D,* pyelogram seventeen years following the initial operation, the anatomic and functional findings being essentially those noted five years previously. The boy's growth has been normal and he is now in college. The only abnormal urine finding is a faint trace of albumin; culture sterile.

356

redundancy is not uncommon and this is treated by excision and oblique end-to-end anastomosis to leave the patient with a straight ureter and unobstructed dependent drainage. Later the opposite ureter is similarly treated if necessary.

The transvesical intubation of the ureter with a large catheter (16 to 26 F. according to age and size of the patient and degree of ureteral dilatation) provides free drainage for ten to thirty days following the ureterovesicoplasty, by which time the ureteral anastomosis is adequately healed. One boy with bilateral ureterovesical junction stricture and widespread dilatation of each upper urinary tract (Fig. 185) and in whom the procedure was started at the age of seven months, was so desperately ill and septic when first seen that he was twice given up for dead his initial night in the hospital. Bilateral nephrostomy was instituted and later 4 and 5 inches of redundant ureter were resected from the right and left ureters respectively, and a congenital valvular obstruction of the prostatic urethra was transvesically relieved. Twenty-one years later his physical development is normal, he engages in full activity, the urine is sterile, but urinalysis reflects the permanent residual nephritic damage consequent to the original grave injury and infection. The urine shows a faint trace of albumin with an occasional hyalin and granular cast while the urograms indicate permanent mild dilatation of the ureters. The left kidney pelvis is moderately dilated but the finer markings are clear while the right pelvis is contracted and shows hydronephrotic atrophy with minimal function. Size 13 F. dilating bulbs and bougies pass readily to each pelvis attesting their respective patency. Another boy whose original condition and subsequent treatment were almost precisely similar is now finishing college. Four and six inches of redundant ureter were removed from the left and right side respectively as part of the surgical treatment.

A transvesical pull-through procedure employed by me offers a relatively simple yet most effective method of eradicating tight, dense ureterovesical stricture, particularly if there is more than a sharply localized narrowing (Fig. 906, Section XV). This operation may have been done by predecessors but I have not seen it described elsewhere. As shown in Figure 906, the bladder is opened through a midline incision or, as I prefer, by a transverse incision. A small curved probe is then introduced into the lower end of the constricted ureter and, using the probe as a guide, the ureter is incised upward 2 to 4 cm. This incision divides the bladder wall and frequently goes into perivesical tissue near the ureterovesical junction. The last is of no moment because free suprapubic drainage subsequently will forestall extravasation.

Having divided the intramural and adjacent ureter on its roof, the thickened mucosa, submucosa and surrounding scar will be readily observed. This ureteral opening is grasped with clamps at four equidistant points, a deep circular cuff incision is made to mobilize the intramural ureter as a tube, these tissues being divided and/or dissected from the musculature of the bladder wall and from its immediate perivesical vicinity. The mobilized low ureteral segment is then gently pulled through into the bladder. In pulling the ureter through it will be noted that the periureteral adventitia dissects away readily; in this maneuver, the tip of the knife handle assists greatly in freeing adhesions, the ureter pulling through much as a finger being withdrawn from an inverting glove finger.

When there is unusual ureteral redundancy this will be eradicated according to the length of ureter pulled through. In some of these cases in the young as much as 6 inches of redundant ureter on each side have been eliminated at one sitting. Occasionally high fibrous periureteral adhesions hold the ureter firmly fixed, usually at a point of angulation or other secondary obstruction. Such interference must usually be later corrected by exposure of the ureter through the loin and ureterolysis. In some of our cases further resection of ureteral redundancy with end-to-end oblique anastomosis or wide ureteropelvic anastomosis has proved necessary.

The condition of the child or the advanced damage of a kidney which must be salvaged frequently demands preliminary ureterostomy or nephrostomy, maintained until such time as the status of the patient and his renal function warrant radical ureteroplastic attack. Many of these young patients are desperately ill when first seen and complicating infection is frequently grave. In the surgical management of bilateral infected hydronephrosis of this causation, it is frequently necessary to employ bilateral nephrostomy as the initial procedure and perhaps even up to a year. When the kidney must be saved and the stricture cannot be adequately treated, make the nephrostomy permanent.

Congenital Ureteral Valves. These are present as transverse folds of redundant mucosa which are made prominent by their circular muscle fibers, rarely if ever cause urinary obstruction and usually disappear as the child grows. The studies of Östling (1942) have splendidly demonstrated the genesis of many of these so-called valves (Fig. 172). In an extensive study of the ureter in the fetus and newborn, Gerard noted the relatively large caliber of the channel at this period and showed that valvelike folds and kinks are not uncommon, especially in the lower portions. These folds usually appear in proximity to the ureterovesical junction, generally within the first 3 cm., but only rarely cause urinary obstruction. They are next most common in the pelvic segment of the ureter, are less frequent in the iliac portion and rarely appear in the lumbar spindle. Wolfart found them in one in five of 100 autopsies in the newborn, but found none in adults thus examined. Probably 10 per cent of newborn children show such formations; in our autopsy series they were found in twelve of 123 children with congenital ureteral obstruction but were not found in 32,834 adults. In short, they are commonly found in the fetus, nearly all disappear by the fourth month of life, and are clearly to be distinguished from pathologic ureteral valves or kinks. Persisting, they may cause obstruction and thus become of clinical importance; Wharton reported such a case in a twelve-year-old girl (Fig. 185) and Wall and Wachter (1952) recognized the condition in a six-month-old boy in whom they resected the involved segment but the infant subsequently died. They could find but seven cases reported, all but one being unilateral.

The *symptoms* of ureteral valve obstruction are those of ureteral stricture; Ostry (1948) reported hypertension caused by congenital ureteral valve obstruction. The diagnosis is rarely made during life, but the uretero-gram may be expected to suggest the condition as it did during life in a seventeen-year-old boy at Bellevue Hospital and had postmortem confirma-tion (Fig. 186, *C*). In this case ureterograms showed several transverse filling defects in the lower segment giving the channel a somewhat sausage-like appearance. Upon this finding the diagnosis was made. Such transverse filling defects may not mean valves but rather (1) plication of the ureter, (2) restricting periureteral bands, or (3) compression by extraureteral blood vessels.

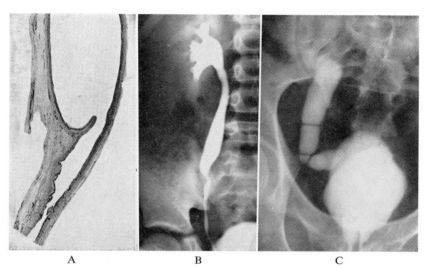

A   B   C

Fig. 186. Congenital ureteral valves causing obstruction. *A*, specimen removed from a girl of twelve years whose reduplicated ureter from the left upper pelvis opened ectopic just beneath the urethra and caused urinary incontinence at birth. The pyelogram was almost an exact duplicate of *B* in a three-year-old boy. Valve specimen histology courtesy of Dr. Lawrence R. Wharton. *C*, congenital ureteral valves in a seventeen-year-old boy in whom the diagnosis was confirmed by autopsy. The peculiar sausage-like appearance noted in the ureterogram was caused by the transverse folds of the valves. (Bellevue Hospital.)

The *treatment* of ureteral valves is largely that of the renal complication, frequently demanding ureteronephrectomy. In one instance plastic surgical removal of the valve itself was successfully performed.

Congenital Dilatation of the Upper Urinary Tract (primary megaloureter, primary ureteral atony, ureteral neuromuscular dysplasia). This reflects faulty neuromuscular development, being distinguished from the large ureters secondary to obstruction. In 1923 Caulk coined the term megaloureter to denote congenital dilatation of the duct without lengthening, angulation or kinking, in the absence of demonstrable obstruction and attended by a relaxed immobile ureteral orifice, altered ureteral dynamics, prolonged infec-tion or neuromuscular disease. Isolated cases alleged to result from neuro-muscular dysplasia of the ureter alone have been reported by many ob-servers. Yet in the personal examination of several hundred patients with dilated ureters, in later years chiefly infants and children, there have been only two cases in which seemed warranted the probable diagnosis of congenital ureteral atony (Fig. 187), and not attended by neuromuscular vesical disease (Section XII) or obstruction. In the personal cases seen and comparable to most of the cases reported in the literature, we have not been able to identify the condition as other than a collateral manifestation of neuromuscular vesical disease, prolonged infection, or obstruction, either congenital or acquired (Campbell, 1952).

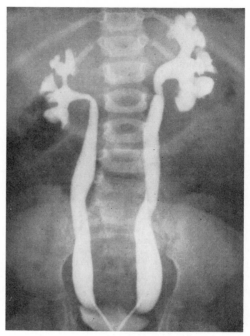

Fig. 187. Atonic neuromuscular disease of upper urinary tract associated with bilateral achalasia at the ureterovesical junction. The ureterovesical junction readily accommodated an 11 F. ureteral bulb without difficulty. Mild secondary infection. The lateral ureteral dilatation in the absence of longitudinal dilatation is believed by some to signify an atonic neuromuscular rather than obstructive (ureterovesical junction) condition. The author does not attach great importance to this observation or distinction.

Etiology. Hinman (1935) has summarized the etiologic theories of megaloureter as follows: (1) persistence of a sausage type of fetal ureter, (2) obstruction by fetal valves which have subsequently undergone normal regression but have left a dilated ureter, (3) neuropathic dilatation, (4) spasm of the ureteropelvic junction (pelvic dilatation), (5) inflammatory dilatation, (6) atonic dilatation (*a*) with, and (*b*) without an insufficiency of the ureterovesical orifice, (7) insufficiency of the ureterovesical valve, (8) spasmodic contraction of the bladder, and (9) ureteral stasis to toxins. One or another of these theories will explain all cases of congenital megaloureter but some are more plausible than others.

Persistence of the disproportionately large fetal ureter may well be due to a faulty neuromuscular mechanism as evidenced by atony and absence of peristalsis (see ureteral atony in neuromuscular vesical disease). As previously indicated, congenital megaloureter is to be distinguished from the massive ureteral dilatation due to congenital ureterovesical junction stricture for example (Fig. 174). Chwalla's theory of ureteral dilatation resulting from obstruction during fetal life and consequent to a persistent vestigial membrane has also been adduced to explain megaloureter. Beer (1912), Braasch (1928), and others offered the explanation of inflammation rather than obstruction to cause the enormously dilated ureter. Opponents of this last theory point out that inflammation causes stricture and not dilatation, despite the fact that dilatation due to chronic inflammation is a commonly observed urologic phenomenon. *In fine,* no explanation fits all cases and with the exception of theories 1 and 3 as given by Hinman, it is difficult to explain the development of megaloureter on the nonobstructive basis although it is possible that at the time the examination is made the obstruction may no longer be demonstrable. Wide dilatation of the ureter without demonstrable cause was recorded in twenty-six (unilateral 5, bilateral 21) of 19,046 autopsies in infants and children (1:907). Yet neuromuscular vesical disease seemed likely in four of these; Hirschsprung's disease was not mentioned. Ureteral overdistention causes pressure anesthesia of the nerve endings in the dilated channel to subdue or disrupt the reflux arc so that the stimulus for strong peristaltic contractions is lost or is ineffectual. Adding to this the effects of the increasing hydraulic pressure of the large mass of urine in the ureter, further dilatation occurs, a situation fundamentally comparable to the ultimate flabby dilatation of the bladder wall in late prostatic obstruction.

Although congenital megaloureter has frequently been thought analogous to congenital megalocolon (Hirschsprung's disease), and similarly to congenital dilatation of the bile ducts (Kelsey, 1948), no suggestive proof of this was offered until the remarkable recent studies of Swenson and his co-workers (1948 et seq.) shed some light on this most important and interesting problem.

Swenson et al. showed that in patients with megalocolon there is a striking diminution of parasympathetic ganglion cells in Auerbach's myenteric plexus in the constricted nonperistaltic rectal or rectosigmoidal bowel segment. As a result, colonic peristaltic waves stop at the aganglionic segment to produce functional obstruction at this point with great dilatation and hypertrophy of the proximal colon above. In proof of this by application of the therapeutic test, resection of this aganglionic segment cures the disease with restoration of normal bowel function. The rectum, rectosigmoid and bladder are embryologically one (gut) with a common parasympathetic innervation through the pelvic nerve (nervi erigentes) distribution in which one major branch goes to the lower bowel and the other branch to the bladder. There is vesical dysfunction in about half of all cases of Hirschsprung's disease and although it may not cause recognized symptoms, the condition is readily demonstrable by cystometry which shows a dilated atonic bladder with a low intracystic pressure until the viscus is well distended. Commonly in Hirschsprung's disease there is associated megaloureter, generally bilateral, an observation made by Swenson and several others including the writer. By comparable histologic study of the bladder wall, Swenson et al. (1951) found a striking diminution or absence of parasympathetic ganglion cells from their usual site, this being chiefly in the vesical adventitia and in the areas adjacent to the entrance of the ureters into the bladder where these cells are normally in greatest concentration, and are in slightly lesser numbers about the seminal vesicles in the male and in the vaginal septum in the female. In this variety of megaloureter not only are parasympathetic ganglion cells fewer in number in the areas just mentioned but they are less well developed and functionally defective. Ganglion cells are found in small numbers in normal ureters and even in megaloureters.

On the basis of these findings Swenson believes that ureteral peristalsis is maintained down to the aganglionic ureterovesical junction area with relative adynamic obstruction (achalasia) and wide dilatation of the tract above. Because of the subnormal parasympathetic nerve function, the bladder is unable to empty itself completely, residuum and intracystic pressure increase, the latter commonly amounting to 30 to 35 cm. of water pressure and affording an increasing hydrostatic force against which the kidneys must excrete and ureteral peristalsis propel. Megalobladder, dilated ureter(s) and hydronephrosis result. The great straining necessary to urinate, employing the abdominal and other accessory muscles, helps to increase the vesical and upper tract dilatation. It is this group of cases of neuromuscular vesical disease in which limited transurethral resection of the vesical outlet is frequently beneficial even though cystoscopically demonstrable obstruction may not be present. Because of this decidedly mixed and overlapping parasympathetic dysfunction, megaloureter should be considered a collateral manifestation of neuromuscular vesical disease rather than an isolated ureteral lesion and distinctly to be separated from wide upper tract dilatation consequent to long-standing infection or non-neurogenous obstruction.

Symptoms of megaloureter may be entirely absent but generally there is persistent pyuria, urinary frequency, hematuria, pain in the back and/or bladder, these symptoms being present singly or in combination. With increasing renal injury the systemic manifestations of urinary toxemia and renal failure ensue.

The diagnosis will be made by cystography, cystoscopy, ureteral chromomeatoscopy, and retrograde pyelography if necessary, demonstrating the features of megaloureter previously described. Cystography generally discloses massive ureteral reflux while cystoscopy and ureteral instrumentation reveal no obstruction. Estimation of the residual urine must be made promptly at the completion of voiding lest inaccuracy occur consequent to the down rush of urine from the greatly dilated upper tract reservoirs. Cystometry will confirm the diagnosis of neuromuscular vesical disease. Although the ureteral orifice may appear snugly constricted, it is not strictured nor even tight in primary megaloureter and will permit the ready passage of relatively large ureteral dilating instruments.

Treatment of megaloureter is at present most unsatisfactory; the procedure which has brought about most improvement has been the establishment of prolonged suprapubic drainage, making sure that it in truth drains the renal pelves as well. Parasympathomimetic drugs, such as mecholyl, acetylcholine, doryl, urocholine, trasentine and so forth, are without substantial value, doubtless because of the paucity of normal parasympathetic ganglion cells for these drugs to act upon. By the use of urine collecting paraphernalia such as a small rubber flounder bag anchored to the upper thigh, patients of all ages on permanent suprapubic drainage are able to be active and carry on comparatively normal lives. Transplantation of the ureter from the variably aganglionic segment to a more normal area has been employed by some successfully, this neuroanatomic explanation being the only logical one under the circumstances and in view of this most recent knowledge. Reduction of the caliber of the greatly dilated ureter by removal of a generous full length strip of the duct proved ineffective in three children as reported by Nesbit and Whithycombe (1953). Hutch (1952) described a technique to bring about contraction of the extremely dilated ureter; through the opened bladder the lower end of the duct is mobilized and pulled through the bladder wall. The intravesical segment of the ureter is left 1.5 to 2 cm. long and its "under" side is sutured to the underlying bladder wall with the notion of simulating the so-called physiologic (elongated) ureteral valve (Figs. 908 and 909; Section XV, Chapter 5). The operation proved most satisfactory in eradicating vesicoureteral reflux in a half dozen children in the hands of both Hutch and Flocks. Occasionally transurethral vesical neck resection will permit the patient to empty his bladder and gain essentially the same therapeutic value as permanent suprapubic cystotomy. The combat of infection remains one of the most important considerations and this must be strictly according to specific bacteriologic indications.

Diverticulum of the Ureter. This may be congenital or acquired. This rare congenital condition is an outpocketing from the ureter and contains the same muscular and mucosal layers as does the ureter. Some fifteen cases of blind ending branches of bifid ureter forming diverticula have been reported including one of mine (1936), while ten cases of segmental hydroureter have been called ureteral diverticula. Yet there have been thirteen cases of true diverticula recorded, one of which described by Culp (1947) was situated at the ureteropelvic junction and held a thousand cubic centimeters. In another case reported by McGraw and Culp (1952), the upper third of the ureter was the site of sacculation. Most of these cases have been found at the juxtavesical area although a few were at the sacroiliac level.

Acquired diverticula developing as ureteral back-pressure blowouts above obstruction or consequent to or following ureterostomy lack some of the ureteral coats and regularly show infection. Forty such cases of ureteral diverticulum have been reported and some of these have been in the young including an autopsy case of Kretschmer's in a child and Rathbun's striking clinical case in a ten-year-old boy, the lesion occurring bilaterally in the juxtaseminal vesicle area. The etiology is not yet clear but doubtless the diverticulum often develops as an accessory ureteral bud; this explanation probably fits most cases. Secondary diverticulum may arise as a blowout formation proximal to obstruction and is characteristically globular in outline.

The ureteral obstruction may be congenital or acquired. In the congenital variety, the process has usually been in operation since the fifth or sixth month of fetal life when urinary renal secretion starts. In the cases reported to date, the sex incidence has been about equal, the lesion appearing slightly more often on the right than on the left; about 5 per cent are bilateral. In two thirds of these the lesion sprung from the lower third of the ureter and chiefly the juxtavesical region.

These diverticula are important as possible causes of ureteral obstruction in which the overdistended sac of the juxta-ureteral diverticulum may com-

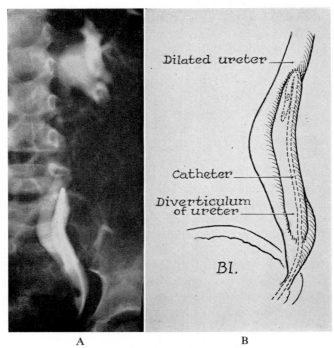

A   B

Fig. 188. Diverticulum of the ureter. This four-year-old girl with recurrent pyuria complained of continuous pain in the left side. A blind-ending ureteral pocket was demonstrated by ureteral catheterization and retrograde pyelography. The distended diverticulum sac compressed the ureter to cause obstruction with mild ureteral dilatation and pyelectasis. The sac was excised with cure. (Bellevue Hospital.) From author's article, courtesy American Journal of Surgery.

press the adjacent "normal" ureter. Pyuria and pain in the loin are the chief complaints; pain was the principal symptom in a man with recurrent pyuria and was the outstanding symptom in a four-year-old girl whose diverticulum of the ureter I removed.

The diagnosis of "chronic pyelitis" is frequently made in these cases; the futility of chemotherapy is noted. Abdominal pain may result from distention of the sac or may be a ureterovesicoenteric reflex manifestation and is apt to lead to needless laparotomy. A diverticulum of clinical importance may be the site of urinary retention, calculus formation, rupture or, as in my case, cause pressure on the adjacent normal ureter (Fig. 188).

The diagnosis is made by retrograde or excretory ureterography or by operation, the retrograde ureterogram being of greatest diagnostic value, as it demonstrates the localized bulbous or sausage-like dilatation. In my patient, from the initial ureterogram, I thought the catheter had been turned back in the ureter by a stricture. Stereoscopic urography will at once demonstrate the lesion and show its precise relationship to the ureter (Fig. 188). The treatment is excision of the diverticulum and is regularly satis-

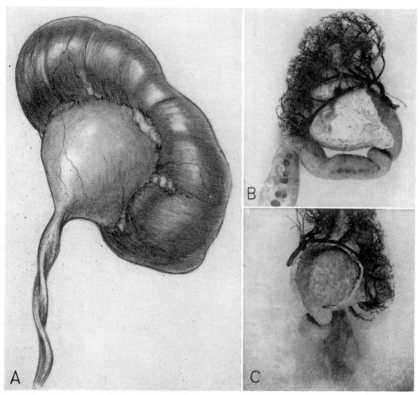

Fig. 189.   Torsion (spiral twists) of the ureter. *A,* as observed in an infant at autopsy at Bellevue Hospital; there is secondary hydronephrosis. Ureteral twists of the ureter of late fetal life; corrosion specimens. *B,* anterior view. *C,* lateral view from pelvic aspect. (Courtesy Dr. Karl Östling.)

factory. In Rathbun's case the bilateral sacs, adjacent to the seminal vesicles, were excised and the ureters were transplanted into the bladder. When advanced isolateral disease or technical difficulties prohibit extensive employment of either of these two methods, ureteronephrectomy must be performed.

Spiral twists or **torsion of the ureter** are extremely rare being noted but twice in 12,080 autopsies in children (Fig. 189). The embryologic explanation is failure of the ureter to rotate with the kidney and when the condition is pronounced, obstruction and secondary hydronephrosis result. In a four-day-old boy with imperforate anus and peritonitis, bilateral ureteral torsion caused advanced hydronephrosis (Fig. 189), and in a two-week-old boy at the Nursery and Child's Hospital, bilateral congenital torsion of the ureter with advanced hydronephrosis was the only lesion found. As Östling's (1942) studies suggest, ureteral twists or torsions are a phase of fetal mucosal redundancy. The lesions may be diagnostically demonstrated by stereoscopic ureterography but I have not encountered a case clinically and apparently the condition with urographic confirmation has not yet been observed.

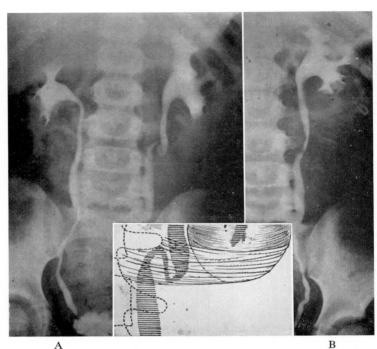

A   B

Fig. 190.   Congenital left ureteral kink in a five-year-old girl with persistent pain in the left loin for three years and normal urine. *A*, urogram was obtained with the child horizontal, upright, and in Trendelenburg position, indicating the firm fixation of the kink. Insert: conditions found at operation. A dense fibrous band passing from the lower pole of the kidney medially transfixed the ureteral kink. *B*, pyelogram two months after mobilization of the kink and high suspension of the kidney. Complete relief from symptoms. A slight narrowing of the ureter at the point of kinking is apparent in the postoperative pyelogram; this was treated by therapeutic ureteral dilation. (Bellevue Hospital.)

Ureteral kinks are seldom congenital but result from secondary angulation consequent to longitudinal dilatation of the ureter and secondary to peripheral obstruction such as ureteral stone or stricture, or stenosis of the external urethral meatus, for example (Fig. 190). Occasionally a true congenital kink is encountered as was observed in the left ureter of a premature boy. In mono-ovular twins observed post mortem at Bellevue Hospital, there was a sharp S-shaped kink at precisely the same point in each left ureter and, oddly enough, also identical transduodenal bands. Kinks high in the ureter are most likely to produce symptoms; the angulation generally appears where the ureter leaves its fixation to the peritoneum to pass to an abnormally mobile kidney. With sagging of the kidney and ureteral twisting or angulation, obstruction develops to be manifested by the characteristic symptoms of ureteral blockage including, with sudden sharp kinking, the renal colic of Dietl's crisis. The symptomatic picture is essentially that of supravesical obstruction in which urinary infection and its train of manifestations are frequent complications.

The *diagnosis* is usually made at the time of complete urologic investigation performed because of pain in or about the course of the upper urinary tract or because of persistent infection. The diagnosis is made by ureterography, preferably stereoscopic, and with the patient in the vertical as well as in the Trendelenburg position (Fig. 190, *A*). The kink remains fixed.

Treatment. Many unfixed kinks will disappear following eradication of a distal obstruction while others will be relieved by a belt to support the kidney. In a five-year-old girl examined urologically because of persistent pain in the left loin, a kink in the upper third of the ureter appeared identical in both the excretory and the retrograde pyelograms (Fig. 190) and at operation was found firmly fixed by a broad band of scar which crossed from the lower pole of the kidney to the spine and produced a mild hydronephrosis. The ureter at the point of obstruction was mobilized, the duct straightened out and the kidney suspended to prevent recurrence of the angulation. Subsequently, ureteral dilation for correction of the ureteral stricture obstruction was periodically performed. In this case, as sometimes happens, a moderately dense stricture was found at the site of kinking and *in utero* undoubtedly caused the obstruction which induced the renal sagging with angulation at the point where the kink existed.

Congenital hernia of the ureter has been previously described (Fig. 170)

Vascular Compression of the Ureter. This blockage by anomalous renal vessels has been discussed under Anomalies of the Kidney. Apparently no proved cases of primary vascular obstruction of the lower ureter have been reported, but secondary vascular obstruction is probably not rare although it generally fails to be diagnostically recognized (Fig. 142). In secondary compression the dilated ureter is compressed against the vessel, ureterovesical junction stricture being the commonest initial cause of the ureteral dilatation in these cases. The condition was clinically recognized in three children; in only one of these, a girl of thirteen months, was operation performed and the diagnosis confirmed. Here an artery and a vein, presumably uterine (the condition of the patient did not warrant extensive dissection), firmly compressed transversely the right ureter which was dilated above a ureterovesical junction stricture. Following division of these vessels the compressed area of the ureter became fully expanded and in subsequent ureterograms, the transverse vascular filling defect no longer could be seen.

The symptoms of vascular obstruction of the lower ureter are indistinguishable from those of ureteral stricture and together with the treatment have been considered elsewhere under aberrant vessel ureteral blockage at

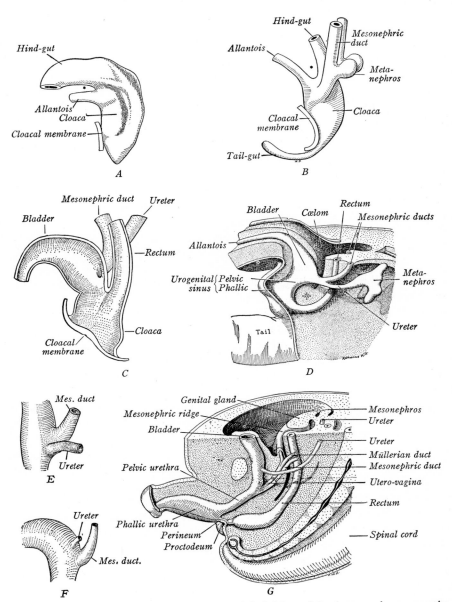

Fig. 191.   Embryology of the bladder. Partial division of the human cloaca, as schematically illustrated as viewed from the left side. *A, B,* at 3.5 mm. and 4 mm. respectively
(Arey after Pohlman; × 50). *C,* in fetus at 8 mm. (× 50). *D,* at 11 mm.; × 25 (Arey
after Keibel). The asterisk indicates the cloacal septum. Completed division of the
human cloaca and associated changes as schematically shown from the left side. *E, F,* at
six weeks (× 50) and seven weeks (× 35) respectively, denoting the absorption of the
left ureter and mesonephric duct into the wall of the bladder. *G,* at nine weeks; × 50
(Arey after Keibel).

the renal level. Having relieved the vascular obstruction, the stricture or other distal blockage must be eradicated, and the urine sterilized before the patient can be considered cured.

Ureteral compression by the vas deferens where it crosses the duct was observed at autopsy at Bellevue Hospital in a four-year-old boy; the ureter was strictured at this point so that the major obstructive factor could not be precisely determined.

EMBRYOLOGY OF THE BLADDER

By the sixth week *in utero* the urorectal septum has separated the cloaca into a posterior rectal segment and an anterior vesicourethral division from the dorsal surface of which emerge the ureteral stalks and wolffian ducts

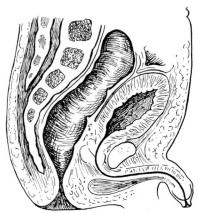

Fig. 192. Normal high position of the bladder in the newborn male. Recognition of this high vesical position in early infancy is clinically important in estimating vesical distention both clinically and for needle, trocar or open cystostomy.

(Figs. 150, 191). The upper portion of this anterior segment becomes the bladder while the inferior segment becomes the posterior urethra in the male, and the entire urethra in the female (Fig. 191). The urachus passes from the uppermost portion of the bladder to the umbilicus and is formed by a condensation and fibrosis of the allantois. Occasionally the urachus fails to close, thus giving rise to a fistula or to cyst formation (Figs. 194, 195). Because of its cloacal derivation, the bladder is primarily an entodermal structure surrounded by coats of mesenchymal muscular and areolar tissue. The trigone, a wolffian duct derivative, is largely mesodermal in origin. Because of its hind gut derivation, it receives blood and nerve supply from the same segmental derivation, a matter of considerable clinical importance in the diagnosis and treatment of neuromuscular vesical disease in particular. As a corollary, the rectal tone as determined by digital examination will usually reflect that of the vesical outlet.

In infancy the bladder is essentially an abdominal organ partly as a result of its tubular derivation from the urachus, and partly because the

distended viscus is too large and long for the comparatively small pelvis
(Fig. 192). As the child grows the bladder settles into the pelvis to assume
the anatomic relationships observed in adults.

ANOMALIES OF THE BLADDER

The principal vesical malformations are

1. Agenesis
2. Hypoplasia (dwarf bladder)
3. Reduplication
4. Diverticulum
5. Exstrophy
6. Urachus cyst
7. Urachus fistula
8. Trigonal folds
9. Cloacal formation

Vesical Agenesis. Absence of the bladder is extremely rare and of anatomic rather than clinical interest. Ten cases have been reported but some
recorded occurrences of the condition do not bear strict scrutiny because
they are simply extreme manifestations of exstrophy, hypoplasia or contracture. The ureters open externally or into a dilated urethral pouch but
commonly they are absent as are the kidneys. When kidneys and ureters
are present, the condition usually leads to an early fatal pyelonephritis. We
found seven instances in 19,046 autopsies; two of these were anencephalic
monsters, but in each of the seven cases other grave anomalies coexisted
including absence of the kidneys and ureters in five, absence of the cervix,
absence of the vagina, malformed uterus, tubes and imperforate anus in
one, absence of the penis in another, and in another polycystic liver and
kidneys, meningocele, polydactylism, split tongue, cor biloculare, and diverticulum of the sigmoid.

Faulty development of the urogenital sinus with or without atrophy of
the allantois produces vesical agenesis. Surviving birth, the infant with
vesical agenesis usually dies of pyelonephritis although the anomaly is not
always incompatible with prolonged life. When the child lives, the dilated
ureters opening into the urethra act as urinary reservoirs and the musculofibrous tissue at the constricted orifices assumes a sphincteric action and
prevents incontinence (Huber, 1936). As in renal agenesis, other urologic as
well as non-urologic anomalies regularly coexist.

Hypoplasia. Dwarf bladder is extremely rare, is usually one of several
anomalies of the urinary tract and its interest is largely academic. Coexisting
anomalies are almost always incompatible with life. A hypoplastic bladder
measuring 2 by 0.8 cm. was found in a stillborn male at the Babies Hospital, with hypospadias and horseshoe kidney (Campbell, 1937).

Reduplication. Vesical reduplication or double bladder may be complete
or incomplete, the complete variety being the more common. Senger and
Santare (1951) proposed the following simple classification of congenital
bladder divisions:

   I. *Sagittal or Longitudinal*
      (A) Complete reduplication of the bladder
      (B) Incomplete reduplication of the bladder (vesica biparta)
      (C) Incomplete sagittal septum
  II. *Frontal or Transverse Divisions*
      (A) Complete frontal septum
      (B) Incomplete frontal septum
      (C) Hourglass bladder
 III. *Multilocular Bladders*

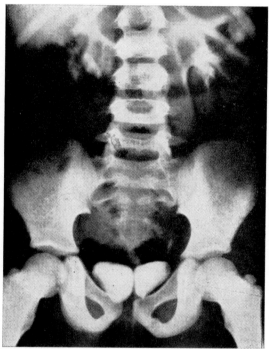

Fig. 193.   Double bladder. Demonstration by excretory urography. Each bladder was joined with its own urethra and penis. (Courtesy of Dr. Reed M. Nesbit.)

In *complete reduplication* there are two separate bladders (vesica duplex, Fig. 193), and frequently in these cases there is rectal reduplication. There may be reduplication of the müllerian duct derivatives such as the fallopian tubes, uterus and vagina. In the male there are commonly two penises and urethras but I have not found a record of more than two testicles (cf. Lanman, 1931; Mezan, 1929; Nesbit, 1933; Wehrbein, 1940; Burns et al., 1947; Senger and Santare, 1951). The embryologic etiology is unknown but obviously a splitting of the vesico-urethral anlagen occurs. Associated rectal anomalies suggest whether this schism occurred before or after the division of the cloaca by the urorectal septum. Thirty-four cases of double bladder have been reported.

In *incomplete vesical reduplication* the organ may be divided by a complete or incomplete sagittal septum into a right and left segment or by a complete or incomplete frontal septum dividing the bladder into an anterior and a posterior division (vesica biparta). With horizontal midvesical constriction, an hourglass bladder may form; sixteen cases were collected by Ockerblad (1940), ten being males, the youngest was eleven years of age. The four prevailing theories of the embryologic cause of incomplete vesical reduplication are concerned with (1) the atavistic relationship of hourglass bladder normally found in some animals (Krasa and Paschkis, 1921), (2) the persistence of ureteric membrane (Chwalla, 1927), (3) unequal growth of two bladder anlagen (Gruber, 1928), or (4) complete or incomplete splitting of the bladder anlage, complete splitting resulting in two separate bladders.

In vesical reduplication the ureter from each kidney drains into the isolateral segment; the urethra may be reduplicated or not. Edwards (1933) noted the reduplicated vesical compartment always contains a ureter and its posterior segment is normal bladder wall, the septal wall is of fibrous tissue with a mucous membrane covering on each side, the absence of muscle fibers from the interlocular septum favoring the contention that initially the ureter failed to perforate the mucosa and submucosa of the bladder while the remainder of the tube is patent and passes through the membrane. The musculature of the bladder appears later than the union of bladder and ureter. In short, it has been suggested by many that these added loculi are akin to ureterocele (q.v.) initially being a variety of blind ending (intramural) ureter into which a communication with the bladder cavity is eventually established (cf. Chwalla). In multilocular bladder there are as many ureters as loculi (cf. Senger and Santare, 1951; also Wehrbein, 1940).

The malformation is usually accompanied by other urogenital anomalies; its chief interest lies in its possible clinical resemblance to vesical diverticulum, a sharp distinction between the two conditions being essential. Although diverticula sometimes contain ureteral orifices, their genesis is usually associated with obstruction and their musculature is seldom as complete as that of the bladder. Because of the gross anatomic similarity to and inadequate conception of the genesis of diverticulum, several cases of diverticulum have been reported as double bladder.

Several bizarre varieties of congenital multilocular bladder have been described, being triple or even quadruple. In some of these reduplications the conformation of the bladder outline suggests the designation hourglass, especially in the vertical variety in which the ureter(s) open into the lower compartment. The diagnosis of vesical reduplication is made by cystoscopy; by cystography the condition may be splendidly shown especially in the oblique and lateral positions.

Treatment consists of excising the diseased segment of the reduplicated bladder or removal of the septum and complicating calculi, obstruction and infection. In some instances ureteroneocystostomy may be required to save the kidney if it is worth preserving or ureteronephrectomy if it is not salvageable.

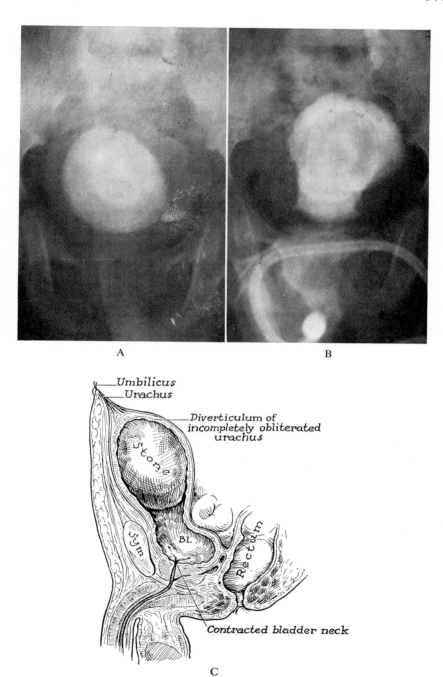

Fig. 194. Diverticulum of the urachus in a two-year-old boy with congenital contracture of the vesical outlet. *A*, large stone in the diverticulum; *B*, the sac is cystographically outlined. *C*, schema of *B*. (Bellevue Hospital.)

Congenital Vesical Diverticulum. When a diverticulum of the bladder is encountered in a child with infravesical obstruction the condition is probably congenital. True congenital vesical diverticulum is extremely rare; the demonstration of vesical neck obstruction in the newborn may be difficult. The condition has been found in the fetus and newborn and constitutes about 5 per cent of all diverticula (Fig. 194). In 1937 I reported uncomplicated congenital vesical diverticulum found post mortem in a boy of seven days, in a girl of five weeks, and in a girl of three months. In the second case the left ureter opened into the diverticulum. Apparently five times as many male children develop diverticulum while in adults the ratio is ten to one. In addition to nine instances discovered post mortem we have observed twenty clinical cases of vesical diverticulum in infants and children but in most the obstructive factor could not be ruled out. Despite the high incidence of diverticulum in adults, in nearly all of these the lesion is acquired, having formed as a back-pressure blowout process consequent to peripheral obstruction.

The *etiology* of diverticulum may be summarized as

(1) Obstruction, which is the usual primary cause (see section on obstruction (Hinman)

(2) Intrauterine conditions (congenital variety)

    a. Retention in the fetus due to temporary occlusion of the urethral mucosa (Englisch)

    b. A superabundance of embryonic tissue in the bladder wall

    c. Formation of excess of epithelial tissue at the fusing edges of the wolffian and allantoic elements of the bladder and a temporary failure of epithelialization between the two

    d. Supernumerary ureteric buds

    e. Patent urachus, the probable cause of all cases found at the dome

Those who believe all diverticula are congenital observe that the lesion generally occurs near the ureteral orifices where the longitudinal bladder muscle fibers are absent and outpocketing is facilitated. Others believe diverticula on or about the trigone represent dilatations of anomalous ureteral stumps, and that diverticulum of the bladder dome is a form of incomplete urachal cyst (Figs. 194, 195). The fact that over 90 per cent of all diverticula in children are found near the posterior angles of the trigone or in the dome lends some weight to these hypotheses of an embryogenic genesis. Yet until proved otherwise, in all cases infravesical obstruction must be assumed to exist (cf. Kretschmer). In short, diverticula may generally be considered as bladder wall blowouts through the separated detrusor muscle bundles and produced by chronic increased intracystic back pressure. The theory of temporary occlusion of the fetal urethra by agglutination of the epithelial lining (Englisch) is the soundest advanced in embryologic explanation of congenital diverticula and implies the obstruction factor. Hyman (1923) observed a juxta-urethral diverticulum in the absence of obstruction in three boys—three months, three and nine years of age.

Infravesical obstruction such as contracted bladder neck, valves of the posterior urethra, or chronic neuromuscular vesical disease with spastic sphincterospasm is not uncommon even in young children, in many of whom the clinical manifestations of the condition appear early (Figs. 194, 250). On this basis the condition must be considered congenital. Diverticulum occurs in 5 per cent of all children with infravesical obstruction and similarly in 10 per cent of adults. The greater delicacy of the bladder wall in infants and young children explains the relatively high incidence of diverticulum secondary to obstruction; in some of these patients the sacculation reaches two to five times or more the capacity of the bladder itself.

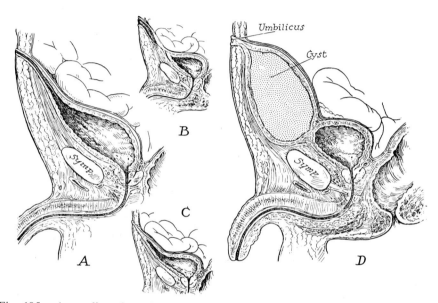

Fig. 195. Anomalies of urachus closure. *A,* patent urachus. *B,* blind external ending urachus. *C,* blind internal opening urachus. *D,* urachus cyst.

In adult males, the lesion is nearly always an acquired manifestation and as a complication of one of the various forms of prostatism, and in the female vesical neck contracture is the usual cause.

Diverticula are usually rounded or oval, communicate freely through their orifices with the bladder cavity, vary greatly in size, and in the congenital form muscle fibers will always be found in their walls, a point of academic differentiation from the acquired variety. A sphincteric action of the muscle about the orifice is sometimes observed cystoscopically. Not only are diverticula likely to be multiple but in 5 per cent are the site of stone deposit or, occasionally in adults, of malignant tumor. Sometimes a stone fills the diverticulum and extends into the bladder cavity in dumbbell formation (Fig. 194). A three-year-old boy with congenital contracture of the vesical neck showed four diverticula, one on each lateral wall behind the ureter, one on the dome, and one on the bladder floor in the midline behind the ureteric ridge. A four-year-old boy with vesical neck contracture showed an enormous diverticulum and another in the midline below—a total of three. As these diverticula enlarge they frequently draw out the ureteral orifice so that the duct discharges into the sac as I have observed in several children and even bilaterally. In a four-year-old boy with congenital contracture of the vesical neck and a residuum of 130 cc. of urine, the left ureter opened into a diverticulum springing from the bladder floor just behind the inter-ureteric ridge and to the left of the midline (Fig. 254). Removal of the obstruction and the diverticulum with transplantation of the ureter to an adjacent portion of the bladder produced a most satisfactory result, completely eliminating the residual urine. Subsequently the urine was sterilized. Recheck examination fifteen years later showed mild dilatation of the transplanted ureter and its renal pelvis but the kidney function was essentially normal.

As the diverticulum enlarges it may compress the ureter to change the course of the duct and produce secondary ureteral obstruction.

Symptoms. Vesical diverticulum is likely to be suspected in children only when, after apparently emptying the bladder, the patient waits a few seconds and is again able to pass several cubic centimeters or ounces more (*pis en deux temps*). When this is performed with regularity in patients of any age, diverticulum should be suspected. This symptom is to be distinguished from the occasional occurring temporary spasm of the vesical outlet, particularly when the patient is attempting to urinate in the presence of another person. Coexisting symptoms are attributable to complicating obstruction and infection with pyuria, frequency, dysuria, hematuria, vesical pain, installment emptying of the bladder, or the passage of extremely foul urine or purulent debris. Urinary decomposition commonly occurs within the sac. Sometimes the urine from the diverticulum passed after first having emptied the bladder is nearly all pus and stinking.

Installment emptying is sometimes simulated in the absence of diverticulum when the upper urinary tract is enormously dilated; here the prompt bladder refill is urine drained down from the dilated upper urinary tract. As a corollary in diagnosis, when there is extensive upper tract dilatation and bladder neck obstruction is suspected, in the determination of the residual urine in the bladder, catheterize at once after urination or an erroneous estimation will be made because of rapid emptying into the bladder of the large dilated upper tract reservoir. Because of the symptomatic manifestations in vesical diverticulum and particularly when pyuria exists, the diagnosis of "chronic pyelitis" too frequently satisfies the physician. The persistence of this symptom picture for more than three or four weeks at the utmost, demands thorough urologic investigation.

The *diagnosis* of diverticulum is readily made by cystoscopy and/or cystography (Figs. 194–196). While excretory cystography may suggest the nature of the condition, the most satisfactory demonstration of the lesion is achieved by retrograde cystography. Here stereoscopic anterior-posterior and lateral-oblique cystograms should be made lest a retrovesical diverticulum be overlooked.

The *treatment* is diverticulectomy, together with the removal of existing obstruction, and eradication of complicating infection. When the ureter opens into the diverticulum, it must be transplanted to the bladder following resection of the sac except when, by a plastic maneuver, the sac can be so removed as to allow the orifice to remain untouched and such vesicoureteral valve function as may exist is left undisturbed. Having removed the sac, the vital consideration is eradication of the infravesical obstruction, whether this means prostatectomy or other procedure. Unless this is done, the operation is incomplete (cf. Section XV, Chapter 5). Finally, the urine must be sterilized.

Congenital absence of the urinary sphincter in an otherwise normal lower urinary tract is extremely rare; the sphincteric deficiency is common enough

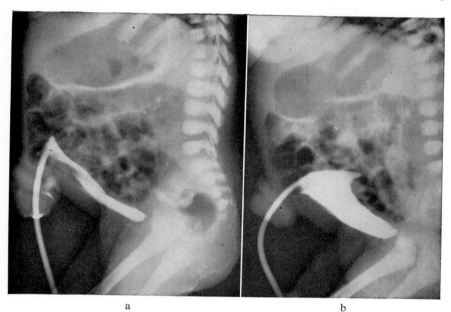

a   b

Fig. 196. Patent urachus in a newborn infant girl. *a,* Catheter has been inserted into protruding redundant umbilicus and contrast medium fills urachus and bladder. *b,* Bladder more completely filled; it appears to be attached to umbilicus. (Courtesy of Dr. R. W. Nichols and Dr. R. M. Lowman.)

with exstrophy and advanced varieties of epispadias. Several operations for its cure have been devised, most of which were based upon the principle of the external rectus fascial sling carried downward beneath the vesical outlet. Doolittle (1952) and Taylor and Berry successfully employed vesicourethropexy, the posterior urethra, vesical neck and adjoining bladder wall being fixed to the symphysis and recti. Yet before undertaking an operation it should be determined that the deficit is due to congenital muscular deficiency and is not a phase of neuromuscular vesical disease.

Exstrophy of the Bladder. Ectopia vesicae is manifested by an absence of the lower abdominal and anterior vesical walls with eversion of the posterior bladder wall (Fig. 197). The ureteral orifices are usually readily found and freely discharge urine externally. The condition is one of the worst congenital afflictions of mankind; the patient is urine soaked, foul smelling, and a social nuisance. Friction of the soaked clothing against the tender, highly sensitive, extruding vesical mucosa and adjacent macerated skin edges produces great discomfort. The chief vital danger in exstrophy is pyelonephritis (ascending renal infection) which is commonly fatal in the early years of life. Untreated, most of these patients die of ascending pyelonephritis before the twenty-first birthday; one half die in early childhood, and two thirds are dead by the tenth year. It was found at autopsy only once, a thirty-year-old male, in 32,834 autopsies in adults.

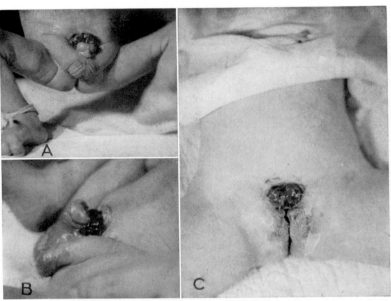

Fig. 197. Exstrophy of the bladder. *A*, in a boy of six weeks; anterior-posterior view. The penis is spadelike and the scrotum is partially cleft. *B*, lateral view of *A*. *C*, bladder exstrophy with excoriation of the perivesical area and vulva by constant soaking in irritating decomposing urine. Female, one year.

The incidence of vesical exstrophy is fortunately low being estimated at about one in forty to fifty thousand individuals. In our study of 19,046 autopsies in children, there were nineteen cases, an incidence of 1:1002 which suggests, by comparison, its relation to an early death. The oldest child was three and a half years of age; fourteen were males and five were females. Higgins (1943) observed the anomaly in twins.

Exstrophy is denoted as (1) incomplete (superior vesical fissure), or (2) complete (lower or inferior vesical fissure). In the rare incomplete exstrophy the defect in the abdominal wall is relatively slight, and the bladder wall protrusion is meager. The pubes are united and the genitals are normal. Incomplete exstrophy is usually readily curable by a plastic closure of the bladder and abdominal walls.

Complete exstrophy is the usual finding; the posterior bladder wall protrudes *in toto*. There is epispadias and separation of the pubis (Figs. 197, 198). The vesical mass appears fiery red, bleeds easily, and is exquisitely tender to touch. Its mucocutaneous margins are sharply defined and sclerotic. The umbilicus is generally located somewhat lower than normal and even may be obliterated by scarring at the upper margin of the exstrophy. If the extruding bladder is reduced, the sharp walls of the hernia ring can be felt. Rarely exstrophy is complicated by intestinal openings in the extroverted area, a condition believed to result from early rupture of the cloacal membrane with exposure of the undifferentiated cloaca, and hence the anomalous enteric orifices (Johnston, 1913). The pubes are widely separated (3 to 8 cm.; Fig. 198) and there is epispadias (Fig. 199). Because

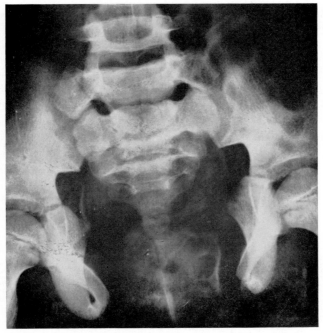

Fig. 198. Exstrophy of the bladder in an eleven-year-old boy showing congenital absence of the pubis which causes difficulty of locomotion in many of these patients; they waddle when they walk. The bones of the pubic girdle in front are joined by a band of fibrous tissue.

of the wide pubic separation, the child commonly waddles or shuffles, due chiefly to the outward rotation of the femurs. Malformations of the rectus muscles and fasciae are reflected in large inguinal and/or femoral herniae (Fig. 199).

Genital anomalies always accompany exstrophy. The penis is a rudimentary broad stump, split or grooved above, as a result of the wide open epispadiac urethra (Figs. 197, 199). The urethral sphincters are incomplete and on the floor of the posterior urethra the verumontanum and the lateral prostatic walls are often seen. The scrotum is smaller than normal, often cleft, and frequently there is cryptorchism. In the female the lesion is similar except that the clitoris is cleft and the labia minora are widely separated anteriorly to expose the vaginal orifice. Coitus, pregnancy and delivery are possible. The urethra is often present, and wide open. The nineteen cases in our autopsy series (one adult) were variously accompanied by ureteral aplasia and ectopia, vesicorectal fistula, absence of the urethra, and aplastic urethra. Ureteral reduplication is frequent in exstrophy and even double penis has been observed. Incomplete exstrophy is in some instances an accompaniment of epispadias.

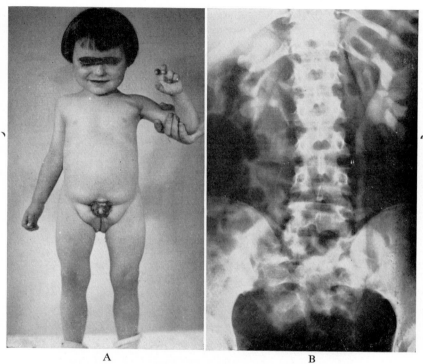

A   B

Fig. 199. *A*, bladder exstrophy in a three-year-old girl. Ureterosigmoidostomy performed employing Higgins' technic. *B*, excretory urogram seventeen years later after the patient had given birth to a child. The upper urinary tract shows remarkably little dilatation. The pubis was absent. The blood Wassermann test was 4 plus at time of initial operation; antiluetic therapy apparently was successful.

Coexisting nonurologic anomalies are also of high incidence. These include spina bifida (Fig. 200), hemivertebrae, clubfoot, absent bones (chiefly pubis), and malformed bones, cleft palate, harelip, malformation of the bowel with vaginorectal fistula, rectal prolapse, imperforate anus, stricture or absence of the rectum; sometimes the rectum is represented only by an anal dimple.

Etiology. The cause of exstrophy remains unknown; several theories have been advanced to explain the condition, the bases of these conceptions being (1) mechanical, (2) pathologic, and (3) embryologic. The mechanical theory invokes (1) rupture of the bladder during fetal life ("Bersten Theorie"), the rupture being caused by bladder wall weakness or urethral obstruction, but this remains unproved (von Geldern, 1924) nor does it explain epispadiac formation; (2) a short or absent umbilical cord has been adduced in explanation, as has (3) transposition of embryologic anlage (ectopia cloacae, a complicated exstrophy) due to a change in position of the vitelline duct. The theory based on pathology advances the notion that intrauterine ulceration of the anterior bladder wall occurs, results from infection or irritation and, by skeletal involvement, there is wide pubic separation (Keith, 1908). The embryologic explanation makes more sense,

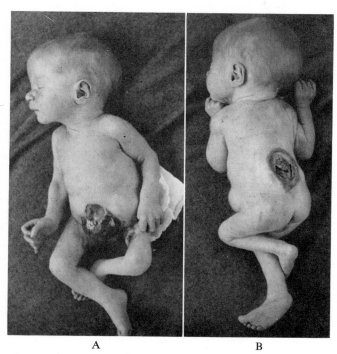

A   B

Fig. 200. *A*, extensive exstrophy of the bladder and colon with large umbilical hernia. Many of these patients have other accompanying malformations, most of which are serious as is the meningocele in this case (*B*). In short, the child was mal-closed both anteriorly and posteriorly. (Bellevue Hospital.)

and is based on failure of the mesoderm to develop locally (Mall, 1908; Wyburn, 1937; see also Patten and Barry, 1952, infra) thus involving the inferior abdominal wall as well as the pubic and spinal skeletal defects (Figs. 201–205).

Of the several theories which have been advanced to explain exstrophy of the bladder, to date the most widely accepted one is that of Gilies (1923) wherein is postulated a forward displacement of the cloacal membrane as a result of which the mesodermal structure comprising the lower abdominal wall fails to develop from the genital papilla to the umbilicus. This theory not only explains exstrophy but also the development of associated anomalies such as epispadias, cleft of the clitoris, labia and scrotum.

The newest interpretation of the probable embryologic mechanism involved in the genesis of estrophy and epispadias is that of Patten and

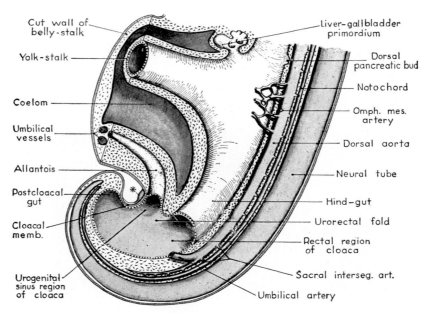

Fig. 201. Primary relations of the cloacal membrane to the unfused primordia of the genital tubercle and to the belly-stalk during the 4th week. The right tubercle primordium is indicated by an asterisk. (Courtesy, Drs. B. M. Patten and Alexander Barry.)

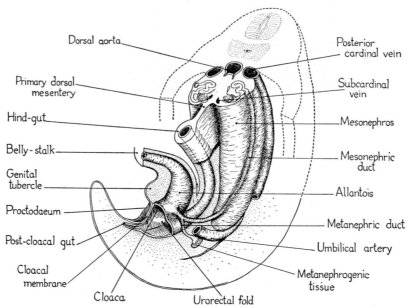

Fig. 202. Sagittal section of embryo of the 5th week showing the primordia of the genital tubercle fused in the mid-line. (After Kelly and Burnam, slightly modified, from Patten "Human Embryology," courtesy of The Blakiston Company.)

Barry (1952). According to them the key to an understanding of exstrophy of the bladder lies in the correct interpretation of the origin of the commonly coexisting epispadias. Although human embryos showing stages in the development of epispadias are wanting, they believe that it is nevertheless possible to postulate a series of hypothetical stages in disturbed development of this region which seem to explain the manner in which these associated anomalies may arise. Their starting point is with embryologic stages young enough to show the basic initially paired condition of the primordia of the genital tubercle. In the primitive streak stage of the human

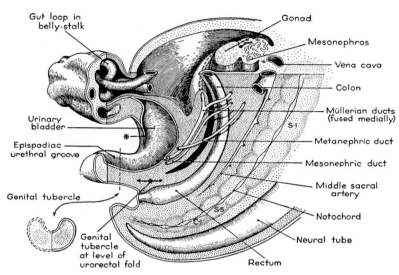

Fig. 203. Hypothetical stage in the genesis of exstrophy of the bladder and epispadias. Compare with Figure 204. Note that the belly-wall in the mid-line (see asterisk) is composed of a thinning plate of ectoderm and entoderm unreinforced by mesoderm. (Courtesy, Drs. B. M. Patten and Alexander Barry.)

embryo, about the end of the second or beginning of the third week of fertilization age, a small midline area—the cloacal plate—can be identified just caudal to the primitive streak and into which the mesoderm has not grown, leaving the ectodermal and endodermal layers in direct contact with each other. Elongation of the tail of the embryo occurs and by the fourth week the easily recognized cloacal plate—now the cloacal membrane— forms the central wall of the urogenital sinus at the base of the allantois (Fig. 202).

Patten and Barry are convinced that the initial developmental disturbance involves the appearance of these paired primordia a little too far caudally with reference to the cloacal outlet (Fig. 203). This displacement is regarded as starting a train of events which could logically account for exstrophy and epispadias and their known variants (Fig. 204). Such a relative displacement could cause the primordia to lie at the level where the urorectal fold divides the original cloacal orifice into urogenital and anal outlets. Under such circumstances the corpora cavernosa would be formed just caudal to the urogenital outlet and the urethral groove would develop in their dorsal angle rather than in their ventral angle as is normally the case. Failure of midline convergence of the displaced paired primordia would account for the not uncommon exaggeration of these associated anomalies in which the penis or the clitoris is represented by separate halves, each molded about a single corpus cavernosum (Figs. 204, 205).

The exstrophy so generally accompanying an epispadiac condition involves a failure to reinforce the ventral body wall by convergent ingrowth of mesoderm. Normally this mesodermal ingrowth first occurs just cephalic to the

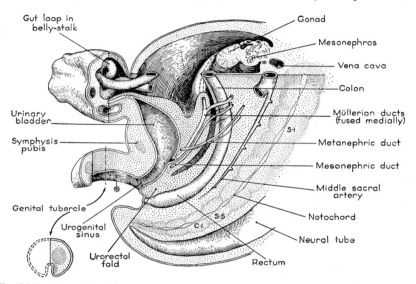

Fig. 204. Normal relations of developing penis in an embryo of the 8th week. Note that the urethral groove (marked by asterisk) is directly in line with the urogenital orifice. In the schematic cross section of the genital tubercle, at the lower left, the developing corpus cavernosum and the corpus spongiosum flanking the urethral groove are indicated by heavier stippling. (Courtesy Drs. B. M. Patten and Alexander Barry.)

urogenital orifice where the paired primordia of the genital tubercle meet each other in the midline. If these paired primordia are caudally displaced, this crucial spot remains overlong without mesodermal reinforcement (Fig. 204). Under these circumstances, when the urogenital membrane ruptures, the opening into the presumptive bladder region will be much larger than normal and tend to extend in the midline all the way to the umbilicus. The likelihood of such an extension is enhanced by the exceedingly rapid elongation of the region between the urogenital orifice and the umbilical cord which occurs at this stage of development. Even slight retardation of mesodermal ingrowth under such circumstances would in all probability mean a delay in reinforcing this region sufficient to account for the characteristic extensiveness of the exstrophic defect.

Symptoms. The chief symptoms are saturation of the clothing by the urine, vesical pain caused by friction of the clothing, the lacerated exposed mucosa often becoming phosphatic encrusted, excoriation of the skin of the abdomen and upper inner thighs, waddling gait when separation of the symphysis is pronounced, high incidence of upper urinary tract infection, and the anal difficulties associated with commonly coexisting rectal prolapse. Renal infection is the usual cause of death.

Diagnosis. This is easily made by inspection; herniation of the exstrophic bladder may contain a considerable mass of intestines. In the examination of these patients it is most important that an excretory urographic study be

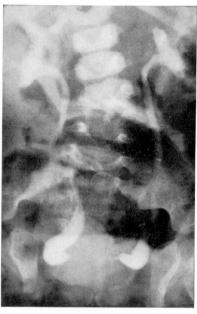

Fig. 205. Congenital bilateral ureterovesical junction stricture in an eight-month-old girl with vesical exstrophy. The resulting ureteral dilatation diminishes the likelihood of a satisfactory result in ureterosigmoidostomy.

made to ascertain if ureteral or renal anomalies coexists and particularly reduplication, and to determine approximately the comparative renal function. It is notable that even in early infancy many of these children urographically show ureterovesical junction stricture with varying degrees of dilatation of the upper urinary tract and particularly of the lower half of the ureter (Fig. 205). Some suffer even graver although surgically remedial upper tract lesions and renal infection is often well established by the time of the initial examination. In some cases the findings will indicate the prospects of a short life at best and this knowledge will spare these unfortunates the futile rigors of major urosurgery.

Treatment. In the past many attempts have been made to close the bladder over and even to construct a vesical neck sphincter but almost without exception they have failed. In many cases a bag of a bladder has been made but the patient had no control and was no better off.

From the standpoint of social relationships and the relative comfort of the patient, ureteral transplantation to the rectosigmoid is the only therapy which has given satisfactory results to date.

Ureterosigmoidostomy is carried out in infants and children primarily because of congenital vesical exstrophy and should be performed by the end of the first year if possible. Physical examination must disclose a normal rectal sphincter; prolapse or other rectal malformations and conditions susceptible to surgical treatment should be corrected prior to ureterosigmoidostomy. When the surgeon is certain that adequate rectal control exists, the transplantation is carried out. In some of these infants rectal prolapse of as much as 10 inches has been observed. Unless a rectal sphincter capable of retaining urine is present, ureteral transplantation only aggravates the condition. Unfortunately many children are not seen until late or, because of medical advice, operation has been postponed until the sixth or eighth year or later. Because of the high mortality of complicating pyelonephritis in these cases, the discovery of vesical exstrophy in adults is most rare.

Considerations in favor of performing ureterosigmoidostomy for exstrophy during the first year of life have been outlined as follows by Higgins (1950), and with these I thoroughly concur:

"1. Just as the infant tolerates the trauma of passing through the birth canal, it tolerates surgical procedures quite well as is attested by the results in other fields of surgery. Delay is not countenanced in plastic operations for harelip or the Ramstedt operation for pyloric obstruction; operative intervention for intussusception or strangulated hernia and other surgical procedures are performed without hesitation.

"2. Recurrent attacks of renal infection may result in sepsis and death before the child is four to six years of age.

"3. The organisms in the bowel of an infant under six months of age probably are less virulent than those in older children and adults.

"4. Because of ureterocystic obstruction the ureter may dilate sufficiently to render its transplantation into the bowel technically impossible. Although one ureter may be transplanted, hydronephrosis on the opposite side may require removal of the kidney.

"5. If the operation is performed early in life, the child may develop normally both physically and mentally.

"6. The operative mortality and morbidity are low.

"7. The tone of the renal sphincter, in my experience, has always been adequate to prevent leakage of urine from the rectum after the sphincter starts to function normally.

"8. Because of the parents' attachment to the child, it is better that if a mortality should result from operation, it should occur before ties are established."

Counseller (1949) and some others feel that operation should be delayed until the child is four or five years of age and has learned bowel control. Counseller states that vesical exstrophy is not a surgical emergency as are pyloric stenosis, tracheobronchial fistula, strangulated umbilical hernia and so forth, and that one can conceivably wait until the fourth or fifth year when anatomic structures are larger and, employing the one-stage Coffey-Mayo technique, anastomosis can more satisfactorily and accurately be done without tension. He further contends that preparation of the bowel for ureterosigmoidal anastomosis can be achieved more easily and completely when the child is older.

Yet experience has shown that young infants do withstand urologic surgery well. Ureterosigmoidostomy, while a highly technical operation, is usually not a difficult one. Preoperative preparation and postoperative care do more to spell the difference between success and failure than does choice of age for operation. Certainly one does not hesitate to carry out on the urinary tract in infancy other operations even more formidable than ureterosigmoidostomy. Because of the considerations of obstruction and infection existing even in infancy, there is no more reason to delay in the surgical treatment of these cases and in the establishment of free drainage than if the patient had the obstruction but not the exstrophy. One does not send away infants and young children with obstructing ureterocele, ureteral stricture, hydronephrosis or renal tumor, to be brought back for surgical treatment when they are four or five years of age; at least, I do not. It is to the patient's advantage to have his operation by the time he is twelve months of age and while it is not necessary to operate during the neonatal period as has been reported by some, most infants nine to twelve months of age will withstand the operation splendidly as they do even more extensive and hazardous urosurgical procedures.

In the past the general operative mortality in ureterosigmoidostomy for exstrophy was relatively high (20 to 25 per cent) but with improved preoperative preparation by bowel cleansing and chemotherapy, the establishment of electrolyte balance, adequate transfusion, gentleness at the operating table, modern chemotherapy and postoperative antibiotic therapy, this mortality has been greatly decreased, even to less than 5 per cent. Moreover, more than fifty consecutive ureteral transplants in infants without a death have been reported (Lanman, 1948; see also Higgins, 1950).

Following ureteral transplantation, dilatation of the upper urinary tract exists in practically every case, even if only as a temporary manifestation (Fig. 199 *B*). In some instances this adds to the morbidity. Refinements and simplifications of operative technic are sharply reducing the incidence and gravity of postoperative ureteral and pelvic dilatation so commonly seen in the past. Formerly the dilated ureter was considered a contraindication to ureteral transplant but, with the technic of suture of ureteral mucosa to bowel mucosa suggested by Nesbit (1948), even moderately dilated ureters can be satisfactorily transplanted to the bowel without great difficulty. Occasionally ureteral reduplication will be found unilaterally or bilaterally and here the Nesbit procedure has served splendidly.

Boyce and Vest (1952) revived by clever modification the Maydl operation of transplantation of the intact trigone to the rectum, this bowel segment having previously been surgically isolated and sterilized by antibiotics; a permanent colostomy of the mid-descending colon takes care of fecal discharge. In their two cases the upper urinary tract remained morphologically normal and sterile. These surgeons advanced the notion that should it seem desirable in later years, the lower bowel continuity may be reestablished and the colostomy closed, bearing in mind this will at once expose the urinary tract to infection.

While no child subjected to the usual ureterosigmoidostomy may anticipate a normal life expectancy, about half of the cases operated upon will survive more than twenty years; a patient of Stevens (1941) lived forty-four years. Yet all late deaths and many deaths occurring in the postoperative period or soon thereafter have been due to renal damage and insufficiency. Yet about as many will live for years without ureterosigmoidostomy as with operation but their lives will be spent largely in social ostracism due to their urinary stench, wishing they were dead, while some will kill themselves. Harvard and Thompson (1951) traced 128 of 144 cases of vesical exstrophy operated on in the Mayo Clinic by the Coffey-Mayo technique. The immediate hospital mortality was 12.5 per cent (eighteen of 144 cases); renal failure is known to have killed twenty-seven of thirty-four who died later; 69.9 per cent of all known survivors had pyelonephritis, and only 12.2 per cent (five of forty-one cases studied by excretory urography postoperatively) showed normal and unobstructed upper urinary tracts.

These and other considerations in ureterosigmoidostomy are splendidly presented by Moore in Section XV, Chapter 4.

If ureteral transplantation is contraindicated by advanced upper urinary tract disease or by the condition of the patient, palliative local cleansing of the exstrophic and surrounding tissues and the liberal protective application of petrolatum must be employed. In many infants at Bellevue Hospital with extensive maceration of the skin and continued bleeding from the excoriated mucosa, cleansing of the parts and periodic exposure (two hours on and two hours off) to electric light—the cradle used in the treatment of burns—has admirably relieved the irritation. Much of this tissue change results from infection which today is more readily controlled superficially by the application of sulfonamide ointments. Yet the application of a very thin sheet of plasticine 6 inches square directly to the raw bladder mucosa and surrounding area minimizes friction, gives symptomatic relief, and is nonirritating. Absorbent cloth or gauze dressings are placed over the plasticine.

Urachal Cysts. These form when the lumen of the allantois fails to be obliterated but the ends of the canal become closed (Fig. 195). These cysts are most often found in the lower third of the urachus and may attain great size to suggest intra-abdominal tumor. Situated posterior to the abdominal musculature, the enlarging cyst is chiefly intra-abdominal and may produce symptoms of intestinal pressure, abdominal pain and, if infected, fever. The cyst fluid is an exudate from the epithelium lining the cyst wall. Begg (1930) has splendidly discussed the anatomy, histology and development of the urachus. Some 111 cases have been reported to date, indicating the condition is comparatively rare. The incidence in males is three times that in females (Sibley, 1950). There were four cases encountered in 19,046 children at autopsy and four in 32,834 adults. In addition, in a forty-five-year-old male there was a *dermoid cyst of the urachus.*

Small cysts usually pass unrecognized but large urachal cysts are manifested by a midline subumbilical protrusion or a palpable mass. Urachal cysts seldom produce symptoms unless they become infected, or intrapelvic or intravesical rupture occurs. Two cases of infected urachus in boys of fourteen months and two and one-half years were reported by Tauber and Bloom (1951). With rupture at the umbilicus, a persistent discharging fistulous tract usually remains. With intravesical rupture a diverticulum of the bladder dome results with persistent discharge into the vesical urine (Figs. 195, 201). Although the lesion is most often found in children and young adults, it has been observed in patients of all ages.

Diagnosis. The presence of a midline suprapubic mass discharging externally or not suggests urachal cyst. The differential diagnosis may be exceedingly difficult particularly when infection has occurred. Urachal cyst may simulate appendiceal abscess, Meckel's diverticulitis, ovarian cyst, tuberculous peritonitis, bursitis, or even a distended bladder. The cyst cavity may be radiologically outlined following its injection with a radiopaque medium but this diagnostic maneuver is unlikely to be employed unless a cyst opening at one end is found.

The usual treatment is excision of the cyst. When the cyst is infected, marsupialization with healing by granulation or subsequent excision may be indicated as in a fourteen-month-old patient of Tauber and Bloom.

Patent Urachus. This results from failure of the allantoic duct to close and is usually consequent to obstruction at the vesical outlet or distally (Fig. 196). When the urachus remains patent throughout, a urinary fistula results; the nature of the underlying pathology is generally recognized. When there is doubt, the discharge may be chemically identified as urine. Dye excreted in the urine may be given, and lateral cystography or injection of the fistulous tract with radiopaque medium is definitive as is cystoscopy. If the urachus is closed only at one end, the open end drains externally through the umbilicus or internally into the bladder according to the site of closure. A persistent discharge at the umbilicus, even though scant and mucoid, at once suggests incomplete obliteration of the urachus but may simulate abscess (cf. Cherry, 1950).

Patent urachus occurred twenty-five times at autopsy in 19,046 children (1 to 761) but is rarely observed clinically. It was noted twice in our adult series (32,843 autopsies). I could find only sixty-seven cases reported in the literature, forty-four of which were patients under four years of age and with a sex ratio of two males to one female. With increased intracystic pressure the blind internal urachal fistula may rupture through and discharge from the umbilicus. Diverticulum at the dome of the bladder is usually a manifestation of a mild degree of patent urachus, and was splendidly demonstrated in a two-year-old boy, the diverticulum being filled with a large stone, as large as the true bladder (Fig. 194).

Excision of the fistulous tract is the treatment, and was performed in six cases I know of.

Redundancy of the Trigonal Mucosa. This forms a valvelike leaflet which, with urination, flaps over the vesical outlet and obstructs. This unusual

condition was found at autopsy at the Babies Hospital in six cases, four
of which were boys (Campbell, 1937). In Harris's (1933) case the mucosal
redundancy formed a cupping at the anterior trigone as occurred also in
Beer's case in an eight-year-old boy. Doubtless in some cases and as observed post mortem, the mucosal flap is in truth an unrecognized ureterocele
redundancy. The cause is unknown. The symptoms and pathologic changes
in the upper urinary tract are those common to obstruction of the vesical
outlet.

The *diagnosis* is made by cystoscopy. As in my first clinical case (Campbell, 1933), if the obstructing leaflet is large, it may block the cystoscopic
field and thus fail to be identified correctly. In a second case, a six-month-old
girl, a triangular fold of mucosa about the size of the trigone was suspended
from lateral anterior bladder wall attachments to comparable attachments
in the posterior urethra. Urethroscopically an opening into the bladder could
be seen both above and below the leaflet and the cystoscope could be
passed through either orifice into the bladder. The best cystoscopic picture
was obtained when the inferior orifice was employed. Overdistention of the
bladder at the time of examination will facilitate the cystoscopic diagnosis
in these cases.

The *treatment* is removal of the obstruction and may be done by transurethral resection when the valve leaflet is small or by excision through the
open bladder when it is large (Fig. 907; see Section XV, Chapter 5). I
have excised these folds in four girls.

Persistent cloacal formation is discussed later in this chapter.

EMBRYOLOGY OF THE URETHRA

The male urethra is derived from two anlagen, (1) the lower narrowed
portion of the vesico-urethral anlagen above the wolffian duct opening,
which forms the urethra down to and including the verumontanum and

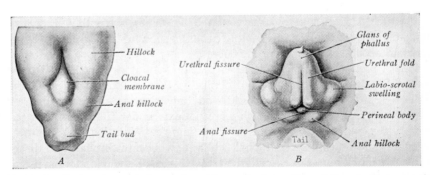

Fig. 206.   Embryology of the urethra. The early formation of the phallic or genital
tubercle and phallic urethra is indicated in Fig. 207. This development from a frontal
viewpoint is shown in the figures above (Arey).

utricle, (2) the urogenital sinus below this opening (Figs. 191, 203–204).
The female urethra is derived from (1) and lacks a verumontanum and
associated structures.

The urogenital sinus begins at the opening of the wolffian and müllerian ducts and extends to the cloacal or urogenital membrane which separates the sinus from the cloacal fossa outside. About the fifth week the tissue bordering the external cloacal fossa anteriorly grows forward bilaterally into a rounded projection, the genital tubercle (Figs. 203, 207). Patten (1952) has stressed the importance of recognizing the dual (bilateral) embryologic derivation of the genital tubercle, particularly in the genesis

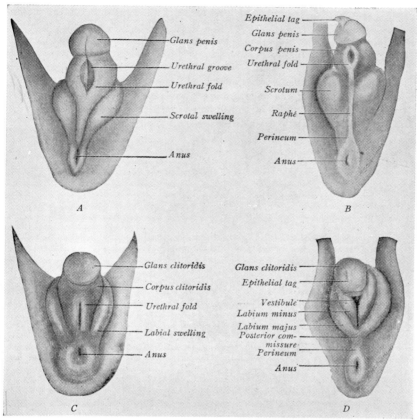

Fig. 207.   Region of the human cloacal membrane. *A*, at 3 mm. (Arey after Keibel; × 60). *B*, at 21 mm. (Arey after Otis). Differentiation of the human external genitalia (× 8) Arey after Spalding. Stages at ten and twelve weeks; *A, B*, male; *C, D*, female.

of hypospadias and epispadias. The genital tubercle rapidly increases in size and soon differentiates into a distal knoblike end, the phallus, and a bulbous ventral expansion (Figs. 206–208). As the genital tubercle grows the urogenital sinus elongates with it; elongation is much greater in the male than in the female. On its undersurface the genital eminence is longitudinally grooved, the first indication of the urethra (Figs. 203, 207). By resorption the urogenital membrane is perforated and the orifice of a ventral sinus— the urogenital opening—appears. The lips of the newly formed urethral gutter and the urogenital membrane of the cloacal fossa closes from behind forward, leaving a urethral tube which opens into the bladder at one end and

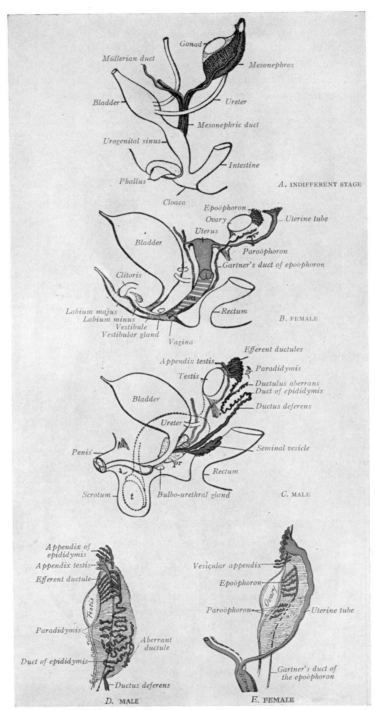

Fig. 208.   Homologues in urogenital development. Diagrams depicting the transformation of the primitive genital system to the definitive male and female types. (Arey after

externally at the meatus at the other (Figs. 195, 204). The anterior part of the groove just proximal to the glans penis is the last portion to be closed over (Fig. 207) and in hypospadias explains the higher incidence of the glandular or balanitic variety.

Development of urethral glands accompanies the formation of the canal. The wolffian duct and the method by which it comes to open into the posterior urethra has been briefly outlined under Embryology of the Kidney, Ureter and Bladder. The development of the müllerian ducts will be described shortly in connection with the embryology of the gonads. The prostate is derived as epithelial outpocketings arranged as five groups: two lateral, the median, anterior and posterior (Lowsley). Skene's ducts are the prostatic homologues in the female; they are seldom of clinical importance in the young but in older women are frequently the site of cyst development or infection and abscess formation.

The question of embryonic formation of the glands in the deep female urethra and in the bladder outlet is still sub judice. This has arisen as a clinical problem in conjunction with the demonstration of gland-like structures in this area in females with persistent urinary infection, the concern being with their origin, whether inflammatory or congenital. While attention has been directed to the fact that the anterior third of the female urethra contains many small scattered glands in which bacteria may seclude and perpetuate urinary infection; Folsom (1945), Deter et al. (1946) and others (Young, 1943; Huffman, 1948) have noted the many tubuloglandular structures of similar importance in the posterior third of the canal (Fig. 798; see Section XIII). Johnson (1922) described these as "homologues of the prostate gland." Normally the posterior urethral glands in the female disappear as such during late fetal life but it is likely that in some instances initial local infection in persistent glands may cause infection of the urinary tract above and, particularly, of the bladder, or by lymphogenous or lymphohematogenous spread, may induce acute renal infection. Not all observers (Cabot and Shoemaker, 1936; Thompson, 1939; McKenzie et al., 1939; Beneventi, 1943; Lisa et al., 1950) are in agreement that in the young female deep urethra there are true glandular structures which may undergo hypoplasia or become infected. Yet the frequent observation of small urethral cysts in this area in cases of persistent vesical irritability in young girls suggests the presence of some glanular or metaplastic gland-like structures. McKenzie (1939) thinks these lesions are the result of vacuolization and cystic degeneration of von Brunn's cell nests consequent to inflammation and fibrosis in the submucosa, the histologic picture being that of urethritis cystica.

In the male the bulbomembranous glands of Cowper bud from the urethra as epithelial nests, branch, acquire a lumen lined with secretory epithelium and open into the deep bulbous urethra. The *female homologues,*

Thompson.) The course of the mesonephric or Gartner's duct is indicated in *B* and *E*. While this structure usually disappears as such, in about 5 per cent of females it persists as a fine patent tube. The persistence of Gartner's duct in its embryonic association with the early kidney structure is advanced to explain the appearance of ureteral ectopia in the vagina and more particularly in the cervix and body of the ureter.

Bartholin's glands, open posterolaterally into the vestibule. Numerous other glands (of Littre) develop in longitudinal rows throughout the length of the anterior urethra. The lacunae of Morgagni are developed in the male as small outpouchings of the fossa navicularis and are lined with nonsecreting epithelial cells. Anomalous development of the periurethral glands (cyst, fistula, etc.) is sometimes clinically important.

Coincident with the development of the urethra, the abdominal wall closes anteriorly as high as the umbilicus. The genital eminence or phallus forms at the junction of the urogenital membrane and of the newly formed lowermost abdominal wall (ninth week, Figs. 206, 207). An undifferentiated sex organ at first, the phallus later becomes the male penis or the female clitoris. By the third month the penis has appeared as such at the tip of the phallus and the urogenital sinus has been drawn out with the formation of the penile urethra (Fig. 207). Simultaneously the penis is covered with skin. Genital ridges, the labioscrotal folds, appear laterally at the base of the phallus. These folds extend posteriorly to unite in front of the rectum and ultimately form the scrotum in the male and the labia majora in the female. The median raphe marks the line of fusion. Thus the pendulous urethra is formed from the genital eminence; the bulbous urethra forms from fusion of the cloacal membrane which also forms the perineum. The prostatic urethra is a wolffian duct derivative.

In the female the urogenital opening remains as a cleft beneath and along the ventral surface of the genital tubercle. Its walls do not fuse as in the male but remain open to form the orifice of the vestibule. Abnormally fusion of the labia minora may occur; this is discussed later in this Section (q.v.). The ventral groove on the female genital eminence closes and the clitoris is formed but without a canal. The sex can be determined in embryos of three months (56 mm., Arey, 1946).

ANOMALIES OF THE GENITAL TRACT

Anomalies of the Penis. Anomalies of the penis as a whole are rare; most are of little clinical importance and are generally associated with defects of the urinary or other system which are incompatible with life. Penile anomalies result from failure of normal development of the genital tubercle (phallus) and the segment of the urogenital sinus concerned with penis formation. In rare instances, the external genitalia are totally lacking as in Kirschbaum's (1950) case but these subjects are shortlived and unlikely to become clinical problems.

Though generally hidden from view, anomalies of the urethra and prepuce are common and have great clinical importance, not only from the standpoint of interference with normal function or as they may produce urinary obstruction, but psychologically as their presence may adversely influence the growing child's outlook upon himself and in his relations to his surroundings and companions. Uncorrected or, occasionally, uncorrectible, the persistence of these genital anomalies generally reflects itself in the personality, behavior and outlook of unfortunate adults, in many of whom the anomaly induces alarming sexual psychoses and not a few resort to suicide.

Through thoughtlessness on the part of the parents, playmates or others, the importance of minor genital defects is frequently and erroneously expanded to produce a genital monomania on the part of the child. Most children are aware of the deformity by the age of five years and, if the condition is not rectified and if he is not made to understand clearly its nature and relative importance, he is likely to become a sexual introvert. Because his abnormal genital condition frequently receives unwarranted attention by his parents and himself, abnormal and unhealthy sex practices are commonly indulged in. Yet the danger of psychologic upset has been greatly overrated and most relatively stable children can, with proper explanation

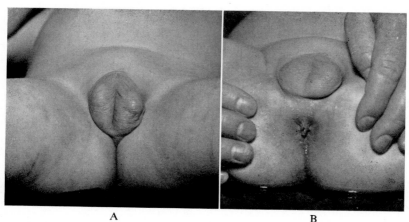

A   B

Fig. 209.   Congenital absence of the penis in a two-year-old boy. *A*, normal testes and partially cleft scrotum. *B*, perineal view showing urethral meatus opening as a tag on the anal margin. The boy's condition was otherwise normal. (University Hospital.)

concerning the anomaly and with sympathetic understanding, be made to endure their malformations in the true light and to the extent that surgical correction does not become an emergency or much dreaded procedure. When the anomaly includes absence of an organ such as the penis and one necessary for reproduction, unless a substitute can be made by plastic surgery, the patient should be surgically unsexed before the age of six. Sexual desire is thereby eliminated and the hardships of congenital sex misfortune are in some measure forestalled.

Congenital Absence of the Penis. This excessively rare condition results from failure of the genital tubercle to develop; the urethra opens in the perineum near or at the anal border (Fig. 209) or, if there is a persistent cloaca, drains into the cloacal rectal cavity. The condition occurs in about one in thirty million males (Harris, 1898). It was not seen in over fifty thousand admissions to the urologic service at Bellevue Hospital and has been noted chiefly at autopsy and in monsters. Twelve cases have been reported to date including two by Gilles and Harrison (1948) and to which three are herewith added. It was observed twice in our autopsy series of 19,046 children: (1) an anencephalic monster with complete absence of the reproductive tract and a greatly dwarfed urinary tract, and (2) in a four-month-old boy whose hypoplastic urethra opened in the midline of the upper anterior scrotum. In the last case there was no corpus spongiosum or other evidence of penis externally and the urethra could be pushed back into the bladder. One testicle was in the inguinal canal and the other was not found nor was the patient an hermaphrodite. There was bilateral clubfoot, accessory lobes of the ears and pigeon breast (Campbell, 1937).

Complete absence of the penis was clinically observed by me in a two-year-old boy in whom the urethra opened as a small nipple at the anterior anal margin (Fig. 209). There was no palpable trace of penile corpora, the

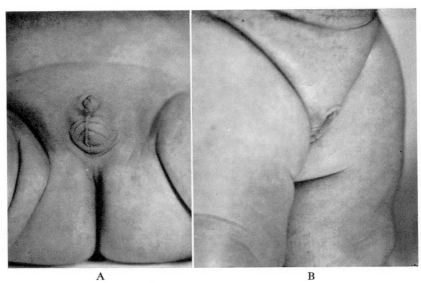

A   B

Fig. 210.   Hidden or concealed penis in a one-year-old boy. *A,* in addition to its con-cealment, the penis also shows congenital torsion with clockwise rotation so that the meatus faces toward eleven o'clock. *B,* lateral view. Scant scrotal development. (Babies Hospital.)

naturally placed testes felt normal as was the scrotum, and abdominal ex-ploration revealed no female organs. There were no symptoms; the upper urinary tract was normal by excretory urography. Construction of a non-erectile penis by abdominal tube plasty was carried out employing the Denis Browne type of procedure used in hypospadias but this structure broke down in its upper midportion when it was later mobilized from the abdominal wall. In the case of Drury and Schwarzell (1935), a thirteen-year-old boy with absence of the penis, urination took place through the rectum but he was unable to distinguish between the desire to urinate and to defecate. The boy was healthy, showed no evidence of urinary infection and both testes were in the scrotum although the scrotal raphe was absent from the back of the scrotum and extended only 2 cm. forward from the penis. The bladder was distended and there was no trace of urethra; excretory urography re-vealed bilateral hydroureter. In Roy's (1932) patient there was abdominal pain from vesical overdistention consequent to stricture of the urethral meatus in the rectum; the retention was relieved by meatal dilation with sounds.

The *diagnosis* of penile agenesis is suggested by inspection but the condition is to be differentiated from concealed penis and pseudohermaphroditism. The diagnosis of penile absence should not be made unless the organ including the corpora cavernosa and corpus spongiosum is entirely lacking. The urethra opens perineally or into the rectum and this predisposes to renal infection which commonly develops and in one reported case caused death. Other urogenital tract anomalies usually coexist and particularly in the upper tract. Strangely enough these were absent in our case.

There is no satisfactory *treatment*. In their patient Gilles and Harrison (1948) attempted to construct a penis with stiffening by the inclusion of

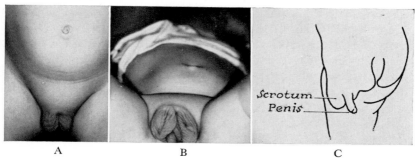

A   B   C

Fig. 211.   Congenital scrotopenile inversion. The penis lies behind a partially cleft scrotum in an eighteen-month-old boy. *A*, anterior view. *B*, perineal view. *C*, anatomic relationships. Treatment: the scrotum was divided in the midline and sutured so that the penis became anterior in the usual relationship.

cartilage (see Section XV, Chapter 11). The two-year-old boy cited previously is undergoing plastic construction procedure by me but the most that can be hoped for is an acceptable cosmetic result with hose action.

Absence of the glans penis has been reported by Atkinson (1898), by Roy (1932) and by de la Peña (1932). The condition is rarely of clinical concern except as the meatus may be stenosed.

Concealed Penis. This may be misdiagnosed penile absence. The rudimentary organ is hidden beneath the skin of the scrotum, perineum, abdomen or thigh (Fig. 210), the fatty subcutaneous tissues of which may be unusually thick. Urogenital development is generally otherwise normal. The condition is of clinical concern in the newborn when urethral angulation causes retention or, in adult life, coitus is impossible. Acute urinary obstruction must be relieved at once. Mobilization and plastic reformation of the penis should not be attempted until growth in size of the organ makes the operation practicable (sixth to eight year) when by dietary or medicinal therapy the excessive obesity of the boy has been reduced so that relatively, the penis is larger and more readily captured. As many of these boys grow and their obesity diminishes, the penis becomes readily visible, although in general the clinical picture is that of genital dwarfism.

Transposition of the Scrotum and Penis. This has been described in six cases (Saunders et al., 1937; Sisto Hontan, 1935; Francis, 1940; a case of Hildebrandt's cited by Francis; Huffman, 1951) to which a seventh is herewith added, an eighteen-month-old boy behind whose partially bifid scrotum the penis dangled from the perineum (Fig. 211). The organ was half size but otherwise normal as were the testes in the scrotum and, as determined by excretory urography, the upper urinary tract as well. The embryologic explanation of scroto-penile transposition is still unsettled. Spalding (1921) and Frazer (1932) advanced the notion that the development of the pars phallica of the urogenital sinus and the genital tubercle is retarded while the ventral labioscrotal swellings now anterior to the tubercle continue to grow normally. Francis believes absence of the urogenital sinus with failure of the scrotal swelling to shift caudad to the penis causes the scrotum to develop anteriorly which is the normal position in the *marsupiala*. The cases reported by Francis and Huffman were each born without a urinary tract. Meyer (1941) found a subcoccygeal penis in a seven-month-old fetus, the retrodeviation of the penis being attributed to pelvic deformity causing embryonal cavernous tissue to deviate backward independent of the urethra. In my patient, the scrotum was surgically divided in the midline and the penis was brought forward to normal position following which the scotum was closed about the base of the penis with eradication of the scrotal cleft.

Diphallus or **reduplicated penis** is more common than the other penile anomalies herein thus far described. Thirty-three cases have been reported elsewhere including two by me (Campbell, 1937). Double penis probably results from lack of fusion of the double primitive anlagen. Other theories include the notion that double penis represents (1) an atavism (some lizards possess two sets of external genitals), (2) a teratoid structure (a double monster), and (3) a simple reduplication like a supernumerary digit. The organs usually course parallel but they may be placed one above the other, with variable degree of separation at the base. The urethra is reduplicated but may join in the prostatic region and maintain separate openings in a common urinary bladder or each urethra may drain a separate bladder. In Pendrino's (1950) case, the double urethra united at a single bladder but the prostate was absent (Fig. 212). The penis may terminate in two glands and, as in Allsner's case, one urethra may be used for voiding, the other for seminal ejaculation.

Associated urogenital tract deformities are nearly always found and include vesical exstrophy, hypospadias, epispadias, improperly descended testes, cleft scrotum, duplication or absence of the bladder, ureter or kidney, fused kidney and so forth and, in many, imperforate anus. Many of these abnormalities are incompatible with life. In a three-week-old male at the Babies Hospital previously reported by me (1937), there were two penises each 1.5 cm. long, the bladder was exstrophic and on the right side there was a large diverticulum (attempt at vesical reduplication) into which the right ureter opened. Only a small urethral dimple was found at the penoscrotal angle of the left penis. The right upper urinary tract was normal; the left kidney was in the pelvis. An enormous left inguinal hernia contained the cecum and appendix. The right testis was in the scrotum but the left was in the pelvis. The vertebral column was reduplicated and there was bilateral clubfoot. In Volpi's (1903) case, in addition to double penis, there was imperforate anus, reduplication of the urethra, bladder and scrotum, together with horseshoe kidney with a single ureter opening into the left bladder. In short, normally reduplicated organs were fused, normally single organs were reduplicated. Reduplication of the urogenital and lower intestinal tracts was reported by Fischer (1952). In an unusual variety of penile pseudoreduplication, Englisch found the organs completely separated in two

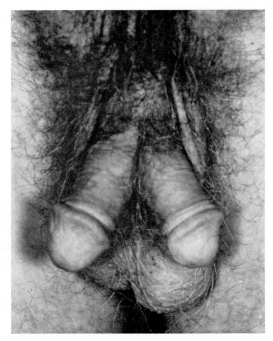

Fig. 212.　Double penis with double urethra leading to a single bladder. Absence of prostate. (Courtesy Dr. J. Pendino and Journal of Urology.)

halves, each corpus spongiosum formed a penis, and the urethra opened between them. Davis (1949) was not certain whether his patient had two, three or four penises. Double penis is to be distinguished from bifid penis and reduplicated or supernumerary glans with a single shaft.

Reduplicated penis rarely requires surgical treatment, especially when the organs drain reduplicated bladders. If one penis is proved thoroughly adequate, its mate may be excised; Lanman extirpated one penis and an extrophic bladder. In any event normal urethral patency must be established and/or maintained.

Torsion of the Penis. Here the frenum and meatus face upward or outward (Fig. 213). The cause of this rare lesion is unknown; it commonly is accompanied by other penile defects, notably hypospadias or epispadias. The penile rotation may be clockwise or counterclockwise; most of the cases I have seen have been counterclockwise, with the penile meatus and median raphe facing toward one, two, or three on the clock face. In five severe cases I have seen the penis twisted to the right in two, to the left in three; the median raphe defines the curve of the twist. The cause of this rare lesion is probably unequal development of the corpora cavernosa. The remainder of the genital tract is usually normal but in about one in three cases the upper

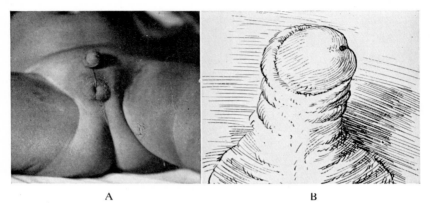

A   B

Fig. 213. Torsion of the penis. *A*, in a two-year-old boy examined because of pronounced dysuria induced by a stenosed meatus. The organ is congenitally rotated counterclockwise with the meatus facing three o'clock. There is scant scrotal development with a deep scrotal midline dimple. The testes were not palpable. *B*, schema of penile torsion.

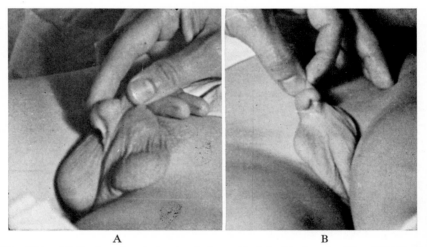

A   B

Fig. 214. Webbed penis. *A,* in association with balanitic hypospadias, lateral view. *B,* with penis retracted upward. Accompanying the webbed penis is extreme congenital penile chordee.

urinary tract is anomalous. The condition seldom causes symptoms except when the external meatus is stenosed as it frequently is, or the urethra is angulated; here the manifestations are those of obstruction and with or without urinary infection. In a three-month-old boy reported by Bland-Sutton (1922) urethral blockage by angulation produced widespread dilatation of the upper urinary tract.

Treatment consists of the establishment and maintenance of free urethral drainage with meatotomy or internal urethrotomy, urethral dilation, or even internal urethrotomy; exceptional chordee may merit correction.

Congenital Adherent Penis. Webbed penis is sometimes found with scrotal hypospadias, the organ being integral with the scrotum and incurved to follow the scrotal form. In adults this may prohibit intercourse. Correction of existing chordee and the hypospadiac urethral defect together with mobilization and plastic repair of the scrotum and penis is the treatment (Fig. 214).

Cleft or **division of the glans penis** is rare, is usually vertical and is to be distinguished from double penis or diphallus (q.v.). Several cases of

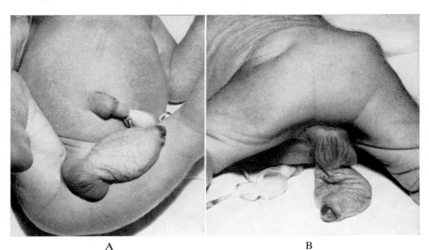

A   B

Fig. 215.   Congenital absence of the corpora cavernosa in a three-day-old boy. The penis is enormous and there is no urethra as such. The external meatus, adjacent 1.5 cm. of urethra and the bladder neck were occluded; the intervening canal was an enormous dilated cavity lined with glistening mucosa of transitional epithelium. The prostate, left kidney, anus and rectum were absent. Aberrant adrenal tissue was present in the left testicle. The cystic right kidney showed marked hydronephrosis. Congenital left hip dislocation. *A,* anterior view. *B,* posterior view showing enormous penis hanging as a flabby bag of skin. (Courtesy Col. J. W. Schwartz, U.S.M.C., Letterman General Hospital.)

vertical cleft have been reported; Hofmokl (1897) reported transverse cleft of the glans in which the urethra opened into the larger and thicker segment below the cleft. The condition is of no clinical concern except as the external meatus is stenosed or the urethra is congenitally strictured. Treatment is not required except when eradication of obstruction, usually by meatotomy, is indicated.

Congenital Absence of the Corpora Cavernosa and the Urethra. This condition which is excessively rare and largely of academic interest has been reported in eight cases, in all of whom there were other severe maldevelopments incompatible with life. It was observed by Schwartz* in a three-day-old male (Fig. 215). The associated malformations included imperforate anus, congenital dislocation of the left hip, abdominal left testis, agenesis of the right kidney, pronounced hypertrophy of the right adrenal, hydronephrotic left kidney with multiple parenchymal cysts, ureteropelvic

* Schwartz, J. W. Personal communication, 1950.

junction fibrous obstruction, aberrant adrenal tissue in the left testis (an example of this last in another boy is shown in Figure 266, and absent prostate.

Megalopenis. Macropenis frequently exists as a manifestation in precocious puberty (Fig. 216), congenital imbeciles, dwarfs, and in certain types

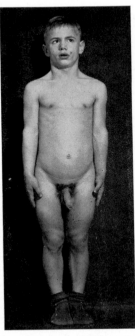

Fig. 216.   Sexual precocity in a four-and-a-half-year-old boy otherwise normal except for an increased output of urinary 17-ketosteroids (9.2 mg. in 24 hours rather than the normal 5.0 mg.). Apparently normal at birth, at one year of age the genitalia were slightly enlarged, and at eighteen months x-rays of the skull demonstrated it to be somewhat large for the stated age. The sella turcica was normal in size and shape and there was no evidence of intracranial tumor. X-rays of the bones disclosed a markedly advanced bone age. One year later exploration of the adrenals disclosed no abnormality nor did biopsy of the rib, testes and epididymides. At four and a half years, he weighed 75½ pounds, was 4 feet 3¾ inches tall (twice the normal size for this age), was well-developed, muscular, presented adult genitalia but without prostatic enlargement. Facial acne, deep voice and pubic hair were present. His mental development was advanced. The metabolic rate was plus 8. He adjusted well to the classroom and has shown no abnormal interest in the opposite sex, being in this respect somewhat different from most "little Hercules" who generally have an abnormal sex drive. (Endocrinology Clinic, University Hospital, and courtesy Dr. Beatrice Bergman and Journal of Pediatrics.)

of endocrine disturbances, especially those of hyperpituitarism and adrenal tumor (Figs. 216–217). Temporary penile enlargement stimulated by the administration of a gonadotropic hormone (A.P.L. substance) in the treatment of imperfectly descended testis is to be distinguished from true megalopenis; the penis returns to former size following withdrawal of the hormone. When megalopenis results from pituitary or adrenal tumor, regression in size has sometimes followed satisfactory eradication of the growth.

Micropenis. The abnormally small organ is seen in infantilism, hypo-

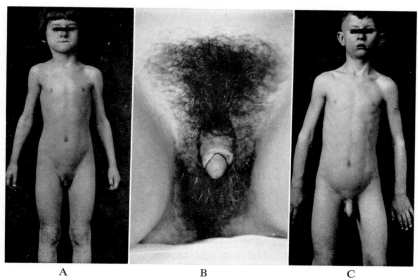

A   B   C

Fig. 217. Macrogenital development in three children in the same family, a brother and two sisters, the two girls having been proved to have cortical adrenal hypertrophy. The parents were apparently normal. *A*, girl at four years of age showed scant growth of pubic and perigenital hair. She was aggressive and had a deep husky booming voice. *B*, genitalia, one year after *A*. Left adrenalectomy. Postoperative death from pulmonary embolism. *C*, brother of girl shown in *A*, five years old. Macropenis with a scant growth of coarse pubic hair. The testicles were abnormally large and penis and prostate were the size of these organs in a boy of fifteen years of age. Unfortunately the study of these children and the sister antedated modern laboratory estimation of hormonal excretion. (Bellevue Hospital.)

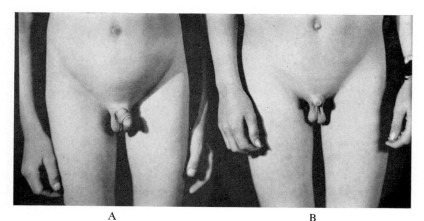

A   B

Fig. 218. Micropenis (right) in a ten-year-old boy compared with normal size penis in a boy of this age. (Bellevue Hospital.)

genitalism, or hermaphroditism and is commonly associated with hypopituitary or hypopineal endocrinopathy, notably Fröhlich's syndrome (dystrophia adiposogenitalis) or there may be failure of development of the corpora cavernosa. Extremely small genitalia are characteristic. In a two-week-old boy seen at Bellevue Hospital the entire penis was no larger than

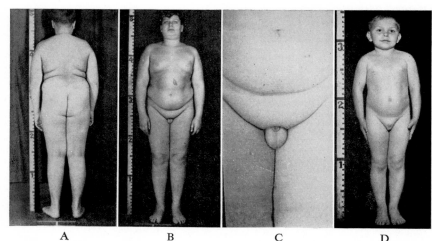

A   B   C   D

Fig. 219.   Sexual infantilism. *A, B,* Fröhlich's syndrome in a thirteen-year-old boy who
is unusually fat, of feminine body contour, and with extremely small genitals including
micropenis (*C*). *D,* in a nine-year-old true pituitary dwarf. (Endocrinology Clinic, University Hospital, and courtesy Dr. Beatrice Bergman.)

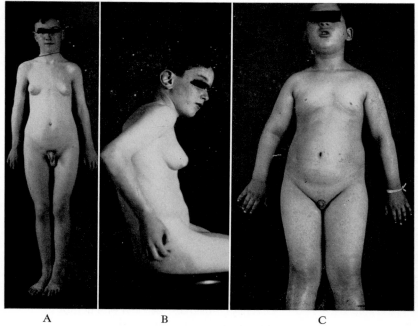

A   B   C

Fig. 220.   *A,* gynecomastia in an eight-year-old boy with right improperly descended
testis. *B,* lateral view; careful study failed to disclose the cause of the condition which
today suggests Kleinefelter's syndrome. *C,* sexual infantilism (Fröhlich's syndrome) in an
eight-year-old boy in whom the characteristic features of the condition are well demonstrated. (Bellevue Hospital.)

the normal corpus spongiosum of this age. The scrotum was absent, the testes could not be found, and neonatal anuria existed for two days. He died of pneumonia at three weeks of age. Micropenis is to be differentiated from concealed penis (q.v.) in which the organ is buried in an excessively fatty subcutaneous tissue and scrotum. The external genitalia are smaller than normal and notably the penis (Figs. 218–220). There may be no scrotum and the testes may not be palpable. The condition is fundamentally a penile hypoplasia in which penile growth is retarded and the prostate also is characteristically abnormally small. The administration of gonadotropic sub-

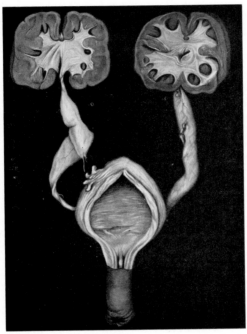

Fig. 221. Congenital stenosis of the prepuce causing death in an eight-day-old male. Urethral dilatation, thickening and trabeculation of the bladder wall with wide dilatation of the upper urinary tract. (Courtesy Dr. C. T. Stepita and University Hospital.)

stances or testosterone may temporarily enlarge the organ but regression to its former unusually small size may be anticipated following withdrawal of the hormone. The administration of testosterone will stimulate genital growth when there is testicular deficiency.

Precocious Puberty. This may occur as early as the second or third year and in boys is generally associated with hypertrophy or neoplasm of the adrenal cortex, tumor of the testicle, pineal or pituitary glands (Figs. 216–217). Disturbances of the pituitary gland as a cause of genital dystrophy are extremely rare. Although sexual precocity usually occurs as an acquired condition, the etiology may be congenital. Clinical aspects of precocious puberty caused by adrenal lesions are discussed in Sections XIII, XIV and XVIII.

Congenital Phimosis. This is the only preputial anomaly of grave concern;

it is characterized by a contracture of the prepuce sufficient to prevent its retraction over the glans, and the preputial opening may be pin-point and permit only a slow discharge of urine (Fig. 221). Physiologic phimosis commonly exists in the newborn and in early infancy. The visceral surface of the prepuce is bound by epithelialization of the glans penis. Separation of the two structures by absorption of the epithelium sometimes occurs *in utero* and normally takes place during the latter months of the first year of life but, persisting, is pathologic. During the early weeks this union is usually so feeble that it can easily be broken up. Sometimes these embryonic epithelial adhesions fail to separate or, as frequently occurs, irritant secretions from the prepuce cause a true fibrous adhesion of the prepuce to the glans. Rarely the prepuce is imperforate.

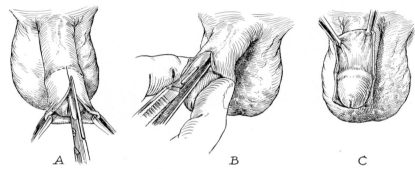

Fig. 222. Dorsal and lateral slits of the prepuce. *A*, dorsal slit employing two Allis clamps and scissors. *B*, employing a knife guided by a groove director. *C*, lateral slits made to obtain wide exposure of the glans and the postcoronal sulcus.

Congenital tight phimosis may retard the growth of the glans or even of the entire penis and, as a rule, the urethral meatus is variably stenosed. Occasionally extreme phimosis produces severe urinary obstruction and grave renal damage results from the urinary back pressure. I know of five cases in the New York metropolitan area in which tight phimosis caused uremic death during the first few days of life and a sixth infant was saved only by prompt circumcision. In a boy of eleven days examined post mortem at Bellevue Hospital extensive dilatation of the entire upper urinary tract resulted from preputial stenosis which was complicated by preputial gangrene and infection (Figs. 221, 223). When the preputial orifice is minute, urination is accompanied by ballooning of the subpreputial cavity. The retention and decomposition of urine in this preputial bladder as well as the excessive excretion of smegma and desquamation of epithelium, commonly causes pronounced irritation, the usual end result of which is ulcerative balanoposthitis. Secondary preputial calculous formation is not uncommon (Fig. 766). Rarely the tight preputial orifice retains stones passed from the urinary tract. Moreover, the local irritant condition may incite masturbation.

In congenital phimosis with phimotic stenosis, each attempt to urinate is likely to be accompanied by straining and crying. Hernia or rectal prolapse may occur. Sometimes an unrecognized stenosis of the meatus hidden beneath the long prepuce is the important obstruction. Even mild urinary blockage here predisposes to urinary infection which is manifested by pyuria, yet the pus from the casually voided specimen may originate in the subpreputial inflammatory process.

A wide variety of reflex disturbances has been attributed to phimosis. This includes malnutrition, epistaxis, convulsions, night terrors, chorea and epilepsy but the etiologic relation is usually unproved. The causal relation of chronic preputial irritation in epithelioma of the penis in adults is well known and in three young boys with phimosis, subpreputial papillomas were found. The complications of phimosis are preventable by circumcision but this is not to be construed as advising that every prepuce which is long or is at first retracted with difficulty should be removed.

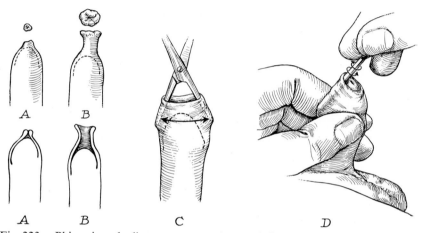

Fig. 223. Phimosis and adherent prepuce. *A*, contraction of the preputial meatus when preputial adhesions exist. *B*, redundant prepuce, schematically showing the elongated collarlike contraction the redundancy frequently presents normal eversion after separation of preputial adhesions. Treatment: breaking down of subpreputial adhesions. *C*, stretching of prepuce with hemostat. *D*, encircling preputial cavity with a probe.

The *diagnosis* of phimosis is made by inspection and the unsuccessful attempt to retract the prepuce behind the glans. Phimosis is to be distinguished from redundant prepuce; in *atrophic phimosis* the prepuce is short but its orifice is tight. Phimosis is commonly accompanied by congenital stenosis of the external urethral meatus.

Treatment. With congenital phimotic stenosis a dorsal slit or lateral slits of the prepuce will at once relieve the constriction and subsequent circumcision will be followed by permanent cure (Figs. 222, 223). Following dorsal slit alone the infection will usually subside and spontaneously disappear as we have frequently observed in boys with the condition and examined because of persistent pyuria or bacteriuria.

Early and periodic retraction of the phimotic prepuce is usually adequate treatment in most cases. There are a considerable number who should be circumcised and the chief indications are: (1) when the prepuce cannot be freely retracted behind the glans, (2) fibrosis of the preputial orifice, (3) recurrent dermatitis of the prepuce, (4) persistent or recurrent balanopos-thitis, or (5) paraphimosis. Although parents cannot be expected to appreciate fully the more unusual indications for circumcision in the young, they all recognize the importance of local cleanliness and genital hygiene and are naturally ready to adopt measures which may avert masturbation. Circumcision is usually advised on these grounds. Stretching of the prepuce with a hemostat (Fig. 223) is an alternative therapy to be combined with periodic retraction of the prepuce. It may be successful in infants but these measures are usually unsatisfactory because they are inadequately performed and may cause as much discomfort as circumcision. When the glandulo-preputial adhesions have been broken up with a probe (Fig. 223) but the prepuce cannot be fully retracted, the points of a hemostat are inserted into the preputial cavity and are passed between the prepuce and glans as far as they will go easily. The forceps is opened gently for a few seconds to stretch the prepuce. If the prepuce cannot be retracted, the stretching is repeated. When the prepuce is dense and resistent, it is often wisest to complete the stretching a few days later. It is undesirable to carry out these genital manipulations over any great period of time. In older boys and adults circumcision rather than repeated manipulation is indicated.

Congenital Absence of the Prepuce. Goddard (1931) reported the occurrence of this condition in a one-legged child stillborn at eight months.

A **short tight frenum** may sometimes cause penile incurvation, especially during erections or may tear easily. Division of the distorting band is recommended, with due attention to the underlying vessels which may bleed copiously.

ANOMALIES OF THE URETHRA

Complete Absence or Atresia of the Urethra. This unusual condition usually kills the fetus *in utero*. The secreted urine distends the bladder and causes pressure upon the umbilical arteries with marked embarrassment of the fetal circulation and has caused dystocia. Renal back-pressure damage during intrauterine development is an added lethal factor.

In a few instances secondary rupture of the bladder into the rectum or a persistent patent urachus has permitted birth of a viable child. Urethral agenesis was discovered four times in 19,046 autopsies in children and urethral atresia in five. An open bladder or one discharging through a patent urachus was present in each and doubtless explains a live birth. In an anencephalic white female, dead at six hours, the urethra was imperforate and the bladder was greatly dilated as was the upper urinary tract. In a male with atresia of the prostatic urethra and dead at one hour, the bladder was greatly dilated, both kidneys were polycystic, the left atrophic and the right enlarged by hydronephrosis. There was a stricture of the lower end of the left ureter with a vesical diverticulum near each ureteral orifice and one between. In the absence of a urethra, the bladder may open through the urachus, directly into the vagina, or into a persistent rudimentary cloaca.

In 1943 Dourmashkin tabulated eighty-eight cases he had collected from the literature and added five of his own in the newborn. An extremely wide variety of urologic, gynecologic, and enteric anomalies coexisted. In fifty living newborn, forty-six were males and four were females, and in half the entire urethra was occluded. An open external urethral meatus may exist but there may be no suggestion of one as in seventy-eight of the eighty-eight cases he reported. Thirty of fifty-five living newborn were successfully treated by *forage* and without mortality. External urethrotomy was employed in seventeen of which one died. Cystostomy, cystotomy and retrograde catheterization of the urethra have also been performed (Ménégaux and Boidot, 1934).

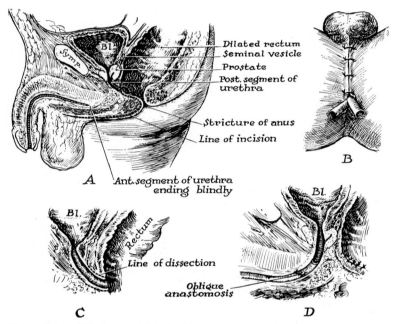

Fig. 224.   Congenital absence of the bulbous urethra in a three-month-old boy in whom the anterior urethra ended blindly in the anterior perineum. A short posterior urethra opened into the lower rectum. The condition was corrected by mobilization of the posterior urethral segment and its anastomosis to the patent anterior segment. Thirteen years later the boy's development is normal.

In some cases of persistent although modified cloaca there is no urethra. The vesical outlet opens directly into the vagina as was observed in an eight-week-old child whose rudimentary ovaries were situated just below the kidney, and it was also seen in a girl dead at five hours.

Although urethral atresia or congenital urethral absence is predominantly a condition of males, several cases of imperforate mucosal diaphragms at the urethral meatus or proximally have been reported in infant and young females. A number of these were born dead with hopeless renal back-pressure injury (Nuñez, 1882; Rochet and Rivière, 1927; Marquardt and Frederick, 1943). May (1949) reported membranous urethral occlusion. In a three-month-old patient of mine, the bulbous urethra was absent, the anterior urethra ending blindly in the anterior perineum; the posterior urethra opened into the rectum (Fig. 224). In some cases of absent or occluded urethra in which the child was alive at birth, the liver is believed to have assumed the urinary (urea) excretory load.

In two clinically observed neonatal males with localized congenital atresia of the urethra and found at eight and twenty-four hours of age respectively

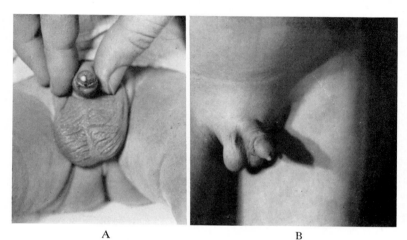

A   B

Fig. 225.   Congenital cyst of the external urethral meatus. *A*, in an eight-day-old boy. *B*, in one of four years. In *A* the white color of the cyst was caused by epithelial debris which was released by opening the cyst. In *B* the cyst was excised.

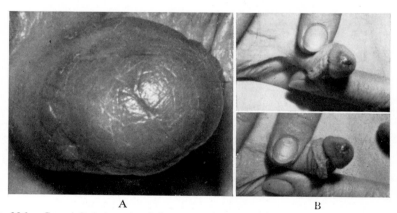

A   B

Fig. 226.   Congenital stenosis of the external meatus. *A*, pinpoint opening without fissures on lateral labia of meatus. Photo about two-and-a-half times normal size. *B*, ulcerated meatus and dermatitis localized to the glans. (Courtesy Dr. Paul Freud and American Journal of Diseases of Children.)

to have solid curtain blockage of the bulbous channel, by gentle urethral instrumentation with small steel sounds, I was able in each case to perforate the obstructive lesion (*forage* of the French) and dilate it sufficiently to permit an 8 F. catheter to be fastened indwelling for twenty-four hours. When this instrumentation is not successful, urinary extravasation may be anticipated and demands prompt external urethrotomy or suprapubic cystotomy with free bladder drainage, adequate incision and antibiotic therapy. The urethral channel is established by plastic surgery at a later date.

Congenital cysts of the external urethral meatus are occasionally encountered in young boys (Fig. 225). The condition rarely causes symptoms except those consequent to the coexisting small meatus. Excision of the cyst is the treatment.

Congenital Urethral Stricture. Stenosis of the external meatus of the pinpoint variety is extremely common and usually exists unnoticed until urinary

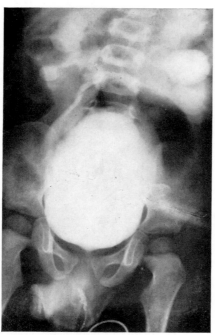

Fig. 227. Stenosis of the external urethral meatus. Cystogram showing the gravely over-distended bladder with reflux outlining the greatly dilated ureters and renal pelves in an eighteen-month-old boy with stenosis of a balanitic hypospadiac urethral meatus. (Bellevue Hospital.) See also Fig. 698.

or urethral infection or dysuria develops or instrumentation is attempted (Fig. 226). The condition is observed in both sexes, it being only slightly less frequent in young females than in young boys. Lattimer (1944) reported tight congenital meatal stenosis with balanitic hypospadias in identical twins. The tight meatal orifice causes dysuria, frequency, urgency and, with ulceration of the meatus, scab formation and bleeding when the scab is wiped off. Ulcerative meatitis is discussed in further detail in Section XIII. The diagnosis of meatal stricture is readily made by inspection. Widespread dilatation of the proximal urinary channel is commonly observed and readily demonstrated urographically. In some of our youngest patients, advanced hydronephrosis and hydroureter and greatly over-distended urethra and bladder have been demonstrated simply by the injection of 20 per cent Diodrast through the incised external urethral meatus (Fig. 227).

Wide meatotomy (Fig. 228) is the treatment of the external meatus, with subsequent periodic dilation as necessary and sufficient to maintain a wide open canal. Unfortunately neither the condition itself nor its potentially grave import is adequately recognized by physicians and especially by pediatricians whose initial opportunity and responsibility it is to relieve the obstruction (cf. Crowell and Anderson, 1950). The early correction of meatal stenosis would unquestionably forestall thousands of episodes of so-called "acute pyelitis" in the young. In my experience urethral stricture accounts for one fifth of urologic disorders in children (1949). In two newborn males, born with projectile vomiting, anorexia and drowsiness (uremia and edema), Cope (1940) discovered tight external urethral meatal stricture to be the

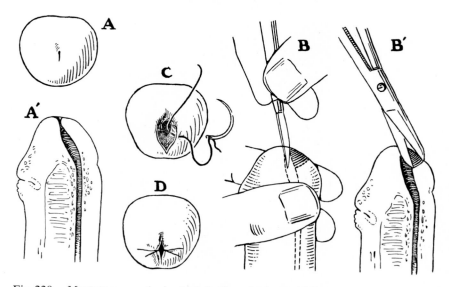

Fig. 228.   Meatotomy employing both knife and scissors. If the tip of the penis is tightly grasped at the time the cut is made, the patient will feel no discomfort. Mucocutaneous suturing as shown in C is unnecessary in young boys.

cause. Simple dilatation of the tight orifice was readily followed by clinical improvement.

Congenital stricture of the urethra other than at the meatus occasionally occurs and notably in the membranous portion or at the penoscrotal junction (Fig. 229). Failing a history of trauma, infection or instrumentation, the stricture is probably congenital. The diagnosis should be suspected by the difficulty of passage of small steel sounds of normal size for the age and development of the patient. Such instruments are firmly grasped by the stricture which may be so tight or dense as to permit only the passage of an extremely small sound or bougie. In many of these cases the diagnosis can be confirmed both by urethroscopy and urethrography. Treatment consists of periodic progressive dilation with sounds but when this fails to achieve the desired result or the canal is impassible, urethrotomy—either internal or external according to the site of stricture—is demanded. The clinical aspects and treatment of urethral stricture in general are considered in Section VI, Chapter 1 and Section XIII.

Unusual urethral deformities such as (*a*) opening on the side of the glans penis, and (*b*) opening in the groin or elsewhere have been described. In a four-year-old boy examined post mortem at Bellevue Hospital, the prostatic urethra described a "Z" course; the resulting obstruction caused by this unique lesion produced wide dilatation of the urinary tract above. I have not found a similar case described nor have we encountered one clinically.

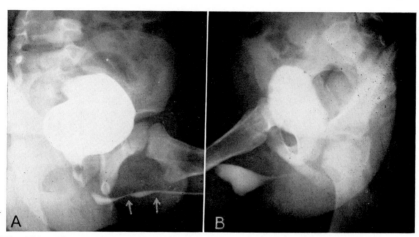

Fig. 229.   Congenital stricture of the urethra. *A*, in a twelve-month-old boy at peno-scrotal junction with slight fusiform dilatation of urethra just behind. In this urethro-cystogram the filling defect of the verumontanum in the prostatic urethra is splendidly shown. Internal urethrotomy. *B*, congenital stricture of external urethral meatus, adjacent anterior bulbous urethra and contracture of the bladder outlet with wide dilatation of the pendulous urethra between in a five-year-old boy. Five ounces residual urine. Treatment: internal urethrotomy; transurethral resection of the vesical neck. Excellent immediate result. Continued periodic urethral dilation is essential to ultimate cure.

Double Urethra. In the male this is a collateral of reduplicated penis (q.v.). Unfortunately the term double urethra is often misapplied to channels which are merely incompletely reduplicated. These accessory channels are situated (1) dorsal to the true urethra or (2) ventral to it being not unusual (Fig. 230). These false reduplicated urethral ducts may be rudimentary or well developed and may even terminate in the bladder or in the prostatic urethra but the true urethra in these cases is essentially normal. Rinker (1943) described double urethra in a two-year-old boy in whom the accessory urethra extended from behind the seminal vesicles to the triangular ligament. Double urethra has been seen in the female with openings side by side or one above the other. In Dannreuther's female case (1923), the true and reduplicated urethras opened through a common meatus; in Deboo's case (1943) the patient was three-legged. The literature of the condition has been splendidly summarized by Coffort (1949) and Gross and Moore (1950).

True double urethra should be distinguished from accessory local urethral canals which may be rudimentary or well developed and even terminate in the bladder or prostatic urethra. Rarely the accessory urethra is ventral. In

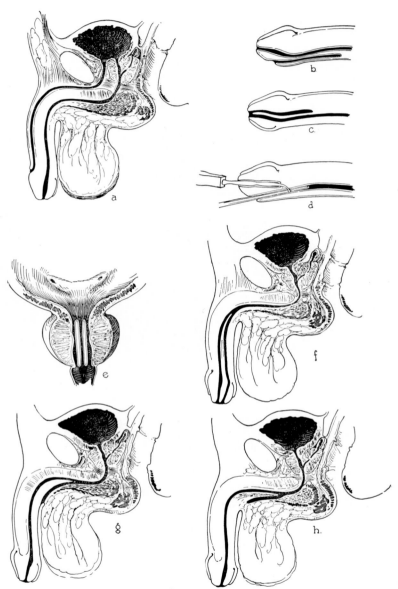

Fig. 230.   Accessory urethral canals. *A*, reduplication; the canal which does not pass through the prostatic urethra is usually incontinent owing to lack of a sphincter. *B*, *C*, blind-ending accessory canals. *D*, method of treatment of conditions *B* and *C* in which the two accessory canals are joined together by scalpel incision against a grooved director in the main urethral channel. *E*, prostatic reduplication. *F*, urethral bifurcation within the penile body. *G*, urethral bifurcation in the bulbous urethra with one opening at the penoscrotal junction. *H*, blind-ending channel in the bulbous urethra (Hinman after Chauvin).

a six-year-old girl with repeated attacks of pyuria and fever associated with double urethra, DeNicola and McCartney (1949) achieved obliteration of the reduplicated urethra by the injection of 0.5 cc. of 5 per cent sodium morrhuate. There was no local reaction and the child remained well.

Accessory Urethral Canals. The various types of dorsally situated accessory urethral canals are indicated in Figure 230. The etiology is still uncertain, the most tenable explanation being that the condition results from a forward continuation of the splitting of the urorectal septum (La Forte, Delbet, Oudard, Jean, Le Brun). When the accessory canals are located on the ventral surface of the urethra, they reflect abnormal closure of the urethral gutter and a *congenital urethral fistula* results. The opening of this fistula may be at any point from the meatus to the triangular ligament but there is no urinary incontinence. The dorsal variety of accessory canal occurs less often than the ventral type, is of the same clinical importance but will not produce incontinence.

Histologically the accessory urethra resembles the normal and causes no symptoms unless by occlusion a cyst forms or by bacterial invasion, especially by gonococci, an abscess occurs or persistent full blown infection results. In some instances extension of the accessory canal to the bladder and unsupplied with a capable sphincter has caused incontinence.

Small *accessory periurethral ducts* opening in or about the meatus are commonly observed in older boys and adult males, vary from 2 to 10 mm. in length, usually end blindly but may join the urethra within the meatus or open externally to produce a fistula. Doubtless they represent imperfect urethral gutter closure and are of importance only as they may harbor infection or be the site of cyst formation. Purcell (1949) reported a male with an unusual reduplication of the prostatic canal, the mucosal wall separating the two channels becoming an obstructing flap or valve when urine struck it. I (1949) encountered a similar finding in the deep urethra and bladder outlet of a six-month-old girl.

The *diagnosis* of accessory urethral canals can sometimes be made by inspection alone but usually requires urethroscopy and/or urethrography which will indicate the caliber and length of the accessory urethra and particularly its relation to the normal duct. Chronic infection or urinary leakage may demand excision of the accessory urethral branch but in some cases I have achieved obliteration by the injection to the point of full expansion of the channel to be obliterated, of 5 per cent sodium morrhuate; other sclerosing agents may be used. In three boys in whom an accessory canal extended backward above a balanitic hypospadiac orifice and with a probe in the accessory canal as a guide to indicate its relation to the true urethra, the intercommunicating tissue was divided to make the two canals continuous (Fig. 230, *d*). After closing the hypospadiac orifice, urine discharged normally from the tip of the glans through the accessory canal.

Epispadias. This is the absence of the upper wall of the urethra (Figs. 231–235). It occurs clinically about once in 30,000 individuals but was observed in four cases in 19,046 autopsies in the young (1:4761). On the other hand, Dees (1949) in a summary of 5,292,212 hospital admissions in

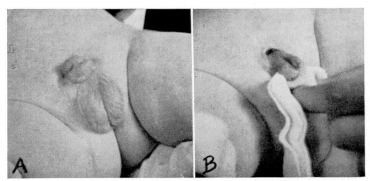

Fig. 231.   Complete epispadias in a 14-month-old boy. *A*, appearance showing stubby, spatulous penis with cleft scrotum and descended testes. *B*, penis drawn forward showing divided corpora cavernosa and funnel-like extension of urethra beneath symphyseal band into bladder. Note pronounced ventral preputial redundancy.

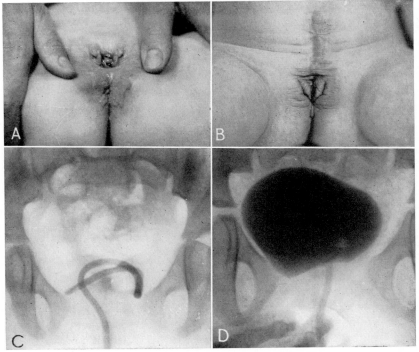

Fig. 232.   Epispadias in a three-year-old female with no urethra and total incontinence. *A*, pronounced excoriation of the perineum. The clitoris is cleft and there is slight protrusion of the vesical membrane. Vaginal opening below. *B*, appearance following surgical correction. *C*, preoperative cystogram with no retention of medium in the bladder; note the wide separation of the pubes. *D*, postoperative cystogram with establishment of normal urinary control and bladder capacity. The operative procedure carried out is that shown in Fig. 927.

several medical centers found there had been only forty-five cases of epispadias in males (1:117,604), and in eleven females (1:481,110). It is notable that a fourth of these patients were admitted to the Johns Hopkins Hospital where they doubtless had been attracted by the special skill of Dr. Hugh Young. The condition is probably not as rare as Dees' survey suggests; I have seen eighteen of these cases myself and have operated on fifteen of them, three of which were males (Campbell, 1952). Gross and Cresson (1952) reported eighteen cases from the Childrens Hospital of Boston, there being fifteen males and three females.

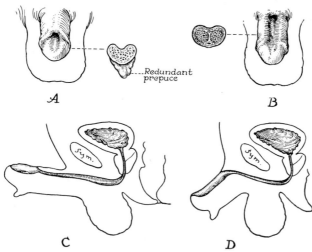

Fig. 233. Varieties of epispadias. *A*, glandular, rarest variety. Prepuce appears as a ventral hood. *C*, lateral view showing slight dorsal chordee; urethra is continuous through superior segment of penis and terminates as a groove in glans. *B*, penile; meatus opens at base of the organ, corpora cavernosa being partially divided. Note absence of corpus spongiosum. *D*, schema of condition in *B;* proximal urethra is normal. (From author's article, courtesy, Journal of Urology.)

Epispadias is a regular accompaniment of vesical exstrophy and even though the bladder is closed, epispadias may always be considered as the first degree stage in the gradation of exstrophy.

Etiology. The embryologic pathogenesis of epispadias is that of vesical exstrophy (q.v.), the difference between the lesions being one of degree. At present, the explanation offered by Patten and Barry (1952) appears to be the most comprehensive to explain this malformation, these investigators considering epispadias as the progenitor in vesical exstrophy (Figs. 201–204).

All stages of epispadias occur and of the incomplete varieties in the male, probably the most common is the glandular or balanitic form (Fig. 233 *A*); the urethral opening is above and behind the glans. A dorsal groove usually indents the glans as far forward as its tip and causes this part to appear flattened out, but the groove may stop at the corona or even proximal.

In penile epispadias the urethral opening may be anywhere from the postglandular sulcus to the suspensory ligament but is most often at the base of the penis. The dorsum of the penis is grooved from the meatus to the tip of the glans; the sulcus is covered by urethral mucosa and is frequently dotted by the orifices of the ducts of the periurethral glands. The prepuce hangs ventrally as a loose tag and leaves the glans uncovered. The organ is smaller than normal, spatulous or spadelike in appearance, incurvated upward, and prostatic development is poor or even lacking. Although these patients in later life may have satisfactory erection and intercourse, reproduction is usually impossible.

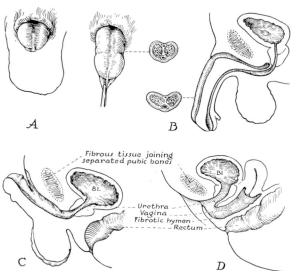

Fig. 234.   *A*, subsymphyseal epispadias. *B*, subsymphyseal epispadias, canal being essentially a reduplicated or accessory urethra ending blindly in a slight bulbous dilatation at triangular ligament. Excision. *C*, complete epispadias in male representing a first degree exstrophy. *D*, complete epispadias in a 13-month-old girl whose bladder was widely open to the outside, there being no true urethra. Vagina was obstructed by an extremely dense, fibrotic imperforate hymen and cervix was lobulated but could not be proved to be reduplicated. Congenital solitary right kidney coexisted.

Complete epispadias occurs in both sexes. *In the male* the urethra is entirely open to the bladder neck as a broad deep funnel and is most commonly associated with exstrophy of the bladder (Figs. 231, 234). The pubic bones are rarely united and often are most rudimentary. Development of the sphincters and control of the urine are poor or absent; incontinence is the rule.

In the female the degrees of epispadias are designated as clitoric, subsymphyseal and complete. Bifid clitoris and prepuce, wide separation of labia (Fig. 232) and separation of the pubic bones are proportional to the degree of the malformation. Especially in the female, should complete epispadias be considered as a first degree of vesical exstrophy. Incontinence exists and may cause the child to be treated for enuresis, to suffer severe urinous excoriation of the skin, and usually social ostracism as well. Urinary incontinence and its sequelae together with the malformation and the clinical manifestations may produce a marked genital fixation complex (cf. Novak, 1948).

In rare instances there may be stenosis of the external meatus of the epispadiac urethra.

Treatment. The therapy of epispadias is surgical and is discussed in Section XV, Chapter 11. In nearly every case, a urethroplastic procedure will usually correct the anomaly and, aided by subsequent surgical stricturization, satisfactory vesical control can be established; see Section XV, Chap-

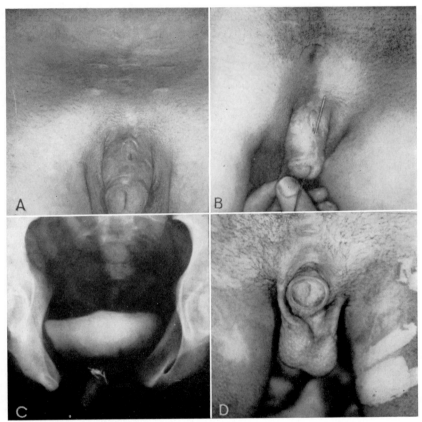

Fig. 235.   Epispadias in a ten-year-old boy. The subpubic epispadias has been corrected but with persistence of a dorsal penile fistula consequent to local suture line breakdown. *B*, probe passed into the newly formed canal. *C*, cystogram showing absence of pubis. *D*, postoperative following closure of the dorsal penile urethral fistula. Normal voiding through the tip of the penis.

ter 5. Experience has taught us to defer the operation until the child is over thirty months of age at which time vesical control normally should be consciously established. Once the repair has been made, the patient is certain to have some difficulty in learning to void and control himself for it is a new and important experience previously denied. Therefore the surgeon should not feel that he has failed simply because the child is unable to control himself normally immediately following operation. In two of my cases the achievement of perfect control took as long as two years after operation. In older cooperative children, control is usually acquired much earlier than in the young and its acquisition may be further stimulated post-operatively by employment of the start-stop-start urination exercise in which the patient, as he voids, starts the stream and stops, starts then stops. Not only does he thereby exercise the new sphincter control but becomes conscious of the sensation of the desire to urinate and of the associated mechanics of bladder emptying (Figs. 232, 235). Among older children in our series, great difficulty in achieving continence was encountered in some instances because of serious behavior problems. Ten of our cases were

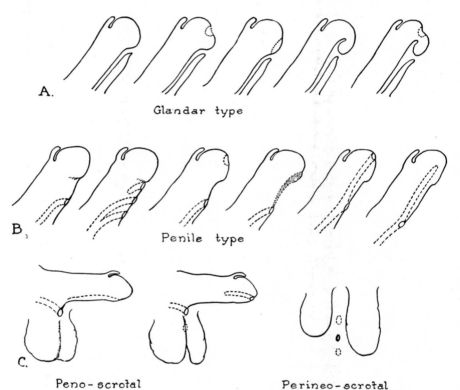

A.

Glandar type

B.

Penile type

C.

Peno-scrotal   Perineo-scrotal

Fig. 236.   Varieties of hypospadias (Hinman after Schmidt).

females; eleven with incontinence were operated upon satisfactorily with the exception of the very young just mentioned. When a sphincter cannot be reconstructed and the rectal control is normal, transplantation of the ureters to the sigmoid should be considered. The patient is entitled to at least two surgical attempts to construct a reliable bladder neck sphincter. Today ureterosigmoidostomy should seldom be necessary and decidedly is to be employed only as a last resort.

Hypospadias. This is a congenital defect of the urethra in which the canal terminates ventral and posterior to its normal opening (Figs. 236–238). The orifice may be at any point from behind the normal site, with backward elongation of the meatus, to as far back as the perineum. Frequently the hypospadiac orifice or meatus is stenosed. Because the posterior urethra is never involved, the sphincters function normally and urinary control exists. The condition occurs in both sexes but predominantly in the male.

Associated anomalies in the male commonly include malformed penis with the glans hooded over by redundant prepuce, absent frenum, chordee with incurvation downward, stenosed meatus in over half of the cases, and frequent abnormal development of the scrotum, notably bifid, and imperfectly descended testicles which themselves are often otherwise anomalous.

Hypospadias is one of the commonest of urogenital anomalies, its incidence being estimated from one in 1800 to one in 160. Schaffer and Erbes

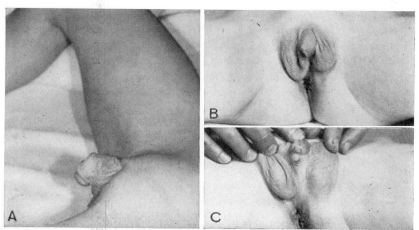

Fig. 237. Hypospadias. *A,* hypospadias at the penoscrotal junction. The redundancy of penile skin and particularly the downward bowing of the organ (chordee) is notable. *B,* hypospadias of the bulbous urethra in a two-year-old boy showing the cleft scrotum and penile incurvation (chordee). *C,* exposure of the urethral opening in *B* corresponds to *C* in Fig. 236.

(1950) found the condition accounted for one in 898 of hospital admissions in Milwaukee. In our autopsy series of 10,700 boys there were twenty-five cases, an incidence of approximately one in 583, but our clinical experience suggests that the condition is even commoner. Among urethral anomalies its incidence is exceeded only by that of congenital stricture of the meatus.

The embryogenesis of hypospadias is an arrest in the urethral development in which the urethral groove, closing ventrally from behind forward, fails to complete closure to the tip of the penis (Figs. 203, 207, 236, 237). In the more marked cases bifid scrotum and accompanying pseudohermaphroditic stigmata are also the result of arrested development; there is failure of proper midline fusion. Hypospadias has been traced through six generations by Moore (1940); I have seen it in three generations. A definite hereditary basis has not been established. This is a point of considerable practical importance, for repeatedly I have encountered young mothers who thought they should not have more children lest genital or other maldevelopment occur. The broad aspects of this problem of recurrent anomalies in offspring have been discussed at the beginning of this chapter. Giving birth to a child with hypospadias by a young mother whose husband is normal of itself is no contraindication to her having further children, and this applies to all types of genital anomalies. When the mother is over thirty-five years of age, the problem becomes more serious and after forty, under such circumstances, subsequent children are most apt to show some type of maldevelopment (cf. Murphy, 1947). So strongly is the laity imbued with the dangers of such hereditary tendencies that, as in one instance in my experience, the father of two teen-age boys with scrotal hypospadias stead-fastly refused them surgical treatment because, as he put it, he does not want any grandchildren with hypospadias! Histories in this instance suggested neither parental nor ancestral maldevelopments.

Hypospadias is not an inhibition of growth but is an hermaphroditic mani-festation in which the urogenital derivatives in the male develop toward the female (cf. Fig. 208). In more pronounced hypospadias, the utricle, a müllerian duct derivative, is usually vaginoform, the depth of the pocket varying from 1 to 10 cm. (Figs. 268-270). The orifice of this dilated utricle may obliterate or replace the verumontanum and not uncommonly the outpocketing terminates in one or two fallopian tubelike structures (Fig. 268). In general the size of the utricular dilatation parallels the severity of the hypospadias and often the boy is more female than male. Hypo-gonadism is frequent and the prostate may be hypoplastic or cannot even be identified. The penis in hypospadias is usually otherwise abnormal and often the scrotum and testes as well, the last chiefly as concerns imperfect descent.

In the anatomic genesis of hypospadias, the terminal or glandular segment of the urethra forms from the terminal urethral plate, is not a part of the urethral gutter proper and, if it does not close, glandular hypospadias results. Sometimes the terminal urethra forms normally but the penile segment does not, leaving a blind-ending glandular canal separated by a variable dis-tance from the hypospadiac opening.

While the precise causes of these changes are unsettled, femininization of the male fetus in the early developmental period (one to eight weeks) logically explains the anomalies and the congenital chordee so regularly seen in hypospadias, an occurrence not satisfactorily explained solely on the basis of faulty urethral gutter fusion. Experimental femininization of preg-nant rats produced in the offspring hypospadias, improperly descended testes, inhibition of prostatic and male duct development with stimulation of female duct growth, conditions precisely comparable to perineal and pseudovaginal hypospadias in the human (Greene et al., 1939). Bifid scrotum and other accompanying pseudohermaphroditic stigmata are usually present in ad-vanced hypospadias and reflect both femininization and failure of proper midline fusion.

Hypospadias in the male has been classified as glandular or balanitic (40 to 50 per cent), penile (25 to 30 per cent), penoscrotal, perineal or pseudovaginal (10 to 15 per cent) according to location, and as many as eleven varieties have been described (Fig. 236). In about 10 per cent the urethral openings are multiple, examples of congenital urethral fistula. Cryptorchism exists in about 15 per cent, and in two thirds of these cases is bilateral.

Balanitic Hypospadias. In this, the commonest form, the urethral orifice opens at the site of the frenum which in turn is rudimentary or absent. The orifice may be a long slit-like continuation of the normal opening or the normal site of the meatus may be identified as a blind-ending pocket with the true pinpoint orifice just posterior. The great clinical import of meatal stenosis in these cases is commonly overlooked and in several cases of this variety we have demonstrated widespread dilatation of the proximal urinary tract (Fig. 227). In balanitic hypospadias the ventral surface of the glans is furrowed in the midline, the channel is lined with urethral mucosa and often the ventral openings of the paraurethral ducts of the lacuna of Morgagni can be seen even in young boys. The glans is frequently flat and spadelike and incurved downward by the ventral chordee. The prepuce is anomalous; absent below, it forms, above, a redundant hood which incompletely covers the dorsum of the glans (Fig. 237).

Balanitic hypospadias seldom produces symptoms other than those due to a tight meatus which usually coexists. There may be urinary difficulty when the meatus is constricted or in the male there is difficulty in the direction of the urinary stream when voiding. Treatment required is dilatation of the small meatus with sounds whenever practicable, but when this fails or is unsatisfactory, a modified meatotomy of the dorsal terminal urethral roof is performed. By incision precisely along the dorsum of the meatal orifice, the ectopic meatus and the ventral dimple on the glans generally can be converted into one compartment without increasing the degree of hypospadias. In carrying out this meatotomy, caution must be exercised not to incise into the vascular portion of the ventral glans or copious bleeding will result. Thereafter, by periodic instrumental dilation the meatus is kept widely patent. Plastic procedures in these cases are seldom necessary and are likely to be meddlesome.

Penile Hypospadias. The urethra opens ventrally at some point between the glandular sulcus and the penoscrotal junction (Fig. 237). The urethra may or may not be grooved from its opening forward to the tip of the glans and when it is, a modified urethral mucosa is found. Sometimes penile hypospadias is a form of congenital fistula; the remainder of the canal proceeds forward to discharge also at the meatus (Fig. 236, *B*). Lacking a second meatus in the glans the urethral canal may extend forward from the anomalous posterior urethral orifice to end in a blind pouch (Fib. 236, *B, C*). The farther posterior the hypospadiac orifice is, the greater are the associated deformities (Fig. 238). Anterior penile hypospadias causes little functional disturbance but the broad flattened incurved glans and corpus penis with the redundant hoodlike prepuce is cosmetically disturbing and later may interfere with insemination. In anterior penile hypospadias there is likely to be little functional disturbance in the absence of urethral stenosis; by elevating the penis, the patient can usually direct the urinary stream although there is often spraying. Congenital chordee, shortly to be described, is seldom pronounced in penile hypospadias but it may give the penis a crescentic shape longitudinally.

Penoscrotal Hypospadias. The penile deformity may be extreme, the organ being dwarfed, flattened, bent downward (congenital chordee), and it may even be attached to the scrotal raphe (webbed penis; Figs. 236 *C;* 237). The urethral orifice is commonly stenosed and often produces the symptoms of urethral stricture. The congenital chordee in these cases results from hypoplasia and fibrosis of the corpus spongiosum which exists as a dense sclerotic band and usually in G-string effect extending from the

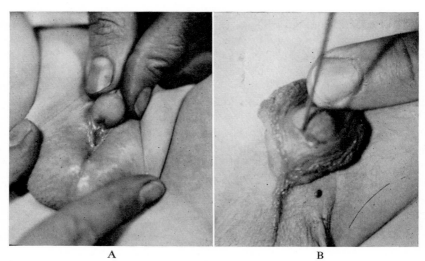

A   B

Fig. 238. Deep scrotal hypospadias of mild pseudovaginal type with short incurvated penis in a seven-month-old boy. *B,* end result following plastic repair by the Browne procedure with the newly established opening at the ventral side of the glans penis.

frenum posteriorly as far as the anterior portion of the penile crura. Excision of this fibrous band is the first step in the operation for correction of hypospadias following which the penis is afforded a chance to grow straight and to more normal size. There is often some malformation or hypoplasia of the corpora cavernosa which after puberty may account for faulty or even absent erections. The scrotum may be cleft or even bifid; in well-developed scrotal hypospadias the bifid scrotum appears labialike, the penis is rudimentary or clitoric, and hypoplasia, cryptorchism, failure of urogenital union or other testicular abnormalities commonly coexist.

Perineal Hypospadias. This is characterized by thoroughly anomalous development of the genitalia; the rudimentary (clitoric) penis is often covered by a preputial hood or is engulfed in overlying bifid scrotum (Fig. 236, *C*). Congenital chordee is extreme, the appearance of the genitalia being that of hypertrophied clitoris and labia. The separated sacs of the scrotum may contain normal, atrophic, or no testes. The urethral gutter is absent, or has a groove, or may extend forward beyond its anomalous meatus to the tip of the glans. The urethral orifice is funnel-shaped, wide open as a rule, and in extreme perineal hypospadias is aptly termed pseudo-vaginal. A great many of these cases have been described, in fact, most persons loosely designated as pseudohermaphrodites merely show pseudo-vaginal hypospadias. More than three fourths of pseudohermaphrodites are of the masculine type (Neugebauer) 722 out of 910, of which 613 were of the masculine external type; cf. Sections XII and XIII.

Most pediatricians and urologists have encountered children in whom determination of the sex was extremely difficult. When the sex cannot be accurately identified by the age of two years, abdominal exploration should be carried out to demonstrate either the female generative organs or the male testes. In a week-old girl whose genitalia at birth seemed unmistakably those of male pseudovaginal hypospadias, vaginoscopy with a small urethro-scope disclosed a normal appearing cervix, the urethral opening was hypo-spadiac, the deep segment showed no verumontanum, and bilateral pyelog-raphy at five days of age disclosed no upper urinary tract anomalies. The enormous labial folds contained no testicles and were fused high beneath the large penile clitoris, leaving only an extremely small orifice. Thus, by the employment of miniature examining instruments, the sex can be satisfactorily determined properly in most newborns when doubt exists. To repeat, when this investigation is not clearly definitive employ lapa-rotomy.

Sexual function is seldom realized by patients with penoscrotal and perineal varieties of hypospadias; because the urethral meatus is well back in penile hypospadias, insemination does not occur because the sperm are ejaculated extravaginally. Because of sterility or low fertility and difficulty of coitus in these cases of advanced hypospadias, reproduction probably never occurs. In order not to spray urine over himself and his clothing, the pseudohermaphroditic male squats or sits to void and in this and many other respects these unfortunate individuals are characteristically more female than male.

Diagnosis of hypospadias is usually readily made by inspection. Adrenal virilism in the female may confuse but here a vagina is present. An hyper-trophied clitoris and fused labia may cause error. A congenitally short urethra exists in the female.

The *treatment* is surgical. The primary reason for operating upon the patient with hypospadias is to enable him to reproduce, and secondly to establish normal controllable urination. These patients should not be operated upon solely to forestall or correct psychologic problems as seemingly impor-tant as these may be to the child's parents. *Glandular* or *balanitic* hypo-spadias requires only the establishment of free urinary drainage by dilatation of the external meatus or meatotomy as indicated. Interference to pretty up the end of the penis is meddlesome surgery and may even leave the meatus farther back than it was before. Any operation for glandular and balanitic hypospadias should be delayed until late childhood or early adult-hood for only then, what with the uncertain growth of the penis and the possibility of a relative change in the distance of the hypospadiac meatus from the tip of the penis, can the desirability of operation be properly determined.

Penoscrotal hypospadias is usually best repaired in two stages, the initial procedure being correction of the congenital chordee by the time the child is one year of age. Later when (1) he is four, five or six years of age or when there is sufficient tissue locally and (2) the penis shows no chordee and is of sufficient size to carry out the urethroplasty satisfactorily, the operation is performed. The importance of early and proper correction of the congenital chordee cannot be overemphasized for, unless the organ can grow to fairly normal size and reasonably straight, there is little point in attempting to make a new canal to the tip of the glans penis. Unless the penis is straightened early, its retarded growth will not only increase the subsequent plastic surgical difficulty, but will mitigate against obtaining the desired end result.

In *perineal hypospadias* the construction of the urethra can be started when the child is four or five years old, building the canal up to the penoscrotal junction from which point more new canal is constructed at a later date. With the Browne technique it is frequently possible to construct a new canal to its full length at one sitting, a fact which highly recommends this procedure. The operations for correction of hypospadias are presented by Cecil in Section XV, Chapter 11; see also Cecil (1951).

Pseudovaginal hypospadias regularly requires a multiple-stage operation which can be begun by the time the child is four or five years old, and after having completed the correction of chordee at an early age. I am aware that some advocate delay in correcting the chordee and the hypospadias even to fifteen or sixteen years of age (cf. Havens, 1949). Pseudovaginal hypospadias is frequently beyond hope for satisfactory cosmetic or functional surgical result.

The psychologic factor in hypospadias should not be permitted to influence either the reason or the selection of time for operation. Most children who do not have their misfortune made the topic of dinner table and household conversation and deprecation are not aware of the momentous problem it is commonly made to become. Unkind playmates will direct attention to the malformation when it is discovered by them, but in my observation more psychic harm accrues to the children through what they hear at home from discussion of the subject between their parents. In short, in the clinical management of hypospadias and similar maldevelopments or of habits such as enuresis and masturbation in the young, the attitude, instruction, and training of the parents merit special consideration.

In summary, early operation is indicated in these cases on surgical grounds rather than psychologic. Before operating for hypospadias the responsible parties should always be informed of the surgical difficulties and high incidence of secondary and other complications which often make necessary several operations before a patent, nonfistulous urethra is obtained. There is no plastic procedure in which the results of infection and breaking down of suture lines are more disheartening. Fortunately, the advent of modern chemotherapy and antibiotic therapy has strikingly reduced these hazards and it is not uncommon now for these wounds to heal *per primam.* The surgical prognosis is far better today than even ten years ago, and the urethroplasty of Denis Browne slightly modified from that described and advocated by Duplay in 1880 and 1886 has been strikingly successful. Yet Cecil's (1951) modification of the Bucknall operation is fully as satisfactory as the Browne procedure and in my hands more foolproof. I know of no operative treatment which brings more psychologic and physical comfort to the patient and satisfaction to the surgeon than successful urethroplasty in hypospadias and epispadias. The resulting personality change is often phenomenal, from shy secretive introspective boys to active, aggressive and happy ones (see Section XV, Chapter 11, for Technique of Surgical Treatment).

Hypospadias in the Female. Here the urethra opens obliquely on the anterior vaginal roof proximal to the normal site of the meatus. The hypo-spadiac orifice is frequently stenosed and causes obstruction. Although only forty-six cases have been reported, predominantly in adult women, I have seen it three times in young girls. The meatus may open abnormally at any point from the usual orifice position to the bladder neck; in the last instance the condition is essentially vesicourethral fistula with incontinence. The congenital nature of this finding is usually overlooked. Associated genital anomalies have included an enlarged clitoris, displacement toward the anus of the openings of all of the urovaginal structures and even opening of the vagina into the urethra. In several adult women with hypospadias, a small vagina and a common outlet, intra-urethral intercourse has been practiced. Urinary leakage is a frequent complaint in all except the mildest degrees of hypospadias in the female. The diagnosis is made by urethroscopy and vaginoscopy.

Dilation of the meatus and urethra with sounds usually suffices to relieve obstruction in mild degrees of hypospadias, but when the orifice is located posteriorly and there is leakage, reconstructive surgery to overcome the defective urethral wall and sphincteric deficiency is necessary, usually employing the Kelly, Kennedy or other methods. In constructing the urethra, sufficiently large and long flaps of lateral urethral wall and vaginal mucosa are brought together over a catheter; suprapubic counterdrainage is advised. These cases may also be treated by suprapubic attack similar to that employed in epispadias in the female.

Congenital Diverticulum of the Urethra. This occurs nearly always as a blowout formation behind peripheral obstruction, notably stenosis of the external urethral meatus, but doubtless is occasionally a limited or modified form of accessory urethral canal (Campbell, 1933; Kretschmer, 1936). It is probable that in many cases of urethral diverticulum alleged to be congenital, only the predisposing obstruction was congenital, the blowout process having evolved as a postnatal development (Figs. 239, 240).

For continuity of presentation, congenital and acquired diverticulum of the urethra in the young can be considered together. Diverticula have been classified as follows:

A. *Congenital diverticulum*
B. *Acquired diverticulum*
    1. From dilation of the urethra due to:
        a. urethral calculus
        b. urethral stricture
    2. With perforation of the urethra resulting from:
        a. injuries to the urethra
        b. ruptures of abscesses into the urethra
        c. rupture of cyst into the urethra

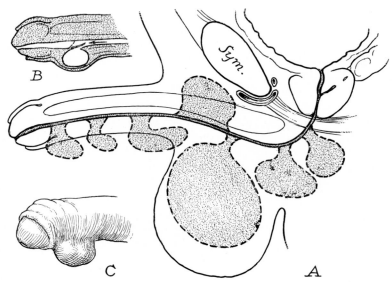

Fig. 239. Urethral diverticulum. Schema: *A*, site of origin of reported cases. *B*, flap valve urethral obstruction in which the distal roof of the diverticulum is elevated in the voiding stream as reported by Gross (see text). *C*, diverticulum of the frenal region.

According to the order of incidence, the site of congenital diverticulum formation is (1) the pendulous urethra, (2) the penoscrotal junction (Fig. 240 *A*), (3) the region of the frenum (Fig. 240 *B*) and (4) the bulbous urethra. Zeringer and Zucker (1939) reported rupture of a congenital diverticulum of the bulbous urethra in a six-year-old boy and followed by extensive urinary extravasation. Two similar cases were reported by J. Bokay (1900) and by Ternofsky (1930) in one. Concealed diverticulum in a young boy as a cause of urethral obstruction was observed by Gross and Bill (1948; Fig. 239) who reported three cases in infants.

Some believe that congenital diverticulum represents an incompleted attempt to form hypospadias. The lesion is most commonly found on the urethral floor and usually springs from the pendulous portion. The youngest reported case was three weeks of age but I saw it in the region of the frenum in a newborn behind a congenitally stenosed external urethral meatus (Fig. 698), and at the penoscrotal junction in a boy four months old (Fig. 240). Peripheral obstruction whether congenital or acquired must be considered the most common and important predisposing factor. Although urethral diverticulum is not rare in adult females, apparently no cases of congenital diverticulum in female infants or young female children have been reported. The pathogenesis, clinical findings and treatment are essentially the same as in the male (cf. Wharton and Kearns, 1950, and Section XII by Wharton in this book).

Symptoms. Urethral diverticulum, whether congenital or acquired, manifests itself as a urethral distention on urination. Usually the sac becomes

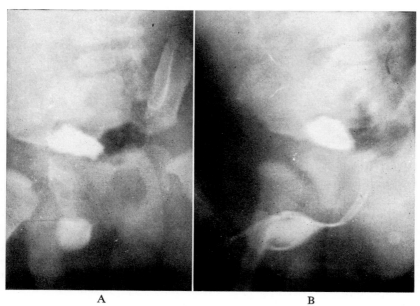

A   B

Fig. 240.   Urethral diverticulum at the penoscrotal junction in a four-month-old boy and forming as a blowout process proximal to a tight congenital stenosis of the external urethral meatus. Following meatotomy and periodic progressive dilation of the external meatus with sounds, the diverticulum gradually disappeared during a three-year period and after ten years shows no trace.

distended with urine before any appears at the external meatus and the subsequent dribbling away of the urine often leads to the erroneous diagnosis of enuresis. The patient voids as much as he can, waits a few minutes and finds he can pass still more (installment emptying; *pis en deux temps* of the French). The last urine passed is generally delivered by stripping the urethra; it represents the contents of the sac and is often thick and foul. Since infection is the rule in these cases, many of these diverticula will be discovered at the time of complete examination because of persistent pyuria. Occasionally there is pain in the urethra or perineum, or a stone may form in the diverticulum or proximal urethra to cause pain and/or persistent pyuria. Children do not suffer sexual disturbances produced by involvement of the colliculus or interference with seminal ejaculation as occurs in many adults with diverticulum of the deep urethra.

Diagnosis. This is suggested by visualization and/or palpation of the distended sac and is confirmed by urethrography and urethroscopy (Fig. 240). In one of my cases, a distended sac in the midline suggested a third testicle. Occasionally the cystoscope can be passed directly into the diverticulum; exploration with a catheter will disclose the depth, and urethrography or radiographic demonstration of the opaque catheter coiled in the sac will indicate its size. In performing urethrography in these cases, lateral, oblique and, preferably, stereoscopic exposures should be made.

Treatment. When the sac does not drain freely it should be excised with plastic closure of the opening of the diverticulum into the urethra. The urine should be diverted by suprapubic cystostomy or perineal urethrostomy drainage until the urethral closure is well healed; an inlying urethral catheter is unsatisfactory as it acts as a foreign body to delay or even prevent urethral closure. When deep urethral sacs cannot be excised, the roof of the diverticulum is widely removed to convert the sac and posterior urethra into a large common cavity. The best approach for the last procedure is through the perineum but in some cases the conversion just indicated can be achieved transurethrally by endoscopic resection of the roof of the diverticulum. Surgical therapy in any variety of urethral diverticulum is incomplete unless treatment of the sac is accompanied by removal of all urethral obstructions such as stenosis of the meatus, stricture, stone and so forth. Postoperatively, and this is most important, periodic dilation of the urethra must be regularly carried out to combat the formation of new stricture either at the site of diverticulum resection or where previously existing obstruction has been eradicated. Finally, the urine should be sterilized.

Congenital Urethral Fistula. The majority of urethral fistulas in children represent congenital or embryonal urethral blowouts behind a distal congenital obstruction. These may persist uncorrected into adulthood. Doubtless congenital stenosis of the external urethral meatus is the commonest etiologic obstructive lesion in these cases, many of which are inadequately diagnosed only as hypospadias (Fig. 236). Ectopic urethral discharge of urine is the principal symptom. The *diagnosis* is made by inspection and by exploration with a probe, it being essential to determine that the patulous urethra progresses forward to the tip of the penis.

The *treatment* requires elimination of the congenital urethral obstruction with excision of the fistulous tract and closure. For this procedure, urinary diversion by perineal urethrostomy drainage is essential. If a large urethral caliber commensurate with the age/size of the patient is maintained postoperatively by the periodic passage of sounds, the fistula may be expected to stay closed.

Urethral Cyst. These rare lesions may occur congenitally at any point from the external meatus (Fig. 225) to the bladder outlet. In all cases of congenital urethral cyst, the pathogenesis is that of occlusion of the duct of structures such as Cowper's gland, the utricle, or anterior urethral glands, or cyst formation in epithelial cell mass inclusions along the urethra and consequent to incomplete urethral fold closure. Urethral obstruction is the usual clinical manifestation; other symptoms consequent thereto are often present. A cyst 2 mm. in diameter springing from Cowper's gland and blocking the membranous urethra of a three-weeks-old boy was reported by Lisansky (1942); chronic complete urinary retention and fatal pyonephrosis resulted. Englisch described four instances in the newborn; the cysts blocked the bulbous urethra and ranged from 3 to 15 mm. in size. Their origin in Cowper's glands was proved by dissection. Bieber reported a similar condition, and Johnson found two cases in the fetus. Wesson described prostatic cyst of the prostatic urethra in a child of twenty-one months. Springer found two cases of cystic dilatation of the utricle (sinus pocularis), a remnant in the male of the müllerian duct, in sixty-two autopsies in children. Cole found a large cyst at the urethral meatus in a female of two weeks and I have seen four clinical cases of congenital urethral meatus cyst, once at eight days (Fig. 225). In Terraneus' patient, an eight-year-old boy, a pea-sized cyst of the orifice of Cowper's gland blocked the bulbomembranous urethra. Dysuria due to the obstruction caused by the cyst was present; frequent catheterization was required as it may be with any urethral cyst, congenital or acquired, when it becomes large enough to occlude the urethra. In a twenty-year-old Negro reported by Johnson, a large mass occupied the midscrotum from infancy, growing from the size of an egg to that of a grapefruit. It arose from a left Cowper's gland, the duct having been congenitally occluded.

These lesions are of interest because of their extreme rarity, but seldom offer clinical problem in children. On the other hand, prostatic cyst and cystic dilatation of the utricle have been observed not infrequently in adults and frequently of sufficient size to cause chronic urinary retention.

The *diagnosis* is made by palpation or urethroscopy, and electrodestruction or incision of the cyst is the usual *treatment* although some large cysts, particularly of the prostate or utricle, may require surgical excision either by transurethral resection or by perineal approach.

Similarly *cysts* may develop *in the median genital raphe,* particularly near the frenum. Knapp reported six cases (1935) and I have seen two frenal cysts in young boys.

Persistent Cloaca. This is characterized by congenital intercommunication between the urethrovesical junction area and the rectum in the male, and between the adjacent vesicovaginal and/or urethrovaginal and rectal segments in the female. The condition is one of the rarest and most severe of urogenital tract anomalies. Fourteen cases have been reported, eight of which were operated upon. Grave anomalies, often incompatible with life, frequently coexist. In a male white child with persistent cloaca and dead twelve minutes post partum, there were congenital absence of the prostate, left leg and foot, left ureter and kidney, meningocele, right hydronephrosis above multiple ureteral strictures (upper, midsection, and ureterovesical junction area) and kinks, with abdominal testes, the left being opposite the third lumbar vertebra and the right adjacent to the kidney. In a stillborn premature boy there was, in addition to cloacal formation, left polycystic kidney, atresia of the anus, clubfoot, atresia of the bladder into which the ureters opened, and persistent urachus. The gravity of the condition is suggested by failure to find it in any of 32,834 autopsies in adults.

The embryologic *etiology* of persistent cloaca is shown in Figures 191 and 202 in which it will be noted how the urorectal septum may fail to join the cloacal membrane, thereby leaving a connection between the bladder and rectum which is recognized as congenital urethrorectal fistula (cf. infra). The *symptoms* are chiefly passage of feces, gas, and urine or even intestinal blood through the rectum, urethra and/or vagina according to sex and which channel opens externally. The incidence of congenital anal atresia in the newborn is about 1 in 6500 infants. Baker and Wilkey (1948) observed cloacal formation in a five-year-old boy with no urethra; in some instances with imperforate anus, urinary drainage occurred through the umbilicus. When the cloacal formation is not directly fatal, secondary renal infection and urosepsis usually kill.

In persistent cloaca, the *diagnosis* is suggested by the history and is confirmed by urethroscopic, proctoscopic and/or urographic investigation. The *treatment* is surgical and consists in separating the malformed channels and establishing a mesially located outlet. This may require the construction of a vesical sphincter or, as in Lowsley's case (1948), construction of both vesical and rectal sphincters.

Congenital Urethrorectal Fistula. This results from failure of the urogenital fold completely to separate the rectum from the posterior urethral segment of the bladder (Fig. 191), but is a less severe malformation than persistent cloaca. In males the fistulous connection is generally in the membranous urethra. The condition is comparatively rare, occurs about once in 7500 individuals, and is twice as frequent in males as in females (urethro-vaginorectal).

As a rule in congenital urethrorectal fistula, the anus is imperforate but when patent there is congenital anal stricture. Twenty-three of the twenty-seven cases I have seen had been operated upon for imperforate anus a few hours after birth at which time the various operating surgeons were amazed to release a gush of urine or, if the urine did not appear at the operating table, it was noted soon postoperatively. The surgeon generally feels he has accidentally perforated the bladder or urethra and fails to appreciate that the anomaly is simply a persistence of mild cloacal formation resulting from failure of complete separation of the urethra and rectum. Rarely, as I observed once, the urethrorectal fistula opens in the anterior trigone but here embryologic aberration must be adduced to explain the finding in the absence of a slip of the surgeon's knife at the time of opening the imperforate anus. Congenital urethrovesical as well as urethrorectal fistula may coexist, together with other anomalies. In a three-week-old boy with rectourethral fistula examined post mortem there was found also horseshoe kidney, imperforate anus and acute prostatitis. In a four-week-old boy the imperforate rectum extended within 5 mm. of the perineum, there being a common opening for the rectum and bladder into the urethra; the upper urinary tract was widely distended.

Symptomatically urethrorectal fistula permits the passage of urine per rectum and/or feces per urethram. Dyes such as methylene blue or indigo carmine injected into the bladder appear in the stool. The diagnosis is most accurately made by cystourethroscopy when the fistulous opening into the rectum will be seen on the urethral floor. Usually the fistulous opening is just behind the verumontanum although it may be just in front of this structure but proximal to the internal sphincter. Moreover, the verumontanum may be dwarfed or even disappear into the fistulous structure. At the time of urethroscopic examination it is wise to pass an instrument such as a sound into the fistulous tract from the rectal side, this orifice frequently being found just within the anal ring. Moreover, one may be able to palpate the fistulous orifice by rectal examination or observe it proctoscopically. When the anus is not imperforate, a tight sphincter regularly accompanies urethrorectal fistula, is situated just below the fistulous opening into the bowel and often is strictured. The treatment consists of excision and closure of the fistulous tract as described in Section XV, Chapter 11.

The various forms of congenital urethrorectal fistula and the accompanying urinary tract anomalies may seriously tax surgical skill. In one of our patients, first seen at four weeks of age, the boy had been operated upon for imperforate anus at the age of four hours (Fig. 224). Later it was found that his anterior urethra ended blindly in the perineum while a short stump of posterior urethra opened directly into the anal stricture. Colostomy was performed initially at six weeks of age. At the age of three months suprapubic cystostomy drainage was instituted and, by perineal exposure, the short posterior urethra was mobilized from its opening in the rectum to the prostate. The fistulous orifice in the bowel was closed by inversion with a row of fine chromic sutures, the colostomy still operating. Dissecting forward in the midline of the perineum with a small sound in the anterior urethra as a guide, the blind ending of the urethral segment in the midbulb was identified and opened. A deep groove was made then in the midperineal line to permit the posterior portion of the urethra to be slung forward and obliquely anastomosed end to end to the distal anterior urethral segment. The wound was closed with a cigarette drain to the deep peripelvic operative fossa. A small catheter was left in the urethra a few days as a splint. Ominously a small urethral fistula developed at the site of anastomosis but subsequently healed spontaneously. Periodically since that time, an ample urethral caliber has been maintained by periodic dilation with sounds. Suprapubic cystostomy was discontinued and two months later the colostomy was closed. Twelve years later this boy's urethral caliber (21 F.) and control were normal, the urine was sterile and the only important reminder of his previous condition is a moderate stricture of the anus which requires occasional dilation.

Congenital Valves of the Posterior Prostatic Urethra. These are identified as deep mucosal folds or redundancies, often paper thin, located in the posterior urethra, and usually attached at one end to the verumontanum (Figs. 241, 242). Rarely the valves are found to be partial or complete diaphragms and show a wide range in location and conformation. Imperforate diaphragms have rarely been found at autopsy, are similar to atresia elsewhere (q.v.) and unrelieved, are usually incompatible with life. Yet the opening in the urethral diaphragm may be no larger than the diameter of a pin and cause practically complete urinary obstruction. In the more usual leaflet type of valves, as the fluid stream strikes the mucosal folds, the valves cystoscopically generally appear to balloon into cusp formation and resemble in action the heart valves. They are to be distinguished from the

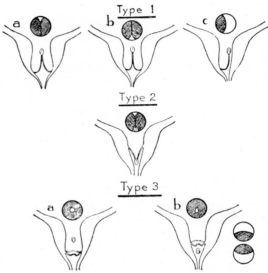

Fig. 241. Congenital valves of the posterior urethra (McKay after Young). Type I: a, two bifurcated valves springing from the distal portion of the verumontanum; b, two fused valves in the same position; c, unilateral valve in the same position. Type II: bifurcated valve extending from the proximal portion of the verumontanum to the lateral sides of the prostatic urethra and roof. Type III: a, iris valve below the verumontanum; b, iris valve above the verumontanum. The shaded circles represent the cystoscopic field seen in the region of the valves. The vesical outlet and the prostatic urethra are shown to be dilated; the region of the membranous urethra is indicated.

low ridges which are merely exaggerations of the normal frenulae of the prostatic urethra and do not obstruct.

Young (1919; Fig. 241) classified valves of the prostatic urethra into three types, the differentiating features being their relation to the verumontanum to which most valves are attached at some point. The most frequent variety passes from the anterior verumontanum to the anterior lateral urethral wall (Type I). Yet valves may extend from the posterior verumontanum into the vesical outlet (Type II). The diaphragm variety is identified as Type III. The valve leaflets may be multiple and particularly is this true of the Type II variety; we have seen as many as seven leaflets (e.g., Fig. 242). Moreover, the valves may be unilateral but these are unlikely to obstruct because the urinary stream can pass along the opposite side of the prostatic urethra. Valves may appear on the urethral roof, but their usual location is on the floor. As in two of our cases, the valves may pass from the midverumontanum laterally to the urethral wall, a modification of Type I (Fig. 242, *E*) and be radiographically demonstrable (Figs. 243–245).

In valvular obstruction the verumontanum is usually anomalous, generally being greatly enlarged and elongated. In some cases we have found it three to four times normal size and to extend from the vesical outlet forward for 2 or 3 cm. and even well back into the vesical outlet. Type I valves

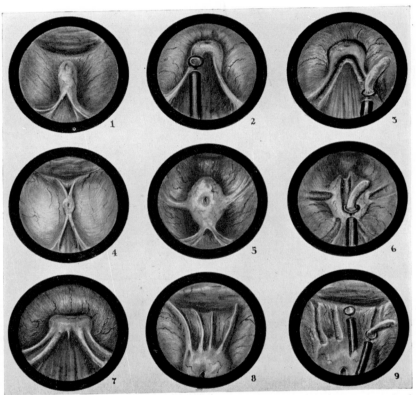

Fig. 242.   Congenital valves of the posterior urethra; various types and methods of treatment. Type I: Moderate dilatation of the urethra behind valves. 2, 3, author's cutting method of valve resection; 4, Type I and II valves. Small verumontanum. Greatly over-distended posterior urethra. 5, 6, Type I valves, also valve leaflets passing from the midverumontanum to the lateral walls. These leaflets caused an hourglass appearance in the posterior urethrogram; 7, reduplicated Type I valves. 8, multiple Type II valves in an eleven-month-old boy, and 9, loop resection in 8.

frequently form a deep pouch or pocket at their bifurcation at the anterior verumontanum and in which pocket urethral instruments are likely to catch. Such a pouch is by-passed by keeping the beak of the instrument firmly against the urethral roof, a requisite which, of itself, is diagnostically suggestive.

The embryologic explanation of urethral valves is unsettled, some observers believing them to be due to (1) enlargement or hypertrophy of the normal urethral folds (Tolmatschew), (2) persistence of the urogenital membrane (Bazy), (3) anomalous wolffian or müllerian duct development

(Lowsley), or (4) fusion of the colliculus with the epithelium of the posterior urethral groove (Watson). But none of these explanations fits all cases; similar valves or cusplike obstructive folds are sometimes seen on the anterior vesical trigone near the outlet as well as in the ureters.

Most of the early reported cases of prostatic valves were discovered post mortem but with present-day miniature instrumentaria the condition should be readily identified urethroscopically, the principal diagnostic difficulty

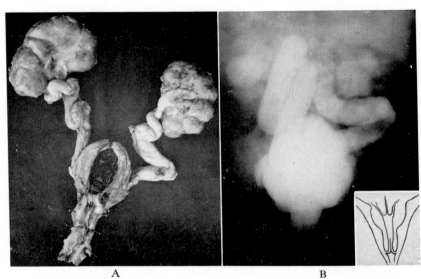

A   B

Fig. 243. Congenital valves of the posterior urethra in an eleven-month-old boy. The verumontanum is nearly four times normal size and length, and bifurcates anteriorly to form Type I valves. Three deep Type II valves are seen extending from the posterior verumontanum to the bladder outlet. There is marked hypertrophy of the bladder wall, four to five times normal thickness, and acute hemorrhagic decompression cystitis due to the sudden evacuation of the chronically overdistended viscus. The patient was admitted to the hospital because of constipation. An abdominal mass was thought to be filled constipated bowels but proved to be greatly distended ureters. The bladder was palpable to the umbilicus. Mechanically the overdistended bladder compressed the rectum to prohibit normal movements. By maneuvering the irrigating fluid, the obstructing valves were cystoscopically observed to balloon into cusp formation. The bladder urine was sterile. Uremic death occurred one week following cystostomy drainage. Extreme dilatation of the ureters and renal pelves with hydronephrotic renal destruction are notable. B, cystogram in A showing extensive dilatation of the entire upper urinary tract and the striking cystographic delineation of the posterior urethra behind the anterior (Type I) valves. (Bellevue Hospital.)

being the differentiation of true obstructing valves from the normal urethral mucosal redundancy and particularly the frenulae passing anteriorly from the verumontanum to the lateral urethral walls. This congenital condition has been observed in newborn twins, and in one of our series was discovered post mortem in a boy five hours old (Fig. 245, A). The relative paucity of reported cases largely reflects diagnostic failure. Because the lesion is obstructive it is certain to be found one or more times in any substantial series of children examined because of persistent pyuria, urinary infection, or so-called enuresis. With recognition before hopeless renal damage has been engendered and the institution of proper treatment, most of these patients can be saved although in the advanced cases irreparable renal damage will have doubtless occurred.

Pathology. Urinary tract changes proximal to the urethral valves are those common to all infravesical obstructions and have been discussed in Section III. With the obstruction unrelieved, the back-pressure damage and dilatation of the proximal urinary channels increase, infection is encouraged, and the clinical picture of so-called chronic pyelitis with recurrent acute exacerbation of the infection develops. Often the ureters are dilated

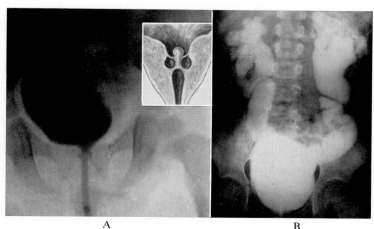

A   B

Fig. 244.   Congenital valves of the prostatic urethra. *A*, in a two-year-old boy examined because of dysuria. The curious valve formation with the proximal leaflet springing from the midportion of the verumontanum caused an hourglass conformation of the posterior urethrogram. Transurethral loop resection of the valves. (Bellevue Hospital.) *B*, advanced injury of the upper urinary tract in a six-year-old boy examined because of chronic pyuria. Marked dilatation of the upper urinary tract with grave renal destruction. Residuum 670 cc. Preliminary cystostomy drainage; six months later transurethral resection of the valves was limited (unilateral) by the poor condition of the patient, yet seventeen years later he appears healthy, is in college, but no urographic follow up has been obtained.

to the size of the colon and longitudinal dilatation may double their length with the formation of numerous ureteral folds, kinks and angulations. Frequently the renal parenchyma is reduced to a thin shell (Figs. 243–245), and with the advent of infection the injury is accelerated and intensified. Coincident with hypertrophy of the bladder wall there is likely to be some hypertrophy of the trigone causing it to stand out in contrast to the coarsely trabeculated bladder wall adjacent. Vesical diverticula and/or stone develop in about 5 per cent of the cases. As in all varieties of obstructive uropathy, prognosis and treatment are considered in terms of renal function.

Symptoms. The symptoms of valves of the prostatic urethra are those common to urinary tract obstruction with renal insufficiency or uremia and in general occur early and are more severe than with other obstructions at or near the vesical outlet. Frequency of urination usually exists from birth and is the most common symptom; with increasing vesical retention, overflow or paradoxical incontinence develops with periodic or continuous wetting. In the absence of infection, these manifestations often cause the erroneous diagnosis of enuresis. Hesitancy in starting the stream and urinary difficulty result from the greatly diminished urethral caliber. Symptoms may be extremely meager until infection occurs, and doubtless this explains why some patients may go to the third or fourth decade of life before becoming sufficiently disturbed to seek treatment. One of our cases was discovered

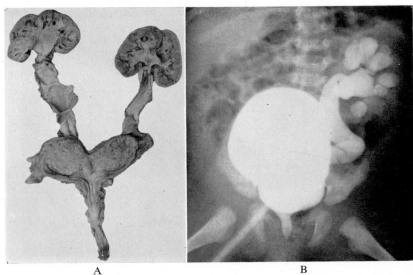

A   B

Fig. 245. Congenital valves of the prostatic urethra in the newborn. *A,* boy dead at five hours of tentorial tears. The verumontanum is enlarged and greatly elongated, bifurcating anteriorly into Type I valves. There is advanced back-pressure injury of the upper urinary tract with moderate bladder wall thickening and extensive ureteral and pelvic dilatation. This back-pressure damage had been operating since the fifth month of uterine life when renal function begins. *B,* this boy was born with an overdistended bladder, was unable to urinate, nor could a catheter be passed. Suprapubic cystotomy was performed when the patient was twenty-four hours old. Urethroscopic study two months later showed Type I valves appearing as indicated in Fig. 241. In the above cystogram the wide dilatation of the bladder and, by vesico-ureteral reflux of the medium, of the ureters, reflects the obstructive effects. Notable is the filling of the posterior urethra down to the point of valvular obstruction. The slight urographic filling defect in the posterior urethra is caused by the verumontanum. In a subsequent cystogram, ureteral reflux on the right side similar to that on the left was also demonstrated. Suprapubic cystostomy drainage was maintained for four months, followed by transurethral resection of the valves through a perineal external urethrostomy opening.

at autopsy in a seventy-two-year-old man. Yet patients with marked valvular obstruction seldom live more than ten years.

Urination in some of these young patients causes them to become purple in the face from straining, to manifest considerable pain, and often to compress the abdomen to force out urine. The chronically overdistended bladder may cause a suprapubic protuberance which sometimes is felt by the patient or parent. An eleven-month-old boy with prostatic urethral valves was admitted to Bellevue Hospital because of constipation and was found to have the rectum firmly compressed by an overdistended bladder sufficient to prevent any bowel movements except following enemas. A five-year-old boy learned to compress his bladder against the seat of a chair.

As the bladder dilates it may fall to one side and give the impression of an abdominal tumor which disappears on catheterization. Vesical retention may produce lower abdominal pain or, with vesicoureteropelvic reflux, there may be pain in the loin or renal region and particularly on straining to void. Because of this generalized abdominal discomfort, the patient may be unable to find a comfortable position in bed.

When infection supervenes, all symptoms are intensified and the clinical diagnosis of "acute pyelitis" is usually made. Occurring with obstruction, acute renal infection is usually severe and unless urinary drainage is promptly established, may be expected readily to convert the kidneys into suppurative pyonephrotic organs with fatal termination. Frequently, however, the acute infection subsides and becomes simply a persistent low-grade pyuria ever likely to flare up in acute exacerbation. With continued renal damage the manifestations of uremia in its progressing stages appear with headache, languor, or irritability because of nervous system disturbance; gastrointestinal manifestations with anorexia, nausea, vomiting, constipation, diarrhea, biliousness, gastritis, failure to gain, or more often, loss of weight, are commonly present singly or in combination. Yet they may be so distressing as to cause the urinary tract condition to be overlooked entirely. It is notable that in these severe urinary obstructions with bilateral renal involvement, gastrointestinal disturbances are outstanding in more than half of the cases.

The terminal picture is urosepsis and intercurrent infection, chiefly pneumonia, or uremic coma. These weakened children are particularly susceptible to acute respiratory or urinary infections which tend to be rapidly fatal. Because of the clinical picture and laboratory findings in valvular obstruction, an erroneous diagnosis of chronic pyelitis, chronic interstitial nephritis, or even polycystic renal disease is sometimes made.

Diagnosis. This is suggested by the history and physical examination. Cystourethroscopy is confirmatory at which time the obstructing valves will be observed (Fig. 242). Physical examination generally discloses the distended bladder and sometimes also distended ureters and kidneys. The urotoxemia is reflected in a dry tongue which becomes boardy and fissured as the uremia intensifies. This drying of the mucous membranes is often accompanied by buccal dysphagia; because of the parched mouth and throat, swallowing is avoided or is impossible, and the patient usually soon dies.

Complicating urinary infection is the rule in these cases, the urinary tract bacterial invaders being chiefly gram-positive staphylococci or streptococci or members of the gram-negative colon bacillary group, either in pure culture or mixed. Pus is found in the urine and sometimes blood together with albumin and casts. Based on these laboratory findings and particularly when infection is minimal, the diagnosis of chronic interstitial nephritis is too often erroneously made, even though it would appear to be confirmed by a high blood nitrogen retention, diminished carbon dioxide combining power of the blood, and reduced phenolsulfonphthalein output. Elevated blood pressure occurs only when there is marked glomerular injury and is seldom encountered in valvular obstruction, in which the renal damage is chiefly tubular. Renal damage consequent to valvular obstruction has sometimes produced the syndrome of renal rickets (q.v. Section XVII, Chapter 2; cf. Derow and Brodney, 1939).

When infection is the principal clinical manifestation and urinary back-pressure damage is less extreme, the diagnosis of chronic pyelitis too often satisfies the physician. Yet valvular obstruction has been found in several boys we have examined because of urinary difficulty or enuresis and in the absence of infection.

Cystographic studies may suggest the correct diagnosis as may excretory urography in which the conformation of the obstructing valves is delineated in the dilated posterior urethra (Figs. 243, 245) and readily distinguishes the condition from the paralytic funneling of neuromuscular origin (q.v.). The outline of the urinary tract above demonstrates the back-pressure dilatation and damage: trabeculation, sacculation, diverticulum formation, ureteral dilatation and angulation, hydronephrosis and so forth (Fig. 243).

Technical difficulty may be encountered in passing the examining cystoscope as it may be blocked by valvular structures. If the tip of the instrument is kept snugly against the roof of the prostatic urethra, its introduction to the bladder is likely to be readily made. It is essential that a forward vision rather than a right-angle prismatic instrument be used to study the urethra and bladder outlet. The previously described back-pressure changes in the bladder wall and at the vesical outlet are seen and, as the instrument is withdrawn into the deep urethra and with a small irrigating stream entering simultaneously through the cystoscope, the obstructing valves can generally be made to distend and balloon into cusps resembling those of the heart as previously described. Supramontane valve leaflets extending into the bladder outlet are usually multiple and deep; the great depth probably results from sacculation produced by continuous urinary distention (Fig. 243). The cystoscopic definition of valves should not be difficult; they are quite different from the normal frenulae of the deep urethra which do not cause obstruction with the severe changes in the deep urethra and bladder so regularly observed in valvular blockage. Contracture of the vesical outlet, spastic neuromuscular disease and hypertrophy of the verumontanum unassociated with valves, congenital urethral stricture, chronic interstitial nephritis, or congenital polycystic disease are ruled out by adequate urologic study. Although some of these conditions may coexist, the valvular obstruction should usually be considered the most important.

Prognosis. This depends upon the degree of renal damage, is always potentially grave, and may advisedly be guarded. The general physical and renal rehabilitation of these patients following the establishment of free urinary drainage and control of infection is often phenomenal. Sterilization of the urine with modern chemotherapy and antibiotic therapy is the co-objective in every case and no patient should be discharged as cured until the urine has been sterilized and all obstruction eradicated.

Treatment. This is best achieved by transurethral resection of the obstructing valves and the administration of intensive chemotherapy and antibiotic therapy as bacteriologically indicated. If the condition of the patient is reasonably good and renal damage is not excessive, it has been our practice to proceed at once with the removal of the obstruction. If these factors are not favorable and there is marked infection, drainage by indwelling catheterization for one to four weeks as necessary has been carried out

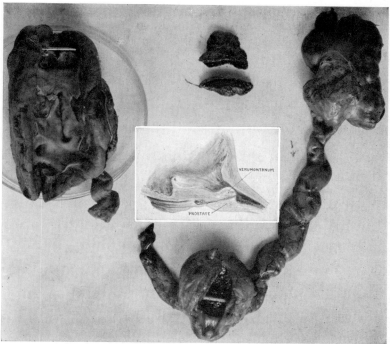

Fig. 246. Congenital hypertrophy of the verumontanum with advanced dilatation of the upper urinary tract and renal destruction in a boy of fourteen months admitted to the hospital in uremia. The urine was sterile; clinical diagnosis; chronic interstitial nephritis. The schematic insert indicates the character and site of the obstruction. (Babies Hospital.)

but with present-day chemotherapy, antibiotic therapy, blood transfusions, and other surgical aids, the number of patients requiring preliminary drainage has vastly diminished as it has in transurethral prostatic surgery in adults. When the renal function and the patient's general condition are extremely poor and prolonged urinary vesical drainage is imperative before transurethral resection can favorably be undertaken, employ suprapubic cystostomy for such period as clinical studies of the improvement process demand. In any event, transurethral resection should be withheld until the patient is in reasonably safe condition and physiologically stabilized.

The introduction of the miniature resectoscope has eliminated the need for removal of valvular obstruction by the perineal, suprapubic or retropubic approaches, by forceful rupture with sounds, the employment of miniature punches or transurethral fulgurating electrodes, each of which was employed in the past. The transurethral resection technique affords excision under visualization with a minimum of surgical shock, tissue injury, bleeding and undesirable sequelae. Postoperatively, fluids are administered freely up to 1200 or 1500 cc. per day with care against overloading the circulation. Acidosis is prevented by the use of normal saline, glucose, or ⅙ molar sodium-r-lactate solution administered as necessary. A catheter is left indwelling postoperatively for two or three days, until all bleeding has ceased, and following its withdrawal free urination may be expected. When the patient cannot void freely during six hours after removing the

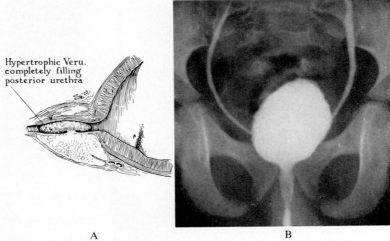

Hypertrophic Veru. completely filling posterior urethra

A   B

Fig. 247. Hypertrophy of the verumontanum with complete filling of the posterior urethra in a seventeen-year-old boy dead of typhoid fever. This lesion caused no pronounced obstruction (Bellevue Hospital.) *B,* urethrographic demonstration of an enlarged verumontanum in a twelve-year-old boy examined because of persistent pyuria and urinary difficulty; the last was caused by the enlarged verumontanum which was partially resected transurethrally.

catheter, the tube should be reinserted for another day or two for a trial period. If the difficulty persists, cystoscopic re-examination and, generally, further resection are demanded. The requisites of urinary antisepsis and blood transfusion as indicated must be observed, mindful that the patient is cured only when the obstruction is completely relieved and the urine is sterilized.

Congenital Hypertrophy of the Verumontanum. In this condition the verumontanum is enlarged two or more times normal size, occupies the greater portion of the transverse lumen of the prostatic urethra, may extend into the vesical outlet posteriorly or into the membranous urethra anteriorly, obstructs urinary outflow and on section shows only hypertrophied normal structure (Figs. 246–248). Frequently superficial inflammatory changes are observed. Hypertrophy of the verumontanum was reported in twenty of 10,712 boys examined post mortem, an incidence of one in 535. Several observers have clinically recognized the condition during the past twenty-five years (Bugbee and Wollstein, 1923; Robinson, 1927; Campbell, 1937; Thompson, 1942; and Johnson and Price, 1949). It has frequently been observed in conjunction with congenital valvular obstruction of the prostatic urethra.

The etiology is unknown. Brody and Goldman (1940) suggested that, in some instances at least, enlargement of the verumontanum and distention of the utricle in the newborn, sufficient to be obstructive, may result from stimulation of circulating estrogens during fetal life.

Symptoms as well as the physical and laboratory findings are similar to those observed in other types of infravesical obstruction and are indis-

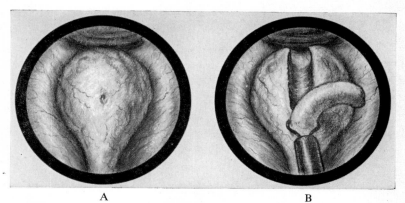

A   B

Fig. 248. Hypertrophy of the verumontanum. *A,* cystoscopic appearance; often the organ fills the entire deep urethra despite liberal dilation with irrigating fluid. Unless the prostatic urethra is well distended at the time of deep urethroscopy, the verumontanum in all boys will appear abnormally large owing to the close proximity of the tissue to the objective lens of the instrument. *B,* author's method of treatment by transurethral electro-cutting loop resection. It is unnecessary to remove the entire organ and as far as possible the ejaculatory ducts should be spared.

tinguishable from those just described under valvular obstruction of the prostatic urethra (see also Section III).

The *diagnosis* is made by cystourethroscopy when an enormous verumontanum is observed to fill the posterior urethra (Figs. 247, 248). The organ may appear as a large ball but more often it is greatly elongated and enlarged and sometimes extends well back into the vesical outlet as a ball valve. The cystoscopic diagnosis should be made with caution and certainty; unless the posterior urethra is well distended with fluid and the verumontanum is well displaced from the objective lens of the cystoscope, a normal verumontanum may appear enormous. Only a panendoscopic or direct vision instrument should be used for this study and unless one is able to obtain a panoramic view of the deep urethra, the diagnosis may be erroneous. If the patient is conscious and will attempt to urinate, the posterior urethral wall will be depressed; this affords better visualization of the verumontanum. Severe congestion and pronounced enlargement of the verumontanum are not infrequent in older boys as the result of chronic masturbation while coexisting inflammatory changes in the adjacent mucosal surfaces, especially over the prostate, should suggest underlying prostatitis. By urethrography the enlarged verumontanum may produce a filling defect in the posterior urethra (Fig. 247, *B*), and when the hypertrophic organ is large, the defect is particularly striking.

Treatment. This demands that sufficient of the hypertrophic verumontanum be removed to permit easy and complete emptying of the bladder (Fig. 248). The preoperative preparation, the technique of transurethral resection,

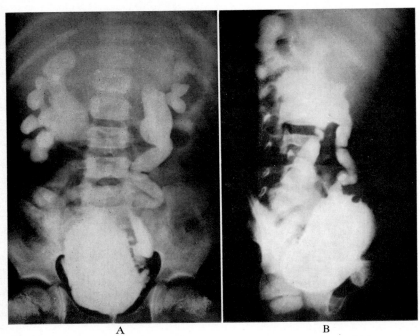

A   B

Fig. 249.   Congenital contracture of the vesical outlet in a five-year-old boy. *A,* cystogram showing bladder enlargement and irregularity with sacculation of the vesical wall particularly on the left; dilated tortuous kinked ureters and moderately advanced hydronephrosis bilaterally. *B,* lateral view of *A* showing the ureteral tortuosity from another angle.

and the postoperative care employed are the same as previously described under valvular obstruction of the prostatic urethra.

Under precise cystourethroscopic visualization as much of the hypertrophic structure as seems indicated is removed, appreciating that by postoperative sclerosis and diminution of edema following eradication of the obstruction, the verumontanum will still further reduce in size. It is unnecessary to amputate the organ completely. As a rule the removal of three or four full length longitudinal strips from the verumontanum is followed by sufficient shrinkage and sclerotic contraction to permit normal bladder emptying. Postoperatively a catheter is generally left indwelling for forty-eight hours. If, on its removal, the boy cannot void freely, further transurethral resection with additional tissue removal is indicated.

While it is possible that sterilization of the patient may result from sealing off the ejaculatory ducts during the transurethral operation, adequate time has not elapsed to determine this personally except in one boy who was found sterile when examined fourteen years postoperative. Follow-up examination of several others has permitted a 3 F. catheter to be passed 1.5 to 2 cm. up the ejaculatory ducts which would suggest that the operation is not always sterilizing but at the time these boys had not achieved the age of spermatogenesis. Removal of the obstruction is the vital consideration and unless this is accomplished early, the problem of reproduction may never arise.

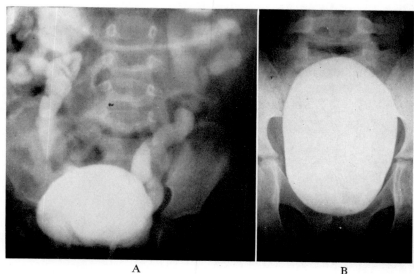

A   B

Fig. 250. Congenital contracture of the vesical outlet. *A*, in a boy of twenty-four months previously treated eighteen months for "chronic pyelitis." Residual urine five ounces. In this cystogram performed through a cystostomy tube, the bladder is seen to be slightly enlarged with outlining of the dilated upper urinary tract bilaterally by vesicoureteral reflux. Suprapubic V-wedge excision from the inferior segment of the vesical outlet. *B*, in an eight-year-old girl with eight ounces residual urine. Although the cystographic outline is still smooth, the bladder is considerably dilated because of the obstruction. Treatment: transurethral resection.

The enlarged verumontanum may also be removed by transurethral punch operation, by suprapubic, retropubic or perineal resection, but these procedures are more traumatic and of greater surgical risk than transurethral electroexcision under visualization; with modern miniature resectoscopic instruments available, these other procedures may be considered obsolete techniques.

Contracture of the Vesical Outlet. This is a form of congenital urethral stricture analogous to meatal stenosis, may be found at any age, has been observed in twin brothers, and about 20 per cent occur in females (Figs. 249–253). This condition has been observed in the fetus and must be recognized as congenital although the clinical manifestations may not appear until the second or third decade of life or even later. Most of the patients with congenital contracture of the vesical outlet that I have seen have been less than six years of age although in several men in their thirties with contracture, both the history and the urethroscopic findings have suggested its congenital nature. A few instances have been described in the female (Fig. 250) but there is no reason why the incidence should not be essentially as high as in the male; the embryologic etiology is simply a congenital narrowing of the outlet canal the same as may occur elsewhere in the urethra or

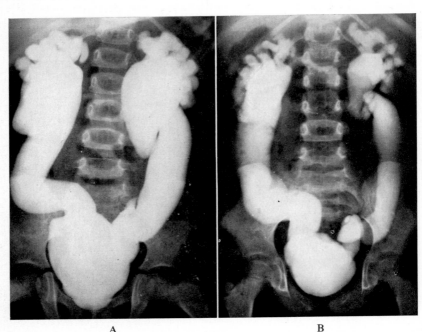

A   B

Fig. 251.   Congenital contracture of the vesical orifice in a five-year-old girl examined because of mild pyuria. No urinary difficulty. There is enormous dilatation of the upper urinary tract; the kidneys were reduced to thin shells. Suprapubic cystostomy drainage was instituted and six months later was followed by transurethral resection of the vesical outlet. B, cystogram six months postoperative indicates considerable diminution of the dilatation in both ureters and renal pelves. Marked improvement in the renal function and general condition of the child followed. The preoperative residuum determined immediately after voiding was five ounces, while postoperative the child emptied her bladder completely. Yet after five minutes, a considerable amount of urine drains into the bladder to confuse the determination of residual urine, hence the importance of catheterization immediately following urination.

in the ureters, biliary passages, vascular system and/or gastrointestinal tract. Moreover, congenital contracture of the vesical outlet and congenital stenosis of the external meatus—a comparable lesion to which contracture ranks second among lower tract obstructions—frequently coexist in the same patient. In both boys and girls I have several times encountered in addition congenital ureterovesical junction stricture with upper urinary tract back pressure damage varying from mild to severe. The upper tract obstruction may be unilateral but is frequently bilateral. In these cases there is obstruction to the passage up the ureter of a 4 F. catheter and cystographic vesical distention shows no ureteral reflux, two findings not present when congenital contracture of the vesicle outlet is the only lesion. Such observations illustrate the need for complete urologic examination in these patients even though the lower tract obstruction is readily recognized.

In 1930 and 1937 I reported a series of these cases under the designation Submucous Fibrosis of the Vesical Outlet, which indicates the local pathology in one group of these congenital obstructions (Fig. 254). It is likely that muscular hypertrophy of the internal sphincter analogous to pylorospasm explains the picture in some cases and may possibly be on a neurogenic

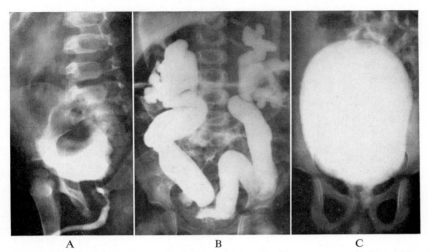

A   B   C

Fig. 252. Congenital contracture of the vesical outlet in a two-year-old boy with persistent pyuria and 750 cc. residuum. *A*, urethrocystogram showing irregularity of the trabeculated and sacculated vesical wall with a tortuous prostatic urethra and tight vesical outlet. *B*, because of extreme ureteral angularity, bilateral nephrostomy drainage gave promise of being more effective than cystotomy. In the above urogram each nephrostomy tube has been injected showing the enormously dilated upper urinary tract. *C*, postoperative cystogram following transurethral resection of the vesical outlet. Note the slight funneling at the vesical outlet and in the posterior urethra consequent to a removal of obstructing tissue at this point. There is also diminution of the irregularity in the vesical outline.

basis (Fig. 254). The term achalasia was first employed by Hurst (1931) in this connection and in 1915 Beer observed that the fibrosis of the vesical neck which exists when the young patient is presented for examination may be a secondary change in the spastic sphincter in neuromuscular disease, and may or may not be associated with inflammation or trophic degeneration. While there is no final proof of this, tissue removed transurethrally from the bladder neck in patients of all ages with neuromuscular vesical disease lends considerable corroborative evidence to bolster Beer's theory. This may exist in older boys but we have not seen it in adults in whom it could be attributed as the primary cause of existent bladder neck contracture.

Contracted bladder neck is of great clinical importance because of the urinary obstruction it produces and it is generally complicated by infection,

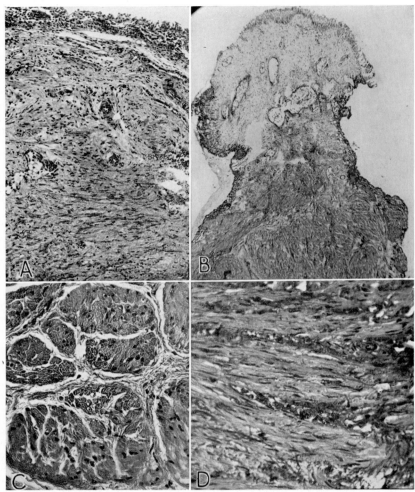

Fig. 253.   Congenital contracture of vesical outlet. Histology. *A*, submucous fibrosis
of the vesical outlet in tissue removed from a two-year-old boy. The absence of inflammation is notable as is the considerably increased fibrous tissue with less muscular hypertrophy than is usually observed. *B*, pronounced muscular hypertrophy in tissue removed
transurethrally from the vesical outlet of a three-year-old boy with congenital contracture
of the bladder neck. There is marked edema of the overlying mucosa. Note the density
of the hypertrophic muscle. *C*, cross section of tissue removed from vesical outlet of a
five-year-old boy with contracture of the bladder neck and showing enormous hypertrophy of muscle bundles in this area. *D*, longitudinal section through the hypertrophic
musculature as shown in *C*. While muscular hypertrophy at the vesical outlet has been
demonstrated in many of our cases of contracture of the vesical outlet in the young, in
about half submucosal fibrosis rather than muscular hypertrophy explains the obstruction.
Yet it is likely that in many cases the muscular hypertrophy is secondary to primary submucosal fibrotic obstruction.

the end picture being that of widespread destruction of the upper urinary tract as described in Section III and as just previously outlined under congenital valves of the prostatic urethra.

The histologic picture in contracture of the vesical outlet is generally an increase in the connective tissue of the submucosa (Fig. 253), this fibrosis involving only a portion of the sphincteric ring or the entire circumference of the outlet with fibrotic extension into the trigonal musculature, adjacent bladder wall, and prostatic tissue. Bundles of hypertrophic smooth muscle fibers will be found coursing through this sclerotic mass and sometimes the connective tissue surrounds the heavy muscle bundles as dense fibrous sheaths (Fig. 253, *C*). Round-cell infiltration is the rule in the event of acute inflammation, while polymorphonuclear cells also may be present. In a thirteen-year-old boy reported by Sisto (1935), there were areas of calcific infiltration in the tissue. The coexisting changes frequently seen in the glandular tissue of the trigone and submucosal glands of adults are generally lacking in children, and not infrequently the tissue removed from the contracted bladder neck in the young shows neither fibrosis nor inflammation but only muscular hypertrophy (Fig. 253).

The entire circumference of the bladder outlet is commonly involved in a collar-like manner but the narrowing may be cystoscopically evident only over the lower segment (5 to 7 o'clock or 4 to 8 o'clock on the clock face) and presenting the cystoscopic picture of median bar obstruction. Because the work of the trigone in opening the vesical outlet is increased by the contracture, trigonal muscular hypertrophy is regularly observed and is of diagnostic import. Changes in the upper urinary tract consequent to infravesical obstruction, the course of the untreated disease, and the terminal picture as previously described in this Section under Valvular Obstruction may be anticipated.

As the vesical neck fibrosis increases, the floor of the orifice is elevated from its usual site with a corresponding sagging of the floor of the supramontane urethra in front of the obstruction and an exaggerated falling away of the bladder floor behind it, the bas fond. The dense constricting ring can usually be palpated with a finger in the rectum, feeling at the bladder neck against an instrument in the urethra. Palpation of the contracted vesical neck through the open bladder discloses an abnormally small tight orifice which can be dilated only with great force or not until sphincterotomy has been performed.

Symptoms. These are similar in all respects to those described under valvular obstruction and usually manifest themselves soon after birth although in cases of lesser severity, the patient may reach the third or fourth decade of life. One of our patients was born in chronic complete retention and so tight was the contracted vesical outlet that not even a catheter could be passed; suprapubic cystotomy tube drainage was instituted at twenty-four hours of age, and six months later the blockage was successfully eradicated by transurethral resection. Frequency of urination, dysuria and hesitancy are the more prominent symptoms and result from the concentric constriction of the vesical outlet by the fibrous infiltration which, in turn, causes it to be opened with difficulty. For this reason, closing of the orifice may be interfered with to produce dribbling. Urgency, crying on urination, straining, passage of an intermittent stream, or enuresis, commonly coexist and with the advent of infection are intensified. Persistent pyuria is noted and with exacerbation of the infection, acute "pyelitis." Chronic complete retention with overflow is manifested by paradoxical or overflow incontinence (pseudo-incontinence). Vesical distention may cause suprapubic or renal pain.

Diagnosis. This is suggested by the history. The distended bladder may be palpable but more often is not. Residual urine is almost always found and may be as much as 16 or 20 ounces, but usually is between 1 and 6 ounces. A residuum of 10 to 15 cc. regularly observed calls for urologic investigation. The diagnosis is accurately made by cystourethroscopy employing a panendoscopic or direct vision lens system. In order to get a panoramic view the deep prostatic urethra should be moderately dilated with irrigating solution at the time the study of the entire vesical outlet is made. Occasionally the cystoscope will be firmly grasped by the tight bladder neck as it is with urethral stricture. In the cystoscopic picture of median bar obstruction, the lower segment of the vesical outlet presents a smoothly rounded elevation with a supramontane bas fond and hypertrophic trigone behind. The urethral floor in front of the obstruction regularly shows sagging but posteriorly rises more or less abruptly to the site of the bar formation. With involvement of the whole circumference of the bladder neck by fibrotic contracture, it appears in the panendoscopic field as a rounded rigid collar-like intrusion of the entire orifice. The hypertrophic trigone often sets up as a high plateau from which the bladder floor sags on its three sides. Trabeculation and often sacculation, with or without cystitis, calculi and/or diverticula are commonly observed. Dilatation of the upper urinary tract may be extreme (Fig. 250).

Differential Diagnosis. Contracture of the vesical outlet is to be distinguished by cystourethroscopy from valvular obstruction of the posterior urethra, congenital urethral stricture, congenital hypertrophy of the verumontanum, sphincterospastic neuromuscular disease of the vesical outlet. The diagnosis of neuromuscular disease may offer difficulties but careful physical and neurologic examinations may be of help as may cystometric study. Associated spina bifida is suggestive of neurogenic vesical disease but is not pathognomonic (see Section XI). Associated anal sphincterospasm is highly suggestive of neurospastic vesical outlet disease. While lesions of the spinal cord are sometimes demonstrable, neuromuscular vesical disease may exist without evidence other than the urologic findings. The spastic vesical outlet of neuromuscular disease lacks the tight firmness or rigidity of contracture or fibrosis as determined by the cystoscope or the passage of other urethral instruments. Moreover, neurogenic atonic bladder and the late atony of chronic infravesical obstruction sometimes are cystoscopically almost indistinguishable, but in the first condition the trigone does not show hypertrophy and in the second it does so regularly.

Prognosis. This is based on the degree of renal damage and the ravages of infection. Long preliminary drainage may fail to result in any striking improvement in renal function and occasionally this failure is also observed following removal of the obstruction. Prolonged dilatation and sclerotic atony of the bladder wall may prevent its adequate evacuation even when the obstruction has been removed. Resection of large segments of the redundant bladder in such cases has been employed (Fish, Kimbrough) and apparently with some success. The prognosis should always be guarded but is regularly improved by adequate relief of the obstruction and control or eradication of coexisting infection.

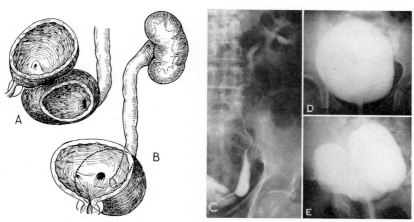

Fig. 254.   Congenital contracture of the vesical outlet complicated by a diverticulum in a four-year-old boy examined because of persistent pyuria. Diverticulum and bladder are of equal size; the dilated left ureter opens into the diverticulum. Five ounces residual urine. Treatment: Diverticulectomy, left ureteroneocystostomy, V-wedge resection of the bladder neck with subsequent sterilization of the urine by the ketogenic diet. Three years later there was no residuum; the urine was normal and sterile. *A, B*, schema of conditions present. *C*, pyelography fifteen years postoperatively shows moderate dilatation of the left lower ureter but the pelvis and renal function are essentially normal. *D, E*, cystographic demonstration of the diverticulum. In the anterior posterior view (*D*) no suggestion of the presence of the diverticulum is given; (*E*) oblique view shows the diverticulum behind and beneath the bladder to be as large as or larger than the bladder itself.

Treatment. The clinical management of contracted vesical outlet consists in removal of sufficient tissue to eradicate completely all obstruction and should be carried out when preoperative preparation as well as clinical and laboratory studies indicate the patient is ready for surgical attack. Preliminary drainage by indwelling catheter or cystotomy may be necessary because of advanced renal damage but in most instances transurethral resection can be employed without great delay.

In some instances dilatation of the vesical neck with sounds or bougies together with installment emptying of the bladder may bring about complete evacuation. In performing installment emptying, the patient evacuates his bladder as well as he can but 1 to 10 or more ounces of urine may be retained. He then waits fifteen to thirty seconds, voids again, and further empties his bladder and reduces the residuum. This process is repeated until no more urine can be expressed and is performed every time the desire to void is felt. Repetition of this practice over a period of time frequently reduces the residuum to only a few cubic centimeters or even zero. I have repeatedly employed this nonoperative treatment when (1) the residuum is only 1 or 2 ounces, (2) infection is negligible or absent, (3) the renal function is not depressed and (4) the patient is cooperative. When these factors are unfavorable or the conservative treatment has failed to eliminate obstruction and residuum, operation is demanded as it is when complicating diverticulum, large stone or other serious surgical conditions exist (Fig. 254).

Today transurethral resection of the vesical outlet is the procedure of choice and has largely replaced all other methods. This is described by Nesbit in Section XV, Chapter 8, and is employed in both males and females. The retropubic approach to these lesions has been advocated by Burns, Lich (1952) and others but to me this seems needlessly radical if one knows how to do a transurethral resection.

If the initial resection proves inadequate, more tissue must be removed; in both children and adults it has been necessary to repeat resection as many as three times before complete bladder emptying was achieved. In the young the removal of five to eight pieces of tissue is usually sufficient and in adults proportionately larger amounts of tissue must be excised, but the obstruction must be removed even if twenty or more pieces are excised. In short, the amount of tissue removed must be enough. Eradication of associated urinary infection completes the treatment (see Cook in Section V, Chapter 1).

Congenital neuromuscular disease of the vesical outlet causing obstruction and/or incomplete emptying of the bladder is discussed *in extenso* by Emmett in Section XI.

Dislocation of the Internal Urethral Meatus. This unusual anomaly has been reported as the cause of obstruction at the vesical outlet (Day and Vivian, 1927). The prostatic urethra enters the bladder lateral to the median line to create a valvelike mechanism, the action of which is encouraged by an overlapping of the right trigonal muscle on the left or vice versa. In a few instances the vesical outlet has been found completely closed over by mucosal membrane while the remainder of the urethral canal has been normal. In a previously reported case, a young male studied post mortem at Bellevue Hospital, the prostatic urethra showed a Z-shaped course (Campbell, 1937).

Absence of the Prostate. This most unusual anomaly is generally associated with other urogenital maldevelopments such as testicular agenesis, bilateral cryptorchism, exstrophy of the bladder, marked epispadias and pseudovaginal hypospadias. It was discovered in three cases in 10,712 autopsies in boys (1 to 3570). *Congenital isolateral hypoplasia of the prostate* and of the associated seminal tract sometimes occurs with unilateral anomalies of the upper urinary tract and notably renal agenesis. Pronounced *hypoplasia of the entire prostate* is observed chiefly in hypopituitary sexual infantilism and corresponds to the underdevelopment of the remainder of the genital tract.

Congenital prostatic cysts are rare and observed generally in middle-aged adults although they have their origin in failure of establishment of the usual communication between the wolffian ducts and vesicourethral anlage. These cysts are to be differentiated from cysts observed in later life and caused by inflammation or trauma (retention cysts) or a new growth. In congenital prostatic cystic disease isolateral ureterorenal anomalies frequently coexist. The symptoms of prostatic cysts are those of obstruction and will vary with the degree of blockage and secondary infection.

Cystourethroscopy discloses the lesion and transurethral or perineal excision of the cyst is the treatment. Most prostatic cysts observed in the young are small, submucosal and disappear on electropuncture but in the adult may be as large as two to three centimeters or more in diameter.

Pseudohermaphroditism. In this congenital condition of the external genitalia, the structures resemble those of the gonadal sex opposite. There were six cases in an autopsy series in children (five less than seven months old), an incidence of about 1:3175; it was also seen in three young adults

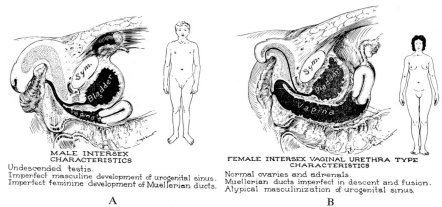

MALE INTERSEX
CHARACTERISTICS
Undescended testis.
Imperfect masculine development of urogenital sinus.
Imperfect feminine development of Muellerian ducts.

FEMALE INTERSEX VAGINAL URETHRA TYPE
CHARACTERISTICS
Normal ovaries and adrenals.
Muellerian ducts imperfect in descent and fusion.
Atypical masculinization of urogenital sinus.

A   B

Fig. 255.   Intersex. *A*, in a male. *B*, in a female. (Courtesy of Dr. Frederick S. Howard.)

(16–40 years), an incidence here of 1:10,944. Pseudohermaphroditism in twins has been reported in ten cases (Collier, 1948). Familial pseudohermaphroditism has been observed and is splendidly discussed by Deming, Goettsch, and Humm (1949). Emmett reported pseudohermaphroditism in a brother and sister. The term intersex is also applied in descriptive identification of pseudohermaphroditism, the anatomic and clinical features of which are here discussed in the light of present-day knowledge.

Pseudohermaphroditism has been classified as (1) complete, (2) internal, and (3) external. In the *complete masculine* variety, the sex glands are male but the external sexual organs are female. In the *complete female* type the sex glands are female and the external genitalia are male (Figs. 255–257). The *internal masculine* type appears in a male with fallopian tubes, uterus and vagina, while the *internal feminine* variety occurs in a female with both male and female sexual passages. In *external masculine* pseudohermaphroditism, the genitalia are male while the sex glands and internal passages are female. In the *external feminine* type, there are female external genitalia but male gonads and inner genitalia.

The male variety of pseudohermaphroditism is the more common (Fig. 255, *A*). Pseudovaginal hypospadias simulates a vulva in which the testes are usually absent and confirms the idea that hypospadias is an hermaphroditic condition. A short cordlike structure represents the uterus and tubes.

In the *external female* type, the lips of the vulva are often adherent and seal over the vagina or the urethral orifice may be common to both vagina and urethra (Fig. 255, *B*). A mild variety of this is seen in congenital fusion of the labia minora of which we have seen twenty-four cases and in advanced

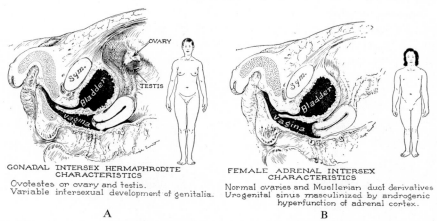

GONADAL INTERSEX HERMAPHRODITE CHARACTERISTICS
Ovotestes or ovary and testis.
Variable intersexual development of genitalia.

A

FEMALE ADRENAL INTERSEX CHARACTERISTICS
Normal ovaries and Muellerian duct derivatives
Urogenital sinus masculinized by androgenic hyperfunction of adrenal cortex.

B

Fig. 256.   Intersex. *A*, gonadal hermaphroditic intersex. *B*, female adrenal intersex. (Courtesy of Dr. Frederick S. Howard.)

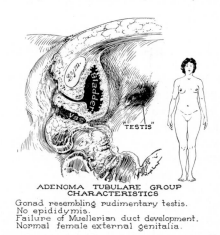

ADENOMA TUBULARE GROUP CHARACTERISTICS
Gonad resembling rudimentary testis.
No epididymis.
Failure of Muellerian duct development.
Normal female external genitalia.

Fig. 257.   Intersex in adenoma tubulare group. (Courtesy of Dr. Frederick S. Howard.)

form in a woman of seventy. The cause is unknown but it is not due to endocrine tumors (adrenal, ovary, pituitary, etc.; cf. Hooks, 1948). Notions as to the etiology include an overabundance of maternal sex-opposite hormone affecting the male or female fetus (Leahy and Butsch, 1948).

Perineal and pseudovaginal hypospadias may offer an extremely difficult or even impossible diagnostic problem in determining the true sex of the patient without surgical exploration. Social and legal problems are of utmost importance in this condition in adults, particularly as to marriage, but the sex of the individual should be accurately determined by the second year of life. When matrimony is anticipated, the partner to be should be apprised of the facts.

External examination is often inconclusive; no gonads can be palpated and the genital morphology is indeterminate. Estimation of the 17-ketosteroid and estrogen outputs may give a suggestive clue but is more likely to be of value in older than in very young patients.

When laparotomy is necessary to establish the true sex, the intra-abdominal gonads should always be seen rather than conclusions drawn as to their presence based on blind palpation alone. Histologic examination of tissue from the gonads should be made not only for determinate reasons but because in the future the observation of the surgeon may be questioned. A uterus may be found in females but in two boys thought to have exaggerated pseudovaginal hypospadias, we found a uterus, ovaries and testes.

The roentgenographic study of the female pelvis in the infant child or virgin adult following *transabdominal pneumoperitoneum* may be adequate to establish the diagnosis in sex endocrine disturbances. This procedure established by Kunstadter, Guterman and Tulky (1952) for the diagnosis of pelvic anomalies and other pathologic conditions when the laboratory and other data are inconclusive, may be expected to spare some of these young patients from exploratory laparotomy. Prior to the pneumoperitone-ographic study, the patient is investigated by: (1) history and physical examination, (2) measurements (weight, height, span, symphysis vertex, symphysis-sole), (3) laboratory (basal metabolic rate (BMR), fasting blood sugar, serum cholesterol, cholesterol esters, intravenous insulin tolerance test), (4) hormone excretion (urinary 17-ketosteroids, urinary pregnanediol), (5) vaginal smear for estrogen activity (Schorr stain), (6) x-ray studies (skull sella turcica, bone age, perirenal insufflation), and (7) endometrial biopsy.

On the morning of the pneumoperitoneal study the patient receives: (1) a high cleansing enema, (2) no breakfast, (3) demerol, intramuscularly, 25 to 100 mg. according to weight, and (4) catheterization of bladder. With the patient on the back of the urographic table, a transabdominal puncture is made 1 inch below and 1 inch to the left of the umbilicus, a 20 gauge spinal puncture needle with a stylet being used. Carbon dioxide gas is then introduced through the needle under 10–20 mm. Hg pressure, using 300 to 700 cc. of the gas (average 500 cc.). The patient is then placed in the modified knee chest position on the radiographic table (Kunstadter et al. prefer the Stein-Arens urologic table with which good pelvic and hip support is achieved) and fast ($\frac{1}{10}$ sec.) stereoscopic x-ray exposures of the pelvis are made. By this method uterus, cystic ovaries, hypoplastic ovaries, and other female pelvic tissues are well outlined in the air filled deep pelvic cavity (Fig. 258). Negatively, ovarian agenesis may also be demonstrated. The carbon dioxide is absorbed in twelve to twenty-four hours.

In cases of bisexuality the surgeon must weigh at the operating table the factors of apparent sex imbalance. These include (1) whether the child has developed more like a boy than a girl or vice versa, (2) the comparative state of development of the two sets of sex structures found, and (3) the past rearing of the child. When these factors are predominantly male, the female sex organs may advisedly be removed and vice versa. To date permanent satisfactory results in these cases have not been achieved by the administration of antagonistic hormones to diminish the effect of the less prominent sex manifestation or by hormones to stimulate the more prominent type of physical and sexual maturation toward which the development of the child appears inclined.

Corrective plastic surgery should not be carried out until the true sex of the patient has been demonstrated. Many penile amputations have been erroneously performed when the organ was thought to be a clitoris and the

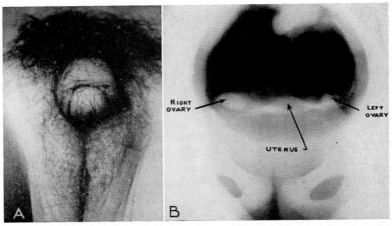

Fig. 258.   Pseudohermaphroditism and adrenogenital syndrome in a five-year-old girl. *A*, abundant pubic hair, penis-like clitoric structure with urethral opening at base of shaft; bifid scrotum-like labia with rugated scrotal folds. *B*, pneumoperitoneogram showing presence of ovaries and uterus. (Courtesy of Dr. R. H. Kunstadter and Journal of Pediatrics.)

removal of masses in the labia majora unwittingly have often been emasculation. In a girl of nine weeks there was atresia of the vagina and marked hypertrophy of the clitoris with a urethral opening at its base; the labia resembled a scrotum but no testes were found (Campbell, 1937). Intraabdominal examination revealed a complete female internal reproductive tract. The adrenals were heavier than the kidneys, the cortex was 4 mm. thick and bluish-red, and the medulla was replaced by mucoid material. This patient doubtless represents a case of intrauterine adrenal endocrinopathy. In a case of similar external morphology, the sex was determined to be female on the fifth day of life by urologic examination and vaginoscsopy.

In pseudohermaphroditism in the male, the treatment of the coexisting vagina will depend primarily upon recognition of the anomaly (Figs. 255–257, 269; cf. Cecil, 1949). Cecil noted that the only difference between male pseudohermaphroditism and perineal hypospadias is that in the former the vagina is discovered although it is present in both conditions. Good results in plastic surgery in perineal hypospadias have been obtained when the presence of a hypoplastic vagina was neither suspected nor treated. In other words, excision of the vagina is unnecessary. No record has been found of obliteration of the vaginal canal by the injection of sclerosing agents such as sodium morrhuate.

Hermaphroditism. In this condition the individual is bisexual, possessing gonads and genitalia of both sexes. The term is derived from the myth that Hermaphrodite, son of Hermes and Aphrodite, when bathing became joined in one body with the nymph, Salmacis. True hermaphroditism is extremely rare and most of the reported cases have been of the false or pseudo-hermaphroditic variety. Four cases of spurious hermaphroditism in one family were reported by Phillips (1886).

Hermaphroditism may be classified:

1. Bilateral: a testis and ovary on each side. I have seen one case clinically, a "boy" of six years proved by abdominal exploration. Because he was predominantly male and had thus been raised, the infantile uterus and ovaries were removed. An instance at autopsy is cited in a succeeding paragraph.

2. Unilateral: a testis and ovary on one side with either a testis or ovary on the other. Bilateral and unilateral hermaphroditism has been reported chiefly in the lower animals.

3. Lateral: an ovary on one side with a testis on the other. There is frequently ectopy of the female organs so that a uterus may appear in the groin and the testes may be ectopic.

4. Ovatestis: present on one or both sides. Twelve cases have been reported to date (cf. Doss and Priestley, 1940).

In true hermaphroditism the individual may be predominantly male or female in body configuration and instincts, but a reversal of sex reaction sometimes occurs whereby a male "subsequently became" female. In a true hermaphrodite, a white male sixteen hours old examined at autopsy, there was atresia of the vagina and external genitalia; scrotum or labia were absent but a pronounced median raphe extended from a knoblike subpubic protrusion to the anus. Both testes were attached to a gubernaculum and the ovaries were in the pelvis. There were also present a small retrovesical rudimentary uterus, four accessory spleens, a Meckel's diverticulum, deviation of the index finger, patent ductus arteriosus, patent foramen ovale and hydronephrosis.

Hermaphroditism is believed to result from a maternal excess supply to the fetus of sex opposite hormones. In the *masculine type* which occurs more often, there is a small short hypospadiac penis, the scrotum is cleft or bifid, the testes are generally in the inguinal canal, and a short small cordlike vagina and the uterus with fallopian tubes are present. The *female type* is characterized by an enlarged penile clitoris, labia formed to simulate a scrotum which may contain one or both herniated ovaries and there is vaginal atresia. Here the precise diagnosis may require abdominal exploration. Treatment consists of plastic reconstruction to preserve the dominant sex.

Young (1937) in his splendid monograph Genital Anomalies, Hermaphroditism and Related Adrenal Diseases presents an extremely complete and interesting discussion of hermaphroditism which is recommended to the reader. Wilkins' (1950) clinical masterpiece—The Diagnosis and

Treatment of Endocrine Disorders in Childhood and Adolescence—presents the present day knowledge of the hormonal factors and treatment in these and other syndromes with hormonal dysfunction and manifestations. See also Section XIV by Drs. Engle and Jailer in the present book.

EMBRYOLOGY OF THE MALE REPRODUCTIVE TRACT

In the fourth week of fetal life the gonads exist as undifferentiated organs derived as mesothelial thickenings on the anteromedial surface of the

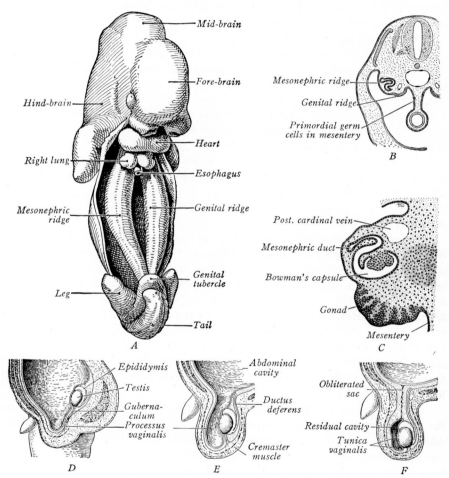

Fig. 259. Derivation and embryology of the testicle. *A, B, C,* urogenital ridge of the human embryo; dissection at 9 mm., ventral view (Arey after Kollman; × 11). *D, E,* schema of descent of the testes; early (*D*) and late (*F*) relationships. Failure of the processus vaginalis to close is of high incidence in young males and gives rise to a variety of congenital hydroceles and hernias.

wolffian bodies (mesonephron; Fig. 259). The mesothelial mass increases in size, becomes the germinal ridge, and contains differentiated epithelial cells imbedded in its connective tissue. These cells arise by a proliferation from the deep surface epithelium covering these ridges (Fig. 259) and from these germinal cells develop the spermatogenic cells of the testis and the graafian follicles of the ovary (six weeks). Failure of the urogenital union at this point causes the testicle and epididymis to develop separately.

During the fifth week, the wolffian and müllerian ducts longitudinally traverse the germinal ridge. It is undetermined whether the müllerian duct originates as an independent development or as an offshoot of the wolffian duct. The müllerian ducts open into the coelum (peritoneal cavity) at their uppermost extremities and unite below in the midline to empty into the urogenital sinus (Fig.191). The lower opening persists in the male as the utricle of the verumontanum. Thus the müllerian ducts form in the female the fallopian tubes, uterus and vagina and in the male the prostatic utricle and testicular hydatids (Fig. 208).

As the developing sex glands enlarge, they separate from the wolffian body to lie free in the abdominal cavity being attached only by a peritoneal pedicle which becomes the *mesorchium* in the male and the mesovarium in the female (Fig. 208). Within the folds of the mesorchium there is a band of muscular tissue known as the *genito-inguinal ligament* or *gubernaculum,* which passes from the lower pole of the testicle to the lowermost scrotum (Fig. 259).

With continued growth of the fetus, the testicle progressively occupies lower levels, and at the third month is near the internal inguinal ring. By now a peritoneal pouch, the processus vaginalis, has grown downward through the anterior abdominal wall (inguinal canal) and toward the scrotum (Fig. 259). Yet it is incorrect to describe as is so often done, descent of the testicle through the inguinal canal for, at this time, a canal is unformed. The processus vaginalis becomes covered with tissue layers derived from the layers of the anterior abdominal wall through which it has passed. Just before birth but occasionally not until neonatal life, the testicle with its vascular, lymphatic, nerve and wolffian duct connections (vas deferens) descends through the peritoneal evagination to reach the scrotum (Fig. 259). Later the processus vaginalis becomes obliterated above to leave the testis lying in the cavity formed of peritoneal derivation. The parietal layer lines the scrotal cavity as the tunica vaginalis, while the visceral layer overlays the tunica albuginea and surrounds the testicle and epididymis except at the head and tail of the last. Failure of the processus vaginalis to close accounts for congenital hernia; segmental closure gives rise to hydrocele of the cord (Section VI, Chapter 3).

At birth the small testes which weigh 0.8 gm. (12 gr.) are normally situated in the scrotum in 90 per cent of males but if not in the scrotum at birth, within a few days or weeks they will be found normally located in 95 to 97 per cent and in two thirds of the remaining cases the organs will descend during the next few years. If the testes are undescended by puberty (about 1.5 per cent), it is unlikely that they will ever spontaneously reach the scrotum (cf. Section I, Chapter 5). With gonadotropic therapy the likelihood of testicular descent at puberty can be anticipated at the age of three or four years.

The cause of testicular descent is still unknown. A long held theory that

atrophic shortening of the gubernaculum (the homologue in the female is
the ligamentum teres uteri) actively draws the testis down, is no longer
generally accepted by anatomists.

Lockwood's (1888) idea that the gubernaculum is a many-tailed fibro-
elastic structure whose component tails terminate (1) in the scrotum, (2)
at the pubic bone, (3) at the root of the penis, (4) in the tissues over
Scarpa's triangle, (5) in the perineum at the tuberosity of the ischium, and
(6) at the sphincter ani, has not been generally anatomically substantiated.

Table 8. Genital Homologues; Derivatives of the Indifferent Urogenital Anlagen

MALE	INDIFFERENT TYPE	FEMALE
Testes	SEXUAL GLANDS	Ovary
Coni vasculosi and ductuli effer-	WOLFFIAN TUBULES	Short tubules of the epo-
entes	(SEXUAL GROUP)	ophoron
Paradidymis		Paroophoron
Duct of epididymis	WOLFFIAN DUCT	Main tube of epoophoron
Vas deferens		Gartner's duct
Seminal vesicle		
Epididymis appendix—upper end		Hydatid of Morgagni
Appendix of testes	MÜLLERIAN DUCT	Oviduct
Prostatic utricle		Uterus
		Vagina
Ureter	RENAL OUTGROWTH	Ureter
	FROM WOLFFIAN DUCT	
Pelvis and collecting renal tubules		Pelvis and collecting renal
		tubules
Bladder	LOWER SEGMENT OF	Bladder
	ALLANTOIS AND PART	
	OF CLOACA	
Prostatic urethra	UROGENITAL SINUS	Urethra and vestibule
Prostate	(OUTGROWTHS FROM	Para-urethral glands
	UROGENITAL SINUS	(Skene's)
	WALL)	
Cowper's glands		Bartholin's glands
Penis	GENITAL TUBERCLE	Clitoris
Lips of urethral groove	GENITAL FOLDS	Labia minora
Scrotum	LABIO-SCROTAL FOLDS	Labia majora

Overaction of bands of (2) and (3), (4), and (5) has been adduced to explain respectively pubic, femoral, and perineal ectopic testis. Wells (1943)
observed that at the seventh month the upper end of the gubernaculum is
attached to the tail of the epididymis and more recent anatomic observations
by Wells and State (1947) have shown that the structure identified as the
gubernaculum probably plays little part in actual descent of the testicle.
Experimentally in rats, even though the gubernaculum was severed, testicular
descent occurred in three fourths (Wells, 1944). This and other experimental
and clinical observations suggest that hormonal influence is probably the
chief factor in testicular descent and without effect on the gubernaculum
(Hamilton, 1941; Wells, 1944, 1946). Others (Hunter, 1926; Curling,
1840; Lewis, 1948) maintain that downward pull of the cremaster is the
impelling force in testicular descent and noted failure of descent in experimental division of the genitocrural nerve. Following section of this nerve

the descended testicle cannot be drawn up into the abdomen, and the gland experimentally placed in the abdomen will not descend. Normal scrotal development and an adequately patent canal are essential to normal descent and growth of the testis.

Seminal Vesicles. About the seventh week of fetal life the seminal vesicles appear as outpocketings of the vas deferens (wolffian duct derivatives). Unusual persistence of a connection of a wolffian derivative, Gartner's duct, with the seminal vesicle, uterus and cervix explains ectopic ureteral openings in these organs (Figs. 150, 207). The derivatives of the indifferent urogenital anlage are indicated in Table 8.

ANOMALIES OF THE TESTICLE

These have been classified as shown in Table 9.

Anorchism or **absence of the testes** is extremely rare, forty-seven cases having been reported. Of these eleven have been bilateral and the remaining

Table 9. Anomalies of the Testicle

A. Anomalies in development..	Anomalies in number...	1. In deficiency:	Absence or anorchism Fusion or synorchism
		2. In excess:	Polyorchism
	Anomalies in size.......	1. In deficiency:	Hypoplasia
		2. In excess:	Hypertrophy
B. Anomalies in position......	Testicle undescended....	At some point in its normal course	Cryptorchism
		Outside its normal course	Ectopia
	Testicle descended......	Upside down	Inversion
		Hindside foremost	Retroversion

unilateral; thirty-six were divided between the two sides. In our series of 10,712 autopsies in boys, the testicle was reported as absent in four each on the right and left sides, and bilaterally absent in twenty-six, an amazingly high incidence suggesting some small glands may conceivably have been overlooked.

Anorchism has been classified according to (1) absence of the testicle only, (2) absence of the testicle, epididymis and a portion of the vas deferens, and (3) absence of the entire spermatic tract. Generally in unilateral anorchism, the other testis is intra-abdominal. In our cases of bilateral anorchism, there were four instances of absence of the seminal vesicles, prostate, and spermatic cord, and two cases in which these structures were absent except for the prostate. In one of the last there was extreme hypoplasia of the penis. Bilateral anorchism was observed in identical twins dead at twelve hours. Although bilateral anorchism is not incompatible with life, the patient is sterile, will grow up in female hormonal imbalance, and bids fair to become a psychiatric problem.

Synorchism. Synorchism designates fusion of both testicles into one mass and may occur within the scrotum (Lenhossek, 1945) or abdominally. Six cases have been reported but there were two in our autopsy series (10,712 boys). In a ten-week-old boy dead of malnutrition and examined post mortem at Bellevue Hospital, a central solidly fused testicular mass was found in the upper pelvis. An elongated epididymis led away on each side from the testicle finally to become the vas deferens and passed to join the ducts of the seminal vesicle. The kidneys were solidly fused (lump kidney; Fig. 260). In St. Hilaire's case, an infant with a solitary kidney, the conditions are strikingly similar. A ten-day-old boy also examined post mortem at Bellevue

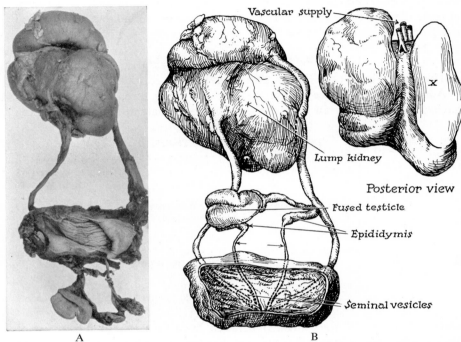

A   B

Fig. 260.   Synorchism in a ten-week-old boy; the condition is one of the rarest of urogenital anomalies. The fused testicle drained by the two epididymides was situated just above and behind the bladder. A lump kidney coexisted, a portion of which labeled X in schema B and as seen from behind, was almost of normal conformation. (Bellevue Hospital.)

Hospital showed testes fused together in the pelvis; accompanying anomalies included horseshoe kidney, rib fusion, meningocele, hydrocephalus, spina bifida (L 2-4), rotation of the bony pelvis, and scoliosis. The testes may be separate and only the epididymides may be fused as Halsted (1907) observed.

Polyorchism (supernumerary testicle) is rare but nineteen cases have been reported. In these cases one or more of the supernumerary testicles showed disease such as torsion of the spermatic cord (Boggon, 1933). The condition has been found more often on the left side. Polyorchism is not to be confused with small firm encysted hydrocele or spermatocele which may appear as an accessory testicle. A testicle-size cyst (spermatocele) was attached to the spermatic cord just above the left testicle in a five-year-old boy seen at Bellevue Hospital and simulated a reduplicated organ on this side.

Splenic rests in the scrotum along the cord have been reported in three instances by Arnheim and Etter (1948), in two cases by Keizur (1952), but should not confuse the diagnosis except as enlargement of the aberrant tissue by systemic conditions causing splenic enlargement might suggest new growth or inflammation in the scrotum. In a two-year-old boy seen at Bellevue Hospital, an aberrant adrenal rest was found in the left testis, and in a one-year-old boy at University Hospital an adrenal rest was found in the right testicle (Fig. 265).

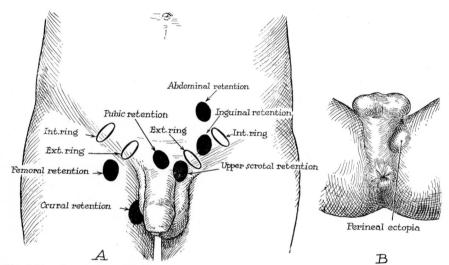

Fig. 261.   Congenital testicular ectopia. The testicle may also be displaced into these unusual positions by trauma.

Hypoplasia or **congenital atrophy of one testicle** is occasionally observed; compensatory hypertrophic enlargement of the mate usually exists. In the young, testicular atrophy is more often the result of trauma than congenital. Right testicular atrophy was extreme in a seven-week-old boy with hydrocele; autopsy also disclosed patent foramen ovale. In a twelve-day-old boy there was torsion of the spermatic cord; necrotic atrophy occurred—one of the earliest observed instances of the condition (see Section XIII concerning torsion of the spermatic cord). Most undescended testes show some atrophy or at least failure to grow and the longer the testis remains imperfectly descended, the more striking will be the developmental failure and/or atrophy. Congenital small testes bilaterally occur in infantilism and are usually associated with or secondary to other endocrine disturbances and notably of the pituitary.

The Improperly Descended Testis. *Cryptorchism* (entomologically hidden testicle) defines the condition of abdominal undescended testicle. It has come to be applied to all forms of the imperfectly descended testes. The organs lie extraperitoneally in the iliac fossa until late embryonic life, but just before or soon after birth the glands descend to the scrotum (Fig. 259). Failure of the testicle to reach its normal destination is the commonest anomaly of the spermatic tract.

Imperfectly descended testicles are classified as (1) abdominal (lumbar or pelvic), (2) inguinal (in the canal), (3) subinguinal (prepubic or upper scrotal, Fig. 261).

The majority of undescended testes are inguinal (70 per cent) while about 25 per cent are abdominal and the remainder are perineal, pubic or are located in other unusual positions (Fig. 261). The condition is often bilateral but the side-incidence, right and left, is about equal. The testes are in the scrotum in about two thirds of newborn premature males.

In a study of 10,852 boys examined post mortem, there were 313 instances of cryptorchism noted, an incidence of one in thirty-four. The right side was involved in thirty-six, the left in forty-three, and the anomaly was bilateral in 234. The testes were intra-abdominal in seventy-one, at the internal ring in twenty-two, in the canal in 170, at the pelvic brim in two, retroperitoneal in one, and at the external ring in twelve. The organs could not be found in forty additional cases. Coexisting urogenital tract anomalies were found in ninety-six or approximately a third of the cases. Nonurologic anomalies were present in 182 or two-thirds of the cases.

When spontaneous descent is to occur it is usually completed by the first year. If normal descent has not occurred by puberty, subsequent descent is unlikely. By comparison with the one in thirty-four incidence in the young, the incidence in males over fifteen years of age was found to be one to 214, based on the observation of cryptorchism in 110 of 23,529 adult males examined post mortem. In these adults the anomaly was on the right in forty-six, on the left in forty-three, and was bilateral in twenty-one, the last being in striking variance with the high incidence of bilaterality in the young.

A high incidence of atrophy of the undescended testis was noted in a series of sixty-four cases in adults examined post mortem. Eighteen of these organs showed pronounced atrophy in contrast to only three in a series of 217 infant and young cryptorchids similarly examined. In the adult group the location of the undescended testicle was intra-abdominal in eight, at the internal inguinal ring in one, at the external ring in eight, and in the inguinal canal in eighteen—this last constituting 28.1 per cent of the total number. These sixty-four adults showed other anomalies, urologic in nine and non-urologic in two.

Etiology. The cause of testicular imperfect descent is unknown. Several theories have been offered in explanation; some of these considerations have been previously indicated on page 460. The following anatomic factors either singly or in combination may predispose to testicular maldescent (cf. Eccles):

1. An unusually long mesorchium (testicular mesentery) which allows the gland undue intra-abdominal freedom and renders engagement in the internal inguinal ring less likely

2. Mesorchial peritoneal adhesions

3. An abnormal persistence of the plica vascularis which may anchor the testicle high

4. Short spermatic vessels or vas deferens

5. The diameter of the testis and epididymis is greater than that of the inguinal canal

6. Testicular fusion

7. Absent, unusually long, or inactive gubernaculum

8. Cremasteric hyperactivity interfering with descent

9. Maldevelopment of the inguinal canal (relative or absolute atresia)

10. Scrotal maldevelopment; absence of a testicular cavity

Adhesions resulting from fetal peritonitis have been suggested as a cause of testicular retention. Whether the peritonitis is the basic factor remains unproved but at operation upon imperfectly descended testes not descending with hormonal therapy, it is regularly noted that they are bound in position by dense adhesions. Elongation or absence of the gubernaculum testis has repeatedly been adduced to explain imperfect descent but what part the gubernaculum plays in the process is unknown; the recent studies of Wells and State (1947) suggest that the gubernaculum is probably of no importance except to guide the descending organ. In the newborn, the testis together with its fascial coverings may be lifted out of the scrotum without tearing anything but a little superficial connective tissue (Hunter, R. H., 1926); this observation casts doubt on the conception of the gubernaculum as a traction band drawing the testicle downward.

Deming (1937) showed experimentally in the immature rhesus monkey that following the injection of chorionic gonadotropin, the testis increased 50 per cent in size because of testicular and interstitial cell enlargement, and tubular enlargement in the epididymis also occurred. The vas deferens becomes doubled in size and elongated, cord vascularity is greatly increased, the cremaster muscle doubles in size, the dartos of the scrotum enlarges as does the inguinal canal but the scrotal skin does not. A paucity or even absence of cremaster muscle in the cryptorchid has been held by some to be the essential factor (cf. Moore and Tapper, 1940; Thompson and Heckel, 1941). Hart (1910) observed the cremaster in marsupials exerts a milking action on the testes while the gubernaculum serves only as a guide. Lewis (1948) in experimenting with rats noted that division of the crural nerve before eight days of age caused isolateral failure of testicular descent and concluded the defect resulted from cremasteric muscle paralysis.

The notion that inguinal cryptorchism results from faulty muscular development in the groin coupled with a failure of the gubernaculum to adjust itself to the muscular growth has also been advanced. When the transversalis and internal oblique muscles and the adjoining tendon are undeveloped, the testicle is retained high in the canal. When the external oblique muscle is anomalous, low testicular retention occurs. Operating room observations disclose that the conditions just cited frequently exist in testicular maldescent.

During the past twenty-five years experimental studies and clinical observations have indicated endocrine factors play an important role in descent of the testicle. The fact that the testes sometimes descend spontaneously at puberty lends weight to the probable relation of endocrine factors to migration of the gland but we still do not know the mechanical agent which directly stimulates and accomplishes the descent (cf. infra, Womack and Koch; 1932; Deming; 1951). The striking structural similarity between the testes of immature monkeys and the human newborn was noted by Engle (1932). Following the injection of prolan A, the monkey testes doubled in weight and the interstitial cell structure increased four to ten times. Accompanying the testicular enlargement there were scrotal edema and turgescence, and the testes descended prematurely from the external ring into the scrotum.

Womack and Koch (1932) determined that before puberty the chorionic hormone is present in greatest amount in the fetus, becoming almost absent in boys from birth to about ten years of age and again becoming present in large amounts during adolescence and continuing so until about the fortieth year when it quantitatively declines. It is believed that the high concentration of this hormone in the fetus is directly responsible for the usual (97 to 99 per cent) normal testicular descent between the seventh and ninth month *in utero*. A "carry over" of high concentration of chorionic hormone probably explains descent during the neonatal period of most testes not down at birth. Not until approaching adolescence with its increased chorionic-like hormonal output is spontaneous testicular descent likely to occur and if the organs are not in the scrotum by this time, their subsequent descent should not be expected. These experimental and clinical observations and studies have widely fostered conservative nonsurgical treatment of cryptorchism in boys but this treatment has not been successful in more than 5 to 8 per cent of the cases in large series.

Migrating Testis. This denotes an unusual free movability of the gland within the inguinal canal; the testis can be pushed freely up or down and/or even into the abdominal cavity. Usually as the child grows, the testicle becomes firmly anchored to the depth of the scrotum. The condition is of high incidence in infants and should be carefully watched as puberty approaches because the condition strongly predisposes to torsion of the spermatic cord. Should pain develop in a migratory testis, perform orchiopexy at once and bilaterally if indicated (see Torsion of the Spermatic Cord).

Inversion and Retroversion of the Testicle. These malformations are rare, are of little importance, are usually unilateral, their causes are unknown, and the condition produces no symptoms. Knowledge of the possible occurrence of this condition is essential in the anatomic localization of the testicle and more particularly of the epididymis.

Ectopic or **aberrant descent of the testicle** signifies that the organ has deviated from its usual course and may be (1) interstitial, (2) femoral or crural, (3) penile, (4) perineal, or (5) transverse (Fig. 261).

1. *Interstitial.* In interstitial testicular ectopy the organ lies anterior to the aponeurosis of the external oblique muscle and is the most common form of aberrant descent. Upon leaving the internal ring, the testis passes upward and outward to lie upon the aponeurosis and the gubernaculum

can readily be identified (Fig. 262). This observation concerning the gubernaculum is offered in explanation of the migration of the gland from its
normal course, but in these cases the scrotal opening is usually blocked by
anomalous development or is otherwise impervious.

2. *In femoral* or *crural ectopy* the testicle lies in Scarpa's triangle (thirteen times in thirty-seven cases of cryptorchism; Burdick and Coley, 1926).
In one of these cases, the passage of the gubernaculum ahead of the testicle
and beneath Scarpa's fascia suggests an etiologic association with the
anomaly.

3. *Penile ectopy* defines location of the testicle at the penile base and
overlying the pubic bone. In a ten-day-old boy at Bellevue Hospital both

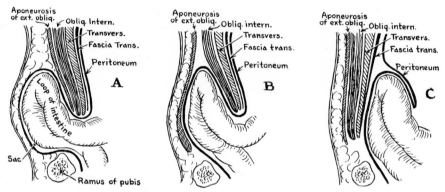

Fig. 262. Interstitial hernia which commonly accompanies imperfect descent of the
testicle. A palpable testicle in the groin is usually in the subcutaneous interstitial tissues
(see text).

testes lay in the upper midpubic margin. Seven other cases have been reported
in the literature including Raspall's (1949) patient with an ectopic testicle
on the dorsum penis.

4. *Perineal Ectopy.* The ectopic testicle is usually attached by the gubernaculum to the spine of the ischium. The spermatic cord overlies Poupart's
ligament (Fig. 263). Only 105 cases have been reported in the literature
but I have seen five, and have operated on three of them. Lockwood's (1888)
theory of overdevelopment of the ischial division or component of the
gubernaculum has been adduced to explain this type of testicular ectopy.

5. *Transverse aberrant testicular maldescent.* Here both organs descend
through the same inguinal canal to the same scrotal sac or the testicle which
has crossed over may be trapped in a hernial sac, as was observed in a
fourteen-year-old boy by Corner. Fourteen other cases of transverse
aberrant testicle have been reported. Hertzler (1916) found both testes
and an infantile uterus in the same scrotal cavity of a pseudohermaphrodite.

The clinical importance of ectopic testicle and the fundamentals of treatment are identical with those observed in the more usual types of cryptorchism.

Pathology of Cryptorchism. While the malposition of the testicle is the
primary observation in these cases, the most striking surgical finding is the

high incidence of congenital hernia, in reported series of cases varying from 70 to 100 per cent. The cause of the congenital hernia here is the failure of the processus vaginalis to close. The detection of hernia by physical examination is of prime concern for if it is demonstrable, the condition is surgical from the start and requires surgical correction of both the maldescent and the hernia. Too often, either failing to recognize or to consider seriously enough the complicating hernia, physicians are content to employ only hormonal therapy which through its inadequacy is to the child's detriment.

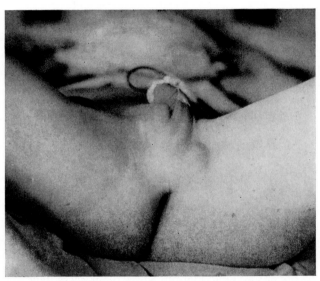

Fig. 263.   Perineal testicle in a seven-year-old boy. Accompanying anomalies included reduplicated left ureter (infected hydronephrosis of the lower half of the kidney), uretero-vesical junction stricture of the ureter of the lower pelvis (ureteroheminephrectomy), six lumbar vertebrae, spina bifida occulta, congenital hypertrophy of the verumontanum, congenital stricture of the midbulbous urethra, and a curious blood grouping which was never accurately matched despite cross matching with more than thirty prospective donors.

While the hernia is usually of the indirect inguinal type, occasionally a sliding hernia is found and even the cecum or sigmoid has been observed to descend through the canal. Interstitial hernia is found in about 15 per cent of the cases (Burdick and Coley, 1926) and here the sac and testis lie (1) between the superficial fascia and the external oblique muscles (subcutaneous), (2) between the external and internal oblique muscles (intraparietal), or (3) between the transversalis fascia and the peritoneum (properitoneal; Fig. 262). Denis Browne (1949) insists that 80 per cent of so-called undescended testes lie anterior to the aponeurosis of the external oblique muscle and in the superficial inguinal pouch. In my experience this percentage is nearer 50.

Congenital malformation of the inguinal canal explains some cases of maldescent, the canal sometimes being completely blocked off by a fascial segment. In some instances the canal is unusually spacious but it is likely that the retained testicle itself may produce this dilatation. The abnormal position of the gland renders it more subject to trauma by direct blow or from muscular contraction of the abdominal wall and there is greater likelihood to undergo torsion. The undescended testis in the inguinal canal may cause compression or even strangulation of herniated bowel as I encountered at operation in a five-month-old boy thought to have torsion of the spermatic cord of an undescended testicle at the internal inguinal ring.

Normally the opening into the scrotum (third inguinal ring of McGregor, 1929) is patent and readily admits the exploring finger. In many cases of cryptorchism this opening is nearly or completely shut off; this finding has been adduced to explain failure of the testicle to enter the scrotum, an interstitial or other ectopic location resulting.

The vas deferens is always of normal length in cryptorchism but the blood vessels of the spermatic cord are short. Sometimes the length of the vas deferens is relatively excessive so that the duct loops back upon itself and may be inadvertently injured or divided at operation. The connective tissues of the cord in the young are fewer and less dense, with less distortion and shortening of the cord than are observed in older patients and, as a corollary, an early operation in small boys requires less intravascular dissection.

The imperfectly descended testis besides being smaller than normal is often attached to the epididymis by a wide or elongated mesorchium (testicular mesentery), a condition which of itself predisposes to torsion of the testis or spermatic cord. In these cases the epididymis is joined to the testis only at the site of efferent ducts (vasa efferentia), the vas deferens may not be continuous with the epididymis, or other forms of failure of urogenital union (q.v.) may exist. In the anatomic examination of 245 undescended testes, Dean, Jr. et al. found an elongated epididymis in seven, anorchia in eleven, absent epididymis and complete separation of the testis and epididymis in three cases each (see Failure of Urogenital Union, p. 478, Fig. 265).

Nearly always the imperfectly descended testis shows atrophy which may be either slight or pronounced; it was extreme in thirteen of the 313 cases in our autopsy series. This change in the gland results principally from anemia caused by interference with the circulation but it may follow trauma or compression within the inguinal canal or blows to the testicle when it overlies the pubis. The soft small atrophic testicle shows both morphologic and functional changes (Fig. 264). The cellular alterations are chiefly atrophy of the seminiferous tubules and involve principally the spermatogenic cells which disappear so that about 90 per cent of testes undescended at puberty are sterile. The endocrine cells of Leydig in the interstitial stroma show little change except an increase in fat but sometimes they hypertrophy. Although these cells are rarely destroyed, occasionally the entire testicle becomes a fibrous mass. Patients whose interstitial cells are preserved are rarely impotent in adulthood even though bilateral cryptorchism exists. The testes of such individuals commonly show marked hyperplasia of the interstitial cells. A hypertrophic fertile organ showing compensatory hypertrophy usually accompanies an atrophic undescended mate.

Although fully 90 per cent of adults with bilateral cryptorchism at puberty are sterile, some amazing instances of fertility have been reported and interesting among these is the small group showing hereditary cryptorchism, in some of whom the condition has been traced through three generations.

The extensive and carefully conducted experiments of Moore (1936) have shown that physiologically the scrotum functions as a testicular radiator in the cooler confines of which the gonad achieves its maximal development and fertility. Employing monkeys in which the normal testes were moved into the abdomen where they showed degeneration, and back to the scrotum

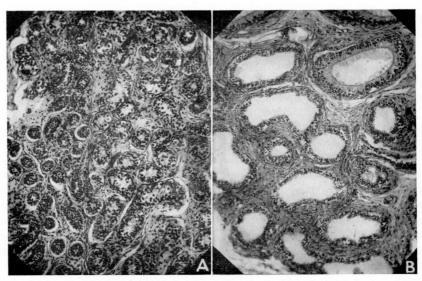

Fig. 264.   Imperfect descent of the testes. Histology. *A,* normal testicle in a ten-year-old boy. Note the rich cellular structure with abundance of tubules and relatively scant interstitial tissues. *B,* inguinal testicle of a ten-year-old boy retained in the inguinal canal. The tubular degeneration and marked increase in interstitial tissue is remarkable and quite in contrast to the normal histology shown in *A.*

where they showed regeneration, Moore conclusively demonstrated that the thermal factors are extremely important in producing the degenerative cellular changes and particularly in the spermatic elements of the improperly placed testicle. Comparative clinical studies of the intratesticular and the intra-abdominal temperatures (Newman and Wilhelm, 1950) confirm the correctness of Moore's dicta. These observations emphasize the advantage of comparatively early operation to correct imperfect testicular descent. The reader is referred to Section I, Chapter 3, by Moore.

In bilateral cryptorchism injury or destruction of the interstitial cells of the testicle commonly causes pronounced endocrine disturbances generally manifested as eunuchoidism or hypogenitalism. The appearance and development of these manifestations usually engender a pitiable inferiority complex in the boy as well as marked psychosexual disturbance.

Symptoms in cryptorchism are local, endocrine and psychologic. These are largely dependent upon the age of the patient and whether one or both glands are involved. Except for the absence of the testes from the scrotum or a complicating torsion of the spermatic cord, the undescended testicle generally causes no manifestations in infancy but in older boys there may be severe cramplike pains in the testicle and even accompanied by vomiting. Often this reflects torsion of the spermatic cord. Inguinal testes may be painful when the legs are crossed or local discomfort may reflect an accompanying hernia. As testicular atrophy occurs and particularly in the ectopic organ, especially perineal, the gland becomes insensitive or may be the site of intermittent dull or acute pain. Epididymitis of an undescended testicle may suggest torsion or, by pain reference, an acute intraperitoneal surgical disease. Meyer (1927) reported three infants with fatal peritonitis secondary to suppurative orchitis (epididymitis) in an abdominal testicle. Chorea, eclampsia infantum or hystero-epileptic attacks have ceased following operation for undescended testes (Meyer). Psychic disturbances rarely appear until late childhood and are often absent, there being no relation to unilateral or bilateral involvement. The mental reaction is characteristically one of depression, of assumed sexual inferiority, and has occasionally led to suicide.

In cryptorchism somatic endocrinopathic changes seldom develop except in bilateral cases.

Diagnosis. This rests largely upon findings by palpation. When (1) the testicle cannot be palpated in the scrotum or in the inguinal canal, (2) there is no history of orchiectomy or testicular trauma, the organ may be assumed to be deep inguinal, retroperitoneal or intra-abdominal.

Careful examination is most essential not only to identify the nature and location of the maldescent but to make sure the organ really is undescended to forestall unnecessary treatment—either hormonal or surgical. An excellent routine for the diagnosis of undescended testes, and one which I have used many years in slightly modified form, has been described by Kunstadter. With the patient standing before the physician, who is seated, to examine the right inguinal region the examiner's left hand is placed on the outer buttock of the patient to give him support. The thumb of the right hand is firmly placed and held above the region of the right internal inguinal ring. The right index finger is now inserted into the inguinal canal, exploring to the internal inguinal ring, if possible. An extra-abdominal testis may be palpable between the thumb and forefinger and, if not, by "stripping," an attempt is made to move the testis downward in the canal by applying descending pressure by the thumb along the course of the canal. A fixed testis will not become noticeably lower but, with this stripping, a migratory gland may be pushed into the scrotum between the thumb and index finger, both being in contact with the testis. This examination will disclose (1) whether a testis is in the inguinal canal, (2) the size, location and consistency of the gland, (3) whether the gland is migratory (pseudocryptorchid) or true cryptorchid and (4) if there is hernia. To examine the left side, the hands and positions are reversed.

A testicle palpable in the groin is most probably in the space between Scarpa's fascia and the fascia of the external oblique muscles (superficial inguinal pouch, Fig. 262); a testis in the inguinal canal is seldom palpable except in boys with unusually thin subcutaneous fat and external oblique fascia. As a therapeutic corollary most inguinal testes alleged to descend to the scrotum following hormone therapy are in fact originally in the superficial inguinal pouch.

In *migrating testicle* the overactive cremaster may withdraw the organ into the abdomen only to have it spontaneously reappear in a few minutes in the scrotum. The differentiation here is made by compression of the canal which will retrieve the mobile testicle but not the true cryptorchid. The diagnosis of intra-abdominal testicle should not be made until the perineum and other sites of testicular ectopia have been carefully examined. Investigation for hernia is the most important consideration in these cases and in at least three fourths of them will be demonstrable.

Complicating disease of an undescended testicle may make the differential diagnosis extremely difficult or it may be achieved only at operation. Acute epididymitis, torsion of an undescended testicle or strangulated hernia accompanying cryptorchism are the more important diagnostically confusing conditions. In epididymitis there is usually a preceding urethral discharge and digital evidence of prostatitis or seminal vesiculitis, together with fever, distressing local pain, reddening and edema of the overlying skin. Gastrointestinal upsets may be severe and, after a day or so, the swollen indurated epididymis can usually be differentiated from the normal testicle except when in high inguinal or intra-abdominal location.

In torsion of the spermatic cord (q.v.), the onset may simulate that of epididymitis with equally excruciating pain but the febrile reaction is less pronounced and local skin reaction may be absent. As the torsion persists and hemorrhagic testicular gangrene ensues, pain nearly or completely disappears. Kelly and Uhrich (1952) collected eleven cases of torsion of intra-abdominal testicles and added one of their own, in a four-and-one-half-year-old boy. In a seventeen-year-old boy seen at Bellevue Hospital, an extremely tender left midinguinal mass was found with reddening of the overlying skin. The isolateral scrotal sac was small and contained no testicle. He had acute gonorrhea, mild fever and no gastrointestinal disturbance. Preoperative diagnosis made by several eminent urologists rested between torsion and gonococcus epididymitis of an undescended testicle, but operation disclosed a neoplasm.

When strangulated hernia complicates cryptorchism, the systemic symptoms usually overcloud the local signs with gastrointestinal disturbances, nausea, vomiting (sometimes fecal), abdominal distention and a low or subnormal temperature. In a five-month-old boy whose history and local findings made the diagnosis of torsion of an undescended right inguinal testicle seem indubitable, exploration disclosed acute strangulated hernia in which the chocolate-colored loop of bowel presenting in the hernial sac was intimately bound by fresh fibrin to the undescended testicle situated at the internal inguinal ring. The hernial opening was surgically enlarged and by relief of the strangulation and the application of hot pads for about fifteen minutes, the circulation was sufficiently restored to warrant closure of the abdomen. His recovery was uneventful and the boy returned home on the sixth postoperative day. In two other cases simulating torsion of the cord in cryptorchism, the testicle was found jammed in the internal ring, half in the abdomen, half out. In short, the gravity of the lesions described calls for immediate operation when the diagnosis will be made or confirmed; especially in infancy and early childhood immediate intervention is imperative.

The *diagnosis* of ectopic testicle is made by discovery of absence of the testicle from the scrotum and its location at the base of the penis, perineum and so forth. Ectopic testicles are nearly always atrophic and may be insensitive. In any patient with cryptorchism the perineum should be carefully examined.

Treatment. The preservation of fertility is the most important consideration in the treatment of imperfect descent of the testicle. Over 90 per cent of the patients with bilateral cryptorchism are sterile after puberty (McCallum, 1935) but following early and proper treatment, satisfactory testicular development generally occurs. Unless androgen or surgical therapy succeeds in bringing the testicle well down into the scrotum, aspermatogenesis becomes almost a certainty.

Logically, bilateral maldescent suggests either bilateral mechanical (anatomic) hindrance or that, *in utero,* there was inadequate chorionic hormone at the critical prenatal time (seven to nine months). When one gland is normally descended, a mechanical factor such as retaining fibrous bands or anomalous development of the gland or canal should be suspected. Since the gonadotropic hormone usually causes not only widening and enlargement of the inguinal canal in preadolescence, so that the possibility of a small passageway for the testicle can be ruled out, failure or hormone therapy to bring about testicular descent must be considered to indicate a mechanical unilateral or bilateral retention of the gland by fibrous bands, a shorter than normal blood supply, or an organ malformed sufficient to be unable to enter the inguinal canal above or pass through it. The employment of hormone therapy does not rest on whether or not the testis is palpable. Scrotal development often gives a clue; in abdominal cryptorchism the isolateral scrotum is usually poorly developed and small; in congenital absence of the testes, the scrotum is not developed. Unless there is at least fair scrotal development, the hormonal treatment of cryptorchism will be unsuccessful.

When visible retraction of the cremaster, ease of manual reduction and reasonably good scrotal development indicate the testicle is merely retractile, surgical treatment may not be required. By this differentiation from mechanical ectopic fixation of the testicle, the therapy is formulated.

When the cause of the maldescent is unsettled and there is no hernia, the employment of *hormone therapy* will be successful only when there is no mechanical retardation of the gland. The therapeutic course to be pursued then depends upon the presence or absence of complicating congenital hernia. When hernia is demonstrable, the problem is patently surgical from the start. When no hernia exists the patient should be given the benefit of endocrine therapy and here we rely upon the intramuscular administration of chorionic gonadotropin (the anterior pituitary like follicle stimulating hormone of pregnancy urine; commercial marketing: Antuitrin-"S", Follutin-S, A.P.L., and others). The dose to be given will usually be relative to the size and age of the patient. A four-year-old boy can usually be given 250 international units two or three times weekly, a ten-year-old boy 500 international units at these intervals. Chorionic gonadotropic therapy is of no value in imperfectly descended testicle associated with pronounced testicular hypoplasia incapable of stimulation or when mechanical factors retain the testis. If satisfactory descent of the testicle is to occur consequent to hormone therapy, progress will nearly always be noted in two to three weeks and, if no benefit is evident with the administration of a maximum of 2500 international units, operation is advisable. The testes which descend with chorionic hormone therapy are the ones which normally would descend during puberty (cf. Thompson and Heckel, 1941). Rea (1949) employed hormone therapy in thirty of 131 cases of cryptorchism, achieving testicular descent in seven. The interstitial Leydig cells of the testis are stimulated by chorionic gonadotropin to secrete increased amounts of androgens. Excess fruitless overtreatment is likely to produce the manifestations of pubertas praecox (q.v.). Even more important, excess hormonal therapy will stimulate closure of epiphyseal bone centers to prevent normal bony development and encourage a variable dwarfism. I have seen many boys thus continuously and expensively subjected to long courses of anterior pituitary-like hormone therapy and in whom a large congenital hernia was readily demonstrable, in some was even visible, and initially demanded prompt operation rather than endocrines. The administration of the gonadotropic hormone may produce temporal headache and/or fever and demand a period of rest, a reduction of the drug or even its complete stoppage.

Testosterone has been similarly employed but it must be recognized that testosterone therapy is replacement therapy, whereas the gonadotropic substance is stimulative. Androgenic hormone is indicated only when the testes transplanted to the scrotum fail to develop. Heckel (1939) and others have shown that androgenic therapy causes reduction in spermatogenesis and if carried far enough experimentally, aspermia and agametocytogenesis. Several boys have been seen who had large doses of testosterone propionate given elsewhere to stimulate testicular descent but caused only an abnormally large genital growth with a cropping out of pubic hair and variable testicular atrophy. A six-year-old boy showed almost complete bilateral testicular atrophy consequent to the administration of enormous doses of testosterone propionate over a long period. The undescended testicle was atrophied as was the normally descended one, a thoroughly expectable result from the overadministration of replacement therapy in which the testicles underwent a variety of atrophy of disuse. Despite advertisements recommending the employment of testosterone propionate in the treatment of cryptorchism in the young, its use for this condition is strongly advised against, in favor of gonadotropic substances which should be employed up to a total of not over 2500 international units.

Chorionic gonadotropin administered for a week preoperatively is frequently technically helpful in inducing engorgement and enlargement of the structures of the cord, thereby facilitating intravascular dissection which is always a delicate and precise procedure and sometimes an extremely tedious one.

Surgical Treatment. When hormonal therapy fails to cause the testicle to descend to the scrotum and stay there, operation is demanded. In more than half of the conservatively treated there will be no evidence of mobilization of the testicle but in many cases thus treated the testicle will descend to the scrotum. It will remain there for a variable period after cessation of treatment, but within two to four weeks will again rise out of the scrotum and often retract back into the inguinal canal. In this last group of cases it is of considerable advantage to repeat the conservative treatment and when the testicle has reached the scrotum, operate, repair the hernia and by orchiopexy, firmly anchor the gland to the lower scrotal pole as described in Section XV, Chapter 12.

Prevention of testicular atrophy and, by the same token, preservation of spermatogenesis is the prime objective in fixing the testicle in its normal site. Even though the testicle thus operated on is hypertrophic, in most cases a striking increase in size will be noted six months to a year postoperatively. By reasonably early treatment, testicular pain, the likelihood of endocrine or psychic disturbances, torsion of the spermatic cord or strangulated hernia are materially lessened.

Where there is complicating hernia, operation rather than a truss should be employed and, parenthetically, *under no circumstances should a truss be permitted with undescended testicle.*

Pronounced local symptoms such as pain, recurring torsion, hernia and so forth, demand immediate operation and here the chief postoperative difficulty is the management of urinary incontinence in the very young. For a number of years I have employed a small indwelling catheter in these cases for five to eight days postoperatively or at least until the likelihood of wound contamination by urine seems unlikely. The administration of small dose of penicillin, Terramycin or Aureomycin largely removes the hazards of surgical infection. Most of these wounds in the young heal surprisingly well, even though occasionally drenched in urine. Especially in children the larger-than-normal doses of vitamins A, B complex, C and D during the preoperative and postoperative period will do much to favor prompt wound healing.

When to Operate. In bilateral cryptorchism, steps to correct the condition should be begun by the age of three or four years. In unilateral cryptorchism one may wait until six years of age, yet early operation is always preferred to late. By placing the testicle in its normal position in the scrotum, (1) atrophy and other undesirable sequels are rendered less likely to occur, (2) the comparative delicacy of the vascular adhesions in the spermatic cord in boys simplifies the operative technique, and (3) in general, a better end result is assured. The administration of chorionic gonadotropin renders it no longer necessary to wait until puberty to ascertain if the testicle will descend because this phenomenon can be anticipated by a test series of injections of the hormone, even at the age of two or three years. The boy with bilateral cryptorchism should be favored by its early correction (third year) and when conservative hormone therapy is neither indicated nor successful, operated without great delay.

It is probable that increased knowledge of testicular and interrelated endocrinology will result in a more conservative surgical attitude among urologists in particular. But the incidence of congenital hernia in these cases is not likely to be altered so that variations and innovations in conservative therapy, particularly hormonal, will not concern more than perhaps 15 per cent of the patients with cryptorchism. The high incidence of associated hernia and the excellent results now obtained by the Torek operation or one of its modifications and the incontrovertible fact that the patient is happier with two testes in the scrotum than with one or none, should lead to more widespread employment of combined endocrine and surgical therapy or surgical therapy alone. The needless anxiety of hopefully waiting for puberty by a boy with cryptorchism is not to be compared with the successful result of operation in which the testes are both in the scrotum, testicular sensation is preserved, the hernia is cured, and as the patient grows the scrotum and its contents develop normally.

Occasionally the imperfectly descended testis cannot be brought down adequately into the scrotum, let alone joined to the thigh; here much will depend on the condition of the opposite gland. With an apparently normal properly descended testis and when its abnormal mate is only moderately hypoplastic but cannot be brought down into the scrotum, it may be left in the inguinal canal for such hormonal value as it may have and where it will be readily examined periodically. Especially should it be preserved if the opposite organ is poorly developed or its condition is unknown. Yet in general, orchiectomy is preferable to leaving the testis in the abdomen or groin, and certainly it should not be left over the pubis to be continually subjected to trauma. Small atrophic undescended testes should be removed. As far as can be done with safety, the patient should keep his abnormal testis although a small fibrotic nubbin of a testicle will serve no purpose and should be excised.

From studies of a large series of tumors of the testicle Dean (1940) found the incidence of these growths in imperfectly descended testes to be twenty-two times greater than in normal testes. Yet, comparatively, new growths of the testicle are so rare as to merit scant consideration in this connection. On a statistical basis, the danger of malignant change in the testicle alone should not be adduced as an indication for operation in cryptorchism, nor should it necessarily cause a relatively good testicle to be removed rather than replaced in the abdomen when it cannot properly be brought down into the scrotum. Such a testicle, though probably sterile, is likely to be sufficiently well developed to elaborate androgenic hormone. Moreover, orchiopexy *per se* does not prevent testicular neoplasm; several cases of neoplasm developing in testes surgically placed in the scrotum have been reported.

Irrespective of the apparent therapeutic success in bilateral cryptorchism, the testes of the patient must be considered spermatogenically subnormal. The chances of procreation will be greatest in the early twenties and, if progeny are desired, an early marriage should be advised. Although it is recognized that in two thirds of the cases of undescended testicle at birth, the gland will probably descend by the end of puberty; in the intervening years the maldescended organ is subjected to the various deleterious factors discussed in preceding paragraphs. We are not doing full duty by our patients when we subject them to unjustifiable hazards such as torsion of the spermatic cord and possibility of aspermatogenesis of the involved testicle through unwarranted and needless delay.

In *abnormally mobile testes,* orchiopexy is the treatment. The gland is securely anchored to the lowermost part of the scrotum and co-existing hernia is simultaneously repaired. Unless the freely movable testicle is firmly anchored, there is grave likelihood that torsion of the spermatic cord will occur with subsequent loss of the gland by atrophy, gangrene, or orchiectomy. The surgical treatment of imperfectly descended testicle is described in Section XV, Chapter 12.

The *treatment of ectopic testicle* is surgical with mobilization of the gland from its ectopic site and emplacement in its normal position in the scrotum. Endocrine therapy is valueless in these cases; unless the condition is causing symptoms, operation may be withheld until after the third birthday.

Perineal ectopia requires transplantation of the testicle to its normal scrotal position before the boy starts riding a bicycle or in active play runs the risk of a straddle injury. The operative treatment is usually simple since the cord is always long enough to permit the testicle to reach the depth of the scrotum.

Prognosis. The degree of testicular damage and the correctness of therapy will determine the prognosis and results in cryptorchism. If (1) the boy is operated upon before the eighth year, (2) atrophy has not occurred, and (3) the testicle is placed at the bottom of the scrotum without injury to the blood vessels of the spermatic cord, it is likely that a thoroughly satisfactory functioning testicle will remain. The male androgenic hormonal elaboration may be expected to continue or increase.

Operations on improperly descended testicles require an unusual surgical expertness, gentleness, patience and experience because of the grave danger of irreparable vascular injury of the spermatic cord and particularly trauma or severance of these vessels which results in subsequent thrombosis and testicular gangrene. Unqualified operators are too often satisfied to achieve lengthening of the cord by undue cutting of vessels; grave impairment of the blood supply with atrophy or sloughing of the gland commonly ensues. Here the spermatic artery is the most important single vessel; if it is divided, the artery of the vas deferens affords a collateral supply but this vessel is small and testicular atrophy or failure to grow is certain even though the gland may not slough.

No recent comprehensive data are offered indicating the fate of the testicle, its function and development following operations for cryptorchism and especially when bilateral. MacCallum (1935) studied the fertility of eighty-nine men previously examined and operated upon for improperly descended testes at the Children's Hospital in Boston. Sixty-one per cent of those who were operated upon were fertile as compared to only 10 per cent of those not operated upon. The striking and encouraging observation of MacCallum's study was that in eighteen patients with bilateral undescended testes on whom orchiopexy had been performed, there was fertility in 80 per cent, and in sharp contrast to the usual estimated 10 per cent of fertile males with bilateral cryptorchism and without orchiopexy (MacCallum). Yet Bishop's (1945) study of his own cases and his analysis of the published reports of many other students of this problem are much less encouraging than MacCallum's observations. The prognosis should always be

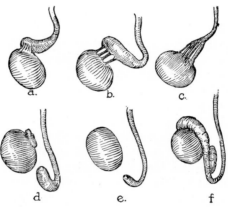

Fig. 265.   Anomalies of urogenital union. Schematic presentation of some of the more common maldevelopments of urogenital union. *a,* epididymis detached from the testicle except at the globus major. *b,* epididymis attached to the testicle only by elongated ductuli efferentes. *c,* direct union of the vas deferens through ductuli efferentes to the testicle; the epididymis is absent. *d,* the body of the epididymis is absent; failure of union of the vas and testicle. *e,* globus major and body of the epididymis are absent. *f,* accessory epididymis forming on the globus minor of its mate. (Hinman after Hinkey and Lubash.)

guarded especially in boys with a strong tendency to eunuchoidism or infantilism, conditions more often encountered in cryptorchid than normal boys.

Failure of Urogenital Union. Anomalies consequent to the failure of urogenital union are frequently associated with imperfectly descended testes and are of far higher incidence than generally recognized (Fig. 265). Only twenty cases have been reported to date and three of these were recently added by Dean, Jr. et al. (1952) but I have seen five cases showing pronounced abnormality. The normal junction between the testicle and the mesonephric derivative, the epididymis, fails to take place and these organs develop separately. The results of this malunion have been classified (Windholz, 1929) in five groups: (1) the epididymis and vas deferens are descended into the region of the scrotum but the testicle is absent (anorchism; in a five-year-old patient of mine this condition was confirmed at operation); (2) the testicle is present but undescended; the epididymis is partially descended into the scrotum; (3) only the vas deferens is present in the scrotum, and (4) the testicle and epididymis are descended but are widely separated by a long mesorchium; the epididymis usually precedes in the descent process (cf. Lazarus and Marks, 1947; Orr et al., 1948). The conditions indicated in group (4) will be found in most cases of high inguinal or abdominal testicle and are rarely significant except as potential predisposing factors in the development of torsion of the spermatic cord (q.v.) or in causing isolateral sterility.

Adrenal rests in the testicle—ectopic adrenal tissue congenitally misplaced—were twice encountered; on the right in a one-year-old and on the

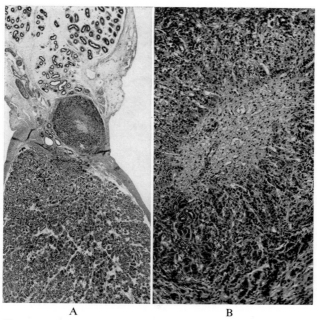

A   B

Fig. 266. Aberrant adrenal rest in the rete testis of a one-year-old boy. *A,* the ectopic adrenal tissue rests between the epididymis (above) and testicle (below). *B,* histologic character of the ectopic adrenal rest in *A.* Note the typical adrenal cortical structure; medullary tissue was not found. (University Hospital.)

left in a three-year-old. Similar ectopic displacement along the spermatic cord has also been noted (Fig. 266).

Congenital hydrocele is often observed in the newborn; its clinical aspects are discussed in Section VI, Chapter 3 and its surgical treatment is considered in Section XV, Chapter 12, together with that of the acquired condition.

Anomalies of the remainder of the spermatic tract (epididymis, vas deferens, seminal vesicles, and utricle) are extremely rare and are seldom recognized before puberty when spermatic function begins unless revealed as a surgical disclosure. A lesion described as a spermatocele above the left testis and attached to the spermatic cord was found at autopsy in a five-year-old boy but lacked microscopic proof—most likely it was simply an occlusion cyst of the cord.

Aplasia or **Agenesis of the Isolateral Spermatic Tract.** This occurs occa-sionally when the urinary tract is similarly involved and is a reminder that when genital anomalies exist, the upper urinary tract is anomalous in about a third of the cases.

Aberrant wolffian duct remnants in the epididymis may become cystic masses to be differentiated from spermatocele. These cystic masses appear chiefly as (1) the hydatid of Morgagni which is a blind duct located near the head of the epididymis, and (2) the paradidymis or organ of Giraldes which is a blind duct located near the tail of the epididymis. Occasionally these cysts grow to sufficient size to be palpable even in young boys and for unknown reasons may become twisted upon themselves (torsion of the testicular appendages) to induce great pain, scrotal swelling and the symp-tomatic picture commonly observed in torsion of the spermatic cord. *Torsion of the testicular appendages* is largely a condition of childhood (Section VI, Chapter 3 and Section XIII). Excision of the involved pedicle is the treatment.

Vas Deferens. The vas deferens is subject to considerable variation in size and occasionally is absent, particularly in isolateral renal agenesis. Bilateral *congenital absence of the vas deferens* has been reported by Keshin and Pinck (1948) and was observed in four cases in our autopsy series (see anorchism); a sixth case of reduplication of the vas deferens was described by Mathé and Dunn (1948) and associated with isolateral renal agenesis. In 1950 Nelson collected twenty-eight cases of congenital absence of the vas deferens including three of his own, and in some of which the condition was bilateral. The testes were present in each but in three the isolateral kidney was absent, and in seven the isolateral seminal vesicle was diminutive or absent. Yet absence of the vas deferens does not imply testicular agenesis because the testis and vasa efferentia are derived from the genital fold while the vas deferens, globus minor and body of the epididymis, seminal vesicles and ejaculatory ducts are of wolffian duct origin.

The anomaly accounts for sterility in some cases. In a fourteen-year-old boy operated upon for right cryptorchism, the small fibrotic testicle was found in the femoral ring; the vas deferens as it left the abdomen was nor-mal and continued so until 3 cm. from the epididymis where it became a fine thread. The spermatic cord in this segment was also markedly hypo-plastic and this doubtless explains the testiculoepididymal hypoplasia and fibrosis. At operation in a three-year-old boy with right freely movable testicle, congenital hydrocele and hernia, a strung-out epididymis was at-tached to the testicle by a long mesorchium; the vas deferens, kinked upon itself in corkscrew fashion, extended upward to the epididymis for 3 cm. to terminate blindly in a rounded club-shaped end near the internal inguinal ring. Michelson (1949) in a study of seventy-four cases of congenital anomalies of the vas deferens and epididymis, found fifty-three cases of aber-rant vasa deferentia (forty-seven unilateral; six bilateral) and twenty cases of absence of the vas (eighteen unilateral; two bilateral); one case of uni-lateral absence of the vas and contralateral vasal aberrancy. There were defects of the testicle in fifteen of the seventy-four cases; bilateral absence in five; unilateral absence in twenty-three and maldescent in thirty. Normal testes were bilaterally present in only sixteen cases. The gland was aberrant in forty of sixty cases of epididymal defects (three bilateral) and absent in twenty (eighteen unilateral; two bilateral). These malformations are of potential clinical interest in young boys and of vital consideration in adults as they concern impaired fertility.

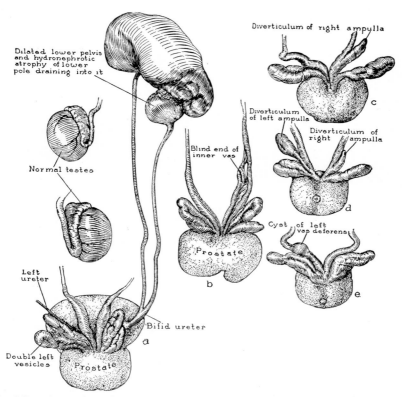

Fig. 267. Anomalies of the vas deferens and seminal vesicles. Schematically showing the more common malformations. *a*, double left seminal vesicle with bifid ureter. *b*, reduplicated right seminal vesicle and vas deferens, the inter-vas ending blindly. *c*, diverticulum of ampulla. *d*, diverticulum of both ampullae. *e*, cyst of the left vas deferens. (Hinman after Preisel.)

Seminal Vesicles. These structures show great variation in size, sometimes with one large and the other small, rudimentary or absent (Fig. 267). Anomalies of the seminal vesicles are comparatively rare; in our autopsy study in 10,919 boys there were six cases. In four male infants there was congenital absence of the seminal vesicle, prostate, testes, and in two the spermatic cord also was missing. In two of these there was bilateral renal agenesis, in two unilateral agenesis (ipsilateral) and in all six the isolateral testicle was absent. Gutierrez (1935) classified sixteen different varieties and combinations of seminal vesicle anomalies. While this condition may seldom present a problem in the young, in adults the anomaly may be of vital concern in failure of reproduction. Rarely the two vesicles may unite into a common opening in the utricle, a condition observed perhaps more frequently in the advanced stages of hypospadias and pseudohermaphroditism or other comparable anatomic manifestations of estrogenic hormonal imbalance. In these more serious urethrogenital anomalies urethroscopic examina-

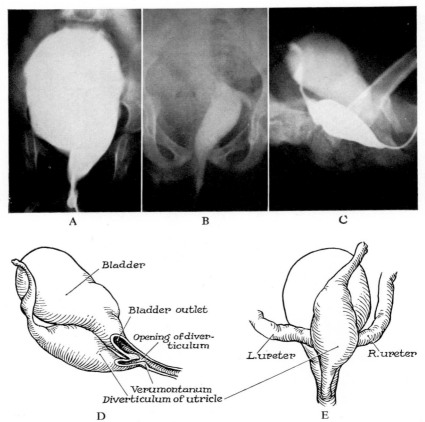

Fig. 268. Congenital diverticulum of the utricle in an eighteen-month-old boy with penoscrotal hypospadias examined because of persistent pyuria of one-year duration. *A*, the distended bladder and utricle are clearly shown; the dilated left upper urinary tract is feebly outlined by cystographic reflux. Urinary distention of the diverticulum caused pressure on the lower ureters and on the urethra, thus producing obstruction. *B*, utriculogram in *A*, anterior posterior view. *C*, lateral view of combined utriculogram and cystogram, a medium of lighter density being injected into the bladder. A curious fallopian-tube-like termination of the utricle is notable, this being the male homologue of the uterus. *D, E*, schema of local pathology.

tion is advised to determine if a verumontanum and/or prostate is present and whether the ejaculatory ducts open normally or are absent, fused, reduplicated or ectopic. By their catheterization and injection with a radiopaque medium (seminal vesiculography), the morphology of the seminal vesicles can be demonstrated.

Congenital cysts of the seminal vesicles have been reported in eight cases (Stewart and Nicholl, 1949), the youngest patient being eighteen years of age. The symptoms are predominantly those of bladder outlet blockage consequent to extravesical or extraurethral pressure. Some of these cysts may be urethrographically demonstrated by contrast medium injected through a catheter passed into the utricle in the verumontanum. The treatment is excision of the cyst.

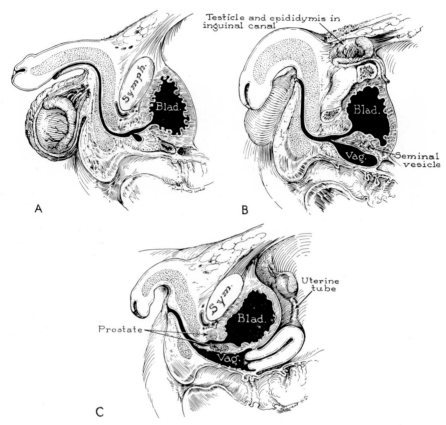

Fig. 269.   Anomalies of the utricle; these are most commonly observed in advanced hypospadias. *A*, in penile hypospadias with slight enlargement of the utricle reflecting a minimal degree of feminization. *B*, greatly dilated utricle in penoscrotal hypospadias accompanied by incompletely descended testes, and hypoplasia of the penis, prostate, and seminal vesicles which reflects greater feminization than in *A*. *C*, extreme feminization in which the penis resembles a large clitoris and the urethral meatus is perineal. An atrophic testis and a rudimentary epididymis lay in contact with the uterine tube in the pelvis, the uterus being well developed and the vagina present. Prostatic underdevelopment with absence of seminal vesicles and vasa. A somewhat similar condition is shown in Fig. 270. (Courtesy Dr. F. S. Howard and Journal of Surgery, Gynecology and Obstetrics.)

Utricle (Uterus Masculinus). This develops by midline fusion of the müllerian ducts and may be extremely deep and even lead to spacious dilatation or diverticulum, or a cyst formation extending up between the seminal vesicles behind and beneath the bladder. Fluid distention of this cyst or a well filled diverticulum of the utricle may produce compression against the urethral floor with obstruction and interference with urination in boys and, in addition, in older males cause sexual dysfunction (Figs. 267–269). Endoscopic studies have revealed a high incidence of malformations of the utricle and associated structures in hypospadias (q.v.; also cf. Howard, 1948). Landes and Ranson (1949) collected fifteen cases including one of their own. The youngest, a three-and-a-half-year-old boy, suffered urinary obstruction; he was cured by excision of the cyst (McKenna and Kiefer, 1939). In many of the more advanced cases, an infantile uterus-like body is roentgenographically demonstrable (Figs. 268, 270). In an eighteen-month-old boy with secondary bladder neck obstruction and persistent

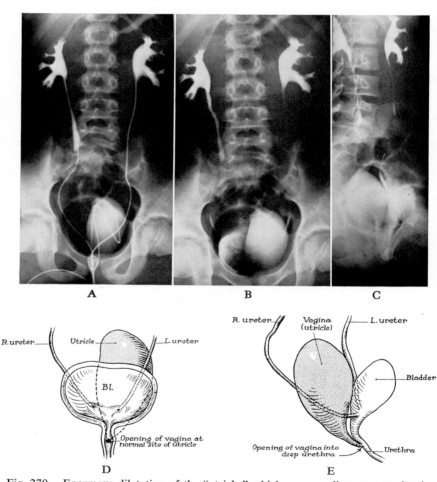

Fig. 270.   Enormous dilatation of the "utricle," which was a rudimentary vagina in a nine-year-old "boy" with an infantile uterus and fallopian tubes. Testes were not demonstrated. Pseudovaginal hypospadiac type of external genitalia (C in Fig. 269). A, catheter coiled in utricle and utriculogram made. B (anteroposterior view). C (oblique view), combined utriculogram and cystogram, the capacity of the former being greater than that of the bladder (C). D, E, schema in this case. D, anterior posterior. E, lateral. The child's clitoris was even larger than normal penile growth for the age. She had been raised as a boy showing predominantly male characteristics, was desexed and correction of the hypospadias was carried out. No excision of the utricle, the orifice of which was in the deep urethra and in the absence of a true verumontanum, appeared hymenlike.

pyuria, we demonstrated an enormous diverticulum of the utricle which extended posteriorly and terminated in a fallopian-tubelike structure (Fig. 268).

Cysts of the müllerian duct are occasionally encountered in older children and adults; they are usually located in the midline and are of variable size but may be large enough to obstruct the lower bowel. They are palpable by rectum and urethroscopically show a variable compression of the bladder outlet with distortion of the trigone and/or bladder floor. Perineal or suprapubic excision is the treatment. Culbertson (1947) reported two cases. Similar cysts have also been observed in the seminal vesicles and prostate (q.v.). The seminal vesicles, utricle and vas deferens may be the site of ectopic ureteral opening as discussed in this chapter under Ureteral Ectopia.

MALFORMATION OF THE FEMALE UROGENITAL TRACT

Persistent cloaca has been previously discussed in this chapter.

Congenital fissure of the clitoris is analogous to cleft glans penis, is rare and of no clinical concern except as it may suggest the presence of other urogenital tract anomalies. The incidence of *absence of the clitoris* is about that of penile agenesis (q.v.). *Congenital hypertrophy of the clitoris* was observed in seven cases at autopsy, in two of which there was pseudohermaphroditism associated with adrenal dysfunction. In an eleven-day-old girl and in a ten-year-old girl there were cystic ovaries, and in the last case pronounced hypospadias. In a one-month-old girl with hypertrophied clitoris, the ovaries were absent.

Fusion of the Labia Minora. Also known as synechia vulvae, this condition is characterized by a midline sealing together of the labia minora, usually leaving a minute unfused area just below the clitoris through which the child urinates and later menstruates (incomplete variety, Fig. 271). Although the twenty-seven cases I have seen were unquestionably congenital, in a study of 110 cases Nalle et al. (1949) concluded that the condition is an acquired rather than a congenital malformation. Acquired fusion is thought by some to be the result of intrauterine inflammation with sealing together of the labia minora or of the vaginal orifice or to result from postpartum inflammation with cohesion of the inflamed tissues (Vakar, 1930). Oschenius (1927) attributed it to local inflammation in acute infectious diseases such as pneumonia, scarlet fever, diphtheria, typhoid, typhus, cholera and smallpox.

Vulvar fusion is seldom recognized until months after birth; the oldest child in whom I have seen the condition was eight years old and was examined because of persistent pyuria which in turn resulted from vaginal collection of decomposed urine and the resulting inflammatory cellular exudate. On the other hand, the oldest adult was a sixty-nine-year-old virgin who presented a labial orifice not over 2 mm. in diameter, 1.5 cm. below the clitoris and through which she had urinated and menstruated during her lifetime. Most of the cases in my experience have been thought to be instances of pseudohermaphroditism or hermaphroditism; the youngest was four months old. Yet to the uninstructed, the lesion may present a most perplexing problem. A mother presented two daughters for examination, five and six years of age, with pronounced fusion of the labia minora in each and for the cure of which she had been told by several physicians that construction of a new vagina in each child would be necessary. In her pocket she had a list of eleven plastic surgeons scattered over the United States whose opinion she anticipated seeking as to treatment for the girls.

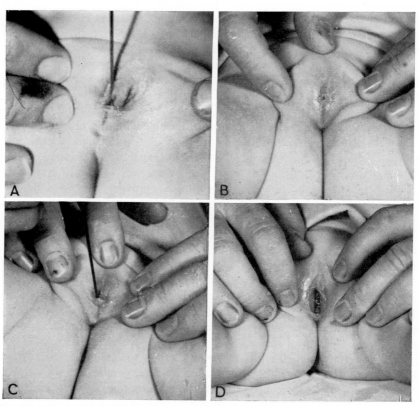

Fig. 271.   Fusion of the labia minora. *A*, the fusion appears as a transparent membrane readily ruptured. *B* extremely small orifice in fused labia minora through which patient must void and in later life menstruate. An even smaller orifice was found in a sixty-nine-year old woman with fused labia minora and through the minute opening she had menstruated. *C*, instrument introduced into introitus preparatory to breaking down the labial adhesions. *D*, adhesions broken down leaving a normal introitus presenting.

Simple division of the labial fusion in the office was promptly curative and disclosed in each child not only a hymen, but normal vagina and other genital structures.

Fused labia minora present a striking appearance, the interlabial vulva region appearing as a smooth, regular, reddish or reddish-blue surface which extends well anteriorly and sometimes the clitoris is completely covered by the midline fusion (Fig. 271). When the labia majora are separated the perineum appears as a solid flat surface up to the subpubic level, usually with a minute opening at or near the underside of the clitoris. The surrounding tissues and especially the orifice show chronic inflammation. When the midline fusion is thin it appears slightly bluish, but when it is dense there is little color differentiation in the tissues. The fusion is disassociated from the hymen. The chief clinical interest and importance of vulvar fusion is concerned with urinary obstruction and in the cases we have seen, infection. Local inflammation has been observed to cause urethrovesical disturbances and particularly frequency and smarting on urination.

The *diagnosis* is made by inspection of the separated labia majora and, once having seen the anomaly, it is unlikely the condition would fail to be recognized again.

Treatment. This consists in separation of the labia minora by a midline cleavage of the line of fusion and is readily performed in the office without anesthesia. Customarily a hemostat is inserted into the small orifice below the clitoris and as the forceps are opened widely the line of fusion will separate toward the clitoris and posteriorly to the body of the perineum. When the line of fusion is dense it is incised with scissors or scalpel. After dividing the fusion, the finger inserted in the introitus will break down any remaining adhesions and will assure that the orifice is widely patent. When the labia are separated, a normal pouting hymen and urethral orifice appear. Clitoric adhesions are broken down to liberate smegmatic debris. Following this treatment a small pledget of cotton can wisely be left in the introitus for a day to keep the divided labia widely separated. The child should be examined again in a month to make sure that refusion has not occurred as it did five times in a six-year-old patient of mine.

The female urethra and prostatic male urethra are homologous. *Hypospadias* may occur *in the female* but is far less common than in the male. *Epispadias* occurs in the female seven times more often than in the male as has been discussed earlier in this chapter.

Wolffian duct derivatives persisting in the female may give rise to cysts and other conditions in the lower female urogenital tract. Embryologically the wolffian tube passes median as *Gartner's duct* in the layers of the broad ligament and downward to the cervix and lateral vaginal wall to an opening near the orifice of Bartholin's glands (Fig. 208). Retention cysts may develop at any point in these duct remnants and notably as vulvar or parovarian cysts. A persistent Gartner's duct was found at autopsy in two middle age females; in one the left ureter was bifid but the other case showed no added anomalies. Johnson (1938) and Parker (1929) respectively reported the appearance of grape-sized cysts formed in the urethrovaginal septum just posterior to the external urethral meatus, the patients being newborn females. Conceivably such cysts may cause urethral urinary obstruction by extraurethral pressure although this did not occur in these two newborns. Parke Smith (1952) excised an infected cyst of this nature from a four-year-old girl, the opening being made just below the urethral orifice on the left. Subsequently this tract was urographically injected and showed a tract dilated upwards for about 4 cm. and into which the right

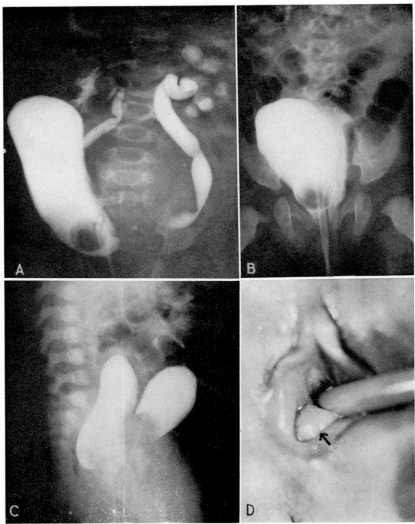

Fig. 272. Pronounced urinary obstruction in infancy consequent to pressure on the urethra by a large hydrocolpos. This eight-week-old girl presented a rounded firm suprapubic mass 10 cm. in diameter. Various intra-abdominal cystic malformations had been diagnostically suggested by the several surgeons who examined the child. Yet urologic investigation disclosed imperforate hymen with a massive hydrocolpos. Suprapubic pressure caused the hymen to bulge for 1 cm. or more as a grayish ballooning (*D*). *A*, cystogram; anterior posterior view showing wide vesical displacement to the right by the central distended vagina, with extreme dilatation and lateral deviation of the ureters. *B*, combined cystogram and vaginogram (anteroposterior view); the bladder is in front. *C*, lateral vaginogram and cystogram indicating the relation of the two structures. Treatment: cruciate incision of the hymen. (Mountainside Hospital.) A similar case in a girl ten hours old was also seen at Bellevue Hospital and radiographically demonstrated.

ureter opened; the left upper tract was absent. Johnson postulates that intraurethral rupture of such cysts may explain some urethral diverticula in the female.

Atresia of the Hymen. This important though rare lesion produces *hydrometrocolpos* before puberty and *hematocolpometra* after puberty. The distended vagina compresses the urethra to interfere with urination; commonly complete vesical retention ensues, which in turn may bring about widespread dilatation of the entire upper urinary tract and often complicated by grave infection (Fig. 272). Thirty cases in children have been reported (Rosenblatt, 1943; Flax, 1946). The treatment consists of wide cruciate incision of the hymen or of hymenectomy. Two unusual cases of this rare condition we observed merit citation. In a girl ten hours old at Bellevue Hospital and weighing 3 pounds 9 ounces, a cystlike mass protruded from the vulva. No vaginal opening could be found and the urethral meatus was located only with great difficulty. Catheterization returned clear urine. The cyst was incompletely aspirated and 18 cc. of thick mucinous milk-colored fluid was obtained. A vaginogram was then made by injection of the cyst with 6 cc. of Diodrast, this showing a greatly dilated genital tract. Wide cruciate incision of the hymen was performed and the subsequent course was normal. In an eight-week-old girl with urinary difficulty, a smooth round mass 10 cm. in diameter was felt suprapubically. Diagnosis was concerned chiefly with congenital ovarian cystic disease and abdominal exploration had been advised by a general surgeon. Cystography disclosed the bladder pushed far to the right and downward by the mass (Fig. 272). Excretory and retrograde urography demonstrated wide dilatation of the upper urinary tract. The bladder floor was cystoscopically observed to be elevated and distorted. Not at first suspecting the nature of the condition despite previous experience with it, I noted that suprapubic pressure caused pronounced bulging of the imperforate hymen (Fig. 272). A wide cruciate incision was made into this structure releasing about 3 ounces of whitish gray purulent sterile fluid. Simultaneous cystograms and vaginograms showed the dilated vagina to be of greater size than the bladder. Emptying the hydrocolpos induced profound *ex vacuo* shock from which the infant soon recovered and her subsequent course was uneventful.

Congenital Absence of the Vagina. This rare anomaly is of urologic interest because urinary tract anomalies and malformations usually coexist, unilateral absence or hypoplasia of the kidney being the most common. *Agenesis of the vagina* was found at autopsy in two newborns with a variety of upper urinary tract anomalies in each instance. A hundred cases were reported by Bryan et al. (1949) from the Mayo Clinic, forty-one of which were urologically examined; twenty were normal. Of the twenty-one with urinary tract anomalies, seven had pelvic kidneys, five had solitary kidneys, ureteropelvic reduplication was found in four. Two had pyeloureterectasis and in one each there was a nonfunctioning kidney, a fused solitary kidney, and nephrectomy for unknown reason. These anomalies were right-sided in ten and left-sided in eleven. Treatment consists in construction of the vagina by one of the several plastic procedures found described in gynecological text-books.

Hypoplasia of the vagina results from improper fusion of the müllerian ducts, the canal being short and narrow. It is regularly accompanied by other anomalies in the reproductive tract and in most cases in the urinary tract as well, notably ureterorenal agenesis.

In a fifty-one-year-old female a bicornuate infantile uterus was accompanied on each side by a rudimentary fallopian tube and vestigial ovary. The ovary was infantile and no cervical canal was found—merely two small dimples. In an adult female the small vagina was only 4 cm. long. Vaginal hypoplasia is constantly found in external female hermaphroditism and in many cases of male pseudohermaphroditism. The hypoplastic vagina may be enlarged, excised, or forgotten.

Duplication of the Vagina, Uterus and Rectum. This most unusual anomaly was reported by Ladd and Chisholm (1943), the condition resulting from incomplete resorption of the müllerian ducts. The septate anomaly may be partial or complete to give one or two vaginal orifices respectively. In our autopsy study of 5,205 female infants and children there were two cases of double uterus and double vagina (ages: eight hours; ten years) and one case of double uterus in a newborn with polycystic kidneys and left ureteral stricture.

Other Anomalies of the Female Reproductive System. In a stillborn female, there was a uterus but no vagina or urethra or rectum; pyometria coexisted.

There were six cases of bicornuate uterus, one (fifteen months) had a Meckel's diverticulum and horseshoe kidney, one (six weeks) with poly-cystic kidneys and a septum which extended to the internal os, one (still-born) with imperforate anus, congenital absence of the bladder, uterus, tubes and ovaries, and a stillborn with no adnexa, absent diaphragm, deformed heart, mongolism and agenesis of the right kidney and ureter. In a stillborn there was absence of the cervix, vagina, bladder, ureters and urachus; the uterus was elliptical in shape. In another stillborn, there were maldescent of the right ovary, horseshoe kidney and skeletal anomalies. A stillborn showed cystic graafian follicles and in a thirteen-year-old girl there were ovarian and parovarian cysts. Aside from the problem in surgicogyneco-plasty and obstetrics these malformations present, they are urologically in-teresting because of the high coincidence of urinary tract anomalies which largely parallels that noted in congenital absence of the vagina.

Anomalies of the Adrenal. These frequently accompany urologic anomalies and notably of the kidney and chiefly agenesis and ectopy. In 6,966 autopsies in infants the adrenal was congenitally absent in seven (1:995; right two, left one; bilaterally four) and all of whom were under six months of age. The gland was hypoplastic in ten other cases, the right and left sides were involved in one case each and bilaterally in eight, all but one (one year) of these being under seven months of age. In 18,394 adults there were eleven (1:1674) which showed absence of the adrenal—presumably congenital—; on the right in two, left in six and bilateral in three. In the children in this series the organ was ectopic in twelve (right four, left one, bilateral seven), being with the kidney in ten of these. In the adult series the adrenal was ectopic in nineteen (right eight, left three, bilateral in seven and unstated one). It was with the kidney in fourteen, apart from it in three, and "other" in two. In one there was an accessory adrenal, and in two boys adrenal rests were found in the testicle (Fig. 266). In an eighty-one-year-old man bone marrow was found in the adrenal. In three infants under six months and in an eleven year-old boy and one adult the adrenal was cystic (male three, female two) and bilaterally so in all. In two infants and one adult only the medulla was cystic and in two the areas of involvement were not stated. Some of these cystic glands were more than twice normal size. In passing, infection of the adrenal was found post mortem in seven infants and children; four were under six months, one each were two and four years of age; five were female and two male; four were definitely bilateral; one involved the cortex only, and in two each, the infection was in (*a*) the medulla and in (*b*) both medulla and cortex. The infection was tuberculous in five, and meningococcic and luetic in one each. The kidney was involved in three; in one abscesses were bilateral.

REFERENCES

ABEL, S. and VAN DELLEN, T. R.: Congenital defects following maternal rubella. J.A.M.A., *140*:1210, 1949.

ABESHOUSE, B. S.: Crossed ectopia with fusion; review of literature and report of four cases. Am. J. Surg., *658*:683, 1947.

————: Rare case of ecoptic ureter opening in uterus and review of literature. Urol. and Cutan. Rev., *47*:447, 1943.

————: Renal aneurysm, report of 2 cases and review of literature. Urol. & Cutan. Rev., *55*:451, 1951.

ALEXANDER, J. C., et al.: Congenital solitary kidney. J. Urol., *64*:230, 1950.

ANDERS, J. M.: Congenital single kidney with report of a case. The practical significance of the condition with statistics. Am. J. Med. Sc., *139*:313, 1910.

ANDERSON, J. C. and HYNES, W.: Retrocaval ureter. Brit. J. Urol., *21*:209, 1949.

ANDREWS, S. E. and ETTER, E. F.: Report of a case of splenic rest in scrotum. J. Urol., *55*:545, 1946.

ANSON, B. J., CAULDWELL, E. W., PICK, J. W. and BEATON, L. E.: The anatomy of the pararenal system of veins, with comments on the renal arteries. J. Urol., *60*:714, 1948.

AREY, L. B.: Developmental Anatomy. Ed. 6, Philadelphia, W. B. Saunders Co., 1954.

ATKINSON, I. E.: Congenital absence of the glans penis. New York Med. J., *68*:668, 1898.

BAGG, H. J. and LITTLE, C. C.: Hereditary structural defects in the descendants of mice exposed to x-ray irradiation. Amer. J. Anat., *36*:275, 1925.

BAYER, L. M.: Pseudohermaphroditism; a psychosomatic case study. Psychosom. Med., *9*:246, 1947.

BAZY, P.: Oblitération de l'urètre par une valvule congénitale en forme de diaphragm. Bull. et Mem. Soc. de Chir. de Paris, *29*:32, 1903.

BEER, E.: Chronic retention of urine in young boys due to bladder neck obstruction. J.A.M.A., *65*:1709, 1915; Ann. Surg., *79*:264, 1924.

BEGG, R. C.: The urachus, its anatomy, histology, and development. J. Anat., *64*:170, 1930.

BELL, E. T.: Cystic disease of kidneys. Am. J. Path., *11*:373, 1935.

BERG, O. C. and KERNS, W. M.: Solitary pelvic kidney (lit.). J. Urol., *62*:275, 1949.

BESSON, H.: Polycystic kidney. J. Urol., *30*:285, 1933.

BIGLER, J. A.: Frequency of pyuria in anomalies of the urinary tract in children. Am. J. Dis. Child., *47*:780, 1934.

BISHOP, P. M.: Studies in Endocrinology. V. The Management of the Undescended Testicle, Guy's Hospital Reports, 194, Nos. 1 and 2, p. 12, 1945.

BLAND-SUTTON, J.: In Rocher, H. L., Torsion congénitale de pénis. J. de Méd. de Bordeaux, *52*:26, 1922.

BOGGON, R. H.: Polyorchidism. Brit. J. Surg., 20:630, 1933.
BOKAY, J. V.: Beitrag zur Kenntniss der Harnröhrendivertickel bei Knaben. Jahrb. f. Kinderh., 3F, 2:181, 1900.
BOOGAARD, A.: Nederl. Tijdschr. v. Geneeskunde, 1:145, 1857.
BOUND, J. P.: Two cases of congenital absence of one kidney in the same family. Brit. M. J., 2:747, 1943.
BOYCE, W. H. and VEST, S. A.: A new concept concerning treatment of exstrophy of the bladder. J. Urol., 67:494, 1952.
BOYDEN, E. A.: Congenital absence of a kidney. An interpretation based on a 10 mm. human embryo exhibiting unilateral renal agenesis. Anat. Rec., 52:325, 1932.
————: Description of a horseshoe kidney associated with left inferior vena cava, etc. Anat. Rec., 51:187, 1931.
BRAASCH, W. F.: Atrophic pyelonephritis. J. Urol., 7:247, 1922.
————: Stricture of the ureter. J.A.M.A., 91:1263, 1928.
BRODY, H. and GOLDMAN, S.: Metaplasia of the epithelium of the prostatic glands, utricle and urethra of the fetus and newborn infant. Arch. Path., 29:494, 1940.
BROWN, A.: An analysis of the developing metanephros in mouse embryos with abnormal kidneys. J. Anat., 47:117, 1931.
BROWNE, D.: Treatment of undescended testicle. Proc. Royal Soc. Med., 42:9, 1949.
BRYAN, A. L., NIGRO, J. A. and COUNSELLER, V. S.: One hundred cases of congenital absence of the vagina. Surg., Gynec., & Obst., 88:79, 1949.
BUGBEE, H. G. and WOLLSTEIN, M.: Retention of urine due to congenital hypertrophy of the verumontanum. J. Urol., 10:477, 1923.
———— and ————: Surgical pathology of the urinary tract in infants. J.A.M.A., 83:1887, 1924.
BUNDESEN, H. N., POTTER, E. L., FISHBEIN, W. I., BAUER, F. C. and PLOTSKE, G. V.: Progress in reduction of needless neonatal death. J.A.M.A., 148:907, 1952.
BURDICK, C. C. and COLEY, B. L.: Abnormal descent of the testicle. Ann. Surg., 84:867, 1926.
BURNS, E., CUMMINGS, H. and HYMAN, J.: Incomplete reduplication of the bladder with congenital solitary kidney. Trans. Am. Assn. Genito-Urin. Surg., 38:97, 1947.
BURSTEIN, H. J.: Double kidney with Y-shaped ureter and ureteral calculus in an infant. Urol. and Cut. Rev., 42:575, 1938.
CABOT, H. and SHOEMAKER, R.: The role of the glands of the female urethra in the production of infection of the urinary tract. Tr. Am. A. Genito-urin. Sugeons, 29:461, 1936.
CAMPBELL, E. W.: Megalo-ureter. J. Urol., 60:31, 1948.
CAMPBELL, H. E.: Incidence of malignant growth of the undescended testicle. Arch. Surg., 44:353, 1942.
CAMPBELL, M. F.: Congenital absence of one kidney: unilateral renal agenesis. Ann. Surg., 88:1039, 1928.
————: Submucous fibrosis of the vesical outlet. J.A.M.A., 94:1373, 1930.
————: Vascular obstruction of the ureter in juveniles. Am. J. Surg., 22:527, 1933.
————: Diverticulum of the urethra: two cases in young boys. J. Urol., 30:113, 1933.
————: Diverticulum of the ureter. Am. J. Surg., 36:385, 1936.
————: Surgical treatment of anomalies of the upper urinary tract in children. J.A.M.A., 116:193, 1936.
————: Pediatric Urology. New York, Macmillan Company, 2 vol., 1937, Ectopic kidney, Vol. 1, p. 188; Dwarf bladder, ibid., p. 294; Vesical diverticulum, ibid., p. 296; Double penis, ibid., p. 324; Hypertrophy of verumontanum, ibid., p. 353; Submucous fibrosis of bladder outlet, ibid., p. 354; Pseudohermaphroditism, ibid., p. 362.
————: The dilated ureter in children. Am. J. Surg., 39:438, 1938.
————: Ureteral obstruction in children. J. Urol., 41:660, 1939.
————: Ureterocele. J. Urol., 45:598, 1941.
————: Congenital bladder neck obstructions. Southern M. J., 41:99, 1948.
————: Urethral stricture in infants and children. J. Pediat., 35:169, 1949.
————: Ureterocele; a study of ninety-four instances in eighty infants and children. Surg., Gynec., and Obst., 93:705, 1951.
————: Clinical Pediatric Urology. Philadelphia, W. B. Saunders Co., 1951.
————: Congenital obstruction of the urinary tract. Med. Ann. District Columbia, 21:123, 1952.
————: Epispadias; a report of fifteen cases. J. Urol., 67:988, 1952.
————: Primary megaloureter. J. Urol., 68:584, 1952.

————: A new ureteral meatome. J. Urol. (in press).

CARLSON, H. E.: Supernumerary kidney: a summary of fifty-one reported cases. J. Urol., *64:*224, 1950.

CARSON, W. W. J.: Solitary cysts of the kidney. Ann. Surg., *87:*250, 1928.

CATHRO, A. J. McG.: Section of inferior vena cava for retrocaval ureter. J. Urol., *67:*464, 1952.

CAULK, J. R.: The importance of the ureterovesical valve. J. Urol., *9:*315, 1923.

CECIL, A. B.: Surgical management of the vagina in male construction in hermaphrodites. J. Urol., *62:*709, 1949.

————: Modern treatment of hypospadias. Trans. Am. Assoc. Genito-urin. Surg., *43:*148, 1951.

CHALKLEY, T. S. and SUTTON, L. E., JR.: Infected solitary cyst of kidney in child with review of literature. J. Urol., *50:*414, 1943.

CHERRY, J. W.: Patent urachus (lit.). J. Urol., *63:*693, 1950.

CHWALLA, R.: Congenital hour-glass bladder. Ztschr. f. Urol. Chir., *230:*200, 1927.

————: Process of formation of cystic dilatations of vesical end of ureter and of diverticula at the ureteral ostium. Urol. & Cut. Rev., *31:*499, 1927.

COCHRANE, W. J. and SAUNDERS, R. L. de C. H.: Rare anomaly of penis associated with imperforate anus. J. Urol., *47:*810, 1942.

COFFORT, L.: Urethral reduplication in a male. J. d'Urol., *55:*954, 1949.

COLLIER, T. W.: Pseudohermaphroditism in twins: report of tenth case. Am. J. Dis. Child., *76:*208, 1948.

CONROY, M. J.: Aneurysm of renal artery; analysis of all cases in literature with report of case and dissertation on etiology, pathology, symptoms, diagnosis, prognosis and treatment of this condition. Ann. Surg., *78:*628, 1923.

COOPER, E. R. A.: Histology of the retained testis in human subject at different ages and its comparison with scrotal testis. J. Anat., *64:*5, 1929.

CORNER, E. H.: Male Diseases in General Practice. London, Oxford University Press, 255, 1910.

COUNSELLER, V. S., NICHOLS, D. R. and SMITH, H. L.: Congenital absence of testis. J. Urol., *44:*237, 1940.

CRAWFORD, R. H.: Polycystic kidney. Surg., Gynec. & Obst., *36:*185, 1923.

CROWELL, W. M. and ANDERSON, R. H.: Congenital urethral stricture. Clinical Proceed. Children's Hospital, Washington, D. C., *6:*68, 1950.

CULBERTSON, L. R.: Mullerian duct cyst. J. Urol., *58:*134, 1947.

CULP, O. S.: Ureteral diverticulum; classification of literature and report of authentic case. J. Urol., *58:*309, 1947.

CURLING, T. B.: Diseases of the Testis. Philadelphia, Blanchard and Lea, 1856.

DALCQ, A. M.: Form and Casualty in Early Development. London, Cambridge University Press, 1938.

DANNREUTHER, W. T.: Complete double urethra in a female. J.A.M.A., *81:*1016, 1923.

DAVIS, D. M.: Intubated ureterotomy: result after four years. J. Urol., *57:*233, 1947.

————: Intubated ureterotomy: experimental work and clinical results. J. Urol., *59:*851, 1948.

————: A case of double, triple or quadruple penis associated with dermoid of the perineum. J. Urol., *61:*111, 1949.

DAY, R. V. and VIVIAN, C. S.: Congenital obstructions in posterior urethra. Tr. Sect. Urol. A. M. A., pp. 65–81, 1927.

DEAN, A. L.: Cancers of the genito-urinary organs in children. J. Pediat., *15:*340, 1939.

DEAN, A. L., JR., MAJOR, J. W. and OSTERHEIMER, E. J.: Failure of fusion of the testis and epididymis. J. Urol., *68:*754, 1952.

DEBOO, S. M.: Three-legged person with two urethral openings. M. Bull., Bombay, *11:* 3397, 1943.

DEES, J. E.: Congenital epispadias with incontinence. J. Urol., *62:*513, 1949.

DE LA PEÑA, A.: Absence of glans penis. Urol. & Cut. Rev., *36:*684, 1932.

DEMING, C. L.: Nephroptosis: causes, relation to other viscera and correction by a new operation. J.A.M.A., *95:*251, 1930; also Am. J. Surg., *9:*218, 1930.

————: Gonadotropic factor as an aid to surgery in the treatment of the undescended testicle. J. Urol., *36:*274, 1936.

————: Hormonal bases for the treatment of the undescended testis. Am. J. Surg., *38:* 186, 1937.

————: Hormonal therapy in cryptorchism. Trans. Am. Assoc. Genito-urin. Surg., *43:* 169, 1951.

————, GOETTSCH, J. B. and HUMM, F. D.: Clinical and hormonal studies in familial pseudohermaphroditism. J. Urol., 61:144, 1949.

DE NICOLA, R. A. and MCCARTNEY, R. C.: Urethral duplication in a female child. J. Urol., 61:1065, 1949.

DEROW, H. A. and BRODNEY, M. L.: Congenital posterior urethral valve causing renal rickets. New England J. Med., 221:685, 1939.

DETER, R. L., CALDWELL, G. I. and FOLSOM, A. I.: A clinical pathological study of the posterior female urethra. J. Urol., 55:651, 1946.

DOOLITTLE, L. H.: Congenital absence of the urinary sphincter. New England. J. Med., 246:266, 1952.

DOSS, A. K. and PRIESTLEY, J. T.: True hermaphrodism: report of a case. J. Urol., 43: 859, 1940.

DOURMASHKIN, R. L.: Herniation of the ureter. J. Urol., 38:450, 1937.

————: Complete urethral occlusion in living newborn; report of five cases. J. Urol., 50: 747, 1943.

DRURY, R. B. and SCHWARZELL, H. H.: Congenital absence of penis. Arch. Surg., 30:236, 1935.

ECCLES, W. M.: The anatomy, physiology and pathology of the imperfectly descended testis. Lancet, 1:569, 1902.

EDWARDS, C.: Multilocular bladder. Med. J. Australia, 2:443, 1933.

ELLIS, A.: Sexual psychology of human hermaphrodites. Psychosom. Med., 1:108, 1945.

EMMETT, J. L., ALVAREZ-IERENA, J. J. and MACDONALD, JOHN R.: Atrophic pyelonephritis versus congenital renal hypoplasia. J.A.M.A., 148:1470, 1952.

———— and LOGAN, G. B.: Ureterocele with prolapse through urethra. J. Urol., 51:19, 1944.

ENGEL, W. J.: Ureteral ectopia opening into the seminal vesicle. J. Urol., 60:46, 1948.

ENGLE, E. T.: Experimentally induced descent of testis in Macacus monkey by hormones from anterior pituitary and pregnancy urine; role of gonadokinetic hormones in pregnancy blood in normal descent of testes in man. Endocrinology, 16:513, 1932.

ENGLISCH, J.: Über angeborene Verschleissungen und Verengerungen der männlichen Harnröhre. Arch. für Kinderh., 2:85, 1880–1.

————: Double penis. Bull Méd. Paris, 9:153, 1895.

FAGARASANU, I.: Récherches anatomiques sur la veine rénale gauche et des collatérales; leurs rapports avec la pathogénie du varicocèle essential et des varices du ligament large (démonstrations expérimentales). Ann. d'Anat. Path., 15:9, 1938.

FELIX, W.: Development of the Urogenital Organs. Keibel-Mall, Human Embryology, ed. 2, Philadelphia, J. B. Lippincott Co., 1912.

FISCHER, H.: Duplication of the urogenital and lower urinary tracts. Zentralbl. f. Gynäk., 73:1561, 1952.

FISTER, G. M.: Fibrosis and submucous calcification of the vesical neck. J.A.M.A., 118: 604, 1942.

FLAX, H. J.: Hematocolpos in young girl causing complete retention. Bol. Asoc. med. de Puerto Rico, 38:453, 1946.

FOLSOM, A. I. and O'BRIEN, H. A.: The female urethra. J.A.M.A., 128:408, 1945.

FRANCIS, C. C.: Case of prepenial scrotum (marsupial type of genitalia) associated with absence of urinary system. Anat. Rec., 76:303–308 (March 25), 1940.

FRASER, F. CLARKE and FAINSTAT, T. D.: Causes of congenital defects. Am. J. Dis. Child., 82:593–603, 1951.

GERINGER, D. and ZUCKER, M. O.: Diverticulum of anterior urethra in male child. Am. J. Surg., 44:463, 1939.

GILLES, H. and HARRISON, R. J.: Congenital absence of the penis. Brit. J. Plast. Surg., 1:8, 1948.

GODDARD, H. S.: Unusual case (congenital absence of leg and foreskin). M. J. and Rec., 133:87, 1931.

GOLDBLATT, H.: Studies in experimental hypertension. Am. J. Clin. Path., 10:40, 1940.

GOLDSCHMIDT, R.: Physiological Genetics. New York, McGraw-Hill, 1938, p. 384.

————: "Progressive heredity" and "anticipation" possibility of genetic explanation of certain odd hereditary phenomena observed in man. J. Hered., 29:140, 1938.

————: The Material Basis of Evolution. New Haven, Conn., Yale Univ. Press, 1940.

GOLDSTEIN, A. E.: A new surgical procedure for the treatment of polycystic kidneys. J. Urol., 34:536, 1935.

GREENE, C.: Bilateral hypoplastic cystic kidneys. Am. J. Dis. Children, 24:1, 1922.

GREENE, R. R., BURRILL, M. W. and IVY, A. C.: Experimental intersexuality. The effects of estrogens on the antenatal sexual development of the rat. Am. J. Anat., *67:*305, 1940.

———, ——— and ———: Experimental intersexuality. Anat. Rec., *74:*429, 1939; J. Exper. Zool., *86:*211, 1941; Physiol. Zool., *15:*1, 1939.

GREGG, N. M.: Rubella during pregnancy of mother with its sequela of congenital defects in child. Med. J. Australia, *1:*313–15, 1945.

GROSS, R. E. and BILL, A. A., JR.: Concealed diverticulum of the male urethra as a cause of urinary obstruction. Pediatrics, *19:*44, 1948.

——— and CHATWORTHY, H. W., JR.: Ureterocele in infancy and childhood. Pediatrics, *5:*68, 1950.

——— and CRESSON, S. L.: Epispadias. J. Urol., *67:*477, 1952.

——— and MOORE, J. H.: Urethral reduplication. Arch. Surg., *60:*749, 1950.

GRUBER, C. C.: Two cases of cystic kidneys. Ztsch. f. urolog. Chir., *15:*246, 1924.

GRUBER, G.: Virchow's Arch. f. Path. Anat., *258:*441, 1923.

———: Entwicklungsstörungen der Nieren, Harnleiter und der Harnblase. Handbuch der Urologie, *3:*1, 1928.

GRUNFELDER, B. and LASCH, W.: Anomalies. Annales Pediatrici, *173:*388, 1949.

GRUENWALD, P.: Mechanisms of abnormal development. Arch. Path., *44:*398; 495; 648, 1947.

GUTIERREZ, R.: The Clinical Management of Horseshoe Kidney. New York, Paul B. Hoeber, Inc., 1934.

———: Anomalies of the Seminal Vesicles. In Cabot's Urology, 3rd ed., Philadelphia, Lea and Febiger, 1936, Vol. II.

HALE, F.: J. Heredity, *24:*105, 1933; Am. J. Ophth., *18:*1087, 1935.

HALSTEAD, W. S.: Ectopia testis transverse. Surg., Gynec., and Obst., *4:*129, 1907.

HAMILTON, J. B.: Therapeutics of testicular dysfunction. J.A.M.A., *116:*1903, 1941.

HAMILTON, W. J., BOYD, J. D. and MOSSMAN, H. W.: Human Embryology. Baltimore, Williams and Wilkins, 1945, Chapter 8.

HARRIS, A. H.: Am. J. Surg., *20:*64, 1933.

HARRIS, R. P.: Congenital absence of penis, the urethra moving its exit into or below the rectum and emptying into the bladder by, or exterior to the anus. Phila. Med. J., *1:*71, 1898.

HARRIS, S. H. and HARRIS, R. G. S.: Renal sympathetico-tonus, renal pain and renal sympathectomy. Brit. J. Urol., *2:*367, 1930.

HART, D. B.: The nature and cause of the physiological descent of the testis. Descent in marsupials. J. Anat. and Physiol., *43:*244, 1909; Descent in man, idem, *44:*4, 1910.

HARVARD, M. B. and THOMPSON, G. J.: Congenital exstrophy of the bladder; late results. J. Urol., *55:*225, 1951.

HAVENS, F. Z. and BLACK, A. S.: Treatment of a hypospadias. J. Urol., *61:*1053, 1949.

HAWES, C. J.: Solitary ectopic kidney. J. Urol., *64:*453, 1950.

HAWTHORNE, A. B.: Embryologic and clinical aspects of double ureter. J.A.M.A., *106:* 189, 1936.

HECKEL, N. J.: Production of oligospermia in a man by use of testosterone propionate. Proc. Soc. Exp. Biol. and Med., *40:*658, 1939.

HELMHOLZ, H. F. and THOMPSON, G. J.: Urinary obstruction and infection among children: the importance of their early recognition. Proc. Staff. Meetings Mayo Clinic, *16:*6, 1941.

HEPLER, A. B.: Solitary cysts of kidney: Report of 7 cases and observations on pathogenesis of these cysts. Surg., Gynec., and Obst., *50:*668, 1930.

———: Etiology of multilocular cysts of kidney. J. Urol., *44:*206, 1940.

———: Bilateral pelvic and ureteral reduplication with uterine ectopic ureter. Trans. Am. Assn. Genito-urin. Surgeons, *38:*115, 1946.

HERTZLER, A. E.: Ectopia testis transversa with infantile uterus. Surg., Gynec., and Obst., *23:*597, 1916.

HESS, E.: Pyelocystostomy in crossed renal dystopia. J. Urol., *22:*667, 1929.

——— and WRIGHT, B. W.: Pyelocystostomosis: Report of two cases. J.A.M.A., *127:*267, 1945.

HIGGINS, C. C.: Exstrophy of the bladder. J. Urol., *63:*852, 1950.

HILDEBRANDT, A.: Weiterer Beitrag zur pathologischen Anatomie der Nierengeschwülste. Arch. für Klin. Chir., *48:*343, 1894.

HINMAN, F.: Principles and Practice of Urology. Philadelphia, W. B. Saunders Co., 1935.

——— and MORISON, D. M.: Comparative study of circulatory changes in hydronephrosis, caseo-cavernous tuberculous and polycystic kidney. J. Urol., *11:*131, 1924.

HINMAN, F., JR.: Congenital bilateral absence of the kidneys. Surg., Gynec., and Obst., *71:* 101, 1940.

HOFMOKL, T.: Ein Fall von angeborener Zerspaltung der Glans Penis. Arch. f. Klin. Chir., *54:*220, 1897.

HOFSTATTER, R.: Cryptorchism: Incidence in newborn. Klin. Jahrb., *26:*155, 1911.

HONKE, E. M.: Ectopic ureter. J. Urol., *55:*460, 1946.

HOOKS, C. A.: Clinical aspects of intersexuality. J. Urol., *61:*52, 1948.

HOWARD, F. S.: Hypospadias with enlargement of the prostatic utricle. Surg., Gynec. & Obst., *86:*307, 1948.

HOWARD, T. L., FORBES, R. P. and LIPSCOMB, W. R.: Aneurysm of the left renal artery in a child 5 years old with persistent hypertension. J. Urol., *44:*808, 1940.

HUBER, H. G.: Nabelkoliken bei Doppelbildung und Verengung des Ureters. Kinderärztl. Praxis, *7:*254, 1936.

HUFFMAN, J. W.: The development of the periurethral glands in the human female. Am. J. Obst. and Gynec., *44:*773, 1943.

HUFFMAN, L. F.: A case of prepenile scrotum. J. Urol., *65:*141, 1951.

HUNNER, G. L.: Ureteral stricture. Bull. Johns Hopkins Hosp., *29:*1, 1918; J. Urol., *18:*21, 1929; Southern M. J., *34:*885, 1941.

HUNTER, JOHN: Treatise on the animal. Economy, 1786.

HUNTER, R. H.: The etiology of congenital inguinal hernia and abnormally placed testes. Brit. J. Surg., *14:*125, 1926.

HURST, A. F. and JONES, J. G.: Case of megaloureter due to achalasia of the ureterovesical sphincter. Brit. J. Urol., *3:*43, 1931.

HUTCH, J.: A new procedure to prevent vesicoureteral reflux. J. Urol. (in press).

HUTCH, J. A.: Vesico-ureteral reflux in paraplegia. J. Urol., *68:*457, 1952.

HYMAN, A.: Diverticula of bladder in children. Surg., Gynec., and Obst., *36:*27, 1923.

JEWETT, H. J.: Scrotal ureter. Urologists' Letter Club, Jan. 13, 1951.

———— and HARRIS, A. P.: Scrotal ureter. J. Urol., *69:*184, 1953.

JOHNSON, C. M.: Diverticula of the urethra. J. Urol., *39:*506, 1938.

JOHNSON, F. P.: The later development of the urethra in the male. J. Urol., *4:*447, 1920.

JOHNSON, S. H., III and PRICE, W. C.: Hypertrophy of the colliculus seminalis in childhood: Report of 18 Cases. Am. J. Dis. Child., *78:*892, 1949.

JOHNSTON, T. B.: Extroversion of the bladder, complicated by the presence of intestinal openings on the surface of the extroverted area. J. Anat. and Physiol., *48:*89, 1913.

JOLY, cited by LOWER, W. E.: Am. J. Urol., *10:*486, 1914.

KAMPMEIER, O. F.: A hitherto unrecognized mode of origin of congenital renal cysts. Surg., Gynec., and Obst., *36:*208, 1923.

KARUFFA-KORBUTT, K. W.: Zur Frage über die Entstehung und die aetiologische Bedeutung der Ureteranatomie. Folia Urol., *2:*167, 1908.

KEIZUR, L. W.: Accessory spleen in the scrotum. J. Urol., *68:*759, 1952.

KELLY, C. M. and UHRICH, G. I.: Infarction of intraperitoneal undescended testicle. Am. J. Surg., *65:*233, 1952.

KELLY, H. A. and BURNHAM, C. F.: Diseases of the Kidney, Ureter, and Bladder. New York, D. Appleton & Co., 1914.

KELSEY, W. M.: Idiopathic dilatation of the common bile duct in childhood. J. Pediat., *31:*211, 1947.

KEMP, T.: Acta Path. Microb. Scand., Supp. *54:*195, 1944.

KESHIN, J. G. and PINCK, B. D.: Bilateral congenital absence of vasa deferentia. J. Urol., *59:*1190, 1948.

KIRSCHBAUM, J. D.: Congenital absence of the external genitals. J. Pediat., *37:*102, 1950.

KJELLBERG, S. R. and RUDHE, U.: The fetal renal secretion and its significance in congenital deformities of the ureters and urethra. Acta Radiologica, *31:*243, 1949.

KOCH, L. A.: Projectile vomiting and intoxication in the newborn infant. Am. J. Dis. Child., *60:*917, 1940.

KORNBLUM, K. and RITTER, J.: Retroperitoneal cyst with agenesis of the kidney. Radiology, *32:*416, 1939.

KRASA, F. C. and PASCHKIS, R.: Trigone of bladder in mammals. Ztschr. f. Urolog. Chir., *6:*1, 1921.

KRAUSS, L. W. and STRAUS, R.: Retroperitoneal cyst arising in persistent metanephros with congenital absence of right kidney and ureter. J. Urol., *34:*97, 1935.

KRETSCHMER, H. L.: Diverticulum of the bladder in infancy and in childhood. Am. J. Dis. Child., *48:*842, 1934.

————: Diverticula of the anterior urethra in male children. Surg., Gynec., and Obst., *62:*634, 1936.

————: Renal rickets and polycystic disease of the kidney. J. Urol., *59:*773, 1948.

KREUTZMANN, H. A. R.: Hypertension associated with solitary renal cyst: Report of two cases. Tr. West. Sect. Am. Urol. A., *13:*39, 1946; also J. Urol., *57:*467, 1947.

KRON, S. D. and MERANZI, D. R.: Completely fused pelvic kidney. J. Urol., *62:*278, 1949.

KRUGLICH, T. and MINNICK, S.: Bilateral hypoplasia of the kidneys with report of case. Arizona Medicine, *4:*34, 1947.

KUNSTADTER, R. H.: Technique for the diagnosis of undescended testis. J.A.M.A., *148:* 117, 1952.

————, GUTERMAN and TULKY: Pneumoperitoneum in the diagnosis of pelvic anomalies. In press, Pediatrics, 1952.

KUSTER, D.: Die Chirurgie der Nieren. 1896–1902.

KUTZMAN, N. and SAUER, H. R.: A consideration of the problems presented by unilateral cystic kidney disease. J. Urol., *63:*34, 1950.

LADD, W. E. and CHISHOLM, T. C.: Double uterus, vagina and rectum. Am. J. Dis. Child., *66:*629, 1943.

———— and LANMAN, T. H.: Exstrophy of the bladder and epispadias. New England J. Med., *222:*130, 1940.

LANDES, R. R. and RANSON, C. L.: Mullerian duct cysts. J. Urol., *61:*1089, 1949.

LANMAN, T. H.: Personal Communication.

————: Urinary incontinence; its surgical significance. Pediat., *1:*776–779, 1948.

LATTIMER, J. K.: Similar urogenital anomalies in identical twins. Am. J. Dis. Child., *67:* 199, 1944.

LAZARUS, J. A. and MARKS, M. S.: Anomalies associated with undescended testes. Complete separation of a partly descended epididymis and vas deferens and abdominal testes. J. Urol., *56:*567, 1947.

LEAHY, L. J. and BUTSCH, W. L.: A study of the beta 17-ketosteroids in a case of pseudo-hermaphroditism due to adrenal cortical tumor. Ann. Surg., *128:*1124, 1948.

LEE, H. P.: Crossed unfused renal ectopia with tumor. J. Urol., *61:*333, 1949.

LEJARS, F.: Les voies de sûreté de la viene rénale, Bull. Soc. Anat. Paris, *63:*504, 1888.

LEVIN, HARRIS: Bilateral renal agenesis. J. Urol., *67:*86, 1952.

LEWIS, L. G.: Cryptorchism. J. Urol., *60:*345, 1948.

———— and KIMBROUGH, JAS.: Megaloureter. South. Med. J., *45:*171, 1952.

LICH, R., JR.: Retropubic surgery in children. Urologists' Letter Club, Nov. 25, 1952.

———— and WAUD, R. E.: Unilateral polycystic kidney in a newborn. J. Urol., *68:*60, 1952.

LIEBERTHAL, F.: Pyelonephritic contracture of the kidney. Surg., Gynec., and Obst., *69:* 159, 1939.

LISANSKY, E. T.: Congenital cyst of urethra in a three-weeks-old male infant causing death and pyonephrosis. Bull. School of Med. Univ. Maryland, *26:*241, 1942.

LOCKWOOD, C. B.: Development and transition of the testis, normal and abnormal. Brit. Med. J., *1:*440, 1887.

LONGO, V. J. and THOMPSON, G. J.: Congenital solitary kidney. J. Urol., *68:*63, 1952.

LOWSLEY, O. S.: Congenital malformation of the posterior urethra. Ann. Surg., *60:*733, 1914.

————: Persistent cloaca in female; report of 2 cases corrected by operation. J. Urol., *59:*692, 1948.

———— and CANNON, E. M.: J.A.M.A., *121:*1137, 1943.

LUDWIG, EUGEN VON: Beitrag zur Entwicklungsgeschichte der Nachniere. Acta Anatomica, *8:*1, 1949.

LUND, A. J.: Uncrossed double ureter with rare intravesical orifice relationship: case report with review of literature. J. Urol., *62:*22, 1949.

LYNCH, K. D. and THOMPSON, R. F.: Unilateral multicystic kidney in infant. J. Urol., *38:* 58, 1937.

MACARTHUR, P.: Anaemia in nephritis. Arch. Dis. Child., *17:*1–22, 1942.

McCREA, L. E.: Congenital solitary pelvic kidney. J. Urol., *48:*58, 1942.

McGRAW, A. B. and CULP, O. S.: Diverticulum of the ureter: report of another authentic case. J. Urol., *67:*262, 1952.

McGREGOR, A. L.: The third inguinal ring. Surg., Gynec., and Obst., *49:*273, 1929.

McIVER, R. B.: Plastic surgery of the renal pelvis. J. Urol., *42:*1069, 1939.

McKENNA, C. M. and KAMPMEIER, O. F.: Consideration of development of polycystic kidney. Tr. Am. Assn. Genito-urin. Surg., *26:*377, 1933; J. Urol., *32:*37, 1934.

——— and KIEFFER, J. H.: Congenital enlargement of prostatic utricle with inclusion of ejaculatory ducts and seminal vesicles. Trans. Am. Assoc. Genito-urin. Surg., *32:*305, 1939.

MACCALLUM, D. W.: Clinical study of the spermatogenesis of undescended testicles. Arch. Surg., *31:*290, 1935.

MALISOFF, S.: Sulfonamide induced anuria associated with congenital solitary kidney in a child. J. Urol., *61:*725, 1949.

MALL, F. P.: Pathology of the Human Ovum. In Keibel and Mall: Manual of Human Embryology. Philadelphia, J. B. Lippincott Co., 1910.

MARCEL, J. E.: Unilateral polycystic kidney. La Semaine des Hôpitaux, *27:*1351, 1953.

———: Grosse hydronéphrose par urétère rétrocave. Arch. Français de Pédiatrie, *10:*1, 1953.

MARQUARDT, C. R. and FREDERICK, A. J.: Congenital imperforate urinary meatus. Urol. & Cutan. Rev., *47:*78, 1943.

MATHE, C. P. and DUNN, G.: Double vas deferens associated with solitary kidney. J. Urol., *59:*461, 1948.

MAY, A.: Absence of urethra. Ztsch. f. Urol., *42:*245, 1949.

MAYNARDT, C. R. and FREDERICK, A. J.: Congenital imperforate urinary meatus. Urol. and Cutan. Rev., *47:*78, 1943.

MAZURSKY, M. M. and SAWAN, E.: Female pseudohermaphroditism due to congenital adrenal cortical hyperplasia with associated Addison-like symptoms (infant). J. Pediat., *36:*789, 1950.

Ménégaux, G. and BOIDOT, M.: Des oblitérations congénitales du méat et de la portion balanique de l'urètre (hypospadias excepté). J. de chir., *43:*641, 1934.

MERTZ, H. O., HENDRICKS, J. and GARRETT, R. A.: Cystic ureterovesical protrusion: etc. J. Urol., *61:*506, 1949.

——— and WISHARD, W. M., JR.: Renal aplasia. J. Urol., *63:*959, 1950.

MEYER, H. W.: Undescended testicle, with special reference to Torek's method of orchiopexy. Surg., Gynec., and Obst., *44:*53, 1927.

Meyer, R.: Transposition of penis and scrotum—subcoccygeal penis in seven-month fetus. Anat. Rec., *79:*231, 1941.

MEZAN, S.: Contribution à l'étude clinique de la vessie multiloculie. J. d'urol., *27:*31, 1929.

MICHELSON, L.: Congenital anomalies of the ductus deferens and epididymis. J. Urol., *61:* 384, 1949.

MOORE, C. R. and QUICK, W. J.: The scrotum as a temperature regulator for the testes. Am. J. Physiol., *68:*70, 1924.

———: Physiology of the testis and application of male sex hormone. J. Urol., *47:*31, 1942.

MOORE, N. S. and TAPPER, S. M.: Cryptorchism: a theory to explain its etiology; modifications in surgical technique. J. Urol., *43:*204, 1940.

MOULON, A.: Révue General. Anatomie et Physiologie Conformation Vicreuse, Arch. Gen. d. Med., *17:*424, 1828.

MURPHY, D. P.: Congenital malformations: A study of parental characteristics, etc., 2d ed., Philadelphia, J. B. Lippincott Co., 1947; also J.A.M.A., *107:*382, 1936; Surg., Gynec., and Obst., *62:*585, 1936.

NALLE, B. C., JR., CROWELL, J. A. and LYNCH, R. M., JR.: Solitary pelvic kidney with vaginal aplasia. J. Urol., *61:*862, 1949.

NATION, E. F.: Renal aplasia. J. Urol., *51:*579, 1944.

NAUMANN, A. F.: Cited by Eismayer, G.: Ueber Uterusmissbildung bei kongenitalem Mangel einer Niere. Ztschr. f. urol. Chir., *11:*191, 1923.

NELSON, R. E.: Congenital absence of the vas deferens. J. Urol., *63:*176, 1950.

NESBIT, R. M. and BROMME, W.: Double penis and double bladder. Am. J. Roentgenol. and Rad. Therapy., *30:*497, 1933.

——— and WHITHYCOMBE, J.: Concerning megaloureter and its treatment. J. Urol. (in press).

NEUGEBAUER, L.: Der Hermaphroditismus, 1912.

NEWMAN, H. F. and WILHELM, S. F.: Testicular temperature in man. J. Urol., *63:*349, 1950.

NORDMARK, B.: Double formations of the pelvis of the kidneys and the ureters. Acta Radiol., Stockholm, *30:*267, 1948.

NORRIS, R. F. and HERMAN, L.: Pathogenesis of polycystic kidneys: reconstruction of cystic elements in four cases. J. Urol., *46:*147, 1941.

NOVAK, E.: Genital anomalies. Surg., Gynec., and Obst., *86:*247, 1948.

NOWLIN, P., ADAMS, J. R. and NALLE, B. C., JR.: Vulvar fusion. J. Urol., *62:*75, 1949.

NUNEZ, J. E.: In Guyon, R. Infiltracion Urinosa; Leccion Recogida per J. E. Nunez, Cron. Med. quir de la Habana, *7:*515; 565, 1881.

OCKERBLAD, N. F.: Congenital hour-glass bladder. Surgery, *8:*665, 1940.

OLSON, R. O. and AUSTEN, G., JR.: Postcaval ureter. New England J. Med., *242:*963, 1950.

OPPENHEIMER, G. D. and NARINS, L.: Unilateral polycystic kidney disease. J. Urol., *61:* 866, 1949.

ORR, L. M., and GLANTON, J. B.: Prolapsing ureterocele. J. Urol., *70:*180, 1953.

⸻, HAYWARD, J. C. and TURNER, A. F.: Failure of the urogenital union. J. Urol., *60:*147, 1948.

OSCHENIUS, K.: Fusion of labia minora. Deutsche Med. Wchnsch., *53:*838, 1927.

ÖSTLING, K.: The genesis of hydronephrosis. Acta Scand., *86:* Suppl. 72, 1942.

OSTRY, H.: Hypertension associated with congenital ureteral valve. J. Urol., *60:*738, 1948.

PARKER, D.: Gartner duct cyst at urethral meatus. Urol. Letter Club, Nov. 8, 1949.

PASQUIER, C. M., JR. and WOMACK, R. K.: Ectopic opening of ureter into seminal vesicle. J. Urol., *70:*164, 1953.

PATTEN, B. W.: The genesis of vesical exstrophy, to be reported: personal communication, 1950.

⸻ and BARRY, A.: The genesis of exstrophy of the bladder and epispadias. Am. J. Anat., *90:*35, 1952.

PEIRSON, E. L., JR. and BARNEY, J. D.: End results of operations for nephroptosis and aberrant renal vessels. New England J. Med., *201:*568, 1929.

PETERMAN, M. G.: Congenital absence of spleen and left kidney. J.A.M.A., *99:*1252, 1932.

PETILLO, D.: Ureterocele; clinical significance and process of formation; report of four cases. Surg., Gynec., and Obst., *40:*811, 1925.

PHILLIPS, J.: Four cases of spurious hermaphroditism in one family. Am. J. Obst. & Gynec., *8:*1108, 1886.

PICK, J. W. and ANSON, B. J.: Renal vascular pedicle; anatomical study of 430 body halves. J. Urol., *44:*441, 1940.

POTTER, E. L.: Facial characteristics of infants with bilateral renal agenesis. Am. J. Obst. and Gynec., *51:*885, 1946.

POWERS, J. H. and MURRAY, M. F.: Juvenile hypertension associated with unilateral lesions of upper urinary tract. J.A.M.A., *118:*600, 1942.

PRENDERGAST, J. J.: Congenital cataract and other anomalies following rubella in mother during pregnancy. Arch. of Ophth., *35:*39, 1946.

PURCELL, H. M.: Another cause of urinary obstruction. J. Urol., *62:*748, 1949.

QUINBY, W. C.: Clinical picture of hydronephrosis in children and young adults. South. M. J., *23:*328, 1930.

RALL, J. E. and ODELL, H. M.: Congenital polycystic disease of the kidney. Am. J. Med. Sc., *218:*399, 1949.

RANDALL, A. and CAMPBELL, E. W.: Anomalous relationship of right ureter to vena cava. J. Urol., *34:*565, 1935.

RASPALL, G.: Rare congenital anomalies of the genito-urinary tract, ectopic testis and urethrocele in a male. J. d'urol. méd. et chir., *55:*265, 1949.

RATHBUN, N. P.: Diverticulum of the ureter. J. Urol., *18:*347, 1927.

RAVITCH, M. M. and SANFORD, M. C.: Unilateral multicystic kidney in infants. Pediatrics, *4:*769, 1949.

REA, C. E.: Treatment of undescended testicle. Tr. West. Surg. Assoc., Chicago, *56:*95, 1949.

REEVES, H. A.: Lancet, *2:*588, 1884.

RINKER, J. R.: Accessory urethra in boy. J. Urol., *50:*331, 1943.

ROBINSON, W. W.: Congenital hypertrophy of the verumontanum as a cause of urinary retention. J. Urol., *17:*381, 1927.

ROCHERT, H. L. and RIVIERE, M.: Congenital imperforate urethra with retention of urine. Bull. soc. d'obst. et de gynéc., *16:*325, 1927.

ROOS, A.: Polycystic kidney; report of case studied by reconstruction. Am. J. Dis. Child., *61:*116, 1941.

ROSENBLATT, M.: Hydrometrocolpos in infancy. Ann. Surg., *117:*635, 1943.

ROY, K. S.: Absence of the glans penis. Indian Med. Gaz., *67:*518, 1932.

RUBIN, J. S.: Supernumerary kidney with aberrant ureter terminating externally. J. Urol., *60:*405, 1948.

SAUNDERS, F. J., et al.: Transposition of penis and scrotum, quoted by Hinman, Practice of Urology, loc. cit.

SCHAFFER, A. A. and ERBES, J.: Hypospadias. Am. J. Surg., *79*:183, 1950.

SCHINAGEL, G.: Bifurcated urethra. Urol. and Cut. Rev., *40*:398, 1936.

SCHWALBE, M. I.: Aneurysm of the renal artery. J. Urol., *63*:74, 1950.

SCHWARTZ, J.: Unusual unilateral multicystic kidney in infant. J. Urol., *35*:259, 1936.

SEIDEL, E.: Complete absence of urinary organs in female infant surviving for 21 days. Praxis, *10*:489, 1939.

SENGER, T. L. and SANTARE, V. J.: Congenital multilocular bladder. Trans. Am. Assoc. Genito-urin. Surg., *43*:114, 1951.

SHANDS, H. C.: Simultaneous occurrence of polycystic kidneys and erythroblastosis fetalis: report of three cases. Arch. Path., *40*:72, 1945.

SHEARER, T. P.: Retrocaval ureter. J. Urol., *62*:152, 1949.

SHUMACKER, H. B., JR.: Congenital anomalies of the genitalia associated with unilateral renal agenesis. Arch. Surg., *37*:586, 1938.

SIBLEY, T.: Urachal cyst. Am. J. Surg., *79*:465, 1950.

SISTO, HONTAN E.: Congenital implantation of penis with hypospadias in perineum between scrotum and anus. Pediatrica Españ., *24*:344, 1935.

SMITH, C. H. and GRAHAM, J. B.: Congenital medullary cysts of the kidneys with severe refractory anemia. Am. J. Dis. Child., *69*:369, 1945.

SMITH, P. G., et al.: Polyorchism. J. Urol., *64*:515, 1950.

SOLEY, P. J.: J. Urol., *55*:46, 1946.

SPAULDING, M. H.: The development of the external genitalia in the human embryo. Contributions to Embryology, No. 61, Washington, D. C., Carnegie Inst., 1921.

SPERMAN, H.: Embryonic Development and Induction. New Haven, Conn., Yale Univ. Press, 1938.

SPILLANE, R. J. and PRATHER, G. C.: High renal ectopy. J. Urol., *62*:441, 1949.

SPOONER, C. M. and LINDSAY, M. L.: Intravesical ureteral cyst associated with embryonic cartilage in the kidney of a newborn infant. J. Urol., *17*:453, 1927.

STEVENS, A. R.: Single pelvic kidneys. J. Urol., *37*:610, 1937.

————: Longevity following uretero-intestinal anastomosis. J. Urol., *46*:57, 1941.

STEVENS, W. E.: Congenital obstructions of the female urethra. J.A.M.A., *6*:89, 1936.

STEWART, B. L. and NICHOLL, G. A.: Cyst of the seminal vesicle. J. Urol., *62*:189, 1949.

SWAN, C., et al.: Congenital defects in infants following infectious diseases during pregnancy, with special reference to relationship between German measles and cataract. M. J. Australia, *2*:201, 1943.

SWENSON, O.: A new surgical treatment for Hirschsprung's disease. Surgery, *28*:371, 1950.

————: The diagnosis and surgical treatment of Hirschsprung's disease. Nebraska State Med. J., *37*:275, 1952.

————, NEUHAUSER, E. B. D. and PICKETT, L. K.: New concepts of the etiology, diagnosis and treatment of congenital megacolon (Hirschsprung's disease). Pediatrics, *4*:201, 1949.

————, RHEINLANDER, H. F. and DIAMOND, L.: Hirschsprung's disease, a new concept of the etiology. New England J. Med., *241*:551, 1949.

TAUBER, J. and BLOOM, B.: Infected urachal cysts. J. Urol., *66*:692, 1951.

TAYLOR, J. A. and BERRY, W. H.: Congenital absence of urinary sphincter with operative cure. J. Urol., *70*:203, 1953.

TEDESCHI, C. G. and HOLTHAM, W. H.: Bone formation in aplastic kidney. J. Urol., *68*:457, 1952.

TERNOVSKY, S.: Congenital urethral diverticula. Urol. and Cut. Rev., *34*:578, 1930.

THOMPSON, G. J.: Urinary obstruction of the vesical neck and posterior urethra of congenital origin. J. Urol., *47*:591, 1942.

———— and GREENE, L. F.: Ureterocele, a clinical study and a report of thirty-seven cases. J. Urol., *47*:800, 1942.

THOMPSON, W. O. and HECKEL, N. J.: Endocrine treatment of cryptorchidism. J.A.M.A., *117*:1953, 1941.

THORN, G. W.: Treatment of renal insufficiency. J. Urol., *59*:119, 1948.

TOLMATSCHEW, N.: Semilunare Klappen der Harnröhre und vergrösserte Vesicula Prostatica. Arch. f. Path. Anat. und Physiol., *40*:348, 1870.

TOMPKINS, P.: The treatment of imperforate hymen with hematocolpos. J.A.M.A., *113*:913, 1939.

TOULSON, W. H. and WAGNER, J. A.: Congenital encapsulated multilocular serous cyst associated with hypertension in 19 months old infant. Bull. School Med. Univ. Maryland, *26:*177, 1942.

TRAUT, H. F.: The structural unit of the human kidney. Contributions to Embryology, Washington, Carnegie Inst., *15:*103, 1923.

VAKAR, N. A.: Fusion of labia minora. Pediatriya, *14:*477, 1930.

VAUGH, A.: Facial characteristics in bilateral renal agenesis. Ann. West. Med. and Surg., *4:*131, 1950.

VERMOOTEN, V.: Dilated ureters in children. J. Urol., *41:*455, 1939.

VIRCHOW, R.: Polycystic disease. Arch. f. Path. Anat., *45:*506, 1869.

VOLPI, R.: Double penis. Policlinico, *1:*46, 1903.

VON GELDERN, C. E.: Etiology of exstrophy of the bladder. Arch. Surg., *8:*61, 1924.

VON LENHOSSEK, M.: Synorchism. Anatomischer Anzeiger, 1845.

WALL, B. and WACHTER, H. E. Ureteral valves. J. Urol., *68:*684, 1952.

WALTERS, W.: Resection of the renal pelvis for hydronephrosis; its complications and results. Surg., Gynec., and Obst., *51:*811, 1930.

WARKANY, J.: Etiology of Congenital Malformations. Advances in Pediatrics, New York, Interscience Publishers, Inc., Vol. 2, 1947.

WARKANY, J. and SCHRAFFENBERGER, E.: Congenital malformations induced in rats by maternal nutritional deficiency. Effects of a purified diet lacking riboflavin. Proc. Soc. Exper. Biol. and Med., *54:*92, 1943.

WATSON, E. M.: The structural basis for congenital valve-formation of the posterior urethra. Trans. Sect. Urol. Am. Med. Assn., p. 162, 1924.

WAY, R. A., JOHNSON, G. D. and WALLACE, F. T.: Pyelocystostomy in infant. J. South. Carolina Med. Assn., *42:*246, 1946.

WEHRBEIN, H. L.: Double kidney, double ureter, and bilocular bladder in a child. J. Urol., *43:*804, 1940.

WELLS, L. J.: Descent of the testis: anatomical and hormonal considerations. Surgery, *14:*436, 1943.

————: Hormones and descensus testiculorum. Bull. Minnesota M. Found., *4:*50. 1944.

————: Descensus testiculorum: descent after severance of gubernaculum. Anat. Rec., *88:*465, 1944.

————: Effects of injections of equine gonadotropin upon the gonads and adrenals of fetal rats. Proc. Soc. Exper. Biol. and Med., *62:*250, 1946.

———— and STATE, D.: Misconception of the gubernaculum testis. Surgery, *22:*502, 1947.

WESSON, M. B.: Incontinence of vesical and renal origin (relaxed urethra and vaginal ectopic ureter); case report. J. Urol., *32:*141, 1934.

WEYRAUCH, H. M. and FLEMING, A. E.: Congenital hydrocalycosis: hydrocalycosis of a single renal calyx in a new-born infant with complete destruction of the kidney. J. Urol., *63:*582, 1950.

WHARTON, L. R. and KEARNS, W.: Diverticula of the female urethra. J. Urol., *63:*1063, 1950.

WHITE, R. R. and WYATT, G. M.: Surgical importance of aberrant renal vessels in infants and children. Am. J. Surg., *58:*48, 1942.

WILKINS, L.: The Diagnosis and Treatment of Endocrine Disorders in Childhood and Adolescence. Springfield, Illinois, Charles C Thomas, 1950.

WILLMARTH, C. L.: Ectopic ureteral orifice within an urethral diverticulum. J. Urol., *59:*47, 1948.

WINDHOLZ, F.: Partielle Verdoppelung des rechten Samensleiter bei einem 54 jährigen Mann. Wien. Klin. Wchnsch., *42:*447, 1929.

WOLFFER, A. : Ureteral valves. Arch. f. Klin. Surg., *21:*294, 1877.

WOMACK, E. B. and KOCH, F. C.: Undescended testis. Endocrinology, *16:*267, 273, 1932.

WYBURN, C. M.: The development of the infra-umbilical portion of the abdominal wall with remarks on the etiology of ectopia vesicae. J. Anat., *71:*201, 1937.

YARMUDIAN, K. Y. and ACKERMAN, M. A.: Congenital polycystic kidneys. Urol. and Cut. Rev., *47:*147, 1943.

YOUNG, H. H.: Genital Abnormalities, Hermaphroditism and Related Adrenal Diseases. Baltimore, Williams and Wilkins Co., 1937.

YOUNG, H. H., FRONTZ, W. A. and BALDWIN, J. C.: Congenital obstruction of the posterior urethra. J. Urol., *3:*289, 1919.

YOUNG, H. H. and McKAY, R. W.: Congenital valvular obstruction of the prostatic urethra. Surg., Gynec. and Obst., *48:*509, 1929.

YOUNG, W. W.: Sclerosing injection of polycystic kidney following surgical exposure. J. Urol., *55:*323, 1946.

Section V

INFECTIONS AND INFLAMMATIONS
OF THE URINARY TRACT

CHAPTER 1

Urinary Infections

EDWARD N. COOK, M.D.

Infections of the urinary tract are of frequent occurrence, both as primary disorders and as complications of other urologic conditions. Formerly, only too often the virulence and magnitude of a coexisting infection precluded institution of an otherwise indicated surgical procedure. In the last twenty years, however, largely because of the investigative work of Clark and Helmholz, which has been carried on by Walthers, Crance, Herrold, Carroll and many others, better understanding has been acquired of the bacteriologic aspects of these infections and of the underlying pathologic conditions.

As the causative agents became known, specific treatment became a fertile field for study. Consequently, today a number of chemotherapeutic and antibiotic compounds are largely successful in eradicating these causative agents. Also, the physician has acquired increased awareness that infection may be accompanied by other pathologic processes in cases in which the usual treatment for a given infection fails. This has made for vast improvement in results.

ETIOLOGY

Patients who have infections of the urinary tract may be of either sex and any age. Furthermore, other pathologic conditions may or may not coexist. Primary interest is in what organism or organisms are present and also in how these organisms reached the urinary tract. These questions cannot always be answered, but in most instances today helpful information can be obtained.

Organisms. Classification of the great variety of organisms which cause infections of the urinary tract is not easy. Reports vary so greatly, moreover, that the relative frequency with which one or another organism is causative is practically impossible to ascertain. This qualification should be kept in mind when some of the following statements are read.

503

The microorganisms usually found in the urinary tract are gram-negative bacilli and gram-positive cocci. The former are found in approximately 75 per cent of cases. Among females and children, bacillary infections assume an even higher proportion.

Escherichia coli is by far the most commonly occurring gram-negative organism that is responsible for infections of the urinary tract. Closely related organisms, the Aerobacter aerogenes among them, account for only about 10 to 15 per cent of cases of bacillary infection. Other bacilli are found in decreasing frequency; namely, members of the genera Proteus, Pseudomonas, Salmonella, Shigella, and Alkaligenes.

Gram-positive cocci are found in approximately 25 per cent of cases of infection of the urinary tract. The members of the genus Micrococcus are of particular interest. Certain nonpathogenic micrococci, such as those which appear in tetrads and Sarcina lutea, frequently are found as normal inhabitants of the male urethra and at times may be confused with the true pathogenic cocci. The greater part of the latter belong to the species Micrococcus pyogenes and are of both varieties, aureus and albus. Infections with these organisms as well as with those caused by various streptococci usually are thought to be blood-borne and secondary at times to foci elsewhere in the body. The hemolytic and green-producing streptococci occur in less than 5 per cent of cases of infection of the urinary tract.

The Streptococcus faecalis is an important, and usually a secondary, invader. Cabot stated that, in his opinion, it rarely occurred unless instrumentation or a surgical procedure had been done previously. This organism has resisted many forms of treatment and today infection with it must be treated in a special way.

At this point it should be mentioned that institution of proper treatment need not always be preceded by identification of the infectious organism. Such identification requires a laboratory and culture of the urine. It entails expense. As will be brought out later, careful microscopic study of the gram-stained urinary sediment will provide the necessary information concerning more than 90 per cent of patients who come to the office with a urinary infection. Repeated study of the sediment while the patient is under treatment will give evidence of progress or the reverse and, when the response is not satisfactory, it calls attention to the need of further urologic investigation: cultures of the urine, cystoscopy and urography, one or all of them.

Route of Infection. Obviously, if infection is to occur in the urinary tract, infecting organisms must reach it (Fig. 273). Through the years it has been thought that infecting microorganisms reached the urinary tract by way of the blood stream or the lymph passages, directly from a source of infection adjacent to the kidney, and also by ascent along the urinary passages. The latter is no doubt particularly true in the female, both young and old, and no doubt accounts for the increased frequency with which infections of the urinary tract do occur in the female.

Many investigators have shown that infection of the urinary tract can be blood-borne. Both cocci and bacilli may reach the kidney thus, but hematogenic infections of the kidney usually are attributable to cocci. Cabot called

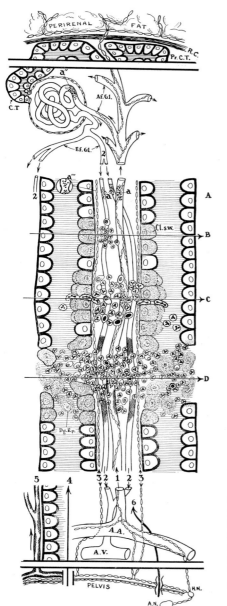

Fig. 273. Schema of renal infection. Routes of invasion of the renal parenchyma. 1,2, hematogenous. *A.A.*, arcuate artery giving off interlobar branches (1) which ultimately pass to the glomeruli as the afferent glomerular arteries (*Af.Gl.*). Leaving the glomeruli, the efferent glomerular vessels (*Ef.Gl.*) pass downward as nutrient vessels of the parenchyma, ultimately to become large veins (2) and finally empty into the arcuate vein (*A.V.*). Retrograde extension of bacteria by pyelovenous or pyelotubular backflow from the pelvis may occur.

3. Lymphogenous. Through lymphatics of the pelvis, or those which surround the arteries and collecting tubules (Kumita), or those which penetrate the renal capsule (*R.C.*) from the perirenal fat. *H.N.*, hilar lymph node; *A.N.*, aortic lymph node.

4. Intratubular. Spread by retrograde extension (reflux) through the tubules from the pelvis. Experimentally this is difficult to produce and the pathway is probably seldom of clinical importance.

5. Extension from the pelvis by vascular thrombosis. Helmholz in particular has emphasized the importance of this process.

6. By rupture through the pelvis with direct intertubular (interstitial) extension or extravasation. This is probably rare. Bacterial invasion of the kidney by irruption from neighboring foci or by surgical attack is not indicated.

Pathologic sequence of infection:

A. Bacterial embolism in interlobular arteriole a, interlobular efferent vessel *a'*, glomerular arteriole *a''* or lymphatic vessel *a'''*.

B. Early cellular reaction to the bacterial invasion. Note that the lesion is at first limited to the interstitial spaces of the kidney and the interstitial reaction is a perivascular leukocytic infiltration. Cloudy swelling (*Cl.sw.*) of the epithelial cells of the adjacent tubules occurs (Fig. 736, *B*). Symptoms are probably uncommon at this stage.

C. An advanced stage of B. Leukocytic infiltration and cloudy swelling increase; polymorphonuclears, lymphocytes, plasma cells, and large mononuclears are the cells regularly found. Histosections of this stage frequently show polymorphonuclears extruding their way between the swollen epithelial cells into the lumen of the tubules.

D. Late stage of C with massive focal suppuration. Vascular thrombosis, extensive leukocytic infiltration, destruction of the adjacent tubules (*Dg.,Ep.*, degenerated epithelium) with discharge of the purulent debris into the collecting tubules and thence into the pelvis (Fig. 738).

The above schema indicates why, in so-called pyelitis, the interstitial lesion is so much more important than mere inflammation of the pelvis. It also demonstrates how most of the pus found in the urine in these cases originates in the interstitial lesions rather than in areas of urothelial inflammation.

C.T., convoluted tubule. *Pr.C.T.*, proximal convoluted tubule.

505

attention to the confusion that exists when renal infection follows instrumentation of the lower part of the urinary tract. Here the problem is whether transient bacteremia develops, with a shower of organisms reaching the kidney through the blood stream, or whether the infection passes directly up

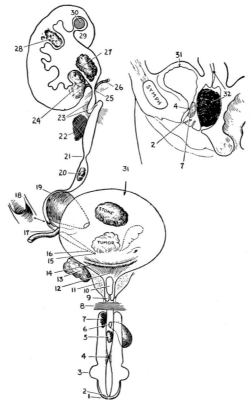

Fig. 274.   Common causes of urinary tract obstruction: 1, phimosis; stenosis of prepuce, 2, stenosis of urethral meatus, 3, paraphimosis, 4, urethral stricture, 5, urethral stone, 6, urethral diverticulum, 7, periurethral abscess, 8, external sphincterospasm, 9, congenital valves of the posterior urethra, 10, hypertrophy of the verumontanum; diverticulum of utricle, 11, prostatic abscess or growths, 12, contracted bladder neck; median bar, 13, periprostatic abscess, 14, mucosal fold at bladder outlet; trigonal curtain, 15, stricture of ureteral meatus; ureterocele, 16, ureterovesical junction stricture, 17, vascular obstruction of lower ureter, 18, congenital ureteral valves, 19, ureteral obstruction by compression by vesical diverticulum, fecal overdistention of rectosigmoid, pelvic cyst, etc., 20, ureteral stone, 21, ureteral stricture, 22, periureteritis or tumor, 23, ureteral kink; periureteral fibrous bands, 24, renal tumor, 25, ureteropelvic junction stricture, 26, aberrant vessel obstruction of upper ureter, 27, pelvic stone, 28, renal tuberculosis (secondary obstructive lesions consequent thereto), 29, stricture of calyceal outlet, 30, calyceal stone, 31, neuromuscular vesical disease, 32, urethral compression by hematocolpometra or hydrocolpos.

the urinary passage; namely, through the bladder and then the ureter to the kidney. No doubt either may occur, and sometimes both in the same case.

Concerning infection through the lymph channels the literature is confusing. Certain anatomic studies seem to demonstrate that the only continuous lymphatic connections along the urinary tract are a few in and around the kidney. In many instances of infection around the kidney, there is little or no evidence to suggest that the infection has extended to the urinary tract. The lymph channels along the ureter have been suggested as a means whereby infectious microorganisms can travel from the lower part of the urinary tract to the kidney. However, experiments seem to show that this is not a direct route but that the channels follow a segmental distribution and drain into regional nodes. Certainly there has been no proof that invasion is always by any one lymphatic route.

In a large group of cases, infection of the kidney cannot be explained by previously suggested methods of invasion. Undoubtedly, many times infection from the lower part of the urinary tract, the prostate gland or the bladder will proceed directly along the urinary tract to the kidney. Helmholz showed that when the bladders of some rabbits were infected, the causative organisms traveled through the ureter to the kidneys. Careful consideration of certain clinical cases, moreover, seems to bear out the impression that this occurs in man. Whether the organisms travel through the muscle or connective tissue layer of the ureter, along the mucous membrane or in the urinary stream is of little importance. Unquestionably such a process would be aided by obstruction at the vesical neck or in the ureter. Obstruction in the urinary tract as a result of congestion may well prepare a fertile soil for the development of infection (Fig. 274). Helmholz observed, furthermore, that if animals were debilitated or had some disease, spontaneous and experimentally induced infection occurs more easily than otherwise.

PATHOLOGY

Study of the pathologic changes in tissue in the presence of inflammation of the bladder and kidney is largely impracticable. First, in the majority of cases the inflamed tissue is not examined at necropsy because the lesion goes on to complete recovery. Second, specimens for biopsy are difficult to obtain and rarely give an accurate picture of the various changes that are taking place as a result of the inflammatory process.

Bladder. In general, acute, subacute and chronic inflammation of the mucosa and submucosa of the bladder is essentially the same as an inflammatory process anywhere. The gross appearance of the tissue noted on cystoscopy is of much greater importance to the urologist than is its microscopic appearance.

As a rule, in acute cystitis resulting from congestion, the whole vesical wall is reddened. The normal, pale, salmon-pink mucosa is not seen. When the lesion involves almost the entire vesical wall, the condition is referred to as "diffuse cystitis." However, more frequently the lesion is localized and the term used to denominate it is "areal cystitis." Edema of the vesical mucosa frequently is associated with acute cystitis. Its presence makes evaluation of the existing lesion difficult at times because of the frequent association of edema with an underlying malignant growth. The patches of edema usually are localized but they may be rather diffusely scattered through the entire vesical wall. Commonly edema occurs over the trigone and around the vesical neck. Many times it consists of nothing more than a fullness of the mucosa but it assumes a bullous appearance in the presence of the more virulent infections. Then the raised portions may form bullae which have the appearance of cysts; their bluish color suggests venous engorgement and their frequent association with malignancy must always be appreciated. With acute cystitis hematuria is commonly found and cystoscopy often reveals ecchymotic, punctate areas which bleed easily on distention of the bladder. Even ulceration may occur in some instances.

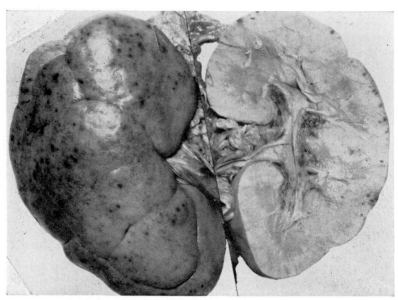

Fig. 275. Kidney in "acute pyelitis" in a four-year-old girl; the renal infection was secondary to pneumonia. On the surface are seen multiple cortical hemorrhagic abscesses and in the cross section of the organ the extent of these grossly visible changes is seen. (Babies Hospital.)

In association with chronic cystitis certain changes commonly are found. The vesical mucosa becomes pale, loses its normal sheen, and its surface frequently is somewhat irregular. The vesical capacity may be reduced and trabeculation may result from the cicatricial changes in the wall. In general the trigone and the area around the neck of the bladder are the most common sites for the greatest changes of the chronic type. In these areas, frequently the mucosa and submucosa undergo proliferation, which produces some granular changes, single or multiple. The resulting condition frequently is referred to as "granuloma." These changes, too, may be confused with those of malignancy but, on overdistention of the bladder, they tend to flatten out and become less prominent, a phenomenon which does not occur in the presence of tumor.

Cystitis Cystica. When small vesicles occur they usually are found particularly at the base of the bladder and over the trigone; usually they suggest vesical inflammation of long standing. The reason for their formation is not known but they seem to be direct results of a proliferation of the mucosa

which takes place in the acute or subacute stage of the disease; in themselves they do not cause symptoms. Frequently they will still be present
long after the existing infection has been eradicated.

Kidney. As has been suggested, tissue available for study usually is limited
to that which displays the end results in fulminating cases unless, by chance,
an individual whose renal infection is of lower grade dies from some inter-

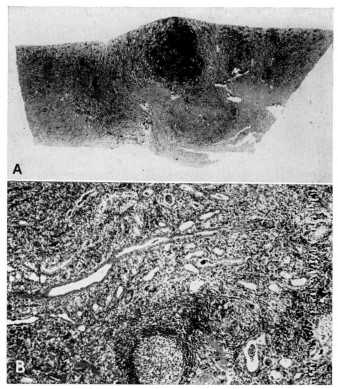

Fig. 276.   Acute renal infection. *A,* focal cortical abscess in kidney with elevation of
the renal surface. To the left are two small subsurface cortical abscesses in generation;
on the right is evidence of still earlier infection. Male, ten years, Bellevue Hospital.
B, histology of marginal area of focal abscess shown in *A.* There are a few remnants
of parenchyma suggesting the normal kidney architecture but these are invaded by extensive areas of suppuration.

current cause. Hematogenous lesions of the kidney, the causative agents of
which usually are gram-positive cocci, are multiple, widespread abscesses
of the cortex and medulla (Figs. 275, 276). Usually they are bilateral and
frequently they form contiguous groups of abscesses which may fuse and
form the so-called carbuncle of the kidney. Associated perinephritis often is
present, the evidence of which consists of the small, yellowish dots of subcapsular abscesses distributed over the surface of the kidney in association
with edema and induration of the perirenal tissue.

Helmholz and others have shown experimentally that the pathologic
process which occurs when ascending infection reaches the kidney is essen-

tially the same as an inflammatory process anywhere. However, the actual site of involvement of the kidney varies, depending on the stage of inflammation when the kidney is examined. Early, only simple pyelitis exists and the inflammation is primarily confined to the surface of the mucosa. As the disease continues, however, the entire mucosal and submucosal tissue becomes involved. Then, by extension along the blood vessels, the inflammatory process spreads throughout the entire renal parenchyma (Figs. 273, 277, 278).

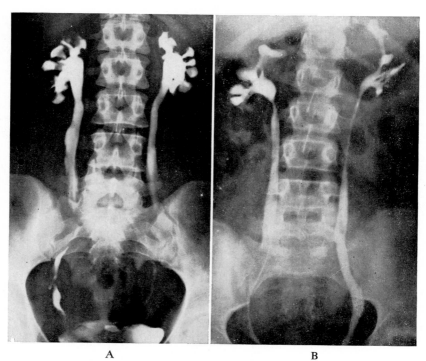

A   B

Fig. 277. Chronic pyelonephritis. Terminal urographic changes. *A,* in twenty-three-year-old girl periodically observed for ten years. The initial lesion was bilateral uretero-vesical junction stricture which responded well to conservative dilation. Progressive decrease of renal function throughout the clinical course. Uremic death. There is contraction of the kidney with narrowing of the calyceal necks and irregular calyceal dilatation with ureterectasis. *B,* pyelography in a five-year-old boy showing irregular renal sclerotic contraction especially on the left, with corresponding pelvic distortion.

In general, bilateral hematogenous infections of the kidneys involve the renal cortex, while ascending renal infections usually are localized to the renal pelvis, the peripelvic tissues and the medulla of the kidney.

Perinephritic Abscess. This process arises as an extension of an inflammatory lesion in the capsular or subcapsular structures. Pyelonephritis develops and an abscess forms in the renal parenchyma. The abscess erodes through the capsule into the perinephric fat which offers an excellent medium for the development of the so-called perinephritic abscess (Figs. 279–281). This mode of involvement seems to me much more likely than that septic emboli lodge in the end arteries of the perinephric fat and produce the abscess.

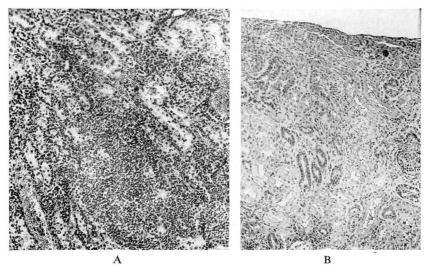

A   B

Fig. 278. Advanced chronic pyelonephritis with massive widespread suppuration. *A,* extensive loss of renal architecture with sheets of leukocytes and inflammatory debris interspersed throughout the tissue. *B,* pyonephrosis with advanced tubular destruction but functioning glomeruli remain along the course of the blood supply.

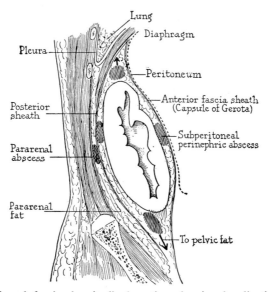

Fig. 279. Perirenal fascia; longitudinal section showing localization and routes of spread of perirenal suppuration. Fused above at the diaphragm, the anterior and posterior sheaths pass downward enclosing the kidney and its perirenal fat. The last, due to lack of fascial fusion below, is continuous with the fat of the pelvis. Because of this, pelvic infections may subsequently become clinically manifest as perinephric abscess or vice versa. The common sites of perirenal abscess are indicated. (From Editor's book, Infections of the Kidney, courtesy Harper and Bros.)

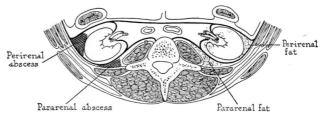

Fig. 280. Perirenal fascia; transverse section showing localization of perirenal and pararenal abscess. It is noteworthy that the anterior fascial sheath (heavy line) passes from side to side in front of the ureters, great vessels, and vertebral column, and fuses laterally with the posterior fascial sheath. The last in turn is attached medially to the vertebral column. Separation of the perirenal and the pararenal fat by the posterior fascial sheath is indicated. (From Editor's book, Infections of the Kidney, courtesy Harper and Bros.)

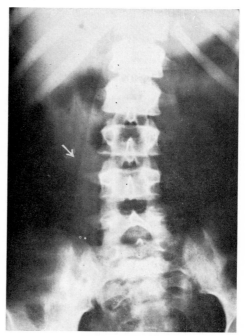

Fig. 281. Perinephric abscess. Suggestive diagnostic findings in the plain urogram: (a) lateral scoliosis away from the side of the lesion (left), and (b) the disappearance of the shadow of the isolateral psoas muscle. Arrow points to the margin of the right psoas muscle which is distinct. Eight-year-old girl. (Courtesy Dr. Charles P. Howze.)

SYMPTOMS

The remarkable advances made in study of the particular etiologic agents of various infections of the urinary tract, as well as in chemotherapeutics and antibiotics, place the physician of today in an advantageous position for management of such infections. However, the erroneous impression may get about that the new therapeutic preparations make unnecessary the old attention to the fundamentals: elicitation of symptoms and care in diagnosis.

Such an impression would result in mismanagement in some cases. It is with this in mind that the following summary is presented.

The Basic Symptoms. Careful taking of the history, in the course of which all symptoms are elicited, is of the greatest importance in properly evaluating a patient who is suffering from an infection of the urinary tract. Burning and frequent urination (the most common symptoms) at times associated with urgency, dysuria of varying degree, and hematuria, may be present in any case, depending on the underlying pathologic entity. It is the relationship of these basic symptoms to accompanying symptoms, as well as their relation to the act of urination, which will give the examiner a true notion of just what is going on in a particular case. If the symptom complex suggests the presence of other pathologic conditions, such as obstruction, stone or tumor, there is no reason to go ahead with chemotherapy. Efforts to eradicate infection are of little avail when such complications are present.

Occasionally suprapubic soreness or distress in the flank, which at times is as severe as colic, may be present. General symptoms such as fever, malaise, anorexia, nausea and vomiting may be noted when involvement is severe and the disease has extended to the kidneys, causing pyelonephritis.

Granular Trigonitis, Granular and Cicatricial Urethritis. The relationship of burning and urgency to the act of urination is sometimes very important in assessing the underlying pathologic process. If the irritative distress precedes urination, subsides during it, and then becomes immediately more severe as urination is finished, granular trigonitis often is present. If burning is worst during urination, granular or cicatricial urethritis, or both, usually are present. Appreciation of this is important because, in many cases, much to the surprise of the examiner, examination of a properly obtained urinary specimen will reveal nothing abnormal. In such circumstances, administration of varied and sundry chemotherapeutic and antibiotic compounds will be of no help.

Interstitial Cystitis. A similar situation is encountered in the presence of another symptom complex characterized by marked frequency and urgency. Usually the patient is a female but not always. In addition to the frequency and urgency there is pain, usually severe and located over the bladder although it may be in the hip, vagina or perineum. Passing of urine is not painful and usually the patient will state that for a varying period after voiding, relief of pain is complete. This symptom complex usually is associated with urine that is free of cellular and bacterial elements and is indicative of interstitial cystitis. Here again antibacterial therapy is of no value. (See also Wharton's discussion of this subject in Section XII.)

Cystitis Per Se. In years past many observers doubted the presence of cystitis per se. They believed that cystitis always was part of an infection of the urinary tract including the kidneys. The experience of most urologists in the past score of years, however, indicates that cystitis per se does occur. It is of more frequent occurrence among females than among males and no doubt explains the subacute, recurrent type of inflammation which is commonly encountered. Here the symptoms of frequency of urination, with urgency and suprapubic soreness, predominate. Rarely will there be any general symptoms but, if there are any, the infection is probably renal as well. Hematuria may or may not be present.

Renal Infection, Vesical Calculus. As has been indicated, proper evaluation of all the symptoms will not only suggest the presence of infection of the urinary tract but it can very well disclose the nature of an underlying primary pathologic process, for this process may come to light only as an associated symptom. Renal or ureteral distress arising in the flank and extending anteriorly and into the groin and genitalia, associated with frequency and urgency, may be indicative of renal infection alone, or of stone or obstruction. Suprapubic distress, associated with disturbances of urinary control such as extreme urgency amounting to incontinence, at times along with sudden stoppage of the stream, may be the sign of vesical calculi.

Hematuria. The complaint of hematuria is of superlative importance. Many times neoplasms of the urinary tract may remain asymptomatic until secondary infection makes the patient aware of trouble. The assumption that hematuria is a result of infection may be justified but it never should be considered confirmed until complete urologic investigation has excluded the presence of a coexisting neoplasm somewhere along the urinary tract.

Amicrobic Pyuria. This condition is attended by symptoms like those of any other infection of the urinary tract but they are more severe than in the usual case. Urinalysis will reveal the cellular elements usually found in the presence of infection but organisms are not demonstrable in the gram-stained urinary sediment or on culture. This condition should be better understood. Too frequently, because of the absence of demonstrable organisms in the urinary sediment, a diagnosis of tuberculosis is made. The possibility of this condition should be kept in mind but the diagnosis must not be made until the tuberculous organism is positively identified.

Obstruction. The symptoms discussed thus far are likely to apply to the various clinical types of infection of the bladder, with ascending infection extending to one or both kidneys. These types of infection may occur with or without obstruction. The various conditions which may give rise to obstruction are well illustrated in Figure 274.

The Coccal Infections of the Kidney. There is another group of infections of the kidney, usually hematogenous, to which special attention should be given. They are usually attributable to the pus-producing cocci, particularly the staphylococci of both varieties, aureus and albus. In general there are three types of such infections, depending on the severity of the disease.

The fulminating type is fortunately of very uncommon occurrence. The patient usually is an adult. Frequently diagnosis is difficult because of the severity of the infection. The condition comes on rapidly, with nausea, vomiting and upper abdominal distress, and frequently it is associated with chills, fever and a rapid pulse. Absence of any particular localizing signs, except for the vague abdominal pain, often causes confusion. In instances in which the pain is severe, the lesion may suggest acute pancreatitis or a perforating ulcer of the intestinal tract. The leukocyte count is high. Paradoxically, the urine rarely is particularly abnormal. Urinary symptoms are absent and the only possible finding in the urine is the regular presence of the coccus responsible for the disease. Examination of the gram-stained urinary sediment may be the only definite clue, in the early stages of the disease, as to the origin of the symptoms. One other physical finding of great importance is that of tenderness, sometimes very severe. This is in the costovertebral angle on the side of the infection if the involvement is unilateral. In this fulminating condition, unless treatment is instituted early, prognosis is very grave.

The acute coccal infections of the kidney present symptoms similar to those of the fulminating type. They are not so severe and the patient generally is not overwhelmed by the infection. Again, costovertebral tenderness on one or both sides is helpful in making the diagnosis. According to Cabot, it is in acute cases that carbuncle of the kidney is most likely to occur (cf. Fig. 752). How this lesion is formed was explained in an earlier paragraph. Necrosis is extensive and frequently there is marked breakdown of all cellular elements.

A third type of coccal infection of the urinary tract has been described as subacute or chronic. This is really only a milder form of the other two types.

Perinephritis and Perinephritic Abscess. Coccal infections of the urinary tract may give rise to perinephritis and perinephritic abscess. Unfortunately, however, the condition presents no definite symptomatology. There may or may not be tenderness in the flank. Sometimes a mass is found in the side and sometimes none is found. The only definite indication of the condition may be recurrent daily fever and accompaning constitutional symptoms, without evidence of localization. I have seen a perinephritic abscess become so extensive as to rupture into the peritoneal cavity before the diagnosis was made. Recent boils or carbuncles elsewhere in the body, or presence of a recent septic wound, may be the forerunner of a coccal infection of the perinephric tissues or, for that matter, of the kidney itself.

DIAGNOSIS

Presence of infection of the urinary tract must be proved before treatment is instituted. This seems self-evident. However, it is necessary to repeat that accurate evaluation of the condition at hand is extremely important if patients are to be treated correctly.

Gross Inspection of Urine. The initial diagnostic step is proper examination of the urine and this requires a properly obtained specimen. If the patient is a male the glans penis is thoroughly cleansed and he is asked to void. The initial portion of the flow is not kept for examination as it contains the washings of the anterior part of the urethra, which may confuse the picture. After approximately 2 or 3 ounces (60 to 90 cc.) of urine have passed, however, while the stream is running, a portion of the flow is collected for study. Examination of a specimen voided by a female is of no value unless the result is entirely negative. Usually the urine of a female is contaminated by vulvar and vaginal secretion and therefore contains cellular elements. For this reason, the external meatus must be thoroughly cleansed and a catheterized specimen obtained.

Gross examination of the properly obtained specimen is perhaps the most helpful single procedure in arriving at a diagnosis of infection of the urinary tract. Any cloudiness or discoloration is observed. These may be attributable to the presence of pus cells, shreds, debris or erythrocytes—any or all of them.

Microscopic Examination of Urinary Sediment. Moderate pyuria and bacilluria, however, frequently are seen in a grossly clear specimen of urine. The next step, therefore, is to centrifuge some of the urine, discard the supernatant liquid, place a drop of the sediment on a glass slide, place a cover-slip over the drop, and examine it microscopically with the high-power, dry objective. If pus cells, debris, erythrocytes and epithelial cells are present, there is an inflammatory process somewhere along the urinary tract. In some instances, if enough bacteria are present, they may be seen floating in the suspended specimen.

Recognition of these organisms is the next important step. Much has been written regarding the relative merits of staining and culturing the urine. Actually the two methods are complementary. In the majority of instances, examination of the gram-stained smear of the sediment gives the desired information immediately, with little or no expense to the patient. It not only demonstrates the presence or absence of organisms but discloses whether they are cocci or bacilli and whether they are gram-positive or gram-negative. Thus it helps in selection of treatment.

Culture of Urine. If treatment has not brought about the desired results, it becomes necessary to determine the particular organism present, and for that, culture of the urine is necessary. Proper interpretation of the findings may be difficult. For that reason the procedure is best carried out by a trained bacteriologist even though a number of techniques have been devised for office practice.

Briefly, three culture media are the most useful in identification of organisms usually found in the urinary tract. The first is the eosin-methylene blue agar plate. On this medium nearly all of the gram-negative bacilli grow so characteristically that they can be identified without further study. If this is insufficient, fermentation studies will reveal the exact nature of the organism present. Eosin-methylene blue agar is not conducive to growth of the gram-positive cocci usually found in urinary infections, with the exception of the Streptococcus faecalis; this presents a characteristic growth, as do the gram-negative bacilli. The other gram-positive cocci are best cultured by inoculating blood agar slants or brain broth media. The pathogenicity of these organisms, or the lack of it, can be determined by the coagulase test. For more detailed consideration of cultural methods, standard texts on bacteriology should be consulted.

Urography and Cystoscopy. After such a comprehensive study of the urinary sediment, certain other measures may be indicated. Treatment of infection of the urinary tract in the presence of stone, obstruction or tumor will be only palliative. If the details of the history are such as to suggest the presence of an associated pathologic entity, complete urologic study immediately should be made. It should include excretory urography, cystoscopy and, if necessary, functional studies and retrograde pyelography. The procedure necessary to obtain an excretory urogram is relatively innocuous and the method can be used in the acute stage of the disease. It gives a relative test of renal function when the rapidity with which the dye is excreted through the urinary structures of one side is compared with that on the other side. The presence of gross abnormalities such as stone, tumor, obstruction or congenital anomaly may be demonstrated, thus suggesting the need of still more detailed study.

Cystoscopy is a very important part of the investigation of any patient with resistant infection of the urinary tract. Many times the presence of vesical neoplasm is entirely masked by symptoms of inflammation. Under such circumstances, patients may be treated with the various drugs now available only to find, following relief of pain, that their difficulty returns. Cystoscopy sometimes is postponed too long.

The value of cystoscopy is enhanced by evaluation of the cystogram. This helps particularly to establish the presence of certain inadequacies of the vesical wall. It gives additional evidence, also, of incompetence of the ureterovesical sphincters, and discloses the resulting reflux and dilatation of the upper part of the urinary tract.

Perinephritic Abscess. A hint previously has been given of the difficulty of diagnosis of perinephritic abscess. The history of infection elsewhere in the body, tenderness in one or both costovertebral angles, the presence of a mass in the side, and recurrent fever are suggestive diagnostic points. Leukocytosis is variable but usually present. As the disease progresses, irritation of the psoas muscle on the involved side is of common occurrence and the patient can gain relief from the pain by flexing the hip joint on the affected side.

A few roentgenographic signs may be helpful in the diagnosis of perinephritic abscess (Figs. 280, 281). In the majority of instances the shadow of the psoas muscle is absent on the involved side. There is slight scoliosis, with the concavity directed to the same side as that of the abscess. Renal markings may be indefinite and frequently there is a homogeneous cast to the entire roentgenogram on the side where disease is suspected. Some observers have called attention to the importance of a full lateral film, which usually shows that the kidney and upper half of the ureter are anteriorly displaced if a perinephritic abscess is present.

TREATMENT

Nowadays, the presence of infection, the type of infection, the site of infection and the pathologic conditions associated with infection can and must be determined before treatment of urinary infection is begun. As has been said, the presence of stone, tumor or obstruction must be recognized and treatment for these conditions must be instituted unless the patient's general state forbids. Treatment of infection in the presence of such conditions is only palliative but at times will be indicated for this reason alone.

Active treatment can be divided into general measures, local measures, and oral and parenteral medication. In many cases all are used.

General Measures. Forcing of fluids by mouth or otherwise flushes many infecting organisms out of the urinary tract. Also, the following may be necessary: Rest in bed, application of heat to the affected region, a soft diet and administration of sedatives for pain. Warm sitz baths, by relieving spasm of the bladder, whether or not it is accompanied by pelvic distress, may be most comforting.

Local Measures. Now that urinary antiseptics are easily administered orally it is easy to forget the value of properly administered local treatment. Many times lavage of the bladder, or instillation of various substances such as mild silver proteinate into the urethra, bladder or renal pelvis, bestows on the patient almost immediate comfort, whereas oral administration of a drug would be followed by a period of time for absorption and secretion of the drug in the urine before the desired effect would be evident. Previous to any of the foregoing, cicatricial changes in the urethra may require dilatation.

Astringent solutions may be applied to the urethra or bladder by lavage or topical application and many times they are beneficial. Tampons impregnated with mild silver protein (argyrol, 5 per cent) or strong silver protein (protargol, 0.5 to 1 per cent), or suppositories containing these substances, are helpful against granular urethritis in the female. Localized granulomatous changes in the posterior urethra of the male are treated with instillations of 5 per cent mild silver protein. This is done with a small, soft-rubber catheter. In some cases silver nitrate, 5 to 20 per cent, directly applied to the granulomatous area by means of a swab inserted through the cystoscope, will give great relief. Fulguration of urethral cysts, through the cystoscope, is beneficial. However, in the majority of cases of urethritis, fulguration of granulomatous tissue with the electric cautery is attended with more postoperative distress than the patient had before.

A number of solutions for lavage are available: potassium permanganate, 1:8,000 solution; saturated boric acid solution; acetic acid, 1:3,000 solution. Undoubtedly any of these solutions exerts a mild antiseptic effect but their greatest value is the mechanical cleansing which attends their use. Following lavage of the bladder, instillation of $\frac{1}{2}$ ounce (15 cc.) of a 5 per cent solution of mild silver protein may give quick relief of acute symptoms.

If vesical tenesmus and dysuria are marked, it may be advisable to hospitalize the patient, place an indwelling catheter in the bladder and use continuous irrigations of a urinary antiseptic. Many times when the infecting organism is capable of splitting urea in the urine and producing encrusted cystitis, continuous irrigation with increasing strengths of silver nitrate solution is of great value. Cystoscopy performed with the patient under anesthesia, previous to the beginning of the continuous irrigations, furnishes an opportunity to remove encrustations with the heel of the cystoscope or with blunt forceps. This allows the silver nitrate solution to come in contact with the inflamed mucosa and recovery is hastened.

Instillations of 1 ounce (30 cc.) of a 5 to 7 per cent solution of silver iodide often is soothing to an irritable bladder. The irritability may be functional or it may be a symptom of postradiation cystitis.

Frequently recurrent distress of the lower part of the urinary tract of the male is associated with chronic infection of the prostate gland and, until the prostate has been massaged, the bacteriuria will not be eradicated. A cardinal principle of surgery is that infection in any confined space requires drainage. Prostatic massage, properly administered, facilitates drainage of the swollen and inflamed prostatic ducts and acini. It must be done regularly and often enough to keep the gland drained. Usually three times weekly at the beginning, and then twice weekly, for a total of eight to ten weeks, should be sufficient.

Before leaving this discussion of local treatment, attention must be called to the dangers of overtreatment. In the female particularly, the urethra and bladder may be rendered hypersensitive by local applications and not infrequently such patients will experience great relief from stoppage of treatment.

Oral and Parenteral Medication. At present, infections of the urinary tract are treated largely by oral administration of various chemotherapeutic and antibiotic compounds. If the patient is unable to take anything by mouth, one or another of these compounds is administered parenterally. The use of the individual drug or group of drugs will be discussed under the heading of each compound.*

After evaluation of the history, the results of physical examination and the laboratory findings, choice of the antibiotic or chemotherapeutic compound to be used becomes necessary. It would be ideal if the presence of a particular causative organism invariably was the indication for use of a particular preparation. The best that can be done, however, is to list the compound that usually is effective in eradicating a particular invader.

Recently studies of the sensitivity of microorganisms to the action of various therapeutic preparations have proved valuable. These studies are not necessary in all cases. If results with certain preparations have been unsuccessful, however, and coexisting pathologic conditions have been excluded, studies of this sort will give a fairly accurate idea of the resistance of the organism under consideration to one or another of the various therapeutic compounds. Thus, also, the physician can determine the compound to which the organism is most sensitive. These studies are best carried out by a skilled bacteriologist.

Sulfonamide. This drug in its many forms is the most widely used urinary antiseptic. It is inexpensive; it can be given in small dosage with few, if any, toxic reactions. In the majority of instances, infections attributable to the gram-negative bacilli, with the exception of organisms of the genus Pseudomonas, will respond to its administration. The sulfonamides have proved to be equally effective against most of the staphylococci and streptococci which are the common invaders in the urinary tract. Only in rare

* The employment and dosage of the various drugs and antibiotics in the treatment of urinary infections in infants and children are discussed in Section XIII and as an adjunct in surgical care, in Section XV, Chapter 1.

instances have sulfonamides been used successfully in eradicating infections owing to the Streptococcus faecalis.

Sulfonamides usually are administered orally. A dose of 2 gm. daily (divided into 4 doses of 0.5 gm. each) for one week is sufficient. Only in isolated instances is a larger dose of increased value. A course of sulfonamide therapy given for five to seven days each month for three or four months may be of great value in eliminating recurring infectious disease of the urinary tract. A program of this sort has proved of value not only with the use of sulfonamides but also with the use of any of the chemotherapeutic compounds. Frequently the first course of medication will eradicate the greatest number of infecting organisms, even to the point of relieving symptoms and the attaining of negative smears and cultures. However, a few organisms may still be present in the tissues which, sometime after administration of the drug has been stopped, may become activated. As a result of intermittent treatment in some cases of persistent infection, the number of recurrent infections has been materially reduced. When, for one reason or another, oral administration of drugs of the type under consideration is impossible, the sodium salt of either sulfathiazole or sulfapyridine may be given parenterally. When given in this manner, the equivalent of 40 to 60 grains (2.6 to 4 gm.) of the drug should be administered daily by vein in 1,000 cc. of physiologic saline solution.

Furadantin. This is a synthetic antibacterial agent which has come into general use in the past 2 years in combating certain bacterial infections of the urinary tract. It is a broad spectrum antiseptic and has proved its greatest worth in combating infections due to the Bacillus proteus when other chemotherapeutic or antibiotic agents have failed. In a few instances it has eradicated organisms of the genus Pseudomonas.

Manifestations of toxicity are relatively few. Nausea and vomiting have been noted but are minimal if the drug is taken in the course of meals rather than before or after. If an additional dose is given at bedtime, it should be taken with food. The amount of the drug to be given has become standardized and usually 100 mg. given 4 times daily for five to seven days will suffice.

Penicillin. Penicillin is a most useful adjunct in management of infections of the urinary tract. Oral administration of the drug in pills of 50 mg. each, using 2 to 4 pills four times daily, occasionally has been of benefit. My experience with oral administration of penicillin, however, has not been good. The desired bactericidal effect in the urine was obtained only occasionally. Certainly the results from parenteral injection far surpass those obtained by oral administration.

Penicillin usually is given in a dosage of 300,000 units daily, by intramuscular injection. It has been of value in treating the usual bacillary infections, except those caused by organisms of the genus Pseudomonas. Injections over a period of three to five days usually are necessary to render the urine sterile.

Experience has shown a great change in the efficacy of penicillin in treating most coccal infections of the urinary tract. When used in combination with sulfonamides, most infections with Streptococcus faecalis have been eradicated. Earlier, most infections with staphylococci responded to administration of this preparation. Recently urologists of the entire country are reporting that treatment of infections with staphylococci by administration of penicillin is not satisfactory in approximately 50 per cent of cases in which it is tried. This is because the staphylococci, more than most other organisms, have the ability to develop resistance to a therapeutic preparation and they have done so against penicillin. This is an excellent example of why dogma or rule of thumb is not applicable in management of infections of the urinary tract. The streptococci usually respond very well to administration of penicillin.

Toxic manifestations are minimal but sensitivity to penicillin does occasionally develop following administration of the preparation and rather severe skin reactions have occurred at times. General opinion today is that the substance should not be used promiscuously but only when definitely indicated.

In cases of a fulminating type of urinary infection, or of bacteremia associated with urinary disease, massive doses of penicillin may be indicated. These should be given only if the organism concerned proves to be sensitive to the drug. If massive doses are indicated, intravenous administration of a solution of penicillin by the continuous drip method will allow the giving of 2,000,000 or 3,000,000 units daily.

Aureomycin and Terramycin. These antibiotics will be considered together because their action is much the same. They usually are given orally in divided doses, 250 mg. every six hours, and administration is continued for four to seven days. Their greatest value lies in the treatment of infections attributable to Streptococcus faecalis and Aerobacter aerogenes. These organisms frequently are found to be resistant to sulfonamides and to penicillin, but Aureomycin or Terramycin has proved highly effective in eradicating them. If infections are attributable to organisms of the genus Proteus or of the genus Pseudomonas, Aureomycin or Terramycin rarely is of value.

Symptoms of toxicity following administration of Aureomycin or Terramycin are similar but they are more severe and of more common occurrence with Aureomycin than with Terramycin. Nausea and vomiting attributable to esophagitis or gastritis may prevent administration of Aureomycin or Terramycin for any considerable period of time. More frequently, watery diarrhea from irritation of the bowel requires the stoppage of the administration of these substances.

It seems wise to call attention to a rather severe complication which has developed in a few instances following preoperative administration of these preparations for sterilization of the bowel before surgical procedures. The ordinary flora of the intestinal tract will be reasonably well eradicated by either Aureomycin or Terramycin but eradication of the common inhabitants of the bowel, which normally overlie a number of other organisms, may allow these other organisms to develop to such a degree that they exert a serious effect on the host. A severe form of staphylococcal pseudomembranous colitis may develop and rapidly produce staphylococcal bacteremia.

The condition is usually of a fulminating character but fortunately it does not occur often. Sensitivity studies of the causative organism of this form of colitis are of great interest. The organism is very resistant to either Aureomycin or Terramycin; frequently it is resistant to sulfonamide, penicillin and streptomycin and at present it has been controlled only by administration of erythromycin. A patient whose bowel has been prepared for surgical operation by administration of Aureomycin or Terramycin should be carefully observed for a period of days in order that any evidence of the development of a fulminating infection may be detected.

Achromycin. This antibiotic has essentially the same pharmacologic and bactericidal properties as have Aureomycin and oxytetracycline (Terramycin). The three vary only slightly in chemical formula. Because of its superior solubility and stability, and the decrease in symptoms referable to the gastrointestinal tract after its administration, achromycin may replace its closely related compounds. The dosage is the same as for Aureomycin or oxytetracycline but can be increased to 2.0 gm. daily with few toxic manifestations.

Chloramphenicol (Chloromycetin). Unfortunately, because of the severe toxic reactions which have occurred in a small percentage of cases, general use of this preparation has had to be curtailed. The reaction referred to is aplastic anemia. Usually this has developed after prolonged administration of the preparation but, in some cases, after a relatively small dosage has been given for only a short time. Apparently there are no other toxic reactions.

Nevertheless, chloramphenicol proved to be, among all the antibiotics, perhaps the most effective in management of urinary infections. The preparation is effective in eradicating almost all of the bacillary infections of the urinary tract, except those attributable to organisms of the genus Pseudomonas and occasionally those owing to the genus Proteus. It also is highly effective against most coccal infections, except those attributable to Streptococcus faecalis. The dosage is 1 gm. daily in four divided doses given orally for a period of five to seven days.

Certainly chloramphenicol should not be administered routinely at present but, when studies reveal that the organism causative of the infection at hand is sensitive only to chloramphenicol and the patient is desperately ill, the physician is justified in using the preparation; it may save life and the hematologic complication is not of common occurrence.

Polymyxin. Experience with this antibiotic is extremely limited because danger attends its use. Reports indicate that it is efficient in eradicating infections attributable to organisms of the genus Pseudomonas but its general use has been curtailed because nephrotoxic and neurotoxic symptoms frequently develop following its use. Again, if sensitivity studies reveal that the preparation is the only effective one, and the patient is seriously ill, it is justifiable to administer it. However, the patient should be watched closely and, if urinary outflow decreases, if the number of red blood cells in the urine increases appreciably and if there is evidence that toxic products are being retained in the blood stream, administration of the drug should be stopped. In some instances the neurotoxic signs become of a convulsive nature and should be regarded as a serious complication, necessitating cessation of administration of the drug.

Neomycin. This is another potentially toxic antibiotic which occasionally is of value against infections of the urinary tract. Its general use must be curtailed, however, because at times it causes disturbances of the middle ear similar to those encountered following use of streptomycin. Again its use is indicated only if the patient is seriously ill and studies show this to be the only substance to which the offending organism is sensitive.

Erythromycin. Another of the newer antibiotics is erythromycin. It is given orally and is well tolerated in the majority of cases. Its great importance is that many staphylococci commonly seen in the urinary tract are developing resistance to the other antibiotics. Use of erythromycin is limited to management of infections attributable to gram-positive organisms. The gram-negative organisms usually found in the urinary tract are not responsive to it. Staphylococci are highly susceptible to this drug. Streptococci are also sensitive. The effect on the Streptococcus faecalis as yet has not been determined.

Streptomycin. Streptomycin has been a useful adjunct in the management of urinary infections but its employment in general has been rather limited. In the first place, administration of this antibiotic has not been such as to bring about the desired result in most instances. Most organisms develop resistance to streptomycin within a few days after administration of the drug has been started. Consequently, if safe, small doses are given over several days, resistance may develop before the organism has been eradicated. On the other hand, physicians have feared to give large doses because, somewhat frequently, the preparation has caused disturbances of the middle ear.

However, since dihydrostreptomycin has been in use these untoward side-effects have been at a minimum. This modified preparation need be administered only a short time, moreover, in order to combat any usual type of infection of the urinary tract. Nevertheless, in general, sensitivity studies concerning the effect of this preparation on the particular infection being treated seem indicated, for many of the usually encountered organisms are resistant to streptomycin. There is no consistency as to which organism will respond to it. There seems to be individual variation within particular strains. If the organism is sensitive to the preparation, however, the recommended dosage is 2 gm. daily given intramuscularly in amounts of 1 gm. per injection for two or three days, followed by 1 gm. daily for an additional three or four days.

Streptomycin has been of considerable value when used in combination with the sulfonamides, particularly in treating infections attributable to organisms of the genus Proteus, and recently both experimental and clinical data seem to suggest increased activity when streptomycin is used in combination with penicillin. The synergistic relationship of many of these substances will be discussed later.

Mandelic Acid. This urinary antiseptic is still most useful against many of the simpler infections of the urinary tract. When renal function is normal it can be given with few, if any, toxic reactions and without other danger. Nausea and vomiting do occur but usually can be kept at a minimum if the dosage is reduced during the first twenty-four-hour period in which the drug is administered. Mandelic acid is obtainable in pills or as a liquid. The equivalent of 10 to 12 gm. of mandelic acid should be administered daily by mouth.

The efficacy of this drug depends on its excretion in the urine. Hence, there is need that both kidneys be functioning within normal limits. Not only must the desired concentration of mandelic acid in the urine be obtained but also, to be effective, the acidity of the urine must be below a pH of 5.5. It has been recommended that certain acidifying drugs be administered in conjunction with mandelic acid but this is not usually necessary when the ammonium salt of the acid is used.

Mandelic acid is of great value in treating many bacillary infections of the urinary tract and also those attributable to Streptococcus faecalis. Staphylococcus aureus and the hemolytic staphylococci do not respond to use of this drug.

Intravenously Administered Arsenic. Before the advent of the sulfonamides and the newer antibiotics, intravenous administration of arsenic held a definite place in treatment of many coccal infections of the urinary tract. Its administration still should be considered, however, when an existing coccal infection will not respond to the usual treatment. Mapharsen is the arsenical drug of choice. It is given intravenously in a dose of 0.03 to 0.04 gm., four or five days apart, for three injections. Many times this will prove to be the only urinary antiseptic of any value in a particular case. It is the drug of choice in treating amicrobic pyuria.

Synergy. A synergistic relationship between many of these preparations exists, as has been said. The combination of the sulfonamides with penicillin or streptomycin or the combination of penicillin and streptomycin frequently has brought about sterilization of the urine in the presence of a particularly stubborn infection. Many times organisms of the genus Proteus have been most resistant to all form of treatment, until streptomycin and one or another of the sulfonamides have been given in combination. One cannot generalize, however, and expect increased benefit from the combination of all of them. Experimentally and clinically it has been shown that penicillin in combination with Aureomycin or Terramycin will decrease the activity of both drugs.

THE MOST IMPORTANT CONSIDERATIONS

A thoroughly taken history and proper evaluation of the role which any associated pathologic entity plays in continuing the infection are the first steps when a case of urinary infection is encountered. Next, when possible, a working knowledge should be obtained of the organisms involved and the efficacy of the therapeutic preparations to be used to combat them. Each case must be studied individually. No set program will be efficacious in every instance. No panacea has been discovered which will be effective against all types of infections. Consequently, there is no place for dogmatism or rule of thumb in discussion of this problem.

CHAPTER 2

Tuberculous Infections and Inflammations

of the Urinary Tract

FLETCHER H. COLBY, M.D.

Tuberculosis is a serious disease. Invasion of the urinary tract by the tubercle bacillus is but one phase of a disease that tends to spread to many parts of the body and tuberculosis of the genitourinary tract is a complication of the disease, tuberculosis.

The organ most commonly affected when tuberculosis of the genito-urinary system exists is the kidney. Renal tuberculosis is a blood-borne condition metastatic from some other focus of tuberculosis within the body. Since both kidneys are equally exposed to infection it is only reasonable that at one time, at least, the disease is present as a bilateral condition.

Tuberculosis in any form is best regarded as a systemic disease in spite of the fact that clinical signs and symptoms often suggest the involvement of only one organ or of one system. The association of the urinary and genital tracts is so close that tuberculous infections are likely to involve organs of both systems. Seldom, if ever, is the disease localized to one organ of either the urinary or the genital tract. Renal tuberculosis is a possibility whenever this disease is present anywhere within the body.

With these facts in mind and others presented later, it is evident that the urinary tract manifestations of tuberculosis are those of a disease that is likely to be widespread, serious, and often eventually fatal. An understanding of tuberculosis as a disease, therefore, is necessary in any study of tuberculosis of the urinary tract.

Historical. Tuberculosis has occurred in man from earliest times. The oldest records of this disease are from India thirteen centuries before the Christian era. Tuberculosis was described by the Chinese about six centuries B.C. and by the Greeks in the Hippocratic writings. These early records describe the condition in almost all of its forms. In Europe, in the eighteenth century, tuberculosis was a scourge. Nearly one quarter of the deaths in England at this time were said to be due to "consumption" and one third of the deaths among infants were from some form of scrofula. Although tuberculosis now is far from the affliction it was in the past, even today this disease is a serious problem (Flick, 1925).

Death Rate of Tuberculosis. Little progress was made in the control of tuberculosis until Koch's discovery of the causative organism in 1882.

Since then the mortality of the disease has consistently declined (Weber, 1948a). In 1890, the death rate in the United States for all forms of tuberculosis was 245 per 100,000 of population (Parran, 1947). In 1900, in this country, the death rate was 194.4 and in 1945 it had fallen to 40.1 per 100,000 of population (Pitney and Kasius, 1947). In 1947, the death rate was 33.5, and in 1950, 22.0. This dramatic decline in deaths from tuberculosis is due largely to the establishment of methods of control by individual physicians, and local, State and Federal organizations. There is no evidence that the human strain of the tubercle bacillus has declined in virulence (Weber, 1948a).

Tuberculosis of the respiratory organs is responsible for most of the deaths from this disease. Of the 52,916 deaths from tuberculosis in the United States in 1945, 92.4 per cent were from tuberculosis of the respiratory tract. The death rate for tuberculosis of the genitourinary tract was only 0.3 per 100,000 of population as compared with a death rate of 40.1 for all forms of the disease (Pitney and Kasius, 1947). As the death rate for tuberculosis of all forms has declined there has been a corresponding, and even greater, decline in the death rate of the genitourinary forms of the disease.

Gratifying as these statistics are in suggesting the effectiveness of control measures against tuberculosis, nevertheless, this disease continues to be a serious socio-economic problem in our country. It is said that today we have population groups and geographic areas in which the mortality from tuberculosis exceeds that in other groups and other areas by as large an amount as the tuberculosis death rate at the beginning of the century exceeds the present-day rate.

Susceptibility to Tuberculosis. Susceptibility to tuberculosis varies with color, race, age, sex, and economic conditions. In 1945, in the United States the death rate in non-whites was 102.1 per 100,000 of population as compared to a total death rate of 40.1. The death rate for the Chinese in this country was the highest, 276.1 per 100,000. Among the Indians, it was 211.9 and among the Negroes 98.0. Of the deaths in the non-whites, however, 91.8 per cent occurred in Negroes. Today, among the Negroes, tuberculosis is in fourth place as a cause of death (Weber, 1948b).

Tuberculosis is a disease chiefly of young adults. Deaths from tuberculosis in individuals under twenty years of age were 8.3 per cent, deaths from twenty to forty-four years of age were 44.4 per cent, and deaths at sixty-five years of age or over were 14.1 per cent.

The disease is more frequent in males than females. Males of all ages accounted for 62.2 per cent of the deaths and females 33.1 per cent (Pitney and Kasius).

It is generally agreed that poor economic conditions, overcrowding, overwork and undernourishment, are important factors in increasing susceptibility to tuberculosis.

Control of Tuberculosis. Since tuberculosis has spread to all parts of the world, control measures to be effective must be world wide. In no nation where tuberculosis exists has the disease been known to die out; on the contrary, tuberculosis spreads. Unless tuberculosis is controlled, it has been said that the disease ultimately will be present in nearly the entire population (Myers et al., 1940). A continual warfare, therefore, is necessary to control tuberculosis in man and animals (Colby, 1950).

One of the most effective measures in the control of tuberculosis has been the establishment of sanatoria for the care and segregation of tuberculous patients. The first private sanatorium for this purpose was erected in Ashville, North Carolina in 1825. The first State sanatorium was established by Massachusetts and opened at Rutland in 1898. The first sanatorium for the poor was established by Trudeau at Saranac Lake in 1884 (Paterson, 1947).

The Commonwealth of Massachusetts is one of the few states that has an institution devoted to the care of patients with extrapulmonary tuberculosis. The Lakeville State Sanatorium, about forty miles from Boston, is a three hundred bed hospital which has afforded unusual opportunities to study tuberculosis of the genitourinary organs.

These early sanatoria demonstrated that tuberculosis could be arrested and by the segregation of tuberculous patients they afforded protection to the public. The cost of sanatorium care of tuberculous patients in the United States is nearly $100,000,000 each year (Parran, 1947).

The decline in the mortality of tuberculosis has been attributed chiefly to improvement in living and working conditions. This has increased individual resistance to the disease. As economic conditions improve there follows an improvement in housing and nutrition, shorter hours of work and less physical exhaustion. Better medical care and earlier diagnosis and treatment of tuberculous patients result from an elevation of the standard of living. With improvements in the diagnosis and treatment of tuberculosis there are fewer opportunities for contact infections.

Other factors that have contributed to the decline of tuberculosis are better hygiene, pasteurization, and the segregation of tuberculous patients in hospitals and sanatoria. If the number of infectious hosts is continually reduced, it is thought that the end result, if this continues sufficiently long, will be the extermination of the tubercle bacillus (Rich, 1944).

In spite of the great decrease in total mortality of the disease, however, it is too early to predict the disappearance of tuberculosis. Even in 1940 tuberculosis still was the commonest cause of death between the ages of fifteen and forty-five (Frost, 1947).

Although the mortality rates for tuberculosis in this country declined in a spectacular manner during the past half century, one should not be too complacent over this fact. It is questionable that these figures alone give a fair picture of the actual effectiveness of the control of the disease. While the death rate for tuberculosis in the United States had fallen from 45.8 per 100,000 of population in 1940 to 33.5 per 100,000 of population in 1947, a decline of 27 per cent, *at the same time the registration of new cases rose from 76.4 to 93.3 per* 100,000, *an increase of 22 per cent.* From 1940 to 1947 while the actual number of deaths from tuberculosis fell from 60,428 to 48,064, a decline of 20 per cent, the number of new cases reported rose from 100,772 to 133,837, an increase of 33 per cent (Fig. 282).

Control measures such as extension of hospital facilities, health education, rest, surgery and antibacterial therapy, have reduced the mortality of the disease but have not necessarily prevented the outbreak of new cases of tuberculosis. The death rate of tuberculosis, therefore, may represent a limited and inadequate index of the prevalence of the disease (Edwards and Drolet, 1950).

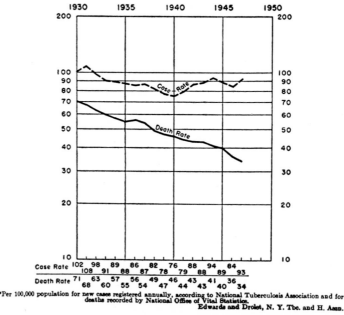

Fig. 282.   A comparison on morbidity and mortality rates* of tuberculosis in the United States, 1930 to 1950. (Reproduced from Am. Rev. Tuberc., 1950.)

The Pathogenesis of Tuberculosis. Tuberculosis is caused by the presence of the tubercle bacillus in the body tissues. The initial lesion is the tubercle. Regardless of the region involved, the tuberculous process is essentially the same. Most infections are from one individual to another or by contact with infected material from persons with open lesions.

Inflammatory exudate, necrosis, and sloughing tissue are prominent features of tuberculosis in man. Sloughing of tuberculous foci and the persistence of necrosis makes the disease relapsing in type and chronic in duration.

In man, tuberculosis is chiefly an air-borne infection of the lungs. The initial lesion is a microscopic focus of lobular pneumonia. By local expansion and necrosis the disease progresses. The discharge of liquefied necrotic material into a bronchus results in cavity formation and allows the bacilli to be spread to other areas. The same process in hilar lymph nodes allows the bacilli to enter the circulation and to be dispersed to other organs. Tuberculosis in other organs is essentially the same as in the lungs with tissue necrosis the most important feature (Edwards and Drolet, 1950).

The Tubercle Bacillus. Tubercle bacilli belong to a large group of bacteria that have a high lipid content and resist decolorization by acids after having been stained by certain of the aniline dyes.

Infections in man are caused by the human and the bovine type of the bacillus. There are no conspicuous morphological differences between these two types of the tubercle bacillus. The differences are cultural and in pathogenesis. The human type of the bacillus is responsible for the great majority of cases of tuberculosis in man. Infection by the bovine bacillus is more common in children than in adults and accounts for most of the instances of tuberculous adenitis. Infections by the human type of the bacillus usually are through the respiratory tract. The gastrointestinal tract is an important route of infection for the bovine type in children (Rich, 1944).

The Formation of a Tubercle. The presence of the tubercle bacillus in tissues causes a tubercle to form. This is the first lesion of tuberculosis. Although the lipid fraction of the bacillus has the power to stimulate the formation of a tubercle, the intact bacillus has a greater power to initiate tubercle formation (Morse and Stott). Koch discovered that the power of the tubercle bacillus to cause the death of tissue and severe constitutional effects depends largely upon the development of a hypersensitivity in the host (Koch).

The presence of tubercle bacilli in the tissues causes first an inflammatory hyperemia. Leukocytes, and particularly lymphocytes, collect at the lesion and tissue cells themselves proliferate. At the periphery of a tubercle is a zone of round cells consisting chiefly of lymphocytes. A zone of larger mononuclear cells, or epithelioid cells, comes next. In the center of the tubercle multinucleated giant cells often are seen (Pottenger). A phagocyte that has ingested a tubercle bacillus becomes transformed into an epithelioid cell and then may become a multinucleated giant cell of the Langhans type. Other mononuclear cells cluster about and become epithelioid cells. This epithelioid cell nodule enlarges progressively. Monocytes also join the cell groups (Rich).

With the formation of a definite tubercle, a network of reticulum fibrils, demonstrable by silver stains, appears between the epithelioid cells. A gradual transition of the reticulum into collagen fibers occurs (Mallory and Parker). Lymphocytes often are present among the epithelioid cells, especially in arrested tubercles. They are most numerous at the periphery of a lesion. If the tubercle bacilli multiply and hypersensitivity develops, the central part of the tubercle becomes necrotic and polymorphonuclear leukocytes enter the tubercle (Rich).

If resistance is high, the tubercle bacilli cease to multiply and are destroyed. There is no further increase in epithelioid cells, the reticulum becomes more dense and there is an increase in collagen. The tubercle becomes more and more fibrous until there is left only a nodule of hyalinized fibrous tissue and the lesion is healed. Healed lesions often are microscopic and may be difficult to detect.

If, however, the bacilli within the tubercle continue to multiply and increase sufficiently in number, they cause death of the cells. Necrosis is seen first in the center of the tubercle where the bacilli are most numerous. As the bacilli multiply, the entire nodule becomes necrotic allowing the bacilli to spread further in the tissues (Rich). Polymorphonuclear leukocytes are attracted to the lesion and an abscess forms. Tubercles may fuse together to form large masses of partly necrotic tissue. If necrotic tissue is discharged to the outside, cavitation or ulceration occurs. If this cannot take place, the tissue disintegrates and assumes a cheese-like consistency called caseation. Giant cells become more numerous and may represent a process of repair. Mononuclear leukocytes and lymphocytes are present in abundance. In more advanced lesions, areas of calcification may be present in a caseous area.

Tuberculosis in man, for the most part, is contracted from individuals who have open tuberculous lesions. The primary focus of tuberculosis in the body usually is in the lungs, tonsils or intestinal tract (Hinman).

Regardless of the manner by which tubercle bacilli gain entrance to the body, eventually they find their way to the lymphatics and usually to the neighboring lymph nodes. For this reason, tuberculosis has been called primarily a lymphatic disease (Pottenger). From its primary focus, tuberculosis spreads to the nearby lymph nodes. When diseased by tuberculosis, the lymph nodes provide a ready method for the entrance of bacilli into the blood stream and their dissemination to other organs of the body. By this method, it is believed, the organs of the genitourinary tract become infected.

When secondary lesions of tuberculosis become evident, the primary focus often has healed or become quiescent. The spread of the disease and its development in other organs such as the genitourinary tract usually is slow (Goldberg).

Sex and Age Incidence of Tuberculosis. The total tuberculosis mortality rate for males is higher than for females but up to puberty and after old age the rates are about the same. At puberty, the total death rate for females rises above that for males and then falls below the death rate for males (Putnam).

Tuberculosis of the genitourinary tract also is more frequent in males than in females. Of 522 cases of genitourinary tuberculosis at the Lakeville State Sanatorium (Massachusetts), 334 were males and 188 were females. This is a ratio of 2:1 in favor of the males.

Genitourinary tuberculosis, as with other forms of tuberculosis, is essentially a disease of young adult life. About 70 per cent of our patients with genitourinary tuberculosis were between the ages of twenty-one and fifty. Fifty-five per cent of the patients were from twenty-one to forty years of age (Fig. 283). In young and elderly patients, the disease was considerably less common. The incidence of genitourinary tuberculosis for patients between the ages of one and ten was 2.5 per cent, and for patients over seventy, the incidence was 1.3 per cent (Colby, 1950). Of 522 cases of genitourinary tuberculosis at Lakeville, twenty-five or 4.8 per cent were under sixteen years of age.

Family History. While a history of exposure to tuberculosis in the family is important information, a great many tuberculous patients give no family history of the disease. Rich found that two thirds of tuberculous patients

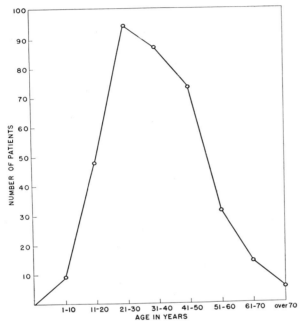

Fig. 283. Age incidence of genitourinary tuberculosis. Lakeville State Sanatorium. (From Colby, F. H., Essential Urology. The Williams and Wilkins Co., Baltimore, 1950.)

came from nontuberculous parents. Seventy-five per cent of our own patients with genitourinary tuberculosis had no family history of the disease (Colby, 1950).

TUBERCULOSIS OF THE KIDNEY

Renal tuberculosis is a metastatic blood-borne infection secondary to a tuberculous focus elsewhere in the body. The tuberculous process within the kidney is similar to that in other organs. With the dramatic decline of all forms of tuberculosis, renal tuberculosis has become considerably less frequent. Nevertheless, tuberculosis is an important renal lesion that is easily mistaken for other less serious conditions. Although many patients who have renal tuberculosis can be cured, the prognosis of the disease is uncertain.

Pathogenesis of Renal Tuberculosis. The method by which the kidneys are invaded by the tubercle bacillus and the pathological histology of early renal lesions of tuberculosis now are well understood. The actual extent of the disease in the kidneys, however, sometimes is impossible to determine. Today, there is a more general appreciation of the fact that renal tuberculosis is a manifestation of a systemic infection by the Mycobacterium tuberculosis.

Infection always reaches the kidney by a hematogenous spread of the bacilli from some other tuberculous lesion. Although a frequent primary focus of the disease is in the lungs, renal infection may be secondary to other tuberculous foci such as the bones and joints or the intestinal tract. From some primary focus, tubercle bacilli spread to the lymphatics and invade a regional lymph node. As a result of softening and necrosis of an infected lymph node, tubercle bacilli readily enter the circulation and are distributed (lymphohematogenous) to the kidneys. Because of the tendency for tubercle bacilli to invade the lymphatic system, tuberculosis has been called primarily a lymphatic disease (Pottenger). When tuberculosis becomes apparent in the kidney, the primary focus of the disease often has healed and is not recognized.

Since renal tuberculosis is a hematogenous infection, the bacilli should be deposited in the vascular system of the kidney. The distribution of the early lesions of tuberculosis is similar to that of other renal hematogenous infections. Early lesions usually are found in the cortex of the kidney, within the capillary tuft of a glomerulus, within capillaries, between the collecting tubules and, at times within the lumen of the tubules (Medlar, 1926). Tiny tubercles form which in some instances heal but which may progress to large areas of tuberculous ulceration and cavitation.

In a careful histological study of the kidneys of patients who died of pulmonary tuberculosis, Medlar found cortical lesions in 75 per cent, medullary lesions in 11 per cent, and corticomedullary lesions in 13 per cent. The most common point of origin was within a glomerulus and the least common in the pyramids. These facts support the vascular origin of renal tuberculosis.

If individual resistance to the tubercle bacillus is high, tubercles within a kidney may heal. Tiny scars representing microscopic areas of tuberculosis were present in many of the kidneys examined by serial section by Medlar. If resistance is low and the individual is unable to overcome the infection, the tuberculous process increases and large portions of the kidney become destroyed by ulceration and necrosis. Tuberculous renal lesions of this extent cannot be expected to heal. Tuberculosis is a chronic disease and the spread of the disease in the kidney usually is slow.

With the dissemination of tubercle bacilli to the kidneys by the blood, it is reasonable to expect that both kidneys receive the infection (Thomas et al., 1941). This is supported by many facts, both clinical and pathological. Histological evidence of bilateral renal disease was present in all of the kidneys of patients who died of pulmonary tuberculosis which were studied by Medlar (1926). Although these patients had no clinical symptoms of renal disease, microscopic areas of tuberculosis were found in the kidneys. Bilateral renal infection was present in 82 per cent of 252 cases of urogenital tuberculosis associated with pulmonary disease reported by Greenberger and Greenberger (1936).

That the lungs are a common primary focus when the genitourinary tract is involved by tuberculosis, is apparent from the fact that 85 per cent of patients who had tuberculosis of the genitourinary system had caseous or cavitating pulmonary foci at postmortem examination. Of patients dying from tuberculosis, caseous or cavitating pulmonary lesions were present in 92 per cent, and tuberculosis of the genitourinary organs was found in 26 per cent (Medlar, 1926).

Clinical statistics, likewise, confirm the frequency of bilateral renal infection. It is not unusual for tuberculosis to become evident in the remaining kidney following nephrectomy although repeated tests and examinations had failed to give any evidence of disease in the apparently normal kidney. This has occurred many times in my experience and shows how inaccurate our methods of evaluation of the extent of renal tuberculosis are likely to be. Disease in the remaining kidney sometimes does not become evident for many years after nephrectomy. In one instance, in my own experience, disease in the remaining kidney only became evident after thirty years of healthy activity following operation.

In 458 cases of renal tuberculosis observed at the Lakeville State Sanatorium, the disease was clinically bilateral in 49 per cent. In 40 per cent, tuberculosis seemed to be limited to one kidney and in 11 per cent we were uncertain as to whether the process was unilateral or bilateral. In ninety-one nephrectomies for tuberculosis, bilateral disease was proven for thirty-five, or 38 per cent, and considered unilateral in fifty-five, or 60 per cent. The status of one patient was not determined.

It is evident from these figures that renal tuberculosis frequently is a bilateral condition. Although clinically the disease often appears to be limited to one kidney, our methods of determining this are inaccurate. In a pathological sense, renal tuberculosis always is bilateral.

Incidence. Although renal tuberculosis is considerably less common than other forms of the disease, especially pulmonary tuberculosis, there is evidence that the kidneys are involved more frequently than has generally been supposed.

At one time, renal tuberculosis was said to account for a third of all surgical renal lesions (Caulk). Today, however, this condition is so infrequent that in large clinics few such patients are seen. With the lowered incidence of all forms of tuberculosis, the renal manifestations of the disease have undergone an even greater decline. Genitourinary forms of tuberculosis now represent a small fraction of the total cases of tuberculosis.

The frequent presence of tubercle bacilli in the urine of patients with other forms of tuberculosis is an indication of the incidence of tuberculous infection of the kidney. Routine urine examinations of sanatorium patients who have various forms of tuberculosis have revealed many unsuspected and symptomless instances of tuberculous disease of the kidneys. Tubercle bacilli were present in the urine of fourteen out of 200 cases of pulmonary tuberculosis observed by Rosencranz. Renal complications in patients with tuberculosis of the bones and joints are more common than in those with pulmonary lesions. Harris reported that the incidence of tuberculous bacilluria in 110 patients suffering from bone and joint tuberculosis was 29 per cent. Genitourinary tract tuberculous lesions were present in 18 per cent of patients who had single bone lesions of tuberculosis and in 32 per cent of those who had multiple bone lesions as reported by McClelland and Davis.

Renal involvement, then, is not an unusual condition in patients who have tuberculosis. Renal lesions occur most frequently in those who have the disease in the bones and joints but this complication also is present in an appreciable number of patients who have pulmonary infections. In many of the patients whose urines on routine examination are found positive for tuberculosis by culture or guinea pig inoculation, there are no clinical symptoms which suggest tuberculous infection of the kidneys. Many times the bacilli disappear from the urine and it must be presumed that small tuberculous foci in the kidney have healed. In others, renal lesions eventually become clinically apparent.

Age and Sex Incidence. The highest incidence of renal tuberculosis is in the years of young adult life. The disease occurs less often in childhood and after middle age.

Seventy per cent of the patients with renal tuberculosis at Lakeville were between the ages of twenty-one and fifty. In patients under twenty-one or over fifty-one years of age the incidence was the same, 13 per cent. Renal tuberculosis seldom was seen in patients who were younger than ten years of age, the incidence being only 2.5 per cent. In elderly patients, likewise, the disease was uncommon. The incidence in patients over seventy years of age was 0.9 per cent. Renal tuberculosis, then, is essentially a disease of youth.

As with other forms of genitourinary tuberculosis, renal tuberculosis occurs more often in men than in women. However, an excess of female over male deaths from all forms of tuberculosis has been said to occur during the ages of five to twenty-four, reaching a maximum between the ages of ten to fourteen when more girls than boys have the disease. The higher mortality in females under twenty-five years of age seems to be associated with the physiological changes which occur at puberty and adolescence (Putnam).

Of 429 cases of renal tuberculosis at the Lakeville State Sanatorium, 254 were males and 175 were females. The ratio of males to females, therefore, is about 2:1.

Tuberculous Bacilluria. It was believed at one time that bacteria could be excreted by a normal kidney and it was thought that tubercle bacilli could be excreted in the urine in the absence of a renal lesion.

This theory, proposed by Cohnheim, is no longer accepted. It is now believed that bacteria do not pass through the kidney by a process of physiological filtration or secretion and that the presence of bacteria in the urine from a kidney indicates the presence of a renal lesion. For tuberculosis, at least, these conflicting points of view were settled by demonstrating that microscopic tuberculous lesions were present in the kidneys of patients who had tubercle bacilli in the kidney urine.

In 1926, Medlar carefully studied the kidneys of thirty patients who had died of active caseating pulmonary tuberculosis. Although none of these patients had clinical evidence of renal tuberculosis, serial sections of their kidneys demonstrated over 300 definite tuberculous lesions, the majority of which contained tubercle bacilli. Scars were present in the kidneys of seventeen of these thirty patients and were interpreted as healed lesions of tuberculosis. Many of the scars were of microscopic size and were detected only by microscopic examination of serial sections.

These studies by Medlar clearly showed that renal tuberculosis, with tuberculous bacilluria, could exist without clinical symptoms and in the

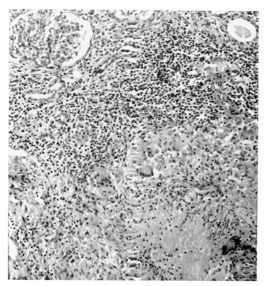

Fig. 284. Renal tuberculosis. Typical tubercle with central caseation, necrosis and surrounding palisades of epithelial cells, Langhans' giant cells and chronic inflammatory infiltrate within the renal cortex. Photomicrograph. Low power.

absence of ulcerating tuberculous lesions in the kidney. It was also demonstrated that small tuberculous lesions in the parenchyma of a kidney could heal. Similar conclusions were reached by Lieberthal and Húth in a study of 1000 cases of renal tuberculosis which had undergone operation. In every one of 240 kidneys whose urines had contained tubercle bacilli, an ulcerated or caseous tuberculous area was found present.

Tuberculous bacilluria frequently has been observed in tuberculous patients who have no clinical evidence of genitourinary tuberculosis (Baggenstoss and Greene, Beach and Shultz, Creevy). The twenty-four hour urines of 287 tuberculous patients were inoculated into guinea pigs by Ordway and Medlar and tubercle bacilli were demonstrated in 7.7 per cent. Most of these patients had no symptoms suggestive of renal tuberculosis. In 300 cases of extra-urogenital tuberculosis studied by Band tuberculous bacilluria was present in 21.3 per cent. These were sanatorium patients who had no clinical signs or symptoms of urinary tuberculosis. The renal lesions evidently healed in many instances, for in 23.4 per cent the tubercle bacilli disappeared from the urine.

When tubercle bacilli are present in the urine of a kidney it is certain that tuberculous lesions are present within the kidney for it appears to be definitely established that tuberculous bacilluria exists only when there is a tuberculous renal lesion, for the normal kidney does not excrete tubercle bacilli.

Pathology. The renal lesions of tuberculosis are similar to those of a tuberculous infection in other organs (Fig. 284). As in other areas, the first lesion is a tubercle. Since the disease is vascular in origin, the earliest lesions are found within or near the blood vessels of the kidney and are most frequent in the renal cortex. The disease progresses by local expansion due to the proliferation of inflammatory exudate and a spread of the bacilli. Necrosis is a feature of the process with liquefaction and sloughing of necrotic material into the pelvis and calyces of the kidney and resulting cavity formation. In these respects, the process is similar to the course of pulmonary tuberculous infections. The essential difference between suppurative tuberculous disease and that caused by other bacteria is that the necrotic tissue of a tuberculous lesion is more difficult to liquify or to become organized by fibrosis (Medlar, 1949). The small microscopic initial lesions within the kidney progress slowly.

The initial tiny tubercles in the kidney may heal leaving the microscopic scars described by Medlar. Healing probably takes place frequently, especially when resistance to the disease is high. If the individual's resistance is low, or for other reasons not understood, the initial tubercles increase in size, necrosis, caseation and liquefaction take place and the bacilli spread to infect new tissue. The vascular distribution of the early lesions of renal tuberculosis already has been described.

Small parenchymal tubercles which have enlarged and become necrotic and broken down, erode into a renal tubule. Tubercle bacilli follow the course of the tubule, and perhaps impelled by the flow of urine or by a process of direct extension of the inflammatory process, they arrive at the surface of a renal papilla. The renal papilla becomes ulcerated and bacilli and leukocytes appear in the urine. The first signs and symptoms of the disease then appear and ulceration of the papilla, if sufficiently large, is the first lesion which can be diagnosed clinically (Lieberthal). These ulcerations tend to progress rather than heal.

Upon reaching the renal pelvis, the tuberculous process spreads. The mucous membrane of the urinary tract is quite susceptible to infection by the tuberculous urine. The mucosa of the renal pelvis and calyces become inflamed. The first lesions of the mucous membrane are isolated tubercles which appear as tiny, pinpoint yellowish raised areas surrounded by a circular zone of red. These small lesions spread and give the surface of the mucous membrane a granular, roughened appearance. The affected areas often are sharply circumscribed with the adjoining mucous membrane normal in appearance.

Tubercles in the mucous membrane eventually caseate, become necrotic and form ulcerations. These tuberculous ulcers have ragged undermined edges. The bases of the ulcerations are covered with gray, necrotic tissue.

At first, the inflammatory process involves only the epithelial layer of the mucous membrane, later there is edema and round cell infiltration of the subepithelial and muscular layers. The tissues then appear thickened and indurated. Ulcerated areas become confluent and the tissues assume a dirty gray moth-eaten appearance.

When the tuberculous process spreads from a renal papilla and affects the calyceal system, the edema, cellular proliferation and fibrosis sometimes are sufficient to obstruct the calyx. That portion of the calyx proximal to the obstruction becomes dilated. Excessive fibrosis and scarring may obliterate one or more calyces. When the same process occurs in the ureter,

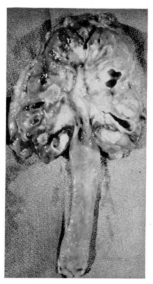

Fig. 285.   Renal tuberculosis. Extensive disease of the kidney and ureter with necrosis and caseation of the renal parenchyma. Gross specimen.

obstruction may take place so rapidly that a hydronephrosis develops which obscures the destructive tuberculous lesions and produces only the picture of a hydronephrosis.

Necrosis is a feature of any tuberculous process. Tubercles in a kidney fuse together and form large masses containing necrotic tissue. If the necrotic tissue can be discharged to the outside through the urinary channels, cavitation or ulceration takes place. When this cannot occur, as in parenchymal lesions with no connection with pelvis or calyces, the tuberculous tissue becomes cheese-like in consistency as areas of caseation. At this stage of the process, giant cells of the Langhans variety become most numerous and are believed to represent repair of the lesion. Mononuclear leukocytes and lymphocytes appear in great numbers.

Many different kinds of lesions may be found in a kidney diseased by tuberculosis; mononuclear tubercles, tuberculous abscesses, caseated areas and scarred areas of fibrosis (Fig. 285). Multiple renal lesions suggest that the kidney may have received showers of tubercle bacilli at intervals.

Areas of calcification often are seen in advanced renal lesions and occasionally the entire kidney becomes a thin walled sac filled with caseous material and lined by extensive calcification (Lieberthal).

An unusual renal lesion caused by tuberculosis is the tuberculoma. This condition easily may be mistaken for a neoplasm of the kidney. Tuberculomas consist of masses of conglomerate tubercles and inflammatory and necrotic tissue which forms a mass in the kidney parenchyma. Microscopically, the lesion has all the characteristics of a tuberculous process with proliferating epithelioid cells, giant cells, lymphocytes and plasma cells. Tubercle bacilli are found in the tubercles (Benjamin and Boyd, Bugbee, Wang and Flaqué).

The rupture of an area of tuberculosis through the capsule of the kidney leads to a tuberculous perirenal abscess.

In summary, the pathological features of renal tuberculosis consist of tubercle formation in the parenchyma of the kidney. The earliest lesions are chiefly in the cortex and have a vascular distribution. Polymorphonuclear leukocytes and especially lymphocytes collect at the lesion. Larger mononuclear cells form a zone about the tubercle which become epithelioid cells. In the center of the tubercle is necrotic tissue often containing multinucleated giant cells of the Langhans type. Tubercles fuse together, necrosis and ulceration occur, and the process involves new areas by direct extension. Eventually, the lesion invades the tubular system of the kidney and a renal papilla becomes diseased and ulcerated. Tubercle bacilli then appear in the urine and infect the urinary tract mucous membrane.

Association with Other Lesions. Multiple lesions in patients with renal tuberculosis are common. They emphasize the fact that the disease often is widespread and serious. Pulmonary, bone and joint lesions and disease of the genital organs most frequently are encountered. Tuberculous lymphadenitis is seen less often than in former years. Other lesions are tuberculous peritonitis and hidden foci in the intestinal tract.

Autopsy statistics have demonstrated pulmonary lesions in the majority of patients with genitourinary tract tuberculosis who died of their disease. Medlar et al. reported that 85 per cent of such patients had caseous or cavitating pulmonary foci. Patients with genitourinary tuberculous lesions also showed a high incidence of miliary tuberculosis. The presence of tubercle bacilli in the urines of patients with pulmonary tuberculosis as an index of renal disease already has been mentioned. Kretschmer (1936) reported that about 72 per cent of patients with tuberculosis in childhood and adolescence had tuberculosis elsewhere; pulmonary involvement was present in 37 per cent and there were bone and joint lesions in 16 per cent.

Renal tuberculosis not infrequently is associated with tuberculosis of the bones and joints. An incidence of tuberculous bacilluria of 29 per cent of these patients was reported by Harris and approximately the same figures were given by McClelland and Davis.

Genital lesions, especially, are frequently associated with renal tuberculosis and most, if not all, are secondary to the renal infection. In a report by Nesbit et al. only 7.1 per cent of patients with genital lesions were free from renal involvement. Many years ago Simmonds found combined renal and genital lesions in 52 per cent of male patients. Lattimer et al. reported that 80 per cent of patients with urinary tuberculosis had other tuberculous foci.

Recent statistics were compiled from the Lakeville State Sanatorium to illustrate the incidence of lesions, other than those of the urinary organs, which were present in patients who had renal tuberculosis. Of 458 patients with renal tuberculosis there were 344, or about 75 per cent, who had

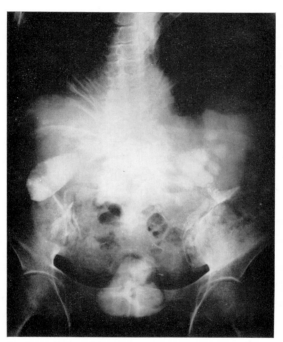

Fig. 286. Renal tuberculosis and tuberculosis of the bones. Unilateral renal disease with tuberculosis of the spine and calcified right sided psoas abscess. Despite the long duration of symptoms, the right kidney showed no evidence of tuberculosis. The diseased left kidney was removed by thoraco-abdominal nephrectomy. Intravenous pyelogram.

tuberculous lesions of organs outside the urinary tract. The genital organs of the male frequently were involved when renal tuberculosis existed in the male. One hundred and thirty-one, or 50 per cent of the 266 male patients who had renal tuberculosis also had the disease in the genital tract.

Evidence of pulmonary infection was found in a considerable number of these patients. One hundred and seventy-three, or about 37 per cent, of our sanatorium patients had x-ray evidence of healed or quiescent pulmonary disease. In many clinics, this percentage of pulmonary infection would doubtless be higher since patients who have active pulmonary tuberculosis are not admitted to Lakeville.

Tuberculous disease of the bones and joints, in our experience, also frequently accompanied renal tuberculosis (Fig. 286). One hundred and sixty, or about 35 per cent, of our patients who had renal tuberculosis also had tuberculosis of the bones and joints. Ninety, or 56 per cent, of them had tuberculosis of the spine. The spine was the most frequent portion of the bony skeleton to be affected when renal tuberculosis was present. In many of our sanatorium patients with tuberculosis of the bones or joints, renal lesions seemed to be a secondary manifestation of the disease and urinary symptoms often were mild or entirely absent.

Other less frequent extra-urinary tract tuberculous lesions were tuberculosis of the lymph nodes (9 per cent) and tuberculous peritonitis (4 per cent).

These data from Lakeville give the incidence of lesions outside the urinary tract associated with renal tuberculosis, and are necessarily lower than similar figures based on autopsy figures since those from the sanatorium are based on clinical evidence. However, they give an approximation of the frequency with which multiple lesions occur whenever urinary tuberculosis is present.

Symptoms. The chief symptom of renal tuberculosis is increased frequency of urination. When frequent urination is associated with discomfort or pain, such symptoms are characteristic of the disease. Hematuria often is an accompanying symptom and this triad of frequency, dysuria and hematuria occur in the majority of patients with renal tuberculosis. Symptoms are likely to be of long duration.

The earliest, and usually the first, symptom is urinary frequency. It is due to an acute diffuse cystitis caused, in all probability, by the presence of the tubercle bacillus since the dramatic relief of vesical symptoms which some patients experience immediately after the removal of a tuberculous kidney is difficult to account for otherwise. When the bladder mucous membrane becomes ulcerated, frequency of urination increases and voiding is painful. The diseased bladder becomes intolerant of the smallest amounts of urine and calls for its evacuation grow increasingly urgent and painful until the unhappy, afflicted individual is miserable by day and has little rest at night. At times, the frequency amounts to incontinence. These are the most distressing symptoms of renal tuberculosis.

Hematuria is a frequent associated symptom and occurs in at least one third of these patients (Kretschmer, 1930). Bleeding may arise from ulcerations in the bladder but more often it comes from the diseased kidney. Blood in the urine may be microscopic in amount but, at times, the urine is grossly bloody. Hematuria almost always is intermittent and seldom is serious enough to require surgical intervention. Although hematuria usually is associated with frequency and dysuria, occasionally bleeding is the only symptom.

Other symptoms that may occur with renal tuberculosis are pain, chills and fever, or nausea and vomiting. Pain usually is in the lumbar region as a dull ache. Severe pain in this area may mean infection of the perirenal tissues. When renal colic occurs, it is caused by the presence of blood clot or calcareous material in the ureter. The pain of tuberculosis of the vertebrae or of a developing psoas abscess may be mistaken for renal pain. Suprapubic pain arises from the diseased bladder.

When chills and fever are present, renal disease is likely to be advanced, as in the development of a tuberculous pyonephrosis or infection of the perirenal tissues. Extension of the inflammatory lesions of the bladder into the perivesical tissues cause a severe systemic reaction with an elevated temperature and chills.

In the late stages of advanced bilateral tuberculosis, nausea and vomiting are evidences of failing renal function and impending uremia.

A tabulation of the chief symptoms of renal tuberculosis as seen in sanatorium patients is given in Table 10 (Colby, 1950).

The most frequent symptoms of tuberculous renal infection in these patients were frequent and painful urinations. Gross hematuria was fairly common. An appreciable number of patients, however, complained of no

Table 10. Symptoms of Renal Tuberculosis

Lakeville State Sanatorium

	PER CENT
Frequency and dysuria	73
Frequency, dysuria and hematuria	38
Renal pain	16
Frequency only	8
Hematuria only	3
Suprapubic pain	2
Chills, nausea and vomiting	1
No symptoms	11

urinary symptoms. For the most part, patients with no symptoms were those who were investigated because of abnormal urinary findings. Advanced renal disease existed in some.

The onset of acute epididymitis has been the initial symptom of genitourinary tuberculosis in a significant number of patients. Its sudden onset often suggests pyogenic rather than tuberculous infection. Thorough investigation of such patients reveals renal lesions in the majority (Wells, 1943). Acute epididymitis was the initial symptom in 20 per cent of our patients.

Diagnosis. The diagnosis of renal tuberculosis depends upon identification of tubercle bacilli in the urine from a suspected kidney. Histological examination of diseased tissue may strongly suggest tuberculosis but lesions of other conditions sometimes have similar characteristics.

Tubercle bacilli are found in stained smears of the urinary sediment or are detected by culture or by guinea pig inoculation. If the urine is heavily infected with the organisms, stained smears may be satisfactory but their accuracy depends upon a long, patient, persistent search. More dependence is placed upon cultures and guinea pig inoculation. Cultures have the advantage of an early method of diagnosis since cultures may be positive within a period of two weeks and so shorten the waiting period of six weeks or more before reports from animal inoculation are considered reliable. Cultural technique has improved in recent years and this test is thought by some to rival the guinea pig in accuracy. However, it is my opinion that animal inoculation is the most accurate test for tuberculosis. The diagnosis of renal tuberculosis is not always an easy one and repeated laboratory and clinical tests may be necessary before it is established.

Renal tuberculosis should be suspected in any individual with urinary symptoms or persistent pyuria who has active tuberculosis elsewhere in the body or who has been treated in the past for a tuberculous infection. The progress of the disease is slow and years may elapse between the initial infection and any evidence of renal disease. Any patient with a persistent pyuria which does not respond quickly to our efficient present methods of treatment, may have renal tuberculosis. If the purulent urine is acid, and sterile on culture for ordinary pyogenic organisms, the likelihood of tuberculosis is increased (Rohrer, 1940). The presence of organisms other than M. tuberculosis in the urine, however, does not exclude tuberculosis since secondary infections occur in from one third to one half of patients with renal tuberculosis (Alkorn and Buchtel, Corbitt, Kretschmer, 1930, Nesbit et al.).

Most patients with renal tuberculosis have positive tuberculin tests. When used in proper dilutions, the skin tuberculin test has always been positive in such cases, in my experience. Negative tests in adults are infrequent, although perhaps more frequent than formerly, and are an evidence of lack of exposure to the disease or an overwhelming infection. All the patients I have seen with renal tuberculosis have had positive tuberculin tests.

In our sanatorium patients, a sign of early renal tuberculosis has been the appearance of albumin in the urine. This has been noticed particularly among those who have tuberculosis of the bones. When the charted urine reports began to show small amounts of albumin in the urine and the urines were inoculated into guinea pigs, an appreciable number were reported positive for tuberculosis although urinary symptoms were lacking and blood or pus was either absent or present in insignificant amounts. We, therefore, came to regard the presence of albuminuria as a possible indication of early renal tuberculous infection.

Cystoscopic and *roentgen examination* aid in the confirmation of a diagnosis of tuberculous renal infection and help determine the extent of the disease. Inspection of the bladder may at once show that the vesical symptoms are caused by lesions other than tuberculosis such as interstitial cystitis, neoplasm, or other conditions. At times, however, the appearance of the bladder leads to no other reasonable diagnosis than tuberculosis because of the presence of submucous tubercles or extensive areas of ulceration. A bladder diseased by tuberculosis is notoriously intolerant of any irrigating solution, or even urine, and is exquisitely sensitive. Cystoscopic examination, however, gives one evidence which leads only to a presumptive diagnosis of tuberculosis and catheterization of the ureters and pyelography are necessary. Specimens of urine from each kidney then are available for examination to see if they contain leukocytes or tubercle bacilli.

Intravenous urography is of considerable value in the study of patients suspected of having renal tuberculosis. Since renal function usually is well preserved, except in instances of advanced disease, this procedure may well

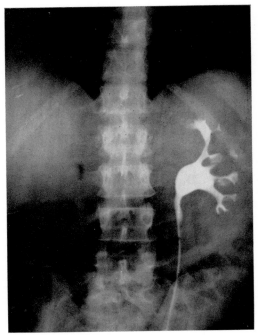

Fig. 287.   Early renal tuberculosis. Irregular filling of the upper calyx of the left kidney. The outline of the calyx has a vague, fuzzy appearance due to tuberculous ulceration as contrasted with the clear outline of the other calyces. Retrograde pyelogram.

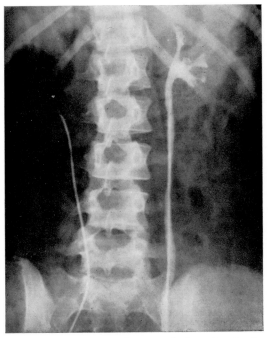

Fig. 288.   Early renal tuberculosis. Small areas of ulceration in the upper and lower calyces of the left kidney. Retrograde pyelogram.

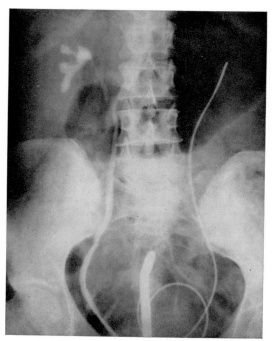

Fig. 289.   Renal tuberculosis. The upper calyx of the right kidney is obliterated by tuber-culosis. Retrograde pyelogram.

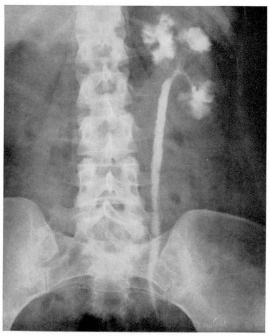

Fig. 290.   Renal tuberculosis. Extensive disease with ulceration and necrosis of all the calyces of the left kidney. Retrograde pyelogram.

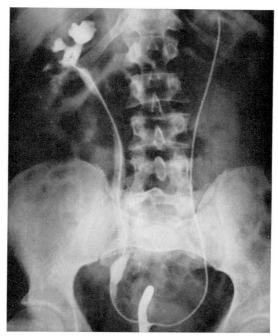

Fig. 291.   Renal tuberculosis. Extensive ulcerating disease of the lower portion of the right kidney with dilatation of the ureter. Retrograde pyelogram.

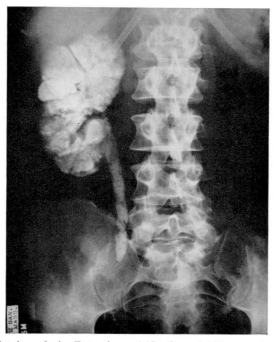

Fig. 292.   Renal tuberculosis. Extensive calcification of kidney and ureter. Plain film. (From Colby, F. H., Essential Urology, The Williams and Wilkins Co., Baltimore, 1950.)

visualize areas of disease in a tuberculous kidney. As a test of renal function, intravenous urography has merit, particularly in demonstrating the presence of a functionless kidney.

More accurate information, however, usually is obtained by retrograde pyelography. There should be no hesitation in employing this procedure when so much depends upon an accurate diagnosis and an appraisal of the extent of the disease. The risks involved usually are overweighed by the information obtained.

Renal lesions of tuberculosis visualized by roentgen examination are chiefly those of the calyces and pelvis. Early lesions appear as areas of irregular filling such as slight irregularities, fuzziness of outline, incomplete filling or slight dilatation (Figs. 287, 288). When the lesions are more advanced, gross alterations in the normal architecture of the kidney become apparent. Portions of the collecting system are obliterated or a calyx communicates with a large abscess cavity within the renal substance (Figs. 289, 290). Since other lesions may give the same pyelographic appearance as tuberculosis, perhaps no deformity can be considered characteristic of the disease. Large areas of tuberculous destruction may be present in the parenchyma of a kidney which have no connection with the pelvis or calyces and which cause no detectable deformity (Fig. 291). A normal pyelogram, therefore, does not exclude the possibility of tuberculosis (Braasch and Olson, Taylor).

A diagnosis of renal tuberculosis, then, is based upon the presence of tubercle bacilli in the urine. Long-standing symptoms and chronic pyuria suggest the disease. Cystoscopic examination and roentgen visualization aid in localizing the lesions and determining their extent (Fig. 292).

Treatment. Renal tuberculosis is one manifestation of a systemic infection and intelligent treatment is based upon this fact. The removal of a tuberculous kidney does not cure the disease. Remaining areas of tuberculosis are healed or arrested by the individual's powers of resistance. As in other forms of the disease, every effort should be made to increase individual resistance to tuberculosis. Generally this is accomplished best in a sanatorium (Colby, 1940; Joly; Thomas et al.).

Not many years ago, preoperative and postoperative care was not seriously considered in the management of patients with renal tuberculosis. Eighteen years ago, when I was appointed consultant at our State institution for patients with extrapulmonary tuberculosis, renal tuberculosis was a surgical condition and nephrectomy was performed as soon as the diagnosis was established. The patient was returned to full activity as soon as possible. In the first year, under this regimen, we had a postoperative death following nephrectomy. With the realization that patients with renal tuberculosis should have periods of preoperative and postoperative care, this was changed and during the past eighteen years there have been no postoperative nephrectomy deaths. Institutions for the care of patients with extrapulmonary tuberculosis are few and other sections of our country would do well to follow the lead of the Commonwealth of Massachusetts.

Seldom is there any hurry about operating upon patients with renal tuberculosis. The disease is slowly progressive, widespread and serious. By preoperative rest and routine care, most patients improve. During a two months or longer period of preliminary care, resistance increases, symptoms abate, and the patient is better able to withstand operation. Although our methods of measuring resistance are not accurate, information in this regard can be obtained during a period of observation. Patients who develop new tuberculous lesions under sanatorium care or who do poorly generally seldom are suitable for surgery. After operation, sanatorium care is continued for several months.

When renal tuberculosis is clinically unilateral and disease is demonstrable by pyelograms, nephrectomy is indicated. There is little evidence that such lesions heal even under the most recent therapy. If no pyelographic deformity is present, operation is not advised, although tubercle bacilli be present in the kidney urine. Such patients are kept under observation to determine whether their lesions heal or progress.

Most patients who are operated upon have clinically unilateral tuberculosis. There are times, however, when it is justifiable to operate on patients who have known bilateral infection. If the disease is considerably more advanced in one kidney than in the other and symptoms are severe, a great deal of benefit may be derived by removal of the badly diseased kidney. Such a procedure seems justified today when the better kidney excretes tubercle bacilli in the absence of any pyelographic deformity.

Uncontrollable bleeding, or excessive pain, may necessitate nephrectomy in bilateral renal disease. When one kidney is removed and there is disease in its mate, there is no evidence that the lesions in the remaining kidney improve following operation. While the results of nephrectomy in bilateral disease are not equal to those when the opposite kidney appears healthy, many such patients have lived more comfortably and for many years after operation. If one kidney is completely calcified, no bladder symptoms are present, and the urine is normal, it may be presumed that the disease has healed (Fig. 292). Operation, then, is unnecessary.

Cutaneous ureterostomy has been performed in many patients who have renal tuberculosis. This procedure is reserved for patients who have advancing tuberculous lesions in the kidney remaining after nephrectomy and who have severe symptoms. Occasionally, it is indicated in the presence of advanced bilateral renal disease. Diversion of the urine to the skin is an irreversible procedure and before it is done the patient should not only be fully appraised of its disadvantages but should be eager to have it performed (Fig. 293). Skin ureterostomy has made many patients comfortable after years of suffering and has added years to their lives by slowing down renal destruction especially in the presence of ureteral obstruction. Cutaneous ureterostomy is preferable to nephrostomy or ureterosigmoidostomy in renal tuberculosis (Colby, 1941).

In 1944 a substance was developed that has been extensively used in the treatment of tuberculosis. The first published report on streptomycin by Schatz and Waksman stated that this agent had a marked bacteriostatic and bactericidal effect in vitro against a human strain of M. tuberculosis. This has been confirmed in subsequent years. Streptomycin was found to be well tolerated in guinea pigs and exerted a striking suppressive effect on the pathologic proclivities of the human tubercle bacillus (Feldman and Hinshaw, 1941). On well-established tuberculosis in guinea pigs, streptomycin showed unprecedented therapeutic effects (Riggins and Hinshaw).

In man, streptomycin seems to lessen or prevent the multiplication of tubercle bacilli in tuberculous lesions. Usually this suppressive effect is of limited duration and resistant bacilli appear that fail to yield to streptomycin

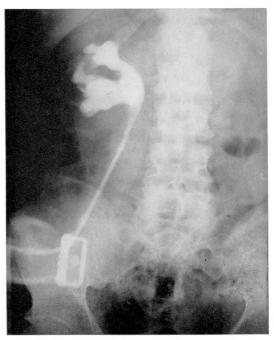

Fig. 293. Renal tuberculosis. Cutaneous ureterostomy. The left kidney had been previously removed for tuberculosis. Distressing symptoms and progressive renal damage in the remaining kidney made skin ureterostomy advisable. Retrograde pyelogram.

therapy (Feldman et al., 1948). During its effective action, streptomycin was found to improve symptoms and to have considerable effect on certain tuberculous lesions. In cases of early miliary tuberculosis and tuberculous meningitis, streptomycin therapy is considered mandatory.

Less encouraging results have been obtained by streptomycin in renal tuberculosis. Renal lesions visible in pyelograms have remained essentially unchanged although tubercle bacilli have disappeared from the urine in over 80 per cent of cases during treatment. Relapses, however, frequently occur (Lattimer et al.; Streptomycin Committee). Streptomycin is of no lasting benefit in advanced destructive lesions of the kidney although temporary improvement often takes place and symptoms often are improved.

It appears evident that although streptomycin is the first drug which has shown promising results in the treatment of tuberculosis in man, nevertheless, its value is limited. Toxic effects arise from prolonged administration, most often disturbances of hearing and equilibrium. Streptomycin alone cannot be counted upon to cure tuberculosis. Relapse rates in treated cases have been high and mortality rates for different forms of tuberculosis over a two to three years period have been from 21 to 67 per cent. The best results in the treatment of renal tuberculosis have been in healing bladder lesions after nephrectomy and in the healing of minimal lesions in kidneys which show no gross pyelographic defects (Nesbit and Bohne, 1948). Streptomycin therapy should be regarded as an aid in the treatment of tuberculosis and should be combined with other agents, such as surgery, in our efforts to cure the disease.

When tubercle bacilli become resistant to streptomycin the effectiveness of the drug is reduced. Para-aminosalicylic acid (PAS) prevents or greatly retards the in vitro emergence of streptomycin resistant bacilli and possibly improves the therapeutic effects (Graessle and Pietrowski; Lehman; Riggins and Gearheart). This drug is of relatively low toxicity in man and its use is advised in combination with streptomycin (Bogen et al.; Carstensen; Dooneief et al.). Before, during and after streptomycin treatment, it should be determined whether or not the tubercle bacilli isolated from a patient are streptomycin-sensitive or resistant (Steenken).

Patients who are in a sanatorium usually have been given streptomycin, gm. 0.5, intramuscularly twice daily. Twelve grams of para-aminosalicylic acid are given by mouth each day in divided doses of 4 gm. each. Many patients are unable to take this amount of para-aminosalicylic acid at first so the dose may range from 6 to 12 gm. It is believed that treatment should continue after leaving the sanatorium for an indefinite period of time, particularly if there is the slightest evidence of an active or dormant tuberculous lesion. Patients at home are advised to continue treatment with 1 gm. of streptomycin twice weekly and para-aminosalicylic acid each day.

Isoniazid (isonicotinic acid hydrazide) is a more recent agent that has been used in the treatment of tuberculosis. This drug has been found to possess a high degree of antituberculous activity. It should be used in combination with other antituberculous drugs since the tubercle bacillus acquires a resistance to isoniazid when used alone. Isoniazid is available under several trade names. The recommended dose is 3 to 5 mg. per kg. of body weight divided into two or three doses. The average adult dose is 150 to 300 mg. three times daily. At Lakeville most patients receive 100 mg. t.i.d. in addition to streptomycin and PAS. Toxic reactions to isoniazid have been few. Only about 0.5 per cent of patients have had reactions of any sort and fatal reactions are reported as extremely rare. The nervous system most often is affected with muscular twitching, restlessness and exaggerated reflexes. Psychoses have been reported. Allergic reactions occasionally occur. Most reactions subside when the drug is stopped. Contraindications are severe renal damage and unstable mental states. The results of isoniazid in the treatment of urinary tract tuberculosis are still to be evaluated.

Prognosis. The outlook for patients with renal tuberculosis is uncertain. The extent of the disease is difficult to determine and the integrity of the remaining kidney after nephrectomy is doubtful. Disease in the supposedly healthy kidney may take many years to become apparent. A patient with tuberculosis requires many months of treatment. In spite of an uncertain future, many patients with renal tuberculosis eventually are cured and have no further symptoms of tuberculosis. Prognosis depends upon the extent of the infection, ability to acquire resistance, and proper treatment. Life expectation for patients with renal tuberculosis is considerably better when there is no clinical evidence of bilateral renal disease.

Statistics from many sources appear to indicate that the five-year survival rate for patients with renal tuberculosis is about 50 per cent. Wildbolz in 1929 reported that 59 per cent of patients were cured after nephrectomy; most of the others died of tuberculosis. A total of 1380 cases in three reports indicated that about 50 per cent of the patients were alive five years after operation (Emmett and Kibler; Nesbit et al.). Best results were obtained when the opposite kidney was free from evidences of infection and in patients who had little or no cystitis. Severe cystitis was considered a poor prognostic sign. Nesbit et al. reported a mortality of 0.82 per cent in 153 nephrectomies and a survival rate of 50.3 per cent eleven years after operation. When no tubercle bacilli were present in the opposite kidney 71 per cent of the patients survived for ten years. Emmett and Kibler reported that if the urine from the "good" kidney was negative for tuberculosis on guinea pig inoculation the chance of death was 13.3 per cent and the chance of cure was 50.3 per cent.

When tubercle bacilli are found present in both kidneys the prognosis is definitely worse. Forty per cent of such patients in Nesbit's series survived 8.2 years and 60 per cent had died. The chance of dying within five years under these circumstances has been given as 41.8 per cent with the possibility of cure 21.8 per cent (Emmett and Kibler, 1938). The rising mortality of bilateral renal tuberculosis with the passage of years is apparent from the statistics of Braasch and Sutton. In 167 cases of bilateral renal tuberculosis with no operation the survival rate of patients traced three years or more was 72 per cent, for five years or more it was 58 per cent, for ten years or more 26 per cent, and for fifteen years was 16 per cent.

One's own experiences are more valuable to him than those of others.

All patients with renal tuberculosis at the Lakeville State Sanatorium have been personally studied and operated upon. These patients have had the advantage of preoperative and postoperative care in an institution devoted to the care of cases of extrapulmonary tuberculosis. Operations are performed under the favorable circumstances provided by the Massachusetts General Hospital. Under these conditions ninety-one nephrectomies for tuberculosis have been performed, fifty-five in patients who had clinically unilateral renal tuberculosis and thirty-five on those in whom we knew the disease was present in both kidneys.

To determine the five-year results, statistics were collected concerning those patients who were operated upon before 1946. During these years, 118 patients with renal tuberculosis were available for comparative study. In fifty-eight patients nephrectomies were performed. Sixty patients with known bilateral disease were not operated upon.

In the fifty-eight nephrectomies, the disease was clinically unilateral in thirty-three patients or 57 per cent. Ninety-four per cent of these patients were alive five or more years after operation and the average duration of life has been nine years. Two, or 6 per cent, have died of tuberculosis. Not all of the survivors are free of disease, however, for tuberculosis in the remaining kidney has become evident in some.

In twenty-five, or 43 per cent, of those patients who had one kidney removed, there was evidence of bilateral renal disease, either the urines were positive on guinea pig inoculation with no pyelographic defect or there were positive urines with obvious renal lesions. Three, or 12 per cent, of these patients died within two years, eleven, or 44 per cent lived over five years and four or 16 per cent lived for over ten years. The average survival rate after operation was about six and one-half years.

Contrast these figures for patients with known bilateral renal disease who were operated upon and sixty cases of bilateral disease seen before 1946 who were not operated upon. Twenty-seven or 45 per cent, of the patients not operated upon who had bilateral disease died within two years or less. Seventy-five per cent died within five years. Fifteen, or 25 per cent, lived over five years and three, or 5 per cent, lived over ten years.

These statistics indicate that the prognosis after nephrectomy for patients under sanatorium care is good when the disease clinically is limited to one kidney and definitely worse when both kidneys are involved. There appears to be some advantage in the removal of a badly diseased kidney when it is known that the other kidney is infected although such a procedure is advised only after careful consideration and with clear indications.

Cutaneous ureterostomy was performed in thirty patients. Almost always, this operation was done on patients who had advanced and progressive disease in the remaining kidney after nephrectomy. The average length of life after skin ureterostomy was three and one-half years. Nine patients lived for over five years. The longest survival after this procedure was thirteen years.

Although renal tuberculosis is a serious condition, the chance of cure by proper treatment is good when there is no evidence of bilateral disease. When both kidneys are infected by the tubercle bacillus, the expectation of life is limited although some individuals survive for many years. Modern chemotherapeutic agents are of great help in the treatment of renal tuberculosis; they supplement surgery and make surgery safer.

TUBERCULOSIS OF THE URETER

The mucous membrane of the urinary tract is very susceptible to infection by the tubercle bacillus and the mucosa of the ureter is no exception. When renal tuberculosis is present, the ureter probably always is affected to some extent. Tuberculosis of the ureter may result in stricture formation with sufficient narrowing of the ureteral lumen to impede the free flow of urine, hydronephrosis develops, and renal destruction then is accelerated. The ureter, diseased by tuberculosis, always tends to stricture. Sometimes, the lower portion of the ureter becomes narrowed by fibrosis and thickening of the bladder wall when tuberculous cystitis has been severe and of long duration.

Pathology. The first changes in the ureter from tuberculosis are inflammatory. Diffuse inflammation of the mucous surface with leukocytic infiltration is the earliest change. At first, the process is limited to the epithelial layer but gradually the submucosa is involved. Isolated tubercles then appear as small nodules which project above the mucosal surface (Fig. 294). They have yellow centers and are surrounded by a narrow, red zone. As the lesion spreads, tubercles fuse together, caseate and break down to form sloughing areas of ulceration. The mucous membrane appears roughened and granular. Gradually, the submucosal and muscular layers are affected by edema, round cell infiltration and tubercle formation. Even the peri-

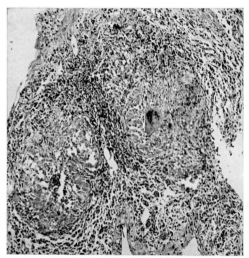

Fig. 294. Tuberculosis of the ureter. Two large tubercles within the submucosa associated with edema of the wall of the ureter and crypt-like ulceration of the mucous membrane. Photomicrograph. Low power.

ureteral tissues may become diseased. The wall of the ureter thickens from inflammatory changes and fibrosis and has the appearance of an indurated, firm cord. As disease in the ureter progresses, the ureter loses its elasticity, the muscular coats are destroyed and the organ becomes a shortened, cordlike structure which retracts the entrance of the ureter into the bladder giving the uretero-vesical orifice a gaping or "golf-hole" appearance.

Encircling tuberculous lesions in the wall of the ureter, with scar tissue formation, narrow the lumen and produce strictures. These strictures are particularly dense and resistant to dilatation. Stricture formation with obstruction to the urine may take place so rapidly that the developing hydronephrosis obscures the tuberculous process in the kidney. Occasionally, the ureter becomes thin walled and very much dilated and tortuous (Lieberthal; Moore).

Symptoms. Since tuberculosis of the ureter is secondary to renal tuberculosis, symptoms are chiefly those of the diseased kidney. Extensive ureteral lesions with stricture formation and obstruction cause lumbar pain due to urinary retention.

Persistent urinary symptoms after nephrectomy often are thought to be due to disease in the remaining portions of the ureter. In my experience, this occurs much less frequently in tuberculosis than in severe pyogenic infections. In several instances in which the retained ureter has been accused of causing persistent urinary symptoms, this structure has been removed and has been found to be a thin, fibrous cord devoid of any evidence of active tuberculosis.

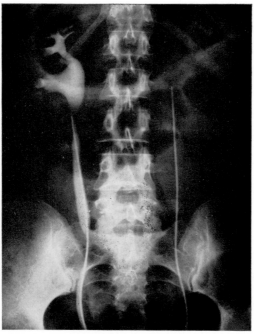

Fig. 295. Tuberculosis of the ureter. Renal tuberculosis with disease at the ureteropelvic junction. There is early ulceration of the upper calyx of the right kidney and the ureter is narrowed where it joins the renal pelvis. Retrograde pyelogram.

Obstruction of the lower portion of the ureter sometimes occurs in patients who have had a kidney removed, particularly when cystitis has been severe and prolonged. After cutaneous ureterostomy, because of progressive dilatation and damage to the remaining kidney, sometimes no tubercle bacilli can be detected in the kidney urine. In such cases it would seem that the severe inflammatory changes and fibrosis in the diseased bladder had resulted in damage and stricture of the pelvic portion of the ureter and that the active tuberculous process had healed.

Diagnosis. Early tuberculosis of the ureter often is most evident at the ureteropelvic junction (Fig. 295). When the tuberculous kidney is exposed at operation, the organ may appear grossly normal to examination but the ureter, at the ureteropelvic junction, feels thickened. This is an encouraging sign to the surgeon that renal tuberculosis is present.

Narrowing of the ureter in early renal tuberculosis may be detected through roentgen visualization of the ureter by intravenous or by retrograde methods (Fig. 296). More advanced ureteral disease appears as irregular areas of dilatation and constriction of the lumen of the ureter. The cystoscopic appearance of the "golf hole" ureteral orifice is characteristic of advanced tuberculosis of the ureter.

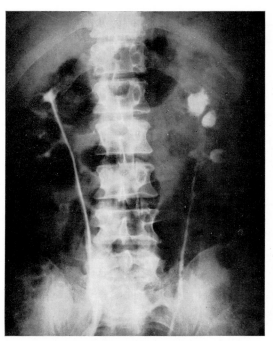

Fig. 296.   Tuberculosis of the kidney and ureter. There is extensive destruction of the renal parenchyma. The ureter is shortened and ulcerated. Retrograde pyelogram.

Treatment. After removal of the infected kidney, most tuberculous lesions of the ureter heal. If the ureter is extensively diseased, the entire ureter should be removed when nephrectomy is performed. Treatment of the ureter at the time of nephrectomy has seldom been a problem in our sanatorium patients. With adequate preoperative and postoperative care, persistent sinuses after nephrectomy have been uncommon. In most of our cases the cut end of the ureter simply has been carbolized and ligated. Early tuberculous ureteral lesions may be benefited by streptomycin therapy but in advanced lesions little help can be expected from chemotherapy. It has been reported that there is a greater tendency for the tuberculous ureter to become strictured as a result of streptomycin therapy. Whether this is true or not, I am not prepared to say but it has not been observed in our sanatorium patients.

TUBERCULOSIS OF THE BLADDER

The bladder is the sentinel which announces the presence of tuberculosis in the kidney. Tuberculosis of the bladder always is secondary to some other focus of the disease and the source of infection usually is the kidney. In the male, however, the bladder may become infected from a genital lesion when the kidneys show no demonstrable tuberculous disease. Direct extension of a tuberculous process in the female pelvic organs to the bladder, also is possible. The extent of vesical involvement in renal tuberculosis is variable and probably depends upon the virulence of the infection and the individual's resistance to the tubercle bacillus. In some instances of early renal tuberculosis, bladder symptoms are severe and inflammatory changes in the vesical mucous membrane are extensive. In other instances of advanced renal disease, bladder symptoms are lacking and the vesical mucous membrane is normal in appearance.

Tuberculous lesions in the bladder usually heal after the source of infection, such as a diseased kidney, has been removed. The process of healing, however, often is prolonged. Renal lesions of long standing may result in permanent damage to the bladder wall with irreversible changes caused by deep ulcerations and extensive fibrosis.

Pathology. Vesical lesions of tuberculosis are similar to those of other mucous membrane surfaces of the urinary tract. The presence of the tubercle bacillus in the bladder causes at first a diffuse inflammation with edema and hyperemia. Tubercle formation follows. The appearance of tubercles on the mucosal surface is characteristic of the disease. Inflammatory changes and tubercle formation often are most marked in the region of the ureteral orifice which leads to the infected kidney.

As the disease progresses in the bladder, tubercles coalesce, caseate and break down and ragged areas of ulceration appear. These ulcerations have irregular, undermined edges, often well circumscribed from adjoining normal appearing mucous membrane. The base of the ulcers is covered with dirty, gray, necrotic material. These areas bleed easily and are exquisitely sensitive.

Tuberculous cystitis of long duration results in a shrunken, inelastic bladder whose wall is thickened, fibrotic and irretrievably damaged (Fig. 297).

Tuberculomas, similar to those in the kidney, may form in the bladder. These solid tumors are easily mistaken for neoplasms.

Symptoms. The bladder diseased by tuberculosis is extremely irritable and tolerates poorly the presence of any urine. Excessive vesical irritability is characteristic of tuberculosis. Bladder symptoms, however, occur in pyogenic infections although they usually disappear under modern treatment while those due to tuberculosis are unaffected by ordinary drugs. Suprapubic pain or discomfort is a common complaint.

Urination in tuberculosis becomes more and more frequent and more and more painful. The unfortunate sufferer has no peace by day and little rest at night. Symptoms may be so severe, and the bladder so intolerant, that urinary incontinence occurs. The contractions of the bladder, inflamed by tuberculosis, in its efforts to expel the last few drops of urine are especially distressing.

Spontaneous rupture of the tuberculous bladder occasionally occurs.

Diagnosis. Persistent cystitis with pyuria and a urine sterile for pyogenic organisms, suggests tuberculosis. Other lesions such as interstitial cystitis.

amicrobic pyuria or Reiter's syndrome may simulate tuberculous cystitis so
that, at times, the presence or absence of the tubercle bacillus in the urine
is the deciding test before an accurate diagnosis can be made.

Cystoscopic examination often aids in the diagnosis of vesical tuberculosis.
In early cases, the bladder is diffusely red and extremely sensitive. Bladder
capacity is small because the bladder is intolerant of any irrigating solution.
If tubercles are present in the mucous membrane, a diagnosis of tuberculosis

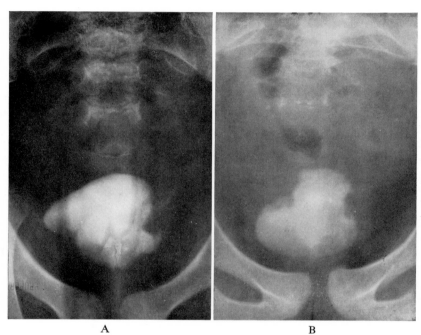

A   B

Fig. 297. Vesical tuberculosis, cystographically demonstrated. *A*, pronounced vesical
irregularity in a three-year-old girl with right renal tuberculosis. *B*, irregular but somewhat symmetrical contracture of the bladder in a nine-year-old boy with tuberculosis of
the left kidney, prostate, and left seminal vesicle, vas deferens and epididymides. (Bellevue
Hospital.) In each of these patients ureteronephrectomy was performed.

is obvious. Ulcerated areas in the bladder strongly suggest tuberculosis although ulcerations occur in pyogenic infections. Neoplasms of the bladder
sometimes appear as shallow ulcers, similar to a tuberculous lesion, and
are differentiated only by biopsy.

The determining factor in the diagnosis of tuberculosis of the bladder is
the isolation and identification of the tubercle bacillus.

Treatment. Many drugs and solutions have been used to treat tuberculous
cystitis. Most of them have little value. Local treatment of the condition has
been generally unsatisfactory. Removal of the source of infection, usually a
diseased kidney, is the most effective treatment.

After nephrectomy, the vesical lesions of tuberculosis usually heal fairly
rapidly. Sometimes, there is prompt relief of bladder symptoms immediately
after nephrectomy. At times, however, tuberculous lesions in the bladder

are slow to heal or disappear and many months may elapse before the patient is again comfortable. Persistent, severe bladder symptoms after nephrectomy suggest tuberculosis in the remaining kidney or extensive disease of the bladder itself.

The vesical lesions of tuberculosis have responded well to streptomycin therapy provided the lesions have not been deep-seated and fibrotic.

TUBERCULOSIS OF THE URETHRA

The urethra seems to have considerable resistance to the tubercle bacillus since instances of tuberculosis of the urethra are uncommon. In spite of the fact that the urethra is continually exposed to infection in the presence of renal or genital tuberculosis, severe urethral infections seldom are encountered. The female urethra is less likely to become diseased by tuberculosis than the male urethra. Severe disease of the urethra becomes evident from stricture formation. Tuberculous strictures resist all forms of treatment.

Pathology. The first lesions of tuberculosis of the urethra are small tubercles just beneath the epithelial surface. As in other areas, tubercles enlarge, coalesce and become ulcerated. The deeper layers of the urethra become involved and dense scar tissue forms which contracts and narrows the lumen of the urethra (Walker).

Symptoms. There are no symptoms from tuberculosis of the urethra until stricture formation takes place. The symptoms then are the usual ones of this condition.

Treatment. Tuberculous strictures of the urethra are notoriously difficult to treat. They are difficult to dilate and after dilatation rapidly tend to close down. Periodic dilatations, however, may be helpful. Dense, impossible strictures or those not helped by dilatation may require diversion of the urine by cutaneous ureterostomy or suprapubic cystotomy.

REFERENCES

ALKORN, K. A. and BUCHTEL, H. A.: The urine in renal tuberculosis; its reaction and associated bacteria. J. Urol., *39:*376–382, 1938.
BAGGENSTOSS, A. H. and GREENE, L. F.: Healed tuberculosis of the kidney. J. Urol., *45:* 165–175, 1941.
BAND, D.: Healed microscopic foci of tuberculosis in the kidney. Post-graduate M. J., *19:* 266–269, 1943.
BEACH, E. W. and SHULTZ, W. G.: Spontaneous healing in renal tuberculosis. J. Urol., *46:* 590–601, 1941.
BENJAMIN, J. A. and BOYD, H. L.: Renal tuberculoma and tuberculous perinephritic abscess. J. Urol., *53:*265–268, 1945.
BOGEN, E., LOOMIS, R. N. and DRAKE, W. W.: Para-aminosalicylic acid treatment of tuberculosis. Am. Rev. Tuberculosis, *61:*226–246, 1950.
BRAASCH, W. F. and OLSON, F. A.: Roentgenographic diagnosis in renal tuberculosis. Surg., Gynec. and Obst., 28:555–561, 1919.
BRAASCH, W. F. and SUTTON, E. B.: Prognosis in bilateral renal tuberculosis. Canad. M.A.J., *45:*320–325, 1941(a).
BRAASCH, W. F. and SUTTON, E. B.: Prognosis in bilateral renal tuberculosis. J. Urol., *46:* 567–578, 1941(b).
BUGBEE, H. G.: Tuberculoma of the kidney: report of a case. J. Urol., *46:*355–358, 1942.
CARSTENSEN, B.: Para-aminosalicylic acid (PAS) in pulmonary and extrapulmonary tuberculosis. Am. Rev. Tuberculosis, *61:*613–620, 1950.
CAULK, J. R. Renal tuberculosis. J. Urol., *6:*97–113, 1921.
COLBY, F. H.: Renal tuberculosis and sanatorium care. J. Urol., *44:*401–405, 1940.

COLBY, F. H.: Cutaneous ureterostomy in active renal tuberculosis. Tr. Am. Assn. Genito-Urin. Surg., *34:*101–114, 1941.

COLBY, F. H.: Essential Urology. The Williams and Wilkins Co., Baltimore, 1950.

CORBITT, R. W.: Secondary bacteriuria associated with renal tuberculosis. J. Urol., *51:*11–13, 1944.

CREEVY, C. D.: An example of apparent healing of bilateral minimal renal tuberculosis. J. Urol., *47:*614–618, 1942.

DOONEIEF, A. S., BUCHBERG, A. and STEINBACH, M. M.: Para-aminosalicylic acid (PAS) in chronic pulmonary tuberculosis. New England J. Med., *242:*859–862, 1950.

EDWARDS, H. R. and DROLET, G. J.: The implications of changing morbidity and mortality rates from tuberculosis. Am. Rev. Tuberculosis, *61:*39–50, 1950.

EMMETT, J. L. and KIBLER, J. M.: Renal tuberculosis; prognosis following nephrectomy based on preoperative observations in the "good" kidney. J.A.M.A., *111:*2351–2356, 1938.

FELDMAN, W. H. and HINSHAW, H. C.: Streptomycin and Dihydrostreptomycin in tuberculosis. 14–20. Riggins, H. M. and Hinshaw, H. C., Editors. National Tuberculosis Association, 1949.

FELDMAN, W. H., KARLSON, A. G. and HINSHAW, H. C.: Streptomycin-resistant tubercle bacilli; effects of resistance on therapeutic results in tuberculous guinea pigs. Am. Rev. Tuberculosis, *57:*162–174, 1948.

FLICK, L. F.: Development of Our Knowledge of Tuberculosis. Wickersham Printing Co., Lancaster, Pa., 1925.

FROST, W. H.: How much control of tuberculosis? Am. J. Pub. Health, *27:*1, 1947.

GILE, H. H.: Tuberculosis of the kidney with special reference to follow-up results in the Squier Clinic. Surg., Gynec. and Obstet., *64:*1046–1050, 1937.

GOLDBERG, B.: Clinical Tuberculosis. F. A. Davis Co., Philadelphia, 1935.

GRAESSLE, O. E. and PIETROWSKI, J. J.: The *in vitro* effect of para-aminosalicylic acid (PAS) in preventing acquired resistance to streptomycin by Mycobacterium tuberculosis. J. Bact., *57:*459–465, 1949.

GREENBERGER, A. J. and GREENBERGER, M. E. Urogenital tuberculosis associated with pulmonary tuberculosis. Med. Clin. North America, *2:*787–810, 1936.

HARRIS, R. J.: Tuberculous bacilluria: its incidence and significance in patients suffering from surgical tuberculosis. Brit. J. Surg., *16:*464–484, 1929.

HINMAN, F.: The Principles and Practice of Urology. W. B. Saunders Co., Philadelphia and London, 1935.

JOLY, J. S.: Editorial. Post-graduate M. J., *117:*261–262, 1943.

KOCH, R.: Fortsetzung der Mittheilung über ein Heilmittel gegen Tuberkulose. Deutsch. Med., Woch., *17:*101, 1889–1891.

KRETSCHMER, H. L.: Tuberculosis of the kidney. A critical review based on a series of two hundred and twenty-one cases. New England J. Med., *202:*669–671, 1930.

KRETSCHMER, H. L.: Tuberculosis of the kidney in childhood and adolescence. Illinois M. J., *70:*119–125, 1936.

LATTIMER, J. K., AMBERSON, J. B. and BRAHAM, S.: The treatment of genito-urinary tuberculosis with streptomycin alone. J. Urol., *62:*875–888, 1949.

LEHMAN, J.: Para-aminosalicylic acid in the treatment of tuberculosis. Lancet, *250:*15–16, 1946.

LIEBERTHAL, F. and HÚTH, F.: Tuberculous nephritis and tuberculous bacilluria: a study of 1000 operated cases of renal tuberculosis. J. Urol., *30:*153–180, 1933.

LIEBERTHAL, F.: Renal tuberculosis. The development of the renal lesion. Surg., Gynec. and Obstet., *67:*26–37, 1938.

McCLELLAND, J. C. and DAVIS, K. F.: The relationship between skeletal and genito-urinary tuberculosis. J. Urol., *47:*320–322, 1942.

MALLORY, F. B. and PARKER, F., JR.: Reticulum. Am. J. Path., *3:*515–525, 1927.

MEDLAR, E. M.: Cases of renal infection in pulmonary tuberculosis. Am. J. Path., *2:*401–414, 1926.

MEDLAR, E. M.: The pathology of tuberculosis in relation to chemotherapy. Streptomycin and Dihydrostreptomycin in Tuberculosis. Riggins, H. M. and Hinshaw, H. C., Editors. National Tuberculosis Association, 1949.

MEDLAR, E. M., SPAIN, D. M. and HOLLIDAY, R. W.: Post-mortem compared with clinical diagnosis of genito-urinary tuberculosis in adult males. J. Urol., *61:*1078–1088, 1949.

MOORE, R. A.: A Textbook of Pathology. W. B. Saunders Co., Philadelphia and London, 1944.

MORSE, P. E. and STOTT, E.: Studies of the tissue reactions to various products of the tubercle bacillus. J. Lab. and Clin. Med., 2:159–167, 1916–17.

MYERS, J. A., HARRINGTON, F. E., SPRAGUE, E. and PEREZ, E.: Epidemiology of tuberculosis. J.A.M.A., 115:1609–1614, 1940.

NESBIT, R. M. and BOHNE, A. W.: A present day rationale for the treatment of urinary tuberculosis. J.A.M.A., 138:937–941, 1948.

NESBIT, R. M., KEITZER, W. A. and LYNN, J. M.: The prognosis of renal tuberculosis treated by nephrectomy and the outlook of the patient who is considered unsuitable for operative treatment. J. Urol., 54:227–234, 1945.

ORDWAY, W. H. and MEDLAR, E. M.: Tuberculous bacilluria. A ten year study. J.A.M.A., 119:937–942, 1942.

PARRAN, T.: The control of tuberculosis in the Americas. Public Health Reports, 62:827–834, 1947.

PATERSON, R. G.: The evolution of official tuberculosis control in the United States. Public Health Reports, 62:336–341, 1947.

PITNEY, E. H. and KASIUS, R. V.: Tuberculosis mortality in the United States and each State. Public Health Reports, 62:487–512, 1947.

POTTENGER, F. M.: Clinical Tuberculosis. C. V. Mosby Co., St. Louis, 1917.

PUTNAM, P.: Sex differences in pulmonary tuberculosis deaths. Am. J. Hyg., 7:663–705, 1927.

Report of the Council on Pharmacy and Chemistry: Current status of the chemotherapy of tuberculosis in man. J.A.M.A., 142:650–653, 1950.

RICH, A. R.: The Pathogenesis of Tuberculosis. C. C Thomas, Springfield, Ill., 1944.

RIGGINS, H. M. and GEARHEART, R. P.: Combined chemotherapy in clinical tuberculosis. Its effect on the emergence of streptomycin and dihydrostreptomycin resistant strains of tubercle bacilli. Streptomycin and Dihydrostreptomycin in Tuberculosis. Riggins, H. M. and Hinshaw, H. C., Editors. 537–545, National Tuberculosis Association, 1949.

RIGGINS, H. M. and HINSHAW, H. C. The streptomycin project of the American Trudeau Society. 29–35, Streptomycin and Dihydrostreptomycin in Tuberculosis. Riggins, H. M. and Hinshaw, H. C. Editors. National Tuberculosis Association, 1949.

ROHRER, P. A.: Renal tuberculosis. J. Urol., 44:871–872, 1940.

ROSENCRANZ, E.: Frequency of tubercle bacillus in urine of chronic pulmonary tuberculosis in relation to urogenital complications. J. Urol., 44:498–506, 1940.

SCHATZ, A., BUGIE, E. and WAKSMAN, S. A.: Streptomycin, a substance exhibiting antibiotic activity against gram-positive and gram-negative bacteria. Proc. Soc. Exp. Biol. and Med., 55:66–69, 1944.

SCHATZ, A. and WAKSMAN, S. A.: Effect of streptomycin and other antibiotic substances upon Mycobacterium tuberculosis and other related organisms. Proc. Soc. Exp. Biol. and Med., 57:244–248, 1944.

SIMMONDS, M.: Ueber Tuberculose des maennlichen Genitalsystem. Beit. 2 Klin. d. Tuberk., 33:35, 1915.

STEENKEN, W., JR.: Streptomycin and the tubercle bacillus. Streptomycin and Dihydrostreptomycin in Tuberculosis. Riggins, H. M. and Hinshaw, H. C. Editors. 39–57, National Tuberculosis Association, 1949.

Streptomycin Committee, Veterans Administration. Streptomycin and Dihydrostreptomycin in Tuberculosis. Riggins, H. M. and Hinshaw, H. C. Editors. 430–458, National Tuberculosis Association, 1949.

TAYLOR, H. K.: Renal tuberculosis. Pathogenesis and roentgen findings. Am. J. Roentgenol., 42:700–708, 1939.

THOMAS, G. J., STEBBINS, T. L. and SANDELL, S. T.: The control and arrest of lesions of renal tuberculosis. J. Urol., 46:579–590, 1941.

WALKER, G.: Studies in the experimental production of tuberculosis in the genito-urinary organs. Johns Hopkins Hosp. Rep., 16:1–222, 1911.

WANG, S. L. and FLAQUÉ, A. V.: Tuberculoma of the kidney. Report of a case. J. Urol., 51:275–277, 1944.

WEBER, F. J.: Decline of tuberculosis mortality. Public Health Reports, 63:161–162, 1948 (a).

WEBER, F. J.: Tuberculosis and the Negro. Public Health Reports, 63:425–426, 1948 (b).

WELLS, C.: The tuberculous kidney. Diagnosis and prognosis. Post-graduate M. J., 217:270–278, 1943.

WILDBOLZ, H.: Renal tuberculosis. J. Urol., 21:145–179, 1929.

CHAPTER 3

Parasitic Diseases of the Genitourinary System

LUIS A. SANJURJO, M.D.

Introduction. Every day throughout the world, thousands of individuals are infected or reinfected by a score of parasites known to be pathogenic to man, but only a few of them affect the urogenital tract. Several noteworthy exceptions are: Schistosoma haematobium and mansoni; the filaria, Wuchereria bancrofti; Trichomonas vaginalis; Taenia echinococcus; Endamoeba histolytica; Eustrongylus gigas, and Strongyloides stercoralis.

It is difficult to explain this striking relative immunity enjoyed by the urinary and genital organs: however, one is compelled to suspect that if a careful and meticulous search were made, and autopsies performed more frequently, interesting findings and more data on human parasitoses would be collected, increasing the proportion of instances in which the genitourinary system is involved by parasites.

The limitation of some parasites to certain countries, mainly tropical and subtropical, is conditioned by temperature and other factors on which depends the presence of intermediate hosts or vectors essential for the transmission of these diseases. The habits of individuals, which vary from one country to another, and the prevailing sanitary conditions, are important contributing factors that must be borne in mind in order to have a clear understanding of the occurrence and mode of transmission of these diseases.

SCHISTOSOMIASIS

Geographical Distribution. Urinary schistosomiasis is endemic and widely distributed in Africa from the Nile Delta to Central and South Africa, Sudan and Ethiopia. The disease is also found in Persia, Cyprus, Mesopotamia, Palestine, Arabia, India, Iran, Iraq, Madagascar, Réunion, and Mauritius. In Australia, Greece and the Southern Coast of Portugal, endemic areas are known to exist. Throughout the world the parasite has been discovered in individuals who left infested areas, sometimes twenty years previously, and in whom reinfestation was considered impossible.

Manson's schistosomiasis is also found in Africa. It was probably introduced in the New World by infected Negro slaves. The presence of a suitable intermediate host in these areas permitted the spread of the disease in Northern Brazil, Venezuela, and the West Indies.

560

Schistosoma japonicum is limited to the Far East, China, Japan, Formosa, and some of the Philippine Islands.

General Considerations and Life Cycle. Schistosomiasis, a parasitic disease that has plagued mankind for centuries, had its origin traced back 3,000 years, B. C., by the finding of calcified eggs in carefully studied Egyptian mummies, and from the descriptions of hematuria found in ancient papyri.

Three species of schistosomes are of clinical importance: Schistosoma mansoni and japonicum produce the hepato-intestinal form of schistosomiasis, and Schistosoma haematobium is responsible for the urinary form of bilharziasis.

These parasites are sexually differentiated trematodes. The female is cylindrical, while the males possess a longitudinal groove (gynecophoric canal), in which the former lies during copulation. These parasites have a similar life cycle, require the presence of a fresh water mollusc during the asexual phase of their development, and are capable of producing identical pathologic lesions in the organs and tissues of their predilection. The flukes average 1 to 1.5 cm. in length; the females have a slender, fusiform appearance, while the male is broader than the female, and is split longitudinally by the gynecophoric canal.

The eggs laid by the parasites are oval-shaped, and the species can be readily identified by the spine on it: terminal for Schistosoma haematobium, and subterminal for the mansonic type, while the eggs of S. japonicum present a small subterminal knob, which is not always visible.

The ova of these parasites are ejected from the human body with the urine or feces, and must reach fresh water for the embryo to hatch and survive. The miracidia contained within the ova leave the egg shell and swim in search of the corresponding intermediate molluscan host, which they penetrate, and within which they multiply considerably. When maturity is attained the cercariae, amounting to several thousand, leave the snail and swim freely in the water, until an adequate mammalian host is found. The cercariae penetrate the skin or mucous membranes of the definitive host who bathes in, or drinks infested waters, entering the dermal lymphatics or veins, and being then carried to the heart and lungs, before reaching the arterial blood, from where they are distributed to all organs and tissues. Only those parasites that reach the portal system survive and attain maturity within interhepatic portal branches.

Copulation takes place within the tributaries of the portal system, following which the female is ready for oviposition. In the mansonic and Oriental schistosomiasis the females migrate against the venous blood flow to reach the venules of the mesenteric and hemorrhoidal plexuses, while the schistosomes of the urinary form wander towards the pelvic, vesiculoprostatic and pubic venous plexuses. The parasites lay their eggs in the fine venules of the submucosa of the intestine in the former species and in those of the bladder, seminal vesicles, prostate and urethra in the latter variety.

When the female withdraws from the venule, after oviposition, many of the eggs remaining within the lumen of the vessel are washed by the venous blood towards the liver, where they are trapped in portal venules or in sinusoids.

Pathology. The disease may be divided into three stages (Koppisch, 1943).

The penetration of the larvae through the skin produces an urticarial reaction manifested by severe itching accompanied by wheal and petechial formation in some instances. These local manifestations may be absent, or so minimal that they may go unnoticed by the individual. Severely infected patients may complain of low grade fever, headaches, general malaise, and pulmonary and gastrointestinal disturbances beginning two to four weeks after exposure.

The effects of the deposition of eggs by the female constitute the second stage of the disease, and begins five to seven weeks following infestation. In the mansonic and Japanese schistosomiasis, episodes of bloody diarrhea, chills, fever, or pneumonic symptoms may be present, accompanied by an increased leukocyte count and a marked eosinophilia. This clinical picture may last several weeks.

In urinary schistosomiasis the deposition of eggs in the submucosa and mucosa of the bladder is manifested clinically by terminal hematuria and bladder irritability, but at times a total or terminal hematuria, more frequently the latter, precedes other symptoms of bladder involvement.

The third stage is characterized by chronic irreversible damage produced in the liver, spleen, bowel, bladder, ureters, prostate, seminal vesicles, urethra, testicle, epididymis, and spermatic cords, whose physiological functions are significantly altered as a result of long-standing irritation provoked by the ova.

The tissues respond to the presence of ova by a more or less diffuse infiltration with eosinophils, lymphocytes, plasma cells, and monocytes. They also provoke the formation of pseudotubercles composed of foreign body giant cells and epithelioid cells centrally, and eosinophils and round cells at the periphery. The embryo dies within some 12 days after deposition of the ovum, and the shells undergo slow dissolution, or else become calcified.

GENITOURINARY SCHISTOSOMIASIS

Schistosoma haematobium and mansoni involve the genitourinary organs, particularly the bladder and lower portions of the ureters, in a markedly different proportion. Thus, in Egypt, according to Abdel Rahman El Sadr, S. mansoni is found in only 4 per cent of the infected cases, whilst, in the remainder S. haematobium is the offending parasite.

Cases of double infection are found in which the ova of both varieties of schistosomes are recovered from the urine. In some of these cases intestinal involvement due to the mansonic parasite may also be present.

The ova of S. haematobium have been recovered from the excreta of individuals also infected with S. mansoni. Khourl reported one case known to have had urinary bilharziasis, and considered cured, in whom twenty years later, and while suffering from Manson's schistosomiasis, eggs with a terminal spine were discovered in the excreta.

Monstestruc (1940) has reported on a patient who always lived in Martinique, where Manson's schistosomiasis is the only variety found. The patient complained of hematuria and bladder irritability accompanied by suprapubic pain. A diagnosis of vesical bilharziasis was made upon finding the eggs of Manson's schistosomiasis in the urine. Recently he saw another patient from Martinique with similar complaints and in whom the same diagnosis was made later on in Paris.*

Kidneys. This organ is rarely affected by either of the three species of schistosomes.

In the renal tissue the ova of these trematodes have been found at autopsy and in operative material obtained from severely infected cases, which

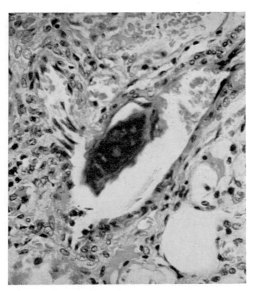

Fig. 298. Manson's schistosomiasis of kidney. An ovum with an embryo are observed within a branch of the renal vein. 360×. (Sanjurjo and Koppisch, School of Medicine and Tropical Medicine, University of Puerto Rico.)

probably result from a hematogenous dissemination of ova, the seriousness of the condition depending on the number of ova.

Significant lesions which could be interpreted as direct deposition of ova by the flukes are extremely rare. Stevens (1940) reported a patient in whom a papillary carcinoma of the renal pelvis was found with implants in the ureter and bladder, accompanied by hydronephrosis. The microscopic study of the tissue revealed ova with a terminal spine.

In severe infestations the ova may be deposited in large numbers within the walls of the renal pelvis, and the consequent irritation leads to papillomatous formations and malignant change. These papillary growths may give rise to hydronephrosis, when obstruction is produced at the ureteropelvic outlet.

Massive deposition of ova within the renal tissues may result in hematuria and, with advanced fibrosis, impaired renal function is to be expected. In the case reported by Sanjurjo and Koppisch, the left kidney was removed

* Monstestruc: Personal communication.

for severe intractable hematuria in a patient suffering from advanced intestinal schistosomiasis of the mansonic type (Fig. 298). In the microscopic sections, a large number of pseudotubercles and ova were found in the renal cortex. No other manifestations of genitourinary involvement were discovered (Fig. 299).

Ureters. The lower portions of the ureter are very vulnerable to urinary schistosomiasis, because of the intercommunications between its veins and the vesical plexus and middle hemorrhoidal vein. The parasites may migrate and deposit their ova within the venules of the terminal ureter, especially

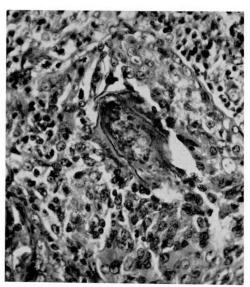

Fig. 299. Manson's schistosomiasis of kidney. Pseudotubercle with egg and embryo in center. 360×. (Sanjurjo and Koppisch, School of Medicine and Tropical Medicine, University of Puerto Rico.)

the intramural segment, or the latter may become involved by extension from the bladder when this organ is severely infected. The middle third of the ureter is less frequently affected, and the upper third, rarely so.

The formation of pseudotubercles in the ureteral wall is followed by fibrosis of the muscular layers, congestion and thickening of the submucosa and mucosa and, later on, by a loss of tonicity and segmental stricture, which may be severe in advanced cases. Ureteral dilatations, sacculations and hydronephrosis are the result of obstruction, and if bacterial infection supervenes, pyonephrosis will be the natural consequence.

Urinary stasis, infection, ulceration, desquamation of epithelium, and the presence of ova create ideal conditions for the deposition of urinary salts and formation of calculi, which often complicate the clinical picture.

When the ureter is incised longitudinally, the mucosa appears congested, sandy-patched and ulcerated in places. Small, pouch-like formations above the strictured segments, and minute blebs or blister-like elevations resembling ureteritis cystica are seen. These cystic formations are microscopic, or may occasionally attain 4 mm. in diameter. On the mucosa these blebs may be pedunculated or sometimes deep-seated in the muscularis. The fluid they contain is clear and watery in some instances, or else viscid. Their color varies from yellowish to red, due to the presence of blood pigment, but no ova have been found within them. Granulomatous lesions and, less frequently, papillomatous growths are also encountered, resulting from the irritation produced by the eggs.

Calcified ova in the ureteral wall are easily recognized in roentgenograms the images obtained being very characteristic. Renal destruction can be

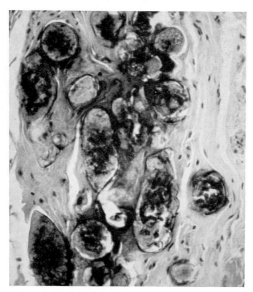

Fig. 300. S. haematobium infection of bladder. Calcified eggs of the bladder in the submucosa. 300×. (Courtesy of the Armed Forces Institute of Pathology, Washington, D. C.)

appreciated in the excretory pyelograms by decreased concentration and excretion of the contrast media and evidences of back pressure.

In the advanced stages of the disease, complete unilateral or bilateral ureteral occlusion may be encountered, with concomitant renal destruction, uremia, and death as the final outcome.

Bladder. The disease takes a heavy toll of victims in Egypt, where in some rural areas 90 per cent of the population is infected.

Symptoms. Following infestation by the flukes, the disease may remain asymptomatic for several months or years.

The foremost clinical manifestation of vesical schistosomiasis is hematuria, which may be terminal or total, and which results from congestion and ulceration of the bladder mucosa due to the presence of the ova. The intermittent passage of bloody urine may be the only symptom of urinary schistosomiasis, but as the infection progresses, or when pathogenic bacteria gain entrance to the bladder, the symptoms of vesical irritability, pollakiuria, urgency, dysuria, and strangury gradually become part of the composite picture of vesical involvement. At a later stage the extensive fibrosis of the vesical wall is responsible for diminished vesical capacity, and consequently the pollakiuria and incontinence become very distressing (Fig. 300).

The formation of calculi, which occurs frequently, contributes considerably to augment bladder irritability (Fig. 301).

Cystoscopy. During the cystoscopic examination the mucosa of the bladder appears congested, velvety, vesicular, and granulomatous. Overlapping the trigone and ureteral orifices, small vesicular elevations of a whitish to brown color can be observed. They have a sandy appearance, and represent ova deposited in the mucosa and submucosa. Sandy patches result from coalescence of pseudotubercles. When the disease progresses, the whole mucosal

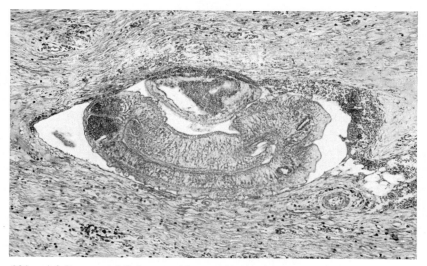

Fig. 301.   Adult worm of S. haematobium within a vein of the bladder wall. (Courtesy Armed Forces Institute of Pathology, Washington, D. C.)

surface is covered by these sandy patches and larger elevations which, when overlaid with urinary salts, have the appearance of pepper-like specks. Ulcers and necrotic areas are quite conspicuous, and soon become encrusted with calcareous deposits. Bilharziomata are rarely seen in the trigone, but the continuous irritation resulting from the deposition of ova gives rise, in about 8 per cent of the cases, to sessile or pedunculated, raspberry growths, single or multiple, projecting prominently around the fundus of the bladder, the apex and the ureteral orifices, which they sometimes obscure (Fig. 302). Rarely, if ever, are they seen in the trigone. These growths may be covered partially or totally with calcium salts. Carcinoma of the bladder is frequently found in patients suffering from schistosomiasis of many years' duration. Malignant tumors of the bladder are found ten times more frequently in individuals suffering from urinary schistosomiasis. Continuous bladder irritation by ova, infection, parasites, and calculi are responsible for the high incidence of malignant degeneration.

Contraction of the bladder, the result of fibrosis and atrophy of the mus-

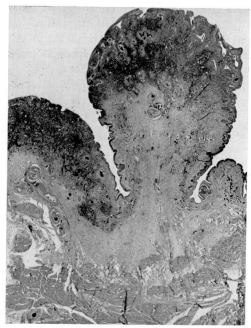

Fig. 302. S. haematobium infection of bladder. Papillomatous growths. 8×. (Courtesy Armed Forces Institute of Pathology, Washington, D. C.)

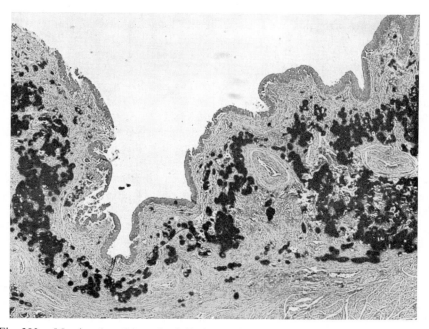

Fig. 303. Massive deposition of calcified ova of S. haematobium in the submucosa of the bladder which are capable of casting "cloud-like shadows" on the roentgen films. (Courtesy Armed Forces Institute of Pathology, Washington, D. C.)

cularis in cases of long-standing infection, is represented cystoscopically by loss of elasticity of the mucosa, trabeculations, and a decreased capacity.

Roentgenographic Studies. The plain films of the bladder assume considerable importance in vesical bilharziasis, especially in latent cases, when ova are not recovered in the urine. The mucosa and submucosa, studded with calcified eggs, cast beautifully characteristic, cloud-like shadows, which may be diagnostic (Fig. 303). A diagnosis in retrospect can be made in certain instances.

Seminal Vesicles, Prostate, Posterior Urethra and Corpora Cavernosa. Bilharziasis of these structures will be considered together, in view of their anatomical and physiological relationships.

Ova are deposited in the walls of the seminal vesicles; some pass into the lumen and may be recovered in the ejaculated semen. On rectal palpation the vesicles are hard, irregular and fibrotic, with marked perivesicular involvement that fixes them intimately to the prostate. Fibrous nodules may be felt here and there among areas of softening resembling, in some instances, cystic formations. Hematospermia and painful ejaculations are an almost constant complaint. Calcification of the seminal vesicles in cases of mixed bilharzial infection has been reported by Smyrniotis.

The prostate is similarly involved. Rectally the gland appears fixed and enlarged, as in benign hyperplasia, and is studded with firm nodules that never have the hardness of carcinoma; however, both conditions may coexist. These nodules represent bilharziomata and areas of fibrosis. Prostatic cysts have been described, resulting from occlusion of glandular ducts.

When inspected with the urethroscope, the neck of the bladder appears deformed and irregular, as a result of the long-standing infection, with the development of fibrosis and contracture of the vesical outlet. The posterior urethral lip is elevated, and the mucosa appears velvety and covered with sandy patches or areas of calcification. The posterior urethra is more roomy than usual; the verumontanum is congested and has a granular mucosa, but around the ejaculatory ducts the mucosa is velvety and has a deep red hue. Very little change is observed in the utricle.

When the deposition of ova in the corpora cavernosa is intense, plaques of fibrosis develop which resemble Peyronie's disease or chronic fibrous cavernositis.

Urethral strictures, accompanied by periurethral abscesses and fistulous formations, are rather frequent complications of urinary bilharziasis, and favor sepsis of the mid and upper urinary tract.

Epididymis, Testis, Spermatic Cord and Scrotum. The ova and parasites of S. haematobium have been found in all these organs and tissues.

Bilharziomata in the epididymis appear as painless small hard nodules, single or multiple, which can be confused with tuberculosis or tumors.

When lesions are found in the testis, a hydrocele is almost always present; the organ is enlarged and, on section, white masses having a gritty sensation due to the presence of calcified eggs are encountered, surrounded by zones of inflammation and fibrosis. In other places, granulation tissue and pseudotubercles in various stages of development are observed.

In the spermatic cord, hard, irregular, painless nodules result from the deposition of eggs of S. mansoni or haematobium. They are round, oval or cord-like fibrous growths that can be shelled out with ease. On microscopic examination they consist of fibrous tissue with a heavy eosinophilic infiltration and multiple bilharziomata. In older lesions these nodes represent hyaline fibrous tissue within which calcified eggs, or the chitinous capsule, may be identified. The flukes may erratically migrate to the scrotum where massive deposition of ova of S. mansoni and haematobium may lead to chronic edema and fibrosis. The resulting elephantiasis never attains a large size, although occasionally partial resection of the scrotum is necessary.

When elephantiasis of the scrotum accompanies peri-urethral abscess formation and fistulae, acute septic infection of the scrotum may occur periodically.

Female Genitalia. Extensive schistosomal lesions may develop in the female genitalia.

The lesions of the vulva consist in polypoid growths that resemble venereal warts, and which occasionally may be very extensive (Barquero Gonzalez). An ulcerative form has been described in which the clitoris and hymen are involved and consequently the external urethral orifice is similarly affected.

At times these lesions resemble carcinoma, from which they must be differentiated, but a great disproportion exists between the extensiveness of the lesions and the relatively good health enjoyed by these patients, which of course is not observed as a general rule in carcinoma.

When the vagina is affected, the mucosa is friable and bleeds easily, it looks thickened, sclerotic and covered with sandy patches here and there. Rarely, vesicovaginal fistulae develop in advanced cases.

The bilharzial lesions of the uterine cervix consist in ulcers, friable polypoid growths and fibro-adenomatous tumors (Gibson). Involvement of the ovary, fallopian tubes and mesosalpynx has also been observed.

Diagnosis. In the presence of hematuria, a history of residence in a country where the disease is known to be endemic must arouse the suspicion of urinary schistosomiasis. The finding of terminal or lateral spiculated ova in the urine is in itself diagnostic; however, in certain instances, eggs cannot be found in repeated samples of urine. Gelfand has employed the biopsy technique of the vesical mucosa that was modified in Puerto Rico by Hernández Morales and Maldonado for intestinal schistosomiasis. Small bites of mucosa are taken with a cystoscopic forceps; the specimen is crushed between two glass slides, and is examined directly under the microscope for ova. Gelfand claims 40 per cent positive results.

This method has two great advantages: a diagnosis may be established when other necessary criteria are lacking, and it can also be determined whether the embryos within the ova are dead or alive. As can be readily surmised, the second point is of great clinical and prognostic significance following medical treatment. Le Gac claims to increase the yield of ova in urine specimens by dilating the urethra with Beniqué sounds, in patients with terminal hematuria in whom vesical schistosomiasis is suspected.

In doubtful cases, intradermal tests can be performed with extracts prepared from cercariae, but the test will be positive in infections produced by any of the three species of schistosomes. A complement fixation reaction devised by Fairley can also be of great diagnostic aid.

Treatment. The treatment of schistosomiasis can be divided into: (1) prophylactic, (2) medical and (3) surgical.

1. *Prophylactic.* Mass treatment of all infected individuals could be considered an ideal solution to the problem of schistosomiasis, but this would constitute a formidable endeavour, far beyond present-day facilities.

The extermination of the snails has been attempted in countries of high endemicity by the drainage of swamps and the utilization of molluscocidals, the latter being the most promising measure.

Instructions and warnings to avoid exposure to cercariae should be periodically distributed among the population living near areas where infestation is possible.

2. *Medical.* For several years some organic antimony compounds have been the drugs of choice in the treatment of bilharziasis. Tartar emetic was first employed by Christopherson with relatively satisfactory results, but the great toxicity of the drug, the unpleasant side effects reported, and the high percentage of failures, moved investigators to continue the search for a safer and more effective agent.

In 1930, Fuadin, another antimony compound, was offered in vials containing 5 cc. which are injected intramuscularly every other day, for a total dosage of 50 cc.

Many investigators are of the opinion that this amount is insufficient, and a double or triple dose has been recommended. Hernández Morales et al. claim 78.3 per cent of apparent cures in one of their series of cases.

Anthiomaline, also an antimony compound, has been used with good results. It is dispensed in 3 cc. vials, and is injected intramuscularly, every other day, for a total of 30 cc. Again, some authors recommend a larger dose. These drugs are contraindicated when there is marked liver and renal damage, and in cachectic individuals.

3. *Surgical.* The surgical complications arising in the course of schistosomiasis consist of obstruction, formation of calculi, and bacterial infection. Surgical treatment will be directed toward the relief of obstruction, removal of calculi, and control of urinary sepsis. The surgical procedures must be combined with medical treatment.

Following treatment with antimony compounds, the absence of ova in the stools and the urine are considered an index of cure. In practice, however, this criterion is misleading when such examinations are not repeated at intervals during a period of at least six months.

FILARIASIS

In 600 B.C. the Hindus and Persians (Douglade) recognized filariasis as a clinical entity, but it was not until 1863 that Demarquay, in Paris, discovered the microfilariae of Wuchereria bancrofti in a chylous hydrocele. In 1865 Wucherer demonstrated the presence of the larvae in chylous urine, and several years later Lewis, in India, discovered the larval form of the parasites in the peripheral blood and lymphatics. Sir Patrick Manson, who observed the nocturnal periodicity of filaria bancrofti, was later able to demonstrate the presence of microfilariae in the stomach of the Culex mosquitoes.

The geographical distribution of Wuchereria bancrofti is very extensive, but it is found predominantly in subtropical and tropical countries where, next to malaria and hookworm, it is the most prevalent disease.

Life Cycle. The parasite is a thin, filiform nematode, the male averaging 45 mm. in length and 0.1 mm. in thickness, while the female may be twice as large. The female is oviparous and viviparous.

Mosquitoes of the genera Anopheles, Culex or Aëdes become infected when, upon biting man, they suck blood containing microfilariae. Upon reaching the stomach of the intermediate host, the microfilariae liberate themselves of the enveloping sheath, and then migrate to the thoracic muscles of the insect, and later on to the neck and head, from where they reach the proboscis. The infection is transmitted to man by the insect's bite. After penetrating the skin, the larvae reach the superficial lymphatics and are thence transported to the deep lymphatic vessels and lymph nodes which constitute the natural habitat of the parasite. The parasites frequently invade lymphatic channels of the spermatic cord, testicle, epididymis, scrotum, upper and lower extremities, and mammary gland. It probably takes the filarial worms not less than one year to reach maturity and to begin to reproduce.

Pathology. The presence of the adult filarial worms within the lymph glands and vessels produces two different types of lesions: a partial obstruction, and a proliferative inflammatory reaction in the wall of the lymph channels and about them.

A granulomatous reaction takes place about dead worms, with the participation of many eosinophils, giant cells, epithelioid cells, and a few polymorphonuclears, surrounding the disintegrating parasites, which at times undergo calcification. This is followed by fibrosis and by proliferative endolymphangitis of neighboring lymph vessels, resulting in their occlusion. The adjacent lymphatics may dilate considerably, which results in edema and the formation of lymphatic varices.

At the beginning, the presence of filariae in the lymphatics is responsible for attacks of lymphangitis. Following repeated episodes of inflammation the tissues of the extremities, scrotum and vulva increase in size due to the presence of chronic edema, which is characterized by both subcutaneous edema and fibrosis, and in time leads to elephantiasis.

Genital Filariasis. The genital manifestations of filariasis vary from one country, or from one section of a city, to another. Thus, while elephantiasis is commonly seen in British Guiana, it is rare in Saigon. In Allahabad, chyluria and lymph varices are frequently observed, yet these are rare in other countries where filariasis is endemic. In Puerto Rico filarial hydroceles are very frequent. There is a great disproportion between the number of patients with microfilariae in the blood and those having complications such as chyluria or elephantiasis. Because of this discrepancy the role of bacteria has been extensively studied and considered a contributing factor. However, McKinley was of the opinion that bacteria should not be incriminated and held responsible for the development of these complications in the early stages of the disease.

Genital manifestations of the disease are not found in infected children until they reach puberty.

Filariasis of the Spermatic Cord. The testis and epididymis possess an abundant lymphatic supply that originates about the seminiferous tubules (Testut and Latarjet) and drains into several lymphatic trunks that ascend towards the body of Highmore, where they unite with the efferent lymph channels arising from the epididymis. They form seven or eight main trunks that join the other elements of the spermatic cord and finally drain into the juxtaortic and preaortic lymph glands.

When the lymphatics of the cord are invaded by the parasites or involved in the reactions set up by their presence, the clinical manifestations of funiculitis, epididymis and orchitis become evident.

SYMPTOMS. In the acute stage, involvement of the spermatic cord is accompanied by severe, sharp pain, simulating renal or ureteral colic, or appendicitis, when the right side is affected. The pain may be felt initially in the spermatic cord or testicle, or in both, with radiation to the corresponding lumbar areas. In our experience, the opposite has been frequently observed. Chills, fever, general malaise, nausea, and vomiting may also be present. When the reaction is severe the patients may become toxic and stuporous.

The spermatic cord becomes the site of an induration that progresses rapidly to complete involvement within a few hours. The epididymis and testicle may become affected also, especially the former.

The spermatic cord is tender and hard; it occasionally is matted to the adjacent cutaneous tissues. In places, one or more nodules, attaining the size of a hazelnut or of a pigeon's egg, may be felt. These nodules are seldom very hard, and usually have an uneven surface. Within these nodes filarial worms are found with relative frequency. Microscopically the worms are seen surrounded by many eosinophils, epithelioid cells and lymphocytes. The vas deferens cannot be differentiated from the other elements of the cord, but even though its lymphatic supply takes part in this inflammatory process, the vas itself is not involved or occluded. Semen obtained following attacks of funiculitis has been found to contain normal spermatozoa.

The acute phase subsides in a few days, but the swelling of the spermatic cord and nodes persists for several weeks or months. After repeated attacks of funiculitis, the edema is gradually replaced by fibrosis.

The frequency and severity of attacks of funiculitis vary considerably, and appear to be directly related to the number of adult parasites present, and on the occurrence of reinfestation. Subsequent attacks are generally more severe than preceding ones, because of the damage already produced to the spermatic cord (Fig. 304).

The attacks of funiculitis sometimes are very mild and evanescent, lasting but a few hours. Occasionally patients complain of dull pain, or of a dragging sensation, in the scrotal portion of the spermatic cord or testicle; still, on examination, no evidence of inflammation may be detected. The pain may last a few weeks or months, and the patients go from physician to physician in search of alleviation.

Filarial nodules with induration of the spermatic cord have been observed by the author in patients without history of pain or malaise in that area.

Varicocele may exist prior to attacks of filarial funiculitis, or it may result from repeated inflammation of the veins of the cord, which may undergo thrombosis. When exposed surgically, the vessels are dilated and

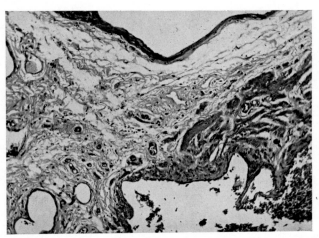

Fig. 304.   Severe dilatation of lymph and blood vessels of the spermatic cord in a patient with chronic filariasis of the spermatic cord. (Author's Case, Veterans Hospital, San Juan, Puerto Rico.)

separated from one another by yellowish or white tissue that represents edema or fat deposition. Varicocelectomy in these cases is fraught with technical difficulties, and severe scarring usually follows the procedure. The author saw one patient who complained bitterly of pain in the left testis following excision of dilated veins; removal of the testicle, with exeresis of the cord up to the internal inguinal ring, was necessary because of the extensive fibrosis.

During an attack of funiculitis, bacterial infection may occur, resulting in suppuration and abscess formation. When suppuration extends upwards to involve the retroperitoneal lymphatics, septicemia (usually streptococcal) and death are the final outcomes (Castellani and Chalmers; Knott).

Carbera and Caridad have reported on a lymphatic cyst of the spermatic cord, within which alive adult filariae were encountered at operation.

Filariasis of the Tunica Vaginalis, Testicle and Epididymis. In the author's experience, filariasis accounts for 80 per cent of hydroceles found in Puerto Rico. In most instances, neither microfilariae are discovered in nocturnal blood samples, nor a history of filariasis is elicited; however, in the great majority of patients who undergo operation, unequivocal evidence of filariasis is present.

Filarial hydroceles may be small or large, and may develop rapidly or gradually, over a period of months or years, usually following repeated attacks of epididymitis (Khalil Bey). The amount of fluid varies from a few cubic centimeters to several hundred: 1,500 cc. in one of the author's cases. Following an acute attack of funiculitis or epididymitis, the hydrocele fluid may be reabsorbed, in a few instances, but as a general rule it persists or increases gradually.

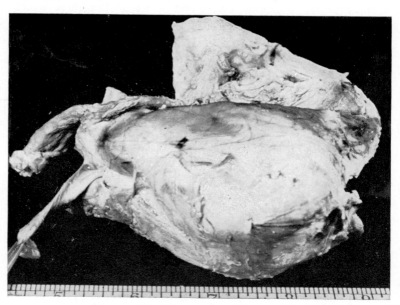

Fig. 305. Severe calcification of the visceral and parietal layers of the tunica vaginalis. The spermatic cord was also involved by extensive fibrosis. (Author's Case, School of Medicine and Tropical Medicine, San Juan, Puerto Rico.)

In early hydrocele the fluid is straw-colored, clear and albuminous, and contains mononuclear cells, lymphocytes and cholesterol. In older cases it is turbid, and when allowed to stand in a tall glass, the surface becomes covered with fat-like globules which are in relation to the amount of cholesterol present. When a lymph varix ruptures into the cavity of the tunica vaginalis, a chylocele is formed. The author has not found microfilariae in hydrocele fluids but has seen them in chyloceles.

Early in the beginning of the disease the tunica vaginalis does not differ grossly from idiopathic or traumatic hydroceles; in older cases it becomes thick and inelastic. Patches of fibrosis may be identified here and there either on the visceral or parietal layer. In some instances there is deposition of cholesterol in the form of plaques of different sizes, and in the older cases these are replaced by calcific deposits that may attain considerable proportions. Several years ago the author had the opportunity to operate on a patriarch with two moderately large hydroceles (Fig. 305). The tunics were almost totally calcified, a concomitant testicular atrophy was present, and the hydrocele fluid had a chalky appearance. Unilateral calcification of the tunica vaginalis has also been observed by the author in six instances (Fig. 306). The hydrocele fluid may be under tension regardless of the amount present, but as a general rule the tension is greatest in the presence of a large amount of fluid.

Transillumination will be positive if the fluid is clear but in old cases, when the cholesterol content is high, or in chyloceles, light will not be transmitted. Spontaneous rupture of the hydrocele sac is very unusual and

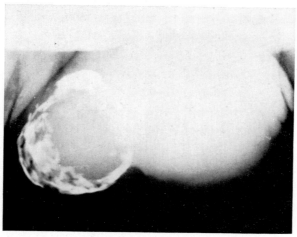

Fig. 306.   Radiograph of scrotum demonstrating total calcification of the parietal layer of the tunica vaginalis. On palpation the vaginalis had the consistency of an egg's shell. (Author's Case, Veterans Hospital, San Patricio, San Juan, Puerto Rico.)

follows injury. At the San Juan City Hospital in Puerto Rico the author had the opportunity to see a patient with a huge right-sided hydrocele of filarial origin. While awaiting admission to the hospital for operation, he sustained a fall, with moderate scrotal injury. Severe pain was experienced, accompanied by a fainting sensation, and the patient felt that something had yielded inside his scrotum. Immediately the skin became edematous, and the scrotum and penis enlarged considerably. The extravasated hydrocele fluid was reabsorbed, but reproduction of the hydrocele took place within a few weeks. At operation, dense adhesions and necrosis were found, requiring extirpation of the testicle and spermatic cord.

Adult worms of Wuchereria bancrofti have been found in sections of the epididymis removed surgically or at necropsy (Fig. 307). The reaction set up in the epididymis by the worms probably depends mostly on the number of parasites present. Small hard nodules may be found without significant clinical manifestations. These nodules most frequently represent lymphocytic and eosinophilic zones of reaction around dead worms. In some instances multiple nodules are found, predominantly in the globus minor. The more acute and severe forms of epididymal swelling are observed in acute attacks of filarial funiculitis. In our experience, all cases of filarial funiculitis have been accompanied by some epididymal involvement.

The parasite has also been found within the testicle. During an attack of acute orchitis the latter is large, tender and boggy; usually hydrocele fluid soon accumulates (Bhaskara Menon). The epididymis is closely bound to the testicle, with obliteration of the sinus epididymidis. In severe and chronic cases, dense adhesions may be present between the scrotum and the testis. The epididymis may undergo necrosis (Ray).

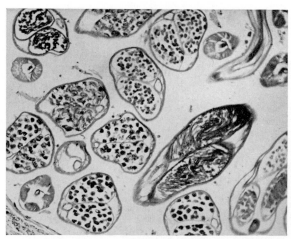

Fig. 307.   Living filarial worm in lymphatic of epididymis. 80×. (Courtesy Dr. E. Koppisch, Dept. of Pathology, School of Medicine and Tropical Medicine, University of Puerto Rico.)

The testicular sensation is preserved in these cases, which sometimes offer serious diagnostic problems. Syphilis, testicular tumors and hematoceles must be differentiated from filariasis.

Filariasis of the Scrotum and Penis. Elephantiasis of the scrotum is one of the most frequent complications of filariasis in Puerto Rico. The condition follows repeated attacks of lymphangitis of the scrotum. After each attack the skin remains thicker than before, and the sac enlarges, due to chronic edema and progressive fibrosis with loss of elasticity and contractility of the tissues (Fig. 308). The intervals between these attacks may vary from a few weeks to several months or years. During the author's service in the Armed Forces in Puerto Rico, one soldier had four episodes of lymphangitis of the scrotum within a period of six months, and about a year later a plastic repair of the scrotum had to be performed for cosmetic purposes.

Huge scrotal enlargements are not seen in Puerto Rico. Elephantiasis of the penis usually accompanies scrotal involvement, but it is rare to find the penis exclusively involved (Fig. 309).

The author has observed that although filariasis of the spermatic cord, testis and epididymis may occur without elephantiasis of the scrotum, the first two organs are invariably involved in all the cases operated upon for scrotal elephantiasis. During surgical exposure the gonads and cords are found surrounded by a moderate amount of a white or yellowish material resembling jello. In many instances the edema is so marked that lymph drips profusely on the operative field. The veins of the spermatic cord appear tortuous, dilated, and surrounded by abundant edema and fatty tissue. The venous engorgement of the scrotal wall occasionally attains monstrous proportions, resulting from the dependent position of the scrotum, drawn downwards by its own weight, and to the burden placed on the venous circulation by the edema and fibrosis.

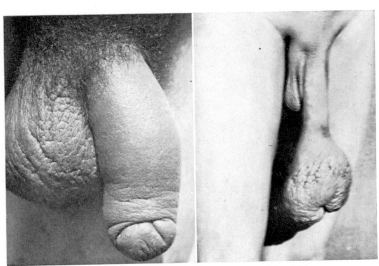

Fig. 308   Fig. 309

Fig. 308. Elephantiasis of penis and scrotum. (Courtesy Dr. F. Hernández Morales, Dept. of Medicine, School of Medicine and Tropical Medicine. University of Puerto Rico.)

Fig. 309. Severe elephantiasis of the distal third of the penis. (Author's Case, Fajardo Charity District Hospital.)

CHYLURIA

The term is applied to the passage of chyle into the urine, whereby the latter becomes milky. W. bancrofti is the most frequent cause of this condition. The incidence of chyluria is low, when one thinks of the large number of patients suffering from filariasis (Yamauchi). A non-parasitic form of chyluria has also been described.

Chylous Urine. The color of the urine varies in direct proportion to the amount of chyle present. The urine may seem normal, but on chemical analysis minimal amounts of fat can be identified. At times the urine is opalescent, while other times it is milky-white or creamy.

In addition to fat, chylous urine contains red and white blood cells, albumin, globulin, and fibrinogen, the latter being responsible for the formation of chylous clots which may obstruct the urinary pathways. Red blood cells may be present in large quantities, and may impart a pinkish tint to the chylous urine.

The fat contained in the urine may be dissolved in chloroform, when mixed in equal parts and shaken. This is diagnostic, since turbid urine due to pus, phosphates or carbonates will not be clarified by the addition of this solvent. If chylous urine is permitted to rest in a glass for some time, three layers are formed: the top one contains the fat, the middle layer contains fibrin and albumin, and the bottom layer is composed of erythrocytes and leukocytes.

Pathogenesis. The gradual obstruction of the retroperitoneal lymphatic vessels and glands seems to be responsible for the dilatation of the lymph channels, with the formation of lymphatic varices. Following a rich fatty meal, a sudden effort, trauma, or the effect of some other unknown factor, a communication is established between the dilated lymph channels and the urinary system, with the passage of chyle from the former into the

Table 11. Patients with Chyluria

	TOTAL 22	MALE	FEMALE
Right kidney		5	
Left kidney			2
Bilateral		1	2
Right ureter			1
Left ureter		1	
Right kidney and bladder		1	
Bladder		3	2
Vesical neck			1
Posterior urethra		1	
Undetermined		2	
		14	8

latter. The rupture may take place at the level of the calyces, renal pelvis, ureters, bladder, or urethra. Several communications may be present in the same individual as, for instance, in both the kidney and bladder. In twenty-two cases (14 male, 8 female) of chyluria studied by the author the site of the communication was tentatively traced, during cystoscopy, as follows: bladder, 5; right kidney, 5; left kidney, 2; bilateral, renal, 3; right ureter, 1; left ureter, 1; right kidney and bladder, 1; posterior urethra, 1; vesical neck, 1; undetermined, 2 (Table 11). Chyluria usually does not supervene until several years after infestation. The author has seen a case in which chyluria appeared 58 years after the first clinical manifestations of filariasis. During that period the patient had a yearly average of eight attacks of lymphangitis of the extremities.

Chylous urine may be passed intermittently or continuously, during periods varying from days to years, or the patient may pass chylous urine only once. During an episode of chyluria the urine may be milky for a whole day, or else at day-time or night-time. In one of our patients chyluria was present between 10 P. M. and 3 A. M. for over a period of six months but one year later was passing milky urine at all times and forming chylous clots frequently. Postural changes may affect the passage of chyle into the urinary system.

Symptoms. A dull pain in the back, a sensation of heaviness in the lumbar region, lassitude, and abdominal discomfort may be premonitory symptoms. Urinary symptoms are generally lacking, and these patients as a rule enjoy good health. In chronic, long-standing cases, or when the amount of fat lost is considerable, the patients lose weight, and their skin becomes dry and thin, as part of the cachexia. The formation of chylous clots in the bladder may produce obstruction of the vesical outlet, with complete or incomplete urinary retention. Ureteral occlusion and renal colic may result from clotting in the renal pelvis. Emotional individuals go through transient episodes of anxiety, because of their belief that chyluria is a serious manifestation of disease, and because of the frequent suspicion of a malignant condition.

Diagnosis. The diagnosis must usually depend on the clinical history, symptoms and physical findings. It is a curious but well-substantiated fact that in most cases with clinical manifestations of filariasis, no microfilariae are found in the blood, and vice versa.

Treatment. *Filarial Funiculitis and Epididymo-orchitis.* Generally, the acute phase subsides within a few hours or days. Bed rest, a scrotal support, local heat, and symptomatic treatment for pain and fever are recommended. Antibiotics and chemotherapy are prescribed on general principles, to prevent and control a concomitant bacterial infection.

Hydroceles. Small asymptomatic hydroceles should be treated conservatively, unless operation is demanded by the patient for cosmetic purposes. Moderate large, or symptomatic hydroceles are best treated by open surgery with inversion of the tunica vaginalis. When the vaginal sac is large and redundant, it should be resected to prevent pocket formation and extensive fibrosis. In large hydroceles, when the amount of fluid is expected to be greater than 500 cc., the author prefers to aspirate a few hundred cubic centimeters of fluid a few days before the excision of the tunica vaginalis. In two instances in which huge hydroceles were operated upon by the author without previous aspiration, the patients went into moderate circulatory shock for several hours. Shock was attributed to the sudden evacuation of fluid, and not to the effects of anesthesia.

Elephantiasis. Scrotal elephantiasis may be a distressing and annoying condition for which resection of the elephantoid tissues and plastic repair are indicated. The operation must be as radical as possible, with resection of all the fibrous and edematous tissue. A line of demarcation is always visible on the posterior and lateral aspects of the scrotum, where healthy skin is present. The scrotal flaps can be made to cover the testicles, but when this is not technically feasible, skin flaps may be obtained from the thighs.

In elephantiasis of the penis the reflected layer of the prepuce seldom becomes edematous or fibrotic, and it may be utilized to cover the penile shaft. When the phallus is unusually large, whole thickness grafts can be used to cover the defect.

Recurrences following scrotal resections occur frequently, because usually extensive lymphatic obstruction is present, and inadequate lymph drainage is not established, as a rule. Lasting satisfactory results are obtained in those cases in which a collateral lymphatic circulation is established, and the progress of the disease is arrested.

Chyluria. The passage of milky urine is a rather alarming sign for which most patients seek prompt medical advice. When the amount of fat lost is small, or when the episodes of chyluria, although repeated, are of short duration, reassurance is the best treatment recommended. In the presence of cachexia, attempts should be made to control the loss of fat. Nephrectomy has been performed in some instances, but this radical measure has proved to be disappointing, because in some instances the remaining kidney became the source of chyluria at a later date. Renal decapsulation is employed in some instances with satisfactory, mediocre and bad results. In our experience the results have been satisfactory in only one half of the cases treated.

Sclerosing solutions, such as 20 per cent sodium iodide and 1 or 2 per cent silver nitrate, have been used with inconclusive results. The author has used these therapeutic agents in a few cases with immediate satisfactory results, but recurrences usually supervened several weeks or months later.

In the past the medical treatment of filariasis has been extremely varied and useless, and was not placed on a firm basis until the discovery of hetrazan (1-diethylcarbamyl-4-methylpiperazine) by Hewitt. In 1947 Santiago Stevenson, Oliver González and Hewitt first demonstrated in Puerto Rico, the low toxicity of the drug, its prompt reduction of the microfilarial count, and its possible action against the adult worms. All of this has been subsequently confirmed, and has put the drug in the rank of the specifics. Far-advanced manifestations resulting from extensive tissue damage may not be expected to regress greatly, however.

Hetrazan is administered orally, in tablet form, in doses of 0.5 to 2 mg. per kilo of body weight, three times a day, for three weeks.

The mass treatment of individuals living in an endemic area is feasible and may prove satisfactory to control the disease.

ECHINOCOCCOSIS

Geographic Distribution. Echinococcosis predominates in sheep and cattle-raising countries, among which Arabia, Algiers, Tunisia, Egypt, Abyssinia, Australia, Iceland, New Zealand, Uruguay, Brazil, Argentina, North China, Japan, the Philippine Islands, and some Central European countries constitute important endemic areas. The disease is infrequently observed in Canada and the United States, where a few hundred cases have been found among immigrants.

Life Cycle. Taenia echinococcus is a minute tapeworm measuring, in the adult stage, 3 to 5 mm. in length. The body is composed of a head or scolex, provided with a row of hooklets and suckers, a neck, and three segments or proglottids. At maturity the last segment contains about 500 eggs, which are ejected with the feces of infected animals, such as dogs, wolves, swine, sheep, and cats, which become infected upon eating the carcasses and offal of infected cattle (Fig. 310).

The close association between man and infected dogs is responsible for human infestations. The ingestion of food and water contaminated with echinococcus ova is the usual manner of infection.

A great number of the ingested eggs are destroyed by the gastrointestinal secretions, but those that escape their action liberate the embryos which, after penetrating the wall of the duodenum, enter venules and are then carried to the liver, where most of them are retained. Some pass through the liver and are deposited in other tissues and viscera, among which are the genitourinary organs. However, the liver is predominantly involved in

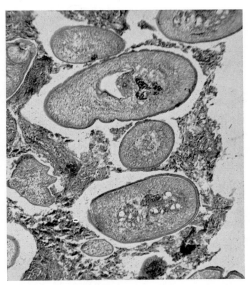

Fig. 310. Taenia echinococcus in the intestine of sheep. 80×. (Courtesy of Dr. J. Bacigalupo, Dept. of Pathology, University of Buenos Aires, Argentina.)

70 per cent of the cases. A great many embryos succumb to the local tissue defences, but those that survive give rise within several weeks to a small spherical mass which constitutes the hydatid cyst.

Although the disease is frequently contracted in childhood, the clinical manifestations produced usually appear in adults, several years after infestation. The slow development of the cyst is responsible for this period of latency. Echinococcus cysts have been discovered in children in several instances.

Evolution of a Hydatid Cyst. Upon reaching an organ the embryo arouses an inflammatory reaction, and later a zone of fibrosis results, which is very dense, and adheres to the cyst, this fibrous shell representing the outer layer of the wall of the latter.

The middle layer separates easily from the surrounding fibrous capsule, and consists mainly of elastic tissue that retracts when a cyst ruptures. This membrane serves the purpose of protecting and nourishing the scolices contained within the cyst. By osmosis it permits the passage of nutrient material inside the cyst.

The innermost layer or germinative membrane gives rise, from its inner aspect, to small spherical growths that represent the brood capsules or daughter cysts. Many of the brood capsules detach from the germinative membrane and float in the crystal clear fluid contained within the cyst, as hydatid sand (Fig. 311). Granddaughter cysts or scolices are derived from the brood capsules.

Renal Echinococcosis. The kidney is involved by hydatid cysts in only 2 per cent of the cases (Borrell and Barnes). Usually the disease is uni-

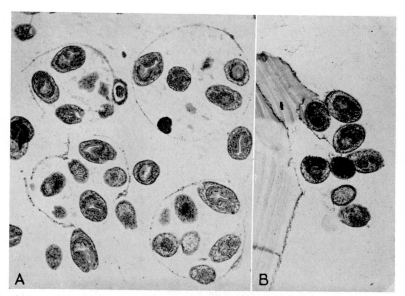

Fig. 311.   *A,* multiple proligerous cyst filled with scolices. 80×. (Courtesy of Dr. J. Bacigalupo, Dept. of Pathology, University of Buenos Aires, Argentina.)
   B, germinative membrane of hydatid cyst with scolices. 80×. (Courtesy of Dr. J. Bacigalupo, Dept. of Pathology, University of Buenos Aires, Argentina.)

lateral, but in some cases both organs are affected. Cysts may be present in one kidney and other organs or several cysts can be found in the same kidney (Fig. 312). The presence of hydatids in the other organs of the urogenital tract are considered medical curiosities.

Symptoms. Although a state of well-being and good health is compatible with echinococcus disease, the presence of multiple hydatids, and the rupture or infection of a cyst, will be responsible for some of the clinical manifestations. A sensation of heaviness or dull pain in the flanks and lumbar area are frequent premonitory complaints, usually present when the cyst has attained a large size. Sometimes the patients discover a movable mass in the abdomen, or the cyst is accidentally recognized in the course of a routine physical examination.

Large cysts compress adjacent viscera, producing an ill-defined clinical picture that cannot be differentiated in some instances from other abdominal conditions. Transient episodes of hematuria, due to renal compression and congestion, are observed occasionally, but they are usually mild and of no serious concern. Attacks of renal colic may supervene, when urinary obstruction is produced by a cyst encroaching upon a calyx or upon the renal pelvis. By compression the cyst is capable of destroying the renal tissues and the mucosal lining of a calyx or of the renal pelvis. It is at this moment that ruptures of the cyst can take place, especially in the presence of trauma. A fistulous communication may be established between the cyst and the excretory passages with evacuation of its contents.

At the time of rupture a sharp, stabbing pain is felt in the flank, accompanied by hematuria. The pain becomes colicky, radiating to the lower

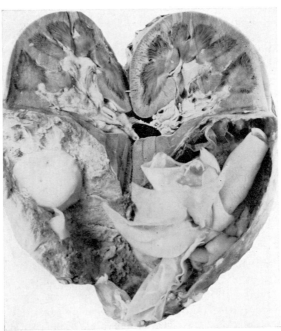

Fig. 312.   Echinococcosis of human kidney. (Courtesy Dr. J. Bacigalupo, Case Prof. P. I. Ilizalde, University of Buenos Aires, Argentina.)

abdomen and genitalia, during the passage of scolices and pieces of membrane, but at times hydatid material is evacuated without pain or discomfort.

The contents of the cyst may obstruct temporarily the site of rupture for a variable number of months or years, and during this period the patients remain asymptomatic. The hydatid material may be discharged intermittently for some time into the renal pelvis. When the communication with a calyx or pelvis persists, infection of the cyst is most likely to supervene. The symptoms of a renal abscess will then be present, and unless prompt surgical measures are taken, the prognosis is grave.

Diagnosis. The presence of hydatid material in the voided urine constitutes a pathognomonic finding. In uncomplicated cysts the diagnosis may prove difficult. Roentgen studies may afford valuable information. Rounded, translucent shadows and calcified cysts are easily recognized in the films, but these findings must be correctly interpreted and differentiated from solitary renal cysts or malignancies that have undergone calcification.

Excretory urograms are informative regarding renal function and the extent of damage to the parenchyma. Very little or incomplete information is obtained in pyelograms when dealing with closed hydatid cysts or when, because of their location and small size, the calyceal pattern is not distorted. But when the architecture of the calyces or pelvis is altered, a differential diagnosis must be established between a hydatid and the different growths arising in the kidney.

In open cysts the opaque medium penetrates and fills partially the cystic cavity, or it may infiltrate the space between the renal substance and the laminated membrane, casting a crescent or wineglass-like shadow in the pyelograms.

The intradermal (Casoni) and complement fixation (Ghedini-Weinberg) tests are valuable diagnostic adjuncts (Kellaway and Fairley). For the former the fresh hydatid fluid is employed, but usually it is not easily obtainable, particularly in non-endemic areas. Positive results are obtained in 90 to 95 per cent of the cases. The complement fixation test is positive in 80 per cent of cases. A negative test does not exclude hydatid disease. Individuals infected by other cestodes may show positive results.

Prognosis. The prognosis is good in the absence of complications, or when the latter are treated adequately.

Treatment. Surgical treatment is the procedure of choice in most cases of renal echinococcosis. When the renal damage is minimal, attempts should be made to remove the cyst or to perform a partial nephrectomy. To avoid spillage of hydatid fluid into the wound, which would produce severe allergic reactions or even death, the wound must be protected with pads, the cyst being emptied by aspiration. The cavity is then injected with several cubic centimeters of a 10 per cent formaldehyde solution, for the destruction of the daughter cysts and scolices, and to prevent contamination of the wall and the formation of new cysts. After five or ten minutes the injected solution is aspirated, and one can proceed with the removal of the cyst in relative safety.

Nephrectomy is indicated in the presence of extensive renal damage. In some cases the operation may be an extensive, difficult, and tedious procedure, especially in the presence of adhesions which may bind the cyst to surrounding structures. When radical operation is impossible, marsupialization should be done, preceded by a careful sterilization of the cyst with formaldehyde solution.

A case may be considered cured when the complement fixation test is found negative one year after excision of a cyst. A positive reaction implies the presence of active echinococcosis, either as a result of a primary multiple infection, reinfestation, or wound contamination during operation.

TRICHOMONIASIS

Trichomonas vaginalis, discovered by Donné in 1837, is a protozoan flagellate widely distributed throughout temperate and tropical countries, and responsible mainly for infections of the female genital tract.

Morphology and Life Cycle. The parasites are ovoid or pyriform, unicellular organisms, about the size of a white blood cell, and provided with four or five flagella, an undulating membrane measuring one or two thirds of the total length of the parasite, and a short axostyle posteriorly. They reproduce by longitudinal division.

Epidemiology. Trichomonas vaginalis is transmitted during copulation, but infection is considered possible by direct contact with soiled cannulas and linen.

Hees (De la Peña) who believes that the infection may be contracted while bathing in the sea, was able to identify in sea water a parasite similar to T. vaginalis. According to this author, there seems to be a greater incidence of Trichomonas infection during the summer season.

The prevalence of Trichomonas vaginitis is exceedingly high, the parasite being found in 40 to 60 per cent of examined cases (Baumeister and Hollinger). Women are considered the parasite's reservoir, whilst men are the transmitters in most instances.

It was formerly believed that the parasite was predominantly a host of the female vagina, and that the male genital tract was but infrequently infected. The clinical evidence accumulated after the observations of Riba, Visher, Miura, Marchard, Feo, Rath, Baumeister and Hollinger, Heckel, Nitschke, De la Peña, Night and Shelanski, Katsunuma, Liston and Lees, and Grim, seems to prove that infections of the male genitourinary system are more frequently encountered than was formerly suspected. During the past ten years the author has found trichomonads in 13 per cent of patients examined and treated for nonspecific urethritis and prostatitis.

Pathology. Several authors believe that trichomonads are nonpathogenic, unless they become associated with bacteria, among which bacilli of the colon group, streptococci and staphylococci are most frequently found.

Rosenthal sustains the theory that trichomonads may remain dormant in the male lower urinary tract, becoming pathogenic when virulent bacteria gain entrance into the urethra.

The author has observed Trichomonas vaginalis in the urine of patients who were free of urinary symptoms, and in whom bacteria were not identified by stains or cultures.

Riba and Perry claim that the parasite cannot be made to grow in culture media that is free of bacteria.

Trichomonas Urethritis in the Male. *Symptoms.* The first clinical manifestations of Trichomonas urethritis may become evident within a period of 24 hours or several days following sexual relations with an infected partner. The severity of the symptoms varies among different individuals. At the beginning there is itching or a burning sensation in the urethral canal between or during micturitions, accompanied or followed later on by a scant white or creamy discharge. Some individuals complain of a clear morning drop, without smarting or painful urination. In very acute cases the discharge is abundant and frothy, and is associated with distressing urethral irritation. When the infection extends to the posterior urethra and bladder there are symptoms of vesical inflammation, strangury and terminal hematuria.

Prostato-semino-vesiculitis. Trichomonas prostatitis and semino-vesicu-
litis are complications arising in the course of urethritis due to this protozoön. Very seldom are acute symptoms present, and the disease is
usually recognized in the subacute or chronic stages. Most patients seeking
medical advice complain of a urethral discharge, mild pollakiuria, terminal
smarting, and of a dull perineal pain, or a sensation of heaviness in the
rectum. Rectally the prostate feels enlarged and boggy, and the seminal
vesicles are distended and painful during the acute stage. Frequently, the
usual physical findings of bacterial prostatic infections are lacking.

Trichomonas Urethritis in the Female. The female urethral meatus is
continuously bathed by vaginal secretions that frequently contain this parasite. Women suffering from Trichomonas vaginitis often complain of mild
transient burning during urination, increased urinary frequency, dysuria,
and a dull suprapubic pain or discomfort. Episodes of acute cystitis are
not uncommon. In our series of cases fifteen patients were referred to the
author for symptoms of acute cystitis, which was their main complaint.
During examination, a severe vaginitis, urethritis and cystitis were found,
due to Trichomonas vaginalis. The parasite was discovered in large quantities in the vaginal exudate, in the urethra, and in the urine.

On examination the urethral meatus is congested, edematous, and very
sensitive to the touch. The passage of a soft rubber catheter, or of a small
sound, proves to be an extremely painful procedure which reflects the degree
of urethral inflammation.

Chronic urethritis is responsible for the formation of small polypoid
growths or cyst-like elevations in the vesical outlet; when large and multiple,
they produce mild symptoms of urinary obstruction.

Urethral caruncles are frequently observed, specially among women in
the fourth and fifth decades of life in whom a history of chronic vaginitis
may be elicited. Salerno claims to have found Trichomonas vaginalis in
all his patients with urethral caruncles. Among five patients with caruncles
seen by the author at the San Juan City Hospital, trichomonads were found
in the vaginal canal, urethra and bladder, but the author does not believe
that Trichomonas vaginalis per se are responsible for the development of
urethral caruncles. These tumor growths are known to result from chronic
urethral infection of different cause, among which trichomonads can be
mentioned.

Vesical Trichomoniasis. Trichomonas infection of the urinary bladder
usually accompanies urethritis and prostato-semino-vesiculitis in the male,
and vaginitis in the female. Trichomonas cystitis is characterized in some
instances by severe symptoms of irritability of the bladder, accompanied by
pyuria, stranguria and hematuria. Several of the symptoms of cystitis may
be absent in mild cases, specially when the vaginal infection subsides.

Cystoscopy reveals a generalized congestion of the vesical mucosa. In
acute and early cases the inflammation may be limited to the trigone and
bladder neck. In chronic cases the trigonal mucosa has a white or pearly
color, and appears covered with multiple small spherical elevations which
resemble those of bullous edema. Sometimes multiple bloody blisters appear

scattered about the urethral orifice and extending into it. These lesions persist for several weeks and disappear gradually. Occasionally the mucosa is pale and whitish, with a fluffy appearance. Rarely, if ever, do these lesions extend beyond the confines of the trigone.

Renal Trichomoniasis. Trichomonads may be transported to the kidney by the blood stream, or may reach the renal pelvis from the bladder. Some authors sustain the theory that trichomoniasis is a systemic disease (Manwell). Experimentally, strains of Trichomonas vaginalis bovis were injected subcutaneously into ten women; in six of them a Trichomonas vaginitis developed. The oral administration of the parasite has also resulted in positive blood and stool cultures within a period of ten days. In the light of these experiments one is tempted to accept the theory that blood-borne infections of the kidney are a possibility. Lewis and Caroll, and Madsen are among those who have reported renal infections due to Trichomonas vaginalis. In these cases the parasite was also present in the bladder and vagina. Renal infections with this protozoön resemble bacterial infections of the kidney in that pyuria, chills, fever, and lumbar pain are present.

Other Genital Manifestations of Trichomoniasis. Trichomonas vaginalis is capable of producing ulcerative lesions of the mucocutaneous membrane of the external genitalia. Soubigou, Duliscouët and Gaudin reported the case of a sailor who, following sexual relations with three women, developed a moderate ulcerative balanitis involving the frenulum. A careful search for B. ducrey, T. pallidum and N. gonorrheae was fruitless, but T. vaginalis was recovered from the ulcer; none were found in the purulent exudate, urine or stools. Local treatment with a ten per cent stovarsol solution proved to be effective in this case. In 1924 Katsunuma also identified trichomonads in the urine of a 3-year-old boy in whom the infective focus was located in the prepuce.

Diagnosis. In view of the high incidence of Trichomonas infection, both in male and female patients, the parasite must be routinely searched for in the exudates obtained for bacteriological examination.

A small drop of fresh exudate is placed on a glass slide and diluted with one drop of warm normal saline solution; the preparation is examined directly under a microscope. The parasites are identified by their motility and lack of progression in a given field.

A fresh sample of urine, preferably the first morning specimen, is adequate when trichomoniasis is suspected and the parasites are not identified in the urethral discharge. When the latter is very scanty or absent, a few cubic centimeters of urine are centrifuged at low speed for one minute, and the sediment examined as aforementioned. Stained preparations are ideal for identification of the flagella and undulating membrane, but wet preparations are time-saving and usually adequate for diagnostic purposes.

Treatment. When a diagnosis of Trichomonas infection is made, it would be ideal to examine both partners. The infection is most likely to recur if sources of contagion are missed, or if the treatment of an infected partner is neglected. Sexual abstinence may be helpful, but when this is not possible, or refused, the utilization of condoms is to be encouraged.

In our experience the sulfonamides have proven of no value in trichomoniasis of the male. We have further observed that the associated bacterial flora is resistant to therapy, and negative cultures are obtained only when the trichomonads are eradicated.

Urethritis in the Male. Irrigations with silver nitrate, acriflavine, mercurochrome, mercuric cyanide, and permanganate of potash have been widely employed by various authors, who claim satisfactory results.* In our hands daily urethral irrigation with increasing strengths of silver nitrate solutions (1/5000 to 1/500) were adequate to obtain 90 per cent of cures. Apparent failures in our series were attributed to reinfestations and to lack of cooperation.

Prostato-semino-vesiculitis. Daily irrigations of the urethra with silver nitrate solution, diathermy, and prostatic messages once or twice a week should be sufficient to control the infection. One or two endoscopic applications to the posterior urethra, of phenol-glycerine 50 per cent followed by 5 to 10 per cent silver nitrate solution, will help intractable cases in which urethral granulations are present. The female urethra should also be treated in cases of Trichomonas vaginitis, since it may serve as a focus of reinfection. Bladder and urethral irrigations with silver nitrate solutions should complement vaginal treatments. San Louis recommends, with apparently satisfactory results, insufflations of the urethra and vagina with parasiticidal powders. Lewis and Caroll, and Madsen, treated their cases of renal trichomoniasis with indwelling urethral catheters and pelvic lavage, utilizing solutions of silver nitrate.

UROGENITAL AMEBIASIS

Amebiasis is a disease produced by Endamoeba histolytica, the most conspicuous lesions of which are found in the large intestine. The parasite is endemic in the temperate and tropical countries, but in the latter the clinical manifestations are more acute and severe. Amebae are found in the vegetative or cystic forms in the excreta of infected individuals. The most frequent source of human contagion is the consumption of infected food, water and, especially, uncooked vegetables. The protozoön is capable of infecting the liver, spleen, lungs, kidney, bladder, testis, epididymidis, vas deferens, vulva, uterine cervix, and the skin.

Pathology. After reaching the small intestine, the amebic cyst gives rise to four amebae which later on reach the large bowel. They are capable of penetrating the mucosa and submucosa by their ameboid movements and by cytolysins.

When they produce ulcers of the colon, the vegetative amebae may enter the portal circulation, and thus reach other organs, especially the liver (Scott). Although the genitourinary system is seldom infected by this parasite, a sufficient number of cases has been reported to warrant mention in this chapter.

*Since this Chapter was submitted for publication we have used Aureomycin to treat Trichomonas infestations of the male genitourinary system with gratifying results. Average recommended dosage ranges between 2000 and 2500 mg. per day for a week or ten days.

Cystitis. Apparently, amebic cystitis is the most frequent genitourinary complication (Franchini; Gascio Rocca; Mattei).

The parasites may reach the urinary bladder from the lymphatic and blood streams, directly from the outside through the urethra, or from the bowel in cases of vesico-intestinal fistula (ascending), and from the kidney (descending).

In most instances a history of intestinal amebiasis is elicited, or symptoms suggestive of this disease are present.

Symptoms. In the acute stage, severe urinary frequency, urgency, and smarting during urination are always present. Tenesmus and a piercing pain in the region of the bladder precede and follow micturition, the latter becoming excruciating and agonizingly painful towards the end. Most patients complain of a continuous sensation of suprapubic weight or fulness, and of hematuria, which is usually present and terminal and consists of the passage of a few drops of blood.

Untreated patients as a general rule may go through periods of well-being during which they are free of urinary symptoms, or the latter are minimal and tolerable; however, recurrences are very likely to occur.

Diagnosis. The urine is acid, and contains pus cells, erythrocytes, mucoid matter, debris, and amebae and cysts. Bacteria also contribute to the severity of the symptoms.

Cystoscopy. In the acute stage, patches of congestion are seen here and there in the mucosa of the bladder; later on the whole mucosa becomes inflamed. Near the dome and lateral walls, small bullae of a yellowish, pink or bloody color are seen. In the chronic stage there are elevations on the mucosa of the bladder resembling polypoid growths which may attain the size of a millet seed or a grain of corn. Superficial ulcerations may be present, their size ranging from a few millimeters to 1 cm. in diameter.

Kidney. Amebiasis of the kidney will be discussed under two headings; amebic pyelitis and perinephric abscess. In the former, the amebae may reach the kidney from the blood stream, or may ascend the ureter to gain the renal pelvis. Both kidneys may be simultaneously infected (Bernardini and Esquivel).

Symptoms. A dull pain in the flank, chills, fever, and general malaise are usually present. There may be prostration, in severe cases. The bladder is frequently involved, and in some instances cystitis dominates the clinical picture. Although a history of amebiasis is usually elicited in these cases, the patients reported by Segurola and Thomas gave a negative history.

Perinephric Abscess. Amebae may reach the perirenal fat and tissues by the blood stream, from ruptured amebic abscesses of the liver, or from perforated amebic ulcers of the colon.

Symptoms. Chills, fever, pain in the lumbar and costovertebral angles, muscle spasm, rigidity, and a palpable mass in the flank are usually present. General prostration and toxemia will be observed in some early cases, or when there is procrastination in treatment. The spontaneous rupture and evacuation of an amebic abscess into upper collecting urinary channels is a possibility (Casco).

Vas Deferens, Epididymis and Testis. The invasion of these organs by E. histolytica has been recognized since Warthin reported the first case in 1922. The patient was a Russian who had contracted amebiasis several years previously and who on admission was suffering from amebic dysentery. There were no symptoms referable to the genital organs, but at autopsy numerous amebae were found in the vas, epididymis and seminiferous tubules.

Seminal Vesicles. In 1923 Hines reported the first case of amebiasis of the seminal vesicles. The patient complained of fulness and pain in the perineum, radiating to the glans penis, and of a creamy urethral discharge.

Amebic Vaginitis. Infection of the vagina is possible in the presence of a rectovaginal fistula or by direct extension from the vulva. Clinically, a profuse vaginal discharge is present, in which the amebae may be identified (Saujeon).

Uterine Cervix. This is an extremely rare condition. The only cases reported in the literature are those of Wu and Chi, and Lee. The mode of infection claimed by these authors was direct extension from the outside or when rectovaginal fistulae are present.

Amebiasis of the Vulva. The lesions produced by this parasite in the vulva may extend into the vagina and be confused with carcinoma (Retrespo and Méndez Lemaitre). The absence of adenopathy, and the state of good health enjoyed by the patient leads one to suspect that the lesions are inflammatory and nonmalignant. The identification of amebae in the smears is diagnostic.

Treatment. Amebic infections of the urinary tract appear to have responded satisfactorily to the administration of the derivatives of ipecacuanha, of which emetine hydrochloride is the most effective. Emetine is administered hypodermically, 1 mg. per kilo of body weight, daily, without exceeding a total of 10 mg. per kilo. Acetarsone and carbarsone are pentavalent arsenical compounds prescribed in tablet form for oral use; carbarsone, 0.25 gm., twice daily for ten days, and acetarsone, 0.25 gm., three times daily for seven days.

STRONGYLOIDES STERCORALIS

This parasite, also known under the name of Anguillula stercoralis, A. intestinalis and Strongyloides intestinalis, is a fusiform round worm which usually parasitizes the small intestine of man.

It is found predominantly in tropical countries but some cases have been reported from temperate countries. In North America, sporadic cases have been found in New York, Ohio, Cincinnati, Pennsylvania, Louisiana and, farther north, in Canada.

Life Cycle. Two cycles are known: the free living generation, during which the parasite lives and reproduces in the soil, and the parasitic generation occurring within the human body.

The worm penetrates the skin of man in the larval form, and enters the venous circulation to reach the right side of the heart; it then passes into the capillaries of the pulmonary alveoli which it traverses and enters the pulmonary alveoli. If female and male worms are present, fecondation may take place here or in the bronchi, trachea or intestine where they are found after being swallowed by the human host. The female enters the mucosa of the small bowel, where oviposition takes place.

Autoinfection may occur if the first stage larvae are transformed into filariform larvae that are capable of traversing the wall of the colon and reach the lungs. The larvae are usually found in the small intestine, less frequently in the large bowel, but they have been also encountered in the mesenteric veins, lymph nodes and lymphatics, liver and pancreatic and biliary ducts.

Fornara in 1923, and Whitehill and Miller in 1944, recovered the larvae and the adults worms from the urine of man. The latter case was very well studied. The patient complained of long-standing lower abdominal discomfort, urinary frequency, urgency, and some incontinence of urine. The finding of the parasite and larval forms in the urine, and the subsidence of symptoms following treatment, make it almost certain that the parasite was responsible for the patient's complaints. Although this parasitosis is found with relative frequency in Puerto Rico, we do not know of a single case of urogenital involvement.

Treatment. The only specific drug is gentian violet, administered in enteric coated tablets (0.06 gm.), before meals, three times a day, to a total of 32.5 gm. Intractable cases may be treated by instilling 25 cc. of a 1 per cent solution of gentian violet directly into the duodenum through a duodenal tube.

STRONGYLOSIS

Eustrongylus gigas (Dioctophyma renale) or giant kidney worm is a cosmopolitan parasite infecting a diversity of animals, such as the wolf, raccoon, mink, skunk, horse, dog, and ox. The parasite is one of the largest nematodes known. The adult male worm measures 14 to 20 cm. in length and the female is twice as long. Ten cases of human infection have so far been reported.

Life Cycle. Very little is known about the evolution of the parasite. The eggs are found in the water and soil, and the contained embryos may remain alive for several years under adverse climatic conditions. Heretofore, experimental attempts to produce the disease in animals have failed. The intermediate host of the worm has not been discovered; however, it is believed that certain fishes may be the source of contagion.

Pathology. The parasites, single or multiple, reach the renal pelvis, which they are capable of distending considerably. Gradually the parasites destroy the renal parenchyma and, after several years, a shell is all that remains of the kidney. Chronic perinephritis is always present in the terminal stages.

Symptoms. The presence of the parasite is not characterized by any special symptomatology. Patients complain of dull lumbar pain or discomfort. At times the pain may be excruciating, and radiates to the lower abdomen and bladder, when the parasites occlude the ureteral lumen. Repeated attacks of hematuria may take place, and renal lithiasis and infection may complicate the clinical picture. Ureteral perforation has been known to occur during the parasite's migration to the bladder. The patient seen by Lisboa complained of vulvar pruritus and vesical discomfort, and volunteered that she had the sensation that something was swimming inside her bladder. Following the expulsion of a parasite, that was identified as a Dioctophyma renale, all symptoms disappeared.

Diagnosis. The recognition of ova in the voided urine, and the passage of worms, are the only means of establishing a correct diagnosis.

Treatment. If the disease is recognized before severe renal damage has been produced, the worms may be removed surgically, but when renal destruction is advanced nephrectomy is recommended.

CATFISH INFESTATION

A small (3 inches long; 3-4 mm. diameter) urinophilous fish Candiru (Vandellia cirrhosa) invading the urethra and bladder of Amazon Indians is discussed in Section VIII, Chapter 2. With phosphatic incrustation, the dead fish becomes an irritating foreign body.

REFERENCES

ABDEL RAHMAN EL SADR: Localized bilharziasis of the ureter. Urol. Cut. Review, *52:*334–339, 1948.

BARQUERO GONZÁLEZ, R.: Un caso de papilomas vulvares y perianales producidos por S. Mansoni. Rev. Policlini, Razetti, *3,*155–160, 1939.

BAUMEISTER, C. and HOLINGER, N.: Trichomonas infection of male genitourinary tract. Arch. Surg., *43:*433–444, 1941.

BERNARDINI, R. and ESQUIVEL, R. B.: Urinary amoebiasis. Semana Médica, *1:*248–256, 1939.

BHASKARA MENON, T. and ANNAMALAI, D. R.: Some pathological changes met with in filarial orchitis and their significance. J. Trop. Med. and Hyg., *38:*18–21, 1935.

BORRELL, J. H. and BARNES, J. M.: Renal manifestations of hydatid disease. New York State M. J., *33:*1390, 1933.

CARBERA Y CARIDAD, J.: Filarial lymphatic cyst of inguinal cord. J. Rev. Kuba, *3:*111–113, 1947.

CASCO, E. D.: Amoebic abscess of kidney with spontaneous elimination by urinary route. Rev. Med. Latino Am., *17:*1165–1167, 1932.

CASTELLANI, A. and CHALMERS, A. J.: Manual of Tropical Medicine. 2nd ed., p. 1429, London, Baillière, Tindall and Cox, 1912.

DE LA PEÑA, A.: Prostato-vesiculitis due to trichomonas vaginalis. Rev. Clin. Española, *2:* 157–160, 1941.

DOUGLADE, J. H. and FITZGERALD, P. J.: Asymptomatic microfilaremia in the Caribbean area. U. S. Navy M. Bull., *46:*193–201, 1946.

FORNARA, P.: Hematuria from Strongyloidosis. Policlínico (Seg. Prot.), *30:*75–80, 1923.

FRANCHINI, G.: Amoebic cystitis. Urol. Cut. Rev., *32:*790–796, 1928.

GASCIO ROCCA, L.: Cystitis from Endamoeba Histolytica. La Reforma Médica, *44:*344–348, 1928.

GELFAND, M.: Bilharzial disease of the bladder as determined at autopsy, with particular reference to its diagnosis by mucosal snips. Am. J. Trop. Med., *28:*563–566, 1948.

GIBSON, W. B.: Bilharziasis of the female genital tract. M. J. South Africa, *21:*44–45, 1926.

HERNÁNDEZ MORALES, F. and MALDONADO, J. F.: The diagnosis of schistosomiasis mansoni by a rectal biopsy technique. Am. J. Trop. Med., *26:*811–820, 1946.

HERNÁNDEZ MORALES, F., SANTIAGO STEVENSON, D., OLIVER GONZÁLEZ, J. and MALDONADO, J. F.: An evaluation of the therapeutic effectiveness of fuadin and anthiomaline in the treatment of Manson's schistosomiasis, Puerto Rico J. of Pub. Health and Trop. Med., *25:*256–260, 1949.

HINES, L. E.: Endamoeba histolytica in seminal fluid in a case of amoebic dysentery. J.A.M.A., *28:*274–275, 1923.

KELLAWAY, C.H. and FAIRLEY, K.D.: Clinical significance of laboratory test in echinococcosis. M. J. Australia, *1:*340, 1932.

KHALIL BEY, B.: The etiological role of filariasis in endemic funiculitis and hydrocele in Egypt. J. Egyptian M. A., *18:*389–395, 1935..

KHOURI, J.: Sur un cas rere d'infestation simultané par Schistosomum mansoni et par Schistosomum haematobium. Bull. Path. Exotique, *21:*772, 1928.

KNOTT, J.:Filariasis of the testicle due to Wuchereria bancrofti. Trans. Roy. Soc. Trop. Med. and Hyg. *3:*335–347, 1939.

KOPPISCH, E.: Manson's schistosomiasis. J.A.M.A. *121:*936–952, 1943.

LEGAC, P.: Procedé pratique d'enrichessement des urines en oeufs de Schistosoma haematobium chez les sujets atteints de bilharziose vesicale. Bull. Soc. Path. Exotique, *29:* 434–435, 1939.

LEWIS,B. and CAROLL,G.: A case of Trichomonas vaginalis. J. Urol., *19:*337–339, 1928.

LISBOA, A.: Estrongilose renal humana. Brazil Médico, *59:*101–102, 1945.

MCKINLEY, E. B.: Role of bacteria in acute filarial lymphangitis. Puerto Rico J. Pub. Health and Trop. Med., *6:*419–427, 1931.

MADSEN,A.C.: A case of trichomonas infection of the renal pelvis. West Virginia Med. J., *29:*356–357, 1933.

MANWELL, E. J.: Urinary symptoms in relation to trichomonas vaginalis infestation. New England J. Med., *211:*567–569, 1934.

MATTEI,A.: Inflammation due to Endamoeba vesicalis. Annali di Med. Navate e Colon. *34:*24–47, 1932.

MONSTESTRUC, E : Bilharziose vesicale à schistosoma mansoni. Bull. Soc. Path. Exotique, *33:*333, 1940.

RAY, P. N.: Chronic epididymo-orchitis or fibrosis of the testicle of filarial origin. Brit. J. Surg., *22:*264–268, 1934.

RETRESPO, R. and MÉNDEZ LEMAÎTRE, A.: Amoebic infection confused with cancer. Rev. Fac. de Méd. Bogotá, *16:*914–920, 1947.

RIBA, L. W. and PERRY, E.: Trichomonas prostato-vesiculitis. J. Urol., *22:*563–571, 1929.

ROSENTHAL, D. B.: Urinary infection with trichomonas vaginalis in the male. M. J. Australia, *1:*782–783, 1931

SALERNO, E. V.: Urethral caruncles and trichomoniasis. Prensa Médica Argentina, *31:* 2554–2558, 1944.

SANJURJO, L. A. and KOPPISCH, E.: Manson's schistosomiasis with unilateral involvement of kidney. J. Urol., *66:*298, 1951.

SANTIAGO STEVENSON, D., OLIVER GONZÁLEZ, J. and HEWITT, R. I.: Treatment of filariasis bancrofti with 1-diethylcarbamyl-4-methylpiperazine hydrochloride (Hetrazan). J.A.M.A., *135:*708–712, 1947.

SAUJÉON, M.: Troubles uro-génitaux guéris par l'hemetine, origine amebienne vraisemblable. Bull. Soc. Path. Exotique, *21:*883–884, 1928.

SCOTT MACFIE, J. W.: Observations on urinary amoebiasis. Ann. Trop. Med. and Parasit., *10:*291–304, 1916.

SEGUROLA, M.: Un caso de amebiasis renal. Vida Nueva, *20:*24–28, 1927.

SMYRNIOTIS, P. C.: Calcification of seminal vesicles revealed by roentgenography in patients infected with mixed bilharzia. J. Egyptian M. A., *12:*231–235, 1929.

SOUBIGOU, DULISCOUET and GAUDIN: Ulcerous balanitis due to trichomonas vaginalis. Bull. Soc. Path. Exotique, *31:*52–55, 1938.

STEVENS, A. R.: Schistosomiasis infestation with involvement of the upper urinary tract. Urol. Cut. Rev., *44:*681–685, 1940.

TESTUT, L. and LATARJET, A.: Anatomia Humana. Salvat Ed., Spain, 1932.

THOMAS, F. D.: Endamoeba histolytica involvement of the urinary tract. Urol. Cut. Rev., *40:*199–200, 1936.

WARTHIN, A. S.: The occurrence of Endamoeba histolytica with tissue lesions in the testes and epididymis in chronic dysentery. J. Infect. Dis., *30:*559–568, 1922.

WHITEHILL, R. and MILLER, H. M.: Infestations of the genito-urinary tract by strongyloides stercoralis. A Case Report. Bull. Johns Hopkins Hosp., *75:*169–174, 1944.

WU, T. T. and CHI, C. K.: Amoebiasis of uterine cervix. Chinese Med. J., *49* 69–73, 1935.

YAMAUCHI, S.: Chyluria: Clinical, Laboratory and Statistical Study of 45 Personal Cases Observed in Hawaii. J. Urol., *54:*319–347, 1945.

Section VI

INFECTIONS AND INFLAMMATIONS OF THE MALE GENITAL TRACT

CHAPTER 1

Penis and Urethra

EDGAR BURNS, M. D. AND IAN THOMPSON, M. D.

CHANCRE

In a discussion of the inflammatory lesions of the male genital tract it seems correct to begin with *syphilis*. Chancre, which in the past has been more commonly the province of the urologist than at present, is merely the pale foreshadowing of the many more seriously generalized tissue reactions which have concerned the field of medicine for many years. It is caused by penetration of the Treponema pallidum, the specific spirochete isolated first by Schaudinn in 1905. It gains entrance through the intact or abraded skin or mucous membrane. The penis is the usual site of primary involvement in the male. The sites of predilection on the penis are the glans and prepuce but other situations, such as on the meatus, within the urethra, and on the shaft, are not uncommon.

The chancre begins as a hyperemic or erythematous spot which develops in a more or less circumscribed fashion followed in a day or two by desquamation with surrounding induration to form usually within a week either the hard papule or the more characteristic ulcerated lesion. The rubbery hardness of the ulcer is due to surrounding vascular sclerosis with pronounced lymphocytic plasma cell and epithelial cell infiltration. Typically, the lesion is a painless, rather clean, shallow ulcer with indurated rolling borders. Usually solitary, it persists in rather quiescent fashion until the secondary stage (Fig. 313) or until treated, whereupon it gradually heals, usually without scarring. The site of the healed chancre may occasionally appear slightly pigmented.

The Treponema pallidum is a delicate parasite which multiplies by transverse fission. Since it does not live long outside of the human body, slide identification is feasible only in fresh material. Under a highly refined darkfield condensor it is easily distinguished from other treponemas by its size, morphology and movements. Its undulations are slow, gentle, forward

595

and backward, so that it is easily kept in the microscopic field. It bends only in the middle and is usually much smaller than other spirochetal denizens of the area. Proper collection of material to be studied is important. The ulcer should be cleansed and serum alone should be expressed from it, for pus and red cells interfere considerably with the examination.

The average interval from infection to appearance of the chancre is ten to twenty-one days. Much longer incubation periods, which have been reported, are open to question. The development of a positive serologic reaction ranges from three weeks to three months after inoculation.

The severity of infection appears to be modified by a number of factors, such as the amount of the inoculum, the time the race has been exposed

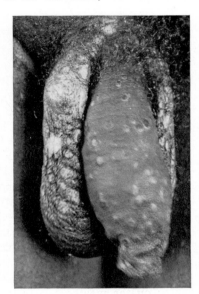

Fig. 313.   Syphilis. Secondary eruption on penis and scrotum.

to it and a certain natural immunity. Estrogens experimentally delay and lessen the severity of the infection. Systemic infections are more common in the primary stage than is generally recognized.

In the *diagnosis* and differential diagnosis of chancre emphasis should be placed upon the value of the darkfield microscope. The clinical appearance of the sore is only suggestive. Serologic tests are usually of no value during the first few days after appearance of the lesion since the amount of reagin present during this period is usually not enough to produce a positive reaction. The lesions from which chancre must be differentiated are chancroid, granuloma inguinale, lymphogranuloma venereum, the balanitides of varying etiology, carcinoma, scabies, psoriasis, lichen planus, leukoplakia, erythroplasia and a host of other entities.

The ulcers of chancroids are soft, dirty, ragged and painful. They spread by apposition and tend to produce early inguinal adenitis with much periadenitis and suppuration. The adenopathy of syphilis is nonmatting and freely movable with no tendency to suppurate unless secondarily infected.

Differentiation may be made by microscopic identification of the spirochete or Ducrey's bacillus. Both infections may be present in the same lesion in as much as 50 per cent of cases. The serologic and Ducrey skin tests are corroborative only when the reactions are positive. Granuloma inguinale is a superficial affliction of the skin with red velvety granulations rolling towards the periphery in serpigenous outline. Buboes are uncommon. Tissue biopsy demonstrates the Donovan bodies. The penile lesion of lymphogranuloma inguinale is usually so insignificant as to escape notice in the majority of cases. The absence of penile lesions, inguinal adenitis, a positive reaction to the Frei skin test and complement fixation reaction with negative serologic reaction for syphilis provide sufficiently conclusive evidence. The balanitides of varying etiologies will be found devoid of spirochetes and replete with the causative bacteria. Carcinoma of the penis has so often been treated as venereal infection that biopsy and tissue analysis should be made a part of the investigation of the majority of indurated or ulcerative lesions upon the genitals of more than two or three weeks' duration. Scabies, lichen planus and psoriasis are usually typical clinically but serologic tests should be routine. The treatment of syphilis is not within the province of the urologist and will not be discussed here.

CHANCROID

Chancroid, or the soft chancre, has been known since ancient times. Prior to identification of the etiologic agent of each it was often confused with the chancre. The coexistence of syphilis and chancroid has been so common that chancroid has often been described as the masker of the chancre. It is much more prevalent universally than syphilis.

Chancroid is a predominantly local and regional disease of rather superficial nature; untoward late systemic morbidity has never been ascribed to it. The causative agent is the Hemophilus ducreyi, a gram-negative, short, plump rod occurring predominantly in parallel chains. The disease is contracted by contact with abraded skin or mucous membrane, usually during coitus, and thereafter is fostered by poor genital hygiene and general unsanitary habits. Further lesions may develop in adjacent areas by autoinoculation.

In the male the initial sites of predilection are the parafrenular areas and the coronal sulcus. The incubation period is relatively short, reported by some as one to two days and usually no longer than one week.

By means of inoculation studies utilizing the bubo fluid of inguinal chancroidal abscesses, Wilcox (1950) had frequent opportunities of observing step by step development of the local lesion. According to him, it appears first as an erythematous area, which blends into a small papule within twenty-four hours, followed by a distinctly inflamed button at forty-eight hours, a pustule at ninety-six hours, and rapid subsequent ulceration. The ulcer may be linear, serpiginous or circumferential and its borders are not indurated. The sore may penetrate deeply; its base may be granular or membranous and is frequently covered with a purulent exudate. The ulcer is painful and bleeds easily. If uncomplicated, it will heal simply by cleansing within two or three weeks, soft cicatrization closing in from the periphery. The pathologic picture is one of lymphocytic infiltration which may undermine for some distance the superficial borders of the ulcer.

The varying types of lesions which have been described result primarily from the secondary infection which may develop in the unattended ulceration, furthered by the presence of a redundant prepuce, instrumental in the retention of infected secretions. Thus, simple ulcerative and inflammatory soft chancres have been delineated. The mixed lesions are frequently the cause of clinical confusion owing to concurrence of syphilitic and chancroidal characteristics.

The secondary manifestations of chancroid may be classified as local, regional and systemic. Phimosis due to inflammatory edema is frequent and propagates increased infectional destruction. Severe paraphimosis may result if unwise manipulation of the prepuce succeeds in its retraction past the corona. Phagedenic chancroid occurred more commonly in the past, for at present earlier treatment has prevented the deep-seated infections which could destroy, partially or completely, the glans penis, resulting in gangrene occasionally and scarring and urethral stricture rather frequently.

Inguinal lymphatic involvement develops reputedly in about one half of the cases (Rowe, 1951). Spread to involvement of the inguinal lymphatics may vary from mild adenitis and peri-adenitis to bilateral abscesses; unilateral involvement, however, is more common. The peri-adenitis distinguishes the chancroidal from the syphilitic, for there is matting of the nodes, together with attachment to the skin, rarely seen in syphilis. The enlarged nodes are tender and will persist either to resolution or fluctuation within one or two weeks. Prolonged chronic adenitis with lymphatic blockage must be ascribed more readily to concomitant lymphogranuloma venereum. A systemic phase usually is dependent upon the extent of inguinal infection and consists in fever, malaise and occasionally anemia.

In the diagnosis of chancroid, despite the suggestive clinical features, the soft, painful, dirty, multi-designed lesions with the typical matted adenopathy and buboes, reiteration of the fundamental tenets of the study of penile lesions is necessary; the organism must be demonstrated. Ducrey's skin reaction, auto-inoculation and cultural characteristics are corroborative only when the bacillus is found. Differential distinction between chancroid, syphilis, lymphogranuloma venereum and granuloma inguinale may be promulgated by the shorter incubation period of chancroid, the multiplicity of lesions, the type of ulceration, the spreading by adjacent inoculation and the character of the adenitis.

Herpes progenitalis and nonspecific ulcerations are usually of little import in differential diagnosis. They may be ruled out by inspection and subsequent smear.

Erosive and gangrenous balanitis demands the anaerobic protection of a long prepuce and the adenopathy seen therein is usually not tender. Difficulty may be encountered in garnering Ducrey's bacillus from the ulcers; Levin (1941) estimated that only 20 to 60 per cent of cases may be diagnosed by smear. On the other hand, others have been able to isolate the organism with methyl green pyronine stains in almost 90 per cent of cases. Many believe that only repeated biopsy will establish the diagnosis in those ulcers which are not identified by simple smear.

Ducrey's skin test, which will give a moderate number of false positive reactions, becomes indicative of chancroid within one or two weeks of the appearance of the lesion, and occasionally more promptly. The reaction remains positive for a varying length of time subsequent to infection. Auto-inoculation and hetero-inoculation techniques (Willcox, 1950), though cumbersome, may more readily allow demonstration of the organism.

Prior to the advent of chemotherapeutic and antibiotic agents the *treatment* of chancroid revolved around attempts at prophylaxis, wherein soap and water and calomel ointment rubs were utilized immediately following suspicious exposure. Subsequent to the appearance of the lesion simple cleanliness allowed the tissues to combat the infection in a great many cases. Weekly cauterization of early lesions with phenol and alcohol was apparently helpful in some instances. A dorsal slit to relieve balanoposthitis is utilized only when necessary. Circumcision is contraindicated during the active stage of the infection because of the spread along the incision. Similarly, when necessary, aspiration is preferable to incision of large inguinal abscesses.

The introduction of the sulfonamides tremendously reduced the frequency of complications incident to chancroidal infection. The sulfonamides are generally agreed to be the best preparation for the treatment of chancroids for two reasons: first, they are as efficacious as any other medication, and secondly, they have no masking effect on the appearance of syphilis, which may coincidentally have been acquired. Each of the antibiotics in small dosage is capable of postponing the appearance of the syphilitic chancre for as long as several months, thus necessitating careful and prolonged follow-up study for not only clinical but serologic signs of syphilis.

Sulfathiazole in dosage of 4 gm. daily for five days followed by 3 gm. daily for five days has been recommended as curative. Sulfadiazine and sulfonamide combinations have been found equally effective in similar dosage. The patient must be carefully observed for evidence of sulfonamide toxicity, granulocytopenia, renal changes and cutaneous sensitization. A large fluid intake and alkalinization are helpful in the reduction of renal toxicity.

Penicillin has been found to be of little or no value in the treatment of chancroid. Whatever effect it may have is upon secondary coccal invaders. Streptomycin, Aureomycin, Chloromycetin and Terramycin have all been investigated experimentally (Willcox, 1951) and have been found preventive against hetero-inoculative bubo material. There is difference of opinion as to the clinical value of streptomycin and many have reported the sulfonamides to be more effective. The use of Aureomycin in dosage of 2 gm. daily for seven to ten days has been found to be quite effective. Terramycin in a dosage of 4 gm. daily for five days has been found to be curative in a few cases. Chloromycetin has also proved effective in the treatment of all manifestations of chancroid.

Since most cases of chancroid may be treated adequately by cleansing and protection of the lesions, with the addition of the sulfonamides, it would seem wise to limit use of the antibiotics to those patients who either are sensitive to or fail to respond to sulfonamides. Moreover, because of the masking power of these drugs, follow-up examinations for evidence of syphilis are imperative.

LYMPHOGRANULOMA VENEREUM

Lymphogranuloma venereum, lymphopathia venereum or lymphogranuloma inguinale are symptoms for a venereal disease which in the past few years has received increasing attention. This is due as much to studies concerning the high incidence of previous infection, or latency, as evidenced by extensive utilization of the complement fixation and Frei skin tests, as to the relatively recent suspicion that the causative organism, a virus of the psittacosis group, may also in some fashion be related to the pleuropneumoniae organisms isolated with fair frequency in the nonspecific urethritis and oculo-mucocutaneous syndrome group.

The inclusion bodies of lymphogranuloma were demonstrated first in 1927 and the assumption that the etiologic agent was a filtrable virus was subsequently verified. Although the disease begins on the genitals, it soon becomes systemic. Morbid manifestations, however, occur essentially in three aggregates: glandular, anorectal and occasionally a persistent genital group. As is true of the majority of such diseases lymphogranuloma is encountered more often in those of the lower income and cultural strata.

Lymphogranuloma is primarily acquired during coitus. The incubation period has been variously described as ranging from two days to three weeks, the discrepancy undoubtedly being due to the frequent evanescence of the primary lesion and the inaccuracy of the history of exposure.

Initially, an erosion, papule or vesicle appears commonly about the coronal sulcus but feasibly anywhere upon the penis. It tends to heal quickly subsequent to its painless, nonindurated and frequently unnoted existence. Occasionally, a mildly febrile systemic reaction is present. Within one to four weeks or perhaps longer the inguinal nodes begin to show involvement. Unilateral adenitis is more common; peri-adenitis with matting of the nodes and fixation to the skin is followed by subsequent suppuration. Unless treated or spontaneous subsidence occurs, sinus tracts are formed as outlets for purulent exudate. If extension continues, infection proceeds to the deep pelvic nodes and thence to the perirectal lymphatics as well as upward along the psoas muscles.

The third clinical type of lymphogranuloma is that which browses slowly in the penile tissues accompanied by subacute chronic involvement in the groin. This results eventually in severe stenosis of the lymphatic channels of the penis and scrotum with subsequent development of elephantiasis.

Following resolution of the acute lymphatic stage of the disease, the condition becomes chronic wherein evidence of activity may be difficult to detect, but secondary invaders, coupled with the virus in a more latent form, are still at work in the perirectal and inguinal tissues. It is here that proctitis, rectal strictures and other granulation reactions take their incipience.

The *diagnosis* and differential diagnosis of lymphogranuloma venereum may be difficult to make, owing to the fact that a laborious search must be made for the inclusion bodies in tissue sections; yolk sac and brain inoculation may be necessary to demonstrate the virus before exact identification is possible. Lack of a primary lesion concomitant with suppurative inguinal adenitis, appearance of the typical herpetiform, papular, or tiny ulcerated primary lesion devoid of the causative organisms of other diseases on smear and culture, and delineation of anorectal involvement are compatible with the diagnosis; these may be quite suggestive of lymphopathia. Utilization of the Frei skin test and the complement fixation test will be of assistance in most instances but biopsy is strongly recommended, especially in inguinal and rectal lesions, not only because the histologic picture is considered almost pathognomonic of the disease, but also because tissue examination may reveal the presence of the virus. Without adequate biopsy, carcinoma of the rectum cannot be ruled out. The Frei and complement fixation reactions are quite specific for lymphogranuloma but in most instances do not become positive early in the disease and after once becoming positive, the Frei reaction at least, remains so, perhaps for life; thus, activity is not necessarily indicated by a positive reaction.

The type of primary lesion as well as the nonsuppurative adenitis will, in addition to the finding of the Treponema pallidum under darkfield examination, declare a lesion syphilitic rather than lymphogranulomatous. The dirty, auto-inoculable lesions of chancroid, concomitant with buboes, both replete with Ducrey's bacilli on smear, will distinguish the soft chancre. Absence of Donovan bodies in the granulation tissues of lymphogranuloma on biopsy rules out granuloma inguinale.

Treatment of lymphogranuloma inguinale has long been confusing owing to the efficacy attributable to one remedy or another, which in reality was achieved through control of secondary infection rather than any virucidal property inherent in the medicament. Therefore, it is with caution that the curative effect of the antibiotics are considered. Spontaneous recovery undoubtedly often occurs, as witness the large number of asymptomatic positive Frei reactors.

Prior to the introduction of the sulfonamides, antimony compounds were used with little effect. Aspiration, irradiation and surgical removal of involved nodes have proved valuable in many instances. Sulfathiazole or sulfadiazine in dosages of 4 to 6 gm. daily to a total of 40 gm. has been and is still declared beneficial in the management of all phases of the disease but most investigators have agreed that the prime effect is upon secondary infection. Penicillin is of value only in similar fashion. Aureomycin has been found to be of distinct value in the early manifestations of the disease, causing the buboes to subside in one to three weeks; aspiration of bubo fluid subsequent to treatment has revealed no evidence of the virus in most instances. In the milder proctitides, results are initially excellent but relapse is moderately frequent. It seems that in many instances rectal stricture can be avoided. In those with severe fibrosis and strictures the subjective improvement is remarkable but it would be illogical to expect dissolution of fibrous tissue, and indeed results achieved here have been as expected. However, often the disease can be sufficiently arrested so that surgical treatment will have a better chance of success. The dosage of Aureomycin recommended has varied from 2 gm. daily for seven to twenty-eight days in the earlier cases to a total of from 80 to 100 gm. necessary in patients with later manifestations. Chloromycetin and Terramycin have been found to produce almost identical results with similar dosage. Streptomycin is not considered effective.

In the treatment of chronic lymphedematous and fibrous changes which occasionally may involve the penis, scrotum and thighs, the antibiotics are useful prior to surgical attack. The Kondolean and Torek principles have been applied (Weinstein and Roberts, 1950), with some success, coupled with plastic reconstructive operations.

GRANULOMA INGUINALE

Granuloma inguinale is included here more because of its predilection for the genitals than because of the actual knowledge as to its mode of transmission. Considered for many years as a tropical disease, it has been found to exist with equal frequency in the temperate zones. Although Donovan (1905) first identified the encapsulated bacillus which bears his name and postulated its etiologic capacity in the granulation reactions typical of the disease, it remained for Greenblatt et al. in 1939 and Anderson et al. in 1945 to indicate through embryonic yolk sac cultivative achievements, the undoubted relationship of the organisms to the entity. As recently as 1950, Packer and Goldberg in commenting upon the enigma of the transmissibility of the disease, noted that even though injection of bacteria-free suspensions of Donovan bodies into a donor will permit their growth and multiplication, the role of the Donovan body in the production of the lesion may not necessarily be primary. From the fact that the mate of a person with clinically proved granuloma inguinale may remain free of the disease despite prolonged cohabitation, it must be assumed that the contagious aspects of the problem are little understood. It is the incipience of the primary lesions upon the genital tract which accounts for its inclusion in the group of coitally acquired diseases. Direct inoculation of a donor will, however, produce the disease at the site of inoculation (Dienst et al., 1950).

The Donovan body is a gram-negative encapsulated, nonmotile, usually intracellular bacillus which has been found to be intimately related to the Friedländer, Klebsiella pneumoniae family of the Escherichia group, emphasized recently by Packer and Goldberg in the demonstration of a common hapten in the capsule of each. About 2500 cases are reported annually. Owing to the tenacious chronicity of the entity, undoubtedly many cases previously reported are retabulated as new cases each year. The incidence of the disease appears to be greater in the Gulf states, but it is apparently not uncommon throughout the United States. It is almost entirely confined to the Negro population to the extent that inference as to inherent susceptibility has frequently been made.

After an indeterminate incubation period the initial lesion appears as a nodule on the penis, groin or perineal areas, which soon ruptures to unfold bright red, velvety granulation tissue of insignificant depth. Daughter lesions may develop and coalesce; the primary one may simply spread circumferentially or progress in one direction or another. Secondary infection, frequently fusospirochetal, almost invariably supervenes to transform the lesion into a fetid accumulation of exuberant granulations, in the crevices of which purulent matter lurks consistently. Exquisite pruritus is fairly constant in the early stages. The lesions roll, almost as waves, gradually onward to involve at times amazing amounts of the body surface. Superficial and profound cicatricial healing occurs as the disease progresses. On the penis may occur erosive changes which can produce extensive destruction, and with scar tissue proliferation, bizarre deformities.

Anyone who has ever seen the disease in its chronic extensive form can realize the magnitude of the disturbance which may arise. We still have with us a few of those exceptional cases of granuloma *en cuirasse* wherein the body from the knees to the chest is a solid wall of chronically infected cicatrization, causing almost complete invalidism.

Untreated, the disease progresses chronically, in individual and varying tempo, until either the secondary infection can no longer be controlled or death from other cause supervenes. Symptomatology is related to the effects of the concomitant infection rather than to the granulations themselves except in the instance of urethral encroachment where obstructive signs may occur. In cases of extensive genito-inguinal scarring lymphatic stasis may supervene with elephantiatic concomitancies.

The *diagnosis* of granuloma inguinale can be most frequently suspected from the typical chronic sclerosing manifestations but mixed infections coexist frequently and microscopic diagnosis is mandatory. Material from clean subsurface areas obtained by biopsy is subjected to Wright's stain; the Donovan bodies in encapsulated, bacillary or occasionally coccoid forms may be seen, taking a deep blue stain with a surrounding pink capsule and ensconced in large mononuclear cells. Careful scrutiny will always reveal the organisms if present.

In the *differential diagnosis,* tuberculosis can be ruled out by the more rapid and deeply destructive elements encountered with the acid fast organisms; demonstration of typical histologic caseation, and the tubercle bacilli either by smear or animal inoculation may be resorted to if doubt exists. Primary and secondary syphilis are seldom other than concomitant offenders and here the darkfield can assure one that the moist, fragile, elevated, easily distinguishable condylomas teem with spirochetes; primary chancres do not show the tendency for peripheral progression nor the sloping everted edges compatible with granuloma inguinale. The darkfield and serologic tests will prove diagnostic. Gumma may necessitate histologic study prior to differentiation. Carcinoma can easily mimic granuloma in its chronicity and its exuberance but depth of ulceration and persistent localization of the primary lesion will suggest neoplasm. Biopsy cannot be recommended too strongly in any chronic genital lesion in order that carcinoma may be ruled out. The typical dirty, rapidly developing and spreading ulcers of chancroid will not be confused readily with granuloma but buboes occasionally do occur in granuloma if secondarily infected; in such cases aspiration and identification of the proper organisms will confirm the diagnosis. Lymphogranuloma venereum only in its initial and late elephantiatic stages will be confused with granuloma inguinale. The usual evanescence of the lymphogranulomatous primary lesion will indicate the proper category to which it may be assigned. In advanced stages the deep lymphatic involvement of lymphopathia would be infrequently indicative of the presence of granuloma inguinale. Biopsy and differentiation of causative organisms can corroborate the impressions garnered clinically and from the Frei and complement-fixation tests.

It is in the relative infrequence of investigation for the Donovan body that the diagnosis has been missed. Clinics where a routine battery of tests for all the common genital lesions is in operation will seldom fail to make the proper diagnosis.

In 1912 the introduction of antimony in the *treatment* of granuloma inguinale marked the first major step in the conquest of the disease. Prior to that time surgical experience had shown that curettage and cauterization made little progress in palliation but was all that could be offered. Tartar emetic was later replaced by fuadin, a less toxic preparation, and in the earlier cases some authors claimed that together with surgical treatment 90 per cent of cases could be cured. Reports of the usage of such cauterants as podophylline, however, continued to appear regularly in the literature and we remember the many who progressed inexorably, despite the mode of therapy.

When streptomycin and later Aureomycin were introduced, the curative powers of these drugs in a disease of such chronicity was hardly believable but as report after report arose in substantiation of complete cure it was believed that total eradication of the disease, regardless of stage, could be achieved. This apparently still pertains, although without long term reports of freedom from relapse, a cautious and alert viewpoint must be maintained. A succinct summary by Novy (1950), relevant to streptomycin, depicted a 10 per cent relapse rate with one course of treatment; 50 per cent of such relapses responded to a second course and further courses of streptomycin or Aureomycin would cure the remainder.

The conclusions ascertained in a compilation of dosage schedules and cure rates, from the work of Dienst and co-workers (1950), Pariser et al. (1950), Kornblith (1949-50) and others are that there is no relationship of response to medication in regard to duration of the disease, sex or previous therapy. An apparently important factor in determining the length of therapy is the extent of the lesion. Customary dosage of the various antibiotics, in the case of streptomycin 20 to 30 gm. in five to ten days, can be repeated or prolonged as necessary. With Aureomycin, 3 to 5 gm. daily for fifteen days is usually needed. Again, longer courses of therapy may be necessary in those with extensive disease. Chloromycetin is curative in a dosage of 20 to 40 gm. in ten days. Terramycin has been utilized extensively in dosage of 4 gm. daily for two weeks. According to Robinson's (1951) experience relapses occur usually within the first six months following therapy and he utilized as criteria for immediate retreatment, perpetuation of recoverable Donovan bodies within a few days of completion of treatment or upon their recrudescence in healed lesions. It is gratifying to note the efficacy of so many therapeutic entities, since fairly extensive follow-ups have demonstrated that few, if any, patients fail to respond to retreatment with the same or different agents. Surgical measures are still applicable in many instances requiring plastic reconstruction and can be approached in conjunction with utilization of antibiotics, with every probability of success. The masking effect of the antibiotics upon the lesions of syphilis should be reiterated, and careful serologic follow-up study is advised. Toxicity to the antibiotics is generally mild, consisting primarily of gastrointestinal disturbances, chiefly nausea, vomiting and mild diarrhea. Occasional cases of severe ulcerative proctitis and colitis have been noted, however. In such instances the medication should be changed.

PRECANCEROUS LESIONS

Paget's disease occurs on the penis as a small erythematous, at times eczematous, patch which over a long period of time becomes ulcerated. The borders of the ulcer are sharp and vividly red with a fine granular base. Supposedly this disease, which primarily confined to the nipple, arises in extramammary regions from apocrine glands, which may be found occasionally on the penile shaft. The diagnosis is confirmed by the demonstration at biopsy of large round Paget cells. Since the lesion has been observed to become carcinomatous, the only successful treatment is excision or amputation, depending upon its extent.

Bowen's disease is an erythroplasia which develops as single or multiple hyperkeratotic papules progressing slowly to a dull red, scaling, serpiginous patch with central atrophy. It may be distinguished clinically from Paget's disease by its rolling, rather sharply defined borders. Owing to the predominant belief that malignancy may supervene, wide excision is imperative.

Queyrat's erythroplasia, another rather rare penile affliction, may be found primarily on the glans, coronal sulcus and prepuce but it also occurs extragenitally. Typically, it is an erythematous, circumscribed, papular lesion with a velvety appearance. Scaling and superficial ulceration may occur. It may be differentiated from the two preceding lesions by its histologic picture of acanthosis and significant edema occurring between the cells of the epidermis. It must be treated by some form of ablation. Merricks and Cottrell (1953) reported erythroplasia of Queyrat in a seventy-nine-year-old white male, said to be the two hundred and sixty-first case in the literature. Here the lesion developed into a transitional cell carcinoma (Figs. 314, 315, *A, B*); approximately a fourth of the cases of erythroplasia show epithelioma in situ; if not, clinical cancer develops in about a fourth.

Leukoplakia of the glans and prepuce, similar to that seen on the mucous membranes of the mouth, is thought to be almost always associated with chronic inflammation. Predisposition may be caused by balanitis, or as a residuum of any of the venereal diseases. It is seen perhaps more frequently in patients with diabetes. The lesion appears as a glistening, opalescent, whitish thickening of the epithelium. Its appearance is usually diagnostic but biopsy and total removal are recommended, as the possibility of malignant degeneration exists. Balanitis xerotica obliterans, lichen sclerosus et atrophicus, and kraurosis penis are now considered as the same disease. In rare instances they have been considered as possibly premalignant. The glans is uniformly involved, becoming thickened, sensitive and scaly; bullous

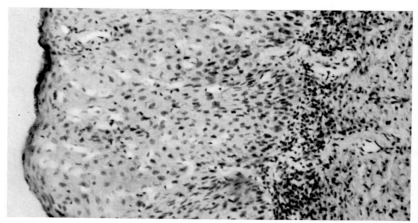

Fig. 314.   Erythroplasia of Queyrat. Histology. (Courtesy of Dr. J. W. Merricks and Journal of Urology.)

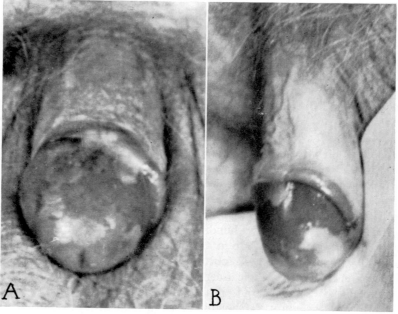

Fig. 315.   Erythroplasia of Queyrat. (Courtesy of Dr. J. W. Merricks and Journal of Urology.)

lesions may supervene but gradually a white scaling membrane arises which may constrict down about the urethral meatus to cause obstruction to the urinary outflow. The diagnosis may be made from the microscopic appearance of atrophy of the epidermis with homogenization of the cutis. Amputation has been recommended by those who think that the condition may lead to cancer.

INFECTIONS

Erosive and **gangrenous balanitis** is mentioned frequently as a venereal disease but it is believed by some to be an uncommon accompaniment of continually unhygienic conditions, wherein a redundant or tight prepuce exists. The etiologic organisms, the spirochete, short and Borrelia-like, and the stubby, fusiform, curved Vibrio, are found to inhabit the mouth, and in many instances the smegma of normal males. Predication is that salivary contact occurs and, alighting upon an already unclean and irritated area, the organisms may produce infection. The incubation period varies from three days to one week. The first signs of involvement may be small red erosions on the glans or undersurface of the prepuce with concomitant development of much preputial exudation; the purulent discharge may be accompanied by phimosis. If the disease is unchecked, confluent ulcerations will develop with considerable edema of the penis. The gangrenous phase appears after a period of much induration, reddening and swelling of the prepuce, which turns black, and may be accompanied by necrosis of the glans and portions of the shaft. In certain instances the entire penis has been destroyed within a comparatively short time. In the advanced stages of the infection, the inguinal nodes reflect the severity of the inflammatory reaction, becoming enlarged, but not tender. Constitutional symptoms of infection are common.

The *diagnosis* may be assumed from the rapid and destructive course of the disease but the organisms are plentiful in smears made from the lesions, and identification of the symbiotic organisms is comparatively easy. The spirochete is a longer, coarser one than the Treponema pallidum and its morphology and movement are entirely different. Since mixed infections may occur, darkfield examination for syphilis must be made as well as inspection of smears for Ducrey's bacillus. The primary lesions of syphilis are hardly ever as exudative, dirty or rapidly spreading. There is no undermining of the erosive and gangrenous ulcers as there is in chancroid, and the adenopathy never matches the chancroidal adenitic involvement in extent or fluctuant course.

Since anaerobic conditions are necessary for the growth of the offending organisms, simple exposure to air and local cleansing has in the past been quite effective. Various peroxide powders and solutions have been utilized and in certain instances arsphenamine has been found helpful. With the introduction of penicillin, control of this rather rare entity was more certain, but in severe cases a dorsal slit with local cleansing is at times necessary.

Late complications of balanitis have been frequently reported. Varying degrees of atrophy of the glans occur, dependent upon the severity of the infection.

Diphtheria of the penis is rare. The disease appears to occur most frequently following ritualistic circumcision, but cases developing subsequent to contact with the laryngeal form of the disease have been reported. Usually edema along the line of circumcision develops, and a necrotic sloughing area is followed by ulceration, with membrane formation. The inguinal nodes are commonly involved. The diagnosis may be suspected from the history of contact with diphtheria or ritualistic circumcision and the gray membrane covering the lesions, when present, is suggestive. Culture of the organism from the affected area is confirmative. Antitoxin with concomitant systemic sulfonamide or antibiotic therapy and local applications of sulfonamide in solution have been recommended.

Tuberculosis of the penis is another extremely rare disease. It occurs either as a superficial lesion of the skin (lupus), as tuberculous cavernositis, or secondary to tuberculosis of the urinary tract, spreading from severe urethritis. It formerly was known to follow ritualistic circumcision. It is believed to occur from coital contact and to be acquired from infected clothing. Whether or not the lupoid forms are the primary and sole manifestations of tuberculosis or whether hematogenous in origin is debatable. Cavernositis is undoubtedly of hematogenous derivation. By contiguous extension severe tuberculous urethritis can become peri-urethritis with subsequent invasion of the cavernous bodies and the glans.

The lupoid forms exhibit induration and subsequent ulceration upon the glans or shaft and inguinal nodes may be involved. The cavernous infection is a hyperplastic, nodular form which can scar and distort the penile shaft; sinus tracts may develop. Stricture from tuberculous urethritis may be noted with subsequent spread to the body of the penis.

The diagnosis is made by biopsy, and exclusion of venereal disease with the appropriate smears and cultures. Evidence of generalized or urogenital tuberculosis should suggest investigations along these lines. The use of streptomycin in the therapy of this condition should be combined with such surgical excision as may be necessary.

Herpes simplex and zoster can occur upon the penis, the former with greater frequency. A viral etiology has been demonstrated. The *simplex* form occurs commonly as a group of tiny vesicles, predominantly on the glans and prepuce. The vesicles rupture and superficial ulceration ensues and may persist for several weeks if cleanliness is not practiced. Symptomatology is slight and confined primarily to pruritus. The possibility of venereal infection must be kept in mind and the fear of it is most frequently the reason why medical attention is sought. The superficial and short-lived nature of the local lesion is significant but if secondary infection has developed, darkfield studies, smears, cultures and biopsy may be necessary to rule out other lesions. It is perhaps wise to perform routinely the serologic and Frei and Ducrey skin tests during and after subsidence of the lesions.

Herpes zoster of the penis, a viral affliction of a nerve root, produces prodromal burning with painful areas which are soon covered by erythematous and subsequently scabrous ulcerations. The typical sequence of events is usually diagnostic.

Great hope was entertained in the therapy of these conditions with the advent of Aureomycin but the course of these diseases is apparently not altered by its administration. Local cleanliness and occasionally sedation are all that can be offered. The condition is self-limited.

Condylomata acuminata or venereal warts, evincing a predilection for moist areas, occur most frequently as granular fronds upon the surface

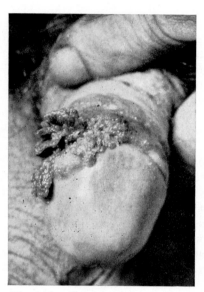

Fig. 316.   Condylomata acuminata.

of the glans or coronal sulcus, but may be seen anywhere, even intra-urethrally (Fig. 316). They are encountered frequently, usually in younger people. More evidence has accrued to support the belief that the disease has a viral etiology than that it is a precancerous manifestation of the results of chronic inflammation. The condylomas may remain in small aggregates or may spread wildly and form almost pedunculated protuberances of large size. Diagnosis is usually certain from clinical appearance but if secondary infection and ulceration have ensued, doubt may arise. Biopsy reveals the typical histologic picture, but examination for venereal disease should be made. Treatment consists in cleanliness and local cauterization; most commonly and successfully employed is electrocoagulation or podophylline, 20 per cent, preferably in an alcoholic solution, to prevent its destructive action from spreading to other areas. When the warts are within the urethra, podophylline or any of the other strong cautery agents is contraindicated for fear of later stricture. Full strength Fowler's solution is preferred and appears to be quite efficacious. Circumcision should be done in patients with a long foreskin.

Condyloma latum is a highly infectious manifestation of secondary syphilis and has been discussed under that heading.

Simple **ulcerations** of the penis may be the result of varied invaders and pathologic conditions. They may be caused by balanitis, which is a superficial inflammation of the glans penis, and balanoposthitis, ascribed to further involvement of the undersurface of the prepuce. These are frequent complications of urethritis, gonococcal or otherwise, but may result simply from unsanitary genital hygiene. Redness, swelling and discharge occur; superficial ulceration or excoriation can result and require smear and perhaps tissue diagnosis to rule out other entities. Cleansing soaks are frequently all that is required in the way of treatment. In severe cases antibiotics may be necessary. Circumcision will prevent recurrence. Paraphimosis, wherein the prepuce retracts proximal to the corona, can develop and produce singular distress owing to the accompanying constriction of the preputial band. Manual expression of edema can usually reduce the inflammation but incision may be necessary.

Other forms of balanitis are occasionally seen in the *oculo-mucocutaneous syndromes of Behçet and Reiter,* and in *ectodermosis erosiva pleuriorificialis.* It is believed that these are all forms of erythema multiforme exudativum, and in many instances are derived from the accompanying urethritis.

The **fungous diseases** may produce inflammation and ulceration on the penis. Reports of actinomycotic, blastomycotic, and histoplasmic involvement occurring primarily on the glans have been described.

Primary penile cutaneous Neisseria gonorrheal infections have been proved culturally (Scott and Thomsen, 1950). They occur usually as abscesses following gonorrheal urethritis and are responsive to penicillin.

Wounds, from contusions to severe lacerations, may be followed by chronic inflammatory ulcerations.

Constriction or **strangulation** of the penis, resulting in inflammation and ulceration are commonly seen. Production by metal rings, string and braided hair has been reported. The rationale is sometimes inebriative but more often superstitious. We saw an instance of almost complete non-suppurative amputation of the glans resulting from hair wound about the coronal sulcus; hypospadias was produced. Vascular injury and bacteria frequently combine to produce a severe ulcerating infection. The necessity of early removal of the constricting band is obvious but highly specialized equipment may be needed in the case of metal objects. Soaks, debridements, antibiotics and plastic procedures may be indicated.

Primary idiopathic spontaneous fulminating gangrene of the penis, in contradistinction to the gangrenous conditions which may involve the penis secondarily or as the terminal picture of many infectious and other pathologic processes, is a distinct entity (Fig. 317). Commonly associated with gangrene of the scrotum, it was first described by Fournier. The loosely contrived cellular structures of the penis and the scrotum in particular are essential factors which allow the sequence of events to occur. Debility predisposes to its onset. It is fortunately not often seen, for the mortality rate has been estimated to be 17 to 27 per cent. The organisms responsible for the majority of cases are the hemolytic streptococcus and staphylococcus, but E. coli, diphtheroids and the Welch bacillus have also been incriminated.

A scratch or unobserved abrasion may be the portal of entry and the characteristic features are soon fulfilled. The onset is sudden in a previously healthy individual and progression to the gangrenous state is rapid. The disease may be confined to the penis with only erythema noticeable on the adjacent scrotum. Usually within twenty-four hours of the onset of redness and swelling of the penis, an exudative, moist desquamation begins.

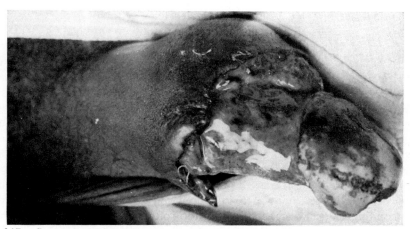

Fig. 317.   Spontaneous idiopathic fulminating gangrene of the penis with considerable loss of tissue.

Crepitation in the pitting surface may be noticed prior to the occurrence of gangrene, which spreads rapidly to involve the entire penis. Spontaneously a line of demarcation appears and within the confines of the gangrenous area sloughing gradually occurs down to the primary fascial planes. The corpora and testicles are not involved. The process may at times be seen to envelop the entire pubic region (see Vest, Chapter 3 of this Section). In a few days the necrosis sloughs away and hemorrhage may occur in the uninvolved base. Granulation tissue soon covers the area and healing proceeds. Systemic symptoms may be severe throughout the course of the disease, chills, fever and pain being common. Complete regeneration of tissue occurs within four to six weeks.

Diagnosis is self-evident from the history, clinical appearance and fulminating course of the process but the organisms responsible must be isolated so that the appropriate chemotherapeutic and antibiotic agents may be utilized, in conjunction with local and general supportive measures. Irrigations with antiseptic solutions and blood transfusions, which were the sole methods of therapy in the past, may be employed subsequent to initial control with one of the antibiotics.

Secondary gangrene occurs in the penis infrequently; diabetes and arteriosclerosis may be productive of it. Somewhat more commonly, the venereal diseases, cavernositis, the balanitides, and local abscesses secondary to the peri-urethral results of stricture and infection, if untreated, may all occasion the development of gangrene. The therapeutic rationale is dependent upon control of the primary disease but extensive surgical repair or amputation may be required.

Sensitization reactions may arise on the glans or penile shaft in a small number of cases. Usually urticarial in form, there may be in addition to edema, a macular eruption. Eczematoid reactions may occur through sensitivity to clothing, contaminants or food. Their appearance may be confusing and require extensive investigation to eliminate the etiologic factor.

Cavernositis is manifested in two forms: the plastic or fibrous cavernositis of de la Peyronie and secondarily in local pathologic processes, such as abscess, extravasation of urine, or as a result of trauma. Occasionally, neoplastic or infectious diseases may give rise to acute cavernositis. Although Kauntze (1950) reiterates Wesson's contention that Peyronie's original cases were in actuality instances of traumatic scar tissue, there is little disagreement as to the existence of a group of fibrous dysplasias of the cavernous sheaths in which no definitive etiologic factor may be promulgated. There are frequent reports of Peyronie's disease in the literature. Theoretical considerations as to etiology have ranged from beliefs that the fibrosis is inflammatory, syphilitic, or due to vascular interference, coital excess, gout, and a multitude of other conditions, to the somewhat more substantiated predication that the mechanism of production may be similar to the fibrous involvement seen in Dupuytren's contracture. Certainly, the two conditions occur concomitantly too often to be only coincidental. Those most familiar with the disease tend to believe that repeated minor trauma may result in fibrosis in a certain percentage of individuals.

The age of discovery of the condition is most commonly in the early fifties but incidents of the affliction have been noted in men of 22 and 80 years. It is a tribute to the disturbance the disease produces during intercourse that the majority of patients seek medical attention early—91 per cent within a year of onset.

The disease is manifested first by a pearly gray fibrous area in the cavernous sheaths which thickens and extends usually in linear fashion, in confluence or as separate infiltrative bodies. Involvement may be cord-like or in wide, flat, plaque-shaped forms. Fibrosis begins preponderantly in the septum between the cavernosa, and thus in the majority of cases reported, the dorsum of the penis was involved. Lateral and ventral locations are much more uncommon. Most frequently the plaques are situated near the glans, next, in the midshaft and least often at the base. Individual plaques have been found measuring 2 cm. by 8 cm. and up to 0.5 cm. in thickness. Microscopically, the relationship of the condition to keloid has been noted; active inflammatory changes have never been found. The discovery of an embryonal type of spindle cell has explained the occasional occurrence of bone or cartilage therein. The tissues within the corporal sheaths are rarely disturbed and the spongiosum has never been found to be involved.

The symptoms produced by the condition in order of frequency are curvature on erection, a lump on the penis, pain on erection, incapability of erection distal to the process and interference with coitus. The gradual onset of these together with the palpatory sensations afforded by the lesion itself are almost exclusively diagnostic but the differential diagnosis may include benign tumors, gouty tophi, traumatic scar tissue following febrile penile wounds, gumma or syphilitic cavernositis, and the residua of inflammatory cavernositis.

In the insidious onset and slow progression of the disease lie the distinguishing characteristics which can exclude trauma and inflammation; the tophi of gout are superficial, irregular in shape, do not produce deformity and are quite rare on the penis. Gumma lies deep in the sheaths, with a characteristic rubbery feel and frequently concomitant draining sinuses. Tumor is hardly ever flat, fibrous or so intimately a part of the covering sheaths.

Therapy has been confined to either radiation or surgery. Surgical removal of the fibrous plaques, with the novel utilization of fat pads in the reparative manipulation of Buck's fascia, to keep the edges apart has been advocated (Hinman, 1935; Lowsley and Gentile, 1947). However, most urologists agree that surgical treatment is not only useless but the deformity is exaggerated by it. Successful results have been reported from the application of radium plaques to the lesions, with repetition of the procedure if necessary, although ulceration at the site of application has resulted in a few cases. Lastly, the use of tocopherol and radium concomitantly has resulted in cure or improvement in a fair number of cases. Roentgen-ray radiation in small doses has also been utilized with some success; the disease is noted for its frequent recurrence, however, since in individuals who tend to scar heavily, efforts to remove the tissues are followed merely by an increase of the fibrosis.

PRIAPISM

Priapism is a condition in which persistent erection occurs, unaccompanied by sexual excitation or desire. Pain quickly supervenes, a fact which even in the transitory cases can serve to differentiate the condition from normal erection. Priapism results from nervous stimulation peripherally, or it may accompany a local pathologic process wherein regional nervous influences are undoubtedly brought to bear. The complex nervous and vascular processes involved in the production of normal erection are little understood and thus much that has been written as to the instigatory mechanism entailed in priapism is essentially theoretic. Priapism may be discussed more rationally, however, if considered as nervous in origin on one hand and mechanical on the other.

Among those resulting from nervous causes may be mentioned cases accompanying cerebrospinal disease and peripheral pudic nerve involvement, and those wherein reflex stimulation occurs as the result of trauma, inflammation, or tumor in nearby locations, such as the urethra. The cases occurring with manipulation of the posterior urethra and those in whom onset follows spinal anesthesia are nervous in origin but of little importance since subsidence is invariably early and complete. Likewise the transitory or recurrent priapism which accompanies local inflammatory disease of the urethra and penis is of little concern, being terminated readily by effective therapy of the conditions involved. It is in cases of severe nervous derangement such as in syphilitic cerebrospinal disease that priapism may be persistent and warrant considerate attention. Fortunately, the majority of instances of priapism are transitory and need no attention, or local or systemic therapy of the instigating cause can successfully prevent recurrence.

Priapism can occur at any age, owing to the varied etiologic factors. The symptoms are confined to pain and exquisite tenderness on manipulation. There may be a short period at the onset wherein the erection is pleasurable but evanescence of this sensation is rapid. Urinary difficulties are more common in cases wherein erection of the corpus spongiosum is included in the process, retention arising fairly often.

The *diagnosis* as to the etiology of priapism may be exceedingly difficult but is nevertheless quite important from a therapeutic point of view. The nervous system must be thoroughly investigated to eliminate the many diseases including tumor and syphilis. The urinary tract and penis must be carefully evaluated for hidden foci of infection as well as for more obvious afflictions. The instances of priapism occurring subsequent to manipulation or anesthesia are not difficult to delineate diagnostically. Mechanical obstructive causes, such as thrombosis and hematoma, will be usually obvious from the history and genital inspection. Priapism as a manifestation of systemic disease, as in leukemia or sickle cell anemia, must be borne in mind and the appropriate blood studies carried out.

Priapism has been known to persist for years without fatality or gangrene ensuing, so that *treatment* of the local condition is in no manner as urgent as determining the mechanism of its production since treatment is governed to a great extent by the causative factors. Neoplasm or inflammation of the nervous system, if treated promptly, will afford relief of the priapism. Therapy of cerebrospinal syphilis may solve the problem. Treatment of disease of the urinary tract or penis may provide relief. In the mechanical forms hematomas must be evaluated and thrombotic elements cleared. In leukemia, radiation, radioactive preparations and leukocidal medications when employed can control the cavernous manifestations. Attempts to relieve the pathologic erection by spinal anesthesia, hypnosis, sedation, oxygen inhalation, estrogen administration, roentgen-ray radiation and parenteral administration of antispasmodics have been only sporadically successful. The actuality of thrombosis has been in many cases doubted, for when thrombus has been suspected, subsequent to aspiration or incision, only thickened grumous material has been found. It has become apparent that only in cases of actual hematoma or abscess should the corpora be invaded. Treatment should be directed toward the etiologic factors responsible and only simple supportive therapy employed for pain and urinary retention. In the approach to frequently recurrent priapisms when diagnosis fails to reveal a correctable lesion, ligation of the dorsal arteries of the penis may provide relief. Priapism is bothersome but will subside in due course, with far better late results, if left alone.

CUTANEOUS DISEASES

Cutaneous afflictions may occasionally be seen as the cause of inflammation or ulcerations of the penis. Of these *scabies* is perhaps the commonest. Caused by Sarcoptes scabiei, a mite, producing pruritic papules in the penile skin, it is acquired by contact or from infected clothing. Its severely pruritic effect and the evidence of other lesions in the surrounding cutaneous creases make the diagnosis probable. The mite can be demonstrated by scraping the papules.

Psoriasis, characterized by silvery, scaling patches distinctive of the disease elsewhere, can occur on the glans or penile shaft. If accompanied by similar lesions in other more commonly affected regions of the body, doubt as to its diagnosis will not arise, but biopsy, darkfield, smear and cultural studies may be necessary to prove that it is not venereal in origin if confined to the penis.

Erythema multiforme may occur on the penis and if arising in that location may at first be confined there. Macules, vesicles and bullae appear which may require differentiation from the venereal diseases. *Eczema, furunculosis, erysipelas, dermatitis venenata, dermatitis medicamentosa, lichen planus* and *molluscum contagiosum* are among many of the cutaneous diseases which have been reported to occur with some frequency on the penis. The existence of similar lesions elsewhere and appropriate biopsy examination will lead to the proper diagnostic assumptions in most cases.

GONORRHEA

Gonorrhea is an infection of the mucous membranes of the genitourinary tract of both sexes, predicated primarily on the basis of coital contact and caused by the gonococcus. Gonorrhea can be innocently acquired, especially in children, as a vulvovaginal, ophthalmic, anorectal or urethral entity from contaminated clothing or pus from other objects harboring the secretion, in which gonococci lurk. In rare instances adult infection may likewise be non-coital. The disease may spread via the blood stream with the possibility of attendant septicemia, arthritis, iritis or endocarditis. Primary cutaneous infection with the Neisseria rarely occurs.

Natural immunity to the infection has never been demonstrated except in the attempts to reproduce pathogenicity in animals, and it is probable that only in the cases of chronic or latent gonorrhea may a healthy coital partner escape infection. Certain factors may affect the severity of the infection and the extent of its effects; alcohol, sexual excess and debility can influence the picture.

The gonococcus occurs usually as a diplococcoid gram-negative organism which in the acute form is most characteristically found intracellularly and when chronicity occurs, more frequently as an extracellular entity. It will grow luxuriantly on media containing animal protein, and aside from various other morphologic and cultural criteria will, alone of the gram-negative diplococci found in the urethra, ferment dextrose and not levulose or maltose. In gonorrhea when in doubt as to the etiologic potential of a certain coccus, the sugar fermentation reaction permits positive identification. Increase in temperature *in vitro* has been found lethal to the organisms but this has not been invariably duplicated by *in vivo* utilization.

The pathologic picture of gonorrhea in men lies in the production of rapidly progressive inflammation of the mucosa of the anterior urethra subsequent to deposition of the organisms within the urethral meatus. The incubation period varies usually from two to ten days with an average of four or five days. Longer intervals prior to clinical onset have been known to occur. Once within the urethra, the gonococci spread over the mucosa in the lacunae, glands of Littre and other anatomic pockets. Subsequent to sufficient proliferation, decomposition of the dying organisms, confronted by body defenses, causes liberation of a toxin which elicits by its irritative effect the outpouring of a purulent discharge, representing acute urethritis. Mucosal destruction occurs in various areas; the organisms reach the more vascular submucosal regions and thus enter the blood stream in quantity if body defense is weak.

Gonococci continue their proliferation in glands, pockets and denuded areas up and down the anterior urethra, producing engorgement and destruction according to the number of organisms and their virulence, until body defenses cause a decline in the rate of proliferation. Reparative processes restore the epithelium completely is destruction has not been too extensive but in the infoldings of a new urethral lining the organisms may be pocketed away from the surface and can lurk there in latency for long periods of time. The barrier which confines the early and the uncomplicated case from extension into the posterior urethra is the external sphincter, the salvation of the remainder of the genital tract in many instances.

Symptomatology related to anterior urethritis may consist in pruritus at the meatus prior to the onset of discharge. Burning on urination may follow and, subject to individual variation, redness and edema or balanitis can occur. The discharge begins as a thin, watery, mucous secretion and within seventy-two hours usually the typical, craemy, purulent exudate is noted. In severely inflamed cases priapism can occur and with proliferative mucosal thickening transient chordee may develop. The acute anterior urethritis may occasionally be accompanied by systemic symptoms, commonly general malaise. Uncomplicated anterior urethritis usually subsides within two or three weeks and a new epithelial lining is present by four to six weeks.

Persistence of the gonococcus in hidden folds and pockets may subsequently and unnoticeably produce soft infiltrations which gradually may be transmitted to the connective tissue narrowing compatible with postgonococcal stricture of the urethra. Other complications, balanitis and balanoposthitis reflect upon the irritative capacity of the secretions. Peri-urethritis with eventual development of abscesses may occur. If the infection persists in the crypts of Morgagni, fofficular urethritis with formation of retention cysts can arise. Involvement of Tyson's glands may produce single or multiple fringe abscesses simulating other venereal diseases. Cavernositis from peri-urethral extension is rare.

The most serious *complication* of acute anterior urethritis is extension to the posterior urethra. This may occur concomitantly with the onset of anterior urethritis or may develop subsequently owing at times to imprudent manipulation or flagrant disregard of the acute anterior infection. The pathologic process in the posterior urethra is similar to that in the anterior portion. The bladder neck, trigone, prostatic glands, ejaculatory ducts and prostatic utricle all become inflamed. Normal increase in intravesical pressure, abetted by such events as coughing or straining to void, can force the infected secretions into the ejaculatory ducts and thence to the seminal vesicles, vasa and epididymes.

In the prostate the abundance of glands and the feasibility of obstruction to their ducts is of profound significance in the establishment of gonorrheal chronicity. The symptomatology heralding the onset of posterior urethral involvement may be more apparent from a urinary point of view. Dysuria, frequency, hesitancy, nocturia, urgency, terminal hematuria and perineal pain are notable. Urethral discharge may be scant but the urine will indicate the presence of infection by an increase in detritus. In some cases, symptoms of prostatitis, vesiculitis and epididymitis follow immediately. Prostatic and vesicular involvement can be established by gentle rectal palpation of the swollen, hot, tender organ. Cowper's glands may become involved and palpable to the examining finger. Bloody ejaculation as well as frequent unexpected seminal emissions may be seen. Systemic symptoms may be severe in gonococcal posterior urethritis; fever and malaise can occur, with occasionally a rather severe degree of prostration.

The incidence of posterior urethral involvement has undoubtedly declined remarkably with the advent of the newer therapeutic agents. Utilization of penicillin has ostensibly caused a further reduction.

Gonorrhea may be said to become *chronic* when sufficient organisms remains reproductive to allow continuous damage to the anterior or posterior urethral mucosa and their appended glandular structures and sinuses. Prolonged infiltration can lead to stricture formation with further pocketing and stasis, comprising the essential elements for perpetuating infection. Poorly drained ducts and other foci can feed the organism either up or down the genitourinary tract, causing continuing symptoms, or periods of exacerbation, leading to severe damage and allowing secondary infection to gain foothold. Systemic flare-ups can easily and frequently result from such nuclei.

The *symptomatology* of the chronic infection is dependent upon the location and severity of the pathologic processes, varying from persistent discharge and urine heavily sedimented with infectious detritus, to chronic prostato-seminal vesiculitis and epididymitis, concomitant with previously enumerated symptoms.

The most frequent cause of acute or chronic urethritis is no longer gonorrhea but a *nonspecific* factor. This had long been suspected but it remained for the application of penicillin to the problem to reveal the many other conditions in which urethritis may arise. Yet, in the differential diagnosis the first assumption must be that the gonococcus is the offender.

The *diagnosis* of gonorrhea depends upon identification of the appropriate organism by smear, culture and fermentation studies. Other causes of urethritis are customarily scrutinized only subsequent to exclusion of the gonococcus. The acute anterior and posterior urethritides, when due to gonorrhea, seldom offer any diagnostic problem, the organisms being plentiful in the discharge or urinary sediment. It is in the discharges secondary to the forms of chronic gonorrhea in which identification of the causative organism may be difficult. The diplococci may not be found in smears and only upon aggravation of the persistent foci, by prostatovesicular massage, urethral stripping or instrumental manipulation may the enfolded pockets or obstructed glands be deprived of sufficient material in which the gonococcus can be identified. If with the previous history of acute gonorrhea, repeated smears and cultures are made of urethral and voided specimens and the gonococcus is not disclosed, then the presence of secondary invaders must be presumed. The complement fixation test as a diagnostic tool has fallen into general disrepute, as the reaction is too variable to be reliable.

Differential Diagnosis. The prime example of nonspecific urethritis is abacterial urethritis, described first by Welsch. The incubation period appears to be prolonged; several weeks may pass prior to onset of a discharge, which is usually not as purulent or profuse as the gonococcal and, although replete with detritus and pus cells, is totally devoid of organisms. The symptoms are less severe and although the posterior urethra and its contiguous genital structure may be involved, the destructiveness seen with gonorrhea is infrequent; however, prostatitis, vesiculitis, epididymitis and strictures can develop.

Trauma is a frequent cause of urethritis, wherein the normal flora becomes pathogenic. Confirmatory of mucosal injury, a history of the traumatic incident, be it instrumental or otherwise, is usually obtainable. Foreign bodies, syringing with prophylactic or contraceptive solutions, rough instrumentation, masturbation, or other external forms of trauma can be productive of varying degrees of irritation and discharge depending upon the accompanying infecting organisms. Within twenty-four hours, usually there appears a purulent or sanguineous exudate which can be differentiated from gonorrhea by careful study of the sequence of events and the absence of the gonococcus. The usual organisms found are the E. coli and the staphylococcus.

Various local diseases may be instigative of urethritis: tuberculosis implanted urethrally from above may be the cause, and penile or urethral neoplasms if productive of discharge should be obvious by palpation or endoscopy. Urethral diverticula may be incriminated from endoscopy, palpation and urethrographic studies. Balanitis may simulate or produce urethral discharge. Such systemic diseases as typhoid, mumps, influenza and smallpox can, if septicemic, produce urethritis. Ingested urethral irritants, canthrides, vegetables rich in oxalates and others may precipitate urethral inflammation. Pellagra, diabetes and gout are responsible in some cases.

Trichomonas vaginalis can be found with fair frequency in abacterial urethritis and is believed by some to be etiologic; wet smears will reveal the protozoan. E. histolytica as a cause of urethral discharge is found almost exclusively in the presence of a recto-urethral or vesical fistula. Bilharzia is a metazoan which produces urethritis rather frequently in endemic areas. Endoscopic appearance and the discovery of the ova in the urine is conclusive. Fungi only rarely produce urethritis.

In summary, management of these patients must begin with the realization that there are various causes of urethral discharge and only routine investigation will determine the etiology. A detailed history will separate acute from chronic conditions. A past history may elicit previous attacks and inadequate therapy. Systemic disease, such as diabetes, gout or tuberculosis, may be discovered and a relationship to the urethritis indicated. The symptoms will frequently localize the condition. Smears and cultures of the discharge will prove diagnostic or reveal the need for further investigation. Inspection and palpation can demonstrate possible venereal ulcerations, strictures or neoplasms as basically important. Studies of the urine voided into two or three receptacles may again by the presence of detritus, by color and by microscopic examination indicate the region of primary importance. Instrumentation may be necessary following subsidence of acute inflammation to reveal pathologic alterations. Endoscopy can then be done.

Treatment. In a consideration of the therapy of gonorrhea too much emphasis has been placed on chemotherapeutic and antibiotic agents. Owing primarily to the rapidity with which acute urethritis subsides under the aegis of such powerful medicaments, cure is frequently assumed without benefit of careful examination of the entire genital tract to verify total ablation of the infection or lack of its involvement of such areas. Frequently therapy is begun without benefit of a single smear, on the assumption that a little penicillin will take care of any discharge. It may be only subsequent to prolonged penicillin therapy and perhaps a trail of one of the other antibiotics that a non-gonococcal etiology is recognized, or chronic posterior urethritis, or prostatitis uncovered. Therefore, of prime importance in the treatment of the Neisserian infection is precise diagnosis.

Local therapy which in the past was the sole recourse, has been replaced completely, except in certain specific instances, by first the sulfonamides and then penicillin. After extensive trial the newer antibiotics have been found for the most part to be effective. Fortunately, the irrigations and instillations formerly utilized have been outmoded, for many of the complications resulted from such therapy in the hands of injudicious practitioners.

The *sulfonamides,* preferably sulfadiazine, should be utilized only in those instances where other agents are not available, for the rapid development of sulfonamide-resistant organisms has made cure uncertain, the rate varying from 30 to 60 per cent of cases. The prime value of the sulfonamides is that they are the sole therapeutic agents which do not mask a concomitantly contracted syphilitic infection, which has been reported to exist in 1 to 3 per cent of cases.

The sulfonamides are best employed in a dosage of 4 to 6 gm. daily for five days accompanied by large volumes of fluid and alkalinization. Attention to signs of toxicity is imperative.

For *acute anterior urethritis,* at present the therapeutic procedure of choice is administration of 300,000 units of procaine *penicillin G* in 2 per cent aluminum monostearate. This provides a higher than necessary blood level, and for a great deal longer time than is essential. Over 95 per cent of gonococcal infections may be cured in this fashion. What undoubtedly affects the cure rate is the repetitive promiscuity occurring immediately subsequent to cessation of symptoms, which is possible within twelve hours; thus reinfection is frequent.

In the treatment of acute gonococcal urethritis with other antibiotics, reports are varied and conflicting. The utilization of antibiotics other than penicillin must depend for the present upon resistance of the disease or sensitization of the patient to penicillin. A combination of penicillin and sulfadiazine orally has proved efficacious.

In acute posterior urethral involvement, heavier and prolonged dosage of penicillin is mandatory; 600,000 units or more of procaine penicillin G should be utilized daily. Such increased dosage is recommended in the case of all acute genital complications.

The *criterion of cure* postulated by Public Health authorities is three weekly negative smears and cultures, but recurring urethritis two to thirteen weeks after treatment may not necessarily mean reinfection. Thus, the absolute criterion of cure in the individual patient is dependent upon careful evaluation of the entire seminal tract. Two to three weeks subsequent to cessation of symptoms and urethral signs of infection, light prostatic and seminal vesicle massage must be carried out, with smear and cultural study of the stripped gleanings of these organs. Careful palpation and inspection must survey the anterior urethra for residual pockets in the glands of Cowper, Littre and Tyson. Search must be made for infiltrations at a subsequent visit, with examination of the urethra over a sound, which by its passage will concomitantly dilate ductile ostia, allowing emergence of such inspissated exudate as may exist. Later investigative sounding for incipient stricture must be readily afforded. Several specimens of urinary sediment subject to culture will add to the evidence of cure or failure. It is in this fashion that posterior urethral residue is made apparent, and in the treatment of such chronic states chemotherapy and antibiotics are not to be depended upon alone. Demonstration of foci of the Neisseria, or of secondary invaders in the prostate or vesicles will frequently be necessary in the chronic phases, owing to persistent symptoms and signs. There may be morning drop, or scanty discharge sufficient to stain the underclothes; bloody ejaculation may indicate existence of the disease; diminution of libido may be experienced; perineal pain or pain referred to the anterior portion of the abdomen or low in the back can be significant. Urinary symptoms, such as frequency, hesitancy, nocturia, or persistently cloudy or even blood-tinged urine may draw attention to the posterior urethra. A boggy, slightly tender prostate or vesicular enlargement will clinically confirm aroused suspicions. Such problems are treated primarily by gentle massage; rectal irrigations, sitz baths and suppositories can be used adjunctively. The sulfonamides, penicillin and other antibiotics have been given in the chronic stages and if accompanied by the establishment of drainage are thought to be helpful.

It is only in the careful and prolonged evaluation of gonorrhea subsequent to its diagnosis and treatment in the acute anterior urethritic phase that many complications of the disease may be successfully avoided. Only those willing and able to undertake such time consuming studies should treat gonorrhea and assess its cure.

NONSPECIFIC URETHRITIS

Nonspecific urethritis is a term which has been utilized to describe any urethritis in which the gonococcus cannot be found to be etiologic. The term thus covers a variety of conditions in which the exact cause is not immediately apparent, but also includes as defined, urethritides in which the provocative element is readily diagnosed. The discussion may thus be separated into two major divisions: the conditions in which no specific cause for the discharge can be found, and those which follow or are the result of a wide variety of bacterial invaders, and may be secondary to a host of pathologic and traumatic instances. In the first category, abacterial urethritis, and Reiter's and oculo-mucocutaneous syndromes, which are accompanied by urethritis, may be grouped.

In a large percentage of individuals with acute or chronic urethral discharge, although suspected of having a gonorrheal infection, demonstration of the Neisseria is not possible. Many of these are treated as gonococcal infections and it is only when they persist, subsequent to a variety of therapeutic measures, that their abacterial nature may be recognized. Subsequent thorough examination of the entire anterior and posterior urethra and upper urinary tract may reveal that the signs of inflammation are present but that structural deformity is not predispositious, and further that etiologic organisms are totally absent.

It has been estimated that 80 per cent of nonspecific urethritides are abacterial in nature. Two forms are prevalent: (1) acute, resembling acute gonorrhea and (2) subacute or Welsch type. Abacterial pyuric conditions of the prostate and upper urinary tract have been known to exist for a long time and occasionally the urethritis is associated with symptoms referable to the upper urinary tract.

The acute *abacterial urethritis* usually has its inception one to five days following intercourse. A profuse purulent discharge occurs with reddening of the meatus and accompanying dysuria. Posterior urethral involvement may be indicated by frequency, urgency and terminal hematuria. The clinical picture is so similar to that seen in gonorrhea that it is confusing when the Neisseria is not demonstrable.

The subacute form may develop primarily or follow the acute stage. In the Welsch type the incubation period subsequent to coitus is customarily longer, but reputedly within one month; discharge is more serous,

and symptoms are milder. In both types, involvement of the posterior urethra may cause prostatitis, seminal vesiculitis and occasionally epididymitis.

Etiologic postulations have finally come to rest, although inconclusively,
in the preponderant belief that a virus causation is distinctly plausible.
Pleuropneumonia "L" type organisms are being studied as possible con-
comitants or transmutants of the inclusion bodies noted with such frequency in the tissue reactions. Inspection of the urethra delineates desquamative, destructive changes, and frequently wedge-shaped gray granulation
projections from the urethral, prostatic and bladder neck surfaces.

The *diagnosis* of abacterial urethritis rests upon exhaustive studies of
the urethral and prostatovesicular secretions and of the urinary sediment.
When no bacteria or other possible causative organisms are found, and tissue
studies demonstrate the possibility of virus invasion then, if disease of the
upper urinary tract, residual foci of bacterial infection in the prostate and
vesicles, and structural alteration of the genitourinary tract have been
ruled out, the diagnosis can be predicated. The *differential diagnosis* rests
upon exclusion of the urethritides appearing in gonorrhea, secondary to
other bacteria, foreign body, trauma, local neoplastic and specific inflammatory diseases, sensitivity reactions, urethral manifestations of systemic disease, and infestation with protozoa, metazoa and fungi.

The salient features suggesting abacterial urethritis are the relationship
with coital contact, and a longer incubation period than that seen in the
gonorrheal infection. The frequent relative benignity of the infection, its
tendency to recur, its lack of response to treatment, and most memorably
the absence of bacteria or other causative factors plus indications of the
presence of virus are all favorably indicative.

The complications which may result are in general similar to those following gonorrheal urethritis but with far less frequence and hardly ever as
severe. Posterior urethritis, prostatitis, seminal vesiculitis and occasional epididymitis have been mentioned. Periurethral or prostatic abscess has not
been found to occur; stricture, however, may follow. Whether or not the
cystitis and abacterial pyelonephritis very occasionally seen are primary or
secondary is not known. Chronic abacterial urethritis occurs with relative
frequency and demands the same attention to the prostate and vesicles, and
foci of infection in the periurethral glands as is necessary in the postgonococcal chronic stages.

That *treatment* of the condition is generally unsatisfactory may be seen
in the perusal of the countless drugs and other therapeutic measures advised.
Neoarsphenamine, 0.3 gm. twice weekly for three or four weeks, has been
utilized. Penicillin is of no use other than as a further differential tool in
the separation of the gonococcal from the abacterial type. Sulfadiazine has
been found by some to be effective predominantly in the chronic form
suggestive of the possibility of its being primarily therapeutic in its action
upon secondary invaders. Streptomycin, Chloromycetin and Aureomycin
have all been shown to affect sporadic cases in a dramatic manner, with
cessation of discharge within twenty-four hours; frequently after a chronicity
of months.

ERYTHEMA MULTIFORME EXUDATIVUM

Reiter's disease and the oculomucocutaneous syndromes vary so little in their urethral manifestations from primary abacterial urethritis that at present they are thought to represent merely varied manifestations of a single virus produced entity. Certainly, the oculomucocutaneous entities vary so little from each other that grouping of them under manifestations of erythema multiforme exudativum is distinctly warranted. Reiter's syndrome perhaps can profitably be included, as well as the abacterial urethritides. In all of these demonstration of inclusion bodies and pleuropneumonia "L" shaped organisms has been mentioned as occurring, at times more than occasionally.

Reiter's disease is described as a primary abacterial urethritis associated with bilateral conjunctivitis and polyarthritis found almost exclusively in males; Reiter's original description included bloody diarrhea. So many subsequent reports of the disease have added to the purportedly diagnostic triad such a multitude of other manifestations, such as balanitis, stomatitis, cutaneous lesions, dysentery and a variety of visceral conditions, that the syndrome in its original description is rarely seen. Frequently, reports are made of cases of Reiter's disease wherein arthritis or conjunctivitis was not found so it is apparent that speaking of it as an entity is rather illogical.

Customarily the urethritis occurs subsequent to coital exposure, and the incubation period is reported to be five to thirty days. The urethritis is most frequently subacute and usually devoid of organisms, the discharge being clear and viscid. A few days later conjunctivitis occurs, first unilateral, then bilateral; usually in ten days to two weeks arthritis supervenes. The urethritis and conjunctivitis may subside quickly and spontaneously, but the arthritis frequently persists for several months.

Other concurrent manifestations are balanitis circinata, which usually accompanies the onset of arthritis, and keratodermia blennorrhagica, consisting of nodules, vesicles and pustules, most frequently found on the soles of the feet. Episcleritis may accompany the conjunctivitis, and other ophthalmic involvements may occur which are more frequently seen in the oculomucocutaneous group, as are the stomatitic lesions occasionally reported in Reiter's disease. Pyelonephritis, cardiac involvement, infarct, and diarrhea have been reported.

The general symptomatology may consist of rather severe pyrexia, and such symptoms as may emanate from the regions involved. Increased sedimentation rates and anemia are frequently noted.

In regard to *etiology,* ever since Reiter postulated a spirochetal causation, owing to the demonstration of spirochetes in his original case, many and varied organisms have been incriminated, but the likelihood of viral causation has been recently strengthened by more frequent isolation of pleuropneumonia "L" organisms in 30 to 40 per cent of all cases, at times from the rectal canal, articular cavities, and from cutaneous lesions as well as from the urethra.

The complications which may arise are dependent upon the severity and location of the lesion. Urethritis may persist in subacute or chronic forms and give rise to prostatitis, vesiculitis and trigonitis, either acute or chronic; epididymitis has not been mentioned. Involvement of the upper urinary tract accompanying urethritis can occasionally occur. Urethral stricture has been reported. Recurrence is notably common in Reiter's disease.

The *diagnosis* and differential diagnosis depend, in the case of abacterial urethritis and the oculomucocutaneous syndromes, in specious argumentation over the percentage occurrence of one lesion or another in each of the syndromes which to our way of thinking is pointless. Other distinct entities in which purpose may be served by differential summation are gonorrhea, in which urethritis, arthritis, ophthalmic infection and other manifestations may occur. The absence of the gonococcus is of the greatest import here, this being demonstrable in the urethral secretions, articular effusions and ophthalmic exudations. Never are the ocular manifestations of Reiter's disease as destructive as in gonorrhea. The arthritis is milder in Reiter's, as is the urethritis for the most part. The incubation period is customarily much longer in Reiter's disease. In the more chronic forms massage and instrumentation may again demonstrate the gonococcus or the absence of it in the discharge.

Acute rheumatic fever may produce many of the manifestations of Reiter's disease and it is only in the absence of the urethritis, the frequent cardiac damage and the response to salicylates, wherein rheumatic fever may be differentiated.

If a meatal chancre occurs with other manifestations of secondary syphilis, then the diagnosis will rest in retrieving spirochetes from the lesions, and corroborative positive serologic reactions for syphilis. Typhoid fever, arthropathic psoriasis, ninth day erythema and the toxic manifestations of the sulfonamides can simulate the picture of Reiter's in its more expanded form.

The treatment of Reiter's syndrome is precisely that utilized in abacterial urethritis and with similar varied success. The dermatologists, who believe that erythema multiforme exudativum responds exceptionally well to intravenous administration of Aureomycin in 2 to 300 mg. dosage or daily oral doses of 2 to 3 gm. recommend its use in Reiter's, as well as the oculomucocutaneous entities.

Stevens-Johnson syndrome, Behçet's disease, ectodermosis erosiva pleuriorificialis and *keratodermia blennorrhagica* are names for syndromes characterized generally by urethritis, stomatitis, balanitis, conjunctivitis, arthritis, diarrhea and cutaneous lesions in mixed forms. Separate names have been given these varied symptoms and signs of erythema multiforme owing undoubtedly to the diversified appearance of the lesions at the time of the practitioner's observation of them, and perhaps through the use of inexact terminology. This, coupled with the undoubted ability of any disease in which variegated symptomatology exist, to exaggerate or suppress one symptom or another, makes usage of the term, oculomucocutaneous variants of erythema multiforme, a more exact one and leaves the field of the urethritides less confused.

The diagnosis, differential diagnosis and management of these manifestations are approached in the same fashion as in abacterial urethritis.

Trauma is the most common nonvenereal cause of urethritis. The traumatic incident may consist of intra-urethral injury from sounds, repeated catheterizations, or use of an indwelling catheter. Foreign bodies, usually infected, may injure the mucosa and produce urethritis. Utilization of irritative chemicals in urethral prophylaxis, or contact with strong contraceptive solutions and creams may cause urethritis. Excessive masturbation or prolonged and rough urethral stripping can sufficiently injure the mucosa to allow inflammation to occur. In most cases, except for infected foreign bodies, the bacterial spectrum of the urethritis is that of the normal urethral flora. The discharge occurs usually within twenty-four hours and varies from serous to purulent and sanguineous; dysuria, burning and tenderness may be severe. The organisms usually involved are the coliform, staphylococcal and streptococcal groups. As in gonorrheal urethritis destruction of the urethral mucosa proceeds apace depending upon the resistance of the host. Unwise manipulation, coital or otherwise, debility, lack of care for the part, and uncleanliness, may foster the entire gamut of urethral complications. Littritis can occur, periurethritis and abscesses may form and stricture may result. Posterior urethritis will develop if the original infection is unattended and prostatitis, seminal vesiculitis, epididymitis, cystitis and pyelonephritis are not at all uncommon. Again if unchecked, prostatic abscesses may develop. The symptoms and signs of bacterial urethritis and its complications parallel equally and virulently the gonococcal types.

The *diagnosis* depends upon the history of trauma and discernment of the nature of the causative organisms by smear and culture. In the chronic forms, massage, sounds and urinary sediment examinations are frequently necessary to find the organism.

Treatment is concerned with identification of the etiologic bacteria and administration of suitable antibiotics; penicillin is preferred for coccal invaders and sulfadiazine, streptomycin or Chloromycetin for the coliform organisms. In the chronic posterior urethral manifestations, again, drainage by massage is far more important than the medicament. Dilation with sounds may be necessary.

Urethritis can be the signal of a great many *structural deformities* and pathologic entities in the upper urinary tract as well as the urethra. Inflammation arising from stricture produces usually a desquamative type of discharge. The diagnosis is dependent upon palpation, urethral instrumentation and endoscopy. Pyogenic disease of the upper urinary tract may so bathe the urethra that posterior and anterior urethritis can develop; pyelographic studies will be indicative. *Urethral diverticula* with or without calculus are at times the cause of discharge, usually purulent. *Carcinoma* of the urethra is customarily heralded by a discharge which is frequently bloody. Chronic prostatitis, seminal vesiculitis and other pocketed infections along the urethra, either postgonococcal or otherwise, are frequently manifested only by a scanty chronic discharge.

Urethral syphilis is uncommon, but chancre occurs more frequently and gummatous formations occasionally. Chancre may arise at the meatus or within the fossa navicularis and, in the presence of concomitant gonorrhea, may be overlooked. Watery discharge and some burning on urination are frequently noted. Palpation will identify the firm induration of the chancre or the nodularity of a gumma. Slight sanguineous discharge may be expressed from the lesions. The inguinal nodes can become enlarged in characteristic fashion. Darkfield examination of secretions and subsequent serologic tests will confirm the diagnosis.

The propagation of urethritis in patients with diabetes and gout is apparently dependent upon a metabolic disturbance of mucous membranes; in the urethra such a change permits the normal bacterial flora to become pathogenic. In pellagra, similarly, deficiency reduces mucosal resistance and urethritis can result.

Urinary bilharziasis, although commonly confined to the bladder, has been noted to involve the urethra, especially with heavy generalized infestation (see also Section V, Chapter 3). The disease is rare in the United States but in global areas where it exists with frequency, the mortality from complications is exceedingly high. Bilharzial infections are discussed by Dr. Sanjurjo in Section V, Chapter 3.

It is doubtful whether the protozoan, *Trichomonas vaginalis,* is an important cause of urethritis, prostatitis and vesiculitis. It is difficult to determine whether the Trichomonas is etiologic for two reasons. First, when it is found in a case of urethritis, most commonly bacterial flora will concomitantly be seen; secondly, the Trichomonas has so frequently been demonstrated to abide in normal male urethras. Trichomonas vaginalis does not penetrate the mucous membrane and thus only surface irritation can be postulated. The Trichomonas is a mandolin-shaped, flagellated organism, somewhat larger than a leukocyte; it can be readily identified by its active motion in fresh secretions. Symptoms purported to occur are of the usual anterior urethritic type; discharge is watery or frothy. If treatment is necessary, lavage of the urethra with quinacrine or zephiran solutions may be employed.

STRICTURE

A stricture of the urethra may be defined as a narrowing or loss of distensibility which is abnormal in the individual urethra under investigation. In general the male urethra varies in caliber from person to person and sometimes within a rather wide range. Again, the various portions of the urethra differ in their customary diameters (at the meatus from 21 to 27 French, in the pendulous urethra 27 to 33 French, in the bulbous 33 to 36 French, in the membranous 27 French, the prostatic urethra 45 French and the vesical neck 36 French caliber). Variation in size can be depicted as abnormal only when a portion of the urethra, except in the rarely seen pipe stem types of infiltration, is abnormally narrow in comparison with other areas. The texture of resistance noted in the passage of instruments can also be diagnostic as to the presence of a stricture in those instances where the stricture may be of wider caliber.

The *incidence* of stricture has seen a change in emphasis rather than a dissolution of the problem in the past twenty years. Although our clinics remain adequately supplied with stricture cases awaiting dilation, most frequently the history of these strictures dates back many years. Strictures of recent origin are encountered chiefly in those males who have undergone transurethral surgical procedures or have sustained some trauma. The sulfonamides and penicillin have reduced the occurrence of postgonorrheal stricture tremendously, as much perhaps from obviation of injury with the irrigations and instillations formerly utilized as from the efficacy of their bacteriocidal properties. Postgonococcal stricture does still occur, however, especially in the Negro.

Strictures may be classified as congenital or acquired. Only the latter will be discussed here; congenital urethral stricture is described in Section IV. The commonest cause of *acquired* stricture at present is trauma. Strictures of the type seen in spasm of the sphincters are not true strictures for relaxation of the spasm will relieve the tension and permit passage of a catheter. The inflammatory narrowings seen during the course of the urethritides are again not true strictures but may later become so.

Traumatic occasions vary from tears to ruptures of the urethra and include instrumental manipulations, such as soundings and transurethral surgical procedures. The use of inlying catheters may be considered as traumatic, for their constant irritative effect, concomitant with infection, can produce a stricture. Instrumentation or operative intervention may superimpose a traumatic stricture upon a previous infectional one. In strictures which develop after transurethral resection the escape of current from the sheath during the procedure has been incriminated as additive in the production of trauma. Lastly, the use of strong chemicals in the urethra, although rarely employed now, can cause sufficient mucosal damage to produce stricture.

Infection, which almost always interacts with trauma to produce strictures, commonly will of itself cause this pathologic picture. Gonorrhea, the abacterial and bacterial urethritides, as well as the rarer ulcerative conditions, such as tuberculosis and syphilis, produce stricture not infrequently. Apparently the incidence of strictures due to infection is in direct proportion to the severity of the infection.

Subsequent to trauma or progression of infection deep into the urethral mucosa, localized thrombophlebitis is set up which, concurrent with abscess pockets and periurethral inflammatory implantations, causes deposition of fibrous tissue in the corpus and surrounding fascial sheaths. It is the later cicatricial deformities of the surrounding tissues which produce clinically apparent stricture. Minor scarring in small areas of the urethra due to infectional erosion of the mucosa rarely produces stricture. At first the scar is vascular and soft but later may become hard and inelastic. Proximal to the strictured area, the force of the urinary stream dilates the lumen and continued infection in scarred pockets may further lengthen the area of fibrous infiltration and resultant stricture. Thus, one stricture leads to the production of others.

Strictures are primary confined to one area or another and usually occur as single entities, meaning that they occur in one locale, or in confluence are restricted to one portion of the urethra. That this clinically apparent single stricture may be made up of a number of stricture pockets is common knowledge. The term multiple strictures refers to those in which widely scattered destruction has permitted several strictured areas to occur. About 11 per cent of strictures are of this multiple type.

Approximately 70 per cent of inflammatory strictures occur in the bulbomembranous urethra, owing to dilation of the urethra here, and the resultant diminution of the flushing potentialities of the urinary stream. The pendulous urethra is next most commonly involved and the glandular urethra least often. Traumatic incidents, especially with transurethral resection, have increased the incidence of pendulous, vesical neck and meatal strictures.

Posterior urethral strictures are uncommon because of the ability of the resilient, highly vascular prostate to absorb the infection without, customarily, any encroachment upon the urethral lumen.

The interval before stricture becomes clinically apparent varies with those of traumatic etiology where production is rapid, frequently within one or two months, to those of infectious nature wherein years may elapse before the occurrence of symptoms. It has been estimated that gonorrheal strictures require an average of twenty years to become apparent. We believe that most infections produce stricture much more rapidly than this.

The *symptoms* of urethral strictures vary with the severity and type of involvement. Rapidly developing strictures scar densely and require constant attention. Others less dense are frequently so modified by treatment as to cause few symptoms. Most commonly noted is chronic discharge, which is due to residual infection in and about the stricture. Urinary symptoms may be present which will signify some type of obstruction. We have not found diurnal frequency to predominate over nocturnal, a supposed differential in the symptoms produced by prostatic hyperplastic obstructions. Dysuria and urgency, as well as changes in the character of the urinary stream, may occur. Frequently, alteration of the force, diameter and appearance of the stream will be indicative of stricture; a split, narrowed or dribbled flow of urine is suggestive of stricture. Acute urinary retention often occurs in the more severe narrowings of long standing. Often retention is only partial, and a large residual urine may exist. Chronic posterior urethral infection involving the prostate and vesicles may be perpetuated by the presence of a stricture. Benign prostatic hyperplasia may coexist with stricture not uncommonly and require endoscopic evaluation.

Symptoms may be referable to the complications of stricture. The effect of back pressure on the upper urinary tract will, in the presence of infection, produce the symptoms of cystitis and pyelonephritis. Frequently, and unfortunately, damage may occur insidiously. The symptoms of abscess and extravasation of urine will couple urinary difficulties with those of infection and absorption of toxic products.

The *diagnosis* is dependent upon the history of urethral infection or trauma, the suggestive urethral symptoms, urethral palpatory indications, and instrumental demonstration of the stricture. The *differential diagnosis* must exclude benign prostatic hyperplasia, which develops in an older age group, infrequently manifests discharge, and necessitates endoscopic inspection for verification in most cases. Symptoms associated with benign prostatic hyperplasia are frequently identical to those of stricture. Physical examination, however, reveals an enlarged prostate, which concomitant with the symptoms of urinary obstruction and the absence of palpatory suggestions of the urethral induration of stricture, is most often sufficiently diagnostic. Chronic anterior urethritis with discharge, and perhaps indurative changes to palpation, will necessitate instrumental diagnosis. Foreign bodies, stones, neoplasms, congenital anomalies, diverticula and other entities will frequently be revealed as distinct from stricture only by endoscopy or urethrography.

Stricture is probably most frequently discovered through attempted passage of a catheter. The hang imparted to the catheter tip at the stricture site can better be investigated, if in the bulb, by the gentle insertion of a curved sound of medium size (20 to 22 F.). In passing a sound the operator should exert only the gentlest force. It is preferable that the operator rather than the stricture yield, in the case of a narrowing exceptionally snug to the probing sound.

Bougies are of more value in the diagnosis of pendulous urethral strictures and are considerably less traumatic. Endoscopy and urethrography should be utilized in the evaluation of some strictures, to rule out neoplasm, ulcerative infection and diverticulum. Often a filiform can be passed in the case of a tortuous stricture of the lumen if it is done under direct endoscopic vision.

The *treatment* of choice for urethral strictures is *dilation*. This necessitates the proper instruments, a maximum amount of patience and gentleness and a minimum of the application of force. The purpose is to dilate the offending scar tissue without producing urethral tears, which can in turn form more scars. Corkscrew tipped filiforms have occasionally been found to pass when the straight ones will not. The concomitant advancement of several filiforms simultaneously will, at times, by blocking the various pockets, finally permit passage of one. Of extreme importance is adequate lubrication of the instruments; injection of jelly or oil under moderate pressure will occasionally dilate the true passage so as to permit a filiform to reach the bladder. Leforte followers will then accomplish the first dilation. Bougies can be utilized with distinct success at times and the possibility of creation of a false passage or perforation of the urethra is lessened in their use. If, after passage of a filiform, even the smallest follower is exceedingly snug or cannot be passed, it is perhaps advisable to tape the filiform in place and allow dilatation to proceed.

In instances complicated by retention of urine we have found that urethral catheters may be useful in evacuating urine while accomplishing dilation. In difficult cases, warm sitz baths as a precursory measure will be of great value. Ample sedation should precede instrumentation in every case.

Subsequent to the initial passage of an instrument, dilation should be repeated within three to five days and if haste is avoided a gradual increase in the urethral caliber can be readily achieved in almost every case. Dilation may then be accomplished weekly or fortnightly, until the time arrives when a 28 or 30 French sound may be passed easily; then instrumentation can be carried out less frequently, until perhaps one dilation every six months, or even yearly, will suffice. This is dependent upon how well the strictured lumen remains patent. Any stricture should be checked at least once a year.

The bladder should be filled with an astringent, antiseptic solution after each manipulation and the urethra cleared of debris in the voiding of it.

In the rare case of impermeable stricture accompanied by retention of urine, after all attempts at urethral manipulation have failed, a trocar or punch cystotomy is indicated. Suprapubic diversion of the stream will allow the strictured area to rest and after the inflammatory edema has subsided passage of a filiform may be extremely easy. If the stricture remains resistant, the suprapubic opening provides access to a sound passed in a retrograde fashion to the stricture. Another sound entering from the meatus will permit definition of the length of the strictured area and subsequent excision and re-anastomosis of the urethra over a catheter.

Pendulous urethral external urethrotomies tend to produce a high incidence of fistulas, which may be bothersome. External urethrotomy and excision of the entire strictured area may be indicated in the instance of constant resistance to dilation or in those which bleed effusively and persistently. It is important to excise all the stricture and deal as far as is possible with healthy urethra. Internal urethrotomy has become almost obsolete although reports of its continued use do occur. The value of an inlying catheter in securing rapid and pronounced dilation of strictures cannot be over-emphasized for frequent urethral manipulation may be followed by urethral fever due to injection of bacteria into the blood stream.

In the management of dense urethral strictures the value of preparatory suprapubic diversion of the urinary stream cannot be emphasized too strenuously. The entire urethra is put at rest, exudate is absorbed, edema and inflammation subside and manipulation and surgical treatment have a greater possibility for successful outcome. It must be carefully explained to the patient that his condition requires continued and regular dilations for the remainder of his life.

The *complications* of stricture are essentially of three types. The first is the obstructive, wherein damage occurs in the bladder and upper urinary tract; hypertrophy of the bladder with subsequent decompensation can occur. The effects of back pressure, if unrelieved, may eventually cause hydroureter, hydronephrosis and pyelonephritis of severe degree.

Periurethral abscess can arise following gonorrheal or nonspecific urethritis, emanating from chronic infection pocketed in the various glands and the lacunae of the urethra, or abscess may occur with a stricture. The infective material of the abscess may burrow deeper and eventually produce swelling evident from without. Most commonly such pus collections are found in the perineum, deriving from bulb or along the course of the urethra from the penoscrotal junction to the bulb. Parafrenular or pendulous urethral abscesses are more frequent occurrences following attacks of acute gonorrhea.

Urinary extravasation subsequent to urethral stricture occurs distal to the triangular ligament and manifests itself as an extension of periurethritis, at times emulating periurethral abscess (see Vest, Chapter 3 of this Section). It occurs when there is erosion of an area of the urethra previously weakened by scar and infection. Urine leaks into the periurethral tissues at each voiding and since the toxicity of the urine itself is added to by the invariable infection concomitant with stricture, a locally destructive process occurs in the tissues which is mirrored by a generalized toxic state. Extravasation of urine from the urethra is governed in its location and progression by certain fascial planes. The superficial layer of the triangular ligament with its attachment to Colles' fascia halts progress upwards toward the periprostatic areas. The further demarcation of Colles' fascia allows bulbous urethral extravasation to proceed into the scrotum, and up over the abdomen, but separates it from anything but superficial penile tissue involvement. In the pendulous urethra extravasation extends along Buck's fascial plane toward the glans. The rapidity of progress of extravasated urine varies remarkably. In certain cases infected urine may spread extensively within twenty-four hours, whereas weeks may elapse in others, merely accompanied by the gradual formation of abscess and slough. In the rapidly extending type the patient is quite toxic and exhibits the usual doughy, unhealthy blushed skin, and perhaps the actual feel of fluid in the tissues.

In a few instances confusion may arise because of the perfect ease with which a catheter is inserted, there being no sensation of "hang." The majority of cases, in fact, will show no evidence of dense or impermeable stricture, and it may not be suspected unless on palpation, indurative indication of the existence of stricture is found.

It is most urgent that the infiltrated areas be drained expediently. There is no substitute for immediate suprapubic cystostomy and wide drainage of all infected areas. The prognosis in these cases has improved considerably with the advent of antibiotics.

Chronic extravasations are still occasionally seen wherein an individual presents himself, usually with the abdominal scars of several previous cystostomies, and a perineum and scrotum replete with draining sinus and abscess pockets. Urine comes from one or several of the perirenal openings and frequently even these pathologic perineal urethrostomies will not allow passage of a filiform. In certain instances where the condition is directly attributable to the patient's apathy and neglect it has been deemed advisable to circumvent the entire lower tract and transplant the ureters to the rectosigmoid, if the upper tracts are structurally compatible with this form of management. In other cases extremely competent perineal urethrostomies, created by the process itself, have been, if adequately patent, allowed to remain. In some instances by diligent manipulation a channel has been reestablished and the fistulas dissected out and closed. The individual problems presented by such extensive complications of stricture allow the full play of a high degree of ingenuity in their solution.

URETHRAL DIVERTICULUM

Urethral diverticulum is not commonly encountered in the male. The preponderant number of urethral diverticula are acquired. Congenital diverticula, commonly limited to the ventral anterior urethra, are caused purportedly by developmental defects, such as absence of the urethral wall with primary atrophy of the spongiosum, faulty union of urethral anlage, cystic dilatation of persistent fetal ducts, embryologic processes similar to those which produce hypospadias and congenital obstruction provocative of diverticula (see Section IV). The diagnostic and therapeutic approaches in the congenital type do not differ from those utilized in the more common acquired variety.

A diverticulum is a tubular or spherical sac-like dilatation which is separate from but communicates with the urethral lumen by means of an ostium. Further classification may pursue, somewhat ephemerally in most instances, the finer differential point as to demarcation of the true from the false or whether all layers of the urethra are or are not present in the diverticulum. Such differentiation would perhaps serve a purpose in etiologic consideration if it were not for the alterations produced in the diverticular wall by the presence of infection, which is almost constant, and stone, which is of very frequent incidence.

Proximal to the triangular ligament acquired diverticulum is by far more frequently encountered whereas distal to the triangular ligament, or in the anterior urethra, the congenital type appears to be somewhat more common. The etiologic factors productive of acquired urethral diverticulum consist of either obstruction in the urethra, or destruction of the urethral wall through trauma or infection. Thus, in the posterior urethra, calculus commonly will be the instigating factor; a stone may lodge in the prostatic urethra, lead to dilatation and subsequent pouch formation, or by ulceration produce a juxta-urethral cavity. Prostatic calculi may by their growth permit a cavity to be a prelude to diverticulum. Evacuation of prostatic abscess into the urethral lumen can lead to diverticular formation. Traumatic incidents, either instrumental, operative or disruptive occurrences concomitant with blows or crushing injuries, may so distort the posterior urethra that pocketing, stasis, infection, stone formation and eventually diverticulum may arise.

In the anterior urethra there is again the same interplay of the two primary factors of obstruction and trauma. Strictures, periurethral abscesses, foreign bodies and injuries couple destruction due to infection with obstruction, to cause diverticula.

Recently reports from the various centers devoted to paraplegic care have revealed the high incidence of diverticula occurring subsequent to the trauma and infection of instrumentation, or the utilization of inlying catheters. Urethral neurogenic dysfunction must be addended as a basic etiologic factor. That trauma may be minimal and yet productive of diverticulum is seen in the occasional case of incontinence subsequent to prostatic operations wherein the pressure of a urinal at the penoscrotal junction allows a large diverticulum to form. Incontinence clamps may also be incriminated in this respect.

The *pathology* entailed is primarily one of distention of a portion of the urethral wall to form the diverticular cavity, or destruction of the wall and extension of the urethral epithelium into the pocket thus created forms the pouch. Usually infection soon obliterates all evidence as to the mechanism of production of the diverticulum. The average age of discovery of congenital diverticulum mentioned in the reported cases is 13 years and of the acquired approximately 35 years.

In the anterior urethra, one half of the congenital diverticula have been found in the penile portion and one half in the bulb. Acquired diverticula of the anterior urethra occur three times as commonly in the bulb as elsewhere. In paraplegics almost all diverticula have been found in the anterior urethra, all gave a history of periurethral abscess and all had undergone some prior urethral trauma, usually in the form of an inlying catheter. The incidence of periurethral abscess has been estimated to be between 5 and 10 per cent among paraplegics and only one half of these resolve without rupture, and subsequent sinus or diverticulum formation.

The *symptoms* are dependent to a great extent upon the size of the diverticulum. Small ones frequently cause no symptoms; the larger ones, owing to the greater tendency to poor drainage and persistent infection, manifest themselves in varying fashion in relation to their situation. Most commonly symptoms will be those of urinary difficulty or of a swelling along the urethral course. In the posterior urethra, prostatitis is simulated and perineal ache, low back pain, dysuria, frequency, urgency, and pyuria announce the chronic infection which is in residence. References to recurrent bouts of cystitis and pyelonephritis are fairly frequent. If the cavity is large, a perineal or rectal fluctuant bulge may be palpated. In the anterior urethra, some form of incontinence is a frequent complaint. Subsequent to micturition urine which has been collected in the diverticulum may be expelled and dribble out the meatus. Frequently the patient will learn to evacuate the diverticulum regularly and only severe infection or disturbance of coitus will send him to the physician. A small diverticulum may produce significant urinary obstruction if one of the ostial flaps is displaced into the urethral lumen by the urinary stream.

The *diagnosis* of male urethral diverticula is in most cases readily made by simple palpation. Compression of the bulging mass allows urine or retained infected material to escape into the urethra. Endoscopy should be accompanied by urethrography in order to ascertain the size and position of the diverticulum and to obviate the lack of recognition of a small ostium or a concealed diverticulum. Palpation of the urethra at the time of endoscopy will be of invaluable assistance in certain cases, for a pin point ostium can more easily be visualized when the diverticular contents are being expressed. In diverticula containing stones a plain roentgenogram is diagnostic.

Treatment. Small diverticula, if their ostia are of good caliber, can probably in many instances be left alone. Larger diverticula, and all wherein drainage is poor, should be excised as soon as local, acute, inflammatory reaction has subsided. Diversion of the urinary stream suprapubically should be a precursory measure in all cases of posterior urethral diverticula although some surgeons rely upon indwelling urethral catheters. Anterior diverticular repair may be preceded by perineal urethrostomy or an inlying catheter may serve adequately. Excision of the diverticulum should be followed by closure of periurethral tissue layers in eccentric fashion so that the suture lines are not in apposition. Frequently, constant suction either via the suprapubic or perineal diversionary tube will prove helpful in effecting tissue union without fistular formation. Urethral stricture at the site of the diverticula must be watched for subsequent to excision.

REFERENCES

ANDERSON, K., DeMONBREUM, W. A. and GOODPASTURE, E. W.: An etiologic consideration of Donovania granulomatis cultivated from granuloma inguinale in embryonic yolk. J. Exper. Med., 81:25–40, 1945.
DIENST, R. B., CHEN, C. H. and GREENBLATT, R. B.: Granuloma inguinale. Urol. & Cutan. Rev., 53:537–543, 1949.
DIENST, R. B., GREENBLATT, R. B. and CHEN, C. H.: Experimental transfer of chemoresistant granuloma inguinale. Am. J. Syph., 34:189–190, 1950.
DONOVAN, C.: Malaria. Indian M. Gaz., 40:411, 1905.
FRIEDMAN, S.: Queyrat's erythroplasia with carcinomatous invasion: report of an unusual case. J. Urol., 69:813, 1953.
GREENBLATT, R. B., DIENST, R. B., PUND, E. R. and TORPIN, R.: Experimental and clinical granuloma inguinale. J.A.M.A., 113:1109–1116, 1939.
HINMAN, F.: Principles and Practice of Urology. Philadelphia, W. B. Saunders, 1935.
KAUNTZE, R.: Peyronie's disease and proctalgia fugax. Guy's Hosp. Gaz., 64:23–25, 1950.
KORNBLITH, B. A.: Lymphogranuloma venereum and granuloma inguinale. J. Insur. Med., 5:30–32, 1949–1950.
LEVIN, E. A.: The diagnosis of chancroid. Urol. & Cutan. Rev., 45:587–590, 1941.
LOWSLEY, O. S. and GENTILE, A.: An operation for the cure of certain cases of plastic induration (Peyronie's disease) of the penis. J. Urol., 57:552–563, 1947.
MERRICKS, J. W. and COTTRELL, T. L.: Erythoplasia of Queyrat. J. Urol., 69:807, 1953.
NOVY, F. G., JR.: The newer antibiotics in dermatology. California Med., 72:201–203, 1950.
PACKER, H. and GOLDBERG, J.: Complement fixation studies in granuloma inguinale. Am. J. Trop. Med., 30:387–395, 1950.
PARISER, H., GOLDBERG, S. Z. and MITCHELL, G. H.: Streptomycin in the treatment of granuloma inguinale. Arch. Dermat. & Syph., 62:261–264, 1950.
ROBINSON, H. M., JR.: The treatment of granuloma inguinale, lymphogranuloma venereum, chancroid and gonorrhea. Arch. Dermat. & Syphil., 64:284–293, 1951.
ROWE, R. J.: Evaluation of chloromycetin as an adjunct to the surgical management of lymphogranuloma venereum and segmental ulcerative colitis. Am. J. Surg., 81:42–54, 1951.
SCOTT, M. J. and THOMSEN, J.: Primary cutaneous neisseria gonorrheae infections. Am. J. Syph., 34:262–264, 1950.
WEINSTEIN, M. and ROBERTS, M.: Elephantiasis and the Kondolean operation. Am. J. Surg., 79:327–331, 1950.
WILLCOX, R. R.: Effectiveness of antichancroidal drugs tested by auto inoculation of bubo fluid. Am. J. Syph., 34:378–382, 1950.
WILLCOX, R. R.: Aureomycin and chloramphenicol in chancroid. Brit. M. J., 1:509–510, 1951.

CHAPTER 2

Infections and Inflammations of the Male Genital Tract

EDWIN P. ALYEA, M.D.

ACUTE INFLAMMATION OF THE PROSTATE AND SEMINAL VESICLE

Occurrence and Etiology. Before the advent of specific chemotherapy, acute inflammation of the prostate was a disease common in urologic practice; now it is a rarity. Acute prostatitis was a common complication of gonorrheal urethritis and it is still seen in the sulfonamide and antibiotic resistant infections. In the past, from 50 to 80 per cent of all gonorrheal infections had an associated mild prostatitis. With the marked decrease in complications, due to specific therapy, acute prostatitis has practically disappeared. The gonococcus used to be the most common etiologic factor in acute prostatitis, whereas, at present, nonspecific infection is most prevalent.

From 1939 through 1950 there were 169,959 patients admitted to Duke Hospital and 244,936 new patients were seen in the out-patient clinic and hospital. In this large group there are recorded 226 cases of acute prostatitis and/or abscess of the prostate. However, on careful study only 31 are considered true acute prostatitis, that is, they had the symptoms, the elevated temperature and the rectal findings of evident acute infection. The vast majority of the 226 cases were patients with gonorrheal urethritis who had symptoms of posterior urethritis and tenderness in the prostate on rectal examination. No doubt, most of them had a mild catarrhal inflammation of the prostate so common when the posterior urethra is involved. This type was discarded and only the patients with probably the follicular or parenchymatous types were selected for study. There were also 10 patients with acute prostatic abscess. Of these 31 cases of acute prostatitis, 15 occurred during the period of 1939 and 1941 inclusive; 10 occurred in the 1942 to 1944 period; 5 in the 1945 to 1947 period and only 1 in the 1948 to 1950 period. This shows a gradual decrease in the incidence of this acute infection since 1945. This is due, of course, to the advent of the antibiotics. The same is true in the incidence of prostatic abscess. During these same periods there were 3 acute abscesses during 1939 and 1941; 4 in 1942–1944, 2 in 1945–1947 and 1 in 1948–1950. These statistics show the remarkably low incidence of acute prostatitis and acute prostatic abscess in both out-clinic and hospital patients. It is only fair to state that these statistics were taken from a clinic

635

which has a relatively low gonorrheal patient rate. In some of the larger city clinics where the percentage of gonorrhea patients is much higher, the relative incidence of this complication will no doubt be increased.

Bacterial invasion occurs in three ways; hematogenous, lymphogenous and by direct extension. Infections of the hematogenous route are usually caused by the staphylococcus or streptococcus, perhaps in small septic infarcts. They frequently have their origin in skin infections, boils, carbuncles or infection of the teeth, tonsils, or the respiratory or gastrointestinal systems. Infections from other diseases such as influenza and other virus diseases occur, but their mode of invasion is unknown. There are certain conditions which cause congestion of the prostate and hence supply a fertile field for the growth of invading organisms—such as excessive alcoholism, abnormal or excessive sexual practices, general body chilling, trauma to the perineum such as received in horseback and bicycle riding or direct trauma as massage. Lymphatics surrounding the lower urinary tract and large bowel furnish a possible path of invasion to the prostate. Invasion by direct extension occurs probably most often. Possibly the vast majority of infections in the posterior urethra have an associated infection in the dilated prostatic ducts, causing a mild catarrhal prostatitis. At the time of urethral instrumentation, infection can be carried into the posterior urethra and hence to the prostate. Infection in the upper urinary tract passes to the bladder and posterior urethra and by direct extension to the prostate or seminal vesicles.

The organisms at the present time most commonly encountered in nonspecific infection of the prostate are staphylococcus, streptococcus, E. coli and diphtheroids. It is difficult to consider acute prostatitis and seminal vesiculitis separately because probably 80 per cent of the infections of the prostate have an associated infection of the seminal vesicles. In the discussion here, they will therefore be considered together. All of these patients have an associated posterior urethritis and probably 40 per cent of patients with posterior urethritis have some grade of prostatitis and seminal vesiculitis. In the Duke Hospital group of 31 patients with acute prostatitis, 11 had a gonococcal infection; 12 had a nonspecific coccus and 7 had a bacillary infection. Since the general use of antibiotics, from 1945 through 1950, there was no case of acute prostatitis in which the gonococcus was the etiologic factor, only one was caused by a stapylococcus and four were of bacillary origin. It is interesting to see practically the disappearance of the coccal infections with chemotherapy. This is true also in prostatic abscess; from 1945 to 1950, all three of our cases were bacillary in origin and none was caused by a coccus.

Pathology. Inflammation of the prostate is the result of injury whether it be due to bacterial invasion or to toxins produced by these bacteria. The reaction against this injury produces the process of acute inflammation. Infection is usually associated with a posterior urethritis and seminal vesiculitis. If the prostatic infection is of hematogenous origin then the urethritis is secondary to it but in all other instances the prostatitis is probably secondary to the urethral infection. It may be localized or diffuse. There is a diffusion of a serofibrinous, a sanguinous or a purulent exudate and the normal content of the gland is replaced by lymphocytes and leukocytes. Blood vessels may rupture causing hemorrhage and resultant necrosis with final scarring and contracture of the gland (Fig. 318). The character of the reaction in the prostate, as in other organs, depends upon (1) particular organism involved, (2) the virulence of that organism, (3) the immune reaction of the patient in general and of the gland in particular to the infection. It may be well localized by protective body forces; or the acinous borders may break down and abscess form.

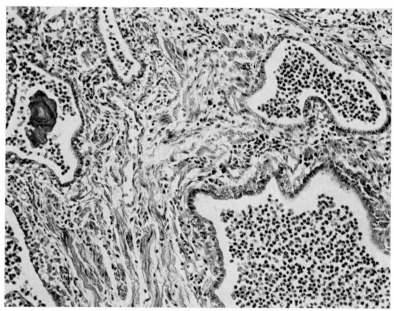

Fig. 318.   Acute prostatitis, showing polymorphonuclear infiltration of the stroma and exudation in the acini. × 102.

There are usually recognized three types of acute prostatic infection: (1) catarrhal, (2) follicular and (3) parenchymatous. Infection spreading from the posterior urethra causes generalized edema, congestion and infiltration of the prostatic ducts and surrounding interstitial tissue with pus cells. Catarrhal inflammation is mild and may produce few symptoms. The infection may progress to the follicular type in which case the prostatic ducts and follicles are inflamed and edematous. This congestion causes enlargement of the gland as a whole. Further extension may form multiple small abscesses with perifollicular infiltration into the parenchymal tissue. It may localize or spread and involve a lobe or the whole gland. Such abscesses are rarely caused by the gonococcus although that may have been the original organism involved. They are usually the result of a secondary invader, the staphylococcus. The infection may continue to spread to the periprostatic spaces or to the ampulla of the vas and into the seminal vesicles. Abscesses may rupture into the ischiorectal fossa and neighboring structures; but this is rare because of the protective covering of Denonvilliers' fascia. They frequently rupture into the urethra, and more rarely into the rectum (Henline, 1943).

Infection and the pathologic changes in the seminal vesicles are similar to those in the prostate. It is rare to have infection in one gland and not in the other. Urogenitogenous or retrograde extension to the seminal vesicles is probably the most frequent mode of spread. Infection passes from the urethra to the seminal vesicles by way of the ejaculatory ducts or from the epididymis by means of the vas. According to Young (1926) it is difficult clinically to separate infection of the prostate from that of the seminal vesicle; pathologic sections of both glands are necessary for proof. Similar to the prostate there is edema and congestion of the mucosa and the lumens of the vesicles are cut off by this inflammatory process. Localized abscesses form. Although usually confined to its border by Denonvilliers' fascia, the abscess may extend into the perivesicular tissues or because of its position on the posterior surface of the bladder, it may rupture into that organ.

Symptoms. *General.* If the acute prostatitis is of hematogenous origin, one may have very few symptoms referable to the genitourinary tract. The onset will be typical of any severe generalized infection; general body aching and debility, anorexia, nausea and vomiting, elevation of temperature, chilly sensations and possibly real chills. If the infection is fulminating in character, the fever may be extremely high and associated with severe chills, marked general prostration and acute toxemia.

Local. (1) Pain. In addition to this general reaction there may be localized symptoms. One may have discomfort in the perineum progressing to perhaps a severe rectal distress or pain on defecation. It is usually a persistent aching, a heaviness or bearing down pain in the perineum. It may be referred to the lower lumbar region of the back, to the genitalia, or to the thighs. There may be pain referred to the abdomen (Freund, 1942) and typical symptoms of acute appendicitis have been reported (Seabaugh, 1946). When the seminal vesicles are involved, there may be severe pain in the groins due to an associated vasitis and peritoneal irritation may be present. Even ureteral obstruction has been reported due to anatomic relations of the seminal vesicles and the lower end of the ureters (Singer, 1946). Suprapubic pain is often present. (2) Sexual Symptoms are rather common. Usually libido is promptly lost as this is a severe acute infection. Even if intercourse were attempted, it most likely would be quite painful due to the activity of the acutely inflamed gland. (3) Urethral Symptoms. If the infection is of retrograde origin, urinary and urethral symptoms probably antedate the acute prostatic infection. There may be burning on urination, frequency, dysuria, urgency, pain on voiding, terminal strangury, terminal hematuria and dribbling. The congestion causes considerable enlargement of the gland and symptoms typical of posterior urethral obstruction occur, with diminution in size and force of the stream, increased frequency, cutting off of the stream and pain on voiding. This not infrequently progresses to complete urinary retention.

If the acute prostatitis lasts for a week or longer with continued septic type temperature elevation, high leukocytosis and rectal symptoms, it is likely that an *abscess* is forming. It is usually ushered in by an increase in all of the above symptoms, particularly with a severe chill, very high fever and rapid elevation of the white blood count; profuse sweating and an increase in the obstructive symptoms with perhaps acute retention. With rupture or drainage of the abscess, all of these symptoms are suddenly relieved and profuse discharge of pus may appear from the urethra, rectum or perineum, depending on the point of drainage.

Diagnosis. The diagnosis of acute prostatitis of urogenitogenous origin is usually not difficult; but the correct recognition of hematogenous infection may be quite puzzling because of entire lack of localizing symptoms. (1) One must consider first the history of primary infection elsewhere in the body; in the skin, tonsils, gastrointestinal, respiratory and genitourinary tracts, etc. (2) The progression of the above-mentioned symptoms is quite suggestive. (3) A urethral discharge must be examined with bacteriologic stains and (4) cultures of urethral or prostatic fluid may be made. (5) Urine examination: the 3 glass test will be of particular significance. Shreds and infection in the voided first glass of urine, perhaps a clear second and then a cloudy third glass is suggestive of prostatic infection. (6) Rectal examination is, of course, of utmost importance. An enlarged swollen, tense, edematous, painful and hot prostate is diagnostic. If abscesses have formed there may be areas of induration alternating with soft boggy spots. These are scattered throughout the gland and give it its irregular surface. (7) One should never massage an acutely inflamed gland but if by examination prostatic secretion is obtained, it will be found full of pus cells. (8) A high leukocytosis, which may increase markedly as the infection spreads to abscess formation is suggestive.

(9) It may be difficult to differentiate from *Cowper's gland abscess* but this should be done. Cowper's gland lies in the anterior perineal body in front of the deep urethra and rectum. Usually infection in one of these glands will start at one side of the midline. The rectal symptoms are not as marked as with prostatitis and early in the disease the normal prostate can be felt above it. However, if the infection in Cowper's gland has progressed to a considerable size or if the prostatic abscess is large, it may be impossible by rectal examination to make this differentiation. It can then be made only at operation. During perineal exposure, a Cowper's gland abscess will be encountered as the ischiorectal fossa is developed, anterior to the prostate and before Denonvilliers' fascia is incised. If the abscess is underneath Denonvilliers' fascia it originates in the prostate and not in Cowper's gland.

(10) Differentiation of prostatic abscess or acute prostatitis from an *infection in a cyst of the utricle* may be made. The utricle is the embryologic remains of the fused müllerian duct in the male and opens into the prostatic urethra in the region of the verumontanum. If, during development, it does not completely close off, a cyst may form. The normal utricle has a central lumen surrounded by complicated racemose tubules lined by epithelium, similar to those in the prostate. These convoluted passageways may become infected and the outlet closed. An infected cyst will form

which may give exactly the same symptoms as acute prostatitis or abscess. The cyst usually arises in the midline, at the midbase of the prostate. Usually the rounded cyst-like mass overlying the midline of the prostate can be distinguished from it. If acutely inflamed there is tenderness and pain on examination and it may be difficult to differentiate from acute prostatic abscess. At urethroscopy, pus may be seen coming from the utricle. As shown in Figure 319, injection of the cyst with opaque media may be made. This cyst was later injected with 10 per cent argyrol and massage was carried out every three days. In two weeks it was almost impossible by rectal examination to distinguish the cyst and the patient was asymptomatic.

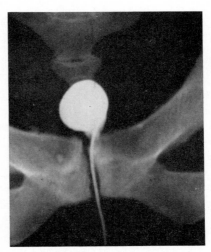

Fig. 319.   Cyst of the utricle injected with iodide, transurethrally.

Treatment. *General.* Treatment of acute prostatitis consists of general medical measures of palliative nature such as bed rest, mild laxative for catharsis, alkaline diuretic and antispasmotic mixtures for urinary sedation, opium and belladonna suppositories for rectal discomfort, and the forcing of fluids. If urinary obstruction is present, fluids should not be forced as this naturally would increase the posterior urethral congestion and irritation. Physical exertion should be avoided and sexual stimulation of any sort entirely prohibited.

Local. Attempt is made to prevent suppuration by applying heat to the prostate by various contraptions. The old-fashioned and simplest method of hot sitz baths or hot enema is probably quite satisfactory. There are several types of rectal applicators using diathermy or electricity, or hot solutions flowing through instruments lying against the gland. Recently the "Elliott machine," in which hot water is run continually through a rubber bag which lies against the prostate has proven a practical and efficient apparatus. By such methods some reports claim definite increase in posterior urethral temperatures (Herring, 1935), others have not obtained any temperature change (Hibbs and Osborne, 1941). Perhaps the hyperemia associated with the treatment and not actual elevation of temperature accounts for the beneficial results from such therapy.

Urinary obstructive symptoms should be treated by mild urinary sedation. If obstruction progresses to retention, a small urethral catheter should be left in for probably two or three days. This is preferred to frequent intermittent catheterizations which may cause further urethral trauma.* Active treatment such as massage or instrumentation of the urethra or prostate in the acute stage is contraindicated.

CHEMOTHERAPY. Without doubt at the present time, the most important form of treatment is specific chemotherapy. There was a time when specific vaccines were most popular but now other therapies are preferable. Before the days of the antibiotics, intravenous neoarsphenamine was the accepted specific drug of choice for coccal infections. At the present time sulfonamides or antibiotics for the specific bacterial infection are of the utmost importance. Cultures of the organism are made and it is tested for its sensitivity to the various antibiotics. These sensitivity tests can now be easily done with the small antibiotic paper discs.

The dosage recommended for the sulfonamides in urinary tract infection, particularly sulfacetamide and sulfadiazine, is 2 gm. a day for a period of one week and then, if desired, 1 gm. a day is given for five days more. Considerable clinical research has shown that the usual urinary tract infection which is not complicated does not require larger doses of the sulfonamides. Infection in the prostate or seminal vesicles requires larger doses; 3 or even 4 gm. a day are given in divided doses with marked increased fluid intake and alkalinization of the urine during this therapy. This treatment should not be kept up longer than a week, and the patient should be carefully watched for toxic drug reaction. Gantrisin, because of its higher solubility, may be given in larger doses of 4 or even 6 gm. a day for four or five days with forced fluid intake. The dose is then reduced to 3 gm. a day for a week or longer.

ANTIBIOTICS. Achromycin and Aureomycin are usually prescribed in doses of 2 gm. a day for two days, and then 1 gm. a day for a week or longer if necessary. Terramycin may also be employed, the usual dosage is 2 gm. a day for four days, and then 1 gm. a day for a period of a week or longer. Streptomycin or dihydrostreptomycin is recommended in doses of 1 gm daily for five to seven days. Penicillin is used in the form of Crystacillin, usually giving 600,000 units per day for at least one week. New antibiotics are continually being made and should be used according to their value against various organisms.

With the administration of any of these various drugs it is necessary to watch the patient for sensitivity or other toxic reactions. The duration of the particular therapy will depend upon the reaction of the infection to the drug. Frequently a medication proved ineffective demands that another be employed.

* Yet acute retention under these circumstances usually means prostatic abscess and demands prostatotomy. Editor.

A chart showing suggested treatment of infections caused by the various organisms would be in order but with the present multiplicity of antibiotics whose popularity changes from time to time such a chart would soon be out of date, and therefore hardly worthwhile. For the ordinary E. coli infection, order of preference of therapy might be sulfacetamide or Gantrisin, then probably Terramycin followed by Furadantin, achromycin or streptomycin. Any of these might be satisfactory clinically, but the one selected would depend on sensitivity tests carried out on the particular organism isolated from the patient's specimen. While we are aware of the apparent discrepancies between the sensitivity tests in vitro and the clinical results, this is still the most intelligent approach in beginning therapy. Clinically, not infrequently an infection will respond quickly to a drug whose in vitro study showed no specific sensitivity, and vice versa. The most obstinate infections are Pseudomonas aeruginosa (pyocyaneus) and Proteus. For the former, at the present time a combination of Furadantin with Terramycin, or Polymyxin B with Terramycin, is recommended. For Proteus infection, a combination of Gantrisin or Furadantin with one of the antibiotics may prove most beneficial. For Staphylococcus or Streptococcus hemolyticus, penicillin is usually the drug of choice; achromycin and Terramycin are also good. This is discussed in detail in Section V, Chapter 1. In this age of chemotherapy, new drugs are continually being synthesized and applied clinically, so that the popular drugs for specific infections today may be replaced by more efficacious ones tomorrow.

COMBINATION OF HEAT THERAPY AND CHEMOTHERAPY. Hyperthermia by various methods was popular several years ago but has been gradually discarded because of the technical help required and the frequent severe reactions encountered. Without doubt, the vast majority of acute prostatic and seminal vesicle infections will be quickly overcome by modern chemotherapy alone.

SURGERY. If the infection should not respond to the above treatment but rather progress to abscess formation, with fluctuation, and often complete vesical retention, operative intervention is necessary. The old method of passing a sound in the urethra or the rectum and blindly forcing it into the abscessed gland is fortunately little used now. Transurethral resection of the intra-urethral bulging prostatic abscess is frequently carried out in the chronic stages and it can also be employed in the acute disease. However, perineal exposure and incision of the abscess is usually the method of choice. The perineal approach is made according to Young's technique, and as Denonvilliers' fascia is incised, the abscess will be encountered. By this method thorough drainage is carried out through the perineum (see Section XV, Chapter 7).

It is noted that no active mechanical treatment of the prostate or urethra, such as massage or passage of urethral sounds or bladder irrigation, have been advised. These procedures should never be used until the acute inflammation has entirely subsided. In the Duke Hospital series, all of the cases of acute prostatitis during the period from 1939 to 1950 were treated by conservative methods including rest, fluids, heat to the prostate usually by

the Elliott machine, retention urethral catheter when required and chemotherapy. None of the patients with acute prostatitis required open operation.
In the abscess cases of this series 3 required perineal drainage by open
operation; 2 were treated by the transurethral resection; 2 ruptured spontaneously into the urethra; 1 ruptured spontaneously into the rectum and 2
were treated by conservative methods. Since 1945, there were only 3 abscess
cases; two of these were treated by transurethral resection and one by
conservative therapy. No perineal operation has been required in the last
five years. It is evident that since the advent of the sulfonamides and antibiotics, acute prostatic abscess has become a rarity and it is now seldom
necessary to resort to open operation.

Prognosis. The prognosis for the vast majority of patients with acute
prostatitis is excellent. They will clear up satisfactorily on conservative
therapy and only an occasional one will require surgical treatment. When
abscess has formed, the majority may require surgical drainage, either
transurethral or perineal. They then usually heal promptly, except for a
residual chronic infection which may persist for a long time.

CHRONIC PROSTATITIS

Etiology and Occurrence. Chronic prostatitis is probably the most common
chronic infection in men over 50 years of age. It can, however, occur at
any age after puberty (and, though rare, before puberty, as well, Ed.). It
very frequently follows acute prostatitis or chronic posterior urethritis. The
majority of these infections are not due to the gonococcus; although
gonorrhea may have been present at the start, the gonococcus is soon replaced by a secondary invader which keeps up the chronic infection (Wesson,
1938). Kretschmer et al. (1937) found only 24 cases of gonorrheal infection in 1,000 patients with chronic prostatitis. According to Pelouze
(1939) 95 per cent of cases of chronic prostatitis are secondary to infection
elsewhere in the body; the most common primary foci are infected teeth
and tonsils. He also states that 35 per cent of all men over 50 years have
chronic prostatitis and 95 per cent of them have dental infection as the
primary focus of their prostatic infection. This is possibly an exaggeration.
The organisms most commonly encountered are: staphylococcus, streptococcus, the colon bacillus and diphtheroids. The infection may be related
to prolonged congestion such as acquired by alcoholic excesses or sexual
abuses in the form of prolonged excitement, frequent masturbation, overindulgence or withdrawal. These practices may cause a fertile field for
bacterial invasion and growth. Perineal trauma from bicycle or horseback
riding, or the army jeep seat may lead to chronic infection. Chronic urethral
infection may easily pass directly into the prostatic ducts. Hematogenous origin
of infection is possible but this more commonly causes an acute infection. Infection in the urinary tract may travel from the kidneys to the bladder, to
the urethra and hence to the prostate. This path of invasion is proven in the
case of the spread of tuberculosis of the urinary tract to the seminal tract.
Other urogenital complications such as urethral stricture, hyperplasia of
the prostate with obstruction, contracture of the vesical neck and prostatic

calculi may cause congestion in the posterior urethral region and with obstruction, lead to infection of the prostate. Chronic infection of the seminal vesicles accompanies prostatitis in the majority of cases and the organisms are the same in each.

In chronic prostatitis, it is difficult to find the specific bacteria in the prostatic secretion. Young (1926) found 40 per cent of smears and 70 per cent of cultures positive. According to Hinman (1935), of 100 cultures taken through the endoscope so as to prevent urethral contamination, 57 were sterile and none was positive for the gonococcus. Delzell and Lowsley, by taking endoscopic cultures of the seminal fluid in 38 patients, found the cultures as follows: staphylococcus, 23; streptococcus, 13; E. coli, 4; miscellaneous, 4. Cummings and Chittenden (1938) in 175 cases; Ritter and Lippow (1938) in 131 cases; and Gardner (1940) found about the same predominant organisms. In the prostatic secretion, the approximate relative frequency of bacteria is staphylococci, 60 per cent; streptococci, 30 per cent; bacilli, 20 per cent, and diphtheroids and others. Many of them contain two or more of these organisms. The gonococcus is rarely isolated. Chronic prostatitis is therefore in the vast majority of cases a nonspecific infection.

Prostatic infection may itself act as a primary focus for metastatic infection, such as endocarditis, iritis, conjunctivitis, myositis, arthritis, etc. Whenever these infections are present, the prostate should always be considered as a possible primary focus. Evidence is very suggestive by the occurrence of an acute flare-up of the metastatic infection when the prostate is massaged. This is not uncommonly seen in arthritis and iritis. The reaction may be either mild or severe with accompanying chills and fever. This phenomenon is thought to be due to the release into the system of specific toxins, to which the patient has become sensitive (bacterial allergy). The reaction is therefore similar to that often obtained by a specific vaccine.

Chronic seminal vesiculitis is usually associated with chronic prostatitis and the etiology and incidence are similar. In addition, congenital anomalies such as stenosed ejaculatory ducts may play a part in vesiculitis.

Pathology. The pathologic picture of chronic prostatitis is chronic inflammatory reaction around the acini with increased polymorphonuclear cells, lymphocytes, and proliferation of connective tissue. The pathology of the chronic infection is quite different from that of the acute. The acute reaction of edema, swelling and deep pain is absent in the chronic form. In chronic prostatitis there is relatively little fluid exudation and a predominance of mononuclear rather than polymorphonuclear cells. There is avascularity as contrasted with marked increase in vascularity in the acute stage. The lumens of the ducts become occluded with pus and epithelial cells and marked periglandular round cell infiltration; dilatation of the acini result (Fig. 320). This causes the soft, boggy prostate which is so often felt in the chronic infections. Fatty tissue is laid down; there is marked shrinkage and distortion of the architecture of the gland. Necrosis with resultant fibrosis and contracture occurs which may involve the posterior urethra, causing vesical neck scarring. If the verumontanum, the utricle and the ejaculatory ducts become infected, chronic inflammation with fibrosis and stricture of the ducts result. Following catarrhal prostatitis, the gland may become slightly enlarged; its consistency soft and somewhat boggy. In the parenchymatous and follicular types, with perhaps resulting abscess, the gland may be smaller and more fibrotic. Clinically it is difficult to differentiate the three types. There are some who think that there may be an aseptic or amicrobic form of prostatitis due only to chronic congestions. This, however, is questionable.

In *chronic nonspecific seminal vesiculitis,* there is thickening of the wall of the vesicle and ampulla. The vesicle may be reduced to a folliculated sac or a fibrous cord. Perivesicular fibrosis and adhesions to surrounding structures may cause contractures of the vesical neck or lower ureteral obstruction.

Symptoms. Chronic prostatitis presents an extremely variegated sympto-

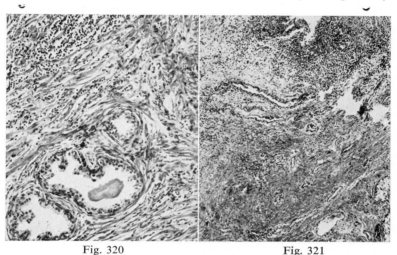

Fig. 320   Fig. 321

Fig. 320.   Chronic prostatitis, showing round cell infiltration of the stroma and fibrosis. $\times$ 184.
Fig. 321.   Tuberculosis of prostate, showing giant cell reaction, chronic inflammation and fibrosis and caseous necrosis. $\times$ 184.

matology. Many patients with a mild infection have no symptoms at all. The usual symptoms may be grouped as follows:

(1) *Urethral.* There is a persistent morning drop or urethral discharge. It is thin, watery, either clear or milky and sometimes sticky in character. It appears at the meatus usually in the morning after the nightly period of no urination or during the day when there is a long time between voidings. It may cause the meatus to be glued shut in the mornings. A chronic urethral irritation may be present.

(2) *Urinary.* There is frequency with a mild urgency, dysuria, burning or discomfort at the bladder neck or in the perineum on voiding. These symptoms are probably dependent upon the associated posterior urethritis and in severe cases may be very distressing. Obstruction may occur as well as severe dysuria, pyuria and terminal hematuria and dribbling. But the severe symptoms are rarely present in chronic prostatitis. The patient may notice shreds in his urine.

(3) *Pain.* a. LOCAL. There is discomfort or a dull aching in the region of the prostate or rectum; a deep urethral irritation and pain at the vesical neck which may radiate down the penis to the glans. b. REFERRED. Pain is common and it appears in various regions of the body according to the dicta of Head. "Surface pains from vesical origin cause a spilling-over of afferent nerve stimuli into areas of the segmental corresponding spinal sensory nerves on the skin." The fibers in the prostate arising all the way from the tenth dorsal to the third sacral segment make it possible to have prostatic or vesicle pain referred to any point innervated by these corresponding spinal nerves. This includes practically the whole body below the diaphragm; the lower lumbar spine, hips, thighs, perineum and suprapubic region are the more common places. An interesting feature of this pain is that often it is present when the patient first arises in the morning and wears off during the day—just the opposite of arthritic pain. According to Young (1926), these areas of referred pain are found in the following order of frequency in his large series of cases shown in Table 12.

Table 12. Referred Pain In Chronic Prostatitis

Lower lumbar region (backache)	64	Like renal colic	10
Perineum	35	Kidney area	8
Suprapubic region	22	Sacrum	5
Groin (one or both)	18	Like sciatica	5
Testicle (one or both)	18	Knees	4
Penis or urethra	14	Legs	4
Rectum	13	Vesical neck	4
Thighs	12	Buttocks	2
Hips (one or both)	10		

(4) *Sexual.* There is frequently sexual dysfunction. There may be loss or diminution of libido or potentia; premature, painful or bloody ejaculation and frequent painful nocturnal emissions. As a rule, severe sexual symptoms are present only in the exceptional case. If the patient is an introspective type individual, he may exaggerate mild sexual symptoms which ordinarily would be ignored. Usually there is a prominently psychic factor in the patients with pronounced sexual symptoms. There may also be prostatorrhea or spermatorrhea in this type of patient; and sexual neurasthenia and/or mental depression may become prominent symptoms.

(5) *Metastatic.* If secondary reactions from bacteria, toxins or allergic sensitivity are present (iritis, arthritis or neuritis), symptoms of these conditions will be apparent. They are often relieved after treatment of the prostate or sometimes may flare up acutely as previously mentioned.

Symptoms from seminal vesiculitis associated with prostatitis are quite similar except that there is a preponderance of the sexual disturbances, such as frequent nocturnal emissions, premature and bloody ejaculations in particular. Functional nervous disorders are frequent; headaches, dizziness and neurasthenias develop which are often difficult to remedy.

Recurrent attacks of epididymitis frequently indicate a chronic infection of the seminal vesicles as the primary focus.

Diagnosis. The diagnosis of chronic prostatitis and seminal vesiculitis is made from the history, the urine examination of the three glass test, the rectal examination, the microscopic examination of the expressed prostatic or seminal fluid, and sometimes by a urethroscopic examination. (1) *History* and (2) *symptoms* are as described above.

(3) Careful examination is made of the *urine* in a three glass test. The first glass contains the washings of the urethra which usually will contain comma shreds; the second glass probably is clear unless there is a posterior urethral or urinary infection, and the third glass will again contain shreds and epithelial cells from the expressions from the prostate at the forceful completion of the act of urination.

(4) *Rectal palpation.* This is of utmost importance in diagnosis. It is advisable to have nearby a rectal prostatic chart so you can draw the outlines of the prostate and indicate the areas of induration or softening as they are felt. The correct procedure of a careful rectal examination and prostatic massage has been described elsewhere in this text (Section II) and will not be repeated here. The chronically inflamed prostate is often irregular in surface outline with areas of induration, cavitation or bogginess and periprostatic adhesions, fixing it in the pelvis. It may be enlarged or a small contracted fibrous gland. A pathologic indurated seminal vesicle is much easier to feel than the normal. It may be irregular, nodular, indurated and not compressible. There may also be perivesicular adhesions extending out toward the pelvic wall.

(5) The normal *prostatic fluid* is grayish opalescent, like milky water but viscous in character. It is thin and sticky, containing a few corpora amylacea, many lipoid granules, epithelial cells, and crystals such as phosphates. There are lecithin bodies which are translucent and smaller than red blood cells (cf. Huggins, Section I, Chapter 4). For normal fluid the white blood cells should be less than 10 to the high power field, an arbitrarily chosen number. The fluid of chronic prostatitis may not be distinguished from normal fluid grossly, but sometimes if the infection is severe, the color and character will be distinctly abnormal. Microscopic examination shows the leukocytes displacing the normal elements of the fluid, particularly the lecithin bodies. The white blood cells are markedly increased, singly or in clumps; as the infection recedes and the white blood cells decrease, the normal constituents return to their correct proportion.

It must be emphasized that one examination of the prostate and its fluid is not sufficient definitely to rule out a chronic infection. If such is suspected, at least three examinations must be made with a day or two of rest in between the examinations. There is disagreement as to whether three massages on alternate days can stir up a latent infection. Some urologists feel that it may, and pus will appear in what was previously normal fluid. There may be discrepancy between the rectal examination and microscopic examination of the prostatic fluid. A normal prostate may be felt by rectal examination but the secretion contains a good many single or clumps of pus cells. Vice versa, there may be an indurated, irregular prostate suggesting chronic infection and the secretion be normal. This is understandable as in the latter case there may be a "burned-out" fibrous chronic contracted prostate without active leukocytes in the acini at that time. Stained smears of the prostatic fluid do not show bacteria nearly as often as one would expect. A fresh specimen should be examined microscopically and then it should be dried and stained with methylene blue or Gram stain. Cultures are also made at the time the specimen is obtained. In getting the specimen for culture care must be taken to prevent contamination from the glans and urethra.

(6) *Urethroscopic examination* of the posterior urethra and vesical neck is not a routine procedure but infrequently may be necessary for an accurate diagnosis. Pus may be seen exuding from gaping prostatic ducts or from the ejaculatory ducts. These may be probed with either the Young or the McCarthy ejaculatory duct catheterizer and strictures of the ducts identified. Signs of chronic inflammation of the floor of the posterior urethra may be seen; the verumontanum may appear granular and enlarged and congested; a chronic inflammatory fibrous bar or contracture of the vesical neck may be present.

(7) A *urethrogram* may show elongation and narrowing of the posterior urethra; if an abscess has opened into the urethra, the opaque solution may fill this cavity. There may be anterior deflexion of the posterior urethra as shown by the contrast media. Injection of opaque media may show abscess strictures or other abnormalities in chronic vesiculitis (Gonzales, 1943; Desson, 1938).

Vesiculography is carried out either by injection of the ejaculatory duct with the McCarthy ejaculatory duct catheterizer or through a vasotomy-incision in the scrotal vas. Either of these will fill the seminal vesicles and the characteristic inflammatory changes in the vas, ejaculatory ducts, ampulla and vesicle are noted (Harlin, 1950).

It may be difficult to differentiate the chronic pyogenic from the gonorrheal or tuberculous infection of the prostate and seminal vesicles. One must correlate the history, the physical and x-ray findings with laboratory data. Prostatic calculi are usually ruled out by the x-ray.

In the differentiation of carcinoma the rectal findings are most important. In carcinoma the surface is usually irregular and nodular and of third degree induration or stony hard; there may be extension of this process into the seminal vesicles or outside of the prostatic capsule. Blood examination for increased acid phosphatase or bone marrow studies for metastatic foreign cells are helpful diagnostic aids. X-ray may show metastasis to the bones or lungs. It has been suggested that the prostate can be vigorously massaged and the secretion examined by Papanicolaou stain for malignant cells. The advisability of this procedure, however, has been questioned; is it advisable to massage so vigorously a prostate, possibly containing malignant cells, as to expel them into the fluid and hence into the urethra? This is certainly contrary to the usual treatment of malignancy anywhere else in the body. A needle biopsy or, better still, open perineal excision and frozen section examination of the suspicious nodule should be carried out. The differential diagnosis of a fibrous chronic prostatitis or an early carcinoma is a most important one.

Prostatorrhea manifests itself by the appearance at intervals of a small amount of urethral discharge resembling prostatic fluid. It is seen most frequently in nervous introspective type individuals who are apt to exaggerate their symptoms and who indulge in excessive or abusive sexual practices. It is thought to be due to relaxation of the prostatic ducts through which an accumulation of fluid escapes. It appears particularly at the end of micturition or when straining at stool. Naturally, it must be differentiated from the discharge of chronic prostatitis. In prostatorrhea the microscopic examination of the fluid is usually normal. Furthermore, one frequently obtains the history of sexual overindulgence or unusual practices and all this usually in a nervous introspective type individual. Treatment for prostatorrhea consists of the correction of sex hygiene, encouragement and reassurance. It must be impressed on the patient that he is not losing all of his prostatic secretion nor will the condition in any way affect his virility. For a while, routine frequent prostatic massage to keep the prostate empty may be of help. It has no serious consequences and usually is easily controlled.

Treatment. Treatment of chronic prostatitis is continually changing. It may be divided into (1) general, (2) chemotherapy, (3) attack on the distant primary focus of infection, (4) eradication of complications which keep up the prostatic infection, and (5) local prostatic therapy.

1. *General.* An hygienic regime is advisable. Diet should be of wholesome character, with plenty of vitamins; the only prohibitions are alcohol and irritative condiments, both of which may cause posterior urethral irritation. Fluids should be forced and constipation avoided. There should be moderation in sexual habits but with regular sexual indulgence; massage is a poor substitute for intercourse in emptying the prostate and seminal vesicles. Overindulgence or sexual habits causing overstimulation are to be strictly avoided. Many patients are benefited by healthy psychotherapy. Stilbestrol has been suggested to decrease the congestion of the prostate but it has not been found particularly beneficial (Cooper and McLean, 1946).

2. *Chemotherapy.* Sulfonamides and antibiotics for chronic prostatitis have been quite disappointing. Bacterial sensitivity tests should determine the drug of choice. Mandelic acid cannot be concentrated sufficiently in the prostate to be of benefit. This is also probably true of the sulfonamides and antibiotics but they may have some beneficial tissue or body reaction. If no improvement is noted in a week or two it is not advisable to continue these therapies longer. Mapharsen or arsphenamine is still probably one of the best drugs for treatment of chronic coccal infections of the prostate. Specific vaccines and hyperthermia have been used for a long time but each of these has limited usefulness at present. Staphylococcus vaccine has perhaps given the best results in this type of therapy as reported by Drummond, (1941).

3. If the primary *focus of infection* is discovered, this should be treated vigorously and eradicated. Pelouze directed special attention to dental foci.

4. There are certain local genitourinary complications which may cause or keep up prostatic infection. *Urethral stricture* is a common offender and

should be progressively and periodically dilated. The use of the Kollmann dilator for posterior urethral dilatations is advocated by many to open the prostatic ducts for better drainage. This instrument need seldom be used and when it is, great care must be taken or trauma may result. Prostatic stones may keep up the infection and these can be removed by perineal operation or transurethral resection. Prostatic valves or a median bar obstruction which causes congestion or posterior urethral granulomatous infection or polyps, or cavities in the prostatic urethra should be appropriately treated by transurethral resection or electrocoagulation.

5. *Massage.* The aim of local prostatic therapy is to drain adequately of all infected material the prostatic acini and ducts. Massage evacuates the pus, bacteria and debris which are plugging the prostatic ducts; this improves the drainage of the gland. It also increases the circulation, stimulates absorption within the gland and thus carries away infection.

(a) Prostatic massage has been used for many decades. Although massage of an inflamed or infected organ is unphysiologic, nevertheless in the case of chronic prostatitis it has proven its worth. There is a difference of opinion as to the manner of carrying out this therapy. Some suggest instilling antiseptics in the bladder before treatment and then have the patient void after massage. Others massage the prostate first and then have the patient void to wash out the secretion from the posterior urethra. Still others pass a catheter into the bladder and inject an irrigation fluid, which the patient voids after the massage. Bladder irrigation and instillation solutions usually suggested are: potassium permanganate 1:5000, 1:3000 acriflavine and recently, 1:5000 to 1:20,000 Zephiran solution.

(b) Two decades ago the most common therapy carried out in a urologist's office was massage of the prostate and irrigation of the urethra and bladder. This has gradually become less and less popular so that now irrigations are reduced to a minimum. Passage of a catheter or the injection of irrigation fluids through the urethra may extend the infection into the prostatic ducts or down the vas and cause acute epididymitis. Probably the safest method is first to massage the prostate and then have the patient void. This gives a natural irrigation of the urethra and no harm can be done to other organs.

There is difference of opinion as to the frequency with which massage should be carried out; some suggest every three days, others every week. Probably once every four to five days is advisable, then decreasing to once a week as the infection clears. If necessary, massage may be continued at once a week for two months. The microscopic findings of the prostatic fluid and other evidence of clearing of the infection are the criteria for stopping massages. After a treatment period of two months it is advisable to discontinue massage for a month or so. If necessary, a second course may then be started. This is better than constant weekly massage for months without rest periods.

By massage, the prostate is emptied of pus and toxins. As toxins are expressed, they may infrequently cause a sensitivity reaction in the patient; this may be mild or severe with chills and fever. It is similar to a vaccine or protein sensitivity reaction. Massage should be carried out carefully at first to find out if the patient is sensitive to extruded toxins. Not infrequently, a massage may cause a flare-up of a general infection such as neuritis, iritis or arthritis. This may identify the prostate as the primary focus of these infections. If this occurs, massage must be continued very gently and cautiously.

(c) Posterior urethral instillations following massage have for many years been a common practice. Instillation is done by gravity or syringe through a catheter, or by the Keyes-Ultzmann syringe directly into the posterior urethra. The most common solutions used for this are mild silver nitrate or silver protein solutions such as 2 per cent Protargol. Such instillations as well as irrigations in the male are becoming less and less popular and now are seldom advisable.

(d) Although heat to the prostate constitutes important therapy in acute prostatitis, it is to a much less extent applicable to chronic infections. The various methods used are the same as have been recommended for acute prostatitis. Shortwave diathermy has been quite popular of late. Hibbs and Osborne (1941) obtained an average increase of 2° F. in the posterior urethra by this method. Subjective symptoms were reduced and objective findings improved. (The use of hot sitz baths once or twice in twenty-four hours is still a simple and usually effective method of applying external heat to the pelvis. The patient sits in the tub with the water not higher than the iliac crests. A temperature of 108 to 110° F. with the patient in the water six to ten minutes is ample; a Turkish bath effect is to be avoided. Ed.)

(e) Intraprostatic injections through a needle inserted in the perineum or in the McCarthy panendoscope have been suggested (Grant, 1938; Ritter and Lippow, 1938). Various antiseptics such as mercurochrome, argyrol or sclerosing fluids have been used. These methods have been shown recently by O'Conor and Ladd (1936) to be of questionable advantage because they cause sclerosis and occlude the normal drainage ducts. Recently injection of penicillin has been advocated (Hatch, 1950) for coccus infections. If specific therapy is found to act locally without causing sclerosis and obstruction, it may serve a good purpose.

(f) Finally, endoscopic treatment of the posterior urethra and the verumontanum sometimes relieves distressing urethral symptoms associated with the chronic prostatitis. Application of 10 or 20 per cent silver nitrate directly to these areas, through the Young urethroscope is a simple and satisfactory procedure. Light fulguration of granulations or inflammatory polyps may be advisable.

The treatment for seminal vesiculitis is similar to that for chronic prostatitis. In addition, dilatation and the injection of the ejaculatory ducts may be advisable. This may be done through the panendoscope with the McCarthy ejaculatory duct catheterizer or through the Young urethroscope using the Young ejaculatory duct dilator. The seminal vesicles can also be injected in retrograde manner by vasotomy, as mentioned previously. Proper massage of the vesicles is probably the most effective therapy. Operative treatment is not to be recommended in nonspecific chronic vesiculitis. Some have suggested seminal vesiculectomy in certain long-standing chronic cases in which there is considerable perivesiculitis, scarring and perhaps obstruction of the lower ureters, or when there is incapacitating neuritis or arthritis associated with vesicle infection. Vasotomy with injection of the vesicles through the open vas has been done for many years. Solutions used for this were usually mild proteins such as 5 per cent collargol or 1 per cent mercurochrome. This method has some strong adherents and others believe its value is questionable (Harlin, 1950).

Prognosis. The prognosis of chronic prostatitis is much less encouraging than that of the acute. A prostate with a long-standing infection probably never will return to normal. It is difficult to say when the patient is cured. The usual criteria of cure are: (a) There shall be no symptoms referable to the infection. (b) The prostatic secretion will contain not more than 10 pus cells per high power field. (c) The first and third glasses of urine in the 3 glass test will have no comma shreds. (d) Prostatic smears, stains and cultures must be negative for bacteria. If there is a metastatic focus resulting from the prostatic infection, that also must remain clear. The most difficult requirement is the clearing of the prostatic fluid and keeping it to less than 10 pus cells per high power field, an arbitrarily chosen number. This may be impossible in many instances even when all other signs of infection have disappeared. The sexual dysfunction may not disappear; and this is most difficult to evaluate, due to the psychic role and irregular sexual habits involved. As a rule, one can say that except for this, the vast majority of these infections will in time leave the patient asymptomatic. It is reported that 50 per cent will clear up and 25 per cent markedly improve. The remainder will drag along for a year or longer, not being able to satisfy, in one way or another, the criteria for a cure.

TUBERCULOSIS OF THE PROSTATE AND SEMINAL VESICLES

Occurrence. The tubercle bacillus is usually inhaled or swallowed so that the primary focus of tuberculosis is most frequently in the lungs, intestinal tract or in glands. The tonsils possibly are a frequent initial focus. Hence, it is probably true that there has never been a primary focus of tuberculosis in the prostate, notwithstanding the reports of approximately a dozen such cases in the literature. To prove a primary focus, there would have to be a most careful and complete autopsy with microscopic sections of every organ in the body. Clinical examination is not sufficiently accurate for such proof.

Genital tuberculosis is usually a manifestation of a more deeply seated primary infection. Medlar (1949) analyzed 5424 autopsies of males over 16 years of age. He found genitourinary tract tuberculosis in 3.1 per cent, 85 per cent of these patients had pulmonary tuberculosis. In the whole group 80 per cent of those with tuberculosis were so diagnosed before death but only 18 per cent of those having genitourinary tract tuberculosis were recognized clinically. This indicates the difficulty in recognizing early tuberculosis of the genitourinary system; not until it is advanced does it present clinical manifestations sufficient for a diagnosis. Thomas (1940) studying 87 patients with genital tuberculosis, found 87 per cent had demonstrable lesions elsewhere;

78 per cent of these were in the lungs. Of 64 patients with genital tuberculosis repeatedly examined over a period of two years, 92 per cent had infection in the kidneys. Moore (1937) also found 90 per cent of his patients with genital tuberculosis had urinary tract infection. In Medlar's series the incidence of tuberculosis was twice as great in the kidneys as in the prostate and three times as great as in the seminal vesicles or epididymis. Only 11 per cent of the cases of genitourinary tuberculosis had no renal lesions and all of these patients had infection in the prostate and one half of them in the seminal vesicles. In our series, 60 per cent of the 25 patients with genital tuberculosis had clinical manifestations of urinary tract tuberculosis, 80 per cent had pulmonary tuberculosis and one had tuberculous osteomyelitis. It is the consensus, therefore, that (1) genitourinary tuberculosis is almost always secondary to tuberculosis elsewhere and (2) that genital tuberculosis is most frequently associated with urinary tract infection.

Pathogenesis. There are several routes of invasion for the tubercle bacillus to reach the genital tract: (1) Hematogenous, (2) descending from the kidney, to the urethra, to the prostatic ducts, to the prostate, seminal vesicles and epididymes and (3) direct extension from local tissues by means of the lymphatics.

(1) *Hematogenous.* In these cases, the infection in the earliest stage is usually found around the blood vessels in the periphery of the prostate. There is no tuberculosis found elsewhere in the genital tract. This is strong evidence of blood stream infection with the genital invasion being primary in the prostate.

(2) *Descending Route.* In Medlar's cases (1949), 65 per cent of renal lesions were of the miliary type and 98 per cent bilateral; of these, 13 per cent showed genital tuberculosis. Twenty-three per cent of his renal lesions were caseous and 86 per cent of them bilateral; of these, 52 per cent had genital tuberculosis. Twelve per cent of the renal lesions showed cavitation and 58 per cent of them were bilateral; of these, all had genital tuberculosis. In tuberculosis of the genital tract, Medlar found the prostate, seminal vesicles and epididymes involved together in 63 per cent. In 29 per cent, the prostate was involved alone and in no case was the seminal vesicle or epididymis alone infected. This again points strongly toward the original genital infection being in the prostate. Of his whole group of genital tuberculosis, 81 per cent had bilateral seminal vesicle involvement and 64 per cent involvement of the epididymes. In our small series of 25 infections by clinical examination there were 22 in the prostate and seminal vesicles; 18 cases with the seminal vesicles and epididymis involved; 16 cases with the prostate, seminal vesicles and epididymis infected. There were only 2 patients with infection in the seminal vesicles and not in the prostate and only 1 with infection in the prostate and not in the seminal vesicles. Most case reports are dependent upon clinical signs and examinations but minor lesions not detectable by clinical means most likely are present in the other genital organs. When complete pathologic examination is made, all three organs are usually found to be involved.

There has never been unanimity among urologists as to where, in the genital tract, the original infection begins. There are now four schools of thought: that it begins in (1) the epididymis, (2) the seminal vesicles, (3) the seminal vesicles and epididymis at the same time, (4) the prostate. Thirty years ago this was a source of heated discussions, with Young, claiming the seminal vesicle and Barney, the epididymis as the primary genital focus. There are good arguments in favor of each view. Barney believes that the infection beginning in the epididymis is most likely blood-borne and spreads from the epididymis to the prostate and seminal vesicles by way of the lymphatics or the vas deferens. Tuberculosis of one epididymis is often followed by involvement of the other. This may be either hematogenous in origin or by way of the seminal vesicles and prostate. Infections in the globus minor are probably by way of the seminal vesicles and vas and those of the globus major are probably blood-borne. Autopsy material may show genital tuberculosis in only the epididymis in some cases and only in the prostate or the seminal vesicles in others. This is rare; most often there is a combination of lesions and at this stage it is impossible to select the original site, perhaps it occurred in all three at the same time (Moore, 1937). Certainly clinical diagnosis of epididymal tuberculosis alone is more frequent than tuberculosis of the prostate and seminal vesicles alone. But this is probably due to the easier physical examination of the former. Furthermore, following epididymectomy, the lesions in the prostate and seminal vesicles, as a rule, markedly regress. Hence one concludes that the epididymis is the primary focus. However, this does not necessarily follow.

The school supported by Young (1922) and others insists just as strongly that the original lesion in the genital tract is in the seminal vesicle. From there the infection proceeds to the globus minor of the epididymis, or to the prostate, urethra and bladder or rarely up to the kidney through the ureteral lymphatics. Young asserts that in every case of epididymal tuberculosis a seminal vesicle is involved and if one's sense of touch is sufficiently acute, the induration may be felt. However this may not always be so and one would need pathologic sections to prove the statement.

(3) The third school holds that the infection begins in the seminal vesicles and the epididymis at the same time. This is quite possible.

(4) The fourth school maintains that it originates in the prostate. At the present time this is probably in most favor. The most recent studies of Medlar, Moore, Thomas and others tend to show that the prostate is the primary genital focus in genital tuberculosis.

During the last thirty years some headway has been made in clarifying the pathogenesis of genital tuberculosis: (1) Tuberculous epididymitis is a disease which can easily be observed clinically while vesiculitis and prostatitis are recognized with some difficulty and are therefore more easily overlooked. (2) Tuberculous epididymitis without evidence of seminal vesiculitis or prostatitis is rare but vesiculitis and prostatitis without clinical involvement of the epididymis may not be uncommon. (3) Tissue studies bear out the clinical findings that the original focus in the genital tract is most frequently in the prostate. (4) By the time the infection is recognized clinically, it generally involves the epididymis, the prostate and the seminal vesicles. This is true in the vast majority of cases subjected to careful pathologic microscopic examination.

Pathology. By clinical examination, tuberculous genital infection may be limited to one side; thus the right seminal vesicle, the right lobe of the prostate and the right epididymis may be involved. However, crossed infections are not rare; the right seminal vesicle and the right side of the prostate and left epididymis may be affected. But on histosection, there is usually widespread infection throughout all three of these organs.

The pathologic changes in the prostate and seminal vesicles in tuberculosis are exactly similar to those in other organs of the body of similar glandular structure. There is formation of tubercles usually beginning near the blood vessels and just beneath the mucosa in the prostate or seminal vesicle, or in the region of the ejaculatory ducts. This process spreads throughout the lateral lobe of the prostate or the vesicle. The tubercle is followed by abscess, caseation and finally cavitation and fibrosis. The caseous abscess may limit itself to one lobe of the prostate or may spread throughout the gland and involve the seminal vesicles in a similar process.

The microscopic picture is one of individual small or conglomerate tubercles with giant cells and extensive necrosis, depending on the stage of disease (Fig. 321, p. 645). According to Walker (1911) the epithelial lining disappears, leaving connective tissue and strands of fibrous tissue. The prostate is converted into cheesy masses interspersed among which are connective and muscle tissues. This later breaks down to form tuberculous granulomatous tissue. Because of the character of the seminal vesicles which are almost blind sacs with complicated cavities and drainage poorly effected through the small ejaculatory ducts, tuberculosis is usually a true chronic granulomatous lesion. Conglomerate tubercles are present with extensive caseation. Obstruction may become so complete as to leave practically no trace of the normal vesicle tissue. There finally results a firm, hard, necrotic, fibrous mass. Scarring in the seminal vesicles may proceed to such a degree as to cause a stricture of the ureter, its close neighbor on the posterior surface of the bladder. Abscess in the prostate or seminal vesicles may rupture into the periprostatic spaces, the bladder, the urethra or the rectum. If it spreads through the periprostatic spaces and into the perineum, persistent perineal fistulae are not uncommon (see Section XIII).

Signs and Symptoms. Tuberculosis of the prostate and seminal vesicles in its early stages is usually asymptomatic. There may be present mild symptoms of chronic prostatitis with perineal discomfort, rectal pain, aching or bearing down feeling in the perineum, and pain in the hips and down the legs. These may be of long duration and increasing in severity.

Attention may first be drawn to the epididymes; it is usually only a mild aching and not the severe pain of acute inflammation like that of gonorrheal and nonspecific epididymitis. There is an indurated, enlarged, hard epididymis with only slight tenderness if any. It is usually irregular and nodular over the surface. There may also be nodules in the vas deferens which is referred to as a "beaded vas" (Fig. 322).

As the disease progresses, symptoms of pain on ejaculation or hematospermia may appear. There may be associated low grade fever. Urinary
symptoms may soon occur due to the involvement of the posterior urethra.
There are urethral and bladder neck irritative symptoms of frequency,
urgency, burning and dysuria. Urinary obstruction symptoms may progress
as the prostate and seminal vesicles enlarge or as the posterior urethra is
strictured by the chronic inflammation.

Diagnosis. When the disease is limited in its early stage to the prostate
and seminal vesicles the diagnosis of genital tuberculosis may be difficult

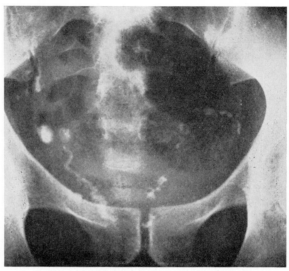

Fig. 322.   Tuberculous calcification of vasa and seminal vesicle. (Courtesy of Dr. T. Leon
Howard.)

and largely presumptive. One must consider the history of general malaise,
loss of weight, low-grade fever, discomfort in the perineum or bladder or
rectum, or sexual symptoms referable to a prostatitis. The history suggestive
of chronic tuberculosis of the lungs or urinary tract is important. One should
always look for (1) concomitant prostatitis, epididymitis, and the signs of
urinary tract tuberculosis as well as (2) the physical signs of tuberculosis
of the lungs or elsewhere. (3) Careful rectal examination of the prostate and
seminal vesicles is imperative. (4) Perineal and scrotal examination for
chronic fistulae often furnish a clue. (5) Study of the urine by routine
examination and by special stains and cultures for tubercle bacilli is essential.
(6) The prostatic and seminal fluids may show acid fast organisms. (7)
Urograms to show soft calcifications and changes in the pyelogram are
a must as are (8) x-rays of the genital tract for calcifications, in prostate for
example. Urethrograms made after urographic injection of the seminal
vesicles may disclose characteristic changes (Fig. 323), as may (9) urethroscopic examination of the posterior urethra and vesical neck. According to

Lattimer (1948) there is a rather characteristic diagnostic picture of the prostatic urethra in tuberculosis (Fig. 324).

In the acute stages the prostatic urethra is beefy red with occasional superficial ulceration. In chronic tuberculous infection, the floor of the urethra is drawn into thick longitudinal folds. There is scarring and contracture near the prostatic ducts which gives a golf-hole appearance similar to that seen in tuberculosis of the ureter. There are three principal characteristics: (a) The dilatation of the prostatic urethra just proximal to the

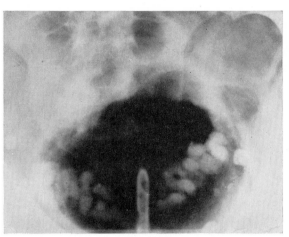

Fig. 323.   Vesiculogram. Seminal vesicles injected through vasotomies plus an air cystogram.

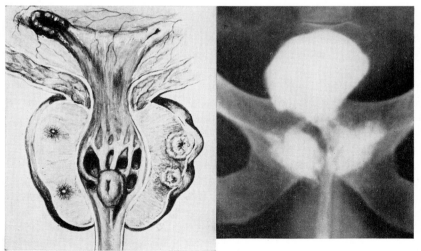

Fig. 324   Fig. 325

Fig. 324.   Dilatation of prostatic ducts and tuberculous abscesses of prostate. (Courtesy of Dr. J. K. Lattimer.)

Fig. 325.   Cysto-urethrogram shows prostatic urea sloughed out from tuberculous abscesses. (Courtesy of Dr. J. K. Lattimer.)

verumontanum. (b) A golf-hole dilatation of the prostatic ducts on the urethral floor. (c) Trabeculation of the prostatic urethra with longitudinal ridges intertwining among the dilated prostatic ducts (Fig. 324). In the differential diagnosis, carcinoma must be considered. Rectal examination may not be diagnostic, but in carcinoma the stony hard, irregular, nodular character of the mass spreading outside the prostatic capsule and into the seminal vesicles is helpful. Roentgenography to show metastasis, blood acid-phosphatase estimations and bone marrow examination may be necessary in making this differential diagnosis. Rarely biopsy through the resectoscope may be required for an accurate differentiation. Granulomatous or fungus disease and syphilis must also be considered in the differential diagnosis of tuberculosis of the prostate.

Treatment. In the treatment of genital tuberculosis the primary focus within or outside of the genitourinary tract must be taken care of as well as the local infection. (1) Conservative or medical treatment includes the administration of complete rest, nutritious food, vitamins, heliotherapy, and chemotherapy: (a) streptomycin, (b) para-amino salicylic acid and (c) isoniazid.

With the advent of chemotherapy and antibiotics, a vast amount of experimental work has been reported on the sensitivity of the tubercle bacillus to many drugs. In animals and man the sulfones, Promine, Diazone, Promizole, and thiosemicarbazones, viomycin, streptomycin, neomycin and Isoniazid show definite evidence of bactericidal action on the bacillus. Evidence is also at hand to show that organisms may become resistant to streptomycin or other antibiotics during prolonged therapy. Of the many drugs tested against the tubercle bacillus in clinical trial, streptomycin and para-amino salicylic acid (PAS) and Isoniazid have proven to be the most effective. The addition of PAS to streptomycin therapy is to prevent emergence of a resistant strain of the bacillus. Tomorrow, another drug to which the organism is much more sensitive may be synthesized; one which will destroy the tubercle bacillus as effectively as penicillin does the coccus. It has been shown by Pulasky (1947) and Lattimer (1948b) that bactericidal concentration of streptomycin cannot be produced in the prostate by either oral or parenteral administration, and that tuberculous nodules still persist in the gland after streptomycin therapy. Notwithstanding this fact, it is still the accepted treatment for genital tuberculosis.

Recently "The Conference on the Chemotherapy of Tuberculosis" reached the following conclusions. At the present time streptomycin, dihydrostreptomycin, para-aminosalicylic acid and Isoniazid are the drugs of choice in treating tuberculosis. Evidence points to the advantage of using them in pairs rather than singly. PAS is used with Streptomycin to enhance its usefulness and circumvent the disadvantages of its toxicity and resistance development of the organism. Combinations of PAS and streptomycin, streptomycin and Isoniazid or Isoniazid plus PAS are all probably of equal therapeutic value. For pulmonary tuberculosis at present the combination of streptomycin and PAS is preferred since it has withstood the test of time well, and the other combinations are so far untested. Other tuberculocidal synthetic chemical compounds are Terramycin, Viomycin and Aldinamide. The conference accepted the combination of streptomycin and Isoniazid as the regime of choice in genitourinary tract tuberculosis. Streptomycin is preferred to dihydrostreptomycin because the latter causes a high percentage of deafness in patients after it has been given constantly for four or five months. In therapies of short duration dihydrostreptomycin is preferred. Suggested dosage of streptomycin is 1 gm. a day for a two week period and then only twice a week. Daily dosage of 12 gm. of PAS is recommended. This combination is given for a period of twelve months with no rest period at any time. Experimentation now is being carried out using one half the dosage of streptomycin and one half of dihydrostreptomycin making an aggregate total of 1 gm. a day. This may prove to be less toxic than either one alone. Dosage of Isoniazid is recommended at 0.3 gm. a day continually with no interruption and given with either streptomycin or PAS. Treatment may be suspended if after a twelve months period the criteria for cure are evident, i.e., negative T.B. cultures of the urine and prostatic secretion, a normal prostatic secretion and urine microscopically and no positive physical signs of genitourinary tract tuberculosis.

Sensitivity tests should be carried out from time to time. Even these may not be of definite significance. One of our patients, whose organism after several years of intermittent treatment became resistant to streptomycin, still is improving subjectively and objectively while she is taking the drug. It is uncertain however if a cure of genital tuberculosis can ever be obtained.

Surgery. This consists of either an epididymectomy or the Young radical operation for tuberculosis of the seminal tract.

(a) An epididymectomy plus the injection of the seminal vesicles through the vas may be done; or an epididymectomy on one side and a prophylactic vasectomy on the other side. The vas may be ligated and carbolized and then dropped back into the wound; or the proximal end may be brought up to the skin and exposed for drainage and subsequent frequent injections. Some recommend always performing a bilateral epididymectomy and there is favorable evidence for this reasoning. A simple epididymectomy usually causes regression of the infection in the prostate and seminal vesicles. This is so constant that it has led the majority of urologists to recommend this operation alone for tuberculosis of the seminal tract.

(b) Radical operation for tuberculosis of the genital tract advocated by Young (1922) has caused a serious debate in urologic circles. This operation includes the removal of most of the seminal tract: the seminal vesicles and the lateral lobes of the prostate, the vasa and the epididymes. The prostatic urethra is left intact and not opened. The seminal vesicles, the parts of the prostate and the vasa, as far as one can reach, are removed perineally. The epididymes and the distal segments of the visa are removed from above through incisions in the groin. For the exact technique of this operation, refer to Young's article. Lewis has recently reported follow-up results of 41 patients who underwent this radical operation. Seven of them are living and well 10 years or more after operation; 27 in all are living and well.

The danger in this operation was the persistent perineal urinary fistulae which not uncommonly occurred whenever the urethra was opened by mistake. It is quite possible that this most troublesome complication now may not be so feared since the fistulae probably would heal on streptomycin and PAS therapy. If this is so, this operation may gain in favor. However, one must remember that these patients have tuberculosis elsewhere which may at any time flare up and progress. Barney (1924) and Braasch claim that Young still has not proven that his late results are any better after the radical operation than those after a simple epididymectomy. Recently, Medlar (1949) showed that 90 per cent of his cases of genital tuberculosis had urinary tract tuberculosis and that only half of the patients with advanced renal tuberculosis presented urinary symptoms so that the status of the renal infection is often not reflected in the genitourinary symptoms. If the intention of the Young radical operation is to prevent the further spread of the tuberculosis, is it not already too late? This is a serious and specialized operation and until it is shown that the late results are much better than simple epididymectomy, the latter plus chemotherapy will probably remain the therapy of choice in the vast majority of cases.

Prognosis. The prognosis of tuberculosis of the genital tract in itself is fair but as stated previously, there is always concomitant disease present; hence the ultimate mortality rate on a differential basis is difficult to estimate. It is said by some that genital tuberculosis in itself is relatively benign and well confined to the genital tract. In a report from the Mayo Clinic of 1200 operations for renal tuberculosis, the late mortality rate of the males in whom the majority also had genital tuberculosis, was no higher than that of the females who did not have genital involvement. Hence, it seems that the genital involvement did not enhance the seriousness of the infection. But the high percentage of urinary tract tuberculosis in patients with genital infection makes this a very serious disease (Ormond and Meyers, 1939).

The immediate prognosis following epididymectomy is usually good; the seminal vesicle and prostatic infection regresses and the glands become smaller and fibrosed. However, one would hesitate to venture the opinion of a cure of genital tuberculosis even with the newer therapies because of the (a) far-advanced infection usually present before diagnosis is made, (b) the concomitant infection elsewhere in the body and (c) the frequency of urinary tract tuberculosis associated with it. Hence, as to the ultimate cure of the genital disease, the prognosis is unfavorable. It is probable that with ever-advancing chemotherapy immediate favorable response will be even better than at present and the late results as to longevity or morbidity much improved.

UNUSUAL INFECTIONS OF THE PROSTATE

These include actinomycosis, blastomycosis, granulomatous disease, coccidioidomycosis, moniliasis, and syphilis. The parasitic infections due to the Tinea echinococcus, Schistosoma (bilharziosis), Trichomonas vaginalis, filaria, Endamoeba histolytica, Eustrongylus gigas and Strongyloides stercoralis are discussed in Section V, Chapter 3.

ACTINOMYCOSIS

Several cases of actinomycosis of both the upper and lower urinary tract are reported. Very few are recorded in the genital organs and most of these are in the testes. Few have been seen in the prostate and seminal vesicles. Hinman (1935) describes a case on which he did a radical seminal vesiculectomy, believing it was tuberculosis.

This disease is a generalized systemic fungus infection, resembling very much tuberculosis. There are two types: (a) Anaerobic, usually producing the so-called "sulfur granules"; 90 per cent of clinical cases are of this type. (b) Aerobic, acid-fast actinomyces, now called Nocardia asteroides, also forming sulfur granules; 10 per cent of clinical cases are of this type. The old name for the latter type was Streptothrix (Benbow et al., 1944).

The pathologic changes characteristic of the disease are chronic infection with suppuration and sinus formation with fibrosis and scarring. The diagnosis is made upon finding microscopically the "sulfur granules" or the mycelium threads. These threads are lobulated bodies of delicate branching filaments, the ends of which appear club shaped due to the gelatinous sheath.

Actinomycotic disease of the prostate presents itself clinically as a chronic infection, markedly resembling tuberculosis. It is distinguished from tuberculosis by the appearance of the mycelia which is usually composed of long-branching threads instead of individual bacilli.

Treatment. This is the only fungus susceptible to chemotherapy. Sensitivity tests should be made with the various sulfonamide drugs and antibiotics and the drug chosen according to these tests. Good results are recorded from the use of both sulfonamides and antibiotics (Benbow et al., 1944; Strauss et al., 1951). General medical care is advisable with rest, nutritious food, supplementary vitamins, etc. Adequate surgical drainage as indicated is essential. Potassium iodide is given together with the specific chemotherapy. The dose of potassium iodide advised for the treatment of actinomycosis is as follows: Five drops of a saturated solution is given three times a day after meals. This dose is increased one drop per dose a day; the second day the patient gets six drops three times a day, and on the third day seven drops three times a day, and so forth. The gradual increase in dose is continued until the maximum of twenty drops three times a day is reached. When this dosage is reached it is again dropped to 5 drops three times a day and worked back again to 20 drops, etc. Penicillin, 1 million units a day, plus 4 to 5 gm. of one of the sulfonamides each day is suggested by Dr. D. I. Smith (personal communication). For the Nocardia infection penicillin is ineffective and large doses of sulfonamides are recommended.

BLASTOMYCOSIS

This is a chronic infection caused by the yeast-like fungi Blastomyces and characterized by the formation of suppurative and granulomatous lesions in any part of the body but most often seen in the skin, lungs and bones. Infection is usually by direct inoculation of the blastomyces. There have been 14 cases of prostatic infection reported (Moore and Halpern, 1948) and all were part of a systemic infection. It is commonly seen at autopsy in the prostates of patients with generalized blastomycosis infection.

The *pathologic* changes of blastomycosis show chronic inflammation with abscess formation, necrosis and fibrosis. There are many small abscesses throughout the prostate with necrosis and fibrosis interspersed. The symptoms are of chronic inflammation and prostatism. These patients are sometimes operated upon for prostatism or prostatic abscess. Diagnosis is made preoperatively by finding the organism in the prostatic fluid or in the urine and by special cultures. The media used are blood agar or beef infusion, glucose agar or Sabouraud's glucose agar slant. The organism may be seen by fresh smear or by mixing the fluid with a drop of 10 per cent potassium hydroxide, a cover glass is added and the slide is gently heated. Round "double-contoured" budding yeast-like cells, 8 to 15 μ in diameter, are then visible.

Treatment consists of potassium iodide to combat the general infection, the dose and method of administration as given under treatment of actinomycosis. If abscess develops and requires surgical drainage, first desensitize the patient and force iodide therapy with the hope that this may prevent spread of the infection when the lesion is opened. Do not incise a lesion unless absolutely necessary because of its grave likelihood and rapidity of spreading. Recently the best results have been reported with the use of intravenous Stilbamidine diluted in saline or glucose. It should be used only by those familiar with its complications which may be serious.

GRANULOMATOUS DISEASE

Granulomatous disease of the prostate closely resembling tuberculosis and tertiary syphilis has been found on pathologic section. The histologic picture is a chronic inflammatory and foreign body reaction. Tanner and McDonald (1943) suggest that this picture is caused by: (1) partial obstruction of the larger prostatic ducts; (2) subsequent secretion in the acini and smaller ducts causing nonspecific inflammatory reaction; (3) destruction of the epithelial lining of the acini and the ducts with escape of fluids into the interstitial tissue; (4) production of chronic inflammation and foreign body reaction; (5) formation of granulomatous circumscribed nodules and, finally, (6) resolution with replacement of fibrous tissue. Some sections resemble caseous tuberculosis without giant cells, but with large numbers of eosinophils scattered through the granuloma. Melicow (1951) suggests that this disease may belong to the allergic granuloma class and be part of a constitutional disease. In old men this chronic inflammation produces obstruction and stasis resembling prostatism. It is difficult clinically to distinguish from prostatism, chronic prostatic infection or tuberculosis. Hence most of these prostates have been removed because of the obstruction. Diagnosis is made only on the microscopic sections of the removed gland (Nesbit, 1949).

COCCIDIOIDOMYCOSIS

This disease, caused by the fungus Coccidioides immitis and primarily invading the lungs, is the most infectious systemic mycosis in man. It was first seen in South America, particularly in Argentina, and from there migrated to California where it became known as valley fever and San Joaquin valley fever. A few cases are now reported throughout the United States. There are two clinical types: (1) primary coccidioidomycosis, a benign self-limited acute respiratory disease which symptomatically resembles pulmonary tuberculosis, (2) progressive coccidioidomycosis, a chronic virulent disseminating disease, involving the skin, subcutaneous, visceral, and osseous tissue.

Genitourinary tract disease due to coccidioidal infection is very rare. There are probably only two cases of epididymal and one of prostatic infection reported in the literature, McDougall and Kleiman (1943). Grossly, the infection in the prostate is a granulomatous process, difficult to differentiate from chronic infections and tuberculosis. Microscopic picture is of tubercle-like formation with abscess and necrosis. In the case reported, a prostatic abscess was aspirated through the perineum. This fluid revealed a double lipoid refractile capsule of the fungus Coccidioides immitis. Careful microscopic identification of the non-budding thick-walled sporule must be made for diagnosis. Entirely unsuccessful treatment in the past has consisted of gentian violet, arsphenamine, copper, antimony and iodides. The present recommended therapy is general medical care and chemotherapy, including the various antibiotics but none are very satisfactory.

MONILIASIS

The fungus of moniliasis, Candida albicans, has been isolated frequently from the stools, vagina, skin and throat in apparently healthy individuals. It is a small oval, budding, thin-walled yeast-like cell which is easily cultured on Sabouraud's glucose agar (Conant and Smith, 1953). It is not so very uncommon to find yeast cells in the urine and probably some strains of monilia are nonpathogenic. These infections of the prostate, however, can be of clinical significance as evidenced by a recent case on our service. This patient had a chronic prostatism which resisted the usual therapy because of definite obstruction and a resistant infection. Following transurethral resection of the vesical neck and prostatic urethra, he improved symptomatically but the infection persisted in spite of chemotherapy and antibiotics. Theoretically antibiotics should be contraindicated since monilia is a yeast cell itself. Such was the case in this patient; there was no response to penicillin, streptomycin, Chloromycetin, Aureomycin and Terramycin. To date none of these infections have been influenced by any antibiotics. The most beneficial treatment in our patient was marked alkalinization of his urine. The accepted treatment is gentian violet locally, and in very severe cases, intravenously. The dosage is 5 mg. per kilogram of body weight daily or every other day for seven to ten days. Vein thrombosis frequently occurs. Desensitization with a specific vaccine may be advisable in a hypersensitive patient. Potassium iodide is also accepted therapy.

SYPHILIS

The tertiary lesion or gumma is the usual syphilitic lesion of the prostate and is rare. Symptoms are those of prostatic enlargement and prostatism.

It is most difficult to differentiate prostatic gumma from benign or malignant growth of the gland. Diagnosis is made on the history, physical findings and Wassermann reaction (Crowley and Thomas, 1947) or biopsy. Treatment consists in administration of antibiotics, notably penicillin, in large doses.

REFERENCES

BARNEY, J. D.: Cabot's Modern Urology. *1:*532, 1924.

BENBOW, E. P., JR., SMITH, D. T. and GRIMSON, K. S.: Sulfonamide therapy in actinomycosis. Am. Rev. Tuberc., *49:*395, 1944.

CONANT, N. F. and SMITH, D. T.: Manual of Clinical Mycology. 2nd ed. W. B. Saunders Co., Philadelphia, 1953.

COOPER, H. G. and MacLEAN, J. T.: Chronic prostatitis associated with nonspecific urethritis. Canad. M. A. J., *54:*136, 1946.

CROWLEY, E. and THOMAS, G.: Syphilis of the prostate: report of case and review of literature. J. Urol., *58:*367, 1947.

CUMMINGS, R. E. and CHITTENDEN, G. E.: Pyogenic prostatitis. J. Urol., *39:*118, 1938.

DAVIES, J. A.: Echinococcal cyst arising from the prostate. Canad. M. A. J., *54:*268, 1946.

DRUMMOND, A. C.: Staphylococcus prostatitis treated with staphylococcus toxoid. Am. J. Surg., *51:*393, 1941.

FREUND, H.: Prostatitis—a cause of acute or recurrent abdominal pain. Ann. Int. Med., *17:*41, 1942.

GARDNER, L. W.: Bacteriology of chronic prostatoseminal vesiculitis. Urol. & Cutan. Rev., *44:*278, 1940.

GONZALES, F.-IMAN: Retrograde seminal vesiculography. J. Urol., *49:*618, 1943.

GRANT, OWSLEY: Treatment of recalcitrant prostatitis by drug injection. J. Urol., *39:*150, 1938.

HARLIN, H. C.: Seminal vesiculitis. J.A.M.A., *143:*880, 1950.

HATCH, W. E.: Intraprostatic injection of penicillin. J. Urol., *64:*763, 1950.

HENLINE, R. B.: Prostatitis and seminal vesiculitis, acute and chronic. J.A.M.A., *123:*608, 1943.

HERRING, J. B.: Therapeutic hyperpyrexia of the pelvic organs. Urol. & Cutan. Rev., *39:*449, 1935.

HIBBS, D. K. and OSBORNE, S. L.: Short wave diathermy in chronic prostatitis. Am. J. M. Sc., *201:*547, 1941.

HINMAN, F.: Principles and Practice of Urology. W. B. Saunders Co., Philadelphia, 1935.

HUFFINES, T. R. and WEBER, W. D.: Results obtained in treating genito-urinary tuberculosis with streptomycin. J. Urol., *62:*6, 862, 1949.

KRETSCHMER, H. L., BARKEY, HECKEL and OCKERLY: Chronic prostatitis, review of 1000 cases. Ill. M. J., *71:*152, 1937.

LATTIMER, J. K.: Tuberculous prostatic urethritis: a suggestive diagnostic sign. J. Urol., *59:*326, 1948.

LATTIMER, J. K. et al.: The streptomycin treatment of genito-urinary tuberculosis: A preliminary report. J. Urol., *60:*974, 1948.

McDOUGALL, T. G. and KLEIMAN, A. H.: Prostatitis due to Coccidioides immitis. J. Urol., *49:*472, 1943.

MEDLAR, E. M. et al.: Post-mortem compared with clinical diagnosis of genito-urinary tuberculosis in adult males. J. Urol., *61:*1078, 1949.

MELICOW, W. M.: Allergic granuloma of prostate. J. Urol., *65:*288, 1951.

MOORE, M. and HALPERN, L. K.: Blastomycosis involving the prostate. J. Urol., *60:*612, 1948.

MOORE, R.: Tuberculosis of the prostate gland. J. Urol., *37:*372, 1937.

NESBIT, R.: Subtotal extirpation of the granulomatous prostate. J. Urol., *61:*766, 1949.

O'CONOR, V. and LADD, R.: Intraprostatic injections. J.A.M.A., *107:*1185, 1936.

ORMOND, J. K. and MEYERS, K. L.: Tuberculous epididymitis. J. Urol., *42:*829, 1939.

PELOUZE, P. S.: Gonorrhea in Male and Female. W. B. Saunders Co., Philadelphia, 1939.

PULASKI, E. J.: Streptomycin therapy of penicillin-resistant and sulfonamide-resistant, specific and non-specific urethritis. J. Ven. Dis. Information, *28:*1, 1947.

RITTER, J. S. and LIPPOW, C.: Pathological and bacteriological processes present in prostatitis and tissue reaction to therapy. J. Urol., *39:*111, 1938.

ROTH, R. B.: Trichomonas urethritis and prostatitis. Ven. Dis. Information. U. S. Public Health, *25:*163, 1944.

SEABAUGH, D. R.: Seminal vesiculitis (congestive) simulating acute abdominal disease. J. Urol., *55:*173, 1946.

SINGER, P. L.: Seminal vesiculitis in the young. Urol. & Cutan. Rev., *50:*328, 1946.

STRAUSS, R. E., KLIGMAN, A. M. and PILLSBURY, D. M.: The chemotherapy of actinomycosis and nocardosis. Am. Rev. Tuberc., *63:*441, 1951.

TANNER, F. H. and McDONALD, J. R.: Granulomatous prostatitis. Arch. Path., *36:*358, 1943.

THOMAS, G.: Genital tuberculosis. Minn. Med., *23:*318, 1940.

WALKER, GEORGE: Studies in the experimental production of tuberculosis in the genitourinary organs. Johns Hopkins Hospital Reports, *16:*1, 1911.

WESSON, MILEY: Symptoms of non-venereal acute and chronic prostatitis. J. Urol., *39:*135, 1938.

YOUNG, H. H.: A radical cure of tuberculosis of the seminal tract. Arch. Surg., *4:*334, 1922.

YOUNG, H. H.: Practice of Urology. W. B. Saunders Co., 1926.

CHAPTER 3

Infections and Diseases of the Scrotum and Its Contents

SAMUEL A. VEST, M.D.

INFECTIONS OF THE SCROTUM

The scrotum is subject to infections by all pyogenic and specific organisms as well as to many rare diseases indigenous to tropical areas. Many of the latter are too unusual to merit recording. In general, infections of the scrotum are not dissimilar to infections of skin and subcutaneous tissues elsewhere in the body, but some differences are manifest because of the nature of the scrotal wall. The scrotal skin is in the form of transverse rugae which tend to render the skin folds inaccessible to air, especially when the dartos is contracted, and this may interfere with resistance to bacteria. The scrotum is situated in a well-protected area, unfavorable for proper ventilation, and, with numerous sweat glands, it is prone to become moist. Bacteria from the rectum and urethra are prevalent on the surface, but there is evidently a local tissue resistance to the organisms so commonly found in this area. Contact with adjacent mesial surfaces of the thighs is often a deterrent to healing processes. The especially loose, fat-free, and contractile scrotal wall reacts to infection with considerable edema. The resulting tenseness leads to excoriation and interference with vascularity, both of which may lower the resistance to infections. In spite of the above, the scrotum heals readily following most infections and after surgery.

Abscess of the scrotal wall as a primary infection is exceedingly rare. Abscess formation usually occurs secondary to an underlying infection such as periurethral phlegmon. For example, in a recent case, an elderly patient could not void until after the passage of sounds to dilate a mild urethral stricture. Following this, the patient voided freely but returned fourteen days later with the scrotum enlarged, red, shiny, and fluctuating at two points. There was obviously pus immediately beneath the skin. Incision and drainage of a large abscess led to urinary fistulae, which frequently develop from such underlying periurethral phlegmon. Cultures of the pus revealed both coccal and coliform organisms. The administration of modern antibiotics, which in this case included penicillin and streptomycin, effected an immediate cessation of the inflammatory process, but the involved scrotal skin area was too devitalized to survive, resulting in loss of scrotal wall. It is remarkable that with the loss of tissue down to the margins of the scrotum, the scrotal wall will regenerate. The partially exposed testes and epididymides were soon covered with regenerating scrotum. With extensive abscess or poor healing hernia testis may occur (Fig. 326).

Abscess not infrequently develops after vasectomy from infection at the proximal end of the divided vas. Tuberculosis and rare specific infections may also cause scrotal wall suppuration. Infecting organisms can metastasize to the scrotum from a distant focus, as in a recent reported case due to Bacillus diphtheriae. Scrotal abscess is more often a result of extension from suppuration in the testis or epididymis, rectum or inguinal regions. Infec-

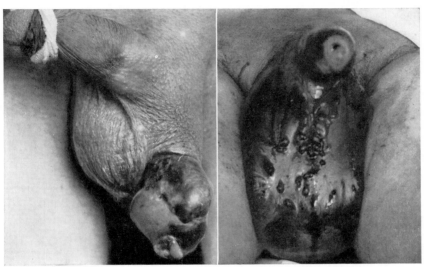

Fig. 326.   Fig. 327.
Fig. 326.   Hernia testis secondary to scrotal abscess in a young adult.
Fig. 327.   Streptococcus scrotal gangrene.

tions of the scrotal wall should be treated with those antibiotics which have a wide spectrum of activity against pyogenic and especially coccal infections. Therapy must also be directed to the underlying disease process which has extended into the scrotal wall.

Infected fistulae before the era of antibiotics were not an uncommon occurrence in the practice of urology. Most cases have multiple sinuses which are the end result of periurethral abscesses developing around the bulbous urethra. They often occur spontaneously in association with a urethral stricture, following trauma, or after the passage of sounds for dilations. Urinary fistulae often heal but usually reopen with episodes of abscess formation. In such fistulae there is considerable granulation and infected scar tissue from the external fistulous opening to the urethra. Treatment is not only excision of the tract but excision of the fistulous opening in the urethra. Single fistula can often be cured with wide exposure of the tract and removal of scar tissue down to the urethra followed by curettage of the urethral opening. In multiple fistulae with more extensive involvement of the urethra, a wide excision of the urethral wall and periurethral inflammatory tissue may be necessary. This often leads to an extensive urethral defect, so that various reconstructive operations are required. It may be necessary to close the urethral defect with whole or split thickness skin grafts. If the urethra is not adequately repaired and considerable scar tissue forms during healing, stricture and periurethral inflammation are liable to recur with reformation of abscesses and the reappearance of fistulae.

Scrotal fistulae were at one time common following tuberculosis of the epididymis in which caseous areas gradually extended to the surface, but tuberculous fistulae are now relatively uncommon (see Epididymitis). Untreated tertiary syphilis with gumma of the testis not uncommonly erodes through the scrotal walls in a manner similar to that in caseous tuberculosis. A case of actinomycosis of the scrotal wall was recently reported by Anderson. This patient had chronic recurring anal fistulae for a number of years. He was seen after a long interval of time during which fistulae had appeared on the side of the scrotum. The wall was thickened, indurated, painless, and with typical chronically infected, draining sinuses. Microscopic section from the margins of fistulae revealed colonies of Actinomyces. Fistulae have also been described following a number of tropical parasitic diseases (see Section V, Chapter 3).

Scrotal erysipelas is a diffuse infection of the scrotal skin and subcutaneous tissue occurring as a result of surgical incisions, wounds, scrotal abscesses, and fistulae. It is seen especially in debilitated and senile individuals. This type of cellulitis may also result from retrograde lymphatic infection into the scrotum from acute inguinal adenitis due to malignancy, chancroid infection, and other conditions. Erysipelas in the lower abdomen or adjacent skin areas may progress into the scrotum. This infection of the scrotum may be so intense as to become gangrenous (see Gangrene). It usually develops from a single area with a definite margin and gradually involves the entire scrotum. The soft, loose tissues of the scrotum become markedly swollen, tense, smooth and warm. Blebs may form on the surface. The infecting organism is usually a streptococcus, and a number of antibiotics such as penicillin, Aureomycin, and Terramycin are effective. The scrotum should always be elevated to enhance the circulation and reduce the complicating edema. Local applications of heat and especially wet solutions, as described in most textbooks, are not helpful or indicated.

Gangrene of the scrotum occurs following a wide variety of inciting conditions (Fig. 327). Gangrenous necrosis of the scrotal skin and wall is relatively common after urinary extravasations. It may also occur in the presence of other underlying urinary tract diseases such as paraphimosis, penile erosions, inguinal adenitis, prostato-seminal vesiculitis, and epididymitis. The connection between the underlying disease and the relatively sudden and generalized gangrenous process is not always obvious. It is known to occur after mechanical, chemical, or thermal injuries to the scrotum. Atrophic disturbances, diabetes, alcoholism, and general debility have led to extensive scrotal gangrene. Embolism of the internal hypogastric arteries from an aneurysm of the aorta has resulted in scrotal gangrene. A recent case has been reported by Meleney due to Endamoeba histolytica. A peculiar form of scrotal gangrene has been observed in the last two decades in association with the rickettsial disease, Rocky Mountain spotted fever, which has become prevalent in this country. Gangrene in these cases is due to proliferation of endothelial cells in the walls of the blood vessels, with necrosis of the smooth musculature. This leads to thrombosis, and in severe cases dependent parts of the body such as the scrotum become gangrenous. Secondary infection may accelerate the gangrenous process.

Before the era of antibiotics, scrotal gangrene was not a rarity. Randall (1920) observed 147 cases at the Philadelphia General Hospital in a period of 16 years. In many of these cases the gangrene also involved the penis. In these modern times, most patients seek medical attention soon after urinary extravasation or the beginning of a periurethral phlegmon, at which time administered antibiotics are usually successful in aborting the development of such extensive gangrenous processes.

A remarkable form of "spontaneous gangrene" involving the scrotum occurs in which there is no evidence of preexisting disease either in the genitourinary tract or elsewhere (Fig. 327). This relatively sudden scrotal gangrene was first clinically described in 1885 by Fournier, and since that time it has been given such terms as "Fournier's gangrene," "streptococcus gangrene," "scrotal gangrene," "spontaneous fulminating gangrene," "essential gangrene," or "idiopathic gangrene." It occurs usually in middle or later life, but 26 cases have been described in children (see Section XIII). In 1945 Mair, in analyzing 240 cases of reported gangrene in the scrotum to that date, found that 125 were of the "spontaneous" type. The onset is dramatically sudden, having been described as "explosive," even occurring in the middle of the night and awakening the patient. An otherwise healthy individual may be suddenly seized with pain in the scrotum, following which edema and swelling soon appear. The scrotum becomes tense, painful, reddened, warm, glossy, and, as mortification develops, it becomes moist. The gangrene is usually limited at the demarcation of the scrotum but has been known to spread under Colles' and Scarpa's fascia to the abdomen and even to the axilla. It is usually accompanied by chills, fever, nausea, vomiting, and prostration. It must be differentiated from erysipelas, which usually begins in a limited area and spreads with a perceptible red, raised margin at the periphery. In the latter, the constitutional symptoms are paramount in comparison with the local symptoms. With careful examination, it should not be difficult to differentiate this acute process from acute epididymitis, acute orchitis, hydrocele, or torsion of the testis.

This spontaneous, relatively rare, and inexplicable gangrene is thought to result from an infection. The redundancy of the scrotal tissues is believed to favor the occurrence of such gangrene. It is thought that ingress of the organisms into the wall of the scrotum can occur by one of several mechanisms. Organisms might enter the skin through minute abrasions, possibly by trauma from the fingernails. Embolic bacteria from remote sites in the body have been considered, even though it occurs without any history of antecedent genitourinary tract or general disease. A logical causative factor in many cases could be minute and unrecognizable periurethral phlegmons, through which bacteria progress from the urethra into the scrotal tissue without abscess formation or extravasation of urine.

In the majority of reported instances there is emphysema of the tissues, and actual gas is often encountered upon surgical incision. From a clinical standpoint, it is significant that those cases which have crepitation usually show more constitutional symptoms, such as high fever and evidences of toxemia. The bacteriology in this remarkable disease is incomplete, but anaerobic streptococci, either alone or with other organisms, have been reported in 28 of 44 cases studied (Mair, 1945). A wide variety of other organisms, including hemolytic streptococci, Proteus, and especially the gas-forming anaerobes, have also been encountered. It is well known that anaerobes normally inhabit the male urethra, and it is believed by some observers that the primary infective agents are the anaerobic bacilli which are usually overgrown by streptococci in cultures from this area.

Treatment of gangrene of the scrotum is two-fold. The first is recognition and treatment of any underlying etiologic disease process of the urinary tract when it exists. In urinary extravasation immediate diversion of the urinary stream may be necessary. The second objective is directed toward the probable bacteria involved. In this respect, the early recognition of the pregangrenous state and the institution of proper antibiotics is extremely important. If there is evidence of crepitation, large quantities of specific polyvalent serum should be administered immediately; administration of 100,000 units of penicillin every three hours is imperative. This should be combined with either Aureomycin or Terramycin, on the assumption that it is likely to be a mixed infection. Prompt surgical drainage of the tense, swollen scrotal tissue in either the pregangrenous or gangrenous states relieves tension and drains the edema (Fig. 328). Multiple scrotal incisions with the insertion of Dakin's tubes, followed by irrigations of the tissue with 1:5,000 potassium permanganate solution or zinc peroxide frequently is of value. Zinc peroxide is more efficacious than hydrogen peroxide because it liberates oxygen more slowly. Inasmuch as this unusual and striking disease process may be similar to the "synergistic gangrene" of cutaneous and subcutaneous tissues elsewhere in the body, it might be well to irrigate the tissues with solutions of bacitracin. Prompt recognition, use of polyvalent serum with antibiotics, and proper drainage by surgery should reduce the previous 30 to 35 per cent mortality. Indeed, the prompt use of antibiotics will probably result in this disease becoming an extreme rarity.

Chancroidal infection (soft chancre) occurs more often in Negroes and is rarely a primary infection of the scrotum. The initial lesion of this acute and chronic ulcerative venereal disease is usually on the penis (see Penis). In either case it may manifest itself in several clinical forms. The acute necrosis or "ulcus molle phagedenicum" may spread rapidly from the penis and destroy large areas of undermined scrotal skin. The process is more likely to be one of chronicity with abscess formation and tissue necrosis beneath the surface, with the formation of undermined, purulent, and foul-smelling ulcers. The Ito-Reenstierna skin reaction test does not always indicate the presence of this infection, and the diagnosis is made by culture of the organism (Ducrey's bacillus). As a result of secondary infection, it may be painful, and the characteristic ulcers may offer a wide variety of appearances. Ulcers may develop in the inguinal areas from abscess formation in the lymph nodes. Chancroid must be differentiated from chancre in the chronic form. It may coexist with lymphogranuloma venereum as well as with syphilis, or all three diseases may be present in a single case. In the acute stage, it may be confused with erosive or gangrenous balanitis, but the latter as a rule does not result in painful inguinal lymph nodes nor do the ulcers have an undermined appearance. Extensive cases of herpes progenitalis, so-called "coccigenous" ulcers, and extensive

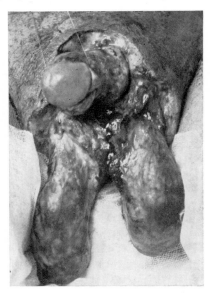

Fig. 328. Streptococcus scrotal and penile gangrene after removing necrotic tissue (cf. Fig. 327). Recovering with ultimate covering with skin; skin grafting not performed.

secondary infections complicating scabies have been mistaken for chancroid. The inguinal adenitis or "bubo" development may lead to lymphatic obstruction and the development of elephantiasic changes in the scrotal skin.

Treatment of chancroid ulcers in the past was primarily surgical, with excision of infected areas and the application of various antiseptics and caustics such as nitric acid, formalin, silver nitrate, phenol, and hydrogen peroxide. Incision and drainage of abscesses is often necessary. The continuous application of 1:4,000 potassium permanganate is helpful. Treatment of this sort usually leads to healing by slow inward growth of the epithelium with scar formation. The use of dmelcos vaccines and foreign protein therapy often expedited recovery by several weeks.

Modern therapy has been attended by considerable success with antibiotics. Various authors have been enthusiastic about Aureomycin, chloramphenicol, penicillin, and the sulfonamides. Experience to date reveals that the relative value of these four medications has not yet been ascertained, as they all seem to be reasonably effective. Sulfathiazole is probably the drug of choice, but it is no longer advocated because of its inherent toxic properties. Aureomycin (0.5 gm. 4 times a day for one to two weeks) has resulted in complete healing of a large percentage of the lesions. It would seem that Aureomycin, chloramphenicol, sulfonamides, and penicillin are all effective and should be used in this order. With these antibiotics, topical treatment of the ulcerative process is no longer indicated.

Granuloma inguinale (granuloma venereum) is a disease characterized by ulcers in the genital regions. This disease is common in the tropics, while in this country it is endemic in the South, with most cases in Negroes. Granuloma inguinale is a nonvenereal disease arising in the genitocrural or genitoanal areas. During the first stage a tiny macule develops, later becoming a

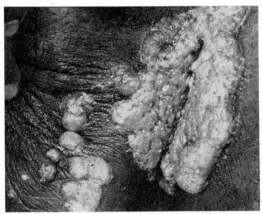

Fig. 329. An early and characteristic lesion of granuloma inguinale involving the scrotum and inner surface of the thigh. The granulations are hypertrophic and exuberant.

papule and finally ulceration. The ulcer is painless and serpiginous in character. The base of the lesion consists of luxuriant granulations, under which there is scar tissue (Fig. 329). The margin of the ulcer has considerable epithelial proliferation. No large abscesses occur, although microscopically minute necrotic areas can be seen. It is not ordinarily accompanied by lymphadenopathy or constitutional symptoms. The scrotum and groin of one side is commonly infected, although it can be bilateral, and in either case it may involve the entire skin of the scrotum. This ulcerative disease must be differentiated from chronic streptococcal ulceration, chancroid, and syphilis. It is important to remember that syphilis and chancroid may occur as a mixed infection with granuloma inguinale. Cases which do not respond to modern antibiotics should be biopsied for carcinoma which may have developed in the ulcers.

A number of organisms have been thought to be the etiologic agent, but it is most likely caused by so-called "Donovan" bodies. Examination of the scrapings from the superficial layers of the ulcer, when fixed by Wright's stain, reveals these protozoan bodies within large mononuclear cells. They are difficult to culture, but the diagnosis is relatively simple from stained scrapings. The vector for the infection has been thought to be the body louse.

Treatment in the past was partially successful with surgical excision of the ulcers followed by compresses, caustics, and antibiotics. Various compounds of antimony (tartar emetic) are fairly effective, although healing often requires repeated courses of the drug. In recent years there has been marked improvement in therapy, with excellent reports following the use of streptomycin, Aureomycin, chloramphenicol, and to some extent Terramycin. They all seem to be much more effective than the time-honored antimony.

Aureomycin has also been reasonably effective in the treatment of this condition, although the Donovan bodies may still be demonstrated in the ulcer until the time of final healing. It is felt that Aureomycin does not have as prompt action as streptomycin, but some observers contend that its effect is more complete with a smaller percentage of recurrences. Aureomycin has been more effective by peroral route in dosages of 250 mg. every 8 hours for twenty to sixty days.

Chloramphenicol* has also been used, and the earlier results were similar to those of Aureomycin, but the occurrence of relapses has not yet been evaluated. Chloramphenicol should be given in dosages of 2 to 3 gm. per day for an average of twelve days. Recently limited reports with the use of Terramycin indicate that it may be equally as effective as the other antibiotics. In one small series, 60 mg. per kilo body weight per day was successful after ten days administration in healing the primary lesions. There is little doubt that all these antibiotics are effective, with evidence at the moment favoring streptomycin. Final evaluation is incomplete, and there is still controversy among various observers as to the superior drug. Experiences with the use of these drugs in combinations are yet unreported.

Lymphogranuloma venereum is an infectious disease caused by a filterable virus. The primary lesion is usually insignificant and is rarely recognized by the patient. It usually occurs on the penis (see Penis) and heals rapidly unless there is a secondary infection. The scrotum may be involved in the later stages of the disease, but primary inoculations here are practically unknown.

Following inoculation, the disease involves the regional lymph nodes and, in the case of genital infection, the inguinal nodes show lymphangitis, lymphadenitis, and perilymphadenitis. The matted lymph nodes in lymphogranuloma venereum may be distinguished from the nodes of syphilis, which are discrete. The localized inguinal adenitis may be self-limiting or may progress into a chronic, persistent infection with necrosis of the nodes, abscess, sinus formation, and finally ulceration. If resolution does not occur, considerable secondary infection develops with thrombo-endolymphatitis, a striking feature.

The *diagnosis* is usually made by the appearance of the chronic ulcerative process in the inguinal area aided by a positive skin test (Frei test) with substances containing antigenic material obtained from cultures of the virus in the yolk sac of chick embryos. Biopsies from the ulcerative areas, either in the groin or scrotum, are not characteristic and show only chronic fibrous tissue infiltrated with leukocytes, occasional giant cells, and minute necrosis. Marked

---

*Additional experiences with chloramphenicol have revealed certain disadvantages due to its inherent toxicity and it is probably unwise to use this antibiotic until other agents have proved ineffective.

perivascular infiltration of lymphocytes and plasma cells is usually present. With long-standing lymphatic stasis and edema, fibrosis and infection of the scrotal wall may occur with elephantiasic changes (pseudo-elephantiasis) of moderate degree.

Treatment is directed at the virus and the secondary invaders. If this results in improved circulation and the scrotal swelling is not too extensive, some reversal of the scrotal enlargement will result. In extensive elephantiasis it may be necessary to remove some of the avascular and hypertrophied scrotal tissue.

There is no specific therapy for lymphogranuloma venereum. The sulfonamide drugs have shown some inhibition, both in vitro and in vivo, upon this virus. Sulfamerazine is the sulfa drug of choice, following which a course of sulfadiazine is usually given. Both Wright and Ridener have reported encouraging results with the use of Aureomycin, although it is by no means specific.

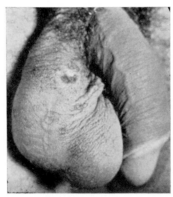

Fig. 330.   Typical chancre, primary on scrotum just below penoscrotal junction.

It is possible that the partially satisfactory response to both Aureomycin and some of the sulfonamides is due to their effect against secondary invaders, thus rendering partial aid to the healing process. Some of the favorable reports following the use of antimony and the newer antibiotics may have been the result of their effect upon granuloma inguinale infections present in combination with lymphogranuloma venereum.

Syphilis of the Scrotal Skin. The scrotal skin is not an uncommon site for a primary lesion of syphilis (Fig. 330). The chancre irrespective of its location is grossly and histologically the same. It may be encountered at the penoscrotal junction in individuals who have used protectives in which case Treponema pallidum are inoculated into the scrotum rather than the penis.

Lesions of the scrotum are much more common in the secondary stage, but they are also encountered during relapses. They appear during relapse within the first two years but rarely occur after this. According to Stokes, the anogenital region is the exclusive site of cutaneous relapse manifestations in 41 per cent of cases. In 25.8 per cent of his cases, the lesions were localized in the scrotum.

Scrotal lesions in secondary syphilis may be part of a generalized cutaneous manifestation, and in this respect they have been encountered in many forms, just as secondary syphilis in general may mimic many cutaneous diseases. These scrotal lesions have been described as papules similar to urticaria pigmentosa. As part of a generalized cutaneous lesion they may resemble the lesions of lichen planus, pityriasis, variola, herpes progenitalis, erythema multiforme, and other skin diseases.

In general, the scrotal lesions in the secondary and especially during the relapse stage of syphilis are more often either papular or annular in character (Fig. 331). Follicular, nodular, and pustular lesions are relatively rare on the scrotum. Moist papules are the most common lesions found on the scrotum in syphilis. Classical annular recurrences are not uncommon in untreated and insufficiently treated patients, particularly in the Negro race. These annular

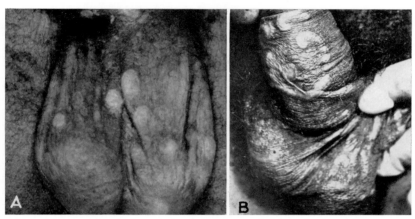

Fig. 331. Syphilis of scrotum in two cases illustrating lesions in secondary and relapse stages. The moist papules in one case are characteristically annular.

lesions are actually moist papules and consist of raised circular ridges about 1 or 2 mm. wide. They are elevated about ½ mm. from the surrounding skin and may be covered by a light scale, from which serum may exude. Later, the papillae appear as slightly glistening or translucent, elevated rings when the skin is stretched. Cases have been encountered with positive serologic tests for syphilis in which the only secondary manifestation consisted of small papular lesions arranged in an annular form on the under surface of the scrotum. These skin lesions are not always apparent because of the marked rugae in the scrotal skin. If the scrotum is pulled outward and put on a "stretch," such annular and papular lesions may be obvious and even striking, especially on the posterior wall. Annular lesions may also occur in the tertiary stage (Fig. 332). It is important to examine the scrotum in any patient in whom there is a history of syphilis. The common annular and papular forms occurring in the secondary stage of syphilis have often been misdiagnosed as dermatophytoses. They may also resemble seborrheic dermatitis, which not uncommonly affects the scrotum.

Papular lesions may sometimes develop into flat condylomas. The latter have an eroded surface representing nonspecific hypertrophy of the cutis and epidermis. They are usually associated with condylomata around the rectum and, in general, result from chronic irritation and uncleanliness, a condition in which a wide variety of saprophytic organisms are present. It is important to stress that scrotal lesions, even in the relapsing phase, are infectious.

Ulceration of the scrotal skin in tertiary syphilis may occur as a result of

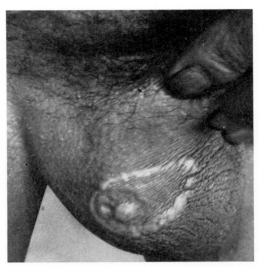

Fig. 332.   Tertiary cutaneous lesions on the scrotum in the form of annular or "target" grouping. In this patient the only cutaneous manifestations were these scrotal lesions. (Courtesy of Dr. Cleveland from Epstein's "Regional Dermatologic Diagnosis," Lea & Febiger, 1950.)

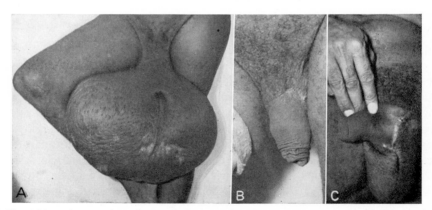

Fig. 333.   *A,* extensive elephantiasis involving the scrotum in South Pacific native. Views *B* and *C* show excellent result following excision of the elephantiasic skin with preservation of the penile skin. (Courtesy of Dr. Perry A. Bonar.)

gumma of the testis and epididymis which has become adherent to the skin, or a gumma of the scrotal skin may develop without involvement of the testes. Such chronic, indolent, and painless ulcers must not be confused with chronic tuberculous ulcers, sarcoma, or necrotic teratoma. All of these diseases may be equally painless. Lymphedema and mild degrees of pseudo-elephantiasis of the scrotum can result as a secondary complication of lymphatic obstruction from syphilis involving the inguinal and femoral lymph nodes.

Elephantiasis of the scrotum is a diffuse enlargement consisting of hypertrophy and hyperplasia of the epidermis and subcutaneous tissues. The skin has the character of the epidermis of a pachyderm—hence the name. It is thick, leathery, coarse, and dry because the sebaceous glands have usually been destroyed. The skin is thickest in the most dependent part of the scrotum, but it becomes progressively thinner towards the top. The scrotal size may range from slightly enlarged to monstrous sizes, some reported as weighing up to 224 pounds (Fig. 333). The consistency of the leathery skin is characteristically that of a nonpitting edema. The condition is due to stasis of the scrotal

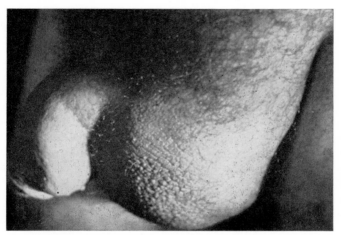

Fig. 334.   Pseudo-elephantiasis or elephantiasis nostra. Area of localized elephantiasis due
to chronic coccal infection of scrotum.

lymphatic system. There are two general types: (1) filarial or elephantiasis tropica, a parasitic disease, and (2) pseudo-elephantiasis or nostra, which results from lymphatic obstruction from a wide variety of causes in both temperate and tropical climates. These are discussed in detail by Dr. Sanjurjo in Section V, Chapter 3.

Pseudo-elephantiasis, or elephantiasis nostra, is occasionally seen in temperate climates and is a result of lymphedema, lymphatic obstruction, and lymphangitis from causes other than filarial infestation. It is usually the result of an inflammatory process with recurrent or chronic streptococcus infection of the lymphatic channels, although a congenital form of pseudo-elephantiasis of the scrotum and penis was reported by Schau in 1935. It may be local or generalized (Figs. 334 and 335). A number of associated conditions in the scrotal lymphatic system can lead to pseudo-elephantiasis. It may occur as a result of multiple scrotal fistulae. Sporadic cases have occurred after hernia operations, metastatic carcinoma, removal of the inguinal lymph nodes, and lymphadenitis due to syphilis, lymphopathia venereum, tuberculosis, or granuloma inguinale. A few instances of unexplained elephantiasic changes in the penis and scrotum have been known to occur. Some cases give a history of episodic scrotal swellings, but in these no evidence of infection or specific etiologic agent could be found. The treatment of pseudo-elephantiasis is elimination of the causal factor plus supportive therapy to the enlarged scrotum. Only on rare occasions will the scrotum become large enough to require surgical excision.

CUTANEOUS DISEASES

The application of any substance or compound to the scrotal skin must be undertaken with care because the scrotal skin is very thin, contains a large number of apocrine glands, and in some respects is dissimilar to other skin areas of the body. It is in constant contact with the clothes and skin of the thighs. It is situated in an area in which evaporation is minimal. Scrotal skin is redundant with many rugae which inhibit proper ventilation, so that it is subject to moisture and denudation. For these reasons, many locally applied drugs and antiseptics are not applicable in strong concentrations to scrotal skin. Agents to combat hyperhidrosis are sometimes beneficial; for example, a mixture of equal parts of zinc oxide and talc is valuable as a drying powder, with the talc rendering a spreading quality to the heavy zinc oxide. Zinc oxide (20 per cent in petroleum or wool fat) as a paste is useful for its drying effect. Aluminum chloride in 10 to 25 per cent solution is another excellent anhidrotic agent. Medicated soaps are not recommended for scrotal skin. The continued use of strong local remedies, whether they be antipruritic, analgesic, antiphlogistic, antiseborrheic, keratolytic, or anhidrotic may produce temporary relief for many uncomfortable scrotal cutaneous diseases, but many of these substances frequently result in a superimposed contact dermatitis (Dermatitis venenata). This is especially true with local applications of sulfonamide drugs and antibiotics, both to the interrupted and intact scrotal skin. Tyrothrycin in 0.1 to 1 per cent concentration in inert lotions or ointments is an exception and does not produce any sensitizing effect. A valuable antiseptic for scrotal skin, with little irritating action, is 3 per cent iodochloroxy quinoline in ointment form. It is superior to ammoniated mercury compounds and various dyes used for superficial coccal infections. Certain esters of fatty acids, such as sodium propionate, are effective fungicidal agents. Addition of keratolytic salicylic acid to fungicidal preparations facilitates the penetration of the fungicide by shedding superficial layers of the skin.

Many of the common generalized skin conditions include the scrotum only in extremely rare instances, although all of the diseases of the skin have, on occasion, spread to involve the scrotum. On the other hand, some diseases not uncommonly have scrotal distribution, while a few have a distinct predilection for the scrotum. The following affections of the scrotal skin occur often enough to merit recording. They are not arranged in the order of their frequency of occurrence or importance but rather with consideration of their general character and etiology.

Dermatophytosis. Fungi affecting the scrotum usually belong to the Epidermophyton and Trichophyton genera and rarely to the genus Microsporum (Fig. 336, see also Section XIII, Fig. 767). Other groups such as favus and monilia may be etiologic agents. Fungous infections, in general, result in scrotal skin changes consisting of deep-seated vesicles containing clear fluid. The vesicles later erode through the skin, followed by desquamation. This condition is seen on the scrotum in patients having ringworm of the hands and feet, although the latter may be entirely asymptomatic. The lesions are accompanied by extreme itching. The diagnosis is established by demonstration of the branching filaments of fungi in fresh potassium hydroxide preparations or by culture on Sabouraud's medium. Another manifestation on the scrotum of fungus disease is the allergic "id" reaction. Fungi cannot

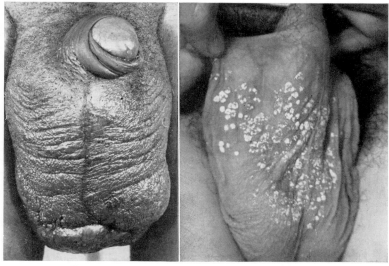

Fig. 335.   Fig. 336.

Fig. 335. Pseudoelephantiasis. Enlargement of the scrotum from chronic infection due to urethritis and urethral stricture.

Fig. 336. Mycotic infection of scrotum. Scrotal skin showing numerous crusts or scutula which are composed of filaments and spores due to infection with Microsporum gypseum. (Courtesy of Dr. E. P. Cawley and the Archives of Dermat. & Syph.)

be found in these "id" eruptions. They may follow therapy of the original scrotal involvement, making it necessary to eradicate the primary focus, which usually is on the feet. Treatment in the acute stage is application of saturated boric acid or a solution of 1:20,000 potassium permanganate every two hours. The keratolytic ointments, such as one half strength Whitfield's, are used later to remove the involved skin. Ointments of sodium propionate or sodium undecylenate (Trydecyl) are reasonably effective. The usual antipruritic agents may give symptomatic relief of such an "id" reaction.

The following clinical entities occur as a result of specific fungus infections.

Tinea Cruris. So-called "jock itch" or tinea cruris usually involves the scrotum and contiguous surfaces of the thigh and intergluteal regions. The etiologic agent is usually Epidermophyton floccosum. The lesion starts with a few superficial reddish-brown and well-defined scaly patches which extend peripherally and coalesce into symmetrical inflamed areas. The brownish-red centers have an elevated edge of deep red. This characteristic margin has suggested the name, "eczema marginatum." The initial lesions may become macerated from secondary infection or moisture, with considerable pain and itching. Active sweating, tight clothing, or obesity favors recurrence of the lesions. Dermatophytons from the feet often provide a reinfecting agent. This fungus can be demonstrated in 20 per cent potassium hydroxide preparations or by culture. If there is an accompanying inflammation, strong fungicidal agents may be contraindicated in the acute stage. Potassium permanganate solution in the proportion of 1:20,000 applied twice daily for fifteen minutes may be all the patient can tolerate. Undecylenic acid or 1 per cent salicylic acid can be applied later. Ten per cent boric acid in equal parts of fuller's earth and talcum may also be helpful. Ointments containing 3 to 5 per cent sulfur and 3 per cent salicylic acid in lanolin and petrolatum have long been used for this disease. Greasy ointments only aggravate the infection. It may be necessary to apply 1 per cent aqueous gentian violet to inhibit superimposed coccal infections.

Erythrasma. This mycotic disease is caused by Actinomyces (Microsporon) minutissimus. It appears as a brown, scaly eruption, somewhat irregular, but finely demarcated and similar to pityriasis, except that it is confined to the scrotum and sometimes the adjoining areas on the thigh and anal region. There is a splotchy spread, which produces no symptoms except those due to contact. The diagnosis is made by staining scrapings from the skin area with a 1 per cent solution of methylene blue. A 10 per cent alcoholic solution of sodium propionate, Schalek's, and Lassar's paste are all efficacious.

Pityriasis (Tinea) versicolor. This superficial fungus disease is due to Malassezia (microsporon) furfur. The fungus can be easily seen in scrapings immersed in 1 per cent methylene blue or 10 per cent potassium hydroxide. It usually occurs in individuals who perspire freely. The lesions consist of slowly enlarging brown macules without evidence of inflammation or subjective symptoms. Other portions of the body covered by clothing may be involved. Application of a 10 per cent solution of sodium propionate usually leads to disappearance of the lesions. Dilute acetic acid or 20 per cent sodium hyposulfite is also recommended.

Pediculosis Pubis (Phthiriasis). This disease is caused by the so-called "crab" louse. Unlike the body louse, which lives in the clothing, it resides on the body parts where there is hair. When the scrotum and pubic areas are infested, the skin has a bitten appearance consisting of small, red points which develop into papules. The associated itching leads to excoriation, bleeding, encrustation, and secondary infection. The original bites may be replaced by brownish discoloration of the skin. Grayish-blue spots measuring up to 1 cm. in diameter (maculae caeruleae) are due to intradermal injection of salivary secretion by the louse. Treatment of pediculosis consists of dusting the affected hair areas of the body with 10 per cent DDT powder, followed by a tub bath the following morning. The ova hatch in seven days, so that it is necessary to inspect the patient at that time for evidence of further infestation. More than two treatments are rarely required. It may be helpful to shave the infected regions and wash the areas with soap and water, after which a 0.5 per cent DDT cold cream preparation can be applied.

Scabies. This is a metazoan infection due to the mite, Acarus (sarcopter) scabiei, var. hominis. The female mite burrows intradermally and deposits eggs in furrows, resulting in intense itching, especially at night when the mites are active. The furrows are readily visible on the scrotum and measure 0.5 to 1 cm. in length. At the distal, closed end of these tiny tortuous channels is an erythematous vesicle in which the female is lodged. Scraping at this end of the vesicle usually produces the mite. Secondary infection, excoriation, pustules, and exudative erosion can distort the appearance of the skin lesion. Even if the mite is not visible, the diagnosis can be established upon examination of scrapings in 10 per cent hydrogen peroxide. Impetigo of the buttocks in children frequently indicates scabies. Treatment consists of bathing the infected region thoroughly with soap and water for twenty minutes and applying one of the following agents: 3 to 10 per cent sulfur, 25 per cent benzyl benzoate, or hexachlorocyclohexane. These ointments and lotions usually eradicate the scabies in one application. The itching may persist for some time after the destruction of the mites. The remaining pink and firm nodules in the skin disappear within several months after completion of therapy and need no further treatment. Persistent treatment over prolonged periods with application of the above agents can result in contact dermatitis, especially if mercury ointments are used.

Dermatitis Venenata (Contact Dermatitis). This form of dermatitis is a hyperergic skin reaction due to contact with various chemicals. It may result in every type of dermatological lesion, such as erythema, papules, vesicles, pustules, etc. Considerable itching usually precedes the erythema, which may be confined to the skin area exposed to the irritating agents, but papule formation with secondary infection of the lesions may spread beyond the original contact area. Dermatitis venenata includes all dermatitides produced by contact with chemical agents. The agent may be irritating to the skin of all scrotums and produce a standard reaction, or there may be a particular sensitizing substance affecting the skin of only some scrotums. Contact may be through dyes in clothing, local medication (e.g., mercury), or it may occur as a result of contact with dust or plant extracts. The agents may reach the scrotum by way of contact with the fingers. Examples of this dermatitis are often seen following operations in which antiseptics are applied to the scrotal skin. In this case, the scrotum becomes swollen, edematous, and painful, accompanied by an intense itching. Scratching and secondary infection may lead to excoriation and cellulitis. In most cases, the diagnosis is relatively easy, but frequently the etiology is difficult to determine. Careful study of all possible contacts to the patient must be made with each recrudescence of symptoms. A tentative etiologic agent may be confirmed if the dermatitis recurs following future contact with that agent. Definitive demonstration of the etiological agent depends upon distinct improvement in the condition following elimination of the causative factor. Treatment is directed toward elimination of the cause. Desensitization is generally of little value. Preventive treatment consists of washing the allergen from the skin or, better still, completely avoiding contact with the known allergen, if it can be determined. Symptomatic treatment is helpful (see Eczema).

Dermatitis Medicamentosa (Drug Eruptions). This dermatitis includes skin eruptions following absorption of chemical substances, whereas dermatitis venenata is the result of contact with chemical substances. The dermatitis, by definition, results from the absorption of a drug by any route: injection, inunction, inhalation, or ingestion. Dermatitis medicamentosa is an idiosyncrasy to a drug and not the result of overdosage of the drug. The eruption may take any form, but the lesions are usually widespread, symmetrical in distribution, and abrupt in onset. It can mimic any skin disease, including even alopecia and pruritus. The diagnosis is made only by the disappearance of the dermatitis when the drug is discontinued and a return of the dermatitis when the drug is again used. Treatment is avoidance of contact with the specific agent along with the use of antihistamines, epinephrine, or calcium gluconate.

Eczema. Eczematoid or atopic dermatitis of the scrotum may be a strictly localized process in distribution. It may appear in patches or as a series of superficially reddened, edematous, and weeping vesicles. The lesions progress from a pale red, nonedematous, dry skin to vesicles with scale formation, and as the condition becomes chronic the skin usually thickens and changes to a brownish hue accompanied by lichenification. There is marked itching, excoriation, and finally pustule formation, with secondary changes in appearance. The underlying cause is usually obscure; however, the condition is known to undergo exacerbations following treatment and after repeated contact with the inciting agent. Therapy consists, first, of exhaustive efforts to determine the etiology, which of course must be eliminated. Treatment otherwise is symptomatic and consists of wet compresses of 2 per cent boric acid or 1 per cent aluminum acetate solution. After the acute stage, calamine lotion is beneficial for its antipruritic and drying effects. Local therapy in the form of various tar preparations has also been helpful. If infection is present, 2 per cent vioform, 10 per cent boric acid ointment, or 2 per cent ammoniated mercury may be advantageous. If coccal infection of the skin is present, 2 per cent gentian violet will usually control this complication. The use of sulfonamides and penicillin is unwise in patients who have a tendency toward sensitization from extract of pollen, dust, or animal products.

Pruritus. Pruritus is a symptom which is commonly noted in skin diseases. As an entity it refers to itching for which no local or general explanation can be found. It is often thought to be of psychogenic origin, after first ruling out any local or general cause. Pruritus may be localized in the scrotum, or it may be part of a generalized disorder as sometimes encountered in systemic, parasitic, allergic, atmospheric, psychogenic, and cutaneous diseases.

Treatment of pruritus is fundamentally treatment of the underlying condition. Allergic and especially mycotic infections must be eliminated. Symptomatic treatment should be considered only after a thorough study has been made to rule out a definite etiology. Such treatment includes analgesic ointments, barbiturates, bromides, calcium gluconate, or tub baths followed by the application of starch, sodium bicarbonate, or oatmeal to the scrotal skin. It may be necessary to use a topical ointment such as calamine with 1 per cent phenol to control the intense itching. If there is any suggestion that the pruritus is allergic in origin, antihistamines are indicated. In severe cases 2 per cent procaine intravenously may be necessary to control the itching. Patients should be encouraged to use a detergent rather than soap for cleansing the scrotum and advised to wear soft underclothes. We recently saw a patient who had severe pruritus of the scrotum for a decade, during which time practically every dermatologic remedy had been tried, including the coal tar products. The scrotal skin had become thickened and leathery, with a beginning elephantiasic appearance. Exhaustive studies did not reveal any allergic or other cause for the persistent and severe pruritus. The patient was seen by a general practitioner who prescribed a coal tar ointment, following which the pruritus immediately disappeared, and the scrotal skin has now almost reverted to normal. The patient stated that the new medicine (coal tar) immediately eliminated the intense itching. This case is an illustration of a psychogenic pruritus.

Prurigo is a chronic skin disorder characterized by an itching, nodular eruption. It rarely involves the scrotum alone, and it is thought to represent a form of neurodermatitis resulting from an autonomic nervous system imbalance. Roentgen therapy, topical application of a mild tar or zinc paste, and 25 per cent Cycloform are all helpful but not specific. N-ethyl-o-crontonotoluidide is helpful in various pruritic dermatoses and is free from many objectionable side effects.

Lichen planus is a chronic inflammatory pruritic disease characterized by pale, bluish, flat-top papules which begin as discrete lesions but in time coalesce to form rings and plaques. The surfaces of the patches are rough and scaly. The lesions may be limited to the genitalia, the inner aspects of the knees and thighs, and the flexor surfaces of the wrists. Focal infection and emotional factors have been suggested as causes. The diagnosis can be made by biopsy. Treatment consists of rest, adequate diet, and elimination of psychological turmoil. Roentgen therapy, vitamins, and elimination of focus of infection are advocated.

Herpes progenitalis is a form of herpes simplex encountered especially on the penis and not infrequently on the scrotum. It is a virus disease which can be transmitted to lower animals. The early manifestation is itching followed by hyperemia and formation of closely grouped vesicles varying in size and filled with clear fluid. The disease is self-limited, but when it appears on the genitalia it is a source of considerable discomfort. An attack does not confer immunity, and we recently saw a patient who had experienced repeated episodes every few months for years. Local treatment consists of a mild astringent such as 1:500 aluminum acetate or spirits of camphor. Two per cent alum has been used, but 2 per cent zinc sulfate has given more relief in our cases. The vaccination of variola apparently increases resistance to this form of herpes. Herpes zoster may, on a rare occasion, affect the scrotum and inguinal areas when it involves the sensory division of the scrotal nerves. Unlike herpes progenitalis, one attack produces immunity. Treatment during the acute stage is the same as with herpes progenitalis. Any herpetic lesion should be watched carefully for inflammation, especially after the vesicles have ruptured. Mild antiseptic solutions such as Zephiran or pHisoderm, applied locally, may prevent the spread of infection.

Deficiency dermatitis, sometimes termed "scrotitis" and "urogenital syndrome," occurred in a considerable number of prisoners during the last war. It is significant that this type of deficiency may appear before any other demonstrable signs of vitamin deficiency. The first symptom is usually itching of the scrotum, noted particularly at night. The skin becomes reddened, with fine desquamation and remains dry with erythematous punctuate lesions appearing where it comes in contact with the leg. It progresses into a wet stage, and the mesial aspects of the legs may become secondarily infected. A second dry stage may follow, during which the skin has a crepitant sensation. It is remarkable that the scrotal skin often acquires an infection of Corynebacterium diphtheriae in these cases. Secondary infection may lead to considerable edema, swelling, and ulceration. By this time, other stigmata of vitamin deficiencies develop. This condition must be differentiated from intertrigo, eczema, chemical dermatitis, and tinea cruris. Intertrigo is not cured by the therapeutic application of vitamins, and the scrotal skin in eczema, unlike this dermatitis, later becomes lichenified. This disease is specifically due to riboflavin deficiency and disappears usually within a week after the addition of sufficient vitamin B complex to the diet. Local applications and antibiotics may be necessary for control of the secondary infection. The moist stage requires considerable attention, including administration of penicillin and local application of normal saline solution. Mild antibacterial and dermatological solutions have been used locally, but the scrotal skin has a tendency to become quickly sensitized to the drugs commonly employed in such chronic dermatitides.

Intertrigo is an erythematous and almost always an inflammatory disease of the skin where surfaces are contiguous and where there is uncleanliness and lack of dryness. It occurs as a result of heat (internal or atmospheric), friction, and especially moisture. Of these, the main factor is either an increased production or retention of perspiration. In children, it has been referred to as "ammoniacal dermatitis" because the voided urine is in contact with the genital skin where it is contaminated by bacteria from the rectal area. This results in the decomposition of urea with ammonia formation. It is further accentuated by the irritative action of secretion from the sweat glands and by the glycosuria present in diabetics. Trauma from clothing further aggravates the condition. It is usually always symmetrical on the scrotum including the inner surface of the thighs. In children, the buttocks and penis are involved as well. It consists of moist, red, oozing patches with sometimes the appearance of vesicles. Moisture with excess sweat or urine leads to maceration. Abrasions of the macerated epidermis usually results in a linear fissure at the junction of the angle formed between the scrotum and the legs. The skin becomes secondarily infected with cutaneous cocci and especially fungi of the Monilia group. Treatment is directed toward the reduction of trauma, infection, moisture, and contamination from either urine or feces. In children, proper cleanliness and hygiene will lead to recovery. It is important to change diapers frequently and to launder them with compounds such as boric acid, which inhibits the bacterial decomposition of urea. The involved skin should be cleansed with mild soap and water, followed by the application of drying powders or mild ointments. A nonvolatile antiseptic methyl benzethonium chloride is combined with sodium bicarbonate and cornstarch in the form of a dusting powder and also in tablets for laundry purposes (Diaperene). Cornstarch is a satisfactory dusting powder, and zinc oxide cream is a mild ointment. The various combinations of zinc stearate, zinc oxide, French chalk, starch, and bismuth make excellent drying powders. Magnesium carbonate is also effective in controlling excess perspiration. Tight clothing must be avoided, and the correction of obesity may eliminate skin friction from contiguous surfaces.

Sebaceous Cysts. One or more sebaceous cysts in the scrotal skin is not an uncommon finding. Cyst formation results either from overproduction of secretions or from an obstruction to the outlet of the gland, or both. These

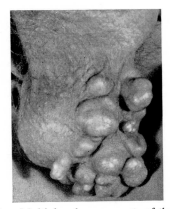

Fig. 336 A.   Multiple sebaceous cysts of the scrotum.

cysts may be present only in the scrotal region. They appear as smooth, round, cystic tumors varying in size from a pea to, in rare instances, a large orange. Inflammation may be present in which case the partially obstructed duct intermittently discharges exudate from the minute orifice. The secretions contain cholesterin crystals and degenerated epithelial cells. The fibrous capsule is lined by stratified squamous epithelium with varying degrees of atrophy. In some instances as many as several hundred cysts have been found in a scrotum, yet they are not considered to be precancerous (Fig. 336 A). They have been known to calcify and in some cases are opaque to x-ray. Because of ossification, some cases may represent an ectodermal disease of nevic origin. Treatment is by surgical excision, and the entire sac must be removed or there will be recurrence.

Psoriasis. This is one of the many skin diseases which occasionally involves the scrotum along with the general body distribution. Psoriasis is a chronic recurrent dermatosis of unknown etiology. The well-demarcated, reddened eruptions covered with dry, silvery scales which appear on the scrotum are similar to those found at other isolated areas of the body. The first appear as tiny, red, flat papules, which enlarge peripherally to coalesce and show desquamation. The lesion may be asymptomatic or mildly itchy; however, in some cases the entire scrotal skin is involved, leading to a pruritic, oozing, and perpetually scaling condition. They tend to disappear in the summertime and to recur in winter. There is no specific treatment, but local agents such as calamine lotion and 1 per cent phenol may allay the itching. Because of the spontaneous remissions, the beneficial results from drugs in this disease are difficult to appraise.

Molluscum Contagiosum. This skin eruption is a viral disease, which occasionally appears on the scrotum. It is seen more frequently in children and is characterized by isolated, waxy papules varying from the size of a pin head to that of a pea. The disease is self-limited and disappears spontaneously. Treatment is not indicated but patients should be observed for secondary infection.

Paget's Disease. Paget's disease has been reported to involve the scrotum on occasions and especially follows chronic eczema-like lesions. The exact nature of Paget's disease is obscure, but it likely represents intra-epidermal metastasis or extension from underlying carcinoma of the ducts of the apocrine sweat glands. Scrotal involvement is usually insidious and at first shows only scaling accompanied by itching. The lesion is usually sharply defined, and the skin at first seems to be thickened and indurated with later denudation, crusting, and the development of an ulcer. Biopsy reveals classical Paget cells, which are pathognomic of the disease. They contain large, deep-staining nuclei with faint protoplasm and are arranged perpendicular to the ulcerative surface. Biopsy of any chronic, persistent edematous lesion in which the skin becomes thickened is imperative. Therapy consists of a wide excision.

Most of the large number of generalized skin diseases do not include the scrotum except on rare occasions. *Pemphigus, xanthoma,* and *erythema multiforme* may have scrotal manifestations, with lesions characteristic of the eruptions elsewhere. *Angiokeratoma* is a rare condition consisting of multiple violaceous lesions which may number up to several hundred. They are minute, slightly elevated areas of venous ectasias. Their appearance is not unlike small, punctate angiomas.

ORCHITIS

Acute infection involving solely the testis is a relatively rare occurrence in clinical urology. The rich blood and lymphatic supply of the testicle gives it a high threshold of resistance with metastatic infection rarely occurring. There are three pathways whereby orchitis may develop: (1) metastatic via the blood stream, (2) lymphatic, and (3) ascending through the vas deferens and epididymis to the testicle. Almost every known infectious process has at times metastasized to the testicle as a primary infection but in the majority of instances the orchitis is secondary to an extension of inflammations existing in the epididymis, so that the process is usually an epididymo-orchitis. Orchitis, in general, may be divided into (1) pyogenic, (2) viral, (3) spirochetal, (4) traumatic, (5) chemical, (6) mycotic, (7) parasitic, and (8) idiopathic, where organisms and a primary focus of infection cannot be demonstrated.

Any pyogenic bacteria causing a septicemia may on occasion result in

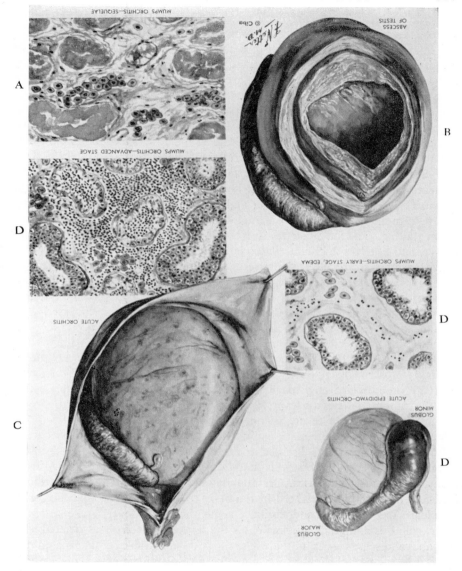

Fig. 337.   *A*, Acute epididymitis. A view illustrating an acutely inflamed epididymis involving the globus minor. There is an area of localized secondary orchitis. (Courtesy of Dr. Samuel A. Vest and The Ciba Co.)

B, Acute orchitis. *Acute hematogenous orchitis* without epididymitis. There is a swelling of the testis with tenseness of the tunica albuginea and punctate hemorrhages on the surface.

C, Abscess testicle. *Abscess of the testicle* from distal pyogenic focus. This usually results in complete destruction of parenchyma.

D, histology of mumps orchitis. Microscopic views show progress from a transitory edematous stage to one in which the interstitial tissue and the lumen of the tubules contain large number of leukocytes and some monocytic cells. A late sequela in some cases is complete atrophy and hyalinization of the seminal epithelium.

pyogenic orchitis. The usual etiologic organisms are Bacillus coli, Bacillus mucosus capsulatus, streptococcus, staphylococcus, Pseudomonas pyocyaneus, and other organisms. In this form of orchitis the testicle is tense, swollen, and bluish in appearance, with many punctuate hemorrhages on the surface (Fig. 337, A-C). Multiple foci of necrosis are found accompanied by considerable edema and interstitial infiltration of polymorphonuclear cells. The seminiferous epithelium is evidently easily damaged as a result of the ischemia. The process may progress to suppuration involving the whole testis, in which event an abscess of the testicle results (Fig. 337, C). The most common cause of suppurative orchitis and abscess formation is epididymitis (Fig. 337, A), complicating prostatectomy, catheterization, or instrumental procedures.

Acute pyogenic orchitis, with or without abscess formation (Fig. 337,B), is usually ushered in with high fever and sudden pain in the involved testicle. The pain radiates to the inguinal canal and is usually accompanied by nausea and vomiting. The involved testis is swollen, tense, sometimes exquisitely tender, and at times fluctuant. There is usually an acute associated hydrocele which becomes a pyocele if the abscess ruptures. The scrotal skin may show some redness and edema. It is frequently difficult clinically to distinguish between acute orchitis, acute epididymitis, and epididymo-orchitis unless the epididymis can be palpated. In children, orchitis may be confused with torsion of the spermatic cord and strangulated hernia, especially if there is a congenital hydrocele or cryptorchidism present. Delineation of the scrotal contents may be difficult even after aspiration of the fluid from the tunica vaginalis.

Acute orchitis also may result in rare instances during such systemic diseases as diphtheria, typhus fever, glanders, influenza, undulant fever, leprosy, dengue fever, typhoid fever, syphilis, paratyphoid fever, varicella, variola, mumps, scarlet fever, tuberculosis, amebiasis, schistosomiasis, sporotrichosis, actinomycosis, rickettsial diseases, malaria, filariasis (see funiculitis), infectious mononucleosis, bilharziasis and, on extremely rare occasions, from many other unusual diseases. Orchitis may occur as a complication of localized foci of infection elsewhere in the body such as sinusitis, tonsillitis, furunculosis, osteomyelitis, endocarditis, acute rheumatic fever, acute articular fever, cellulitis and gout. In some cases the testicular necrosis associated with the above diseases does not always show demonstrable organisms in the testis, and the pathological process may be a result of the action of bacterial toxins on the testicle. Epidemics of obscure orchitis, usually epididymo-orchitis, have occurred in Malta and elsewhere, with as many as 60 cases having been seen during a single epidemic. The clinical picture is one of prodromal fever associated with mild constitutional symptoms without evidence of urinary tract infection. Urologists have observed sporadic cases of epididymo-orchitis of a similar nature. We have recently seen two such obscure cases: one a boy of 8 years and another, a young man of 21 years of age. These cases of orchitis were not due to mumps. In the first case, orchitis recurred after an interval of several months, while in the second case, mumps orchitis was known to have existed five years previously on the opposite testis. Both cases were refractory to streptomycin, penicillin, and other antibiotics.

Traumatic orchitis (see Traumatic Epididymitis) is considered by most urologists to be the result of an infectious process resulting from a lowered resistance of the injured tissues to bacteria. Enlargement of the testis (also spermatic cord and epididymis) may follow trauma, vas ligation, and surgical manipulation, without a history of preliminary disease or inflammation. Histologic studies in some cases reveal a nonspecific granulomatous reaction evidently due to proteins from extravasated sperm following obstruction or traumatic procedures. The tissue reaction includes giant cells and resembles that of tuberculosis. It is probable that granulomatous orchitis in the past has sometimes been confused with tuberculous infection of the testicle. Chemical substances such as iodine, thallium, lead, carbon disulfide, and alcohol have been alleged to cause on occasion destruction of the seminiferous tubules.

Treatment of orchitis is essentially medical, including specific treatment of the underlying disease process. The patient is maintained at bed rest with adequate elevation of the scrotum (Fig. 776). Application of hot or cold compresses is used only for symptomatic relief. Extent of involvement depends upon the intensity of the inflammatory process and the virulence of the infecting organism. Aspiration of the symptomatic hydrocele may give considerable relief. Abscess of the testicle is extremely rare, and usually requires orchiectomy. Incision and drainage only result in sloughing and gradual extrusion of the parenchyma. Antibiotics are indicated according to the nature of the specific etiologic agent. With almost routine use of antibiotics early in all infectious processes in medicine today, there is less suppurative epididymitis and subsequent orchitis. Under the influence of antibiotics an infected epididymis is now safely removed, allowing the secondary inflammatory process in the testis to subside. In any orchitis, except mumps, secondary atrophy and sterility from fibrosis and destruction of the tubules and excretory system frequently occurs.

Mumps Orchitis. Orchitis in mumps, because of its frequency, merits especial consideration. Mumps is a highly incapacitating but self-limited viral disease complicated by orchitis in approximately 18 per cent of cases. It is exceedingly rare before puberty. Onset of the orchitis is usually four to six days after the appearance of parotitis, but, indeed, it may occur without parotid involvement. We have observed a small epidemic of mumps orchitis without parotitis. In about 70 per cent of cases, the orchitis is unilateral, with 50 per cent atrophy of the involved testicle to some degree (Fig. 337, *D*). Inclusion of the epididymis in this process is not rare. Impotence and sterility are infrequent sequelae of mumps. Baumrucker found only 7 cases of sterility in 95 patients with testicular atrophy following mumps orchitis.

The signs and symptoms are essentially those of other interstitial types of orchitis. Nausea, vomiting, and chills may be present in severe cases. Testicular swelling is a prominent feature, although it is not remarkable in the first 48 hours. Mumps orchitis usually subsides in seven to ten days.

Treatment of mumps orchitis is (1) medical and (2) surgical. Bed rest, scrotal support, and either hot or cold application are advised, although the value of these procedures is unsubstantiated. Considerable enthusiasm has been registered in recent years in the use of gamma globulin, diethylstilbestrol, and convalescent serum from individuals who have had mumps within a period of three to four months. Pooled plasma may result in temperature reduction within twenty-four hours in an occasional instance, but it is doubtful that it alters the general course of established orchitis. There is some evidence that it may reduce the incidence of orchitis from 65 to 75 per cent. Gamma globulin, given after the onset of parotitis, has been reported to reduce the incidence of orchitis. Early reports of the effectiveness of diethylstilbestrol in reducing the incidence of orchitis and favorably affecting the course of the disease has not been substantiated by more extensive studies. It is possible, however, that diethylstilbestrol in adequate dosage (3 to 5 or more mg. a day) may diminish the degree of pain, swelling, and fever. There is little evidence that there is any effect on the subsequent degree of testicular atrophy. Cortisone is presently being evaluated as a therapeutic agent for mumps orchitis. It evidently relieves the acute swelling in some cases and alters the course of the disease but the late results are unknown.

Surgical treatment of severe mumps orchitis has consisted of tapping the hydrocele to reduce the pressure in the tunica. Simple needle aspiration of the testicle is of no value. Many urologists advocate an "H" type of incision into the tunica albuginea after exposing the testicle to release intratesticular tension. Follow-up reports are too few in number to be of value in appraisal of this procedure, but there is evidence that if it is done within the first two days of acute swelling, it not only results in relief of symptoms but also in a marked reduction of subsequent atrophy. The difficulty is in deciding which cases will respond favorably to radical therapy. The majority of cases begin to show improvement during the period when this type of therapy would be valuable. It should be reserved for those severe cases in which it appears there is going to be considerable persistent swelling of the testicle.

Syphilis of the Testicle. This has been considered to be common because it has been long known from animal experimentation and from study of testicles in the acute stage of syphilis that they are a favorable depot for the spirochete. Recent autopsy studies in syphilis by Rosahn (1946) have thrown considerable doubt upon the high frequency of syphilitic orchitis. Warthin found many pathological changes at autopsy in the testicles of individuals who had syphilis early in life, and he thought they were a result of early unrecognized syphilitic orchitis. On the basis of Rosahn's studies, these lesions of fibrosis and round cell infiltration occur as frequently in nonsyphilitics as in syphilitics, and there is substantial evidence that these changes are a result of an aging process or other factors and not the result of an earlier unrecognized syphilitic orchitis. There is an acute but rare form of syphilitic orchitis (or epididymo-orchitis) that does occur during the secondary stage of syphilis. It mimics mumps orchitis and pyogenic orchitis and responds to antisyphilitic treatment. Congenital syphilitic orchitis is not un-common, and it usually occurs with other stigmata of syphilis.

Syphilitic orchitis occurs ordinarily in two chronic forms. One is the inter-stitial or fibrous type, and the other is that of necrosis or gumma formation (Fig. 338). It may be unilateral or bilateral. It is significant that these

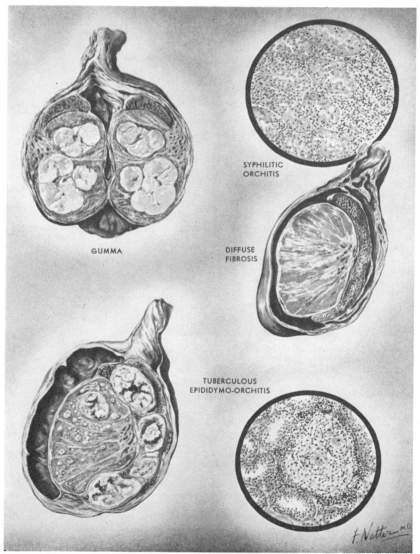

SYPHILITIC
ORCHITIS

GUMMA

DIFFUSE
FIBROSIS

TUBERCULOUS
EPIDIDYMO-ORCHITIS

Fig. 338. Gumma of the testicle. Syphilitic necrosis consisting of coalescing gum-matous areas in the testicle without extension into epididymis. Second view illustrates testicle with diffuse fibrosis resulting in "billiard ball" type of syphilitic orchitis.

Tuberculous epididymo-orchitis. Tuberculous epididymitis with secondary involvement of the testicle and tunica vaginalis. There are extensive caseous areas which will result eventually in a single large indolent and necrotic mass. A microscopic view depicts a typical early tubercle showing giant cells with round cell infiltration. (Courtesy of Dr. Samuel A. Vest and The Ciba Co.)

lesions may be entirely painless and unnoticed both by the patient and by the physician. An accompanying secondary hydrocele is the rule. In the interstitial type, the testicle is hard, smooth, and of wooden consistency, so that it has been described as a "billiard ball." The epididymis is not usually involved in the initial lesion. Pathologically, there is an infiltration of plasma cells and lymphocytes between the seminiferous tubules, with great proliferation of fibrous tissue. The entire testicle eventually becomes fibrotic or progresses to gummatous formation.

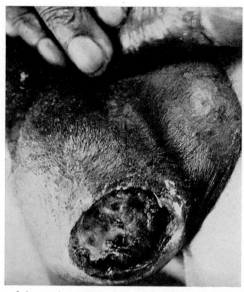

Fig. 339. Gumma of the testis eroding the scrotal skin. This patient gave a history of a painless penile lesion five years previously followed by ulceration and discharge one week before admission. A painless scrotal swelling had been present for three months. The testicle and epididymis was one smooth, firm, painless mass. Prompt healing followed antiluetic therapy.

The less frequent gumma of the testis occurs late in the course of the disease, whereas the interstitial type may occur during the early and late stages. Gummata are usually unilateral and may consist of either one large area of necrosis or of a conglomeration of nodules in the testes. The surrounding fibrous tissue results in hardness of the individual or coalesced nodules. The tunica albuginea and epididymis are eventually involved. The process becomes adherent to the subcutaneous tissue and the skin of the scrotum, which eventually sloughs and ulcerates (Fig. 339). There are few subjective symptoms in gumma, but it is usually accompanied by enlargement of the inguinal nodes and other evidence of syphilis. Any type of syphilitic orchitis responds well to antiluetic therapy. Gumma must be differentiated from tumor and tuberculosis. Tuberculosis always originates in the epididymis, with secondary extension into the testicle. In tumors, the epididymis may be palpated as distinct from the testicular enlargement. Tumors are usually more rapid in development and without attachment to the scrotal skin.

EPIDIDYMITIS

Epididymitis is the most common of all the intrascrotal inflammations. It is mainly a disease of adults, but all forms, especially in conjunction with orchitis, have at times affected children. In general, and for practical purposes, epididymitis may be classified into (1) gonorrheal, (2) non-specific, which is actually specific and usually pyogenic, yet no effort is made to identify the causative organisms, (3) traumatic, (4) specific, or inflammation due to known and identified etiologic agents.

Organisms reach the epididymis commonly through the lumen of the vas from previously established infection in the urine, posterior urethra, prostate, or seminal vesicles. Infections rarely spread to the epididymis through the wall and sheath of the vas by retrograde lymphatic pathways, or as a result of direct extension from a pre-existing orchitis. The hematogenous or metastatic route is a more rare mode of infection.

Gonorrheal Epididymitis. Before the advent of modern chemotherapy, gonorrheal epididymitis, as a complication of gonorrheal urethritis, was a common occurrence in urological practice. It has been known to occur in as high as 25 per cent of patients with gonococcal urethritis. The incidence of gonorrheal epididymitis varied according to the cooperation of the patient and the skill of the urologist in the use of pressure irrigations, instillations, and instrumentation. Straining with a full bladder predisposes to gonorrheal epididymitis. With the advent of the antibiotic era, such local therapy is unnecessary, and epididymitis is now a rare complication of gonorrheal infection. In a community of 5,000 college students, we have not treated a case of gonorrheal epididymitis in three years. It is now encountered only after neglect in treatment or when some complicating factor is present, such as resistance of the organism, urethral stricture, or other local pathology.

Gonorrheal epididymitis rarely involves the testis. It appears first in the globus minor along with some tenderness and swelling of the vas. There may be all degrees of swelling of the epididymis (Fig. 337, *A*) from slight to extreme enlargement. The pathological process is due to accumulations of polymorphonuclear cells in the tubules and throughout the peritubular spaces. In acute cases small abscesses may develop, and, in very rare instances, complete suppuration of the epididymis with abscess of the testicle and scrotal wall has occurred. Scar tissue formation results in sterility in approximately 50 to 80 per cent of cases with extensive involvement.

Symptoms are marked pain and tenderness in one or both epididymides with or without fever. Acute hydrocele is a common complication. It is a self-limited disease, which usually recedes in severity after several days, followed by gradual recovery over one or two weeks. The residuum may be a slightly enlarged and indurated globus minor, with or without obstruction of the duct system.

Treatment up until a decade ago was directed mainly toward avoiding further prostatic massage, sexual intercourse, urethral instrumentations, and irrigations. In the acute stage, local treatment to the scrotum is essentially the same as that described for acute orchitis (see Orchitis). A wide variety of nonspecific local treatments have been used, but they are all of equivocal value. These include, among other measures, intravenous calcium gluconate, needling the epididymis, or incising the vas. Pain may be relieved temporarily by injecting the spermatic cord with Nupercaine, procaine, and other local anesthetics in which arterial spasm is reduced and the recovery phase aided. Modern treatment consists of penicillin administration, but if the lesion is unaffected by adequate dosages, careful search should be made for complicating factors such as urethral strictures, followed by trials with streptomycin, tetracycline, and Aureomycin, in that order. If these drugs also fail, it is likely that the epididymitis is not gonorrheal or that the antibiotics are not reaching the organisms in sufficient quantities because of abscess formation.

Nonspecific Epididymitis. This unscientific term denotes epididymitis not due to gonorrhea, tuberculosis, or any of the rare and unusual organisms. It occurs as a result of epididymal invasion by common pyogenic organisms such as staphylococci, colon bacilli, and occasionally streptococci. Nonspecific epididymitis is usually a complication of infected urine containing pyogenic bacteria, but in rare instances it is a metastatic infection from septic foci, such as pharyngitis and furunculosis. It appears in the course of urethral stricture, cystitis, prostatitis, and seminal vesiculitis and is not an uncommon complication of urethral instrumentations and operations. Straining, which may force infected material or urine into the lumen of the vas, is a precipitating factor. Young men undergoing strenuous physical exercise in the last war experienced localized, sometimes slightly painful or painless thickening in the epididymis, especially at the end of a day's exercise. Careful examination of the urethra, urinary tract, and prostate led to negative bacteriological results, making the etiology of this form of epididymitis obscure. In rare instances, epididymitis has been known to occur on occasion without any demonstrable inciting cause other than the reflux of sterile urine (Graves).

The incidence of nonspecific epididymitis has precipitously decreased in modern urological practice for three major reasons: (1) widespread use of antibiotics during the pre- and postoperative period; (2) rapid cure of gonorrhea without posterior urethritis; (3) use of a Foley (balloon) retention catheter, which eliminates obstruction of the urethra by constricting adhesive tape and the retention of exudate within the lumen.

Symptoms are essentially the same as those with gonococcal epididymitis. The degree of enlargement and tenderness is quite variable. It may be mild in the chronic state, and every urologist encounters patients in whom there is induration and slight enlargement of the globus minor and in whom there is only a faint memory of pain in the affected organ or none at all. It is probable that some cases of this indolent type are due to "specific" infections, such as tuberculosis and melitensis. So-called nonspecific epididymitis often assumes an acute course with suppuration, abscess formation, and extension into the testicle. In some cases the pathological picture is complicated by sperm invasion of the epididymal tissues and foreign body reaction to their presence (see Orchitis). Chronic epididymitis on rare occasions may progress to complete calcification and the formation of minute calculi. Accompanying hydrocele is common. In children, epididymitis is usually diagnosed as orchitis, but it can also be confused with torsion of the spermatic cord and strangulated congenital hernia. After the acute stage has subsided, a thorough search must be made for the initiating focus, especially investigating the genitourinary tract. Many cases result from chronic and sometimes asymptomatic prostatitis acquired earlier following gonorrhea or urinary tract infection in which pyogenic organisms remain as a residuum.

The local *treatment* of acute nonspecific epididymitis does not differ from that of the gonorrheal variety, in which rest, scrotal support (Fig. 776), and observation for abscess formation are of prime consideration. It does not respond to antibiotics as dramatically as does gonorrheal epididymitis. Penicillin is the drug of choice, and in acute cases large doses will usually relieve the pain, although the swelling may be slow to subside. Streptomycin, Aureomycin, Terramycin, and sulfa drugs, either alone or in various combinations, are used when the response to penicillin is unsatisfactory.

The chronic form may result in an annoying, painful condition. Subacute and chronic epididymitis are liable to episodes of recurrence, especially if there is associated infection in the prostate and seminal vesicles which cannot be readily eradicated or improved. Epididymectomy is the procedure of choice in such instances, provided fertility is not a consideration. Sterility, in any event, is almost an inevitable consequence.

Postoperative epididymitis complicating all varieties of prostatectomy and urethral catheterization deserves special comment. Patients may develop epididymitis weeks or months following operation, with subsequent episodes of recurrence. Besides discomfort, it leads to considerable morbidity, mental depression, general debility, and lack of ambulation, which in turn may lead to complications such as atelectasis, embolism, and pneumonia. There is also the economic aspect in the longer postoperative hospitalization. Epididymitis may be acute, subacute, chronic, and recurrent, and at times refractory to all antibiotics with progression to diffuse or localized abscess formation in the testis and scrotal wall. We promptly remove the epididymis in this age group under local anesthesia in any case not responding to antibiotics. If the testicle is involved, epididymo-orchiectomy should be performed. Prompt improvement usually follows such surgery, and hospitalization for the complication is lengthened only a few days.

The value of prophylactic vasectomy before surgery has been debated for the last half-century. Preoperative vasectomy is believed by most urologists to lower the incidence of epididymitis. With a completely divided vas, infection of the epididymis following operation could not take place through the lumen, and would therefore occur only by the more rare routes, such as metastatic and lymphatic or as a result of organisms already in the epididymis at the time of vasectomy.

The routine use of modern antibiotics and development of transurethral resection has unquestionably reduced the incidence of epididymitis from the former 20 to less than 4 per cent. If epididymitis does occur, it is likely to be less acute and a limited disease under the influence of antibiotics. Preoperative vasectomy should be done only in the absence of infected urine and before catheterization or instrumentation. The resulting sterility is usually not important in this age group.

Modern practice has reduced this complication in our own clinic to such a low magnitude that we believe preoperative vasectomy unnecessary. In the past three years, we have noted only 6 cases of postoperative epididymitis to occur in cases with uninfected urine on admission in a total of 903 prostatic operations of all types. In only 2 of the 6 cases was the epididymitis of enough severity to merit surgery, and prompt epididymectomy in these cases led to immediate recovery. We believe that the morbidity and disability in these 6 cases was far less than the sum total of expenditure of energy and time, had we done many hundreds of preoperative vasectomies. The latter is disturbing to the patient, requiring expense, sedation, and, furthermore, it is sometimes followed by hematoma, infection, and abscess formation (Hinman and Nesbit).

Traumatic epididymitis (sometimes epididymo-orchitis) has long been an enigma in urological practice. The question has revolved around whether traumatic epididymitis is a distinct clinical entity or whether the incidental trauma (injury to the epididymis or undue strain) has initiated a dormant infection already present either in the epididymis or from other previously infected genitourinary structures, such as the prostate. Another possibility is that the traumatic incident has only served to direct the patient's attention to an already existing chronic, asymptomatic epididymitis. Those who argue for an "entity" contend that the strain either forces urine back through the vas into the epididymis or else the trauma lessens the resistance of the tissues to infection from some distant focus. It has also been suggested that the infection may be due to saprophytic organisms which are normally present in the posterior urethra or seminal vesicles without pathological reaction but which become pathogenic when forced backward into the epididymis.

The relationship of trauma to the appearance of an epididymitis poses a difficult problem in relation to compensation. There is little doubt that on occasion sudden straining, tugging, or strenuous lifting can aggravate a pre-existing asymptomatic condition or else cause infections to extend to the epididymis from inflammation present in the prostatic urethra or prostate. Since causal relationship between trauma and this type of epididymitis seems definite, we have taken the attitude in this clinic that the degree of strain or trauma should be considered a vital point in the calculation of compensation. In instances of unusual trauma and excessive strain, we have assumed that epididymitis would not have necessarily occurred as a complication of the pre-existing infection without the superimposed trauma. In mild strain or trauma, it is our feeling that the benefit of doubt should be given to the employer.

Cases have been recorded of trauma to the scrotal contents in which no evidence of infection existed and surgical aspiration revealed no organisms. A thrombosis of the pampiniform plexus has been found (see Funiculitis) in a rare case. Instances have been described of acute fat necrosis following chronic trauma (bicycle riding) to the spermatic cord (see Funiculitis), and they may account for some obscure cases of scrotal trauma.

Specific Epididymitis. Besides the common pyogenic bacteria, a variety of well-known and sometimes rare organisms have infected the epididymis either by way of the metastatic route during a systemic infection or extension from a focus present in the genitourinary tract. An example of metastatic epididymitis is that occurring as a complication of meningococcal septicemia as well as with pneumococcal pneumonia. Blastomycosis has affected the epididymis on a number of occasions, either as a result of a systemic infection or, in a few cases in which the foci were unknown, with the patients only complaining of recurrent chronic epididymitis. Brucellosis of the epididymis (and also testicle) has been reported as occurring in 4 (abortus) to 20 (melitensis) per cent of individuals having undulant fever. Indeed, epididymitis of moderate severity may be the first sign of this disease. Brucellosis should be considered if epididymitis of obscure origin is accompanied by malaise and general systemic symptoms. Appropriate agglutination and skin tests with cultures of the urine and blood may clarify the diagnosis.

Epididymitis has been described by Coutts as a result of the virus of lymphogranuloma venereum. In these cases, it is usually an ascending infection from the prostate and seminal vesicles. The clinical findings are not dissimilar to tuberculous epididymitis, with necrosis of both the epididymis and testis and the formation of a scrotal sinus.

Almost every other known organism has at one time infected the epididymis, such as the bacillus of Friedländer, B. influenzae, various fungi (sporotrichosis), and parasites, such as amebae, schistosoma and filariasis (see Funiculitis). The general course of symptomatology recapitulates the symptomatology of either the acute, subacute, or chronic phase of the so-called nonspecific epididymitis. The pathology may vary from a diffuse inflammation to abscess formation with or without involvement of the testicle and sinus formation. Specific treatment is directed toward the underlying disease with the indicated antibiotic.

There are two forms of specific epididymitis which merit special comment: (a) syphilitic and (b) tuberculous.

Syphilitic Epididymitis. It is believed that syphilis of the epididymis occurs more frequently than is generally recognized by patients and physicians, because in the majority of cases there are no symptoms, and there is failure to examine the epididymis. Syphilitic epididymitis without orchitis may occur early in the secondary stage of the disease, or as late as eight or nine years following the onset. Congenital syphilitic epididymitis has been reported as early as two years of age. There is a diffuse thickening of the globus major of the epididymis, but in some cases rubbery nodules can be palpated. This form corresponds to the interstitial type of syphilitic orchitis and is insidious, indolent, and entirely asymptomatic. An acute painful type has been known to develop, not unlike the so-called nonspecific acute and subacute epididymitis, with the striking exception that it involves the globus major. Primary chronic gummatous epididymitis as a late tertiary lesion of the epididymis is extremely rare.

The diagnosis of syphilitic epididymitis is usually presumptive because other evidence of syphilis is present in the absence of urethritis, prostatitis, seminal vesiculitis, or urinary tract infection. Furthermore, all degrees of the above involvement disappear immediately on antiluetic treatment. An accompanying secondary symptomatic hydrocele is a frequent complication. Secondary extension into the epididymis from the testicle is a common complication of gummatous orchitis.

Tuberculous Epididymitis. The incidence of tuberculous epididymitis in the general male population has never been accurately assessed. Statistics as to epididymal tuberculous involvement have usually been a part of complicated data on the entire genitourinary tract. According to both Lowsley and Medlar, some part of the entire genitourinary tract is infected with tuberculosis in 2.1 to 3.1 per cent of all males coming to autopsy. In a healthy male population (Army) Chute found 0.003 per cent had some form of genitourinary tuberculosis. In patients dying of tuberculosis in a general hospital, Medlar has stated that 26 per cent had tuberculosis in some part of the genitourinary tract.

Tuberculous infection in the epididymis occurred in 0.8 per cent of Medlar's 5,424 male autopsies in a general hospital. In 5,476 males with known active tuberculosis, Borthwick made the clinical diagnosis of tuberculous epididymitis in 7.3 per cent. In 579 male autopsies of tuberculous deaths in the U. S. Army during World War II, Aronson found epididymal tuberculosis in 4 per cent. When the genitourinary tract is involved with tuberculosis, there is epididymal involvement in approximately 63 to 75 per cent. The incidence of tuberculous epididymitis is greater in the presence of extensive tuberculous lesions elsewhere in the body, especially in the kidneys.

Epididymal tuberculosis in only a part of constitutional tuberculosis. In Borthwick's series of 402 cases of tuberculosis epididymitis in a sanatorium, the disease was present elsewhere in the body in 88.3 per cent, while in the remaining 11.7 per cent no search for foci was made. When epididymal involvement is present, Medlar found tuberculosis of the lungs in 74.8 per cent of his autopsy cases, while clinical studies have revealed pulmonary disease in 30 to 50 per cent. The kidneys are involved in practically all cases of genitourinary tract tuberculosis, with the prostate and seminal vesicles second, and the epididymis last in the order of incidence.

It has been concluded from such data that tuberculous epididymitis always implies renal tuberculosis. There is strong evidence that the primary focus in the genitourinary tract originates in the kidneys. Sixty per cent of all genitourinary tuberculosis is limited solely to the kidneys, while in the other 40 per cent with genital tract tuberculosis 73 per cent have also obvious renal tuberculosis. It is highly probable that healed renal lesions could be found in the remaining cases of genital tract involvement if serial sections were made. In 44 cases of tuberculous epididymitis studies at autopsy, Medlar found no instance without renal involvement, and the prostate or seminal vesicles were found to be infected in 63 per cent.

When genital tract tuberculosis is present alone, either the prostate or seminal vesicles or usually both are involved in 100 per cent of the cases, while the epididymis is infected in only 62 per cent. In autopsies of soldiers dying of tuberculosis, Aronson found that involvement of the kidney occurred 10 times more frequently and involvement of the prostate 4 times more frequently than that of the epididymis. Further clinical evidence indicating that tuberculous epididymitis represents a late development in genitourinary tract tuberculosis has been ascertained recently by Borthwick. He selected 200 male patients with pulmonary and other forms of tuberculosis in whom, on careful examination, there was no evidence of tuberculous epididymitis. In 30 of these, or 15 per cent, a definite diagnosis of tuberculous prostatitis could be made even though no symptoms existed. In the succeeding year, 12 of these patients with tuberculous prostatitis developed epididymitis. The preponderance of modern evidence indicates that epididymitis is a later manifestation of established tuberculous disease, which in the case of epididymitis is always present in the kidney and likely in the prostate or seminal vesicles. Urological literature in the past is replete with the argument as to whether the epididymis is the primary focus in the genital tract, with secondary extension to the prostate and seminal vesicles or, conversely, whether the epididymis is secondarily infected from the latter, as contended by Hugh Young. The pathogenesis indicates a primary tuberculous bacilluria in the vast majority of cases. The prostate and epididymis may be infected at the same time from this bacilluria or the epididymis may become involved at a later date. The epididymal infection probably occurs from a retrograde flow of infected urine through the lumen of the vas, but lymphatic spread or contiguous infection through the wall or sheath of the vas from prostatic infection may also account for a rare case.

Tuberculous epididymitis is essentially a disease of young manhood and middle life, although it is by no means a rarity in children. It has occurred within the first few months of life, usually accompanied by a hydrocele which may mask the underlying indolent condition. The clinical course is one of considerable variety. It is occasionally ushered in with an abrupt onset of pain, swelling and tenderness, with redness of the scrotal skin just as in gonococcal or pyogenic epididymitis. Most cases develop gradually with little tenderness or pain. Indeed, many patients have an early enlargement of the epididymis without any symptoms or recognition until it is discovered in the course of a general medical examination. In Medlar's autopsy series the tuberculous nature of the epididymis was not suspected clinically in 55 per cent of the cases, as there was no complaint directed to the epididymides. Undoubtedly, many cases of tuberculous epididymitis are mistaken for chronic nonspecific infections. Besides the acute and insidious forms, some run a middle clinical course in which there are episodes of slight enlargement and tenderness. About 60 per cent of the latter have mild or aching pain radiating to the groin.

The progress of the disease varies greatly, depending upon the general resistance of the patient, the extensiveness of the primary process elsewhere, and the virulence of the organism. Tuberculous orchitis as a primary infection is extremely rare, but practically all tuberculous epididymitis eventually involves the testicle with caseation at a later stage in the disease. It has been estimated that the testicle is infected in 60 per cent of cases within six months and in 85 per cent within twelve months following onset of the epididymitis.

Tuberculous lesions in the epididymis microscopically do not differ from those encountered elsewhere in the body. The pathological findings reveal destruction of normal tissue and its replacement by caseous material and scar tissue (Fig. 338). The process may be dormant for long periods of time, only to gradually progress to subacute and acute stages. It usually begins in the globus minor and later extends to the entire epididymis and testicle (Fig. 338). The vas deferens is usually involved either as a firm, smooth cord, or it may be slightly beaded especially near the epididymis. Coexisting hydrocele is not uncommon. It is unilateral when discovered in about two thirds of cases, with the opposite epididymis showing involvement in 75 per cent of cases within twelve months and 100 per cent within 108 months (Borthwick).

The diagnosis is usually suspected by the history of a slowly increasing, relatively painless, and nontender epididymal mass which on examination is indurated, slightly irregular, and firm. With caseation, one or more scrotal fistulae may occur. Cutaneous fistulae formerly occurred in as high as 70 per cent of cases. The resistance of the body in genital tuberculosis is undergoing considerable change so that extensive caseation and fistulae are becoming less frequent. Indeed, two decades ago at two local sanatoria of approximately 400 male beds, there were always patients with tuberculous epididymo-orchitis with fistulae and caseation, whereas at this date there is not a single patient with clinical evidence of any active epididymitis on the wards. This apparent reduction may be only a part of increased general resistance to tuberculosis, but it also may be due to the fact that pulmonary infection is treated much earlier, both by surgery and streptomycin, with the result that there is less chance for this later complication to occur.

Treatment. Any treatment of tuberculous epididymitis should begin with a full awareness of the tuberculous processes elsewhere in the body.* This entails a search for all possible foci, especially in the kidneys. Specific measures consist of streptomycin and para-amino salicylic acid. Streptomycin has been generally unsuccessful in curing epididymitis and orchitis. An occasional sinus tract will close under streptomycin therapy with some reduction in the induration, but the underlying infection is not eradicated, with almost surely a recurrence of activity later. Tuberculous epididymitis does not tend to undergo the fibrous reaction necessary to healing that inherently occurs in the prostate and to some extent in early renal lesions. Its response to modern antibiotics is far inferior to results of treatment in these organs and elsewhere. Neomycin in its present form is too toxic an agent to prove valuable. In a few instances the use of Thiosemicarbazone (TB-1)

* The clinical and therapeutic aspects of tuberculosis of the urinary tract are discussed in Section V, Chapter 2, and of the prostate and seminal vesicles in Section VI, Chapter 2.

has been reported as successful, but it is too early to appraise the permanency of the results. Isoniazid is also reported to be of value in the treatment of genital tuberculosis and is currently being investigated.

Conservative surgical methods include simple epididymectomy with removal of the vas deferens to the level of the external ring, epididymo-orchiectomy when the testicle is involved, and radical incision of sinus tracts which may have appeared. Such surgical extirpation may be combined with removal of an infected kidney and, in rare cases, the removal of an infected prostate and seminal tract. Because of the rarity of spontaneous healing in the epididymis, even with antibiotics, surgical extirpation is distinctly the treatment of choice in this condition. The resulting sterility is of secondary importance to elimination of a disease, which may be a hazard to life. Eventual loss of the testicle is possible in any event.

The greatest value of streptomycin has been as an adjunct to surgery. Patients occasionally develop tuberculous meningitis following simple epididymectomy in spite of greatest care with surgical manipulation. We had two patients die of this complication ten years ago, but in one recent case streptomycin was promptly administered, and the patient recovered from an early meningitis. It is imperative to remove the epididymis under the influence of streptomycin, and it is our policy to administer the drug for one to two weeks preliminary to surgery. Prophylactic vasectomy is always advisable on the uninvolved side and should include not only the vas but the surrounding sheath. Some urologists believe that it is important to carry out prophylactic epididymectomy, because even with vas ligation epididymitis will occasionally develop later, probably as a result of an unrecognized focus of infection present in the epididymis at the time of the ligation.

DEFERENTITIS AND FUNICULITIS

Inflammation of the spermatic cord may primarily involve either the vas or one of the other major structures of the cord (vessels, lymphatics, and connective tissue). In many instances all or a combination of these structures are involved. Acute, subacute, and chronic inflammations may be encountered without evidence of disease elsewhere in the genital tract, but the vast majority of infections of the spermatic cord result as a complication of prostatitis, seminal vesiculitis, and especially infections of the epididymis and testicle (see Epididymitis). The infectious process reaches the cord from the above organs either through the lumen of the vas or by way of the lymphatics, although in rare instances funiculitis is a metastatic process from disease elsewhere in the body.

Before modern antibiotics, gonococcal vasitis caused the greatest number of cases. This produces tenderness of the vas usually in association with gonococcal prostatitis, seminal vesiculitis, and epididymitis. Rare instances have been reported in which solitary gonococcal abscess formations have occurred in the cord without epididymitis but with evidence (induration) of infection in the ampulla of the vas. The most common infectious process today in the spermatic cord is vasitis following trauma or operative procedures to the prostate and posterior urethra. Most funicular infections are due to the ordinary pyogenic organisms. Several categories of acute inflammation of the spermatic cord constitute clinical entities worthy of recording.

Deferentitis, or inflammation restricted to the vas deferens, as a segmental infection unassociated with infections elsewhere in the genital tract, is rare, but has been reported on a number of occasions. Usually there develops a variably tender, indurated, fibrous, and nodular enlargement of the vas from the epididymis to the inguinal area. The surgical exploration and removal of chronic segmental lesions in certain cases has revealed the presence of tuberculosis. Some segmental lesions have been known to appear with gonococcal urethritis and to disappear with treatment and improvement in the latter. *Granulomas* of the spermatic cord and testis have been recognized following trauma and vas ligation. They occur as a painful mass in the cord resulting from the extravasation or penetration of sperm into the tissues, around which a histologic reaction containing giant cells develops. *Vasitis nodosa* has recently been described by Benjamin as a peculiar beading and nodularity involving the vas deferens just above the epididymis. These tiny, firm nodules on the wall of the vas show epithelial-lined spaces. They are probably the result of a previously unrecognized vasitis of unknown origin.

Funiculitis generally refers to inflammations of the tissues of the cord except the vas deferens. It should be stressed that most acute inflammations, especially tuberculosis and pyogenic infections associated with epididymitis, frequently involve all tissues of the cord and especially the lymphatics. Funiculitis may be acute, subacute, or chronic, and there are several well known varieties. *Endemic funiculitis* has been thoroughly reviewed recently by Paul. It is an entity which has been known since the eighteenth century and on occasions has been epidemic in character. This acute inflammation occurs as a cellulitis of the cord. It may be associated with fever and symptoms of general toxemia; however, in other instances the symptoms are extremely mild. There is slight thickening and induration of the cord which may progress to a size several inches in diameter and in which abscess formation and necrosis occurs. In subacute and chronic cases the cord contains fibrous nodules. The pathological findings are striking, consisting of thrombosis of the veins in the pampiniform plexus, sometimes with pus formation. The testicle, epididymis, and other tissues of the cord where infections ordinarily occur are usually normal. The vas in these cases, as a rule, cannot be palpated because it is obscured by the general enlargement of the entire spermatic cord. The etiology is entirely unknown, but from incomplete bacteriological studies it is thought to be a streptococcus. This type of funiculitis occurs sporadically in temperate climates. We have observed one case in which there was a fusiform tender enlargement of the entire spermatic cord without epididymitis, prostatitis, or infection in the urinary tract or elsewhere. In our case, administration of modern antibiotics resulted in immediate resolution, and no insight as to the etiology was gained.

Filarial funiculitis is essentially a disease of the lymphatics and may take one of several forms and clinical courses, depending upon the degree of secondary infection and whether or not the patient is subject to continual reinoculation with filaria.* There may be a secondary hydrocele containing the parasites, and at times involvement of the testicle and epididymis is present. Late changes as a rule in the testicle, epididymis, and spermatic cord do not always occur in well developed scrotal elephantiasis because of the difference between testicular and scrotal lymphatic drainage. This funiculitis is characterized by swollen semi-solid masses in which alive or

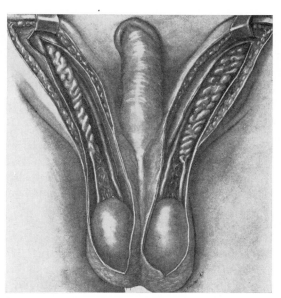

Fig. 340. Filarial funiculitis, illustrating asymptomatic lymphangectasia in the spermatic cord discovered at operation for hernia. The soft structures exuded lymph on rupture. Probable diagnosis was filariasis with lymphatic obstruction but without secondary infection and concomitant fibrosis. (Courtesy of Dr. Bradley L. Coley and the Amer. J. Surg.)

dead parasites can often be found. Funiculitis due to filarial infections when seen in this country takes one of three forms:

(1) The first is somewhat similar to lymph scrotum (see Lymph Scrotum) in that the enlarged lymphatics in the spermatic cord are either discovered at operation (Fig. 340) or can be palpated as soft compressible vessels. They differ from varicocele by the absence of the blue appearance, and if interrupted they contain opalescent milky fluid (lymph).

(2) The cord may contain thick and rubbery masses without any history of previous recurrent lymphangitis, funiculitis, or indications of filaria infection. This type is evidently a later manifestation of the earlier form mentioned above in which the parasite is probably dead. Young and others have described cases in which there were fibrous and nodular enlargement throughout the spermatic cord distinct from the vas deferens. The patients usually complain of a lump in the scrotum, and in most cases the epididymis, testicle and vas deferens are normal. Most of these patients usually give

* Urogenital filariasis is also discussed by Dr. Sanjurjo in Section V, Chapter 3. (Ed.)

a history of having lived in tropical areas. Because of the wide dispersion of young men in our population during the last war, any chronic induration in the spermatic cord and groin must be considered as possibly filarial in nature. At this date enough time has passed since the original infestation to expect such late manifestations. They may be accentuated by secondary infection superimposed on a damaged lymphatic system in the spermatic cord, even though the original parasites have died as a result of the pathological reactions that they stimulated in the tissue. Eosinophilia and a positive intradermal skin test (see Mumu) may be diagnostic.

(3) Mumu is considered a definite clinical entity and is probably filarial in nature. During the last war a number of our troops in filarial areas developed a syndrome characterized by swelling and "doughy" edema of the spermatic cord (95 per cent of cases). It is sometimes accompanied by swelling of the scrotum, epididymis (53 per cent), and testicle (15 per cent), and the appearance of a hydrocele. The swelling is definitely of the centrifugal type, appearing first in the inguinal canal and within twelve hours spreading to the region of the epididymis. The cord is greatly swollen, rubbery, tender, and approximately the size of a finger. Each acute episode is liable to be followed by recurrent attacks which gradually subside in one or more years after leaving the endemic areas. The concept of this disease is that it is an allergic manifestation which develops following inoculation by filaria. Most textbook descriptions of filariasis only describe the late manifestations of the disease. The demonstrable damage is usually negligible although 23 cases with permanent changes are recorded in army personnel. In the few pathological specimens obtained there is only diffuse edema and cellular infiltration of the spermatic cord, epididymis, and testis. The lymphatic vessels were thickened, dilated, and surrounded by leukocytes and eosinophils. No parasites have been seen on tissue biopsies or examination of the hydrocele fluid. Filaremia is absent in Mumu and was rare in the troops in these areas. Positive skin tests to intradermal injections with the antigen Dirofilaria immitis extract have produced a similar lymphangitis. It remains to be determined whether further pathologic changes will be encountered by urologists in the spermatic cord and other scrotal structures in later years in individuals with this variety of funiculitis.

Lymphogranuloma venereum funiculitis has been encountered on a few occasions. It is usually a retrograde lymphatic involvement of the cord, apparently from infection of the deep iliac nodes by this virus. In the largest number of instances, the vas along with the other structures of the cord is involved. There is also a peculiar and characteristic involvement of the veins and arteries of the cord which are evidently secondarily infected by passage of the virus through the wall of the primary lymphangitis.

Syphilitic funiculitis is a rare disease, there being only 7 acceptable cases up to 1920. It occurs four to nine years following the primary lesions and is characterized by irregular masses in the spermatic cord, having the firm and elastic consistency of gumma. There is not anything pathognomonic of this condition, and the diagnosis can only be suspected with the findings of syphilis elsewhere in the body and the rapid disappearance of the tumors after the application of specific antiluetic therapy.

Spontaneous Thrombosis of the Pampiniform Plexus. The signs and symptoms of acute thrombosis of the veins of the pampiniform plexus resemble those of subacute or acute endemic funiculitis. McGavin reported three cases in 1935, in which there was a history of sudden pain in the scrotum, following which the spermatic cord became enlarged with palpable nodules. The etiology is unknown.

Disorders involving the arteries in the spermatic cord have been observed. Buerger and Mathé have described thrombo-angiitis obliterans of the internal spermatic artery resulting in partial infarction of the testicle. In most cases this disease involves the spermatic artery alone without affecting the veins. The degree of the infarct in the testicle is unpredictable. Acute fat necrosis of the cord following mild constant trauma has been recognized by Hinman. A lumpy mass which can be palpated distinct from the testes and vas, develops in the cord. They are resorbed in a few weeks.

INFECTIONS OF THE TUNICS

In most instances the tunics become directly infected from an underlying epididymitis, epididymo-orchitis, or funiculitis. An acute secondary or symptomatic hydrocele usually develops, which later becomes inflamed. All degrees of inflammation of the interior of the tunica cavity have been encountered. The contents may vary from clear fluid which contains only a few lymphocytes to that in which the tunica vaginalis is filled with frank pus (pyocele). Infection may occur as a result of a wide variety of organisms, including syphilis, but more commonly from tuberculosis, gonorrhea, and the ordinary pyogenic bacteria causing epididymitis. The symptoms depend upon the intensity of the infection and the nature of the process. Pain and tenderness may be absent in purulent accumulations within the tunica from tuberculous and syphilitic epididymitis. When a preexisting hydrocele becomes secondarily infected, the hydrocele fluid ceases to transluminate, and it usually becomes tense to palpation. In cases where the process is self-limited or resolves as a result of antibiotic therapy, there is a late hypertrophy of the wall of the tunica. The cavity may become obliterated by fibrinous adhesions with rigid walls. Fibrinous bodies may be formed and discovered subsequently at operation.

Treatment is by proper recognition of the underlying disease and the application of the indicated antibiotic. We do not hesitate to aspirate acute hydroceles, and on rare occasion surgical drainage may be necessary. This usually relieves the symptoms, permits a more complete examination of the scrotal contents, and aids in recovery. *Any infected tunica surgically explored should be drained.* With removal of the infected epididymis or testis, the process in the tunica vaginalis becomes self-limited and proceeds to rapid healing. It must be remembered that in children acute infections of the hydrocele cavity may result from the extension of a peritonitis through a patent processus funicularis (congenital hydrocele) or, by the same mechanism, a peritonitis may develop as a result of extension from an infected tunica vaginalis.

A vegetative type of proliferous periorchitis of the tunics has been known since the time of Virchow. In this condition, the lining of the tunica is studded with vegetative papillary-like growths, which on pathological study are composed of fibro-hyaline tissue which sometimes becomes calcified. These lesions represent the end result of a chronic inflammation, especially following chronic gonorrheal epididymitis.

OTHER SCROTAL CONDITIONS
HYDROCELE

A hydrocele may be defined as an accumulation of serous fluid greater in amount than the few drops normally present within the two layers of the

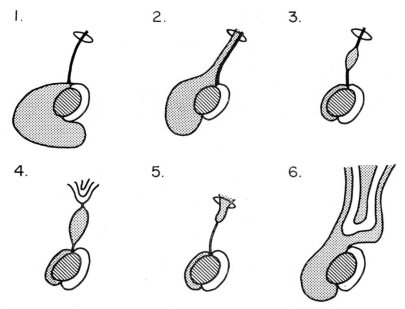

Fig. 341.   Hydrocele: 1. Simple hydrocele. 2. Congenital hydrocele. 3. Hydrocele of the cord. 4. Hydrocele of cord with hernia. 5. Hydrocele (cord) of a congenital hernia. 6. Hydrocele with hernial sac.

tunica vaginalis (Figs. 341, 342). As the testis descends from its retro-peritoneal position in the abdominal cavity to its final site in the scrotum, it carries with it two layers of the peritoneum. The portion which covers the testis and epididymis proper is known as the visceral layer of the tunica vaginalis, while the portion in contact with the interior of the scrotum and continuous with the visceral layer is termed the parietal layer. The communication between the tunica vaginalis and the peritoneal cavity becomes a small canal known as the processus funicularis, which before or soon after birth becomes atresic, thus closing the connection with the abdominal cavity. Abnormalities of these coverings and of the funicular process lead to the several varieties of hydrocele (see Congenital Hydrocele, Section IV).

The incidence of hydrocele has never been determined, but it is a common urological finding. It is said to be present in 1 per cent of all male admissions to general hospitals. In tropical countries it is far more common in occurrence (7.5 per cent of males), probably as a result of parasitic disease and the greater instances of lymphangitis, epididymitis, and orchitis. It is encountered at all ages, but 90 per cent occurs after the age of 21.

Forms of Hydrocele. (1) *Hydrocele of the Testis:* The most common type of hydrocele is the *simple hydrocele* of the testis, in which the normally formed tunica vaginalis is distended with fluid (Fig. 341, *1*). It usually appears as a pyriform or globular mass. Another type of hydrocele of the testis is the so-called *infantile hydrocele,* in which the fingerlike funicular process has failed to close. In these cases, the processus funicularis remains open and extends to various levels, even to the internal ring; however, the upper end is closed, and there is no communication with the peritoneal cavity. Hydrocele of the testis may exist in the *congenital form,* in which the processus funicularis has a small lumen communicating with the abdominal cavity (Fig. 341, *2*). In this type, the fluid in the tunica may ascend or can be forced upward into the peritoneal cavity. *Inguinal hydrocele* is very much like a simple hydrocele of the testis, with the exception that the testis is undescended, and its position may be within the inguinal canal or in the pubic area. In this respect, hydrocele has been known to occur in intra-abdominal testes.

Rare types of localized hydroceles have been known to occur, involving either a portion of the epididymis or testis. The posterior surface of the testis and epididymis has no tunica covering. At the point of the reflection of the tunics, small encysted serous cavities have been known to develop. They are termed *encysted hydroceles* of the epididymis or of the testis. Accumulations of fluid have been known to occur between the visceral layer of the tunica vaginalis and the underlying tunica albuginea of the testis.

(2) *Hydrocele of the Cord.* Hydrocele may occur as a collection of fluid in an encysted sac of peritoneum localized in the cord (Fig. 341, *3*). These fluid-containing sacs are usually long, oval, or fusiform in shape and lie in the upper portion of the scrotum or inguinal canal. They are closed at each end, without communication with either the tunica vaginalis or peritoneal cavity.

(3) *Hernial Hydrocele.* An accumulation of fluid within the tunica vaginalis may be associated with inguinal hernia in several different ways. In one type there is merely a small and limited projection of the processus funicularis into the scrotum (Fig. 341, *5*). This closed hernial pouch terminates above the testis and does not communicate with the tunica vaginalis surrounding the latter. Bowel and omentum are usually not present in this sac because of its small lumen, but the communication with the general peritoneal cavity is apparent because as a rule the hydrocele fluid can easily be expressed back into the peritoneum. In this type there is an impulse and

hernial defect in the structures within the inguinal canal. Another variety is that in which a large communication exists between the cavity of the tunica vaginalis and the peritoneal cavity. This is actually a complete congenital hernia, in which bowel and omentum have descended partially into the scrotum, with fluid present distal to the bowel in the cavity of the processus vaginalis below (Fig. 341, 6).

(4) *Combination Hydroceles.* There are a number of combinations of the above described hydroceles such as a simple hydrocele of the testis associated with an inguinal hernia. Another example is simple hydrocele of the testis associated with hydrocele of the cord, without communication between the two. Hydrocele of the cord may also occur with an inguinal hernia in which the peritoneal or hernial pouch above does not communicate with the hydrocele of the cord (Fig. 341, 4). The true situation in these combined types can usually be discerned after careful examination of the patient in the upright and supine positions. It may be difficult in infants to determine the exact combination because of the small size of the structures.

Etiology. Hydroceles have been classified with regard to etiology into symptomatic (or secondary) and idiopathic (or primary). The symptomatic may be acute or chronic, while the idiopathic is always chronic in character.

Acute symptomatic hydrocele is frequently a complication of orchitis or epididymitis. It results also from generalized disease processes such as typhoid fever, febrile reactions, and cardiovascular insufficiency. Trauma not infrequently results in an acute hydrocele. In this respect, hydroceles often occur and may persist for several days or weeks in the newborn following obstetrical trauma. In acute symptomatic hydrocele, the fluid may be admixed with fibrinous, purulent, or hemorrhagic material, depending upon the underlying disease. The fluid, after the acute stage of the hydrocele has subsided, may gradually disappear or it may not be absorbed, leading to a chronic, symptomatic hydrocele. Therapeutic aspiration after the acute stage, followed by rest and elevation of the scrotum may expedite absorption and lead to cure.

The chronic form of symptomatic hydrocele is usually secondary to any chronic pathological process in the epididymis, testis, or spermatic cord. Tuberculosis, nonspecific epididymitis, syphilis, and malignant tumors have often resulted in insidious accumulations of fluid within the tunica vaginalis. Chronic hydrocele is common in the Far East and in many instances results from filarial infestations.

The greater majority of hydroceles are the so-called "idiopathic" or primary variety. They develop slowly, without evidence of pre-existing disease of the genital or urinary tract. Regardless of this fact, it is thought by most urologists that the etiology is based upon some undisclosed or healed infectious process. Shah has concluded that there is no direct etiologic relationship to climate, diet, nutrition, or occupation. There is some evidence of obscure relationship between trauma and chronic idiopathic hydroceles. For example, in the East, certain tribes prone to hydrocele formation wear a type of loin cloth (dhoti) which may result in constant mild trauma to the scrotum. Shah has studied the pathology in 15 instances of chronic idiopathic hydrocele and states that biopsy shows evidence of chronic inflammation in the subserous layers of the tunica. These changes may be a result of repeated trauma. Hydroceles often follow known trauma and especially herniorrhaphy, involving manipulation of the cord. They may also appear as a complication of varicocelectomy or any other scrotal operation. They are not uncommon after the use of trusses to correct a hernia. Because of the appreciable incidence of hydrocele occurring after surgery, *a prophylactic hydrocelectomy should be performed in all intrascrotal operations.* Allen has concluded from a study of the parietal tunica removed at operation or autopsy that there is a congenital lymphatic defect associated with hydrocele formation. There is evidently a constant changing of the fluid in all such serous cavities, with a balance between secretion and absorption. In hydrocele formation, there is either an overproduction or fluid or an impairment of resorption due to insufficiency of the lymphatics. It is felt that spontaneous disappearance of congenital hydrocele occurs with later development and accelerated function of the lymphatic system. Winsbury-White and Posner feel that idiopathic hydroceles in older men are distinctly associated with prostatic hypertrophy, but there is no conclusive evidence to support this assumption.

Pathology. In symptomatic hydrocele, secondary to chronic infection, the contained fluid usually has a higher specific gravity, and in some cases it is an inflammatory exudate of varying degrees. In acutely infected cases, the fluid may be cloudy or brownish in color, especially if hemorrhage has occurred.

The fluid in uninfected idiopathic hydroceles is clear, amber in color, and resembles blood plasma. It is neutral in reaction and has a specific gravity of from 1.010 to 1.025, which is indicative of an exudate rather than a transudate. The albumin content varies from 3 to 6 per cent with total proteins varying from 4.0 to 6.3 per cent. The fluid contains electrolytes, fibrinogens, cholesterol and usually a few lymphocytes and epithelial cells. Fibrous plaques are frequently found on the walls of the tunica. Hydrocele fluid may also contain free bodies composed of fibrin. In some instances, complete calcification of the tunica has been reported. The latter can be diagnosed by the presence of crepitation upon palpation and confirmed by x-ray.

In hydroceles of long duration, the tunica may be 0.5 cm. in thickness, especially when the underlying process is epididymitis or orchitis, present for some time. Formation of fibrin in idiopathic hydroceles may result in adhesions between the two layers of the tunica, which in some cases results in multilocular cyst formation. Atrophy is not uncommonly found in association with hydroceles. It is probable that a greatly thickened tunica vaginalis may by exerting pressure interfere with the circulation within the testis. The atrophy also may be due to a disturbance in the heat-regulating mechanism or to increased tension of the hydrocele fluid.

The *symptoms* of hydrocele depend upon the size of the mass and the amount of tension created by the fluid within the sac. Slowly forming hydroceles are usually painless until they reach sufficient size and weight so as to pull on the spermatic cord. They can produce a dull ache or pulling sensation when the patient is in the upright position. Fluid which accumulates rapidly as a result of underlying inflammatory process is usually accompanied by considerable tension in the parietal tunic and severe pain. Large hydroceles may partially obstruct urination and make catheterization difficult. As much as five gallons of hydrocele fluid has been found in a single case.

Diagnosis. Diagnosis is usually simple in the adult. Unless very large, hydroceles occur as a pear-shaped mass, with the smaller end located in the upper part of the scrotum. They are smooth, elastic, and feel cystic on palpation. An outstanding characteristic is translucency, except in cases in which

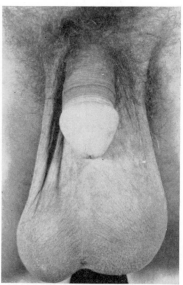

Fig. 342. Hydrocele. Left hydrocele of moderate size with the testicle in a posterior and somewhat inferior position. The cystic hydrocele mass above the testicle was translucent to light.

the parietal tunica has become so thickened that it no longer transmits light. The testicle is situated in the posterior and lower portion of the hydrocele cavity (Fig. 342). The differentiation of hydrocele from hernia may be difficult if the hernia cannot be reduced. In such instances, bowel sounds may be present on auscultation, and the mass may be tympanitic at certain points. In infants, with either a congenital or infantile type, there are no sure signs that will differentiate hydrocele from congenital hernia. An inguinal impulse on straining and coughing or a history of a disappearing swelling is strongly suggestive of hernia.

Hydrocele may be confused with spermatocele, chyloceles, hematocele, and solid tumors of the testis such as malignant growths, and gumma. In chylocele and hematocele, the contents are not translucent to light. Hematocele may be associated with the presence of cutaneous ecchymoses. Without diagnostic aspiration, these cannot be differentiated in the case of a thickened tunica. Spermatocele is usually easy to differentiate unless it is extremely large, in which case it may coexist with hydroceles. Spermatoceles are usually distinct masses situated above and behind the testis, with an attachment to the region of the upper pole of the epididymis. Solid tumors do not have an elastic or resilient sensation to palpation. Gumma does not transilluminate light and is usually more doughy to palpation. Chylocele is more likely to be associated with changes in the inguinal nodes and with elephantiasic changes in the scrotal skin.

Diagnostic aspiration was formerly advocated with caution because of inducing hemorrhage, secondary infection, or the possibility of puncturing a malignant tumor, inflammatory process, or the bowel in the case of hernia. With modern antibiotics and aseptic technique, there should be little chance of introducing infection. Diagnostic aspiration in obviously cystic conditions has served readly to differentiate hydrocele from large spermatoceles, hematocele, or chylocele, and we do not hesitate to employ this procedure in instances in which it is difficult to establish a correct diagnosis.

Treatment of Hydrocele. Treatment of acute secondary or symptomatic hydrocele is either palliative or aspirative. The patient should be at bed rest. Elevation of the scrotum for improvement of circulation and relief of pain may be indicated. Aspiration is used in acute hydrocele for the relief of pain or for the procurement of fluid, to clarify the diagnosis by allowing palpation of the scrotal contents. In the hydrocele of mumps orchitis and other forms of orchitis, aspiration is said to be helpful in preventing testicular atrophy. The course of acute hydrocele is usually a reflection of the underlying inflammatory process in the testis or epididymis. If the infection is acute, proper antibiotics are indicated for any underlying disease.

Treatment of chronic hydrocele may be (a) general, (b) aspiration, (c) aspiration and injection of sclerosing agents, and (d) surgical.

(a) The older general treatments for chronic hydrocele, such as vaccines and nonspecific protein therapy as well as subcutaneous injection into the patient of fluid aspirated from the hydrocele, are all a matter of history and for practical purposes are not worth recording.

(b) Aspiration is often curative in young children during the first year of age, but one must be sure that no hernia is present. Aspiration in the adult results in reaccumulation of fluid within several months. Aspiration. in general, is a palliative procedure and rarely leads, except in the young. to cure of the hydrocele.

(c) Aspiration and injection of sclerosing solutions is a treatment of choice by many. It has been tried for many centuries, and a variety of solutions including port wine, ether, chloroform, mercury and silver nitrate have been used. In the last two decades, correctly performed aspiration and injection has led to cure in approximately 90 to 95 per cent of cases. In the idiopathic variety, Ewell experienced no recurrences in sclerosing 179 hydroceles. Injection therapy is best performed with either sodium morrhuate or quinine hydrochloride and urethane. We have used the latter with a satisfactory degree of success, although most patients at our clinic come from long distances and prefer to have their hydrocele operated on and cured at one visit. The objection to sclerosing treatment of hydrocele is that success is not always obtained with one injection. This is especially true if the walls of the hydrocele cavity are very thick, i.e., as in symptomatic hydrocele. The 5 per cent sodium morrhuate employed is more painful and apparently more irritating than the quinine and urethane. If this substance is preferred, the tunica can be anesthetized by a preliminary injection of 2 per cent procaine.

The technique of the sclerosing procedure is simple and is as follows: A 1 per cent procaine solution is used to make a weal on the anterior upper aspect of the scrotal skin, because the testis usually resides posteriorly near the bottom of the scrotum. An aspirating needle is carefully directed downward through the anesthetized skin until the hydrocele cavity is entered. The fluid is gently expressed so as to remove as much as possible, thus not allowing dilution of the sclerosing solution. One to four cubic centimeters of quinine urethane (quinine 13.33 per cent, urethane 6.66 per cent) is slowly injected, following which the scrotum is thoroughly massaged to distribute the solution throughout the cavity. The patient is then sent home with a rather firm suspensory. There is usually only mild discomfort. It is felt that the solution of quinine hydrochloride and urethane is only a mild irritant and is more ideal for the treatment of hydrocele rather than a true sclerosing solution. With such a relatively mild irritant, there is formation of fibrous tissue beneath the surface of the intact tunica. According to examination of the tunics at a later date following successful injection treatment, this combination evidently does not produce a reaction in the mesothelial lining of such a magnitude as to result in fibrous union between the opposed surfaces. This solution probably interferes with or depresses the fluid-forming function of the tunica so that the imbalance between excess formation and absorption is counteracted. The fluid usually reaccumulates in the tunica vaginalis along with some edema of the scrotal skin following this procedure. It should again be aspirated at the end of each week for three to four weeks, with reinjection each visit. Less fluid accumulates after each injection. Following this, the patient is then seen every few weeks until a decision can be reached whether subsequent injections are necessary. With careful aseptic technique, there should be no infection introduced. Considerable reaction may occur if the solution is injected outside the tunics and into the tissues.

If the hydrocele is secondary to an active inflammatory process, the use of sclerosing solutions is *not* indicated because of the possibility of igniting a quiescent infection. This form of therapy is contraindicated with demonstrable hernia and especially in children in which an open processus funicularis may communicate with the general peritoneal cavity. We reserve this method of treatment for patients who refuse surgery or in instances in which hospitalization is impossible or economically not feasible. It is also valuable in senile patients and in those with severe cardiovascular disease, where any surgical procedure is contraindicated. The advantages of this therapy have at times been offset by the occurrence of transient orchitis or epididymitis. This may be due to injury to the testis by the needle. Swelling of the testicle commonly follows such an injection, but it is probably reaction in and beneath the tunica and not, as formerly thought, epididymo-orchitis. Some urologists have felt that the injection treatment of hydrocele might lead to the overlooking of some existing pathology, such as tuberculous epididymitis and malignancy of the testicle. Hydrocele rarely occurs with malignancy, but careful palpation of the scrotal contents after aspiration should lead to suspicion of a tumor or other pathology. If such is found, injection therapy should be abandoned, and surgical exploration is recommended. Cases have also been reported in which there was abnormal sensitivity to quinine, but in these cases sodium morrhuate can be substituted.

(d) Surgical excision of hydrocele has become popular with the development of modern antibiotics and asepsis, and present-day operations are followed by almost uniform success. Many operative techniques have been devised over the past several centuries for the radical cure of hydrocele, but in general only two are now favored (see Section XV, Chapter 12). The first is the Andrews or so-called *"bottle" operation.* Local anesthesia is satisfactory in this procedure. The tunica vaginalis is exposed and incised in the upper scrotum. After evacuating the fluid, the parietal tunica is carefully everted around the cord. The cut edges of the tunica, which have been passed upward around the cord, are next secured with one or more sutures. None of the everted tunica is removed. This operation is only applicable for the simple hydroceles in which the tunica is not thickened and the sac is not unduly large.

The most satisfactory procedure, especially applicable to large hydroceles and to those cases in which the tunicas are greatly thickened, is the *Winkelmann operation.* In this technique, the tunica is entered in the upper aspect of the scrotum and the parietal layer dissected free from the inner wall of the scrotum and from around the cord. The parietal layer is excised and removed down to within approximately one quarter of an inch of its reflection from the margins of the testis and epididymis. The cut edges, particularly in chronic hydrocele with greatly thickened walls, are liable to bleed, and meticulous hemostasis is necessary. The incisions in both these operations can be closed without drains only if hemostasis has been obtained. Atrophy of the testis occasionally follows hydrocelectomy and may be due to injury of the vessels of the cord or to immobilization of the testis. A properly performed operation, especially of the Winkelmann type, should lead to cure in practically all cases.

SPERMATOCELE

A spermatocele is an intrascrotal cyst resulting from a partial obstruction of the tubular system which transports sperm (Fig. 343). The exact anatomical disturbance is not known. Sexual excitement, chronic inflammation of the epididymis, gonorrhea, and trauma have all at one time or another been thought to be the probable basis for this condition. Obstruction may not be a factor because vasectomy does not subsequently increase the size of the spermatocele. Other cysts of the appendix testis, organ of Giraldès, vas aberrans, and other structures occur within the scrotum but do not contain spermatozoa.

A spermatocele is lined by pseudo-stratified epithelium surrounded by a thick layer of connective tissue. The membrane has a selective permeability, in that the fluid does not contain phosphates from the blood plasma, and phenolsulfonphthalein is absorbed much more rapidly than from a hydrocele cavity. The fluid is turbid or milky in color, and on microscopic examination it contains immobile sperm, fat bodies, and an occasional epithelial and lymphocytic cell. The aspirated sperm usually become active after a short period at room temperature. In elderly individuals with cessation of spermatogenesis, spermatozoa may not be present. Spermatocele does not occur until after puberty.

Spermatoceles transmit light and present on palpation a round mass distinct from the testis, giving the impression of an additional testis (Fig. 343).

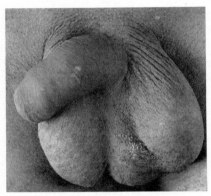

Fig. 343. Spermatocele in scrotal midline below suggesting a third testicle. Patient 40 year old. It is recognized that the location of the lesion here is unusual and does not convey to the student or general practitioner the appearance of the common variety of spermatocele which lies above the testis.

They are ordinarily located within the tunica vaginalis, although an extra-vaginal variety outside the tunica can occur. They displace the testis anteriorly and downward and can often be palpated, if not too large, as arising from the globus major. They may occur with hydroceles, in which case they are not recognized until operation, if study of the aspirated contents is omitted.

Most spermatoceles are asymptomatic, but many patients seek medical attention because of cancerphobia. In approximately 10 to 20 per cent of cases, there is slight pain or dragging sensation within the scrotum. Spermatoceles of large size are annoying because of their deformity. Except for possible discomfort, treatment is unnecessary for smaller spermatoceles. Treatment, when indicated, is either surgery or x-ray. Aspiration and injection of sclerosing solutions is not satisfactory or permanent. A small incision is made in the scrotum and the spermatocele delivered and completely excised. It is usually wise to perform a prophylactic Andrews' "bottle" operation for hydrocele. If the patient is beyond the fertile age, x-ray in small dosage (600 roentgen units given over several days) is all that is necessary for cure (Huggins). Roentgen therapy apparently suppresses testicular function just enough to abolish the seminiferous secretion, so that the epithelial-lined sac of the spermatocele remains collapsed. The testes may atrophy slightly or not at all, and usually there is no change in the sexual potentia following this treatment.

EDEMA OF THE SCROTUM

Edema of the scrotum may result from either a localized or general pathological condition. Extensive edema of the scrotum can occur in chronic cardiovascular disease and cause great distress (Fig. 1077). Indeed, edema may appear first in the scrotum rather than in the extremities or other areas. Local causes of edema are trauma and inflammation of the scrotal wall. Adenitis, malignancy, or other diseases of the inguinal nodes may, by obstructing the lymphatics, result in a nonpitting type of scrotal edema. Edema may be the first sign of elephantiasis and other tropical diseases which involve and obstruct the lymphatic system of the scrotum. Trauma or any surgical incision into the scrotum is usually followed by a considerable amount of edema for several days, and one must always be careful not to compress the upper portion of the scrotum with tight adhesive bandages or suspensories.

Edema as a result of inflammation occurs frequently in the scrotum. The loose structure of the scrotal tissues reacts with edema from the slightest inflammatory reaction or disturbance in the vascular or lymphatic system. It may occur as a result of cellulitis or other necrosing infections. Any underlying acute epididymitis or epididymo-orchitis frequently is accompanied by scrotal edema. Torsion of the spermatic cord and other acute intrascrotal conditions may be complicated by edema. We noted marked edema involving the entire scrotum on one occasion from a spider bite. In another case, a young teen-age boy was subject to recurrent, sudden attacks of angioneurotic edema involving at times only the scrotum which would suddenly become greatly swollen, while at other times attacks would be restricted to the face.

In most cases, scrotal edema is self-limited and depends upon the extent of the causative process. The treatment of scrotal edema, especially that associated with inflammation, is directed toward correction of the basic infectious process. If the edema is massive, as with cardiac failure, the dependent portion of the scrotal skin may become moist, with denudation of the epithelium and formation of ulcers. Patients with considerable edema should be confined to bed and the scrotum properly supported by an adhesive tape bridge, a small pillow, or bath towel folded between the legs. This accelerates venous and lymphatic drainage. Remarkable relief can sometimes be gained in the edema of cardiac failure by the subcutaneous insertion of one or more Southey tubes into the dependent portion of the scrotum. In a few hours, one or more liters of fluid often escapes, affording considerable relief. Premature babies are prone to develop scrotal edema during the first few months of life. In edema due to general causes, the penis is usually involved, and in massive edema it may be obscured. In such instances, the irritative action of urine on the tense, fragile skin easily leads to cellulitis and ulceration.

VARICOCELE

Varicocele may be defined as an abnormal dilatation and tortuosity of the veins of the pampiniform plexus in the scrotum. It is usually described as a "bag of worms," which presents a bluish appearance through the scrotal skin. In the supine position, they disappear. If the onset is sudden and the veins do not disappear on recumbency, it is probably a secondary varicocele due to obstruction of the internal spermatic veins near their terminus by renal or retroperitoneal tumors, hydronephrosis, or aberrant renal vessels. The sudden onset of varicocele after the age of 30 is apt to be indicative of retroperitoneal disease.

The incidence of varicocele has never been accurately determined. It has to be governed by the examiner, who determines in his mind what does and does not constitute a pathological dilatation of the pampiniform plexus. The definition is not one of sharp demarcation, and for this reason statistics have varied considerably. In general, it is believed that approximately 10 per cent of young men have a varicocele. Recent data from the Army by Lewis indicate that varicocele occurs in 16.5 per cent of men. Most instances occur between the ages of 15 and 25 years. It is estimated that 35 per cent of those having varicocele seek medical advice. Much has been written about varicoceles being the result of either sexual excesses or unfulfilled desire. Reflex vascular mechanisms resulting in venous congestion have been described. The most reasonable conception is that there is an increase of arterial blood flow to the scrotal contents during youth. In support of this, it has been noted that varicoceles often tend to disappear, or at least the symptoms tend to vanish, after marriage. The symptoms of varicocele are increased by exertion, and it was a difficult problem for military physicians in the last war to differentiate between legitimate complaints and malingering.

The *symptoms* of varicocele are some of the most difficult to evaluate in urology. The main complaint is a constant pulling, dragging, or dull pain in the area of the scrotum and sometimes in the testis. In the supine position, the symptoms should promptly disappear. Acute exacerbations of pain are more apt to be due to complications such as hernia, epididymitis, and localized venous thromboses, which are known to occur (see Funiculitis). Careful examination in every case is necessary for evidence of hernia and especially for tenderness in the epididymis and testis, in which case the symptoms may not be due to the varicocele. Individuals have various thresholds for pain, which may account for the variability of response in this condition. Patients with varicocele often have a wide variety of unrelated complaints such as impotence, nervous instability, lassitude, and general disability, which is certainly not related to the varicocele. Some patients complain of a small testis on the side of the varicocele, and an unknown percentage of patients with varicoceles do have a smaller testis on the involved side.

Varicoceles have been classified into small, medium, and large, but this does not serve any particular purpose because symptoms are notoriously unrelated to size. A greater percentage of larger varicoceles, however, are more apt to have somatic complaints. When large varicoceles do not lead to symptoms, it taxes the ingenuity of the examiner to appraise the symptoms from the minimal varicocele. In our practice, we are convinced that all patients complaining of general symptoms, of which varicocele is but one, should have psychosomatic consideration. We must be convinced that there is no constitutional neurasthenia and that the pain and discomfort directed toward the scrotal venous enlargement is reasonably bonafide before contemplating surgical therapy. Patients must be studied as a whole, or else unnecessary operations will be performed on maladjusted individuals.

The *indication for operation for varicocele* is as follows: (1) A voluminous and marked deformity, (2) scrotal pain, which on thorough study reveals no constitutional or psychological basis, (3) when herniorrhaphy or hydrocelectomy is indicated, (4) rapid increase in size of the varicocele, (5) secondary varicocele which does not disappear in the supine position, (6) definite evidence of testicular atrophy usually associated with a large size varicocele. It should again be emphasized that complete urological investigation is indicated when secondary varicoceles are discovered.

Treatment of Varicocele. The treatment of varicocele is either conservative or operative. Conservative therapy begins with proper psychosomatic appraisal. The use of suspensories may be worthwhile for a therapeutic trial. The injection of sclerosing solutions may lead to necrosis and complications and is to be avoided.

A brief description of the pampiniform plexus is pertinent to any discussion of surgical therapy. The veins in the pampiniform plexus gradually coalesce, and in 60 per cent of cases a single trunk is formed in the inguinal canal. In the remaining cases, two or more trunks may be present in the inguinal canal. The right internal spermatic vein enters the vena cava obliquely below the right renal vein. On the left, the vein terminates in the renal vein at a right angle, apparently without valve formation at this junction. As a result of this, 99 per cent of varicoceles are left-sided and 1 per cent bilateral. Varicocele is not reported occurring on the right alone, except when secondary to pathological intra-abdominal obstructions. The pampiniform plexus consists of three general groups of veins: the anterior or internal spermatic vein emerging from the testis and accompanying the spermatic artery, the middle group of veins of the ductus deferens, and the external spermatic veins (cremasteric, funicular, or posterior veins) running a course on the posterior aspect of the spermatic cord. The latter leave the pampiniform plexus distal to the external ring, where they empty into branches of the superficial and deep inferior epigastric veins and also into the superficial and deep pudendal veins. This external or posterior group affords a route of collateral circulation for the return of blood other than through the main internal spermatic veins. All three groups freely anastomose with each other near the testis. With varicocele formation, there is a reverse flow of blood in the main trunk of the internal spermatic vein, thus adding to the volume of blood flowing away from the testis to be transported by the middle deferential veins or by the anastomosis between the posterior group of veins and inferior epigastrics.

The literature is replete with various operations for the surgical treatment of varicocele. Over half a century ago, Lydston in his monograph on the subject discussed 24 leading operations at that time. The present-day surgical procedures, of which there are many variations, are as follows:

(1) *Intrascrotal Excision.* The veins are exposed in the scrotum and carefully dissected from the vas, with the hope that the spermatic artery is spared. Sections of the plexus 2 to 5 cm. in length are removed, and the two ends of the ligated plexus are brought together by means of a catgut suture in order to suspend the testis. This operation is unsatisfactory and has been followed by an appreciable incidence of testicular atrophy, postoperative orchialgia, and secondary hydrocele. The spermatic artery has evidently been divided on many occasions, and this, together with ligation not only of the spermatic group of veins but also the posterior group, has led to secondary vascular changes and testicular atrophy.

(2) *Suspension Operations.* Various techniques have been utilized to suspend the testicle. The most successful has been an incision above Poupart's ligament and over the external ring, following which the fascia of the external oblique muscle is reflected downward and sutured to the upper pole of the testis so that the latter is suspended well in the upper portion of the scrotum. The results from this procedure are fair, but they are probably better than intrascrotal excision of the varicocele. This operation does not remedy the retrograde flow of blood in the internal spermatic vein, but it may expedite blood flow in the collateral circulatory system. Excision of a portion of the scrotal wall for support of the varicocele has also been practiced but without significant success.

(3) *Compression Operations.* The principle of these procedures is to give added support to the pampiniform plexus. One type of operation consists of an incision into the scrotum and exposure of the testicle, with special care to preserve the parietal layer of the tunica vaginalis. The tunica is opened in the most dependent portion and is carefully reflected upward around the varicose pampiniform plexus. If there is a hydrocele present, then more tunica is usually available. The everted tunica is then sutured tightly around the spermatic cord, so that it actually encases and compresses the pampiniform plexus. This operation is actually a modification of the Andrews eversion operation, with particular attention to suturing the reflected parietal tunica around the cord for vascular support.

(4) *High Ligation of Veins.* As early as 1906, Dean Lewis reported ligation of the internal spermatic veins, including the spermatic artery, high in the inguinal canal for cure of varicocele. Ligation of the artery at this point did not result in testicular atrophy because the testis evidently received adequate blood supply through the deferential and cremasteric arteries. His report was evidently overlooked, but the principle has recently been rediscovered, especially by surgeons in South America. A number of variations in the technical procedure of high ligation have been devised in which the

veins have been ligated at the level of the external inguinal ring, within the inguinal canal, and also above the internal ring.

The first procedure has the disadvantage of usually including the collateral posterior or external spermatic veins where they anastomose with the inferior epigastric and pudendals. Ligation within the inguinal canal is a relatively simple procedure. An incision is made just above Poupart's ligament and the external oblique fascia divided as in hernioplasty. The veins are carefully separated from the internal spermatic artery, if the latter can be identified. There may be one, two, or three veins encountered at this point. From reports in the last war, a hernial pouch of some degree was found in 25 per cent of such varicocelectomies, although as a rule it was not recognized preoperatively. It is possible that the hernial pouch is the basis of symptoms in many patients with varicocele and that the continued symptoms following intrascrotal ligation have been due to the overlooking of this factor. Ligation within the inguinal canal may be combined with several types of testicular suspension. The distal stump of the divided internal spermatic vein can be pulled upward and sutured to the internal oblique muscle. A second method is to open the cremasteric fascia in a longitudinal manner when exposing the veins and then closing the fascia transversely so as to produce shortening. In a third variation, the cord is elevated above the conjoined tendon, with the latter sutured to the inguinal ligament below the spermatic cord, thus resulting in an elevation and shortening. With the high ligation techniques, most patients are allowed up within the third postoperative day and are hospitalized for a total of only five to six days.

Radical cure of varicocele can also be accomplished by ligating both the veins and artery of the spermatic cord above the internal ring. A small oblique incision is made through the abdominal wall in the region of the internal ring and the vessels of the cord easily separated from the peritoneum just above the point where the vas deferens and the deferential vessels leave the spermatic vessels. The undisturbed deferential and external spermatic vessels in such cases are adequate for circulation. With the small incision necessary for this complete ligation of the cord, there is little risk of postoperative hernia. It can be performed under local anesthesia without hospitalization.

These operations of high ligation have the advantage of exposure in an area of cleaner skin. They have led to far superior results, and the pessimism formerly exercised by surgeons in the treatment of varicocele is not justified. One must continue to caution, however, against operation in cases in which the symptomatology, though directed to the varicocele, is but a part of a general hypochondriacal state.

TORSION OF THE SPERMATIC CORD

Axial rotation or volvulus of the spermatic cord results in infarction or complete gangrene of the testicle (Fig. 342). The condition is not infrequently encountered in urological practice, but the true incidence is unknown because many cases are unreported. It predominantly occurs in childhood and adolescence, but this may be due to the fact that cases occurring later in life are mistaken for episodes of acute epididymitis. The condition in infants and children is also considered in Section XIII. It occurs in an approximately equal number of cases on both the right and left sides and in childhood about as frequently in cryptorchids as in completely descended testes. The latter would indicate that cryptorchidism is a predisposing factor. A few cases have been reported in intra-abdominal testes.

Most cases are initiated with a history of sudden and excruciating pain in the testicle, followed by extreme tenderness. The pain is localized within

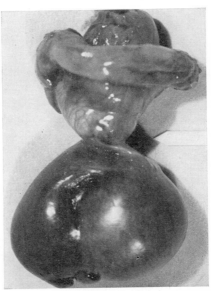

Fig. 344.   Torsion of the spermatic cord. Complete 360 degree rotation of the spermatic cord with gangrene of the testis and epididymis in a four-year-old boy. The child was awakened in the night with nausea, vomiting and pain across the abdomen. It was diagnosed as a gastrointestinal upset and the swelling and redness in the scrotum was not recognized until eight hours later at which time a diagnosis of acute epididymitis was made.

the scrotum but may be referred up along the cord and lower abdominal areas on the affected side. If the torsion is intermittent, the patient will give a history of repeated episodes of short duration, with discomfort disappearing after palpation or manipulation of the testicle by the patient, who actually is performing an external detorsion or unwinding. A mild form does occur with a gradual onset and only moderate pain lasting but a few minutes or a few hours. The testicle is tender, and the epididymis cannot be palpated in its usual posterior position. Within a short period after onset, edema and hyperemia of the overlying skin appear. The testicle is characteristically elevated to the upper part of the scrotum by spasm of the cremasteric muscles. As time progresses, there is a gradual swelling of the scrotal contents and the formation of fluid in the tunica vaginalis. After several days, it is impossible to delineate or outline the epididymis as distinct from the testis. In untreated acute cases, the pain gradually subsides after several days and finally disappears, with atrophy of the testis and epididymis resulting.

Acute torsion of the testis, especially in young children, has been confused on occasion with many acute intrascrotal emergencies and even with appendicitis (see also Section XIII). In undescended testis, it may be difficult to distinguish torsion from a strangulated hernia. Suppurative inguinal adenitis, especially in young children in which a history is not obtainable, has been confused with torsion. Elevation of the testis in cases of torsion fails to relieve the pain (Prehn's sign), which is contrary to the case in epididymitis, but this sign is not infallible.

The main predisposing factor is abnormal mobility of the testis. Normally, the visceral layer of the tunica vaginalis does not fully cover the testis and epididymis. The mesorchium is the portion of the tunica reflected from the fixed surface of the testis. With the usual short mesorchium, it is difficult for the testis to rotate on a vertical axis. Certain deviations in embryological development can result in a long mesorchium and a completely free testis within the tunica. There also may be a high insertion of the tunica on the spermatic cord. As a result, it is possible for the testis to rotate from 90 to 360 degrees, with reported cases having rotated four complete turns. An extravaginal type has been described, especially in children, in which the entire parietal tunica revolves within the scrotal tissue. For this to occur, there must exist a loose attachment between the parietal tunica vaginalis and either the inner surface of the scrotal wall or inguinal canal, as in the case of undescended testis. Other predisposing factors that have been suggested are a strong cremasteric muscle, faulty development of the gubernaculum, a voluminous scrotum, excessive length of the spermatic cord, and various other intrascrotal abnormalities. Torsion usually occurs from an outward to an inward direction. Torsion has occurred during sleep, but a wide variety of inciting circumstances has been encountered, such as following sudden muscular effort and trauma.

If the torsion persists for as long as three to four hours, complete infarction is inevitable, and it is rarely that a patient is encountered in which detorsion results in salvage of the testicle. Successful results will vary directly with the time between the onset and the detorsion. Patients with recurrent or intermittent attacks have learned successfully to perform detorsion upon themselves, but as a rule gradual atrophy of the testicle has ensued. If surgical detorsion is feasible, the testis should be fixed to the parietal tunica with one or more sutures through the tunica albuginea, while in certain cases a simple hydrocelectomy may suffice. In most cases, epididymoorchiectomy for impending gangrene is necessary. Because of the high incidence of bilateral abnormalities, it is imperative to carry out a prophylactic hydrocelectomy, with or without fixation of the testis to the scrotal wall, on the opposite side. Some urologists even recommend prophylactic orchidopexy in unusually hypermobile cryptorchid testes on one or both sides to preclude the possibility of torsion. If there is any question as to the diagnosis, one should err on the side of safety, explore the mass in question, and not chance the loss of a testicle. The condition is far too important as balanced against exploration of an acute epididymitis, should the latter be found. Operation in any case is necessary if strangulated hernia has been mistaken for torsion.

TORSION OF THE APPENDIX TESTIS

The appendix testis, sometimes termed the hydatid of Morgagni, is a small, pedunculated, ovoid structure (0.1 to 1.0 cm. in diameter) attached to the tunica albuginea. It occurs in about one third of normal individuals and embryologically is a vestigial structure. It may contain gelatinous and connective tissue and, rarely, epithelial-lined tubules. Some 80-odd cases of torsion have been reported to date, but it is believed that it has been masquerading under other diagnoses and probably occurs more frequently (Fig. 783). The greatest incidence is during childhood, particularly between the ages of 10 and 14, although a few cases have occurred in the fourth decade of life. The condition in the young is discussed in Section XIII.

The main symptoms are similar to torsion of the testis or spermatic cord. The pain may not be severe, although in some cases there has been extreme pain. The slight elevation of temperature and constitutional symptoms associated with torsion of the testis are usually absent. Symptoms have also been referred to the lower abdomen, and on occasion a preliminary diagnosis of acute appendicitis has been made. As in torsion of the testis, a secondary hydrocele may quickly develop, interfering with accurate palpation and a correct diagnosis. Some overlying redness and edema of the scrotum may occur. There is no disturbed relationship between the cord and testis with elevation of the latter, as is present in torsion. A small pea-sized mass is often palpated distinct from the testis near the upper pole, and it is remarkable that the symptoms are out of all proportion to the minute size of this lesion. As a result it has been confused with acute epididymitis, orchitis, and even torsion of the spermatic cord. Episodes of transient rotation of this structure may occur. Torsion of the appendix testis is usually not associated with sudden exertion or trauma, as in torsion of the spermatic cord. Treatment is surgical excision of the small, pedunculated, and usually gangrenous mass, followed by prophylactic hydrocelectomy.

CHYLOCELE AND LYMPH SCROTUM

This unusual condition is one in which lymphatic fluid accumulates within the cavity of the tunica vaginalis. Chylocele is not too uncommon in the tropics as a result of filariasis, but it is rarely encountered in this hemisphere. It only occurs in obstruction to those lymphatics draining the scrotum and especially the tunica vaginalis. Evidently the lymphatics of the tunics in some way rupture, resulting in an open communication between the lymphatics and the interior surfaces of the tunica. Chylocele has the general contour and appearance of a hydrocele except that it is not translucent, and on aspiration the milky fluid contains many fat droplets which collect on the surface. Active filariasis may be present, or the chylocele may represent the end stage of a quiescent filarial infection.

Idiopathic dilatation of the scrotal lymphatics or so-called "lymph" scrotum has been observed in temperate zones. The etiological factors in these idiopathic cases are obscure, but there is probably a defect in the lymphatic system of the scrotum, either congenital or post-inflammatory in nature. The scrotal skin in lymph scrotum may exude chyle following rupture of the cyst-like structure present on the surface. Such cases are said to be amenable to roentgen therapy.

SCROTAL CALCULI

Scrotal calculi or "pearls" are usually loose calcified bodies in the tunica. They are usually spherical in shape, white in color, of rubbery consistency, and have at times an appearance not unlike pearls from oyster shells. They are actually composed of fibrous tissue in concentric layers around a central calcified nucleus. They are thought to occur after scrotal trauma or mild inflammation. They are a curiosity and have no known clinical significance. Fibrous adhesions are not uncommon within the tunica (see Infections of the Tunics).

HERNIA OF TUNICA ALBUGINEA

Gray has described minute hernias containing seminiferous epithelium through the tunica albuginea of the testes. They are located at either pole and usually protrude about 2 mm. through defects of about 1 mm. in diameter in the tunica. There is no evidence of other abnormalities in the testis or scrotal cavity associated with these tiny unexplained hernias.

EMPHYSEMA OF THE SCROTUM

Gas and air within the lax tissues of the scrotum are usually observed under two general circumstances. Gas results from infection by gas-forming organisms. There is redness and tenderness of the scrotal skin, tachycardia, and evidence of toxemia. It is urgent to recognize this type immediately and to institute proper antibiotics and polyvalent serum therapy accompanied by multiple incisions and drainage (see Gangrene of Scrotum).

Emphysema or air in the scrotum may occur as a result of injuries to the pleura and lungs. The air apparently dissects retroperitoneally to reach the scrotum. We have observed marked emphysema of the scrotum following renal surgery. In such cases, the drain in the wound permits an air-sucking arrangement to be established. There is usually some accompanying subcutaneous emphysema in the lower abdominal wall below the renal incision. Rupture of the rectum (extraperitoneal) after inflation for examination and following industrial compressed air accidents may force air into the scrotum from the ischiorectal space. Emphysema has occurred after pneumoperitoneum. If a hernial sac is present, a "scrotal pneumocele" results rather than air in the tissues or emphysema.

ORCHIALGIA

Orchialgia, irritable testis, or neuralgia of the testis (and epididymis) as a clinical entity has long been a perplexing problem in urology. In his treatise in 1845, Sir Astley Cooper stated that "the patient has an unnatural sensibility in a part or whole of the testicle or epididymis: it is extremely tender to touch and rendered more painful by exercise. Generally it is not equally tender in every part, but there is a point in which the morbid sensibility particularly resides that the complaint occasions in some instances so much distress of mind it completely incapacitates its victims from amusement and pursuit of his profession or business." A few years later Curling stated that "the persons subject to it are those of a weak and irritable habit, who are dyspeptic or hypochondriac, and unequal to much bodily exertion. In severe cases of this defection, all enjoyment of life and its pleasures disappear; the sufferers concentrate their thoughts upon their maladies; they fancy they shall never get cured; and while some become uneasy as to the effect of their complaint in comparing the integrity of the gland and rendering them impotent, others urgently desire castration as a sole means of relief from their distress." In the interim there has not appeared any better descriptions or understanding of this condition. Astley Cooper was impressed by the similarity of this clinical condition to tic douloureux. The point of tenderness may be in the testis, epididymis, or various portions of the spermatic cord. This tenderness varies in individuals and may or may not be accentuated by work, rest, or contact with clothing. The symptoms in some cases, however, may be alleviated by proper scrotal support with a suspensory or by recumbency and rest. Some patients have an associated constant dull ache which rarely radiates up into the groin and low back area. Orchialgia is known to occur in children, although the vast majority of cases usually occur in men past middle life. It has also been known to follow scrotal trauma.

In true orchialgia there is no evidence of any local disease in the testicle, epididymis, adnexa, or spermatic cord, either on surgical exploration or pathological study in cases where castration has been performed. True orchialgia must be distinguished from the erotic form of orchialgia that occurs in young men following ungratified sexual excitement. The latter type probably results from increased blood flow to the testicle and epididymis, together with increased intratesticular tension from an excess of retained spermatic fluid. Suppression of secretions with estrogenic therapy is not helpful in true orchialgia, indicating that increased tension is not a factor. Orchialgia must also be differentiated from so-called "secondary neuralgia," in which there is a definite palpable or demonstrable lesion in the testis, epididymis, or spermatic cord. In such cases, abnormal mobility of the testis, varicocele, and unexplained scars in the tunics have occasionally been found. We have observed several cases of this variety in which the point of tenderness was a calcified appendix testis or appendix epididymis. Surgical exploration was not performed, and the discomfort in these instances may have been a result of chronic incomplete torsion of these structures. True orchialgia must, in addition, be differentiated from projected pain to the testicle or scrotal area from a disease process at a distant site. A general urological examination should rule out any associated diseases, such as prostatitis, posterior urethritis, semi-vesiculitis, hernia, disturbances in the bladder, and especially pathological conditions of the lower ureter, which can result in pain referred to the scrotal area.

The question of testicular pain in general has recently been reviewed by Brown with data that tend to disagree with many of the long-accepted ideas. His clinical observations lead to the assumption that testicular pain is never perceived in the scrotum. The testicle originates as an intra-abdominal organ and later migrates to its final site in the scrotum. The testicle originates not in the region of the kidney but in the lower portion of the abdomen which is innervated by segments of the lumbar nerves. In view of this, Brown believes that testicular pain should theoretically be perceived only in the lower abdomen, just as is pain from other viscera in this area. This is contrary to the concepts of testicular pain being referred to the region of the kidney.

In support of Brown's contentions, he has recently made the following observations. If the contents of a hydrocele cavity are aspirated and the tunica vaginalis anesthetized with procaine to eliminate sensibility of the tunics, fluid can then be injected into the testicle under pressure without the patient receiving pain in the scrotum. The pain is not felt in the region of the kidney but deep in the lower abdomen beneath the internal inguinal ring. This corresponds to the site of the embryological origin of the testis. The tunica vaginalis is supplied by the genital branch of the genitofemoral nerve from L-1 and L-2. Following cryptorchidopexy, the genital branch of the genitofemoral nerve is generally divided, making the tunica covering the testis insensitive. With the testis in its new site following the orchidopexy, pressure on the testicle refers the pain to its original intra-abdominal site above Poupart's ligament. A third observation along this line was made during removal of ureteral calculi situated in the lower ureter. The genitofemoral nerve pierces the psoas muscle above the external iliac artery and courses downward under and in contact with the ureteral wall. By leaving a temporary rubber band around this nerve, Brown could tug on the band and stimulate the intact nerve following operation, with the result that acute pain was referred to the area of the testicle. The discomfort was evidently perceived in the tunica vaginalis, which is innervated by the genitofemoral nerve. According to these observations, pain referred to the scrotum from such intra-abdominal regions as the lower ureter is perceptible by the patient in the tunica vaginalis, although it generally is expressed as in the "testicle."

The wall of the scrotum must also be considered in the differential diagnosis of pain in this region and especially in regards to referred pain from disease elsewhere. The scrotum is innervated by S-2 to S-4. Tenderness and pain involving the scrotum could, therefore, be referred from disease in the prostate, posterior urethra, or seminal vesicles. If Brown's assumptions are correct (and our clinical observations tend to support his conception), a local painful stimulus to the testicle is never perceived in the scrotum, and there is no entity such as true scrotal orchialgia. When there is tenderness and discomfort within the scrotum, the painful stimulus either originates in the tunica vaginalis or else is referred to this structure from disease of those intra-abdominal organs supplied by L-1 and L-2.

Orchialgia without demonstrable organic disease is considered in the realm of "sexual neuroses." This inexplicable pain is intimately connected with the state of the genital and mental functions, with most cases being encountered in individuals who have failing sexual potentia and advancing age. The patient should, therefore, be considered as a whole and a search made for psychoneurotic traits, for which orchialgia is only a leading symptom.

Unfortunately, treatment has progressed little since Astley Cooper's recommendations in 1845. He states that he attained success by the use of "Peruvian bark . . . iron therapy . . . blistering the skin at five different times . . . applying leeches to the amount of 200 to the affected part . . . employing various lotions, opium and belladonna." His most valuable suggestion as to therapy in sexually neurotic cases is generally followed today by most psychiatrists. Cooper recommended "a sea voyage to a warm climate, probably from the rest which the ship enforces and from the improvement which sea air and change of climate sometimes produce in general health."

In lieu of success with the psychosomatic approach—and we have experienced failure in most instances—the only local therapy worthwhile is surgical exploration and denervation of the spermatic cord. We have carried out this procedure on a number of occasions with indifferent success. In no case have we discovered on exploration any abnormality, even though careful search was made for minute neuromas or glomus type tumors, which might theoretically account for such discomfort. In one patient, recently, following denervation of the spermatic cord there was entire relief of pain for two months, after which the pain recurred in the operative scar in the midscrotal region. Reexploration of the wound and spermatic cord in search of neuromas was without success. Repeated procaine injections into the spermatic cord below the inguinal ring has been alleged to be effective, but in our experience it is futile. Orchiectomy as a last resort is severe therapy for a fundamentally psychopathic disease, if the latter is the basis of the condition. In one of our cases of secondary orchialgia, the division of unusually strong cremasteric muscles (see Cremasteric Spasm) gave complete relief. In most cases of orchialgia, however, the testis is at the bottom of the scrotum, and there is no evidence of such spasticity.

CREMASTERIC MUSCLE SPASM

Obscure spastic contraction of the cremasteric muscles has been known to traumatize the testes by pulling them against the pubic bone. The spasm has been reported as due to psychic or neurasthenic reflexes, brain or spinal cord injuries, and locally to idiopathic hypertrophy of the cremasteric muscle. A remarkable degree of muscle hypertrophy has been described in some cases. The attacks of spasm may be clonic in character and last for approximately several minutes, but in the majority of cases the episodes are tonic with a duration of several hours. Treatment is psychotherapy, diathermy and hot sitz baths, sectioning of the spermatic nerves, and excision of the cremasteric muscle and fascia. The cremasteric muscle is supplied by T-12, and this nerve can be blocked by procaine. If the spasm is relieved by injection, the nerve can then be injected with alcohol. We have encountered one instance of this condition where division of the cremasteric fascia and musculature led to relief of the testicular pain and tenderness.

PIGMENT DISTURBANCES IN THE SCROTAL SKIN

Scrotal skin may participate in any of the large number of generalized cutaneous pigment disturbances of the body, with the exception of carotenemia. Of the five normal pigments of the skin, the scrotum contains all but carotene. There are no pigmentary disturbances that have a predilection especially for the scrotum. Vitiligo not uncommonly affects the scrotum along with other areas of the body. This is a peculiar benign disease in which the normal melanin disappears from the skin. Newborns, especially those with dark hair and white skin, may occasionally exhibit a dark scrotum at birth. This is evidently due to the marked deposition of melanin as a result of some increased adrenal cortical function in the mother or to an adrenotropic stimulation in the child from the mother's hormonal system.

REFERENCES

Infections of the Scrotum

ACTION, H. W. and RAO, S. S.: Causation of lymph-scrotum. Indian M. Gaz., *65:*541–546, 1930.

ALLEN, L. and RINKER, J. R.: The lymphatics of the tunica vaginalis with special reference to hernia and hydrocele. Anat. Rec., *94:*446, 1946.

BEGG, R. C.: Scrotal pearls. Brit. J. Urol., *22:*132–134, 1950.

CAMPBELL, M. F.: Streptococcus scrotal and penile gangrene. Surg., Gynec., & Obst., *34*: 780–786, 1922.

COUTTS, W. E.: Genito-urinary lesions in lymphogranuloma venereum. J. Urol., *49:*595–599, 1943.

FITTS, W. T., JR. and WELLS, E. J., JR.: Case of fatal arterial occlusions due to aneurysm of abdominal aorta. Am. J. M. Sc., *214:*252–254, 1947.

GIBSON, T. E.: Idiopathic gangrene of scrotum. J. Urol., *23:*125–153, 1930.

LIVERMORE, G. R.: Pseudo-elephantiasis of the scrotum. J. Urol., *51:*170–173, 1944.

MAIR, G. B.: Idiopathic gangrene of scrotum. Lancet, *1:*464–466, 1945.

RANDALL, A.: Idiopathic gangrene of scrotum. J. Urol., *4:*219, 1920.

ROBINSON, R. C. V.: Newer antibiotics in the treatment of venereal diseases. Am. J. Syph., Gon., & Ven. Dis., *34:*273–288, 1950.

RONCHESE, F.: Calcification and ossification of steatomas of the scrotum. Arch. Dermat. & Syph., *49:*12–15, 1944, with correction *49:*304, 1944.

STOKES, JOHN H.: Modern Clinical Syphilology. Philadelphia, W. B. Saunders Co., 1946.

STOKES, J. H., BESANCON, J. H. and SCHOCH, A. G.: Infectious recurrence and mucocutaneous relapse in syphilis. J.A.M.A., *96:*344–351, 1931.

WEBER, F. PARKES: A note on supposed "calcinosis" of the scrotum. Brit. J. Derm. & Syph., *48:*312–313, 1936.

Cutaneous Diseases

CAWLEY, E. P. and GREKIN, R. H.: Parafavus restricted to the scrotum. Arch. Derm. & Syph., *60:*435–436, 1949.

EPSTEIN, ERVIN: Regional Dermatologic Diagnosis. Philadelphia, Lea & Febiger, 1950.

FRANKLAND, A. W.: Deficiency scrotal dermatitis in P.O.W.'s in the Far East. Brit. M. J., *1:*1023–1026, 1948.

GREENBAUM, S. S.: Scrotum: Dermatologic Lesions. The Cyclopedia of Medicine, Surgery, and Specialties. Philadelphia, F. A. Davis, 1940.

NEUMANN, H.: Neurodermatitis circumscripta venenosa scroti. Zbl. Haut u. Geschlechtskr., *62:*617, 1939.

PINKUS, H. and GOULD, S. E.: Extramammary Paget's disease and intraepidermal carcinoma. Arch. Dermat. & Syph., *39:*479–502, 1939.

SEMON, H. C. G.: An Atlas of the Commoner Skin Diseases. Williams & Wilkins Co., Baltimore, Md., 1947.

SUTTON, R. L. and SUTTON, R. L., JR.: Handbook of Diseases of the Skin. C. V. Mosby Co., St. Louis, 1949.

VARIOT, G.: Nigritie congénitale du scrotum et hyperpigmentation des petites livres chez des enfants nouveau-nés. Bull. et Mém. Soc. d'Anthrop. de Paris, 6s, *i:*76–77, 1910.

Orchitis

BAKER, W. J. and RAGINS, A. B.: Actinomycosis of the testicle. J. Urol., *56:*547–553, 1946.
BAUMRUCKER, G. O.: Incidence of testicular pathology. Bull. U. S. Army Med. Dept., *5:* 312–314, 1946.
BROWN, F. R.: Testicular Pain. Lancet, *1:*994–999, 1949.
BURHANS, R. A.: Treatment of orchitis of mumps. J. Urol., *54:*547–548, 1945.
CALLOMON, F.: Metastatische Hodenerkrankungen bei akuten Infektionskrankheiten, ihr Vorkommen und ihre Erkennung. Dermatologische Zeitschr., *67:*193–201, 1933.
CANDEL, S.: Immune serum globin (gamma globulin) in prophylaxis of orchitis. Mil. Surgeon, *99:*199–202, 1946.
CANDEL, S., WHEELOCK, M.C. and GRIMALDI, G. J.: Mumps orchitis, with discussion of plasma prophylaxis. U. S. Navy M. Bull., *45:*97–107, 1945.
FRIEDMAN, N. B. and GARSKE, G. L.: Inflammatory reactions involving sperm—spermatic granuloma and granulomatous orchitis. J. Urol., *62:*363–374, 1949.
GALL, E. A.: The histopathology of acute mumps orchitis. Am. J. Path., *23:*637–651, 1947.
GELLIS, S. S. and McGUINNESS, A. C. and PETERS, M.: Study on prevention of mumps orchitis by gamma globulin. Am. J. M. Sc., *210:*661–664, 1945.
GILFAND, M. and DAVIS, G. B.: Bilharzial lesions of the testis. South African M. J., *14:*332, 1940.
HERMAN, L. and KLAUDER, J. V.: Studies of the prenatal transmission of syphilis. I. Syphilis of the testicle. Am. J. Med. Sc., *159:*705–722, 1920.
HOYNE, A. L., DIAMOND, J. H. and CHRISTIAN, J. R.: Diethylstilbesterol in treatment of mumps orchitis. J.A.M.A., *140:*663–665, 1949.
ISAAC, A. G.: Orchiditis and epididymitis due to undulant fever. J. Urol., *40:*201–207, 1938.
MACKAY-DICK, J.: Infective mononucleosis. J. Roy. Army Med. Corps, *82:*279–282, 1944.
MATHE, C. P.: Suppurative orchitis. Its diagnosis and treatment. J. Urol., *34:*324–335, 1935.
McCORD, C. P. and MINISTER, D. K.: Lead orchitis. J.A.M.A., *82:*1104, 1924.
NIXON, N. and LEWIS, D. B.: Mumps orchitis; surgical treatment. J. Urol., *56:*554–560, 1946.
NORTON, R. J.: Use of diethylstilbesterol in orchitis due to mumps. J.A.M.A., *143:*172–174, 1950.
PIERI, G.: Sulla cura dei dolori del testiculo. Policlinico (Sez. Prat.), *45:*1629–1636, 1938.
PINCK, B. D.: Surgical treatment of mumps orchitis. Urol. & Cutan. Rev., *51:*257–258, 1947.
RAMBAR, A. C.: Use of convalescent serum in the treatment and prophylaxis of orchitis. Am. J. Dis. Children, *71:*1–13, 1946.
ROSAHN, P. D.: Autopsy studies in syphilis. J. Ven. Dis. Inform., *27:*293–301, 1946.
ROSENBERG, WM.: Abscess of the testicle. J. Urol., *34:*44–54, 1935.
SERRI, F.: Le orchioepidimiti da pneumobacillo di Friedlander. Giorn. Ital. Derm. Sif., *87:* 291–301, 1946.
SMITH, R. G.: Plasma treatment of mumps orchitis. U. S. Navy M. Bull., *44:*159–160, 1945.
STENGEL, ALFRED, JR.: Mumps orchitis. Am. J. Med. Sc., *191:*340–356, 1936.
TRASOFF, A. and GOODMAN, D. H.: Rheumatic orchitis associated with rheumatic pericarditis and effusion. M. Ann. District of Columbia, *13:*149–150, 1944.
TUNBRIDGE, R. E. and GAVEY, C. J.: Epidemic epididymo-orchitis in Malta. Lancet, *1:* 775–779, 1946.
WESSELHOEFT, C. and VOSE, S. N.: Surgical treatment of severe orchitis in mumps. New England J. Med., *227:*277–280, 1942.
WEYRAUCH, H. M. and GASS, H.: Urogenital complications of dengue fever. J. Urol., *55:* 90–93, 1946.

Epididymitis

a) SPECIFIC EPIDIDYMITIS

ARONSON, J. D.: The occurrence and anatomic characteristics of fatal tuberculosis in the U. S. Army during World War II. Mil. Surg., *99:*491–503, 1946.
BAND, DAVID: Tuberculosis of the genito-urinary tract. The Practitioner, *165:*245, 1950.

BARNEY, J. D.: Genital Tuberculosis. Chapter XIV. Cabot, Modern Urology, Lea and Febiger, Philadelphia, 1936.

BORTHWICK, W. M.: Pathogenesis of tuberculous epididymitis. Edinburgh M. J., *53:*55–70, 1946.

BOTHE, A. E.: Primary tuberculosis of the prostate. J. Urol., *18:*494–503, 1927.

BUCKLEY, T. I.: Brucellosis of the male genitalia. Calif. & West. Med., *48:*175–179, 1938.

CHUTE, R.: Tuberculosis of the genito-urinary tract among soldiers in World War II. New England J. Med., *235:*586–589, 1945.

COUNCIL ON PHARMACY AND CHEMISTRY: Current status of the chemotherapy of tuberculosis in man. J.A.M.A., *142:*650–653, 1950.

CRONQVIST, STEN: Spermatic invasion of the epididymis. Acta Pathologica et Microbiologica Scandinavica, *26:*786–794, 1949.

HINSHAW, H. C. and McDERMOTT, W.: American Trudeau Society: Thiosemicarbazone therapy of tuberculosis in humans. Am. Rev. Tuberculosis, *61:*145–157, 1950.

JACOBSON, C. E., JR. and DOCKERTY, M. B.: Blastomycosis of the epididymis; report of 4 cases. J. Urol., *50:*237–248, 1943.

LAIRD, S. M.: Meningococcal epididymitis. Lancet, *1:*469–470, 1944.

LATTIMER, J. K., AMBERSON, J. B. and BRAHAM, S.: Treatment of genito-urinary tuberculosis with streptomycin alone. J. Urol., *62:*875, 1949.

LISSER, H. and HINMAN, F.: Syphilis of the epididymis without involvement of the testicle. Am. J. Syph., *2:*465–471, 1918.

LOWSLEY, O. S. and DUFF, J.: Tuberculosis of the prostate gland. Annals Surg., *91:*106–114, 1930.

McDONALD, J. H. and HECKEL, N. J.: Acute pneumococcal epididymitis. Ill. Med. J., *95:* 304–306, 1949.

McLACHLAN, A. E. W.: Syphilitic Epididymitis. Brit. J. Ven. Dis., *14:*134–137, 1938.

MEDLAR, E. M., SPAIN, D. M. and HOLIDAY, R. W.: Post-mortem compared with clinical diagnosis of genito-urinary tuberculosis in adult males. J. Urol., *61:*1078–1088, 1949.

MICHELSON, H. E.: Syphilis of the epididymis. J.A.M.A., *73:*1431–1433, 1919.

ROLNICK, H. C.: Syphilis of the epididymis. J. Urol., *12:*147–152, 1924.

THOMAS, G. J., KINSELLA, T. J., PETTER, C. K. and STEBBINS, T. L.: Surgical Treatment of urogenital tuberculosis. J. Urol., *39:*766–783, 1938.

THOMAS, G. J., STEBBINS, T. L. and RIGOS, F. J.: Tuberculosis of the testicle. J. Urol., *44:* 67–73, 1940.

THOMPSON, L.: Syphilis of the genital organs of the male and the urinary organs. Am. J. Syph., *4:*706–724, 1920.

WELLS, C. A.: Tuberculous epididymitis. Brit. J. Urol., *10:*114–130, 1938.

b) NON-SPECIFIC EPIDIDYMITIS:

ABESHOUSE, B. S. and LERMAN, S.: Vasectomy in the prevention of epididymitis following prostatic surgery. Urol. & Cut. Rev., *54:*385–391, 1950.

GARROW, I. and WERNE, J.: Metastatic epididymitis. Urol. & Cutan. Rev., *51:*3–6, 1947.

HANDLEY, R. S.: Non-specific epididymitis. Lancet, *1:*779–781, 1946.

IANNUZZI, G.: Le Epididimiti e Orchiti Specifiche e Aspecifiche, Roma, 1942.

LYNN, J. M. and NESBIT, R. M.: Influence of vasectomy upon the incidence of epididymitis following transurethral prostatectomy. J. Urol., *59:*72–75, 1948.

McGAVIN, D.: Chronic non-tuberculous disease of the epididymis. Brit. J. Surg., *26:*800–808, 1939.

SCHMIDT, S. S. and HINMAN, FRANK: The effect of vasectomy upon the incidence of epididymitis after prostatectomy. J. Urol., *63:*872–878, 1950.

SLESINGER, E. G. and McGAVIN, D.: Joint Discussion No. 3: Sections of surgery and urology: discussion on non-specific epididymitis. Proc. Royal Soc. Med., *36:*323–326, 1943.

SMITH, DON R.: Treatment of epididymitis by infiltration of spermatic cord with procaine hydrochloride. J. Urol., *46:*74–76, 1941.

STEINBERG, J. and STRAUS, R.: Sperm invasion of the epididymis. J. Urol., *57:*498–503, 1947.

c) TRAUMATIC EPIDIDYMITIS

AMDUR, M. L.: Industrial epididymitis and epididymo-orchitis. Industrial Med., *12:*371–373, 1943.

EWELL, G. H.: Traumatic Epididymo-Orchitis. J.A.M.A., *113:*1105–1109, 1939.

GRAVES, R. S. and ENGEL, W. J.: Experimental production of epididymitis with sterile urine; clinical implications. J. Urol., 64:601–613, 1950.

HENLINE, R. B. and YUNCK, WM.: Epididymitis; its relationship to trauma and compensation. New York State J. Med., 43:1325–1327, 1943.

HINMAN, F. and JOHNSON, C. M.: The differential diagnosis of acute fat necrosis in the scrotum. J. Urol., 41:726–732, 1939.

SLOTKIN, G. E.: Industrial epididymitis and epididymo-orchitis. New York State J. Med., 39:1096–1101, 1939.

WESSON, M. B.: "Traumatic orchitis"; a misnomer. J.A.M.A., 91:1857–1861, 1923.

Deferentitis and Funiculitis

BENJAMIN, J. A., ROBERTSON, T. D. and CHEETHAM, J. G.: Vasitis nodosa: a new clinical entity simulating tuberculosis of the vas deferens. J. Urol., 49:575–582, 1943.

COLEY, B. L. and LEWIS, B.: Filarial funiculitis. Am. J. Surg., 76:15–22, 1948.

KREUTZMANN, H. A. R.: Symposium on pyogenic prostatitis; studies of infections of vas deferens. J. Urol., 39:123–127, 1938.

MATHE, C. P.: Thrombo-angiitis obliterans (Buerger's disease) of the spermatic arteries: report of case. J. Urol., 44:768–776, 1940.

McGAVIN, D.: Thrombosis of pampiniform plexus. Lancet, 2:368–369, 1935.

PAUL, MILROY: The blood and lymph pathways in the spermatic cord. Ann. Royal Coll. Surg. of Eng., 7:128–150, 1950.

MURRAY, D. E.: Genito-urinary aspects of early filariasis. J. Urol., 61:967–971, 1949.

OECONOMOS, N.: Deferentitis considered as a clinical entity. Urol. & Cutan. Rev., 52:388–390, 1948.

WILENSKY, A. O. and SAMUELS, S. S.: Acute deferentitis and funiculitis. Ann. Surg., 78:785–794, 1923.

WOLBARST, A. L.: The vas deferens, a generally unrecognized clinical entity in urogenital disease. J. Urol., 29:405–412, 1933.

YOUNG, H. H.: Some unusual cases of filariasis of the scrotum and groin. J. Urol., 32:383–415, 1934.

Infections of Tunics

GOODWIN, W. E. and VERMOOTEN, V.: Multiple fibromata of tunica vaginalis testis or proliferative type of chronic periorchitis. J. Urol., 56:430–437, 1946.

VAN DUZEN, R. E.: Periorchitis prolifera. Urol. & Cutan Rev., 36:94–96, 1932.

Other Scrotal Diseases

ABESHOUSE, B. S.: Torsion of the spermatic cord. Urol. & Cutan. Rev., 40:699–714, 1936.

ANDERSON, C. W. and JENKINS, R. H.: Actinomycosis of the scrotum. New England J. Med., 219:953–954, 1938.

BRUSKEWITZ, H. and EWELL, G. H.: The end results of the injection treatment of hydrocele. J. Urol., 59:67–71, 1948.

BUERGER, LEO: The Circulatory Disturbances of the Extremities. W. B. Saunders Co., Philadelphia, 1924.

CAMPBELL, M. F.: Hydrocele of the tunica vaginalis. Surg., Gynec. & Obst., 45:192–200, 1927.

CAMPBELL, M. F.: Torsion of the spermatic cord in the newborn infant. J. Pediat., 33:323–327, 1948.

CAMPBELL, M. F.: Varicocele due to anomalous renal vessel: an instance in a thirteen-year-old boy. J. Urol., 52:502–504, 1944.

COTRIM, E. and BARBOSA, DE BARROS, J.: Estudo radiológico in vivo da circulacão no varicocéle por meio de liquidos de contraste. Rev. Paulista de Med., 19:341–351, 1941.

GRAY, D. J.: Hernias through the tunica albuginea testis. Anat. Rec., 94:464, 1946.

HABERLAND, H. F. O.: Kremasterspasmophilie. Ztschr. f. Sexualwissensch., 17:191–195, 1930.

HUGGINS, C. and NOONAN, W. J.: Spermatocele including its x-ray treatment. J. Urol., 39:784–790, 1938.

JAVERT, C. T. and CLARK, R. L., JR.: A combined operation for varicocele and inguinal hernia. Surg., Gynec., an dObst., 79:644–650, 1944.

KICKHAM, C. J. E.: Calcified hydrocele of the tunica vaginalis testis. New England J. Med., 212:419, 1935.

LEWIS, E. L.: The Ivanissevitch Operation. J. Urol., 63:165–167, 1950.

LIVERMORE, G. R.: Torsion of the testicle and its appendages. Urol. & Cutan. Rev., *52:* 1–3, 1948.

MAKAR, N.: An operation for varicocele. Urol. & Cutan. Rev., *50:*27–29, 1946.

MOULDER, MAX K.: Bilateral torsion of the spermatic cord. Urol. & Cutan. Rev., *49:*354–355, 1945.

MUSCHAT, M.: Cremasteric spasm. Arch. Surg., *43:*609–614, 1941.

OLSON, R. O. and STONE, E. P.: Varicocele. New England J. Med., *240:*877–880, 1949.

PALOMO, A.: Radical cure of varicocele by a new technique. J. Urol., *61:*604–607, 1949.

REES, H., B. A. U. S. Annual Meeting: Hydrocele. Brit. J. Urol., *20:*182–183, 1948.

ROGERS, W. W. and GARRETT, J. V.: Pneumocele as a transient complication of artificial pneumoperitoneum. Brit. J. Tuberc., *41:*70–73, 1947.

SCOTT, R. T.: Torsion of appendix testis. J. Urol., *44:*755–758, 1940.

SHAH, K.: Aetiology of idiopathic hydrocele. J. Indian Med. Assn., *18:*184–188, 1948–49.

SPEED, K.: Aerocele of the scrotum. Surg. Clin. North America, *11:*29–40, 1931.

VERMEULEN, C. W. and HAGERTY, C. S.: Torsion of the appendix testis. J. Urol., *54:*459–465, 1945.

VEST, S.: Atlas of the Genital System, in press.

WILSON, W. W.: Injection treatment of hydrocele. Lancet, *1:*1048, 1949.

WYNN-WILLIAMS, N.: Artificial pneumoperitoneum and scrotal pneumocele. Brit. Med. J., 318–319, 1949.

ZUCKER, M. O.: Newer concepts of surgical treatment for varicocele. Mil. Surgeon, *95:* 515–517, 1944.

Section VII

INFERTILITY IN THE MALE

ROBERT S. HOTCHKISS, M.D.

The problem of barrenness is as old as recorded history of man, yet it was usually the wife who bore the burden of blame and it was she who was often despised, hated, and maltreated for the offense of not bearing children. The ancients, however, were aware of inadequacies on the part of the male, and codes and laws provided remedial measures for overcoming barrenness due to the male factor. For centuries, prayer, incantations, mystic measures, and symbolic worship were employed to overcome the curse of infertility. Many primitive tribes and races of today employ the same measures in their quest for begetting children. The invention of the microscope may be regarded as the dawn of the modern era of scientific investigation for, as related by Antonj van Leeuwenhoek, a Dr. Hamm was the first to see a spermatozoon in 1677. The mists of the era of potions, folklore, and idolatry were soon to be lifted.

All prejudices did not vanish, for as late as the beginning of this century the eminent Dr. Marion Sims found cause to defend his belief that the husband should be considered a cause for barrenness. He stated, "I was misrepresented, maligned, and positively abused both here and abroad; for dabbling in the vagina with speculum and syringe was considered to be incompatible with decency and self-respect" (Sims, 1868).

The spectacular advances in medical knowledge of the first half of the twentieth century have permitted much to become known about the intricate processes of reproduction. The husband could no longer be overlooked for his share of responsibility in infertile marriage and the urologist was called upon to assume more and more interest in the joint investigation of the infertile couple. Consequently, the urologic horizon has broadened rather remarkably to include these new responsibilities. Not only are we concerned with the patients confronted with inability to conceive, but it has become necessary to compile and to collate information relating to the physiology of the male genital system. Furthermore, we have become aware of many unsolved basic and clinical problems which challenge the ingenuity and skill of urologists. The resources for the solution lie largely in his domain.

DEFINITION OF "INFERTILITY"

It is appropriate to restate several definitions of "infertility" for the sake of clarity.

(1) *"Absolute infertility"* indicates that there is a complete inability to produce a conception.

(2) *"Relative infertility"* is the term applied where there are certain positive degrees of fecundity, yet the sum total of these elements is below the threshold required for conception.

(3) *"Primary infertility"* pertains to couples who have no living children.

(4) *"Secondary infertility"* is the designation given to couples who have one child but who are unable to beget additional offspring.

Total absence of sperm is therefore classified as "Absolute Infertility" whereas "Oligospermia" is considered as "Relative Infertility."

It is important that these distinctions be borne in mind for they paraphrase the objectives in the investigation of the fertility of the involuntary barren couple. The examination of the husband is begun in the hope that it may be determined whether he is the sole or the contributing factor in the barrenness, or whether he is without demonstrable faults. At the conclusion of the examinations the urologist summarizes all the material in the history, physical examination, and that gained from the laboratory tests, and these in turn are appraised with similar information obtained from the investigation of his wife. The ultimate diagnosis involves two individuals considered as a marital unit. This compounds the difficulties and affords a unique experience in medical procedures, for with this exception we are accustomed in medical practice to deal only with the disorders of a single person.

ANATOMY AND PHYSIOLOGY

A review of the fundamental concepts of the anatomy and physiology of the male genital tract is warranted, for it furnishes a basis for the rationale of the clinical procedures. One is impressed by the many hiatuses in our knowledge of some of the fundamentals but, with due deference to these deficiencies, the following account is related.

The male sexual apparatus consists mainly of four parts:

(1) *Testes,* for the production of spermatozoa and internal secretions.

(2) *Epididymides and ductus deferens,* designed for the conduction and storage of spermatozoa.

(3) *Prostate and seminal vesicles,* producing the vehicle for the spermatozoa.

(4) *Penis, urethra and accessory glands,* the organs for delivery of the semen.

A disturbance in one or all of these subdivisions may affect the fertility of the individual.

TESTES

The development and ultimate fate of the testes may be decided in the prenatal, prepuberal, or the postpuberal period of life. Let us consider the male gonad from its inception to its maturity.

Prenatal Period. Genetic inheritance may decide the eventual value of the testes even before its embryonic construction. There are a number of examples in nature where the male individuals of the species are sterile. The male ass is perhaps the most familiar. The complexities of human inheritance are such that true comparisons with other species are inadmissible. It is apparent that genetic faults follow close inbreeding among humans and sterility of the men is a characteristic of one family having the Klinefelter syndrome (Klinefelter et al., 1942). It is possible that the disturbances of mitosis, discussed in the section on testicular biopsy, have their origin in a genetic defect thereby prohibiting the development of spermatozoa.

During the fifth month of fetal life, there is an enormous hyperplasia of the interstitial cells of the testis. This is maintained until the time of birth and then involution occurs rapidly. This prenatal hyperplasia is due to the mother's gonadotropins elaborated during the pregnancy, rather than to any hormones secreted by the fetus. Sexual differentiation takes place about the fiftieth day of the embryo's life. A controversy has long taken place regarding the influence of circulating hormones as a sex determinant. The weight of evidence favors that the sex of the individual cannot be reversed by any hormonal control even though such is artificially magnified. As the sixtieth day approaches, the gap between the mesonephros and the rete tubules is closed thereby forming the union between the epididymis and the testis. A failure of this urogenital connection accounts for the defects occasionally seen in adult life, resulting in a separation of the testes and the ductal system (cf. Section IV).

The descent of the testes is a result of the straightening out of the body of the embryo and a degeneration of the cranial portion of the testes rather than an actual downward migration of the parts into the scrotum. By the eighth month the testes have descended to the scrotal sac. Permanent bilateral testicular ectopia within the confines of the abdomen or inguinal canals produces the well-known consequence of sterility.

Prepuberal Period. Physiologic control of the testes is established after birth through the gonadotropic activity of the pituitary (cf. Section I, Chapter 5). The bulk of the testicle in the boy is occupied by seminiferous tubules and little space is given to the interstitial cells. The seminiferous tubules of the young boy require a period of ripening before spermatogenesis can be induced. Precocious spermatogenesis has never been stimulated in any immature human or animal by the administration of any androgen or gonadotropin. Small amounts of both androgens and estrogens have been found in boys, indicating that either interstitial or adrenal cells (or both) function in early life.

The diseases, deficiencies and conditions which affect the adult testes, mentioned in the following section, may also injure the preadolescent testes. Gonadal failure in the young, however, without actual testicular destruction, cannot be diagnosed until after puberty since the infantile status is the norm before that event. The signs and symptoms of primary prepubital gonadal failure are, then, only apparent when the gonad fails to make the complete transition from the infantile to the adult structure. Werner (1950) has presented statistics to show that mumps orchitis occurs in one fifth of all cases of mumps occurring in males after puberty. Mumps is one of the commonest infections of childhood, yet clinical mumps epididymo-orchitis is almost unknown before the age of twelve years. This striking immunity and susceptibility of the epididymides and testes to the virus of mumps, strictly according to the individual's age, cannot fail to cause speculation. Can it be that some of the unexplained atrophy of the germinal epithelium in adult life be due to unrecognized damage from mumps occurring during adolescence? There is no proof, and therefore, the consideration is purely speculative.

Postpuberal or Adult Period. Under the control and influences of the other endocrine glands, the secretory and spermatogenic activity of the testes are instigated during adolescence. Both of these processes may continue to death, even though the individual becomes senile. Engle (1939) reports that about one half of men examined after the age of seventy had abundant spermatozoa in the testes.

Nutrition. The proper nutrition of the testes is essential to normal functions. Utilization and absorption of proteins, fats and minerals may be inadequate although there is a sufficient intake of these substances, for there is a recognized distinction between the minimal and the optimal nutritional requirements. The body economy is directly dependent upon the intermediary metabolism of foodstuffs. The liver is a key organ, for when it is damaged not only may the gonads be directly affected, but they may be influenced as well by subsequent alterations of the endocrines. Mulinos and Pomerantz (1941) were able to restore spermatogenesis by the use of chorionic gonadotropins, despite the continuation of an inadequate diet which had caused failure of the germinal epithelium. Their conclusions were that sterility was due primarily to an insufficiency of gonadotropic hormones resulting from a depression of the pituitary gland due to inadequate nutrition. In man, and in the laboratory animal, in the event of liver damage, the inactivation of estrogen may be lost. Consequently there is an elevation of the circulating endogenous estrogens which may affect the gonads directly or cause an imbalance of the pituitary secretions.

Laboratory experiments have shown that a deficiency of vitamin A causes a reduction in spermatogenic activity which is reversible by adequate replacement.

Vitamin B deficiency causes testicular damage in birds but not in mammals.

Vitamin C is not clearly identified with normal testicular function.

Although vitamin D is closely related to cholesterol of the androgens, there is no experimental evidence that a lack of this vitamin causes testicular injury.

Vitamin E deficiency causes profound testicular damage without affecting the interstitial cells. The damage caused by vitamin E deficiency is irreparable.

Three of the amino acids have been shown to be essential to spermatogenesis, but the significance of this fact is questionable since it is difficult to formulate a diet without including these three amino acids.

Temperature. There is an abundance of convincing evidence that elevated temperature has an adverse effect upon the testes. A high elevation of body temperature may cause a transient depression of spermatogenesis (McLeod and Hotchkiss, 1941). Experimental subjection of testes to body heat can produce spermatogenic failure as proven by transplantation of testes from the scrotum to within the body cavity. Dr. Carl Moore has discussed this *in extenso* in Section I, Chapter 5.

Irradiation. The harmful effect of irradiation is recognized from experiments in animals, fish, and observation on man. Engle and Robinson (1948) have described the damage and repair from atomic irradiation in man, using sequential biopsies of the testes over an extended period. This and other information from the Japanese permits a more optimistic attitude to one of the terrors of atomic warfare.

Diseases, Injuries and Anomalies. The various lesions which affect the testes of man will not be enumerated here because they are discussed in other Sections of this book. It may be germane, however, to recall that any inguinal operation may have impaired the circulation of the testes to the detriment of the germinal epithelium, without causing appreciable gross atrophy.

The Endocrines. The pituitary gland exerts an extremely formidable effect on the physiological function of the body. The somatic domains over which

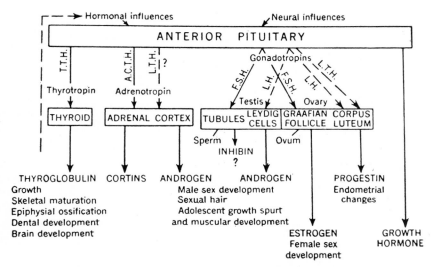

Fig. 345. Hormones of the anterior pituitary. (From L. Wilkins, Endocrine Disorders in Childhood and Adolescence, C. C Thomas, Springfield.)

this "master gland" has sovereignty is vividly demonstrated in the accompanying schema (Fig. 345). Many controversial aspects of the interrelationships, reciprocal and synergistic actions of the endocrines confront the reader of this vast literature. Simplification, with its attendant risks, is therefore a justified maneuver for the interests of clarity.

There are four fundamental links to a chain of events involving the pituitary and its hormones:

(1) Initiating forces must arise in the hypothalamus of the brain where the impulses are passed to the pituitary.

(2) Among the six or more hormones elaborated by the pituitary, there are four tropic hormones which may bear on this subject. Follicle-stimulating hormone (FSH), the luteinizing hormone (LH), and the lactogenic hormone (LTH) are collectively known as the gonadotropic hormones. FSH is intimately connected with the testicular tubules and stimulates both the germinal cells and the Sertoli cells. LH controls the secretion of testicular androgens produced by the interstitial Leydig cells. It may also act in conjunction with

FSH in stimulating spermatogenesis. The role of the lactogenic hormone (LTH) is less clearly defined in the male but may be coupled with LH and have influence upon the Leydig cells. The adenocorticotropic hormone (ACTH) plays an important role in the stimulation of the reticular cells of the adrenal cortex to produce the steroid hormones.

Pituitary hormones are thrown into the blood stream in various concentrations where they circulate throughout the body and are subject to influences before they are utilized by the target glands which in this discussion are the testes, ductal system, prostate, seminal vesicles and adrenals.

The testes are the only organs in the male reproductive tract which secrete hormones. They consist essentially of three divisions, germinal epithelium (G), the cells of Leydig (L), and the cells of Sertoli (S).

The Leydig cells are closely akin to the cells of the adrenal cortex. Both have a common embryologic origin and both produce steroids which are the precursors of the urinary 17-ketosteroids. Testosterone is considered to be *the* male sex hormone because of its potent androgenic properties. It is able to reverse regressive procedures in the secondary sexual characteristics consequent upon castration. It prevents or repairs atrophy of the seminal vesicles and the prostate in a castrate animal. It usually prevents testicular atrophy in the hypophysectomized animals. It produces masculine distribution of the hair, acne, increased musculature, and mobilizes the skin pigment. It causes growth of the accessory male genital organs. It promotes nitrogen retention. Its exact role in the maintenance of spermatogenesis is not, however, entirely clear.

The Sertoli cells which lie in intimate apposition to the germinal cells, have been called "supportive" and "trophic cells." They contain lipids and the mature spermatozoon attaches itself to the Sertoli cell before leaving the seminiferous tubule. A controversy exists concerning the ability of the Sertoli cell to produce a hormone under the influence of FSH. Some evidence is at hand to suggest that this hormone is an estrogen. Others believe the hormone to possess a distinct action of its own, and have designated the product as "X" hormone and also "inhibin." Viewed in the latter light it is nonandrogenic and has the power to retard or inhibit the production of FSH by the pituitary. Likewise the theory has been advanced that it stimulates LH production and in itself supports spermatogenesis. The proponents of the "single" testicular rather than the "dual" testicular hormone theory point out that the "X" hormone has not been isolated and that FSH excretion will be depressed by sufficiently large amounts of testosterone.

ADRENALS. The sexual development of the normal male is dependent on the steroid androgenic hormones which are provided both by the testes and adrenals.

Twenty-eight or perhaps thirty steroids have been isolated from the adrenal cortex. Eleven of these compounds have proven to be biologically active. The remainder are either inactive or have properties that remain unrecognized. It is yet to be determined to the satisfaction of all whether these compounds are derived from one parent hormone or whether they are built up separately.

The physiologic active steroids contain 21 carbon atoms (cortins), with the exception of the three androgenic steroids (androgens), which have 19, and esterone which possesses 18 carbon atoms. The 21 carbon substances are concerned with salt, protein and water metabolism. The neutral urinary steroids are derived from the androgens and are recoverable for assay.

The urine of a normal woman contains two thirds of the amount of 17-ketosteroids as compared to that of a man so that it is apparent that the adrenal of the male contributes more androgenic activity than do the testes.

The administration of ACTH increases the salt-retaining, glyconeogenetic, and androgenic activities of the adrenal so it is assumed that the needs of the body are mediated through the pituitary. Cortisone (compound E) suppresses the activity of the adrenal and decreases the excretion of the 17-ketosteroids.

THYROID. There is a paucity of information regarding the role of the thyroid and its influence on the male reproductive tract. The thyroid hormone, also probably solely regulated by the pituitary, controls many metabolic processes such as consumption of oxygen, rate of circulation, mobilization of cholesterol, conversion of carotene to vitamin A, rate of growth and maturation of body tissues and development of the brain. The direct relationship to the testes remains obscure despite the similarity of function exemplified by the rate of growth in adolescence which is presided over by a combination of thyroid, androgenic and growth hormones.

Summary. The rate and functions of the testicles are then at the mercy of the endocrines of which they are a part. Much more needs to be known of the exact role of the various components of this hypothalamus-pituitary-adrenal-gonadal-thyroid relationship. There is reason to believe and hope that research will unlock some of these mysteries and furnish explanations for cause and a means for treatment.

EPIDIDYMIDES AND DUCTUS DEFERENS

The purpose of the epididymides and vasa (other than that of a conduit) is not known. If a true function can be assigned to the epididymides and vasa, it is probable that they both operate in a similar manner. Presently, the belief is held that there is a period of ripening during which the spermatozoa pass through the epididymides and vasa deferentia. Munro's (1938) experiments with rooster sperm would indicate that a purposeful function is served by the ductal system. He found that spermatozoa possessed higher fertilizing potentials when aspirated from the more distal sites of the efferent seminal tract of the rooster. Only 3.5 per cent of eggs were fertilized by epididymal sperm whereas those from the ductus deferens caused 62 per cent of the eggs to be fertilized.

PROSTATE AND SEMINAL VESICLES

Seminal Vesicles. It would appear that the seminal vesicles have a more definite vital role in fertility than does the prostate. Huggins and Johnson (1933) have demonstrated that the seminal vesicle fluid contains phosphates, reducing substances, protein, nitrogen and chlorides (cf. Section I, Chapter 4). Mann's (1946) experiments have demonstrated that the seminal vesicles have the remarkable capacity of forming fructose, which comprises a large portion of the reduceable substances. From evidence gained through observations on humans by depressing the function of the prostate or seminal vesicles through endocrine manipulations, it has become apparent that the bulk of the semen is produced by the seminal vesicles, rather than by the prostate.

Prostate Gland. The prostatic fluids are low in reducing substances but contain fibrinogen and fibrinolysin which accounts for the liquefaction of the semen after discharge from the body. The role of acid phosphatase remains unknown.

The *semen,* therefore, is a mixture of spermatozoa and the combined secretions of the seminal tracts and prostate and seminal vesicles. The spermatozoon has a unique biological role, for it is a self-sufficient cell which is destined to perform its function independent of any connection with the parent tissue. The spermatozoon is essentially a glycolytic organism in contradistinction to most body cells which obtain their energy by respiration. A spermatozoon utilizes the sugars required for energy by metabolizing them into lactic acid. Under experimental conditions, they prefer an anaerobic environment and, in general, have a type of metabolic activity that is quite similar to that of cancer cells (MacLeod, 1939).

The seminal fluid is an extremely complicated substance containing a large number of elements to which no known function can be assigned. The most important material in the fluid portion of the semen are the carbohydrates which are present in an average of 300 mg. per cent. Only 50 mg. per cent is actually required to sustain metabolism and motility. If the spermatozoa are resuspended in a sugar-free Ringer's solution, motility will cease in about two hours. Both motility and metabolic activity will be revived promptly by the addition of a proper amount of glucose.

METHODS OF EVALUATING THE FERTILITY OF MEN

The investigation of fertility in men utilizes no equipment or specialized apparatus that is not found in the average doctor's office. The main requirements are time and inclination. The procedures are similar to those pursued in any type of clinical investigation and cover the usual three points of (1) history, (2) physical examination and (3) laboratory procedures.

History. A detailed history is a vital part of the examination, for the cause may be discovered therewith for the lack of conception.

Occupation. The occupation should be noted, for such pursuits as radiology or working in an atomic laboratory or plant carry important implications.

Past History. CHILDHOOD DISEASES. Childhood diseases are to be noted together with complications. On occasions, some children have been subjected to x-ray exposures, such as might be the case if there were an osteomyelitis of the hip or a congenital dislocation of the femur. Prepuberal mumps is apparently of little importance before the age of twelve.

CRYPTORCHIDISM. Each patient should be asked whether there had been a failure of one or both testicles to descend and, if so, at which age did they reach the scrotum and whether such event occurred with or without treatment.

ADULT ILLNESSES. The diseases of adult life should be noted on the history, particularly such illnesses as tuberculosis with or without involvement of the genitalia, jaundice or prolonged febrile states. At this point it is well to inquire if there had been any unusual disturbances in the transition from boyhood to manhood, such as marked obesity or retardation in the transition from the preadolescent to the adolescent and mature states. Such questions as: age of shaving, growth rate, and excessive fat give indications of the normal or abnormal developments at this period.

TRAUMA. Any serious injuries to the genitalia should be noted in detail, together with their complications, if any.

OPERATIONS. All operations should be recorded and, in particular, those involving the genitalia and groins. If a hernia repair has been done it is wise to inquire whether the testis was swollen or whether the wound had been infected.

VENEREAL DISEASE. A chronological and detailed report of gonorrheal and syphilitic infections is to be recorded in detail, together with a record of treatment received. Complications, particularly epididymitis, should be clearly established.

HABITS. The dietary habits of the patient should be ascertained. Special attention should be given to the intake of fruit juices, fresh and cooked vegetables, milk, meat, etc. Some patients are accustomed to use vitamin tablets regularly and this should be included in the record. An account of general habits such as hours of work, use of alcohol and tobacco should be obtained.

SIBLINGS. The number of siblings is recorded by sex, and notations are made regarding the fertility of those who are married.

MARITAL RECORD. A detailed account of the marital history of the patient is of utmost importance.

> 1. *Previous marriage,* if any, should be described in detail as to contraceptive practices, conceptions or issues, and in the event a divorce has taken place, whether the ex-spouse has remarried and if she has had children from her present husband.
>
> 2. The *present marriage* should be described in terms of months or years of duration. The period of contraceptive practices either by the husband or wife should be noted and deducted from the length of the marriage. Military duty, or type of occupation, may further reduce the chances of pregnancy by reason of separation. Often the period during which pregnancy might have occurred is only a fraction of the total time of marriage.
>
> 3. The *frequency of intercourse* during the time when no contraceptives have been used is of obvious significance. The average couple is accustomed to relations once or twice a week. Not infrequently the patients are in error of the probable time of ovulation and it becomes evident from the history itself that coitus is limited to a period when pregnancy is very unlikely to take place.
>
> 4. Complete notations should be made of any *previous pregnancies,* miscarriages or probable conceptions that might have occurred during the marriage. If a previous conception has taken place it is important to note the lapse of time during which no contraceptives were used prior to the pregnancy.
>
> 5. Such *fundamental questions* as complete penile penetration, or whether ejaculation takes place, might seem to be too obvious but on some occasions only direct questioning brings forth the fact that

ejaculation has not occurred, or that the husband has never consummated intromission. Occasionally, artificial lubricants such as large quantities of Vaseline, or even contraceptive jelly, have been employed during the time when pregnancy was desired.

6. *Previous semen examinations.* Direct questions should be asked whether previous examinations of this nature have been done, how the specimen was collected, whether part of the specimen might have been lost, and the conclusions reached from previous tests. Likewise, an outline of any treatment that might have been given previously should be recorded in as much detail as the patient can give.

7. *Report on the wife.* A short summary should be recorded concerning the wife: her age, previous marriage, if any, together with the report of such specific tests as pelvic examination, tubal patency tests, and post-coital spermigration tests; her weight, general health, and whether or not she has kept temperature charts.

Physical Examination. The physical examination should be done with the trunk and lower extremities completely exposed. Only in such a way can one judge the distribution of body hair and axillary hair; the type, adiposity, and development of the breasts, and general contour of the body.

(1) The abdomen should be palpated. (2) The external genitalia should be inspected. (3) The penis should be examined for hypospadias. (4) The testes should be carefully palpated and notations made about the size, position and consistency of each. (5) The epididymides should be palpated throughout and notations made about the presence of any nodules which might indicate an area of occlusion. The epididymides may be absent or only partially developed. (6) The vasa should be carefully palpated in the exposed portion. (7) The prostate and seminal vesicles are examined by the rectal digital method and the expressed secretions should be collected for microscopic examination. (8) A summary of the important facts in the history and physical examination serves a useful purpose at this point for it affords the information which is to be assembled along with the laboratory tests.

Laboratory Procedures. A distinction is made between laboratory tests that have a proven and accepted usefulness and those which are of value in research. The latter are often expensive and have not yet proven to be of value in clinical practice.

The *routine tests* are: (a) Urine analysis, (b) microscopic analysis of the prostatic secretions, and (c) semen analysis.

Desirable tests, if indicated, are: (a) Blood Wassermann, (b) post-coital spermigration tests, (c) basal metabolic rate, (d) blood count and (e) endoscopy.

Tests sometimes indicated include: (a) X-ray of the sella turcica, (b) blood sugar tolerance, (c) urine assays for gonadotropic substances, and (d) 17-ketosteroid assay.

SEMEN ANALYSIS

(1) There are several items in the *semen analysis* which have been utilized to determine the fertility index. They are: (a) Volume, (b) viscosity, (c)

be used. This is obtained by drawing the semen to the top of the stem of the pipette or the point "one" mark. All the sperm in five blocks of 16 squares (80 small squares) are obtained as above. Six ciphers are added and the result is divided by two, which will constitute the sperm count per cc.

      Example 2.   30 sperm in 5 blocks, 16 squares
                     30,000,000
                     Divide by 2
                     15,000,000 sperm per cubic centimeter

If only a few cells are sparsely distributed in the counting chamber, it is best to count all the cells present on the entire red blood cell field (400 small squares). Count per cubic centimeter is then obtained by adding five ciphers to the number providing a 1:10 dilution is used.

      Example 3.   25 cells in 1 square millimeter of the counting chamber
                 x 10 for dilution equals 250
                 x 10 to convert to cubic millimeter equals 2500
                 x 1000 to convert to cubic centimeters equals 2,500,000

(2) *Differential Count for Morphology of Spermatozoa.*

(a) *Technique.* Preparation of the smear.

1. Prepare smear for stain similar to method used for computing differential blood count.

2. Shake the specimen thoroughly and place a drop on the slide.

3. If many spermatozoa are present a small drop is used.

4. If few spermatozoa are present a larger drop is used.

5. Place a second slide in contact with the drop and run over the top of the slide.

6. The thickness of the smear can be regulated by the angle between the two slides. The smaller the angle the thinner the smear. Thin smears are desirable if the cell count is about 25 million per cubic centimeter or more.

(b) *Stains.* Numerous stains have been advocated and used for visualizing cell contours. A suitable one should differentiate the nuclear material from the cytoplasm and stain the tail. A stain should be used which permits the cellular portion of the semen to be removed thereby, leaving the spermatozoa only on the slide. The following stains are suggested, for each will accomplish the above and personal preferences will decide which one is more popular.

1. *Stain Composition*

    1. Schaudinn's solution .... 60 cc.
       Mercury bichloride 7% .... 40 cc.
       Alcohol 100% .... 20 cc.
      Time: ½ minute.

This fixing solution permits adherence to the slide without heating the smear, and insures preservation of cell structure. The wet smear is immersed immediately in this solution for the time specified.

    2. Alcohol 50% .... 60 cc.
      Time: ½ minute.
    3. Wash in water .... 60 cc.

    4. Eosin aqueous 1% .... 60 cc.
       Time: ½ minute.
    5. Acid Alcohol .... 60 cc.
       Alcohol 50%
       Concentrated HCl. 3 ggts.
       Time: ½ minute.
This solution removes some mucus but leaves the cells intact. If sperm are
also washed off, weaken the solution by adding water. Wash.
    6. Harris' hematoxylin .... 60 cc.
       Standard formula plus 3 ggts. HCl.
       Time: 2 minutes.
If solution is alkaline, nuclear material will not accept stain. Wash.
    7. Dilute acetic acid .... 60 cc.
       Distilled water .... 60 cc.
       Concentrated acetic acid .... 3 ggts.
(This solution need only be used if nuclear material appears over-stained.
Its purpose is to withdraw excessive hematoxylin. Wash, dry and examine
with oil immersion lens. If desired, mount in balsam with thin cover slip.)
    2. *Stain*:
       1. Air dry smear
       2. 10% formalin
          Time: 1 min.
       3. Wash.
       4. Stain: Meyer's hematoxylin
          Time: 1½ min.
       5. Wash in lukewarm water.
Some experience and practice are required to perform a morphologic
count. A simple classification is to be preferred over the more complicated
ones, which apparently serve no useful purpose, for the main objective is
to enumerate the "normal" from the "abnormal" sperm. It is best to classify
200 to 300 cells. (See Fertility in Men, Chapter 7; Hotchkiss, 1944.)

No description is made herewith of the other techniques required for the
other tests, most of which are well known.

The methods for assay of the androgens, 17-ketosteroids, and the gonadotropins can be found in the references cited for those who are interested
(Wilkins, 1950).

THE EVALUATION OF THE SEMEN ANALYSIS

The value of the semen analysis rests on the assumption that it affords a
means of prognosticating the likelihood of conception. The evidence that
such a value may be given to semen analysis is based on a comparison of
the seminal specimens of a large number of men who are fathers, with
specimens of husbands who have no children. If the semen of these two
groups were without significant differences, conclusions could be drawn
that the quality of the semen was not a representative factor in the fertility
of one group as compared to the infertility of the other. On the other hand,

definite variations in the semen of these two groups would be meaningful provided the groups were sufficiently large enough to give statistical value to the comparison.

The following data on two thousand marriages have been gathered by Dr. John MacLeod (1950). In order to insure that the result would be completely unbiased, Dr. MacLeod was unaware whether the semen specimens were from husbands whose wives were attending the antenatal clinic or whether the semen was procured from husbands faced with the problem of sterility. One thousand individuals of each group submitted specimens for these examinations. The first will be designated as the "fertile semen," and the second as the "infertile semen." The statistical analysis of this large mass of formidable material is in progress. For that reason, and because of the limitation of space available here, a partial treatment of his analysis will be presented. It is, by far, the largest and most comprehensive study of its kind yet undertaken, from which to establish the clinical use of the semen analysis.

There is no cause for debate about specimens of semen which are devoid of spermatozoa. The only precautions required for the evaluation of such specimens is that the sample is a true ejaculate and that the azoospermia is not a transient deficiency due to a febrile state existent previous to collection. Therefore, it is well to collect three samples of semen before the diagnosis of azoospermia is made. In Dr. MacLeod's series there were no samples without any spermatozoa in the fertile marriage group but 10 per cent were found in the "infertile" men.

If any sperm are found in the seminal discharge, it is dangerous and incorrect to assume that the man is completely sterile. If a marked deficiency is found in any, or all, of the categories of the analysis the only conclusion which is justified is that the fertility is reduced. Using this premise as a basis for further discussion, let us turn to the 2000 semen analyses in the hope that there will emerge some standards for deciding what is a subnormal specimen. To receive the designation it should have qualities common to the "infertility group" and not found in the fertile group. The azoospermic semens were not included in the "infertile group," for it was thought that the values would be depressed unfairly. Accordingly, only semen that have some or many spermatozoa, made up the 1000 specimens from husbands concerned with barren marriage.

Volume. The mean (average) volume for the "fertile group" was 3.3 cc. The "infertile" marriage mean volume was 3.5 cc. It is to be seen that the infertile group actually has a larger volume than the "fertile" group. There was no disproportion between the two groups, as regards to a considerable percentage of each having very high or low volumes.

A study of the volume as related to cell count showed a difference between the two groups. The higher volumes are associated with poorer sperm count in the "infertile" group. This is illustrated in Figures 346 and 347 showing the sperm count per cubic centimeter as related to four categories of volume.

Volume	Count per cc.
Under 2.4 cc.	under 40,000,000
2.4 cc.–3.3 cc.	40– 75 million
3.4 cc.–4.4 cc.	80–139 million
4.5 cc. and over	140 million and over.

There are no striking dissimilarities between the groups as far as the volumes of the ejaculates are concerned, which offer leads of clinical value. For reasons presented in a subsequent section it would appear that individual allowances should be made for very small volumes.

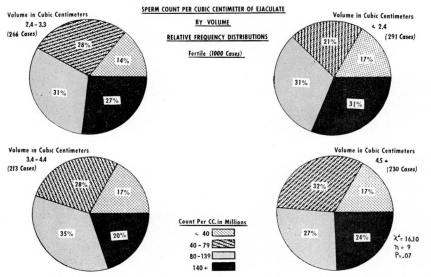

Fig. 346.   Relationship of sperm count to volume in fertile group. (Courtesy Dr. John MacLeod.)

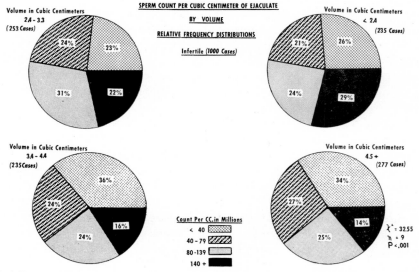

Fig. 347.   Relationship of sperm count to volume in "infertile group." (Courtesy of MacLeod.)

Cell Count. The relationship of the spermatozoa count to fertility has been a much debated subject for many years. The observations of Meaker (1934). Macomber and Saunders (1929), and more recently by Farris (1950), have led workers to believe that 60 million count per cubic centimeter or above was to be regarded as compatible with good fertility. Hotchkiss et al. (1938) in a study of 200 fertile men, found 25 per cent of the cases below 60,000,000 per cc. Falk and Kaufman (1950) in a series of 100 similar cases listed 15 per cent below this level.

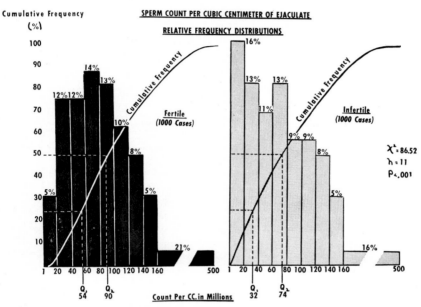

Fig. 348.   A comparison of sperm counts per cubic centimeter in fertile and "infertile" marriage. (Courtesy of Dr. John MacLeod.)

MacLeod's data confirm the latter standards. The conception records of the 1000 fertile men indicated that they may be regarded as a highly fertile group. Twenty-five per cent of the wives were involuntarily pregnant in spite of contraceptive practices. Fifty-five per cent of the women became pregnant within six months after the time contraceptives were not used. A small percentage of these cases had a sterility problem prior to the pregnancy.

The accompanying frequency distribution graph (Fig. 348) of the two groups shows a significant contrast at the 20,000,000 per cc. level. The Q-1 and Q-2 represents the first and second quarters of the two groups. It will be seen that one fourth of the "infertile" groups had counts under 32,000,000, while 25 per cent of the fertile men had counts under 60,000,000 cells per cc., which is to be recalled as a figure commonly used as the dividing line between normal and subnormal specimens. Five per cent of the fertile group had counts between 1,000,000 and 20,000,000 per cc. whereas 16 per cent of the "infertile" group had counts in this range. A comparison between the two groups is further illustrated by dividing the counts per cubic centimeter into graduated categories of 20,000,000 each (1–20 million; 20–40 million; 40–60 million, etc.). The men from each group were then assigned to each 20,000,000 category according to their sperm count per cubic centimeter. The greatest number of men in the fertile group were found in the 60,000,000 to 80,000,000 category whereas the "infertile" men had their greatest representation in the 1,000,000 to 20,000,000 category (Fig. 348).

Total Sperm Counts in the Fertile and the Infertile Groups. No additional information was gained by a comparison of the total sperm counts. The

	Group I (2000 Cases)			Group II (925 Cases)			Group III (925 Cases)		
	A. Fertile Marriage (1000 Cases)			A. Men in infertile marriage with history of conception(s) prior to semen exam (241 Cases)			A. Men in infertile marriage with conception(s) prior to or after semen exam (319 Cases)		
	B. Infertile Marriage (1000 Cases)			B. Men in infertile marriage with history of no conception prior to semen exam (684 Cases)			B. Men in infertile marriage with no conception prior to or after semen exam (606 Cases)		
Count per Cubic Centimeter in millions	No. of Cases in Count Class	Proportion Contributed by A	Difference from 50.0%	No. of Cases in Count Class	Proportion Contributed by A	Difference from 26.1%	No. of Cases in Count Class	Proportion Contributed by A	Difference from 34.5%
All Cases	2000	50.0%	——	925	26.1%	——	925	34.5%	——
Under 20	211	21.8%	Signif.	152	13.2%	Signif.	152	19.1%	Signif.
20 – 39	248	47.1%	Not Sig.	118	26.3%	Not Sig.	118	37.3%	Not Sig.
40 – 59	237	52.7%	Not Sig.	104	26.0%	Not Sig.	104	30.8%	Not Sig.
60 – 79	271	52.4%	Not Sig.	120	21.7%	Not Sig.	120	35.0%	Not Sig.
80 – 99	220	59.1%	Signif.	81	34.6%	Not Sig.	81	43.2%	Not Sig.
100 – 119	191	49.7%	Not Sig.	83	37.3%	Mod. Sig.	83	44.6%	Mod. Sig.
120 – 139	157	52.2%	Not Sig.	69	20.3%	Not Sig.	69	30.4%	Not Sig.
140 – 159	96	52.1%	Not Sig.	45	28.9%	Not Sig.	45	37.8%	Not Sig.
160 – Over	369	57.7%	Signif.	153	33.3%	Mod. Sig.	153	40.5%	Not Sig.

Significant – probability less than .01
Mod. Signif.– probability between .01 and .05
Not Signif. – probability greater than .05

Fig. 349. A comparison of groups I, II and III. (Courtesy of Dr. John MacLeod.)

main points can be briefly summarized: Seven per cent of the fertile men had total counts under 50,000,000, while 15 per cent of the "infertile" men fell into this category.

The group of men listed as "infertile" obviously contain members who are not subnormal and the lack of children may well be due to a sterile wife. Also, in the group are those husbands who have produced conception ending in miscarriage, stillbirth, or husbands who have "one child sterility." In a group of 1000 "infertile" men, 241 have produced one or more conceptions prior to the semen examination, and in 75 cases the history is incomplete. Frequency distribution graphs were made of these two groups of patients, which it is to be recalled, were included in the "infertile" group because all were now concerned with barrenness with their present wives. The two distribution graphs demonstrated the same relationship of each of these segments as the original fertile and "infertile" marriage groups (Fig. 349).

Figure 349 illustrates in another manner the difference between these 2000 cases of barren and fertile marriages.

Group 1. One thousand fertile and "infertile" marriage cases.

Group 2. This is the subdivision of the "infertile" group which has just been described.

Group 3. Husbands who caused a conception prior to or after the semen analysis.

If the count per cubic centimeter were *not* a discriminating factor in fertility, one would expect the number of cases falling in each count classification to be equal to the proportions contributed. In the first group, 50 per cent was contributed by the fertile marriages, and 50 per cent by the infertile marriages. However, the fertile marriage group contributed only 22 per cent to the 211 cases under 20,000,000 per cc. This group should have contributed 50 per cent if the cell count was of no importance. This equalization is arrived at in the next two categories. Similarly, group 2 and group 3 contributions are 26 per cent and 34 per cent respectively, showing again this significant deficit. In counts under 20,000,000 per cc., only 13 per cent of the cases in group 2 are contributed by the "conception group."

Motility. The evaluation of motility was based on the "percentage of active cells" and the "quality of motility." For statistical purposes MacLeod combined the two observations to obtain a value for these two qualities which he designated as "motility index." For example, 50 per cent active cells exhibiting grade 3 motility would earn a motility index of 150. This allowed a single figure for mathematical calculations of the combined values as well as each separately.

He found that 13 per cent of the fertile men had 30 per cent or less active cells whereas 32 per cent of the "infertile" men had poor motility. The importance of good motility was illustrated in the follow-up of the men in the "infertile" group who eventually produced a conception as compared with those who did not. Two and one-half times as many men eventually produced conception with a good fertility index as did the men with a poor index. An exhaustive analysis of the "ease of conception" brought forth the information that where both the percentage and quality of motility was poor, relatively few wives conceived, whereas conception was produced far more rapidly if motility was good. When the percentage of active cells was below 40 per cent, the conception time was longest but if the percentage of active cells was 60 or above, conception took place significantly sooner. The strongest relationship between any aspect of semen quality and ease of conception is that of quality or the aggressiveness of motility.

Morphology. MacLeod and Gold have attacked the difficult problem of evaluating the significance of sperm morphology and the relation of cell structure to fertility. Their material is again drawn from three sources; fertile men, men whose problem was infertile marriage, and the time required to produce a conception, when, and if, such occurred in the second group. Using their criteria there appeared to be three levels of percentage of normal cells that were related to the fertility: 60 per cent, between 60 and 80 per cent, and above 80 per cent normal forms. There were sharp distinctions between fertile and "infertile" men at these points which allowed them to conclude that an estimate of the chances of conception could be made according to morphology as poor, adequate, and good, respectively, as applied to these three percentile groups. It was amply demonstrated again that if the semen exhibits good counts and motility, the odds heavily favor a normal compliment of morphologically normal cells. Conversely, low counts and poor motility carry with them a higher percentage of atypical cells. However, a comparison of the two groups of men demonstrated the fact that at lower count levels (from under 20 million to 80 million per cc.) the fertile group maintains the same proportion of cases with 80 per cent or more normal forms whereas in the "infertile" group, at the same corresponding levels, the proportion of cases with the same number of normal cells more than doubles. Thus even with low counts consistently better morphology prevails with those who cause a conception. It was MacLeod's conclusion that there is a rising fertility potential with uniform normal structure of the spermatozoa and that fertility declines if the number of normal cells fall below 60 per cent.

The following table is useful in summarizing the experience of MacLeod and Gold as their impression of evaluating semen specimens on the basis of three important aspects of semen analyses:

	Count/cc. in Millions	% Active Cells	% Normal Cells
Poor	<20	<40	<60
Adequate	20 — 39	40 — 55	60 — 79
Good	40 +	60 +	80 +

Summary. The evidence gleaned from this vast study indicates that the sperm count, motility and morphology considered individually and collectively differ in fertile and "infertile" men. The subnormal qualities are preponderantly found in men who fail to produce a conception. This fact is verified by a study of a population of sufficient size to warrant statistical comparison of the two large groups and subdivisions within these groups. It would appear that the semen analysis coupled with other data relative to marital habits affords a means of general evaluation of the chances of conception. This appraisal is not absolute in the sense that a boundary line between fertility and infertility can be drawn. Such an absolute decision is warranted only at the point where the semen is devoid of spermatozoa. Presently there is justification to lower the standards as far as count per cubic centimeter to a level of 20,000,000 before concluding that the specimen is subnormal. The percentage and type of motility appears to have definite influence on the probability of conception. Incompleted statistical evidence points particularly to the importance of a good grade of activity as a requisite for good fertility. A combination of a low count and poor motility is definitely disadvantageous to the likelihood of conception.

BIOPSY OF THE TESTES

Biopsy of the human testis has become an accepted procedure for ascertaining the state of cellular activity with the testis. In turn, certain inferences may be raised concerning the general physiologic processes governing spermatogenesis. Nelson (1950) has commented that "testicular biopsy serves a role in the diagnosis of defects of the male gonadal function which is even superior to the endometrial biopsy in the female. The latter reflects the character of ovarian endocrine function without revealing defects of gametogenesis, whereas the testis biopsy furnishes an exact observation of the male sex cells." Testicular biopsy is now currently employed for three specific purposes:

1. It is used to differentiate between azoospermia due to obstruction or incomplete spermatogenesis.

2. To diagnose and evaluate disturbances in the endocrine systems.

3. For research on the normal and abnormal processes that characterize the testis, in puberty, adolescence, maturity and in senility.

A biopsy of the testicles serves a most useful and precise purpose in establishing a diagnosis between obstructive azoospermia and absence of sperm in the ejaculate due to faulty spermatogenesis. The clue to the correct diagnosis may be obtained from the history or the physical examination but often there is no guide. A history of bilateral epididymitis strongly suggests that an obstruction has caused a block preventing the escape of the spermatozoa. Small, soft, testes may be discovered during the physical examination and little doubt remains to account for the azoospermia on the basis of arrested or absent spermatogenesis. It is not uncommon to find a well-developed and otherwise normal man having semen devoid of spermatozoa and without a report of an illness to indicate a probable cause for the azoospermia. There is no controversy about the rationale of a biopsy in such instances.

Testicular biopsies are advocated by many when marked oligospermia is present. It is extremely rare to find an important discrepancy in spermatogenesis when one testis is compared to the other. However, a unilateral occlusion can occur blocking a normal testis and a deficient opposite testis may be the sole contributor of a few spermatozoa to the semen. Testicular biopsy may bring to light a progressive disease such as peritubular fibrosis and permit an unfavorable prognosis in men with oligospermia.

Testicular biopsy has been a most important tool in research where it has been extensively employed to elucidate the various alterations in spermatogenesis and abnormalities in the interstitial cells. Valuable aid to the study of endocrinology has resulted from the testis biopsy and it is clinically employed to advantage in the evaluation of endocrine disorders in which fertility is not the primary or sole consideration (Howard et al., 1950).

Our knowledge has not advanced to a point, however, that permits one to choose or select a type of effective therapy based on specific changes in the testis revealed by study of the excised tubules. Therefore testicular biopsy of men with oligospermia has a limited clinical or practical usefulness for it does not often further the diagnosis or indicate corrective measures to be employed. At least it may serve to avoid useless treatment which in itself is no small virtue.

The classification shown in Table 13, suggested by Engle (1947), correlates possibilities of testicular aberrations with semen examinations.

A description of the various types of tubules seen in tissue removed from the testes is as follows:

1. *A Normal Tubule.* The peritubular membrane is presented by a thin line separating the interstitial from the spermatogenic cells (Fig. 350). All of the blood vessels are found in the interstitial areas and it is presumed that the nutritive elements must pass through the membrane to reach the germinal cells. Likewise the waste products of metabolism must pass out of the tubule by perfusion through the peritubular membrane. Spermatogonia are found in the single row of cells that rest on the basement membrane.

2. The oval or fusiform cells are *Sertoli cells* located just above the spermatogonia, and project radially into the lumen of the tubule. They have the only oval nuclei to be found in the cells of the germinal epithelium.

Table 13. Testicular Biopsy and Semen Analysis

SEMEN ANALYSIS	TESTIS BIOPSY
1. Normal sample	
2. Azoospermia	*a.* With demonstrable occlusion
	1. Normal tubules
	2. Disturbed spermatogenesis
	b. Without demonstrable occlusion
	1. Normal tubules
	2. Progressive tubular fibrosis
	3. Germinal aplasia
	4. Spermatogenic arrest (to spermatocyte I)
3. Oligospermia	*a.* With high frequency of abnormal spermatozoa
	1. Incomplete maturation
	2. Progressive tubular fibrosis
	b. Inflammation and infection

Primary spermatocytes have the largest nuclei around a chromatin network which is clearly visible. Primary spermatocytes are larger than the secondary spermatocytes. The spermatids are recognized by small dark nuclei near the border of the lumen. One often sees the spermatozoa imbedded in the cytoplasm of the Sertoli cell which are therefore considered to be nutritive or trophic cells.

3. *Germinal Aplasia.* Tubules are usually uniform in size but the striking feature is a complete lack of germ cells (Fig. 351). The only epithelial cells present within the tubules are the Sertoli cells. The cytoplasm of the Sertoli cells is rather vague in outline and faintly acidophilic. Occasionally a few tubules may show a sprinkling of germ cells, but mitosis does not go beyond the spermatogonia or primary spermatocyte stage. The Leydig cells are usually normal.

4. *Spermatogenic Arrest.* Spermatogenic arrest is characterized by a failure of spermatogenesis to go on to completion (Fig. 352). The tubules are of normal size, the spermatogonia are normal in numbers, and the Sertoli cells are not unusual. Arrest may occur at the level of the primary spermatocytes, the secondary spermatocytes, or at the spermatid stage. In any event the results are the same. Few, if any, mature spermatozoa are produced. If in-

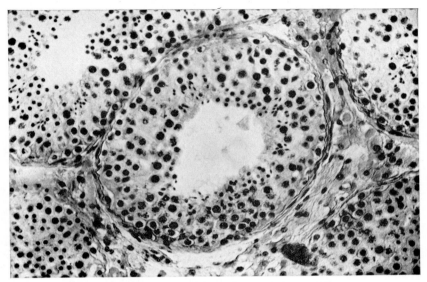

Fig. 350.   Normal seminiferous tubules. × 300.

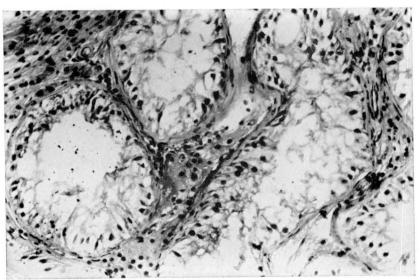

Fig. 351.   Seminiferous tubules. Germinal aplasia. × 300.

sufficient cells are present in the germinal layer there will be an abundance of cellular debris in the lumen of the testis.

5. *Generalized Peritubular Fibrosis*. The testis tubule varies in size in relation to the degree of fibrosis (Fig. 353). When a heavy layer is laid down in the periphery of the tubule, there appears to be a consequent shrinkage in size. Likewise spermatogenesis is often proportionate in degree to the replacement of the tubules by the connective tissue (Fig. 353). The process is probably a progressive one and continues until all germ cells are

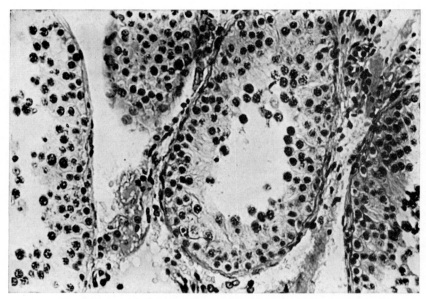

Fig. 352.   Seminiferous tubules. Spermatogenic arrest. $\times$ 300.

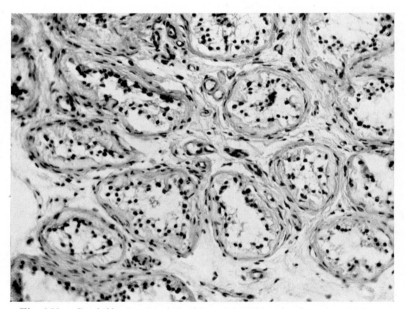

Fig. 353.   Seminiferous tubules. Advanced peritubular fibrosis. $\times$ 100.

eliminated by the thickening of the peritubular connective tissue. Eventually complete sclerosis of the tubule occurs.

6. *Incomplete Maturation and Disturbed Spermatogenesis.* The tubules of such testes are to be found in men who have very few sperm, or cell count below the average. Usually the diameters of the tubules are normal or somewhat smaller than usual. Peritubular fibrosis may be present in varying

degrees so that the testis which produces a small number of sperm may have all the components of the normal and abnormal testis. The commonly recognized defects in this classification are a sloughing of the immature cells, atypical mitosis, particularly at the reduction stage of the division, abnormal nuclei, mature sperm and immature sperm present in the lumen of the tubules rather than being confined to the sustenacular cells of Sertoli, as in the cases of the normal (Fig. 354). A distortion of the cell division of abnormal nuclear construction may be seen. In summary, the most common histologic pattern is one of disorganized spermatogenesis. Aberrations in cell division

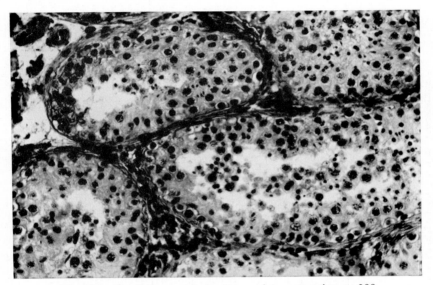

Fig. 354. Seminiferous tubules. Incomplete maturation. × 300.

and chromosomal behavior are correlated with increased atypical forms in the spermatozoa in the ejaculate. Nelson's report (1950) of 623 men whose testicular biopsies were studied in detail is tabulated in summary in Tables 14 and 15 correlating the gonadotropic assays with the condition of the azoospermic and oligospermic.

Much speculation is given to the causes for these abnormalities, since histological evidence for inflammation in the testis is not common.

Other causes are x-ray, toxins, genetic influence and nutritional disturbances, either due to deficiencies or faulty intermediary metabolism. It is evident that the causes for the various disturbances are obscure. Peritubular fibrosis is common in the aged.

MEDICAL TREATMENT

General Considerations. There are only two standards for appraising the efficacy of treatment of men with reduced fertility. The semen might become improved, or, secondly, pregnancy might take place. It is equally apparent that neither one offers conclusive proof of the usefulness of treatment, for it has long been recognized that physiological fluctuations in the

Table 14. Testicular Conditions in Men with Azoospermia

LEYDIG CELLS USUALLY IN NORMAL RANGE

(Nelson, 1950)

CONDITIONS	NO. CASES	SPERMATOGONIA	SPERMATOCYTES	SPERMATIDS AND SPERM	PERITUBULAR CONNECTIVE TISSUE	GONADOTROPINS
Germinal cell aplasia	46	None	None	None	Usually normal	High
Germinal cell arrest	27	Numerous	Increased primary; usually few secondary	Few	Usually normal	Low normal to normal
Generalized fibrosis	24	Reduced numbers	Reduced numbers	Few	Marked increase	Usually high
Obstructed or absent ducts	22	Numerous	Usually numerous	Usually numerous	Variable	Normal

Table 15. Testicular Conditions in Men with Oligospermia

LEYDIG CELLS AND GONADOTROPINS USUALLY IN NORMAL RANGE

(Nelson, 1950)

CONDITION	NO. CASES	SPERMATOGONIA	SPERMATOCYTES	SPERMATIDS AND SPERM	PERITUBULAR CONNECTIVE TISSUE
Sloughing and disorganization	152	Numerous	Numerous, much sloughing	Reduced numbers	Variable
Incomplete germinal cell arrest	74	Numerous	Increased primary; numerous or reduced secondary	Reduced numbers	Usually normal
Regional fibrosis	58	Numerous except in regions of fibrosis	Numerous except in regions of fibrosis	Numerous except in regions of fibrosis	Marked increase in some regions
Germinal cell atrophy	30	Reduced numbers	Reduced numbers	Reduced numbers	Variable
Abnormal mitosis	64	Numerous	Usually numerous, but many abnormal	Reduced normal cells; increased abnormal forms	Variable

character of the semen might take place and that pregnancy, although it is the desired objective, may sometimes occur if only a few spermatozoa are present in the semen. The skeptic, however, has equal difficulty in refuting the possible benefits of therapy should either or both events occur. It is equally apparent that, if each were rejected as a means of evaluation of treatment, there would be no conceivable method to measure the effect. The dilemma could be satisfied if some acceptable point of reference could be established from which all deviations could be analyzed. Thus, the emergence, or the lack of a response, could be made definitely chargeable to treatment. Finally, the difficulties of evaluating therapy are compounded by the fact that two individuals, not one, are the subjects of the test. Thus, a pregnancy may very well be due to an improvement in the wife and unrelated to a shift, or lack of change, of the status of the husband.

The problem of evaluating treatment is by no means confined to the study of sterility. Elsewhere in the medical scene are innumerable examples of disorders where uncertainties are to be found concerning the management of the patients. Nevertheless, efforts are properly being made to find, and to evaluate, therapy, for advancement and progress are dependent upon interest and trial. Resignation in the face of uncertainties leads only to stagnation of thought and knowledge.

A variety of treatments have been used to improve the possibility of conception in instances where men have subnormal but not azoospermic semen. These procedures range from correction of body weight, adoption of proper health habits, eradication of focal infection, instruction for timing coitus during the period of ovulation, to specific medicinal agents. None of these methods can withstand attack of severe scientific criticism, for the results are not often repetitious and cannot be predicted with a satisfactory assurance. Presently, there is only one point of reference upon which we may rely. Complete and persistent azoospermia represents a state from which spontaneous improvement rarely, if ever, takes place. Therefore, any therapy which results in spermatozoa appearing in the semen, where none formerly were found, constitutes acceptable evidence of a therapeutic response. Such an event is afforded by the surgical correction of an occlusion by vaso-epididymal anastomosis. There is no proven system of medical treatments which have stimulated the azoospermic testis to produce adequate numbers of spermatozoa. When, and if, this is done we shall have undisputed evidence of a response and a well established base line. There is a valid objection to insisting that such a demonstration must be made before any attempts at therapy are justified. The oligospermic testis may well be more responsive to therapy than the refractory azoospermic gonad and the two may not be comparable. Consequently, treatment of the subnormal but not totally sterile male, is based on a different premise. The base line or point of reference for the subnormal male may lie in group studies where the erratic behavior of the single individual is lost in the general pattern of the group. Significant changes in a group of treated patients compared to a controlled group might furnish the desired means of comparison.

With these considerations and reservations in mind certain phases of treatment merit attention.

General Measures. The solution of the problem of barrenness may be made apparent during the course of the history. The couple may be misinformed as to the probable time of ovulation, or are accustomed to such infrequent coitus that conception is improbable. Detailed questioning may bring forth the information that a seminal discharge has never taken place. The value of the specific question has already been alluded to in the notes on the taking of the history and the inferences are obvious.

Volume of the Semen. A reduction in the amount of semen may result in an inadequate seminal pool. The buffering capacity of the semen is proportionately reduced and the vehicle may be so scant that the sperm do not reach the cervix. Inadequate expulsion of the semen may be due to a defect in the urethra, or in the glands and ducts of the seminal vesicles and the prostate. A urethral diverticulum may trap all, or most, of the ejaculate. It is not uncommon to discover that retrograde ejaculation into the bladder may follow a transurethral resection of the prostate. Likewise, a hypospadias may cause inadequate deposition, or even ejaculation outside of the vagina.

The volume of the ejaculate may be reduced because the seminal vesicles and the prostate are not secreting the full complement of seminal secretions. Accessory glands are not fully developed in certain cases of hypogonadism, and endocrine disorders, but usually there is no spermatogenesis in such extreme cases, and so the azoospermia precludes much concern about the small volume. Pre-existing infection in the seminal vesicles may cause a cicatrix of the ejaculatory ducts and consequent loss of fluid.

Methods of correcting strictures and diverticula of the urethra, hypospadias, and infections of the prostate and seminal vesicles are recorded in other chapters. If the semen is discharged into the bladder rather than through the urethra, sperm can be recovered and used for artificial insemination. The patient is instructed to empty the bladder after which a catheter is passed and the bladder is washed with Ringer's glucose solution. About 2 cc. of Ringer's glucose solution are then instilled. Ejaculation is produced manually and the patient may then be able to void the solution, or it may be withdrawn by catheterization. Large numbers of very active spermatozoa may be procured by this method for artificial insemination.

Increased Viscosity. The significance of increased viscosity has not been settled to the satisfaction of all. Commonly, viscid semen exhibits poor motility. The cells may be agglutinated or may appear to have difficulty traversing through the thickened media. On the other hand, a viscid specimen may show no impairment in the type, percentage, or duration of activity.

The exact cause of increased viscosity is not known. An infection in the prostate and seminal vesicles may exist but this is not a requirement. The lysis may be incomplete due to faulty action on the part of the enzymes secreted by the prostate. The blood serum, however, will not reduce the viscosity if added to a specimen. It would seem that if the postcoital spermigration test showed active invasion of the cervical canal by the spermatozoa, the viscid semen is not materially detracting from the possibility of conception. Treatment has not been gratifying in correcting increased viscosity of the semen agglutinization of spermatozoa. Massage of the prostate and seminal vesicles would seem a logical method of approach, for it is to be assumed that the difficulty lies in these glands. Testosterone propionate has been used on the basis that it has an action on the accessory sexual gland. The results are not rewarding. Furthermore, the addition of Ringer's glucose solution to the viscid semen does not cause dispersal of the agglutinated islands of cells.

Motility. Poor motility is usually associated with oligospermic specimens. It is unusual to find large numbers of spermatozoa in the ejaculate and to discover only a few or none of the cells are motile. Should this situation be encountered it is well to inquire whether the directions concerning the collection of the specimen were carried out. The commonest error is to use a condom rather than collect the ejaculate in a dry, clean, jar.

Absent or marked reduction in the percentage of sperm that are motile has been designated as "necrospermia." It has been shown, however, that the sperm are not dead as the term implies. When placed in a Warburg apparatus, the cells may be found to be metabolizing reducible substances much in the manner of cells that are very active since they are living cells but are not demonstrating activity. The cause of the defect may be due to testicular abnormality or to a failure of the mechanism which initiates motility. The site of the latter defect would implicate the prostatovesicular secretions. Support for the belief that the spermatozoa may be incapable of being stimulated by reason of faulty spermatogenesis is derived from the fact that, when only a few cells are present, poor motility is often a concomitant factor.

The uncertain results which seem to influence the process of spermatogenesis makes this type of therapy for poor motility an unreliable one. However, if the numbers of sperm are increased it is not uncommon to find that the motility is likewise improved.

If congestion, infection or incomplete drainage is found in the prostate or seminal vesicles these organs should be treated in the hope that an improvement in motility will follow.

The amount of reducible substance in the semen from which the spermatozoa obtain their nutrition responsible for their motility was not found to be reduced in a number of instances when analysis was made. Therefore, the rationale of supplying the Ringer's glucose douche prior to coitus cannot be made on the assumption that a deficiency in glucose is supplied by this medium. If the motility is poor the use of a Ringer's glucose douche may wash away material from the cervical os, or elevate the pH of the vagina. This may serve to minimize the loss of motile sperm and increase the likelihood of penetration into the cervical canal.

Several types of cervical applicators and caps have been advocated to insure insemination. The semen is placed therein and brought into contact with the cervical canal and isolated from the vagina. Whitelaw (1950) reports that motility is retained longer in such a cervical cap and that the pregnancy rate was increased on a group of sterility cases so inseminated.

Oligospermia and Abnormal Morphology. A reduced number of cells or an increased percentage of abnormal spermatozoa implies that the site of the deficiency is in the testis. Testicular biopsies (q.v.) have given the observers much information of the cytological disturbances that take place. It is probable that the difference in spermatogenesis of oligospermic testes as compared to that of the azoospermic testes is mainly one of degree. Peritubular fibrosis, atypical mitosis, particularly at the reduction stage of division, and complete fibrosis of portions of the testis are the common histologic changes that are to be found with oligospermia.

If more information were at hand regarding the cause of these testicular changes, it is obvious that therapeutic efforts would have better design and purpose. The present inferences are that these faulty mitoses might be due to hereditary influences, nutritional deficiencies, faulty intermediary metabolism, disorder of the connective tissue system, or an aberration in the endocrine systems. One might infer that all but the first cause could be attacked by a system of treatment. This theoretical inference is of course subject to severe limitations, both from the standpoint of serviceable knowledge of treatment and likewise from the unavailability of agents to correct a so-called deficiency. Certain simple methods of treatment have, on occasions, produced responses that satisfy the requirements of efficacious therapy.

A basal metabolism test may indicate that thyroid substance may be given. The diet may be altered and reinforced with vitamins A, B complex and E. Weight reduction and correction of excesses in alcohol and tobacco may very well improve the general health. A period of six to eight months may be required to evaluate the effects of such treatment. Several samples of semen must be examined to determine the constancy or the lack of improvement.

In the recent past, considerable interest has been aroused by the findings of Heller (1950) and his report may merit mention here, for it is one of the first which implies that spermatogenesis may be influenced by testosterone propionate. Heller treated a group of patients, whose fertility was judged poor by testicular biopsies. In all, the spermatogenesis was markedly defective and peritubular fibrosis was a nearly constant finding. An assay of the gonadotropic hormones showed a high output of FSH. The patients were given 25 mg. of testosterone propionate daily for a period of ninety days. A biopsy at the end of the treatment showed what appeared to be marked injury to the already defective spermatic tissue. However, a third biopsy taken approximately one and a half years later, revealed that spermatogenesis was immeasurably better than was the case before any treatment was given. From this work the author acknowledges that confirmation is to be desired before his observations can be generally accepted. The implications from this unusual study are obvious and the experience of others with this regimen will be awaited with great interest.

Heckel reported that the administration of testosterone propionate depressed spermatogenesis. In 1951 he and his co-authors described the "rebound" phenomena in five men with subnormal spermatozoa counts.

Each was given 50 mg. of testosterone three times a week for periods from twelve to eighteen weeks. At the conclusion of the treatment, all had either no spermatozoa in the semen or were at near-azoospermic levels. Observations during the subsequent six months revealed that the sperm counts of all exceeded the pretreatment levels. Heckel has extended his work and recently reported upon thirty-eight men so treated and observed for eighteen months or more. Two thirds exhibited this "rebound" to levels in excess of the spermatozoa counts prior to treatment. One third were not improved or were below the sperm concentration before treatment. Testicular biopsies were secured before and after treatment in some of the men. Although improved spermatogenesis was noted in those benefited, the authors were not able to select, or predict, those capable of response from the pattern of the seminiferous tubules.

Other hormones than testosterone and thyroid have been used with disappointing results. The occasional case which seems to have responded to the gonadotropins has maintained an interest in their use, but the over-all opinion is that the gonadotropins are not reliable, and should be used only as a method of last resort. Extracts of the anterior pituitary gland, pregnancy urine extract, pregnant mares serum all have been given to patients with oligospermic semen. It was hoped that, if the gonadotropic assays were low, the substitution of these substances might have the effect of a replacement that would result in better spermatogenesis. The hope has not been substantiated by a sizeable series of cases which have been so treated.

Some direct their therapy toward methods to correct liver deficiencies or to improve the function of that organ. The use of large doses of vitamins, plus the gonadotropins, has been the essence of this treatment to correct faulty spermatogenesis.

It is well to reiterate at this point that one of the greatest difficulties is to appraise therapy, due to the physiologic fluctuations. Therefore, these approaches to the problem are not documented in any satisfactory way, and opinions fall in that vague classification of "clinical impressions." One redeeming feature of therapy is that it need not be expensive. The patient can manage to administer treatment, including the use of hormones, at his home after a brief instruction by the office nurse or by the doctor. Frequent semen analyses need not be done, for, if changes occur, a considerable length of time is required before an improvement is noted.

SURGICAL TREATMENT

Prophylaxis. The correction of testicular ectopia before the age of twelve should be done if a functioning testis is to be preserved for adult life. Orchidopexy does not insure that the ectopic testis will produce sperm, for some individuals having bilateral operations at an early age are sterile even though the testes occupy a normal position in the scrotum in adult life. Spontaneous descent may occur before full adulthood is reached but if this does not transpire, spermatogenic function is lost even though operation is done in the late teens. The reports of McCollum (1935) offer good evidence that orchidopexy at ten or eleven years of age will secure spermatogenesis in adult life in many instances whereas delay to the age of fourteen results in failure of the spermatic tissue to develop.

Vaso-Epididymal Anastomoses. A complete and persistent absence of spermatozoa is irremediable, unless the azoospermia is due to an obstruction. This statement might be modified in the future should therapy improve or if the new principle of androgenic treatment becomes verified.

Testicular biopsy has been previously discussed. If large numbers of mature spermatozoa are found in the testicular tissue, an exploration of the scrotum should be done in the hope that an obstruction, if one is found, can be circumvented. There is no surgical hazard involved in the procedure and complications are remote, but it is proper to inform the patient that the prognosis for success is not favorable, and that there is no assurance of success. His plight is not worsened even with failure.

A microscope with suitable illumination should be installed in the operating room before the procedure is begun. The surgeon should provide himself with sterile slides, small ocular forceps, and gauge 20 and 22 hypodermic needles which have been honed so that the sharp edge is blunted. About 30 cc. of hydrogen peroxide with 10 drops of methylene blue should be available.

Each side of the scrotal sac should be opened and both testes delivered through the wound. At this point, it may be discovered that there is a congenital absence of all or part of the epididymides or ductuli deferentes. Should this congenital anomaly be bilateral, there is no hope of cure unless enough of the head of the epididymis is present and spermatozoa are found therein. If the vas is present and patent at that level, an anastomosis can be done.

A puncture is made with a number 11 Bard-Parker knife at the lower portion of the epididymis and the fluid obtained therefrom is examined for spermatozoa. If sperm are not recovered, additional incisions are made toward the head of the epididymis until an adequate number of spermatozoa are found. The vas is identified at the corresponding level and a transverse incision is made therein. The lumen of the vas is just within the range of vision permitting the blunt pointed needle to be introduced into the distal portion. Ten cubic centimeters of hydrogen peroxide–methylene blue solution is injected. If an obstruction exists distal to this point the fluid will not flow through the tube. Silkworm suture can be inserted into the lumen of the vas and passed distally to discover the site of the obstruction. Should patency be proven and spermatozoa found, vaso-epididymo-anastomosis may be performed.

The epididymal tubule is elevated by small forceps and a window is cut therein. An opening in the vas can be conveniently made, using the point of the needle which has been inserted into the lumen as a guide for a number 11 blade (Humphreys and Hotchkiss, 1935; see also Section XVI, Chapter 12).

The surgeon may elect to follow one of several different plans at this point. He may use number 30 wire or arterial silk for suturing the two openings together. Six sutures are usually required to afford a good approximation, care being used to have the knots lie outside of the anastomosis. The surgeon may elect to insert a silver wire (size 22–24) into the distal vas and thread it into the fenestra made into the epididymis before closing the anatomosis. The free end of this internal splint may then be brought out through the lower pole of the epididymis and thence to the surface of the skin where a lead shot is attached. After six to eight days this splint can then be withdrawn. No drains are required. The procedure is repeated on the opposite side. Bilateral operations are desirable, for the chances of success are accordingly improved. A scrotal suspensory is applied. The patient is given antibiotics and kept in the hospital for four or five days (Michaelson, 1946).

Successful results have occurred in about one out of five cases. The semen is examined every month for one year. It is unusual to find spermatozoa in the ejaculate earlier than the second month, and in one instance more than a year elapsed before spermatozoa appeared. At times spermatozoa may disappear after they have been regularly found in the semen for three or four months, but the usual course is a permanent cure when spermatozoa are to be found following operation. As sequential specimens are examined it is customary to see the quality of semen improve during the next few months following the time the sperm are first seen.

REFERENCES

ENGLE, E. T.: Male Reproductive System. Problems of Ageing. Biological and Medical Aspects, Chap. 15, Baltimore, Williams & Wilkins Co., 1939.

ENGLE, E. T.: The testis biopsy in infertility. J. Urol., *57:*789–799, 1947.

ENGLE, E. T. and J. N. ROBINSON: Effect of neutron radiation of human testes. Trans. Am. Assoc. Genito-Urin. Surg., *40:*129–132, 1948.

FALK, H. C. and S. A. KAUFMAN: What constitutes a normal semen. Fertility and Sterility, *1:*489–503, 1950.

FARRIS, E. J.: Human Fertility. Author's Press, 1950.

HECKEL, N. J., W. A. ROSSO and L. KESTEL: Spermatogenic rebound phenomenon after testosterone therapy. J. Clin. Endocrinol., *2:*235–246, 1951.

HELLER, C. G.: Improvement of spermatogenesis following depression of human testes with testosterone. Fertility and Sterility, *1:*415–421, 1950.

HOTCHKISS, R. S.: Fertility in Men. Chap. 7, Philadelphia, J. B. Lippincott, 1944.

HOTCHKISS, R. S., E. K. BRUNNER and P. GRENLEY: Semen analyses of two hundred fertile men. Am. J. Med. Sci., *196:*362, 1938.

HOWARD, P. A., R. C. SNIFFEN, F. A. SIMMONS and F. ALBRIGHT: Testicular deficiency. J. Clin. Endocrinol., *10:*121–186, 1950.

HUGGINS, C. B. and A. A. JOHNSON: Chemistry of fluids of seminal tract. Am. J. Physiol., *103:*574, 1950.

HUMPHREYS, G., and R. S. HOTCHKISS: Vaso-epididymal anastomosis. J. Urol., *42:*815–820, 1935.

KLINEFELTER, H. F., JR., REIFENSTEIN, E. C., JR. and ALBRIGHT, F.: Syndrome characterized by gynecomastia, aspermatogenesis and increased excretion of follicle-stimulating hormone. J. Clin. Endocrinol., *2:*615–627, 1942.

MACLEOD, J.: The metabolism of human spermatozoa. Proc. Soc. Exp. Biol. & Med., *A2:* 153, 1939.

MACLEOD, J. and GOLD, R. Z.: Sperm morphology in fertile and infertile marriage. Fertil. & Steril. *2:*394–414, 1951.

MACLEOD, J. and GOLD, R. Z.: Semen quality and certain other factors in relation to the ease of conception. Fertil. & Steril., *4:*10–33, 1953.

MacLeod, J. and Gold, R. Z.: Effect of continence on semen quality. Fertil. & Steril., 3:297–315, 1952.

MacLeod, J. and R. S. Hotchkiss: Effect of hyperpyrexia upon spermatozoa counts in men. Endocrinology, 28:780–784, 1941.

MacLeod, J.: The male factor in fertility and infertility. Fertility and Sterility, 1:347–361, 1950.

Macomber, D. and M. M. Saunders: The spermatozoa count. New England Med. J., 200: 981, 1929.

Mann, T.: Fructose—a constituent of semen. Biochem. J., 40:481–491, 1946.

McCollum, P. W.: Clinical study of spermatogenesis in undescended testicles. Arch. Surg., 31:290, 1935.

Meaker, S. R.: Human Sterility. Baltimore, Williams & Wilkins, 1934.

Michelson, L.: Vaso-epididymal anastomosis. Surg., Gynec. & Obst., 82:327–331, 1946.

Mulinos, M. and L. Pomerantz: Reproductive organs in malnutrition. Endocrinology, 29:267–275, 1941.

Munro, S. S.: Effect of dilution and density on fertilizing capacity of fowl sperm in excretory ducts. Canad. J. Research, 16:281, 1938.

Nelson, W. O.: Testicular morphology in eunuchoidal and infertile men. Fertility and Sterility, 1:477–489, 1950.

Sims, M. J.: The microscope as a aid in the diagnosis and treatment of sterility. New York State Med. J., 8:399–413, 1868.

Werner, C. A.: Mumps orchitis and testicular atrophy. Ann. Int. Med., 32:1066–1071, 1075–1085, 1950.

Whitelaw, J. M.: Use of the cervical cap to increase fertility. Fertility and Sterility, 1: 33–39, 1950.

Wilkins, L.: Endocrine Disorders in Childhood and Adolescence. Chap. 4, Springfield, C. C Thomas, 1950.

Section VIII

URINARY LITHIASIS AND FOREIGN BODIES

CHAPTER 1

Urolithiasis

CHARLES C. HIGGINS, M.D.

GENERAL CONSIDERATIONS

Geographic Distribution. It has long been recognized that urinary calculi are observed in some countries or localities more frequently than in others, and investigations in relation to these "stone areas" (Fig. 355) have led to theories that diet, water, climatic conditions or geological formations may be the influencing factors. Most of the statistics describing the geographic distribution of calculi refer to vesical stones and the data dealing with renal lithiasis are less reliable.

Fujimaki (1926) called attention to the prevalence of calculi in southern China in contrast to their relative rarity in the northern part of the country. In India, McCarrison (1931) noted the frequency of calculi in the Punjab, or northern part, as contrasted with the much lower incidence in southern India. Guersel (1936) charted the existing stone areas in Turkey. Additional stone areas have been reported in Madagascar, Egypt, and the valley of the Volga in Russia. Joly (1931) reported that in Great Britain stone areas are to be found along the east coast, in North Wales and in a part of Derbyshire and Westmoreland. He also mentioned that calculous disease was rare in Ireland, South America and comparatively uncommon in North America. The findings in Joly's extensive study indicated that lithiasis was more prevalent in the old world than in the new, and that the three important stone areas, India, Mesopotamia and South China were regions of defective sanitation and hygiene. He attributed a progressive decrease in the incidence of calculi among Europeans to improved hygiene and nutrition.

A survey of the so-called stone areas yields no common denominator to which the cause of stone formation in these regions might be attributed; it is obvious that considerable variation exists among the different groups displaying a high incidence of urinary lithiasis as regards diet, climatic conditions, etc. The evidence indicates that at present the incidence of vesical

767

calculi is lower in some areas where it was unusually high in the past. This is not true of renal calculi; in fact, there appears to be an increase in the incidence of renal and ureteral calculi in the United States. This apparent increase, however, may be influenced by more accurate diagnosis.

Causes of Urinary Calculi. According to our present concepts of calculous disease, it appears that no single causative factor is responsible for the formation of the various types of renal calculi. Prominent among current theories as to pathogenesis are: disturbances in the protective mechanism of the colloids, deficiency of vitamin A, focal and local infection, urinary stasis, recumbency and immobilization, hypercalcinuria, hyperparathyroidism and certain metabolic disturbances.

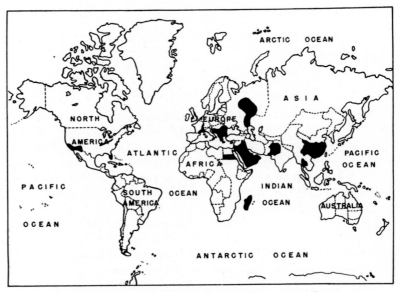

Fig. 355.   World map showing "stone areas."

Chemical Factors. The formation of urinary calculi is a complex process, requiring two distinct substances, the colloid and the crystalline. Thus a calculus is a concretion composed of crystalloids bound together by a colloidal substance. The crystalline constituents of urinary calculi may be composed of substances normally found in the urine, as calcium oxalate or uric acid, or substances which result from disorders of metabolism, such as cystine, and finally, salts which may be present in the urine owing to bacterial activity (ammonium magnesium phosphate).

It has long been known that urine contains small amounts of colloidal substances. Lichtwitz stated that there are 0.83 gm. of colloid per liter of urine. This quantity may be increased by a diet rich in proteins. The colloids obtained by dialysis are a mixture of mucin, nucleic acid, chondroitin-sulfuric acid, glycogen and perhaps other substances. From his investigative work, Lichtwitz concluded that the abnormal solubility of stone-forming salts in the urine depends upon the colloids which prevent precipitation and agglutination of salts and other colloids.

Schade (1923) noted that the requisite for stone formation consists of the precipitation of crystals from a supersaturated solution containing an organic colloidal material, such as fibrin or mucin.

Butt, Hauser, Seifter and Perry (1953) observed that the urine is a highly saturated solution because of the presence of certain colloids. They stressed that the protective action of the urinary colloids is of prime importance in preventing the precipitation and clustering of crystalloids. They noted that if the concentration of such protective colloids was not sufficient, stone formation might ensue. Clinically, they observed that the subcutaneous injection of hyaluronidase creates a pronounced increase in the protective urinary colloids. The clinical application of this therapy was effective in preventing formation or recurrence of urinary calculi for periods of nine to twelve months in fifteen patients with a tendency to rapid stone formation.

As a result of his investigative work, Flocks (1940) stated that the pH of the urine is not the most important single factor in the formation of urine which keeps calcium salts in solution. Substances are present in the urine which form soluble complexes with the calcium and are negatively charged. The ability of the urine to form such calcium complexes (negatively charged) may assume importance in relation to the formation of calcium stones. Flocks found that many patients who have or have had urinary calculi may show a high content of urinary calcium, while the calcium and phosphorus levels in the blood are normal. The exact cause of this increased excretion of calcium is obscure. In Flocks' series, these cases comprised 60 per cent of the group with calcium stones. As a rule, 35 to 50 per cent of patients with calcium stones show a normal or low urinary calcium. Riegel et al. (1947) observed that fourteen of fifteen patients with urolithiasis had an increased excretion of calcium. Seven of the fourteen patients had impaired renal function; in the others, renal function was normal. Davalos (1945) stressed the role of the concentration of urine in the formation of calculi in tropical areas.

Dietary Factors. Numerous clinical and experimental observations have stressed the relationship between stone formation and the absence or deficiency of certain essentials in the diet. Fujimaki, McCarrison, Noble, Boshamer and others stressed the dietary deficiencies of persons residing in the stone areas. In the laboratory, calculi have been produced in animals maintained on a diet deficient in vitamin A (Osborne et al., 1917; Mendel, 1917; Higgins, 1936, 1943). By maintaining white rats on diets deficient in vitamin A for extended periods, and by varying the constituents of the diet, we have produced renal and vesical calculi composed of phosphates with traces of carbonates, and carbonates with traces of phosphates. In rabbits, oxamide calculi and calculi composed of acetyl salts of the sulfonamides were obtained. In dogs, stones containing calcium magnesium ammonium phosphate and, in the Dalmatian dog, uric acid calculi were produced. Finally, a renal calculus composed of cystine was produced in a man with cystinuria (Higgins, 1936). While the clinical significance of such experimental studies is not entirely clear, it does indicate that dietary deficiency may be one of the causes of urinary calculi.

Infection. Rosenow and Meisser, in 1921, inoculated the pulp of the teeth of six dogs with streptococci isolated from the urine of patients with urinary calculi and thereby produced calculi in the animals. Keyser (1923) also produced calculi by infecting the bladder of rabbits with streptococci isolated from the urine of patients with urinary calculi. Hager and Magath (1925) performed similar experiments, utilizing Proteus ammoniae organisms.

Several observers, including Braasch (1917), Bugbee (1932), Keyser (1934), Scholl (1936), Quinby (1933) and others, have discussed the apparent relationship between infection of the urinary tract and calculous formation. In his critical review of twenty-nine patients, Bugbee elicited a history of a preexisting pyelonephritis in twenty-three instances. Randall (1937) found calcium plaques in the renal papillae in 140 of 609 cases in which postmortem studies were made. In forty-nine instances, there were stones adherent to the renal papillae. Randall concluded that, in the absence of pelvic obstruction, a renal calculus would require an initiating lesion for its growth and that such a lesion would have to occur on the renal papilla.

Although there is some apparent connection between renal infection and the formation of urinary stones, this is not the whole story, for many patients who have chronic pyelonephritis do not have kidney stones, or stones may be present in one kidney only. Furthermore, in many cases of urolithiasis, no infection can be demonstrated. In a review of 589 cases of lithiasis, Rovsing (1923) observed that the urine was sterile in 276. In a series of 419 cases, reported by Lett in 1936, the urine was sterile in forty-nine. In 480 cases of urinary lithiasis, including renal, ureteral and bladder stones, Harrington (1940) could elicit no evidence of infection in 26 per cent, and pointed out that the true percentage of sterile cases was undoubtedly considerably higher than this. In a personal series of 800 consecutive cases of renal lithiasis, I found (1943) that the urine was sterile in ninety-eight or 12.2 per cent.

There is considerable evidence that urea-splitting organisms may play an important role in the formation of renal calculi. The organism possesses the power of splitting the urea in the urine into ammonia and carbon dioxide with the resultant formation of ammonium carbonate. This combines with the magnesium salts and phosphates to form ammonium magnesium phosphate, which is insoluble and, by rendering the reaction of the urine alkaline, results in the precipitation of the equally earthy phosphates. The chief offenders are the Staphylococcus, Streptococcus, and Proteus organisms. Cahill has stressed the role of urea-splitting organisms, especially the Staphylococcus and Proteus, in the production of renal calculi.

Infections of the urinary tract which result in the splitting of urea occur more frequently than is usually presumed. Brown and Earlam (1933) have stated that 18 per cent of the bacilli and 40 per cent of Staphylococcus strains possess this power. There appears but little doubt that in recurrent renal lithiasis, infection assumes an important role, especially in the presence of stasis. Keyser (1934) observed that recurrent renal calculi composed of phosphates and carbonates are frequently associated with coccal or bacillary infections. According to Rovsing (1923), 68 per cent of recurrent calculi in his series were infected primarily or secondarily with urea-splitting organisms. In 15.9 per cent of cases, the urine was found to be sterile. In 100 consecutive cases of recurrent calculi, I found infection was present in fifty-four of seventy-two patients with recurrent unilateral stones, and the culture was sterile in eighteen, a relatively high proportion (1938). In several of these cases, the recurrent stones were very small, and urinary antiseptics had been administered in nine instances. In the group of twenty-eight patients with bilateral recurrent stones, infection was present in the kidneys in twenty-three cases and the culture of the urine was sterile in five. Staphylococcus in pure or mixed cultures was the predominant organism, and Proteus organisms were second in frequency.

Twinem (1937), in a review of forty-four cases of recurrent calculi reported from the Brady Foundation of the New York Hospital, stated that the organism present most frequently was the colon bacillus. Bacillus proteus and staphylococci were second and third, respectively. Although the foregoing reports make it evident that renal calculi are frequently associated with renal infection, it is equally evident that aseptic calculi are often observed; hence infection cannot be considered a prerequisite for the formation of stones.

Stasis. Stasis, which often is reported in association with renal calculi, renders the field suitable for bacterial growth and may be instrumental in shifting the pH of the urine to the alkaline side. Hunner (1924) emphasized the importance of ureteral stricture in the formation of renal calculi and recommended dilation of the ureter to eliminate stasis, stagnation and persistent infection. Keyser (1923) emphasized how stasis was instrumental in the retention of crystals and their growth and confirmed his theory in the experimental animal.

Immobilization. According to Lowsley and Kirwin (1940), immobilization acts in two ways to influence the production of urinary calculi: (1) by impairing renal drainage and (2) by producing changes in calcium metabolism. They concluded that renal lithiasis in immobilized patients is the result of skeletal decalcification. Infection may also play an important part in the formation of calculi in this group of patients. Rarely fibrin calculi associated with fibrinogenuria are observed, or bacterial concretions, as observed by Scholl (1936), are reported. The etiology in these instances is obscure.

Hyperparathyroidism. Barney and Mintz, and also Albright and Bloomberg have noted the relationship between hyperparathyroidism and renal lithiasis. In 1934, Barney and Mintz reviewed a series of eighteen cases of hyperparathyroidism and observed that calculi were present in the urinary tract in eleven, or 61.1 per cent. The youngest patient was aged thirteen

years; the oldest, sixty-two years, with the average forty-three years. Twelve
of the patients were women and six were men. Bony changes were evident
in twelve cases, and in six instances, involvement of bone and urinary calculi
were associated. Bilateral renal calculi were present in four, or 36 per cent
of the eleven cases. Their conclusion was that hyperparathyroidism is responsible for about 4 or 5 per cent of the cases of renal calculi. Sangree
(1948) reviewed fifty consecutive cases of renal and ureteral calculi; this
series included one patient with a parathyroid tumor. Braasch (1926) noted
that hyperparathyroidism was the etiologic factor in less than 0.2 per cent of
a series of cases seen at the Mayo Clinic. Beard and Goodyear (1950)
decided that hyperparathyroidism, which was present in 8 per cent of their
series of 150 cases, is a significant cause of renal lithiasis. In a series of
cases I studied, hyperparathyroidism was confirmed by operation in 0.6
per cent (1943). I believe evidence is accumulating to indicate that the
actual incidence of hyperparathyroidism as a causative factor in the formation
of renal calculi is higher than most urologists have presumed in the past.

Metabolic Disturbances. In various metabolic disturbances, there may be
an excessive excretion of urinary crystalloids which become a factor in the
formation of renal calculi. *Cystinuria* is a familial disease said to be caused
by a derangement of intermediate protein metabolism, in which cystine may
be found in the urine partly in solution and also as a crystalline deposit.
Under normal conditions, cystine is oxidized completely and the sulfur is
excreted as sulfate. It has been estimated that 2.5 per cent of patients with
cystinuria develop urinary calculi. Seeger and Kearns (1925) found a
much higher incidence; they collected a series of 181 cases of cystinuria,
and co-existing calculi were present in 124.

Kretschmer (1937) collected a series of fifteen cases of *xanthine* calculi
from the literature and added another. In a review published in 1950, Pearlman found twenty-two reported cases of xanthine calculi of the urinary
tract and added one of his own. I have observed two patients with xanthine
renal calculi.

Uric acid is the most important purine in the urine, but 30 to 50 mg.
of the purine bases, xanthine, hypoxanthine, guanine and adenine, are also
present. Mathews (1930) estimated that 16 to 60 mg. of purine base are
eliminated in the urine daily. In gout, excessive amounts of crystalloids in
the form of urates and uric acid may be present in the urine. Normally,
0.3 to 1.2 gm. are excreted in the urine daily. Patients with this disease may
experience attacks of renal colic owing to the passage of showers of crystals
or small stones.

Oxalic acid, which accumulates from both exogenous and endogenous
sources, is excreted daily in the amount of 12 to 30 mg. Oxaluria may play
a role in the formation of oxalate calculi, while a persistent non-infected phosphaturia may act similarly.

The foregoing reports, which represent only a sampling, demonstrate obviously that many factors may be associated with the formation of renal
calculi and that no single etiologic agent can be held accountable as a common factor in every type of calculus.

Chemical Composition of Calculi. *Classification.* There are two types of calculi, the pure, in which only one crystalloid is present, and the mixed, in which two or more crystalloids form the constituents of the stone. Calculi are also classified as amorphous or crystalloid. However, it has been my experience that true amorphous types are unusual; as a general rule, crystalloid patterns are demonstrable. Prien and Frondel (1947) have also pointed out that examination of apparently amorphous material under the petrographic microscope reveals that the fragments demonstrate the optical properties of crystalline substances and present characteristic x-ray diffraction patterns. Accretions of bacteria and fibrin and urostealiths are the exceptions. The organic framework of calculi apparently is composed of an albuminous material, which some chemists state is fibrin, and appears more abundantly in mixed calculi.

Phosphatic Calculi. Joly stated that phosphatic calculi are composed of crystalloids or amorphous calcium phosphate and, as the name implies, are composed of phosphatic salts. Ammonium magnesium phosphate may be present. Those described in the past as crystalline stones are white, hard calculi in which the crystalline structure may be demonstrable, on section. Radial striations may be evident. Microscopic study reveals the elongated, needle-like crystals in some instances; in others, these are not evident. In contrast to the so-called crystalline calculus, the amorphous type, as classified by Joly, is soft, friable, breaks easily and has a rough, granular surface. On section, the stone appears to be composed of a homogeneous granular mass which does not reveal crystalline structure microscopically. Additional study of this apparently homogeneous material will, however, reveal its crystalline nature. Prien found three different phosphates, while a fourth was identified by Jensen; magnesium ammonium phosphate, apatite, calcium hydrogen phosphate dihydrate, and tricalcium phosphate.

Calcium Carbonate Calculi. Calcium carbonate calculi are infrequently observed. Scholl noted that they have a chalky appearance and powder readily. In his analytic study of 700 calculi, Prien did not observe calcium carbonate; cholesterol, xanthine and indigo also were lacking in the stones he studied.

Uric Acid Calculi. Uric acid calculi have a yellowish or brown color, are ovoid or round in shape and firm in consistency; the surface may be smooth or roughened. They are most often observed in the pure state; when the stones are of mixed type, the uric acid is associated with calcium oxalate monohydrate or apatite. The nucleus is crystalline and the crystals cuboidal in shape, and, according to Shattock, intermingled with the coarse crystals are masses of elongated crystals described as "bacilliform." The body of the calculus is composed of alternate layers described as spongy and compact "tissue."

Urate Calculi. Urates are unusual calculi, although Scholl stated that they are the most common stones found in infancy and childhood. They are described as yellowish-brown in color, smooth and soft. Such calculi may be composed of ammonium urate or sodium acid urate. Errors in chemical interpretation are due, as I previously reported and as Domanski has also noted, to the questionable validity of the chemical test for ammonium urate. I believe such calculi are extremely unusual. Jensen, utilizing chemical diffraction methods, did not observe this type of calculus in a study of eighty-four stones. Prien found sodium acid urate in only one of the 700 urinary calculi he examined.

Oxalate Stones. According to my own experience, the incidence of oxalate stones is increasing in the United States. This substance is observed far more frequently as a constituent of urinary calculi than any other crystalloid. Ord and Shattock, in 1895, classified four types of oxalate stones on their gross appearance: (1) small, shining, smooth, reddish-gray stones, of spherical shape, and usually multiple; (2) mulberry type; (3) those with thorny projections, the jackstone type; and finally (4) the small stones, light brown in color, whose surface is covered with sharp, glistening crystals. Nakano detected the presence of two hydrates in oxalate stones: calcium oxalate dihydrate and calcium oxalate monohydrate. Prien made similar observations and said that he had observed some patients with stones composed of pure monohydrate or dihydrate, while other individuals formed stones which were a mixture of the two hydrates. Because of their rough surface, the calculi may induce bleeding in some instances and then the surface of the stone may be covered with blood or blood pigment.

Cystine Stones. Cystine calculi are yellow or light yellowish-green and usually occur in the pure state. Their surface may be smooth or granular and they can be either soft or firm. Microscopic survey demonstrates the crystalline structure well and the hexagonal tablets are radially arranged, constituting the typical radial striation. The individual crystals vary in size. The color of the calculus may deepen and assume a greenish tint, on exposure to light.

Xanthine. Xanthine stones are rare; they are yellowish-brown, smooth, round and hard. Chemical analysis reveals the presence of xanthine, which must be differentiated from urate. Xanthine may also be present as the nucleus in a uric-acid stone.

Unusual Calculi. Indigo calculi are recognized by their color and are rarely observed. *Fibrin stones* are likewise unusual; those reported have been mixed with calcium phosphate. They vary in size from that of a pea to a concretion that may completely occupy the pelvis of the kidneys and the calices. Fibrin stones are very soft and friable.

Bacterial calculi are rarely observed. They are small, round or ovoid in shape and deposits of calcium phosphate are usually present on their surface. Scholl stated that they are composed of B. coli and claimed that positive cultures may be obtained from them.

Urostealiths are rare and are composed of fat and fatty acids. Such calculi have not been observed in the Cleveland Clinic.

RENAL CALCULI

Etiologic Factors. *Age.* As a general rule, it may be stated that renal lithiasis is predominantly a disease of the third and fourth decades, but it may be observed in patients of all ages.

Sex. Renal calculi occur slightly more frequently in men than in women.

Position. The place of origin of a calculus may be in the pelvis or the calyx of the kidney. The minute calculi are usually observed first in the lower calyx of the kidney. They form at this site primarily or migrate to this dependent position.

Joly classified renal calculi into five groups: (1) calculi free in the pelvis of the kidney or a calyx; (2) stones impacted at the ureteropelvic junction; (3) stones completely occupying the renal pelvis; (4) stones which have become a mould of the renal pelvis and calices; (5) giant calculi which have destroyed and taken the place of the renal parenchyma.

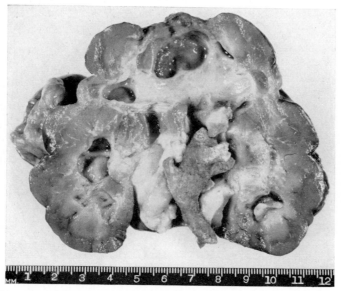

Fig. 356.   Calculous hydronephrosis (localized) and pyelonephritis.

Size. Phosphatic calculi may enlarge very rapidly, while the growth of oxalate stones is quite slow. The growth of cystine and uric acid calculi is somewhat more rapid than that of the oxalate group. The rate of growth of renal calculi is influenced by the rate of crystalloid excretion. In the absence of renal infection, aseptic stones are frequently single and relatively small in caliber; if infection and stasis are present, larger stones develop. Multiple stones often are found in the presence of stasis and infection.

Bilaterality. Bilateral calculi are almost always observed in the presence of infection of the kidneys and, as a general rule, bilateral and multiple stones are found late in the course of the disease. I observed bilateral calculi in 14.9 per cent of 1500 cases (1943); H. P. White (1929) reported 13.8 per cent of bilateral cases in his series; Young, 17 per cent, and Braasch (1926) 10 per cent. Braasch also stated that cases of calculi were multiple in 40 per cent and ureteral stones were associated with renal calculi in less than 5 per cent of the Mayo Clinic series.

Pathology. *Factors Influencing Renal Lesions.* The presence of calculi in the kidney is conducive to the production of damage influenced by the size and position of the stone, by its contour and surface characteristics, by the presence or absence of infection, and by the extent to which it produces obstruction. Locally there may be desquamation of epithelium, ulceration of the tissue contiguous to the calculus, and fibrosis. When a larger stone occupies a thickened pelvis, interstitial fibrosis, leukocytic and round-cell infiltration are evident microscopically. Additional changes are influenced by the degree of obstruction of the outflow of urine from the renal pelvis.

Generally, the obstruction produced by the calculus at the kidney outlet is incomplete and conducive to the formation of intrarenal hydronephrosis (Fig. 356). As the calculus enlarges, its configuration tends to assume that

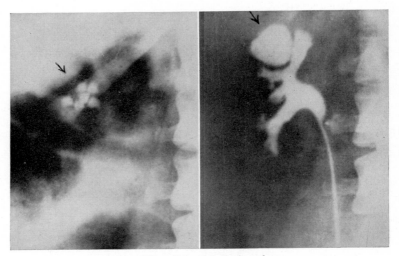

Fig. 357.   Calculi in hydrocalyx.

of the renal pelvis and the urine usually courses around it into the ureter. This adaptability, along with the fibrosis and hypertrophy of the walls of the pelvis, explains the relative infrequency of pelvic dilatation.

The pathologic lesion which develops in the kidney is influenced by the presence or absence of hydronephrosis. The intrarenal nature of hydronephrosis is evidenced by blunting of the calices, and later, by varying degrees of dilatation of the individual calices (Fig. 357). Atrophy and destruction of renal parenchyma follow, and as this process progresses, the dilated calices may reach practically to the kidney capsule.

Usually infection is superimposed, when renal calculi are present, and various lesions may develop, such as calculous pyelonephritis (Fig. 358), calculous pyonephrosis, and perinephritis. With the introduction of infection, the stones may become multiple, renal function is rapidly impaired, and the renal parenchyma is destroyed. Bilateral calculi may then appear.

Calculous Pyelonephritis. In the absence of hydronephrosis, calculous pyelonephritis becomes the prominent lesion (Fig. 359). The gross appearance of the kidney is influenced by the degree and virulence of the infection. The pelvis of the kidney is thickened, miliary abscesses may be observed in the swollen, vascularized cortex of the kidney; with the further ravages of infection, the cortex becomes thin, the infundibula of the calices are obstructed, and localized areas of pyonephrosis are discernible as the calices become dilated. The kidney as a whole becomes adherent to the adjacent

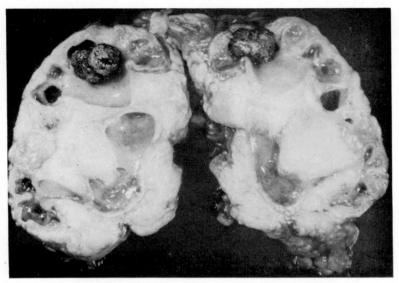

Fig. 358.   Calculous pyelonephritis and ureteritis.

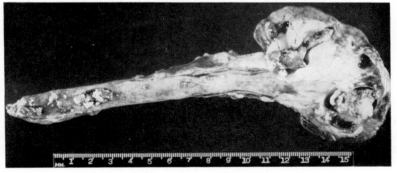

Fig. 359.   Calculous pyelonephritis.

tissue. When the infection is less pronounced, the kidney is smaller and paler, owing to the fibrous tissue reaction.

Microscopically, the wall of the pelvis of the kidney is thickened, the mucous membrane is edematous; desquamation of the epithelium and ulceration may occur. The tubules are filled with debris and blood cells. Many of the tubules may be destroyed as the renal cortex is thinned out. There are interstitial fibrosis, round-cell infiltration, and localized areas of polymorphonuclear white cells.

Calculous Pyonephrosis. Calculous pyonephrosis may develop when infection is superimposed on a kidney which is the site of calculous hydronephrosis. Three types are described: (1) the atrophic, (2) the giant, and (3) the intermediate type.

The *atrophic kidney* is grossly small, densely adherent to the adjacent perinephric fat. Most of the renal parenchyma is destroyed, leaving a shell of tissue attached to the pelvis. On microscopic study but little normal tissue is visible; interstitial fibrosis and round-cell infiltration are evident.

The *giant type* consists of a large multilocular sac which may fill the entire flank. The surface is irregular, owing to the varying size of the tremendously

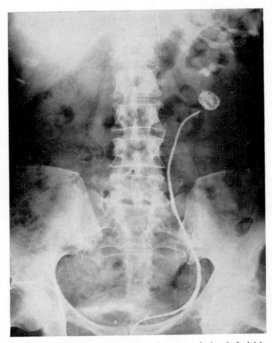

Fig. 360.   Calcification on carcinoma of the left kidney.

dilated calices. Multiple stones or a solitary calculus may be present in the pelvis which may be of normal size. Again, microscopic examination shows but little normal renal parenchyma. The walls of the calices are fibrotic, perhaps thickened, or, in many instances, thin tubular structures are decreased, and the large dilated calices are separated by fibrous tissue septa. The perirenal fat is thickened and especially adherent in the region of the renal pelvis.

Varying pictures may be presented in the *intermediate type,* according to the degree of pyonephrosis. The kidney is not so large as that of the giant type. The surface is nodular; the elevated areas are fluctuant because of the dilated calices and the thinning of the cortex. The capsule is thickened and adherent. Microscopically, more recognizable parenchyma, including glomeruli and tubular structures, are present, the caliceal walls are thin and separated from the renal capsule by fibrous tissue. In other areas, round-cell and leukocytic infiltration occurs. The perinephric fat is thickened.

Nephrocalcinosis. Nephrocalcinosis is a term applied to small, diffuse calcifications distributed throughout the renal parenchyma, usually observed in the pyramids.

Replacement Lipomatosis. A kidney damaged by calculi may be the site of replacement lipomatosis. In 1938, Roth and Davidson collected a series of seventy previously reported cases and added thirty-seven new cases from a museum of pathology. Lower and Belcher (1927) cited an additional case; and in 1950, Simril and Rose added two additional cases. Roth and Davidson concluded that neither calculi nor inflammation was specific or necessary for the development of replacement lipomatosis. Of thirty-three cases reviewed by Kutzmann in 1931, the coexistence of calculi and pyelonephritis was present in 79 per cent. Destruction of renal parenchyma appears to be a requisite for replacement lipomatosis; the fatty masses replace the destroyed tissue.

Squamous-cell Carcinoma. A striking relation between renal calculi and squamous-cell carcinoma of the renal pelvis has been observed (Fig. 360). Gilbert and MacMillan presented a collective review of fifty-five cases of squamous-cell carcinoma of the renal pelvis in 1934. In 1939, I collected fifty-nine cases and added five others, three of which were complicated by renal calculi. In a later collective review (1949) of 106 cases of squamous-cell carcinoma of the renal pelvis by Gahagan and Reed, calculi were present in 48 per cent of the cases and infection was found in most instances.

Perinephritic Abscesses. Perinephritic abscesses with perforation into the intestines or bronchi may result from renal lithiasis, but such cases are of extremely rare occurrence.

Symptoms. The symptoms associated with a renal calculus are of great diversity and are influenced by obstruction, by the presence or absence of infection, by local irritation producing edema of the mucous membrane of the pelvis, with subsequent obstructive and reflex phenomena.

Pain. Pain is caused by increased pressure in the pelvis, owing to obstruction. The so-called "silent stone" may attain considerable size in the kidney, without producing symptoms. Its presence may become evident only through detection in routine roentgenologic survey. At other times, patients with the symptoms of cystitis may have a calculus in the kidney whose presence was not suspected prior to complete urologic examination, because of the absence of clinical symptoms referable to that organ. Most patients with renal lithiasis complain of discomfort or a dull ache in the renal region, punctuated at times by sudden twinges which may radiate down the ureter. The soreness on the affected side may be influenced and aggravated by exercise, manual labor and by activity. The discomfort is not disabling and medical consultation frequently is not sought.

Renal Colic. An attack of renal colic often has an acute onset without prodromal or premonitory symptoms. The pain is severe, intense and may be increased from time to time by excruciating acute paroxysms. Subjectively it is described as a very sharp stabbing sensation, and the patient moves and writhes ceaselessly in an attempt to attain a position which will afford some relief. The pain is usually confined to the renal region, starting in a localized area around the costovertebral angle whence it radiates along the ureter. In the male, it may be referred to the testicle, which is retracted and tender. In women, it may radiate to the vulva. It may be referred down the anterior surface of the thigh or the entire side and abdomen may be painful.

The attack may last for hours or subside within a few minutes. Usually the pain is relieved abruptly, leaving residual soreness for several days. Following the attack, the patient is weak and exhausted. The suffering during such a severe attack is intense, but all degrees of severity may be observed.

The patient with renal colic is cold and clammy; the face is bathed with cold perspiration. The pulse is weak and rapid, and is accompanied by a fall in blood pressure. There is usually only slight or no elevation of temperature unless infection is present in the kidney, in which instance chills and fever are evident.

Nausea and vomiting are usually present, and the abdomen may be distended, suggesting an intra-abdominal catastrophe. In some instances, all the symptoms may be referred to the gastrointestinal tract. The patient is constipated; there is a decrease in the amount of urine excreted, followed by polyuria after the attack subsides.

The incidence of colic in nephrolithiasis varies usually between 40 and 50 per cent. Morris reported colic in 43 per cent of his cases; Cabot, in 54 per cent; Joly noted a history of acute pain in slightly under 50 per cent of septic cases, a figure slightly less than for aseptic stones. In our series (1943), 41 per cent related a history of attacks of pain varying in duration and severity.

Hematuria. Gross hematuria or microscopic blood in the urine is frequently observed in patients with renal calculi. The bleeding is seldom sufficiently profuse to cause alarm, and if it *is* massive, suggests the possibility of another pathologic lesion in the kidney. Herman reported moderate hematuria in 57 per cent of the cases in children, and in 40 per cent in adults; in Joly's and Morris' series, the incidence of hematuria was also 40 per cent. In our own patients, a history of hematuria at some time in the course of the disease was elicited in 43 per cent. In 20 to 25 per cent of the cases, neither gross nor microscopic blood is observed in the urine. After an attack of colic, however, a varying number of erythrocytes may be found in the urine.

Diagnosis. With our present diagnostic procedures, there is usually no difficulty in establishing an accurate diagnosis. It does not suffice, however, merely to arrive at the conclusion that kidney stones are present. The correct diagnosis should include the size, number and position of the stone, or stones, the functional capacity of both kidneys, and whether renal infection is present or absent. Erroneous or inadequate diagnosis may generally be attributed to sins of omission.

History. A carefully elicited history may impart valuable information; the type of pain, its nature, location and radiation are all significant factors. The patient may have experienced a previous attack of colic and have passed a stone. There may be a history of metabolic diseases, such as gout or cystinuria, or cystic lesions of the long bones which immediately focus their attention on the possibility of renal lithiasis. However, such leading signs are often absent. It is estimated that in 35 to 40 per cent of cases, indefinite symptoms may be present, and the history is confusing in many instances.

Physical Examination. Physical examination may reveal a large, firm mass in the renal area when the kidney is the site of a large calculous pyonephrosis. In the absence of perinephritis, the kidney moves with respiration, while lateral movement may be evidenced by palpation. In instances in which the kidney is atrophic, the organ may not be palpable, while tenderness is elicited upon deep pressure in the renal area. The kidney is usually palpable in the intermediate type, is firm, usually regular in outline, and tender to palpation. In the presence of pyelonephritis, its mobility is impaired. When infection is absent, fixation to the adjacent perirenal fat does not occur. Therefore, vertical and lateral mobility are demonstrable; the size of the mass depends on the degree of hydronephrosis, varying from only slight enlargement of the renal mass to a large tense mass occupying the renal area.

During the attack of colic, the pain is provoked and aggravated by pressure of the examiner's hands and renders palpation difficult. Muscular spasm and rigidity and protective guarding of muscle are present on the involved side. Usually gentle percussion in the region of the costovertebral angle or deep pressure anteriorly over the kidney will elicit pain and tenderness.

Differential Diagnosis. An attack of colic on the right side must be differentiated from biliary colic or acute appendicitis, while symptoms simulating acute intestinal obstruction or other acute intraperitoneal catastrophes may be produced by an attack of colic on either side. Biliary colic may be differentiated by the history and absence of tenderness in the right renal area. The pain in gallbladder colic is usually referred to the back or right shoulder. Local examination reveals tenderness over the gallbladder with spasm of the rectus muscle. Microscopic examination of the urine will not reveal blood cells.

Acute appendicitis, at times, may be more difficult to differentiate from a calculus which is coursing down the ureter. Again, significant data are elicited from the history. Locally, in acute appendicitis, the point of maxima tenderness is, as a rule, over McBurney's point; muscular spasm and rigidity, and sometimes rebound tenderness, are present. Tenderness may be absent over the kidney. The general constitutional symptoms are more pronounced, the pulse is rapid, and there may be a higher degree of elevation of the temperature. The white cell count is usually higher than with urinary lithiasis. There are usually no blood cells in the urine, but these may be present. A retrocecal appendicitis is usually more difficult to diagnose than when the appendix occupies the normal position.

In the presence of general distention of the abdomen, failure to pass gas by rectum, and vomiting, acute intestinal obstruction may be suspected. If these symptoms are due to calculous disease, the point of maximal tenderness is in the renal area, blood cells usually are present in the urine, and a carefully elicited history, both past and present, furnish important conclusions. The history of the onset of the attack with its progression produces particularly valuable information. As a general rule, it may be stated that constitutional symptoms are usually more pronounced in intraperitoneal lesions.

Nephrocalcinosis. The numerous small calcifications distributed throughout the renal parenchyma in nephrocalcinosis are usually demonstrated by roentgenologic study (Fig. 361). The disease may occur either in children or adults, and there are no pathognomonic symptoms early in its course.

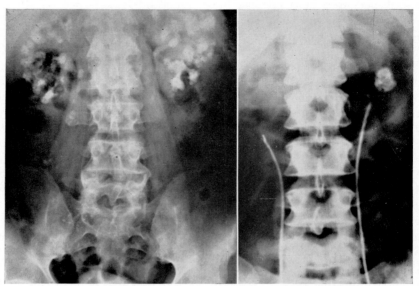

Fig. 361.   Fig. 362.
Fig. 361.   Nephrocalcinosis.
Fig. 362.   Extrarenal calcification.

A history may be elicited of the spontaneous passage of a small calculus. This may be associated with, or followed by, gross or microscopic hematuria. In the presence of renal infection, chills and fever may occur. Later the patient may complain of weakness, lassitude, loss of appetite, nausea, vomiting, polydypsia, or oliguria. Acidosis and hyperchloremia are usually present.

The glomerular function appears to be unimpaired, as indicated by the inulin and urea clearance studies and the relatively normal values of the blood urea. An adequate phenolsulfonphthalein test, the diodrast clearance, and the absence of glycosuria indicate satisfactory functions of the proximal tubules. However, the inability to concentrate the urine, the inability to secrete acid urine, and systemic acidosis indicate impairment of function of the distal tubules. The systemic acidosis results from involvement of the distal tubules which impairs the ability of the kidneys to make ammonia or excrete acid urine. There is also increased loss of calcium in the urine.

Calcifications in the renal tubules of children have been described by Lightwood (1935) and by Anderson (1939), in postmortem studies. Other reports have been contributed by Butler, Wilson and Farber, in 1936, and by Albright and his collaborators (1940) who discussed the etiologic factors. They noted the disturbance in calcium metabolism and cited a case associated with rickets and dwarfism. While rickets may be present, it need not be evident and is a late manifestation of the disease. They concluded that the disease is associated with damage to the distal convoluted tubules, and this view seemed to be confirmed by laboratory investigations. Engel reported a series of seven patients, three of whom he had observed personally; he reviewed roentgenologic and laboratory data in four additional cases. He cited evidence indicating that the sulfonamides exert a toxic and deleterious influence on the distal tubules. He raised the question as to whether it may be more than coincidental that the reporting of these cases, which seems to be occurring with greater frequency, coincides chronologically with the introduction of sulfonamides.

Calculous Anuria. Calculous anuria is a grave complication of nephrolithiasis and may be the first symptom of calculi in the upper urinary tract. Joly cited four types of obstruction that may be associated with calculous anuria: (1) obstruction of both kidneys and ureters; (2) obstruction of the only functioning kidney; (3) obstruction of one kidney, when the opposite kidney is diseased; (4) obstruction of one kidney when the other is healthy. Hinman classified three groups and stated that oliguria or anuria may be caused by mechanical obstruction at some point of the tract, cessation of secretion, and a combination of obstructive and secretory factors. W. White (1929) stated that anuria may occur "as a climax of a gradual but progressive renal failure resulting from long-standing and extensive bilateral calculous disease, occurring quite independently of renal occlusion."

In the obstructive type of anuria associated with nephrolithiasis, the calculus precipitating the attack may be present in the kidney or the ureter. A small stone in the renal pelvis may become impacted in the outlet, producing complete obstruction to the outflow of urine. Stones producing anuria from obstruction in the ureters will usually be found in the upper third, and with secondary frequency, in the lower third of the ureters. When the obstruction is bilateral, in the majority of instances, the anuria is associated with ureteral calculi.

There is considerable controversy as to whether anuria may develop in the presence of complete obstruction on one side and an apparently normal kidney on the opposite side, the so-called reflex anuria. Although temporary arrest of the excretion of urine may occur, the excretion of urine from the normal kidney is restored as the patient's pain and discomfort are relieved. In every instance I know about in which a stone completely blocking the ureter resulted in anuria, followed by uremia and death of the patient, microscopic examination of the apparently and supposedly healthy opposite kidney revealed pathologic findings.

The clinical features may vary from a complete absence of symptoms until the time when the patient observes he is not passing urine, to dull ache and pain in the groin for varying periods, to an attack of acute colic. For a time, the patient's health may seem unimpaired and, except for the inability to pass urine, he feels perfectly well. Gradually signs of uremia are noticeable and unless relief is afforded, death eventually ensues. Physical examination may reveal almost no significant local findings in the renal area, or it may be possible to elicit pain and tenderness over the kidneys. An immediate stereoscopic roentgenogram is always advisable.

Catheterization of the ureters in an attempt to by-pass the obstruction and to restore the excretion of urine is advisable, and if this is accomplished, the immediate emergency is relieved. If urinary excretion is reestablished soon after the onset of the anuria, nitrogen retention disappears, with pronounced improvement in the patient's general health. This allows time to evaluate the

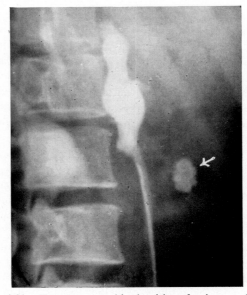

Fig. 364.   Roentgenographic densities of urinary calculi.

condition and to decide on the future management, as the symptoms of the anuria subside.

A critical period occurs when the ureteral catheters are withdrawn; usually, however, the excretion of urine continues and in 50 to 55 per cent of the cases, the calculus is expelled. Even if anuria recurs after withdrawal of the catheter, the patient is in better condition for surgical intervention as a result of the removal of accumulated nitrogenous waste products.

Roentgenography. Roentgenographic examination is the most valuable and important procedure in establishing the diagnosis of a renal calculus. A stereoscopic roentgenogram is always advisable. Satisfactory films may reveal the renal outline, and the size, number and position of the calculi. Roentgenographic study should include the entire urinary tract to rule out coexisting calculi in the opposite kidney, in either ureter, in the bladder, and in the prostate gland (Fig. 363). In a similar manner, lesions involving the bony structures may be detected.

Lateral roentgenograms are extremely useful and are not employed as frequently as they should be. When a question arises, in reviewing the anteroposterior film as to the position of a shadow in relation to the kidney, a lateral film will furnish additional information.

The opacity of a calculus is influenced by its size, thickness, structure, and its chemical constituents (Fig. 364). The high incidence of visibility is due to the presence of calcium, a common constituent of the majority of renal calculi. The most opaque calculi are composed of calcium oxalate, then carbonate stones, and third, phosphate calculi. Calculi composed of urates or

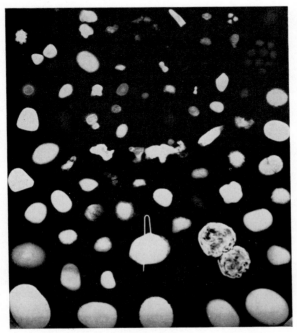

Fig. 364.　Roentgenographic densities of urinary calculi.

uric acid cast fainter shadows. Some authors have stated that cystine calculi are transparent to roentgen rays, but in eleven patients I have observed with cystine stones in the kidney, the calculus was well defined and radiopaque. Since the pure type of calculus is less frequently observed than the mixed, variations in degree of opacity are inevitable.

Herman stated that approximately 5 per cent of renal stones are not visible (Fig. 365). In our series, 97 to 98 per cent of the calculi cast a shadow on the roentgenogram.

Excretory Urography. Excretory urography is a valuable diagnostic procedure. The renal shadows may be outlined, the position of the stone or stones in the pelvis or calices of the kidney may be revealed, the status of the opposite kidney is determined, and it may serve as a test of renal function. The pelvis may be well visualized and conclusions may be drawn as to whether it is

extrarenal or intrarenal. In the presence of adequate function, excellent roentgenograms may be secured. With the presence of impaired renal function,
insufficient concentration of medium may occur to permit satisfactory visualization of the pelvis and calyceal systems, while in complete ureteropelvic
obstruction, visualization of the medium is not possible. This does not imply
the absence of renal function, but only its temporary suspension. Visualization
will be possible again when the obstruction is relieved, unless marked destruction of the renal parenchyma has resulted from the obstruction produced by
the calculus.

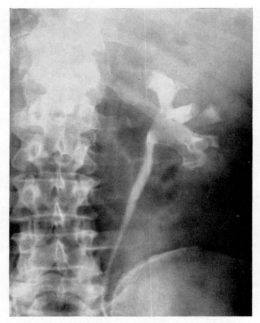

Fig. 365.   Nonopaque renal calculus (left).

Cystoscopy. The cystoscopic picture is influenced by the presence or absence
of infection. In cases in which renal infection is present, there may be a coexisting cystitis, the severity of which is influenced by the duration and by the
virulence of the offending organism. In the absence of infection, cystoscopy
may present a normal picture. The ureteral orifices are observed and the rate
and character of the efflux are noted. The urine spurting from the orifice may
be clear, hazy, smoky or blood-tinged. At times pus, appearing like tooth paste,
may be observed exuding from the orifice.

Following inspection of the bladder, catheters may be passed to the renal
pelves and specimens secured from each kidney for bacteriologic and cytologic
study and pH determinations. If surgery is contemplated, it is important to
determine the function of each kidney prior to operation. At the time of ureteral
catheterization, retrograde pyelograms should be secured.

Retrograde Urography. Retrograde roentgenograms usually permit clearer delineation of the renal pelvis and calyceal system than can be noted in the excretory urogram. Various solutions have replaced the older contrast media and these newer substances are less irritating to the mucous membranes of the ureter and the renal pelvis. Excretory urography, which has already been carried out, furnishes information as to the quantity of medium to be injected in the retrograde procedure. The injection of solution into the catheters should be performed slowly and only to the point at which the patient begins to experience slight discomfort.

Bilateral retrograde pyelograms may be secured, if care is exercised in the injection of the contrast media. In instances in which the calcification is only faintly delineated or is obscured by the contrast media, pyelograms are made after air injection. Although this procedure has been condemned by some urologists, we have never observed any untoward effects from it in the Cleveland Clinic.

By the use of complete roentgenographic studies, renal calculi may be differentiated from other extrarenal shadows, as gallstones, bowel contents, calcified glands, calcifications arising in a tumor of the kidney, and tuberculosis of the kidney with calcifications. Pyelography, either by the excretory or retrograde technique, or both, permits localization of the shadow and visualization of the anatomic status of the kidney. Fluoroscopy, although it is less reliable than the roentgenogram, is utilized by some urologists, especially during operative procedures, to make certain that all of the stones in the kidney have been removed. In selected cases, aortography is a valuable procedure, supplying information as to the blood supply of the hydronephrotic kidney. The findings of this special test may aid in determining the surgical procedure to be employed.

Laboratory Tests. *Examination of the Urine. Routine urinalysis* is helpful in making the diagnosis of renal calculus. During an attack of renal colic or following it, gross hematuria may be present, with microscopic investigation revealing the possible presence of crystals or red blood cells. In the presence of renal infection, the stained smear of the urinary sediment demonstrates bacteria.

Determination of the *urinary pH* is always indicated in cases of suspected lithiasis, and this test is used as a guide to therapy when special diets and/or medication are used. The pH of the urine from the bladder does not provide adequate information, and it is necessary to determine the pH of the urine from the kidneys by means of catheterization, especially in the presence of unilateral stasis or infection. The hydrogen ion concentration of the urine from the kidney harboring the stone may be different from that of the opposite kidney or of the bladder, an observation that has been confirmed by Herrold[*] and also by Randall (1935). Table 16 shows the disparity in urinary findings in the two kidneys in a patient with renal lithiasis.

The *calcium content* of the urine is determined on each patient with renal lithiasis. The patient receives a neutral diet of low calcium content for three days prior to the collection of urine, and the same diet is continued for an

[*] Personal communication.

additional three days while the urine is collected and the calcium output per twenty-four hours is recorded.

When *phosphaturia* is present, it is necessary to extend the investigation to determine whether this is temporary, and whether or not infection is present. Determination of the twenty-four-hour urinary output of inorganic phosphorus (method of Fiske and Subbarow) is advisable.

When infection is an important factor, *bacterial cultures* of the urine and the determination of the presence of *urea-splitting organisms* are indicated.

Renal Function Tests. Excretory urography furnishes a preliminary index to renal function. In cases in which a renal stone has been demonstrated roentgenologically, the function of each kidney is determined separately, at the time of ureteral catheterization. The two functional tests which are most widely

Table 16. Microscopic Examination of Urine from Catheterized Ureters

	LEFT	RIGHT
Turbidity	+	0
Gross blood	++	+
Red blood cells	++	++
Pus	+++	0
Epithelial cells	0	0
Casts	0	0
Crystals (triple phosphate)	+	0
pH	7.2	5.6
Other organisms	Cocci	0

used for this purpose are the indigo carmine test and the phenolsulfonphthalein test, the technical and interpretative details of which are given in Section II.

For the *indigo carmine test,* indigo carmine (5 cc.) is injected intravenously, and as the dye appears in the urine from the ureteral catheters, the time and concentration are observed. This test furnishes a gross estimate of kidney function. Concentrations are estimated as 1+, 2+, 3+ and 4+. The normal time of appearance of the dye is four to five minutes.

The *phenolsulfonphthalein test* is subject to more accurate interpretation than the indigo carmine test and may be graphically recorded. The drug (6 mg.) in 1 cc. of water is injected intravenously. The appearance time of the dye in the urine from the catheters is recorded. Normally, the dye appears in two to three minutes and the percentage of dye eliminated in a given time is estimated. As urine containing the dye may also pass along the sides of the catheters into the bladder, the dye retained in the bladder should also be recorded. According to Shaw, in normal persons, 40 per cent of the dye is eliminated in the first fifteen minutes; 17 per cent in the second; 8 per cent in the third, and 4 per cent in the fourth quarter hour.

Examination of the Blood. Determinations of various constituents of the blood, particularly to rule out the presence of vitamin A deficiency and certain metabolic diseases, are carried out according to the indications in the individual case.

The dependability of the biophotometer test in determining the presence or absence of vitamin A deficiency is questionable. The *antimony trichloride test* on the blood is a more reliable procedure, and hence is recommended.

In the investigations for hyperparathyroidism, *calcium and phosphorus determinations* on blood plasma alone do not suffice. The calcium in the serum is composed of two fractions. Approximately 50 per cent is able to pass through a membrane impermeable to proteins, and 50 per cent remains with the proteins in the serum. Thus, the nondiffusible fraction is bound to the protein. McLean and Hastings (1935) stated that the total calcium of the serum or plasma is nearly all accounted for as calcium ions and the calcium bound to

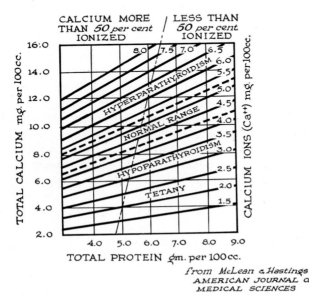

Fig. 366.   Chart for calculation of Ca^{++} ion concentration from total protein and total calcium of serum or plasma. (From McLean, F. C. and Hastings, A. B.: Am. J. M. Sc., *189*:602–612, 1935.)

protein. Of these two forms, the ionized calcium is of primary and clinical importance. In renal lithiasis, it is wise to recall that the calcium ion concentration of the plasma is normally maintained within a limited range by a process of physiologic regulation. As the parathyroid glands assume an important role in this function, an increase in the calcium-ion concentration of the plasma implies hyperfunction of the glands.

It is significant that the calcium-ion concentration of the plasma, as stated by McLean and Hastings, is the resultant of an equilibrium between the total calcium and the total protein in the plasma. The chart in Figure 366 presents a method for the clinical estimation of the calcium-ion concentration from the total protein and the total calcium concentrations of the plasma. The total serum proteins, the fractions, the serum calcium and the serum phosphorus should be determined in all patients suspected of having a disturbance in calcium-phosphorus metabolism.

Analysis of Urinary Stones. Whenever a stone or fragment of stone is available for analysis, this procedure occupies an important place in the diagnosis and planning of the therapeutic schedule for a patient with renal lithiasis. Optical crystallographic study is probably the best method available. Prien and Frondel emphasized its value in correlating pathogenesis with composition and structure of the various types of calculi. At present, my associates and I are comparing the results of the optical procedure with the methods of chemical analysis that have been used heretofore.

Chemical methods in general use today may be traced back almost without change to the work of Hammarsten, in 1896. Although many "modifications" have been devised, in general these have involved no basic change in analytic procedure. Keyser's modification (1948), the modification which Randall (1934) attributed to his co-worker, J. S. P. Beck, the method suggested by Hawk and Bergeim in their textbook, and the original Hammarsten method are identical. This repetition wrongly imparts to others in this field a feeling of confidence in the accuracy of the analytic procedures involved. To Domanski (1937) belongs the credit for suggesting that the procedure is not perfect. For example, in the method of Hammarsten-Heller, Beck-Hawk and Bergeim-Keyser, the identification of the urate radical, followed by the identification of the ammonia which had been liberated by a strong base, was accepted as proof that ammonium urate was present. Domanski found that he was unable to liberate ammonia from pure ammonium urate by this method and hence conclusively proved that the evolution of ammonia could not be used to indicate the presence of this compound. He admitted that he was unable to identify the organic compounds which might be present in the calculus by the odor which resulted from the ashing of the pulverized material. This statement can be appreciated only by those who have actually attempted to use this method. Another obvious point of weakness in the existing method of analysis was the necessity for proving that the carbonates were entirely absent before the oxalates could be identified. Thus, in the presence of carbonates, the reactions used in the identification of oxalates were not specific.

In attempting to correct these errors which had existed almost unnoticed for the past fifty years, Domanski made the following changes: (1) After pointing out that there was no reason to differentiate between ammonium urate and uric acid, he called attention to the method of Boston which was suggestive of, if not absolute in enabling this differentiation to be made. (2) He completely avoided any attempt to identify the organic compounds by the odor of the burned stones. (3) He precipitated the oxalate as calcium oxalate, removed the crystals by centrifugation, examined them microscopically, added sulfuric acid, and noted their ability to decolorize potassium permanganate.

In routine examination of a large number of calculi, it has been found that even the method of Domanski leaves much to be desired. As previously noted, in order to identify the oxalate radical, the procedure was considerably lengthened to avoid the interference of the carbonate radical. Also, in avoiding the interference of carbonates, a new source of error was introduced, since it is possible to imagine that organic constituents might be precipitated under the same conditions as calcium oxalate, and these would serve to decolorize potassium permanganate solutions, even in the absence of the latter.

Table 17. Sodium Fusion Test

	USE PULVERIZED STONE			EVAPORATE PULVERIZED STONE TO DRYNESS WITH HNO_2				
Sodium fusion	Add conc. aq. KOH	If S test was positive add NH_4OH	Add dil. HCl	Add HNO_3	Mix well with resorcinol	If red report	If yellow add NH_3	If yellow add KOH sol
N test S test	Test for NH_3 evolved Evap. to dryness with excess of KOH Sodium fusion on residue N test	Filter Use filtrate to identify cystine	Test for CO_2 evolved If positive, report carbonate	Ammonium molybdate reagent If yellow, report phosphates	Add H_2SO_4 If blue, report oxalates	Uric acid or urates	Red color indicates trace of uric acid or urates	Red color indicates xanthine

In their work with pinene, Dorronsoro and Fernandez (1913) discovered that a blue or greenish-blue color in their material after the addition of resorcinol could be traced to the presence of very small amounts of oxalic acid. This process reversed could offer a specific test for oxalic acid. Thus, it is necessary only to place a small amount of the pulverized stone in the depression of a spot plate, add a drop of concentrated sulfuric acid to dissolve the stone, and at the same time liberate oxalic acid from any oxalate that might be present, and then add a small amount of purified resorcinol. A blue or bluish-green color will develop immediately if an oxalate is present in the original stone. The test is specific and its accuracy in no way depends upon the other constituents of the calculus.

In the scheme of analysis suggested by Hammarsten, the following method of distinguishing between the ways in which nitrogen may occur is presented. Magnesium ammonium phosphate was said to be present if any gaseous ammonia could be liberated from the pulverized stone by treatment with a solution of potassium hydroxide. If, after some of the stone had been evaporated to dryness with nitric acid, ammonia could still be liberated in the same manner, ammonium urate was said to have been present in the original stone. The source of experimental error is obvious. If magnesium ammonium phosphate were present, it would not be destroyed by evaporation to dryness with nitric acid, and ammonia would be liberated in the absence of ammonium urate. Domanski reported that ammonia is not liberated from ammonium urate by this treatment, and hence the results of this test are necessarily erroneous.

For this reason, the following experimental procedure is suggested: A sodium fusion test for nitrogen is carried out on the original material and a positive or negative result is reported. Another portion of the stone is treated with an excess of potassium hydroxide and the liberation of ammonia detected by the filter-paper spot method. If an evolution of ammonia occurs after a positive nitrogen test has been obtained on the other sample, it is then necessary to add a few drops more of the saturated potassium hydroxide solution and to evaporate the contents of the crucible to dryness over a water bath. An elementary analysis by the sodium fusion method is then made on this residue. A positive test will indicate the presence of organic nitrogen compounds, while a negative test will indicate the presence of the ammonium salts of organic acids (Table 17).

These facts were verified in the following way:

1. Ammonium phosphate gave a *negative test for nitrogen* by the sodium fusion method even in the presence of organic material, but liberated ammonia upon treatment with potassium hydroxide.

2. Ammonium oxalate gave a *positive nitrogen test* by the sodium fusion method. This must have been due to a molecular rearrangement by means of which the nitrogen became directly bound to carbon. Ammonia was liberated by potassium hydroxide, but no nitrogen could be detected in the residue obtained by evaporating ammonium oxalate to dryness with an excess of potassium hydroxide.

In tabular form this might be presented as follows:

	A N TEST ON ORIGINAL STONE	B EVOLUTION OF NH3 BY KOH	C N TEST ON RESIDUE FROM B
Ammonium salts of inorganic acids..............	—	+	—
Ammonium salts of organic acids................	+	+	—
Compounds containing organic nitrogen..........	+	—	+

By the foregoing method, it is possible to differentiate between nitrogen as it occurs in the ammonium radical and as it occurs in organic combination. In the absence of organic nitrogen, it is possible to distinguish between the ammonium salts of inorganic and organic acids.

Analysis for sulfur. Because of the limited quantities of cystine which occur in the urinary stone, Hammarsten and others found it convenient to use a method involving the microscopic examination of the crystals, obtained by adding a portion of the stone to concentrated ammonium hydroxide, filtering, and then evaporating a drop of the filtrate to dryness on a microscopic slide. Unfortunately, the appearance of the flat hexagonal crystals is not absolute proof of the occurrence of cystine, nor is the absence of these crystals in a single drop proof of its absence. Since cystine is one of the few sulfur-containing compounds reported as occurring in renal calculi, it has seemed advisable to include an elementary analysis for sulfur. Although a negative sulfur test does prove the absence of cystine, it must be remembered that a positive test does not prove, but merely suggests its presence. If a positive sulfur test is followed by a failure to detect the crystals of cystine, it is advisable to report the presence of unidentified sulfur-containing compounds.

The procedure is as follows:

A. *Elementary analysis.* A small piece of clean metallic sodium is placed in the bottom of a clean 3-inch test tube. To this is added a small amount of the pulverized stone. The test tube may then be heated not only until the sodium has melted, but also until the sodium vapors begin to rise in the tube. Another portion of the pulverized stone is again added, with special care taken to have the powder fall directly on the molten sodium. Heating is continued until all the sodium has been burned off. The red-hot tube is then lowered into a small beaker containing about 10 cc. of water. The tube is merely touched to the surface of the water and raised out of the liquid, but held in such a manner that the heavy glass of the beaker is always between the tube and the eyes of the worker. After any excess sodium has been destroyed, the bottom of the test tube is broken off, and the interior is carefully washed with the water in the beaker. The broken glass and insoluble material are placed in the beaker so as to be completely covered with the water, the solution is heated to boiling and filtered. The filtrate should be clear. This filtrate, or stock solution, may be used in the following manner to detect the presence of both nitrogen and sulfur in the original stone.

SULFUR TEST. One cubic centimeter of the stock solution thus obtained is placed in a test tube and acidified with acetic acid. A few drops of lead acetate reagent are added and the presence of sulfur indicated by a black precipitate of lead sulfide.

NITROGEN TEST. Three cubic centimeters of the stock solution are placed in a test tube, and five drops each of a freshly prepared ferrous sulfate solution, a potassium fluoride solution and a dilute solution of potassium hydroxide are added. The test tube is shaken so as to insure thorough mixing and then allowed to stand for five minutes. A few drops of ferric chloride solution are added and the resulting precipitate of iron hydroxide is dissolved by adding, dropwise, hydrochloric acid. A few additional drops of hydrochloric acid will then produce a brilliant Prussian blue color if the original stone contained organic nitrogen or compounds which by molecular rearrangement may form compounds containing organic nitrogen. This method, as given by Kamm, has been found to be very satisfactory.

B. *The Detection of the Ammonium Radical.* To a small portion of the original pulverized stone which has been placed in a porcelain crucible is added approximately 1 cc. of a concentrated potassium hydroxide solution. The crucible is quickly covered with a large circular filter paper, and 2 drops of Nessler's reagent are placed on this paper. The drops should be so placed that one will be over the open mouth of the crucible, while the other, the control spot, should be placed as close as possible to the edge of the paper. The evolution of ammonia which has been liberated from ammonium compounds will be indicated by the fact that the center spot turns brown much more quickly than the control spot.

C. *The mixture of aqueous potassium hydroxide and pulverized stone* is evaporated to dryness on a water bath, and the resulting mixture analyzed for nitrogen by the sodium fusion method, as described in A. The interpretation of the results of this test will be described later.

D. If a positive sulfur test has been obtained by elementary analysis, about 2 cc. of concentrated *ammonium hydroxide* is added to a small amount of the original stone. The solution can be transferred to a circular filter paper which has been folded in the conventional manner and which is held by placing the fingers over the triple fold. A series of spots may be placed on a clean microscopic slide by contacting the tip of the paper filter and the glass. *Cystine,* if present, will crystallize into characteristic flat hexagonal plates as the filtrate evaporates to dryness. These crystals can easily be identified under the low-power magnification of a microscope.

The following alternative method for the identification of cystine has proved to be more convenient. A portion of the pulverized stone is placed in a depression of a spot plate, and a drop of ammonium hydroxide is added. A drop of a 5 per cent solution of sodium cyanide is then added, and the material is allowed to stand for about five minutes. A few drops of a 5 per cent solution of sodium nitroprusside—$Na_2 Fe(CN)_5 NO \cdot 2H_2O$—are added. If cystine is present, a deep purplish-red color will develop and remain.

E. A small amount of the pulverized stone is placed in a small glass cylinder or in a short wide test tube. To this is added dilute *hydrochloric acid,* about

5 cc. The test tube or cylinder is then covered with a glass microscope slide from which a clear drop of barium hydroxide solution has been suspended. This can be done conveniently by folding a circular filter paper in the conventional manner and adding to it about 1 cc. of the stock solution of barium hydroxide. The filter paper is not placed in a funnel, but held so that a drop of the clear filtrate may be placed on the microscope slide by touching the tip of the paper to the glass. The slide is quickly inverted and placed over the cylinder in such a way that the suspended drop of liquid is over the mouth of the cylinder. This drop, protected as it is from atmospheric contamination, can be clouded only by carbon dioxide liberated from a *carbonate* present in the original material. This method, adapted from the original work of Gutzeit, has been found to be more sensitive than that suggested by Hammarsten.

F. A small amount of the pulverized stone is placed in one of the depressions of a porcelain spot plate, and a drop or two of concentrated *nitric acid* is then added. As soon as the solid material has gone into solution, a drop of ammonium molybdate reagent is added. *Phosphates,* if present, will cause a brilliant yellow color to develop immediately.

G. A small amount of the pulverized stone is then transferred to a porcelain spot plate and mixed intimately with carefully purified *resorcinol.* A drop of concentrated sulfuric acid will produce a green or bluish-green color if *oxalates* are present.

Place in the bottom of a porcelain crucible a thin layer of the original stone. Cover with a minimal amount of *concentrated nitric acid* and evaporate on a water bath to dryness.

H. If the residue is red, *urate* is present. This may, of course, be uric acid or one of its salts. Additional sensitivity may be obtained by allowing the fumes of ammonia from a bottle of ammonium hydroxide to pass over the residue.

I. If the muroxide test is negative, *xanthine* may be identified by the ability of aqueous potassium hydroxide to change the color of the residue from yellow to red.

The reagents are as follows: glacial acetic acid; lead acetate; concentrated and 6-normal hydrochloric acid; concentrated nitric acid; concentrated sulfuric acid; 6-normal potassium hydroxide; concentrated ammonium hydroxide; 10 per cent solution of barium hydroxide; metallic sodium; 10 per cent solution of ferrous sulfate (freshly prepared); 10 per cent solution of ferric chloride; 5 per cent solution sodium nitroprusside (freshly prepared); sodium cyanide in 5 per cent solution; ammonium molybdate reagent; Nessler's reagent.

Method of Recording Analytic Results. Perhaps the greatest source of error in the interpretation of analytic results may be traced directly to the method of recording the data. Any routine method of analysis is necessarily limited to reporting the presence or absence of a given number of possible constituents. Thus, in reporting results, it has seemed essential that both the constituents shown to be absent, as well as those shown to be present, be recorded. For this reason, it is convenient to use a standard form of report, an example of which, with the analytical results included, is shown.

STONE ANALYSIS REPORT

Name_____

Date_____

Record No. _____Analysis requested by Dr._____

Source of stone_____
Analytical data

N in original stone	Trace
S in original stone	Trace
NH$_4$ radical	+++
N after liberation of NH$_3$	Trace
Carbonates	—
Oxalates	+++
Phosphates	+++
Uric acid—urates	—
Xanthine	
Cystine	—

Addtional data

Unidentified sulfur-containing compound	Trace

Interpretation

The stone as received for analysis was about 15 mm. × 8 mm. × 5 mm. It was dark brown in color; individual layers but faintly defined.

Oxalates and phosphates largest part; carbonates and uric acid absent. Relatively strong evolution of ammonia suggested that ammonium magnesium phosphate was present. Positive nitrogen and sulfur tests suggested presence of cystine; microscopic examination failed to identify the compound.

Analysis performed by

_____

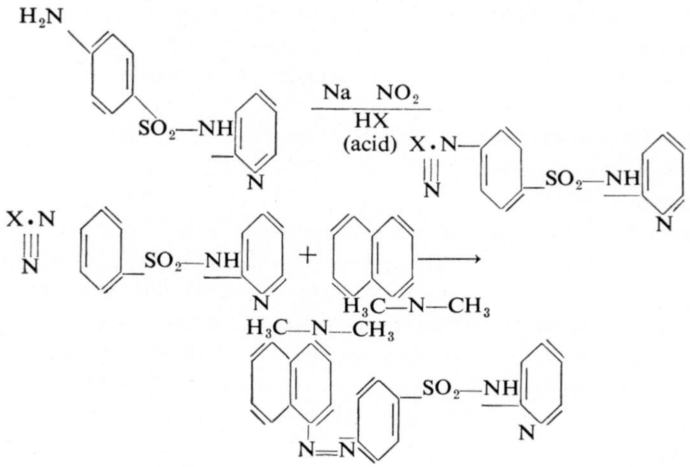

Fig. 367.   Chemical reactions involved in analysis of urinary stones.

Sulfapyridine, 2(p-aminobenzenesulfamido) pyridine, and its derivatives. In view of the recent work in the experimental production of urinary calculi by means of the administration of sulfapyridine, it seems advisable to add to the method of stone analysis a test for this compound and its simple derivatives.

In the routine schedule for analysis of stone, the use of the sodium fusion method of elementary analysis was suggested for the detection of nitrogen and sulfur. If negative results are obtained at this point, the following test may be safely omitted. If, however, positive results are obtained, the following spot plate test should be carried out.

A small quantity of pulverized stone is placed in the depression of a spot plate and covered with two drops of 20 per cent paratoluenesulfonic acid. The solution is then allowed to stand for at least one minute. One drop of freshly prepared 0.5 per cent sodium nitrite is added, and after another minute, 3 drops of dimethyl-α-naphthylamine are added. In the presence of sulfapyridine or one of its simple derivatives, a red color will develop and remain. The chemical reactions involved are shown in Figure 367. These equations show that the reactions involve the diazotization of an aromatic amine with the subsequent coupling necessary to synthesize the colored compound. For this reason, the reaction is not absolutely specific. This limitation is of slight importance, however, when it is remembered that compounds capable of undergoing diazotization reactions are not to be found in normal urine.

Treatment. The treatment of renal lithiasis falls into three categories, expectant, medical and surgical. Dietary management has become an important phase of expectant, or conservative, treatment.

Expectant Treatment. A silent small calculus or one producing negligible symptoms, occupying a position in the renal pelvis or calyx may be treated expectantly, with the anticipation of its spontaneous expulsion. The nature of the stone and its chemical constituents are also important in planning the details of treatment.

In the presence of a mild infection, the appropriate medication, following sensitivity studies, should be prescribed in an attempt at its eradication. It is advisable also for the patient to drink large quantities of water. As a general rule, I believe dietary and medical treatment should also be included, in an attempt to promote dissolution or to prevent further enlargement of the stone. This type of management requires close supervision of the patients. Roentgenograms should be secured every three months, and more frequently if any pain or colic occurs. In instances in which the calculus increases in size, with appearance of infection or incapacitating pain or colic, surgical removal is usually deemed advisable.

Many patients who expel uric acid calculi, associated with colic, are observed to pass progressively larger stones. I have also observed patients with cystine calculi who demonstrated the same characteristic course until the process was arrested by dietary measures.

Dietary Adjustment. For the past several years, we have been interested in studying the role of diet administered in conjunction with other procedures recommended in the past in securing the dissolution of renal calculi and in minimizing the incidence of recurrent renal lithiasis.

The fundamental purpose of the diet is to adjust the pH of the urine to a point where the salts are held in solution, so that precipitation does not occur. By reducing the pH of the urine to the acid side, that is, to a pH of 5.0 or 5.2, the phosphates and carbonates of calcium and magnesium

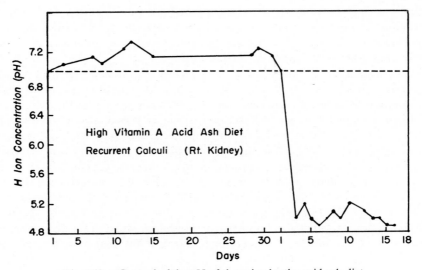

Fig. 368.   Control of the pH of the urine by the acid-ash diet.

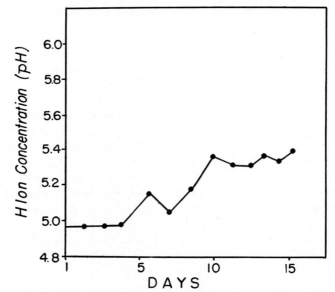

Fig. 369.   Control of the pH of the urine by the alkaline-ash diet.

are held in solution (Fig. 368). Similarly, by shifting the pH of the urine slightly to the alkaline side by the use of the alkaline-ash diet, cystine and uric acid are held in solution (Fig. 369). Care must be exercised that the pH is not shifted too strongly to the alkaline side, so as to cause precipitation of phosphates and carbonates, and *vice versa*. Frequent examination of the urine for crystals is essential.

When no stone is available for analysis, the pH of the urine from the kidney containing the stone and the types of crystals present determine the diet to be utilized and the total acid or alkaline ash necessary. If the reaction of the urine from the kidney harboring the stone is alkaline, the high-vitamin A, acid-ash diet is used; if, however, the reaction of the urine is acid, the high-vitamin A, alkaline-ash diet is employed.

If a stone has been passed previously, it should be analyzed in addition to the determination of the pH and the urinary crystals. Such an analysis demonstrates whether the salts present precipitate in urine that is acid or alkaline. When the stone is composed of phosphates or carbonates, the high-vitamin A, acid-ash diet is recommended. When the calculus is composed of oxalates, the high-vitamin A, low-oxalate diet is employed. It is

Table 18. High-Vitamin Acid-Ash Diet

(25 cc. Excess Acid Ash)

The purpose of the High-Vitamin Acid-Ash Diet is to furnish an adequate high-vitamin diet in which the total acid ash exceeds the total basic ash.

The following *foods* in the designated *amounts* must be included in the diet *daily*.

A. ACID-ASH FOODS:

   1. CEREAL—any one of the following measured servings—

	Amount		*Amount*
Cornflakes	1 cupful (heaping)	Puffed wheat	1 cupful (scant)
Cornmeal (cooked)	⅔ cupful	Puffed rice	1 cupful (heaping)
Farina (cooked)	⅔ cupful	Ralston (cooked)	½ cupful
Oatmeal (cooked)	½ cupful	Rice (cooked)	½ cupful
Rice Krispies	⅔ cupful	Shredded wheat	⅔ biscuit
		Wheatena (cooked)	½ cupful

   2. MEAT—any two of the following measured servings—

	Amount		*Amount*
Beef, loin (med. fat)	4 ounces	Lamb roast	4 ounces
Chicken (broiler)	One half	Liver (beef)	4 ounces
Chicken (stewed)	Breast or thigh plus leg	Mackerel (fresh)	4 ounces
		Oysters (medium)	4–6
Codfish (fresh cooked)	¼ cupful (2 ounces)	Pork chop (medium)	2
Eggs	2	Pork roast	4 ounces
Frankfurters (large)	2	Salmon (fresh)	4 ounces
Halibut	4 ounces	Salmon (canned)	4 ounces
Ham (smoked)	4 ounces	Trout	4 ounces
Heart (beef)	4 ounces	Turkey	4 ounces
Kidney (veal)	¾ cupful (cubed)	Veal chop (medium)	2
Lamb chop (E.P.)	3 medium size	Veal roast	3 ounces
		White fish	4 ounces

   3. BREAD—whole wheat—5 slices.

   4. EGGS—2.

   5. MISCELLANEOUS—any one of the following measured servings—

	Amount		*Amount*
Macaroni	½ cupful	Rice	½ cupful
Spaghetti	½ cupful	Corn	½ cupful
Noodles	½ cupful	Plain cake	2″ cube

B. ALKALINE-ASH FOODS:

   1. MILK—one pint.

   2. CREAM—¼ cupful.

   3. FRUITS AND VEGETABLES—see page 802.

C. CONCENTRATED VITAMIN FOODS:

   1. YEAST—2 cakes.

   2. COD LIVER OIL—2 tablespoonfuls; or HALIVER OIL, 2 capsules before each meal.

   3. WHEAT GERM—2 tablespoonfuls to be added to cereal.

Table 18 continued

HIGH-VITAMIN ACID-ASH DIET

Fruits and vegetables should be chosen from the following list only. Any combination of fruits and vegetables may be selected, but the total excess basic ash must not exceed 17 cc. daily.

FRUITS	AMOUNT	CC. OF EXCESS BASIC ASH
Blueberries (fresh)	⅔ cupful	2.7
Watermelon	2½″ x 2½″ x ½″	2.7
Grapes	½ cupful or 24 grapes	2.7
Pear (fresh)	1 medium	3.6
Apple	1 small	3.7
Grape juice	½ cupful	3.9
Lemon juice	½ cupful	4.1
Grapefruit	½ medium	4.2
Cherry juice	½ cupful	4.4
Orange juice	½ cupful	4.5
Peach (fresh)	1 medium	5.0
Lemon (E.P.)	1 medium	5.5
Tangerine	1 large	5.5
Banana	¾ cupful or ½ large	5.6
Orange	1 medium	5.6
Nectarines	2 medium	6.0
Cherries (fresh) sour	½ cupful	6.1
Cherries (fresh) sweet	15 large	6.2
Strawberries	10 large	6.6
Raspberries (fresh) red	¾ cupful–1 cupful	6.7
Apricots (fresh)	2 medium	6.8
Pineapple (fresh)	⅔ cupful (diced)	6.8
Blackberries (fresh)	⅔ cupful–1 cupful	6.8
Muskmelon or cantaloupe	⅓ of a 4½″ melon	7.5

VEGETABLES	AMOUNT	CC. OF EXCESS BASIC ASH
Asparagus	12—5″ stalks	1.0
Squash (summer)	½ cupful (cooked)	1.1
Green peas	¾ cupful	1.3
Onions	½ cupful	1.5
Pumpkin	½ cupful (cooked)	1.5
Green pepper	1 shell	1.7
Eggplant	½ cupful (cooked)	2.2
Squash (winter)	½ cupful (mashed)	2.8
Radishes	10	2.9
Mushrooms	½ cupful (canned)	4.0
Broccoli	½ cupful (cooked)	5.2
Cauliflower	⅔ cupful (cooked)	5.3
Tomato juice	½ cupful	5.3
String beans	½ cupful (cooked)	5.4
Tomatoes	½ cupful or 1 medium	5.6
Cabbage	⅔ cupful (cooked)—1½ cupful (raw)	6.0
Sweet potato	½ medium size	6.7
White potato	1 potato 2½″ in diameter	7.0
Lettuce	¼ head (16 leaves)	7.4
Celery	4 stalks	7.8
Rutabagas	½ cupful (mashed)	8.5
Carrots	⅝ cupful	10.8
Beets	⅔ cupful	10.9

Table 18 continued

HIGH-VITAMIN ACID-ASH DIET

In addition, the following *acid* and *neutral* foods may be used as *desired*.

ACID FOODS	NEUTRAL FOODS	
Cheddar cheese	Butter	Kaffee Hag
Bacon	Candy (no chocolate bars)	Tea
Flour	Cornstarch	Postum
Plain cookies	Lard	Honey
Pastry with custard or allowed	Olive oil	
amounts of fruit fillings	Salad oil	
Peanuts—Popcorn	Mayonnaise	
Crackers	Sugar	
English walnuts	Tapioca	
Pecans	Coffee	

OMIT:

Dried fruits and vegetables. Highly seasoned foods, spices, condiments such as mustard, pepper, catsup, horseradish. Carbonated beverages such as coca cola, ginger ale; beer, wine, alcoholic beverages; molasses, olives, pickles.

HIGH-VITAMIN ACID–ASH DIET

SUGGESTED PLAN OF MENU:	SAMPLE MENU:
BREAKFAST:	
Fruit	Orange juice—½ cupful
Cereal and wheat germ	Oatmeal—½ cupful with 2 tb. wheat germ
Eggs	Eggs—2
Whole wheat bread	Whole wheat toast—2 slices
Butter	Butter
Beverage	Coffee or tea
Cream	Cream—¼ cupful
Sugar	Sugar
LUNCHEON:	
Meat	Veal chops—2
Rice or substitute (see miscellaneous)	Steamed rice—½ cupful
Vegetable or salad	Green peas—¾ cupful
Whole wheat bread	Whole wheat bread—1½ slices
Butter	Butter
Fruit	Baked apple—1 small
Milk	Milk—1 glassful
DINNER:	
Meat	Roast beef (see list)
Two vegetables (cooked or raw)	Hubbard squash—½ cupful
	String beans—½ cupful
Whole wheat bread	Whole wheat bread—1½ slices
Butter	Butter
Dessert	Tapioca cream pudding
Milk	Milk—1 glassful

also important when dealing with oxalate calculi to reduce the soluble oxalates formed in the intestines by fermentation. The soluble oxalates are derived from the fermentation of sugar, and hence carbohydrate intake must be reduced. In patients whose calculi are composed of urates, uric acid or cystine, the high-vitamin A, low-purine, alkaline-ash diet is recommended.

The treatment of each patient must be individualized, and the pH of the urine must be adjusted to the point at which the salts essential for

Table 19. High-Vitamin Alkaline-Ash Diet

The purpose of the High-Vitamin Alkaline-Ash Diet is to furnish an adequate high-vitamin diet in which the total alkaline ash exceeds the total acid ash.

The following foods in the designated amounts should be included in the diet daily:

A. ALKALINE-ASH FOODS
   1. MILK—one quart
   2. CREAM—½ cup
   3. FRUITS AND VEGETABLES—Any combination of fruits and vegetables may be selected from the following list, but the total excess basic ash must total at least 38 cc. daily:

FRUITS	AMOUNT	CC. OF EXCESS BASIC ASH
Watermelon	2½″ x 2½″ x 1″	2.7
Grapes	½ cup	2.7
Pears	1	3.6
Apples	1 small	3.7
Currants (dried)	¼ cup	3.7
Lemon juice	½ cup	4.1
Orange juice	½ cup	4.5
Peaches	1 medium	5.0
Dates	7	5.5
Bananas	½ large	5.6
Oranges	¾ cup or 1 med.	5.6
Cherries	⅔ cup	6.1
Apricots (fresh)	2	6.4
Pineapple	2 slices	6.8
Cantaloupe	⅓ melon or ½ cup	7.5
Rhubarb (cooked)	½ cup	8.6
Raisins (cooked)	½ cup	21.3
Fig chips (dried)	½ cup	80.7
VEGETABLES		
Asparagus	12—5″ stalks	0.8
Peas (fresh)	¾ cup	1.3
Onions	½ cup	1.5
Pumpkin	½ cup	1.5
Turnip	½ cup	2.7
Squash	½ cup	2.8
Radishes	10	2.9
Beans, canned, kidney	½ cup	3.0
Potato chips	10–12 large	3.6
Mushrooms	½ cup	4.0
Cauliflower	⅔ cup	5.3
Peas (dried)	½ cup	5.4
Beans (snap)	⅔ cup	5.4
Tomato	½ cup or 1 med.	5.6
Beans, canned, baked	½ cup	6.0
Potato, sweet	½ med.	6.7
Potato, white	1 med.	7.0
Lettuce	¼ head	7.4
Celery	4 stalks or ¾ cup	7.8
Cucumber	⅓ cup	7.9
Rutabagas	½ cup	8.5
Carrots	⅝ cup	10.8
Beets	⅔ cup	10.9
Parsnips	½ cup	11.9
Beans, lima, green	½ cup	14.0
Chard	½ cup	15.7
Beans, navy, dried	¾ cup	26.1
Spinach	½ cup	27.0
Beet greens	½ cup	27.0
Beans, lima, dried	⅔ cup	41.6

Table 19 continued

B. ACID-ASH FOODS

1. MEATS—any two of the following measured servings:

Beef, loin, med. fat	4″ x 4¼″ x ½″	Lamb roast	5″ x 5″ x ¼″
Chicken, broiler	one half	Liver, beef	3″ x 6½″ x ½″
Chicken, stewed	breast or thigh	Mackerel, fresh	2″ x 4″ x 1″
	plus leg	Oysters, very	
Cheese, cheddar	3½″ x 2″ x 1″	large	3
Codfish, fresh, cooked	¼ cup	Pork chop, thick	1
Eggs	2	Salmon, fresh	3″ x 4″ x ¾″
Frankfurters, large	2	Salmon, canned	½ cup packed
Halibut	4″ x 2″ x 1″	Trout	2½″ x 3″ x 1″
Ham, fresh	4½″ x 3″ x ¼″	Turkey, 2 slices	2″ x 3″ x ¼″
Heart, beef	2½″ x 3″ x 1″	Veal chop	1
Kidney, veal	¾ cup	Veal roast	3″ x 2½″ x ⅛″
Lamb chop	3 med. size	White fish	2¼″ x 3″ x 1″

2. EGGS—one
3. BREAD—whole wheat—2 slices
4. CEREAL—any one of the following measured servings:

Cornflakes	1 cup heaping	Puffed wheat	1 cup scant
Cornmeal (cooked)	⅔ cup	Puffed rice	1 cup heaping
Farina (cooked)	⅔ cup	Rice (cooked)	½ cup scant
Oatmeal (cooked)	½ cup	Shredded wheat	½ biscuit

C. CONCENTRATED VITAMIN FOODS:

1. YEAST—2 cakes
2. COD LIVER OIL—2 tablespoons; or HALIVER OIL, 2 capsules before each meal.

D. *In addition,* the following *alkaline* and *neutral* foods may be used as desired:

ALKALINE FOODS	NEUTRAL FOODS	
Dairy products including all cheeses.	Sweet butter	Coffee
Soups, except when made from meat stock.	Candy (no chocolate)	Tea
Almonds	Cornstarch	Kaffee Hag
Molasses	Lard	Postum
Olives	Salad oil	Olive oil
	Sugar	Mayonnaise
		Tapioca

The following list contains a few striking examples of foods which must be omitted because of their extremely high acid-ash content:

Meat broths and soups	Cranberries
All breads and crackers	Peanuts
except as listed above	Walnuts
All pastries and rich desserts	Popcorn
	Flour

HIGH-VITAMIN ALKALINE-ASH DIET

SUGGESTED PLAN OF MENU	SAMPLE MENU
BREAKFAST	
Fruit	Orange juice—½ glass
Cereal	Farina—⅔ cup, cooked
Egg	Egg—1
Whole wheat toast	Whole wheat toast—1 slice
Butter	Butter
Cream	Cream—½ cup
Milk	Milk—1 glass
LUNCH	
Meat	Cold sliced lamb—1 serving
Potato	Baked potato—1 serving
Vegetable	Celery—1 serving

Table 19 continued
HIGH-VITAMIN ALKALINE-ASH DIET

SUGGESTED PLAN OF MENU	SAMPLE MENU
LUNCH (*continued*)	
Bread	Whole wheat toast—½ slice
Butter	Butter
Milk	Milk—1 glass
Fruit	Canned peaches—1 serving
DINNER	
Meat	Roast beef—1 serving
Potato	Sweet potato—1 serving
Vegetable	Cauliflower—1 serving
Bread	Whole wheat toast—½ slice
Butter	Butter
Milk	Milk—1 glass
Dessert	Vanilla ice cream
8:00 P.M.	
Milk	Milk—1 glass

Table 20. Low-Oxalate Diet

FOODS OF HIGH-OXALIC ACID CONTENT (0.1% or over)	FOODS OF MODERATE-OXALIC ACID CONTENT (0.02% or over)
To be avoided—	To be eaten sparingly—
Beets	Beans (green and wax)
Beet tops	Blackberries
Black tea	Blueberries
Chenopodium	Carrots
Chocolate	Celery
Cocoa	Coffee (roasted)
Dried figs	Concord grapes
Ground pepper	Currants (red)
Lambs quarters	Dandelion greens
Lime peel	Endive
Nuts	Gooseberries
Parsley	Lemon peel
Poke	Okra
Poppy seeds	Onions (green)
Purslane	Oranges
Rhubarb	Orange peel
Sorrel	Peppers (green)
Spinach	Raspberries (black)
Swiss chard	Strawberries
	Sweet potatoes

All other foods may be used as desired.

A well balanced diet includes each day:

Meat, cheese, fish, or fowl	1 or more servings
Eggs	1
Milk	2 or more glassfuls
Vegetables	2 or more servings beside potato; 1 green or yellow; "greens" often
Fruits	2 or more servings; at least 1 raw; citrus fruit or tomato often
Cereal and bread	2 or more servings; whole grain value or enriched
Butter	2 or more tablespoonfuls

Other foods to satisfy appetite and to complete growth and activity needs.

the formation of a calculus remain in solution and are not precipitated. The basic diet contains an excess acid or alkaline ash of 17.3 and the constituents of the diet are varied daily until the pH is at the desired level. The diet instructions to be followed by the patient according to the requirements of his individual case are shown in Tables 18, 19, 20 and 21.

Table 21. Low-Purine Diet

C—223   P—89   F—115   Cal. 2283

BREAKFAST:

Fruit	1 serving
Cereal (no oatmeal)	1 serving
Eggs	2
Toast	1 slice
Butter or margarine	As desired
Beverage	Sanka, Kaffee Hag, or Postum
Milk	As desired
Cream	As desired
Sugar	As desired

LUNCHEON:

Soup	1 serving (see list)
Cheese	2 ounces
Vegetable (cooked)	1 serving
Vegetable (raw)	1 serving
Bread	1 slice
Butter or margarine	As desired
Dessert	1 serving (see list)
Milk	1 glassful

DINNER:

Allowed soup	If desired
Meat, fish, fowl	2 ounces (twice weekly)
Potato	1 serving
Vegetable (cooked or raw)	1 serving
Bread	1 slice
Butter or margarine	As desired
Dessert	1 serving (see list)
Milk	1 glassful

SPECIAL INSTRUCTIONS:

1. Avoid liver, sweetbreads, brains, and kidney. A 2 ounce portion of any other meat, fish or fowl may be served twice weekly.
2. Serve cheese and eggs as meat substitutes. Fish roe and caviar may be used as desired.
3. Use 1–2 pints of milk daily.
4. Omit all meat extracts, broth soups, and gravies.
5. Eliminate the following vegetables entirely from the diet:
   Dried beans, lentils, dried peas, spinach.
6. Avoid coffee, tea, chocolate, and cocoa.
7. Omit alcoholic beverages of all kinds.
8. Use fruits of all kinds—fresh, canned, and dried.
9. Allow cereals of all kinds except oatmeal.
10. Soups allowed are milk soups made with any vegetables except those forbidden.
11. Desserts allowed are fruit, puddings, cake, ice cream, gelatin desserts or pie.
12. Beverages allowed are milk or buttermilk and any decaffeinated coffee or cereal coffee.

By means of a LaMotte pH apparatus, the patients make their own daily analyses of the urine. The first specimen voided in the morning is discarded to avoid the effects of respiration on awakening and the second specimen is examined before eating breakfast. The reports are recorded and presented to the physician at monthly intervals, so that the diet may be adjusted if the desired pH level is not being maintained adequately and consistently.

The results of dietary management in various types of cases may be summarized as follows: In patients with *bilateral renal calculi,* conservative treatment by means of diet has not been satisfactory, as a general rule. In the majority of cases I have observed, infection, stasis and impaired renal function were also present. The culture of the urine frequently showed Bacillus proteus and it was impossible to shift the pH of the urine to the acid side (Fig. 370). If this cannot be accomplished, the calculi continue

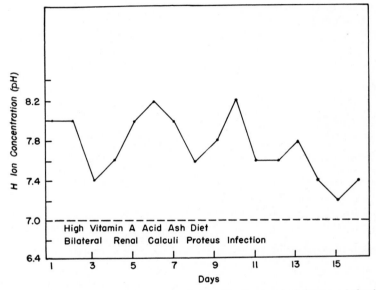

Fig. 370.   Failure to control the pH of the urine because of Proteus infection.

to enlarge, owing to the deposition of alkaline salts. In a few instances in which the pH of the urine was controlled, gratifying results were obtained.

Unfortunately in many cases of *nonobstructive calculus in the pelvis or calyx,* stasis and infection are present. Since these conditions may be causing damage to the renal parenchyma, conservative treatment usually is not indicated. In a smaller percentage of cases in which stasis and infection are not present, the diet may be utilized in an attempt to secure dissolution, or at least to minimize the chances of enlargement.

In patients who *pass stones at frequent intervals but without a demonstrable calculus in the kidney,* satisfactory results may usually be secured with dietary treatment, if infection is absent. The incidence of calculus formation in these cases may be definitely minimized.

Medication. Albright, Suby and Sulkowitch observed that citric-acid mixtures would disintegrate calcium stones, not only because of their acid reaction, but also through formation of a complex calcium-citrate ion.

Subsequent to the introduction of the "buffered" citrate solution by

Albright, solutions "G" and "M" were later developed by Suby. Solution "G" contains citric acid monohydrate, 32.5 gm.; magnesium oxide, anhydrous, 3.84 gm.; sodium carbonate, anhydrous, 4.37 gm., and distilled water, 1000 cc. The reaction of the solution is pH 4. Solution "M" is less acid than solution "G" and is made by adding to 1000 cc. of distilled water 32.5 gm. citric acid monohydrate; 3.84 gm. magnesium oxide, anhydrous, and 8.84 gm. of sodium carbonate, anhydrous.

Keyser, Scherer and Claffey (1948) suggested an attack on the organic matrix of urinary calculi, treating them *in vitro* with ferments prior to irrigation with solvent solutions. So far, 0.5 per cent urease has proved

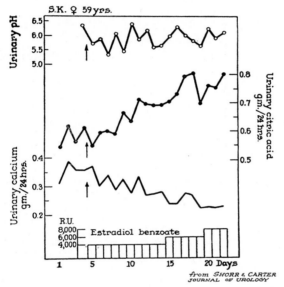

Fig. 371.   Influence of estradiol benzoate on urinary calcium, citric acid and pH.

effective. Startling results have been reported in some instances by the use of the solvent solutions, attacking the renal calculi directly by irrigation of the renal pelvis and calices with the solutions administered through ureteral catheters. Undoubtedly additional solutions which serve the same purpose will be introduced in the near future.

Shorr described the possible usefulness of estrogens and aluminum hydroxide gels in the management of patients with renal lithiasis. The rationale for the use of estrogens rests on the concept that citric acid is a useful urinary constituent by virtue of its capacity to enhance calcium solubility and on the ability of estrogenic hormones to augment the excretion of citric acid and to reduce that of calcium. This is used as an adjunct in the management of stones composed of calcium phosphate, magnesium-ammonium phosphate, or calcium magnesium-ammonium phosphate. In men, in order to achieve increases in citrate excretion of 250 to 350 mg. each twenty-four hours, it is necessary to administer 5000 to 10,000 R. U. of estradiol benzoate intramuscularly daily, or Premarin, 4 to 8 tablets daily, by mouth, may be prescribed; each tablet contains 1.25 mg. of estrone sulfate (Fig. 371).

The side effects of the drug, namely, tenderness of the nipples and the reduction of libido may be complained of by the patient. In women, disturbance in the regularity of the menstrual cycle or endometrial hyperplasia may develop. In menopausal women with intact uteri, Shorr recommended withdrawal of the hormone therapy at varying intervals, to avoid endometrial hyperplasia and bleeding. If a hysterectomy has been performed for other pathologic lesions previously, it is obvious that such complications cannot ensue. In these groups, he recommended an initial dose of 4000 R. U. of

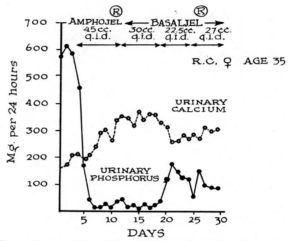

Fig. 372. Effects of amphojel and basaljel in various doses four times daily, with a constant diet, on excretion of urinary phosphorus and calcium. Phosphorus, 1.012 gm.; calcium, 0.489 gm.; nitrogen, 10.48 gm. per day.

estradiol benzoate daily for three weeks, or 4 or 5 tablets of Premarin for the same length of time. This may be repeated after a ten-day rest period. In younger women, the disturbance of the menstrual regularity may be avoided by administering the estrogens from the fifteenth through the twenty-fifth day of the menstrual cycle. Estradiol benzoate (2000 R. U.) is administered intramuscularly, or 2 to 3 tablets of Premarin are prescribed orally during this period.

The rationale for the use of aluminum gel was stated by Shorr as follows: "In passing through the gastro-intestinal tract, the aluminum combines with phosphate ions to form an insoluble aluminum phosphate. This insoluble aluminum phosphate is entirely excreted as such in the stool, thereby diminishing the amount of phosphate available for resorption through the intestinal tract. The serum inorganic phosphorus is therefore lowered, which favors a more complete tubular resorption of phosphate, and thus reduces the urinary excretion of phosphate."

The amount of aluminum gel required to maintain the desired level of excretion of urinary phosphorus is approximately 30 to 60 cc. three or four times daily (Fig. 372). With this amount, the phosphorus excretion may be reduced to 200 mg. or less per twenty-four hours. This is valuable in the presence of renal damage and in instances in which the pH of the urine cannot be controlled by dietary means.

Treatment of Anuria. The treatment of the obstructive type of anuria consists primarily in relief of the obstruction and the reestablishment of free urinary drainage. Cystoscopic investigation, even in the absence of pain, is essential to differentiate the obstruction from the secretory type of anuria. Peritoneal lavage is rarely indicated as peritonitis constitutes a major complication.

The artificial kidney may be utilized in instances in which the patient's condition is critical, along with relief of the obstruction.

When the outflow of urine from the kidneys cannot be reestablished by conservative measures, surgical intervention is necessary. If a stone is present in the ureter, it may be quickly removed by ureterolithotomy. When the stone is in the pelvic portion of the ureter, some surgeons prefer to perform a nephrotomy. If the calculus is in the pelvis of the kidney, a pelviolithotomy is the preferable procedure, with drainage of the kidney either through the pelvis or by means of a separate incision through the renal parenchyma.

In contrast to the secretory type of anuria, in which the prognosis may be grave, the obstructive type caused by renal lithiasis usually responds promptly to treatment, once the obstruction is removed, unless irreparable damage has been done to the kidney, accompanied by a pronounced loss of kidney function. The end results of the treatment of calculous anuria are influenced by the status of the kidneys before the calculi produced a blockage of urine, the duration of the anuria, and the general condition of the patient.

Treatment of Nephrocalcinosis. The objectives in the medical treatment of nephrocalcinosis are to relieve the acidosis, to reduce the hyperchloremia and hypercalcinuria, and to improve the absorption of calcium.

The "citrate mixture" (60 cc. of a mixture of 140 gm. of citric acid and 98 gm. of sodium citrate in 1000 cc. of water) is prescribed daily, to correct the acidosis and to reduce the blood chlorides. Because of the inability of the kidneys to excrete acids, including the chloride radicals, salt should be restricted in the diet. The "citrate mixture" corrects hypercalcinuria by adding base, thus counteracting the necessity for the utilization of calcium as a base.

Brown and Vineberg pointed out that in acidosis there is a reduction in gastric acidity; this is followed by a decrease in the absorption of calcium from the gastrointestinal tract, which is instrumental in the production of the changes in the bones (osteomalacia and rickets). The intestinal acidosis induced by citric acid corrects this reaction. Albright suggested also supplemental vitamin D, stating that this improves calcium absorption and results in a reduction in the fecal calcium. The calcium content of the diet should be relatively high.

Prophylactic Treatment for Prevention of Recurrent Calculi. The incidence of recurrence of renal calculi following surgical procedures for their removal has been considerably reduced in recent years by medical and dietary treatment. Cabot and Crabtree, in 1915, found that renal calculi recurred in 56 per cent of patients treated by nephrotomy and in 51 per cent following pyelotomy. Barney (1922) reported an incidence of recurrence of 32 per cent; Braasch and Foulds (1924), 10.7 per cent; Oppenheimer (1937) cited the incidence of recurrence following pyelolithotomy, pyelonephrolithotomy and nephrolithotomy as 14.9 per cent, 32 per cent and 29.4 per cent, respectively; in Herbst's series the rate of recurrence was 15 per cent. Since 1932, by employing the dietary routine in conjunction with other therapeutic procedures employed in the past, we have reduced the incidence of recurrence following operation from 16.4 per cent to 3.6 per cent (Higgins, 1936, a, c; 1938, b; 1939, d; 1943). Twinem (1937), using the same postoperative regimen, reported a reduction of recurrence from 28 per cent following nephrotomy and 20.9 per cent following pyelotomy, to 5.3 per cent.

In view of the foregoing, I believe that a carefully planned dietary regimen plays an essential part in the management of patients with renal lithiasis. The same management is instituted in the case of the patient in whom the objective of treatment is to prevent a recurrence as for those cases in which an attempt is made to produce dissolution of the calculus. At present, we have a collected series of eighty-four cases in which complete dissolution of a calculus has occurred.

The formation of *renal calculi associated with recumbency* is another factor to consider in planning prophylactic treatment of lithiasis. Military hospitals dealing with orthopedic and neurologic problems requiring the patient to be confined to bed for extended periods have furnished interesting reports which have increased the awareness of the association of renal lithiasis in these cases. Three factors, stasis, infection and hypercalcinuria, are usually present in bedridden patients and play a role in the formation of stones; in some cases, additional causative agents may be operative.

In a review of cases of 800 patients with bone injury who were required to maintain a recumbent position, Kimbrough and Denslow (1949) cited an incidence of calculus formation of 2 per cent. Prather (1947) reported renal calculi in 31.5 per cent of patients with complete transection of the cord and in 20 per cent of those with partial transection; the higher incidence in cases with complete transection was probably due to a longer period of bed rest, which averaged fifteen months from the time of injury. Riba (1945) and Raines* cited an incidence of renal lithiasis of 13 per cent in cases of this type.

Harrison and his collaborators (1945), Kimbrough and Denslow (1949), Leadbetter and Engster (1945), and others, have discussed measures to be utilized to prevent the formation of stone in these patients. The treatment is primarily preventive, with application of the general measures used for the prevention of recurrent stones, but also including frequent changes in the patient's position, during the period of confinement.

To summarize, the procedures utilized in conservative treatment attempt-

* Personal communication.

ing to produce dissolution of a calculus or to prevent recurrence are (1) fluid intake of 3000 cc. daily; (2) eradication of foci of infection, especially in the teeth, prostate and cervix; (3) elimination of infection of the urinary tract by chemotherapy after sensitivity tests; (4) correction of stasis; (5) correction or treatment of metabolic diseases, such as gout or cystinuria; (6) in case of a clinical diagnosis of hyperparathyroidism substantiated by laboratory findings, surgical exploration for a parathyroid tumor; (7) dietary adjustment according to the individual indications.

Surgical Indications. Proper selection of cases is an important factor in the success of conservative treatment; the corollary to this is that definite indications for surgical treatment should be constantly kept in mind. Several features, including the size, situation and composition of the stone, the presence or absence of infection, and the severity of the subjective symptoms, influence the decision in favor of surgical intervention and the choice of the procedure to be used.

Although a stone may be silent, from the clinical standpoint, slowly and insidiously it destroys renal parenchyma; this destructive process is accelerated by the advent of infection. For this reason, operation is advisable when the calculus is impairing renal function by the destruction of renal parenchyma, unless some general disease contraindicates surgical intervention. Many urologists affirm that a calculus over 1 cm. in diameter occupying a position in the pelvis of the kidney requires operation. A smaller stone impacted in the ureteropelvic junction or a larger stone producing symptoms owing to a ball-valve mechanism requires extraction from the renal pelvis. Although the renal pelvis increases in size to accommodate an enlarging stone, sooner or later infection will supervene and necessitate the removal of the calculus. If the stone is small and situated in a calyx, and is not accompanied by pain or infection, conservative medical and dietary treatment may be instituted. When, however, subsequent roentgenograms reveal that the calculus is enlarging, extending into the infundibulum, producing a localized hydrocalyx or pyocalyx, operative intervention is indicated. Obviously, a small stone in the renal pelvis, producing only meager symptoms, especially if it is composed of uric acid or cystine, should be observed in the hope of its spontaneous passage.

Calculi too large to pass spontaneously, varying from 1 cm. in size to large staghorn stones occupying the renal pelvis and calices, usually require surgical removal. It is true that occasionally in an aged individual in poor general health, a staghorn calculus may be discovered during the course of examination, accompanied by practically no clinical symptoms. In such instances, the function of the sound kidney is such that a conservative policy of observation may be advised, always appreciating that in case sepsis appears, operation may be required. I have followed several such patients in this conservative manner without regret. Usually, however, the presence of a calculus in the kidney too large to pass spontaneously is a potential hazard. Eventually infection will supervene and procrastination in regard to surgery may lead to the necessity for a nephrectomy. Even with our newer chemotherapeutic agents, eradication of infection is usually not possible until the calculus is removed. Individualization of cases is necessary, and clinical judgment may be taxed to the utmost in some instances to determine whether to pursue a policy of watchful waiting or to advocate immediate surgical intervention.

Bilateral renal calculi present additional problems. In the majority of instances, infection is present, although occasionally, even with multiple calculi, the urine is sterile. I do not believe surgical intervention is advisable in all cases of bilateral stones. I have observed aged individuals with bilateral renal calculi who live fairly comfortably and succumb to intercurrent disease. In such patients, operation would have been a hazardous procedure. In a younger individual with the same type of bilateral lithiasis, surgical intervention might have been advised, hoping for some restoration of renal function, the elimination of infection in the urinary tract, and prevention of renal failure and sepsis.

In case surgical treatment of both kidneys is necessary, the usual dictum is that operation should be performed on the better kidney first. This, however, is not always the best policy. In the presence of a calculous pyonephrosis associated with sepsis, it may be necessary to operate upon this kidney first, although the opposite kidney has better function. If one kidney is producing severe or acute pain, it implies active injury to a kidney whose function is already impaired, and immediate relief is advisable. Scholl (1936) summarized the accepted view succinctly: "The question of which kidney to operate upon first may be difficult. If either kidney is causing acute pain or is badly infected, this usually will require relief first. If neither stone is causing acute symptoms, the kidney which is least involved should be operated upon first and this is usually the one which has recently caused symptoms."

Multiple bilateral calculi may be dislodged from the calices, to find a new situation in the pelvis or ureter, and thus may be instrumental in the production of anuria. Frequently such calculi are observed in the presence of dilated kidneys. Usually the calculi are not of the same size and the stone in the pelvis is larger than the calculi in the calices. Infection is usually present and operation is advisable.

The opinion has been advanced that in some instances in which calculi of moderate size are present and the functional value of the kidneys is approximately the same, a simultaneous bilateral operation may be performed. I believe this is a radical, hazardous procedure, and rarely, if ever, advisable. In some instances of bilateral renal lithiasis in which one kidney is the site of a pronounced infection, a nephrostomy may be necessary, as the function of the opposite kidney alone is not sufficient to maintain life. In those cases in which one kidney is fairly normal, with the opposite kidney functionless and producing disabling symptoms, a nephrectomy is probably the procedure of choice.

Treatment for the removal of stones from fused kidneys presents the same surgical problems, except that some surgeons advocate a nephropexy when the isthmus of a horseshoe kidney is divided.

It is important to reiterate, for emphasis, that individualization of cases is essential in planning surgical and other treatment for renal lithiasis. Factors may exist in a given case which require treatment different from that which would be instituted if such complications were not present. As a general rule, it is well to lean toward conservatism in regard to surgical treatment.

Types of Operations. (See Section XV, Chapter 3 on Renal Surgery by Dr. James Priestley.)

URETERAL CALCULI

Etiologic and Physical Factors. *Age.* Stone in the ureter is essentially a disease of middle life; it is rare in childhood and unusual in old age. In a series of 857 cases which I reviewed in 1939, 69 per cent occurred in patients aged twenty to fifty years. The youngest patient was twenty years old and the oldest, seventy-two years. The age incidence was similar in a series reported by Mathe (1932) and by Bumpus and Scholl (1925).

Sex. The incidence of ureteral calculi is much greater in men than in women. Jeanbrau reported the ratio as 61 per cent men, 39 per cent women; Bumpus and Scholl, 68 per cent men and 32 per cent women; Ravich, 69.8 per cent men and 30.2 per cent women. In my series of 857 patients, 79 per cent were men and 21 per cent women.

Site of Origin. It is now generally conceded that ureteral calculi are originally formed in the kidney and then pass into the ureter. Their etiology is thus the same as that of renal lithiasis. Calculi which develop primarily in the ureter are rare, as the smooth mucosal lining is constantly bathed with urine and accumulations of crystalloids are washed into the bladder. Available reports indicate that in those rare instances in which ureteral stones may be termed primary, these have been formed in connection with ureteroceles, neoplasms, ureters with blind endings, ectopic ureters, sacculations, or dilated segments of the ureter proximal to a stricture.

Site of Impaction. In migrating down the ureter, certain anatomic characteristics determine where the stone may become impeded in its progress. The points of narrowing are (1) at or just below the ureteropelvic junction; (2) where the ureter crosses the iliac vessels; (3) at the base of the broad ligament in the women and the vas deferens in the men; (4) where the ureter enters the external muscular coat of the bladder; and (5) the vesical orifice (Fig. 373). Between these points of constriction, the ureters are widened into the spindles. The abdominal spindle has an average diameter of 10 mm.; the pelvic spindle, 6 mm.; and the intramural ureter 3.5 mm. Thus, the average diameter of the spindles becomes progressively less from above downward. Two points of angulation also are present: (1) where the ureter crosses the iliac vessels and enters the true pelvis, and (2) at the point where it enters the bladder. These normal anatomic findings explain the frequency with which calculi are observed in various portions of the ureter.

In my series of 251 consecutive cases (1939, b), the calculus was at the ureteropelvic junction and in the upper third of the ureter in thirty-nine, in the lumbar portion or middle third in twenty-three, in the pelvic portion in 155, and in the intramural portion in thirty-four cases. Thus, 61.7 per cent were in the pelvic ureter when first seen and if the stones in the intramural portion are added, 75.3 per cent were in the lower one third of the ureter. In a second series of 350 consecutive cases (1939, e), the corresponding figure was 77 per cent. Geraghty and Hinman (1915) reported a combined incidence of stones in the pelvic and intramural portion of the ureter as 73.4 per cent. Joly (1931) stated that half the stones impacted in the ureter will be found in the pelvic portion, and if those in the intramural portion are included, approximately 70 per cent occur in

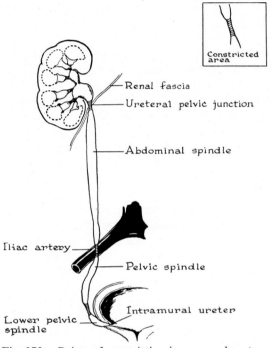

Fig. 373.   Points of constriction in a normal ureter.

the pelvic portion. It is evident, then, that the majority of impacted ureteral stones are found in the pelvic portion of the ureter and this high incidence is satisfactorily explained on an anatomic basis.

Size, Weight and Shape. The size of the ureteral calculus is of considerable importance clinically, but of equal importance is the caliber of the ureter below the stone. The calculi may vary from a few millimeters in size to 1, 5 or 6 inches in length. Heath removed a calculus measuring 6 in. by 1 in. and weighing 65.8 gm. Tennant removed a stone weighing 66 gm., while Joly noted that one reported by Federoff weighed 52 gm. Despite occasional reports of such giant stones, ureteral calculi are rarely more than an inch in length, and the shape varies according to the length of time the stone has occupied a position in the ureter. A calculus recently expelled from the kidney is usually round or ovoid and becomes elongated as it remains in the ureter. Then the longitudinal diameter is usually greater than the transverse, owing to the deposition of crystalloids, chiefly on the proximal end, that is, the upper end of the stone.

In the presence of a large dilated ureter, the stone may remain round, moving freely in the ureter, and acting as a ball valve. Multiple calculi may likewise remain round or ovoid in a dilated ureter, while they may be faceted in the absence of dilatation, or with minimal degrees of dilatation of the ureter. Greatly elongated calculi in the pelvic portion of the ureter may assume the curvature of this segment, as in a case cited by Herman.

Multiple stones may be present but in the vast majority of cases a single stone is observed (Fig. 374). In a series of 350 cases of ureteral calculi seen at the Cleveland Clinic, Higgins (1939, e), noted the presence of multiple stones in the ureter in seven instances and bilateral ureteral calculi in six cases. Braasch and Moore (1915) observed multiple stones in seventeen cases in a series of 278 cases of ureteral stones.

Laterality. Ureteral calculi occur on the left and right sides with approximately equal frequency. Kretschmer (1942), in a review of 500 cases, stated that 45.8 per cent were on the right and 51.8 per cent on the left. Bumpus and Scholl reported that ureteral calculi were observed with equal frequency on the two sides; in our series 47 per cent were present in the right, and 53 per cent in the left ureter. It is estimated that bilateral ureteral calculi occur in 1.7 to 3.6 per cent of cases.

Composition. Since ureteral calculi originate in the kidney, they obviously are of the same chemical types as renal stones. Clinically, however, it is observed that calculi composed of uric acid, cystine, or xanthine are rarely found impacted in the ureter. Such calculi are usually round and smooth and progressively larger stones may be expelled spontaneously into the bladder. Stones impacted in the ureter may be divided into two groups: (1) the septic type in which the calculus is usually composed of phosphates, and (2) the aseptic type in which the chemical constituents may be uric acid, cystine, xanthine, but are usually calcium oxalate. In the septic type, the nucleus may be composed of oxalates but when a urea-splitting infection is introduced into the kidney, phosphates are deposited on the calcium oxalate nucleus. If the calculus is not expelled after it passes into the ureter, continuous deposition of phosphates continues, chiefly on the upper end of the ureteral stone.

Pathology. The presence of a calculus impacted in the ureter produces various pathologic changes influenced by the degree and duration of the obstruction, and the presence or absence of infection. In instances in which a small calculus passes readily or with moderate delay down the ureter, no lasting pathologic changes are discernible and the caliber of the ureter returns to normal.

In the absence of infection and when obstruction is incomplete, the time factor assumes considerable importance. In cases in which the impaction is of recent origin, the ureter is dilated above the calculus, while if the partial obstruction has been present for a considerable period, the wall of the ureter may be thinned out, the ureter elongated and dilated, possibly to the size of the small intestine. In other instances, hypertrophy of the muscular coat is evident. The ureter below the stone is usually normal. With the introduction of infection, peri-ureteritis and ureteritis may be pronounced in the area about the calculus. In one instance I have seen, the calculus ulcerated through the ureter. The ureter at the site of impaction is fixed to the fat and contiguous structures. The degree of dilatation of the ureter above the calculus may be more pronounced and the tortuosity more evident, while in the late stages the ureter is thickened from fibrous tissue infiltration. Microscopically, round-cell infiltration and fibrosis are observed. In infected cases, stricture formation is more prevalent below the calculus than in the absence of infection.

When infection is lacking, varying degrees of hydronephrosis ensue, but when infection supervenes, destruction of renal parenchyma is rapid. The appearance of the kidney may vary from that of chronic pyelonephritis to a huge pyonephrotic sac, the picture varying with the degree of retrograde pressure on the kidney and the virulence of the infecting organism.

Symptoms. A calculus passing down the ureter may present the symptoms of colic previously described (see Renal Colic). The patient may experience an attack of colic followed by the expulsion of the stone, or several episodes may occur as the calculus traverses the course of the ureter more slowly. The first pain is severe and situated in the back, in the region of the costo-vertebral angle; the pain later is more severe in the region of the umbilicus and may follow the course of the ureter to the genitalia. As the stone nears the bladder, the patient may complain of frequency, urgency, and strangury, which occurred in 31.3 per cent of our cases. Dysuria and tenesmus may be pronounced. The pain may be referred to the perineum, bladder, penis or testicles. In our series it was interesting to note that the pain was referred to the lateral aspect of the thigh in two cases, to the knee in one instance, and to the hip in two cases.

A stone impacted in the ureter may present atypical symptoms. In our series, 56 per cent gave a fairly characteristic history of a previous attack of colic, and subsequently a decrease in intermittency of the pain or discomfort which became relatively steady and fixed, although possibly aggravated by exertion. On the right side, the chronic pain may be suggestive of cholecystitis or chronic appendicitis. Bumpus and Thompson found that the appendix had been removed in 26.8 per cent of 138 cases of ureteral calculi prior to the establishment of an accurate diagnosis. In a series of 910 cases of stones in the lower ureter cited by Dourmashkin, an appendectomy had been performed or a diagnosis of appendicitis had been made in 11.8 per cent. Braasch and Moore, in a review of 230 cases of stone in the ureter, stated that the pain was referred to the kidney region in 67 per cent; in 15 per cent, to the upper quadrant of the abdomen, and in 9 per cent, to the lower abdominal quadrant. In five cases, the patient did not complain of pain. In a series of 256 consecutive cases that I reviewed (Higgins, 1948), pain was the predominant symptom. Colic occurred in 59 per cent; pain, chiefly in the back, in 20 per cent; while indefinite abdominal discomfort was present in 22.7 per cent of the cases. In 36 per cent, nausea and vomiting were present. In 350 cases reviewed previously (1939, e), pain was referred to the upper quadrant of the abdomen in 14 per cent and in 6 per cent was referred to the right or left lower quadrant. In seven cases there was no complaint of pain. Twenty per cent presented symptoms not referable to the urinary tract; in the later series of 256 consecutive cases, the corresponding figure was 22.7 per cent.

In our series, the urine examination revealed the presence of red cells in 82.8 per cent, while the patient had detected the presence of blood in the urine in 26.7 per cent. Braasch and Moore cited the incidence of gross hematuria as 14 per cent, while Kretschmer found this symptom in forty-five of 140 cases of ureteral calculi. It is estimated that the urine is sterile in approximately 50 per cent of cases. There was no pus or blood cells in 11 per cent of our series.

The blood count in patients with ureteral calculi has been the subject of considerable discussion. Carp (1937) stated that in a study of 100 patients with ureteral calculi, 93 per cent developed a leukocytosis; of this group, 20 per cent had a white cell count from 15,000 to 30,000; 42 per cent from 10,000 to 15,000; and 31 per cent from 7000 to 10,000. He believes this finding is of great significance and that it should be incorporated in the classical picture of ureteral calculus.

Diagnosis. Many of the pertinent points regarding the physical examination are presented under the discussion of renal lithiasis. Instances have been reported in which a large calculus has been palpated in the ureter on abdominal examination. I have never encountered such a case. Emphasis has also been laid on the significance of pain elicited by pressure over so-called pressure points, but as similar observations may be elicited in lesions extraneous to the ureter, they are not pathognomonic of a ureteral calculus. It is of considerable significance, however, that a calculus in the lower portion of the pelvic ureter may be palpated on rectal or vaginal examination, and hence these procedures should never be omitted.

Roentgenographic Examinations. The shadow cast by a calculus in the ureter presents the same characteristics as that of a stone in the kidney. Again, the chemical composition influences the roentgenographic findings. Oxalates cast the most dense shadows, then carbonates, phosphates and cystine. Pure acid or urate calculi are nonopaque. The bony structure of the pelvis may obscure a calculus which casts a faint shadow. According to Peterson and Holmes (1937), the most frequently overlooked calculi are those located in a small area medial to the spine of the ischium and just above a line joining the lowest part of the ischial spines.

Reports as to the roentgenologic visibility of ureteral stones show considerable variation. Past statistics cited an incidence of 11 to 22 per cent in which the stone was not discernible. However, statistics cited years ago are of little value, since modern equipment has greatly increased the percentage of ureteral calculi visible on stereoscopic films.

Hinman has stated that in the United States approximately 10 per cent of ureteral stones are missed by roentgenographic examination. Herman stated that 3 to 5 per cent of ureteral calculi are invisible, while Peterson and Holmes (1937) found in 100 cases that 96 per cent were diagnosed by roentgenologic study. In our last 250 cases, 4.5 per cent did not cast a shadow or were not observed on the roentgenogram. The roentgenogram usually reveals a single shadow, but in some instances, multiple stones may be seen. As a general rule, the shadow cast by a stone that has been in the ureter for some time is elongated and fusiform, with the long axis in the course of the ureter. A stone recently lodged in the ureter may be round and, when the ureter is greatly dilated, may remain so.

Nichols and Lower (1933) have stressed the value of stereoscopic films in determining the relative anteroposterior position of all calcareous deposits

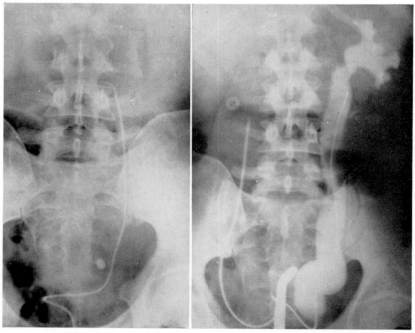

Fig. 374.   Fig. 375.
Fig. 374.   Stone in the ureter.
Fig. 375.   Diagnosis confirmed by ureteropyelogram (same case as Fig. 374).

seen along the course of the ureter. They are also important in ruling out areas of increased density in the pelvic bones, enterolithiasis in the intestines, or dense areas on the external surface of the body. Introduction of the opaque catheter up the ureter is frequently a valuable procedure. If the catheter passes beyond the obstruction, an anteroposterior and an oblique film may be taken with the catheter in place, or two exposures may be made on the same film with the tube shifted according to the Kretschmer technique. This will demonstrate the relation of the stone to the lumen of the ureter, unless the ureter is dilated, in which instance the calculus may be a considerable distance from the catheter and still be in the ureter (Fig. 374). In the presence of a dilated or tortuous ureter, the shadow cast by the stone is some distance from the position occupied by a normal ureter.

The shadow cast by a ureteral stone must be differentiated from intestinal contents, mesenteric glands, phleboliths and atheromatous plaques on the iliac vessels (see Figs. 363 and 364). Lesions on the skin may at times present a similar shadow. Intestinal contents rarely cause confusion if the patient is properly prepared before roentgenographic study. The mesenteric glands shift in position and usually do not have a uniform density. Phleboliths in the pelvic veins may be confusing, especially when multiple. As a general rule, they are round and cast a dense shadow, lateral to the course of the normal ureter.

An accurate diagnosis is usually possible by stereoscopic roentgenogram with anteroposterior and oblique exposures, combined with the introduction of an opaque catheter up the ureter and the injection of an opaque dye in instances in which the catheter passes the obstruction. Failure to meet an obstruction and nonvisualization of a calculus on the initial film does not always exclude the possibility of a small stone in the ureter, which may be too small to obstruct the passage of the catheter, or the stone may be dislodged by the introduction of the catheter.

Renal function tests, the obtaining of urine for bacteriologic cultures and pyelograms may be made at this time. In other instances, if the ureteral catheter fails to pass the obstruction, the stereoscopic roentgenogram will show the tip of the catheter in contact with the stone.

At the time of the cystoscopic examination, a calculus may be visualized in the ureteral orifice. If the calculus has recently passed into this position, submucous hemorrhage is evident about the orifice and marginal tears may be seen. When a calculus occupies a position in the intramural portion of the ureter, the orifice may be gaping and surrounded by an area of bullous edema.

If the procedure is not contraindicated by some general condition, I prefer securing an excretory urogram after the stereoscopic initial films are made. The status of both kidneys is determined, the degree of hydronephrosis, and the integrity of the kidney, as evidenced by the dye elimination on the involved side, is interpreted (Fig. 375). The degree of obstruction produced by the stone, and the status of the ureter above the calculus are visualized. Failure of the dye to be visualized when obstruction is complete does not signify that the kidney is destroyed and functionless, for excellent renal function may be evident as soon as the obstruction is relieved, especially if the obstruction has occurred recently. In many instances, satisfactory information is imparted by the excretory urogram and this may be sufficient for the immediate management of the case. This opinion is confirmed by Dourmashkin, who stated that routine instrumental pyelography should be avoided in cases of ureteral obstruction which present no diagnostic problem. In a series of 1550 cases of ureteral calculi, it was resorted to in 118 cases, chiefly in patients with uric acid calculi, or in patients in whom the stone was not recognized at first, for various reasons.

Treatment. *Factors Influencing Choice of Treatment Procedures.* Few urologic problems require the consideration of so many factors as does an obstructing calculus in the ureter. Whether or not operation should be performed for immediate relief of the obstruction, or whether manipulation should be done, possibly subjecting the patient to a period of disability, painful attacks of colic and perhaps febrile reactions, are the questions which arise in each case. Additional questions are: Should a period of watchful waiting be pursued? What are the most significant factors in this individual case to be considered in making the choice of the procedure to be instituted?

The *economic status and occupation* of the patient may influence the type of treatment to be carried out. A sudden attack of colic in individuals working with machinery, or in engineers and pilots may not only endanger their own lives but also those around them or dependent upon them. A laborer in whom a stone in the upper ureter is passing slowly downward, with arrest of its progress from time to time occasioning severe attacks of colic, may frequently be restored to his gainful occupation, and with less financial burden, if the calculus is removed through a muscle-splitting incision.

Duration of symptoms is an important factor. The patient who has had repeated episodes of severe colic requires relief. Temporizing when the symptoms are of long duration may lead to irreparable renal damage. A relatively short duration of symptoms may imply the possibility of spontaneous passage of the stone. In a series of 350 cases of ureteral calculi, 54.1 per cent of the stones which passed spontaneously did so within a period of sixteen days after examination.

The *size of the calculus* has an influence on the clinical course and the choice of treatment. Generally, the larger the calculus, the less likely that it will pass spontaneously and the greater the possibility that manipulative efforts will fail. Joly advised medical treatment for patients who pass gravel or in whom the shadow is not larger than 5 to 10 mm. in diameter. In our series, calculi larger than 1 cm. in diameter rarely passed spontaneously. In patients with multiple or recurrent calculi, progressively larger calculi may be expelled spontaneously, owing to a gradual dilatation of the ureter itself.

The state of the *renal function* is a prime consideration in making a decision about the treatment for ureteral stones. When the excretory urogram reveals but little hydronephrosis or dilatation of the ureter above the calculus, it signifies that the urine is coursing around the stone or through a groove on one surface, causing but little obstruction. If repeated roentgenograms reveal little or no progress in the descent of the calculus and a progressively enlarging hydronephrosis, the obstruction must be relieved. In the presence of infection, more prompt relief must be afforded. An aggravation of symptoms with a rise in temperature is a danger signal that cannot be ignored. Manipulative procedures must be attempted with caution in such instances. Cessation of pain does not always mean that the obstruction has been relieved, but may be due to the development of a complete obstruction.

The general acceptance of any method of treatment for ureteral calculi should have as its prime objective the prevention of destruction or loss of function of the kidney on the affected side. Clinical evidence of renal back pressure confirmed by intravenous urograms indicating complete ureteral obstruction, or a progressively enlarging hydronephrosis signifies that conservative methods of treatment are unwarranted and surgical intervention should be instituted promptly.

The *degree of impaction* is significant. A stone remaining in the same position week after week probably will not pass spontaneously. According to Joly, if the stone has not moved downward within a period of a month or six weeks, watchful waiting should be abandoned and other methods of treatment instituted. The status of the opposite kidney is extremely important, while in case of a solitary kidney, any continuing obstruction is grave and demands relief.

The *age and general condition of the patient* may influence the procedure to be advocated; elderly, debilitated men may not tolerate instrumentation well, and severe febrile reactions may result. In children, because of technical difficulties, inability to secure good cooperation, and the necessity for repeated anesthetics, I believe open operation is frequently the procedure of choice.

Moore advised that if *infection* is acute, severe, and characterized by repeated rigors, hyperpyrexia and leukocytosis in the presence of an obstructing calculus, prompt surgical interference with well-established free drainage may become a life-saving measure. However, to prepare a patient with ureteral calculus for operation, I have used an indwelling ureteral catheter which is of inestimable value in bringing about the quiescence of a septic course. In elderly men, associated disease, such as prostatic hypertrophy, may make manipulative procedures technically difficult and febrile reactions more likely to occur. In such cases, operation may be the procedure of choice.

In general, a small stone in the ureter accompanied by attacks of colic which are not too frequent or disabling and not accompanied by infection and progressing hydronephrosis, may be observed expectantly with the hope that it will pass spontaneously. The descent of the calculus and the status of the kidney are followed by means of roentgenograms.

In our series of 251 cases, 17.1 per cent of the stones passed spontaneously; in a second series of 350 cases, 18.9 per cent did likewise. If impaction occurs, then more active measures must be resorted to.

Various drugs have been used to facilitate the passage of the calculus, such as prostigmine, the antispasmodics, e.g., atropine, and now banthine. The results are inconsistent and vary considerably in the reports of different urologists.

Manipulation. In my experience with manipulation, the use of single or multiple catheters has been most successful, with minimal complications. There is a divergence of opinion regarding the employment of mechanical stone removers. I agree with Coppridge who believes that their use should be restricted to stones in the lower third of the ureter. In instances in which the ureter is completely obstructed at any level, one or more catheters should be passed, if possible, to establish drainage from the kidney. These may be withdrawn in twelve to twenty-four hours. It has been recommended that 2 per cent Novocain solution, olive oil or avertin, 2 per cent, be left in the ureter above the calculus. I believe this measure is of doubtful value.

Braasch stated the following contraindications for the manipulative treatment of ureteral calculi: (1) when the caliber of the stone exceeds 2 cm.; (2) when there is considerable periureteritis; (3) when the kidney is either hydronephrotic or pyonephrotic; (4) when the stone is known to have been present for a long time; (5) when several unsuccessful attempts have already been made to remove it; (6) when cystoscopy is poorly tolerated; (7) when congenital anomalies of the genital organs are present; (8) when a severe reaction or acute pyelonephritis follows the first manipulative procedure.

If the stone is not removed with one or two manipulative attempts, repeated manipulation should be avoided and operation may be advisable. The several disadvantages of cystoscopic manipulations are well known. Repeated manipulations cause real suffering to the patient, for the trauma may be more pronounced than that produced by surgical intervention. The period of disability may be prolonged, severe reaction and introduction of infection may ensue, and the failure of manipulative procedures still leaves the necessity for surgery.

Various instruments have been devised for manipulative removal of ureteral stones. Dourmashkin advocated the use of metallic dilators for calculi in the lower third of the ureter and rubber-bag dilators for calculi in the upper third; the purpose is to facilitate the downward passage of the calculus by dilation of the ureter at or below the level of the calculus, the dilatation conforming to or exceeding the size of the stone. In his series of 1550 cases of stones in various portions of the ureter and renal pelvis, 1253 received cystoscopic manipulation which resulted in expulsion of the stone in 1171 or 93.5 per cent.

Councill (1945), in a review of 504 cases in which the Councill stone extractor and dilator was used, stated that 364 stones were successfully removed from all parts of the ureteral tract, as follows: upper ureter, twenty-six; middle ureter, sixty-seven; and lower one third of the ureter, 271. In instances in which he was able to pass the extractor beyond the stone, 84.8 per cent was removed and 9.2 per cent passed spontaneously after manipulation. He concluded that success depends upon (1) location of the stone; (2) size of the stone; (3) size of the tract above and below the stone; (4) the possibility of passing the extractor beyond the stone.

Various other mechanical contrivances have been recommended and the large number of instruments available today for the removal of stones in the ureter attest that no one instrument or method is suitable in all instances. Likewise, serious complications may result from the use of such instruments. Perforation of the ureter has been reported by Councill; Rusche and Bacon; and Vickery, while Wishard reported a case of incarceration of a stone basket in the ureter owing to a broken wire.

The current procedure that my associates and I use in the treatment of upper and middle ureteral stones is, in the absence of complications, a policy of watchful waiting. If the calculus is 1 cm. or less in diameter and is moving spontaneously down the ureter, manipulative treatment is delayed until the stone is in the pelvic portion. Then, if manipulation is advised, multiple catheters or a basket extractor are employed. If the stone in the upper or middle portion of the ureter is producing complete obstruction as evidenced by intravenous urography, then surgical intervention is advocated. In the intramural segment, if the calculus does not pass spontaneously, a meatotomy may be performed and the stone removed with an extractor. Dilation may also be recommended to facilitate expulsion of the stone. When manipulative procedures are not to be recommended for reasons previously mentioned, and spontaneous expulsion cannot occur, surgical intervention is advisable.

In 1939, a series of 251 cases of ureteral stones was reported, in which spontaneous expulsion occurred in 17.1 per cent; 14.7 per cent were expelled after manipulation and 68.4 were subjected to surgical intervention. In contrast to these figures, in 1946, 256 consecutive cases were reported in which 11.3 per cent were expelled spontaneously, 58 per cent were expelled after manipulation and 30 per cent required surgical intervention.

Surgical Indications. Certainly dogmatic statements specifying indications may be unwarranted, but in our practice, operation has been resorted to for the following reasons: (1) repeated failure of manipulative efforts; (2) impassable obstructions caused by stones that cannot be moved; (3) renal infections which endanger the life of the patient by temporization; (4) associated disease which renders instrumental attempts technically impossible, such as urethral strictures, hypertrophy of the prostate, etc.; (5) calculi more than 2 cm. in diameter; (6) disease of the upper urinary tract which itself requires surgery; and (7) lack of tolerance to manipulation.

In cases in which open operation was recommended in 1939, Engel observed that when the stone was removed from the lower ureter, the average number of days in the hospital was 10.5, and when the stone was situated in the upper and middle thirds, this period was 11.8 days. The length of time in the hospital has been further reduced during recent years.

Recurrence. The end results of operation for ureteral stone are, as a rule, quite satisfactory. Instances have been reported of a recurrence of a primary stone in the ureter, associated with deposition of phosphates on a suture which had been passed into the lumen of the ureter during its closure after ureterolithotomy. Bumpus and Scholl cited an incidence of recurrent ureteral calculus of approximately 10 per cent. Most of the recurrent ureteral calculi originate in the kidney and again lodge in various portions of the ureter.

After the removal of the calculus and the establishment of free urinary drainage from the kidney, pronounced improvement in renal function will occur, unless the stone has been impacted for an extended period, and marked destruction of renal parenchyma has occurred. Following the removal of a recently impacted stone, the function of the kidney may return to normal. In cases of longer duration, the recovery of the kidney is usually more evident in instances in which there was no coexisting infection. In instances in which a stone has been impacted in a ureter for a long period, causing irreparable renal damage, with development of compensatory hypertrophy of the opposite kidney, there may be no return of function of the kidney on the operated side.

Six weeks after ureterolithotomy an excretory urogram is secured to rule out the possibility of a ureteral stricture at the site of impaction. If impaired drainage is demonstrable, the ureter should be dilated.

The important features, then, in the management of patients with ureteral calculi are prompt diagnosis, early removal of the calculus, whether spontaneously, by manipulative procedures, or open operation, followed by an adequate postoperative regimen, and these measures are usually followed by gratifying end results.

Surgical Treatment. (See Section XV, Chapter 4, on Surgery of the Ureter by Dr. Thomas D. Moore.)

VESICAL CALCULI

Classification. Stones in the bladder have been classified in two groups: primary and secondary. This classification has been unsatisfactory and confusing because various authors have presented different interpretations of these categories. Herman stated the opinion that the nuclei of secondary stones are foreign bodies in the bladder and that stones which have been expelled from the ureters into the bladder should not be considered as secondary vesical calculi. Other authors consider as primary vesical calculi those which have developed in the bladder in the presence of sterile urine, and that secondary groups form in the presence of infected urine. Lowsley and Kirwin believe that probably most vesical calculi originate in the kidney and state that, in the United States, primary stones in the bladder form about foreign bodies in the bladder. Approximately 18 to 20 per cent of the patients having bladder calculi have coexisting stones in the upper urinary tract.

Etiology. As mentioned in the introductory discussion (p. 787), in certain parts of the world the incidence of vesical calculi is quite high, while in others where vesical calculi were unusually prevalent in the last century, there has been a steady and pronounced decrease in incidence of stones in the bladder. In Europe, this decrease has been attributed to dietary and nutritional progress. Joly stated that most instances of bladder stone are the result of deficiencies in the diet, especially in the fat-soluble vitamins.

Age. In considering age as an etiologic factor in calculi of the bladder, variation in the age incidence is influenced by the part of the world in which the patient lives. Denos and Minet, and Civiale observed that, in England and France during the last century, calculous disease was one of childhood. Now, however, it is a disease of adult life. They agreed that the decrease in vesical calculi in childhood is due to progress in diet and nutrition.

In India and China, where pronounced dietary progress has not yet occurred, vesical calculi in children are still relatively prevalent. Calculous disease is also still prevalent among children in Russia. Assendelft, in a review of 630 collected cases, stated that 77 per cent occurred in patients under the age of ten years and 86.5 per cent were younger than twenty years. In China, 25 per cent of cases occur in patients less than ten years old.

Thompson (1921) in England, in a review of 2583 cases, noted that 0.4 per cent occurred in patients under sixteen, 11.7 per cent in those from sixteen to fifty years, and 66 per cent in elderly patients, aged fifty to seventy years.

In the United States, vesical calculus is a disease of adult life. Caulk stated that the majority of patients were aged forty to seventy years. Barney found that 60 per cent occurred in patients from fifty to eighty years of age, while in a series of 606 cases of vesical calculi reviewed by Crenshaw, 418 were present in patients aged forty to seventy years. This agrees closely with our own statistics. The change in the incidence of vesical calculi relative to age was well illustrated by Twinem, in a review of 306 patients, operated upon in the New York Hospital from 1820 to 1937. He observed that the percentage of patients under thirty years of age decreased from 83.3 per cent during the first twenty-five years of the period surveyed, to 10.9 per cent during the last quarter century.

Sex. Vesical calculus is predominantly a disease of the male sex, regardless of the country from which the statistics are being presented. In the review of calculous disease of the bladder in the Canton Hospital, Thompson stated that 2 per cent of cases occurred in women. In this country, the increased frequency of vesical calculi in men is explainable by the age period in which they are encountered. They appear definitely associated with obstruction of the bladder neck, owing to prostatic enlargement, stricture of the urethra, and diverticula of the bladder. In women, they are more frequently observed in instances in which the nucleus is formed by a foreign body.

As to why vesical calculi are more prevalent in male than in female children in the Far East, is a matter for speculation, and although it is attributed to the longer urethra and the tonicity of the vesical sphincters, such a presumption is debatable.

Pathologic Conditions. Various pathologic changes in the bladder conducive to the development of urinary stasis are predisposing factors toward stone formation. Factors giving rise to retention such as stricture of the urethra, prostatic hypertrophy, diverticula of the bladder, cystoceles, or injuries of the spinal cord, are abnormalities which may be associated with the formation of vesical calculi. The majority of vesical calculi are observed at the age when obstruction of the bladder neck occurs. The second group of cases of bladder stone which may not be associated with residual urine are those forming on foreign bodies, such as sutures or catheters or on objects introduced into the bladder via the urethra by the patient.

The role of infection in the production of vesical calculi has been a controversial subject. Calculi which form in the presence of sterile urine are common and, conversely, infection may persist in the bladder for an extended period without stone formation. In Egypt, it is said that bilharziasis is frequently associated with calculous disease, but that an ovum acting as a nucleus is observed in only 10 to 12 per cent of the cases. Certain organisms, such as the B. proteus and staphylococci possess the power of splitting urea, and enhance the possibility of stone formation. In the experimental laboratory, vesical calculi may be produced by introducing such organisms into the bladder. Alkaline decomposition occurs, accompanied by the precipitation of calcium, ammonium and magnesium phosphate. Some individuals may, however, have a persistent phosphaturia for years and never develop calculi. In the presence of infection, changes in the bladder wall with ulceration and inflammatory exudation add another factor prominent in stone formation. As in the case of renal calculi, stones composed of uric acid, urate and oxalate (the latter precipitating in a wide range of urinary pH) are formed in urine with acid reaction, while phosphatic calculi form in the presence of alkaline urine. The shifting of the pH of the urine accounts for the mixed and laminated character of the calculi.

Composition of Stones. The composition of the calculus in the bladder is influenced by the pH of the urine. A calculus may be composed of salts, precipitating in acid or alkaline urine, or a mixture may be present. In the United States, calcium oxalate is the commonest constituent of calculi, while reports from Europe made available years ago, indicated that uric acid and urate stones were more prevalent.

Owing to the more frequent involvement of the bladder than the kidney with urea-splitting organisms, phosphatic calculi in the bladder are of higher incidence than in the kidney. Obstructive lesions of the urethra associated with residual urine and urea-splitting infections occur in later life. Thus, phosphatic calculi predominate in this age group. In children, obstructive lesions associated with stagnation of urine in the bladder are relatively uncommon and, therefore, the stones are more likely to be composed of salts which precipitate in acid urine. Again, "aseptic calculi" are usually composed of urates, uric acid and calcium oxalate, while so-called "septic calculi" are composed of calcium phosphate, triple phosphates, or calcium carbonate. It is of extreme importance to investigate not only the bulk of a calculus but also the nucleus. The central portion of a bladder stone may be composed of uric acid, and when a urea-splitting infection is introduced into the bladder, the uric acid core develops an outer coating of phosphates.

The consistency of the calculi varies with their chemical constituents. Oxalate calculi are hardest, then urate calculi, then uric acid calculi, while the softest stones are composed of phosphates. When mixed calculi are present, the consistency varies with the predominating crystalloid forming the stone.

The calcium oxalate stones are brownish in color, hard, spherical in shape, and frequently the surface is covered with small nodular projections producing the so-called "mulberry calculus." In other instances, the projections are pointed and narrow, resembling jack stones. The growth of pure calcium oxalate calculi is quite slow. The uric acid calculi, when small, are round or flattened, assuming an ellipsoid shape as they enlarge, and are yellowish-red. They are quite hard. Phosphatic calculi are grayish-white, frequently soft, and friable, varying in shape, and their growth is rapid. Cystine vesical calculi are more unusual. They are yellowish-green in color, firm in consistency, and may enlarge quite rapidly. Pure calcium carbonate stones are of unusual occurrence. They are grayish and of hard consistency. Occasionally dumbbell-shaped stones are observed, one portion occupying a position in the bladder and the other in a diverticulum, with the narrow portion of the stone extending from the bladder into the diverticulum.

Usually a single stone is observed in the bladder, but in the presence of retained urine, multiple stones, varying from two or three to 100 or more may be present in 25 to 30 per cent of the cases. It has been noted also that when there are diverticula of the bladder, multiple stones are more frequently observed. Multiple stones may become faceted, and the size of the stones varies tremendously. They may be extremely small, or a large calculus may weigh 1000 grams or more (Fig. 376). Randall described a calculus weighing 1816 grams. The longitudinal circumference was 48

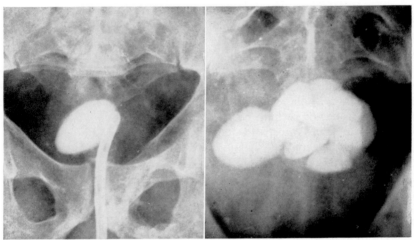

Fig. 376.   Fig. 377.

Fig. 376.   Stone in the bladder.
Fig. 377.   Bladder stone and stones in diverticulum.

cm. and the transverse circumference was 40 cm. The bulk of the calculus was composed of calcium phosphate.

Pathology. In the absence of infection, a smooth stone may be present in the bladder for some time without producing inflammatory changes in the bladder wall. As a general rule, the calculus produces sufficient mechanical irritation to cause chronic inflammatory changes. The earliest cystoscopic change is usually increased vascularity, followed by development of areas of congestion and a reddening of the mucosa. With the introduction of infection, bullous edema, pronounced congestion and ulceration appear.

In instances in which the calculus obstructs the urethral orifice, signs of back pressure are evident in the form of coarse trabeculation, cellule and saccule formation. When there is a coexisting prostatic obstruction, mucopus may be noted on the floor of the bladder and covering the stone. The same signs of back pressure are noted and a diverticulum of the bladder may be seen. The bladder wall is thickened and fibrous tissue reaction occurs in the muscular layer.

In cases of long duration, pericystitis may occur, with adherence of the bladder to the adjacent fat in the pelvis; perforation of the bladder may occur.

A single calculus or multiple calculi may be observed, on roentgenographic study, in a diverticulum (Fig. 377). When the calculi are multiple, they may be faceted. The epithelial lining of the diverticulum may be destroyed by the calculi, the wall is replaced by fibrous tissue, and the wall of the diverticulum is very adherent to the adjacent fat in the pelvis. The quantity of residual urine in the diverticulum depends upon the space occupied by the stone.

A calculus obstructing the urethral orifice produces obstructive and infective changes in the upper urinary tract similar to those associated with prostatic obstruction. In the absence of urethral obstruction, if the calculous cystitis has been present for an extended period, pyelonephritis is usually present.

Symptoms. In some cases of vesical calculus a history of previous renal colic may be elicited; the patient states that the stone apparently had never been expelled. In the majority of instances I have observed, this finding is lacking. In some patients, especially those with prostatic enlargement and residual urine, there may be no symptoms referable to the calculus or calculi. In such instances, the complaints are predominantly those of prostatic obstruction and the calculi are found during the course of urologic examination.

The typical symptoms of vesical stone consist of pain, hematuria and changes during the act of urination. The discomfort may be dull aching or sharp pain, aggravated by exercise and sudden movement. The pain is produced by the movement of the calculus irritating the base of the bladder, which may be ulcerated. Relief may be afforded by assuming the recumbent position. The pain may be more pronounced at the end of urination when the bladder is empty, and terminal hematuria may occur.

The pain, especially in children, may be referred to the tip of the penis, along the course of the second and third sacral nerves, to the scrotum in a similar manner, or to the perineum *via* the third and fourth sacral nerves. Other parts may be the sites of referred pain, such as the back, hip or the heel or sole of the foot.

Besides terminal pain at the end of micturition, there may be an interruption of the urinary stream, owing to encroachment of the stone on the internal urethral orifice or to spasm of the sphincter. Diurnal frequency and dysuria are usually present. The frequency of urination is influenced by activity, and urgency is present in 40 to 50 per cent of cases, while interruption of the stream occurs in approximately 30 to 40 per cent. In the presence of infection, the usual symptoms of cystitis are introduced; nocturia occurs, urgency is increased, and terminal pain is pronounced. Priapism and nocturnal enuresis may occur in children.

Diagnosis. Although a presumptive diagnosis may be tentatively made from a history of pain aggravated by exercise, interruption of the urinary stream, and terminal hematuria, they are not pathognomonic of this disease, since these symptoms may be produced by other lesions in the bladder.

Physical examination is rarely of value in establishing a diagnosis, but instances have been cited in which a large stone was palpable on rectal, vaginal, or abdominal examination.

Albumin, red cells and pus cells are usually to be observed, upon microscopic examination of the urine, but these laboratory findings, of course, are present with other lesions of the urinary tract.

Roentgenographic Study. Many vesical calculi are not visualized by the roentgenogram because of the presence of uric acid in many of them and also because of overlying prostatic tissue. It has been stated that over 50 per cent of bladder stones are not discernible on the roentgenogram, and in Hyman's series, 61 per cent were not disclosed. Nichols found that cystoscopic examination was the surest method for detecting vesical calculi, while if the calculus or calculi were in diverticula, the roentgenogram furnished the most reliable procedure for their detection.

Stones in the bladder, as seen on the roentgenogram, are frequently ovoid in shape, the long axis occupying a horizontal position. The density is usually uniform unless lamination is present. The shadow must be differentiated from phleboliths, masses in the intestines, and calcified glands.

Certainly, however, the most accurate means of diagnosis is cystoscopic survey, and the absence of a shadow on the roentgenogram does not preclude the possibility of a vesical calculus.

Treatment. Since obstructive lesions and infection seem to play a role in the formation and enlargement of vesical calculi, their correction will minimize the incidence of stone formation. Enlargement of the prostate gland, strictures of the urethra, cord lesions with stasis, and superimposed urea-splitting infections, diverticula with retention of urine, or cystoceles with residual urine demand attention if stone formation is to be minimized.

With the judicious use of the newer chemotherapeutic agents, after securing individual sensitivity studies, many infections of the bladder may now be eradicated which were, in the past, classified as drug resistant. Certainly relief of the obstruction and the eradication of infection of the bladder are valuable prophylactic procedures.

Since there is considerable evidence to support the concept that the formation of vesical stone may be associated with a deficiency in the diet, dietary adjustment and added vitamins should be recommended if there is any indication that this might be a causative factor in the individual case. While satisfactory end results have been reported by the use of "G" or "M" solutions, treatment with these agents is protracted and I have rarely employed it.

From the surgical standpoint, two methods of treatment are available, namely, litholapaxy and suprapubic lithotomy. The choice of operation is influenced by the age and physical condition of the patient, the size and hardness of the calculus, and the presence or absence of coexisting pathologic lesions involving the urethra, the bladder neck, or the bladder itself.

Litholapaxy. The modern operation of litholapaxy was introduced by Bigelow, in 1878, and varied opinions are offered regarding indications and contraindications for this procedure. The contraindications are as follows:

(1) The calculus is too large and too hard. Joly said that a calculus up to 5 cm. in diameter may be crushed, while Herman's opinion was that a stone more than ½ inch in diameter should not be treated by litholapaxy. Lowsley and Kirwin believed that suprapubic lithotomy is the preferable procedure if the calculus is 2 centimeters or more in diameter. In some instances, it has been recommended that a large calculus may be crushed in more than one attempt. Such multiple operations cause considerable trauma, and generalized reactions may occur, and I do not believe that they are advisable. (2) When a calculus or calculi are present in a diverticulum, open operation is preferable as it permits removal of the diverticulum at the time of operation. (3) In the presence of a pronounced or acute cystitis, a contracted bladder, or a tumor or calculus adherent to the bladder wall, I believe litholapaxy should not be employed. (4) Congenital anomalies or strictures of the urethra not permitting the easy introduction of the instruments speak for open operation. (5) Prostatic hypertrophy or vesical neck obstruction is present in over 55 per cent of cases. In the presence of a large prostate gland which interferes with manipulation of the lithotrite, the procedure is attended by considerable trauma to the prostate, and suprapubic litholapaxy is the preferable procedure. In the presence of a small gland or a contracted vesical neck, the litholapaxy procedure may be recommended.

Obviously, experience and personal preference will influence the procedure to be advocated. In small children, open operation is usually preferable. Some urologists believe that litholapaxy is contraindicated when the calculus has formed around a foreign body. This is a general statement, and whether or not litholapaxy may be recommended depends upon the size and nature of the foreign body. I have removed calculi from the bladder by litholapaxy in which a hair pin, wax, and a small sliver of wood acted as the nucleus. Lowsley regards the presence of advanced renal disease or poor physical condition of the patient as contraindications to a lengthy procedure, and considerable time may be required to remove a large stone from the bladder when litholapaxy is performed.

Cabot stated, in considering the procedure to be recommended, that three points must be considered: (1) the relative safety of the operation, (2) the certainty of a cure, and (3) the comfort of the patient, length of confinement and the possibility of complications.

COMPLICATIONS. Complications which may follow litholapaxy are prostatitis, urethritis, and epididymitis. More serious complications may be observed, such as acute pyelonephritis, perforation of the bladder and septicemia. In general, it may be stated that litholapaxy may be utilized when the urethra easily accommodates the instrument, and there are no complicating conditions in the bladder which require relief by open operation. I have a preference for spinal or caudal anesthesia when performing a litholapaxy. The bladder capacity is increased, and sudden movement of the patient which might lead to serious complications, is avoided.

Lithotomy. Suprapubic lithotomy should be employed in the group of cases in which contraindications to litholapaxy exist, and if conditions requiring open operation are present in the bladder.

MORTALITY. Barney cited a mortality rate of 7.23 per cent in a series of 392 cases of vesical calculi treated by litholapaxy and of 25 per cent in those treated by suprapubic lithotomy. However, the total series of 455 cases from the Massachusetts General Hospital were treated in the period from 1870 to 1919, that is, before the introduction of the newer chemotherapeutic agents.

Joly cited a mortality rate of 2.2 per cent following litholapaxy. Our mortality rate from 1921 to date is 1.2 per cent at the Cleveland Clinic. Caulk, in a review of 112 cases treated by litholapaxy, reported a mortality rate of 0.89 per cent. Review of the published statistics indicates that the mortality is higher following suprapubic lithotomy, but frequently in these cases, operations of greater magnitude are performed. Caulk cited a mortality rate of 3.1 per cent for suprapubic lithotomy only, while the mortality rate increased to 13.4 per cent when the operations included procedures for prostatic hypertrophy, diverticulectomy, or similar additional surgical measures. In recent years, there has been a pronounced decrease in the mortality rate through adequate preparation of the patient and the introduction of the newer drugs to combat infection.

As a general rule, eradication of the causative factor, usually obstruction of the bladder neck, and elimination of the infection of the urinary tract, are followed by gratifying end results. Recurrence is unusual if there are no retained fragments of stone. However, the reported recurrence rate is about 5 per cent. These statistics, as a rule, are based on cases collected from clinical material in which treatment was carried out before the introduction of the modern drugs. In instances in which infection is eliminated, recurrence is unusual following either litholapaxy or suprapubic lithotomy.

Surgical Technique. (See Section XV, Chapter 5, on Surgery of the Bladder.)

CALCULI OF THE PROSTATE AND SEMINAL VESICLES

Classification. True prostatic calculi are those which develop in the acini of the gland and are not to be confused with so-called false calculi which may be urinary calculi lodged in a dilated prostatic urethra or in a pouch off the urethra. Similarly, a calculus present in an abscess cavity communicating with the urethra should not be considered as a true prostatic calculus.

Etiology. Prostatic calculi are formed by the deposition of calcareous material on the corpora amylacea. Gentile, in a review of forty cases, observed at the New York Hospital from 1920 to 1946, stated that the corpora amylacea obstruct the prostatic ducts, transforming the acini into closed cavities. This is followed by infection of the prostatic secretion within the acini, owing to stasis, with an alkaline or neutral reaction. The infection results in inflammatory changes in the mucous membrane of the acini and the irritated mucosa casts off inorganic salts (calcium phosphate and carbonate). These salts impregnate the corpora amylacea, converting them into calculi. In the cases reviewed by Gentile, infection of the prostate gland was present in every instance. Hinman observed that some prostatic calculi probably arise from precipitation of salts found in normal prostatic fluid,

that is, calcium and magnesium phosphates, while others have held that
the corpora amylacea may serve as nuclei.

The corpora amylacea are small, round or ovoid bodies present in the
alveoli of the prostate gland. They are rare in children and increase in
frequency in older individuals. Corpora amylacea are composed of lecithin
and a nitrogenous substance of an albuminous nature. They are apparently
formed around desquamated epithelial cells and present a laminated structure. In older individuals, they tend to become impregnated with lime salts,
the inorganic constituents being calcium or magnesium phosphate and
carbonate.

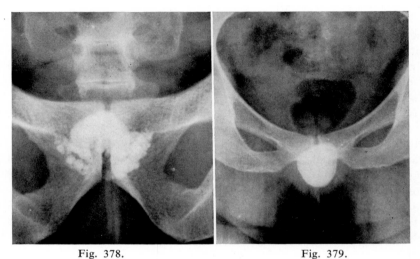

Fig. 378.   Fig. 379.
Fig. 378.   Prostatic calculi.
Fig. 379.   Calculus in a diverticulum of the urethra (female).

Incidence. The frequency of prostatic calculi is questionable, since, in
many instances, they are discovered during routine roentgenographic survery.
In considering their relative frequency, Joly observed thirty-four cases of
prostatic calculi in a series of 636 cases of urinary calculi, representing an
incidence of 5.3 per cent. Stone in the seminal vesicles is a very rare condition. White, in 1928, reported a case in a patient, aged forty-eight years,
and he found only one additional case in the literature. White's case was
not confirmed by vesiculotomy.

Prostatic calculi are rarely observed in children and are infrequent in
men under forty to forty-five years of age. The majority are detected in
men, aged fifty to sixty-five years. Calculi in the seminal vesicles are reported
in elderly men.

Physical Characteristics. Prostatic calculi vary in number from a single
calculus to several hundred. In the majority of cases, they are multiple,
varying from 1 mm. to 3 or 4 cm. (Fig. 378). They are brownish-gray,
round or ovoid. Smaller stones are usually smooth, but larger and multiple
calculi occupying a cavity may be definitely faceted. They are usually firm
in consistency but readily crushed.

Calculi in the seminal vesicles may be single or multiple and are of brown color. The nucleus is composed of epithelial cells and a mucoid substance; this is covered with lime salts. The stones are smooth and hard and vary in size from 1 to 2 millimeters to that of a lima bean.

Composition. While most observers have stated that stones in the prostate are usually composed of calcium phosphate, in the series cited by Kretschmer, a preponderance of calcium oxalate was found. Huggins observed that the organic components, about 20 per cent, include proteins, 8 per cent; cholesterol, 3.7 to 10.6 per cent; and citrate 0.17 to 2.9 per cent. The principal inorganic constituent was tertiary calcium phosphate, presumably with an apatite constitution. The amount of carbonate is somewhat less than in bone; otherwise, the chemical and roentgenographic analysis demonstrated close similarity between the inorganic constituents of prostatic calculi and bone salt. Huggins stated also that corpora amylacea may occasionally be seen in the anterior segment of the prostate, but they occur mostly in the posterior segment, where calculi of the prostate are also primarily found.

Pathology. In the presence of minute calculi, the only pathologic change in the prostate may be chronic inflammation with areas of round-cell infiltration. The acini may be filled with debris and desquamated epithelial cells and the acini themselves may or may not be dilated.

When larger calculi are present, the ducts and acini may be dilated and cavities which vary in size and shape are found. The epithelial lining is absent and round-cell infiltration and fibrosis are observed between the acini. Occasionally in the presence of a large calculus, but little prostatic tissue is identifiable. The calculi are frequently in the mouth of the ducts or deep in the gland. They are not observed in the adenomatous element of the gland but are adherent to the adenoma, resting in the thinned-out prostatic tissue about the adenomatous mass. This explains the finding of calculi at the time of suprapubic prostatectomy. When there has been infection or suppuration of long standing, a periprostatitis may occur, and in case of abscess formation, rupture into the urethra may follow.

With a calculus in the seminal vesicle, chronic inflammatory changes with fibrosis are usually present, and the duct may be completely blocked.

Symptoms. There are no symptoms pathognomonic of calculous disease of the prostate gland and in many cases there may be no suspicion of its presence. Symptoms, when present, may be due to prostatic hypertrophy, stricture of the urethra or chronic prostatitis. In some instances, small prostatic calculi have been passed spontaneously in the urine. The patient may complain of a dull aching pain in the lower back, perineum or penis. Difficulty in voiding, lack of force of the stream and dribbling will be observed in the presence of a urethral stricture or prostatic hypertrophy. Some individuals may note the presence of a urethral discharge.

Hematuria usually is not observed, but terminal bleeding may be present. Abscess formation, owing to calculi, is uncommon, but may occur with the patient complaining of severe deep pain in the perineum and rectum, aggravated at the time of defecation. The temperature is elevated and general constitutional symptoms may be pronounced. The prostate gland is exquisitely

tender to palpation. In the presence of cystitis, dysuria, nocturia and frequency occur. A stone in the seminal vesicle may be silent, producing no
symptoms. In the cases reported, hemospermia, painful erections and
perineal discomfort at the time of ejaculation have been noted.

Diagnosis. The diagnosis is established by rectal palpation of the prostate
gland, roentgenographic study and endoscopy. On *rectal examination,* the
prostate gland may be enlarged or there may be no findings suggestive of
the presence of calculi. About 70 per cent of cases reveal prostatic enlargement. In instances in which small calculi occupy a position in the ducts
or, acini deep in the gland, crepitation may not be elicited. The prostate
will be firm, movable and the borders are well defined. When the calculi are
larger, occupying cavities and dilated acini, crepitation may be elicited.
This is present in 18 to 20 per cent of the cases. The crepitation is usually
more evident near the base of the gland. The consistency of the gland and
its contour vary. It may be smooth or nodular, firm or hard. In the presence
of a large calculus, a localized area of stony hardness is noted. In 18 to 22
per cent of cases, nodules are palpable, while the intervening tissue is of
normal consistency.

In instances in which a calculus is present in a seminal vesicle, the
prostate is usually of normal consistency, while the involved vesicle is
stony hard and fixed. When multiple calculi are present, crepitation is
elicited.

Calculi in the prostate gland must be differentiated from tuberculosis,
which is more frequently observed in younger individuals. One or both
vesicles may be involved and tuberculosis of the epididymis may be present.

Carcinoma of the gland must also be differentiated from prostatic calculi.
The prostate gland with carcinomatous involvement is usually fixed but
may be quite movable in the presence of calculi. In carcinoma of the prostate,
the gland is stony hard and extension toward the seminal vesicle is frequently demonstrable. Crepitation is absent in carcinoma, and usually the
tissue between the nodules is not of normal consistency. Determination of
acid phosphatase and roentgenographic study may confirm the diagnosis of
carcinoma.

Urethroscopic study may reveal only the presence of prostatic enlargement, in case of prostatic calculi. Occasionally a grating is felt in passing
the urethroscope. Rectal palpation of the prostate with the instrument in
the urethra may elicit crepitation. A small calculus may be observed
protruding into and obstructing the urethra.

Roentgenographic study usually confirms the diagnosis. Three characteristic types of shadows may be observed. Diffuse shadows may be generally
distributed throughout the gland, the calculi being very small and occupying the gland. In the types most frequently observed, there are the so-called
horseshoe or ring arrangements. In the ring type, the shadows surround a
clear central portion which is formed by the urethra. In the horseshoe type,
the stones are present on both sides of the gland, while there are no stones
in front of the urethra, as evidenced by the clear space, and the opening is
directed downward. In other instances, a large solitary calculus is observed,

or the prostate gland appears to be completely replaced by calculous formation.

A diagnosis of stone in the seminal vesicle is made by rectal palpation, which demonstrates a hard, tender, smooth nodule in the vesicle. Large calculi may be revealed by roentgenographic study, showing a mottled shadow in the region of the vesicle.

Treatment. In the so-called silent cases of prostatic calculi, when symptoms are absent, no treatment is indicated. Three methods of treatment are available when surgical relief is necessary (see Section XV, Chapters 6 to 9 inclusive).

In recent years, enthusiasm has been expressed for the transurethral removal of prostatic stones. This may produce temporary relief, but does not imply the removal of all the calculi, and recurrent stone formation may ensue. It may be utilized in the younger patients, to avoid impairment of sexual activities, or in the aged patient who is a poor risk. Suprapubic removal may be advocated in the presence of a stone or stones, when there is severe prostatic hypertrophy of the intravesical type. Perineal prostatotomy may be indicated for the removal of a stone in the prostate, while in the presence of multiple calculi, perineal prostatectomy and bilateral seminal vesiculectomy will afford a cure.

Mortality. While the mortality rate in past years for prostatotomy was cited as 5.8 per cent, we have had no mortality following removal of calculi by transurethral resection or perineal prostatotomy. The mortality of the removal of the hypertrophied gland containing calculi, in our hands, has been similar to that of suprapubic or perineal prostatectomy in cases without this coexisting pathologic process.

Recurrence. A recurrence of prostatic calculi may follow prostatotomy, with new stones forming in the cavities of the gland. False recurrences, that is, stones overlooked at the time of operation, may be observed. Therefore, after operation, roentgenographic examination should be secured before the patient is dismissed from the hospital. True or new calculous formation may also occur following transurethral resection. The best results follow suprapubic or perineal prostatectomy.

URETHRAL CALCULI (MALE)

The majority of urethral calculi in man consist of stones expelled from the bladder into the urethra. Their progress through the urethral canal may be temporarily arrested, followed by expulsion spontaneously or by impaction in the canal. Rarely, a calculus may form primarily in the male urethra when stricture is present, or in a pouch or diverticulum opening into it.

Incidence. In oriental countries, where vesical calculi are frequently observed, urethral calculi are not uncommon in children. In the United States, urethral calculi are seldom observed in this age group, because stones of the bladder are so infrequent. In our series, most of the urethral calculi occurred in patients between the ages of forty-five and fifty-five years in whom prostatic hypertrophy acted as a barrier to the passage of the stones.

Position and Composition. In the passage of a stone through the normal urethra, its progress may be arrested in the prostatic urethra, the bulb, in the anterior portion of the perineal urethra, and the fossa navicularis or the external meatus. It may also become impacted at the site of a urethral stricture. Englisch, in a review of 361 cases, stated that 41.2 per cent were in the posterior urethra; 18.8 per cent in the bulb; 28.4 per cent in the scrotal and penile portion; and 11.3 per cent in the fossa navicularis.

The migratory calculi in the urethra obviously have the same constituents as bladder or upper urinary tract calculi, as they originate in either the kidney or bladder. In the case of primary urethral calculus, there is associated infection, and the stone is composed of phosphates. Usually a single stone is encountered.

Symptoms. The patient with urethral calculus usually experiences, during the act of urination, a sudden stoppage with inability to empty the bladder, or mere dribbling. The pain occasioned by the stone in the urethra may be quite severe and radiate to the head of the penis. If the calculus is lodged in the posterior urethra, the pain is referred to the perineum or rectum. When the calculus is lodged in the anterior urethra, the pain may be localized at the site of impaction and the patient will be aware of the palpable mass. With increasing effort to void, the calculus may be expelled, or complete obstruction may occur, which requires catheterization.

A stone may be present in a diverticulum of the urethra for an extended period without producing symptoms, although a urethral discharge may be observed, owing to infection in the diverticulum. The patient may be aware of the presence of a lump on the undersurface of the penis, which has gradually increased in size and hardness, and which may at times become exquisitely tender. There is usually no change in the caliber of the stream of urine, and no dribbling.

Diagnosis. Diagnosis may be established by palpation of the penis or perineum. Rectal palpation may disclose the presence of a calculus in the posterior urethra. The tentative diagnosis may be confirmed by urethro-scopic examination or roentgenography. Likewise, a grating may be felt upon attempting to pass a sound.

Treatment. The treatment to be instituted is influenced by the size, shape and position of the calculus and the status of the urethra. At times, a stone in the anterior urethra may be grasped with forceps, with exertion of pres-sure simultaneously above the stone so that it is not forced into the bladder. A small stone may sometimes be gently massaged or milked forward, so that it may be expelled. Removal of a stone through the urethroscope may be advisable. When a stricture is present, an internal urethrotomy may be per-formed. In instances in which a larger stone has been present in the urethra and impacted for some time, an external urethrotomy may be required. A calculus lodged in the fossa navicularis may be removed by meatotomy.

A calculus recently impacted in the posterior urethra frequently may be pushed back into the bladder and then crushed. When the stone is large and definitely fixed, it may be removed by the perineal or suprapubic route, depending upon the personal preference of the surgeon. A urethrovesical calculus is best removed by the suprapubic route. External urethrotomy of the penile urethra should be avoided, if possible, because of the danger of fistulous formation.

In instances in which the calculus occupies a position in a urethral diverticulum, diverticulectomy should be performed.

Mortality and End Results. While in the past a relatively high mortality rate has been reported, confined chiefly to the group of patients in whom urethral obstruction has been of long duration, with consequent impairment of renal function and pyelonephritis, today, with adequate means of investigating renal function, adequate preoperative preparation, and a choice of newer chemotherapeutic agents, the operative mortality and morbidity are extremely low.

In past years, recurrence was frequently reported, with many of the stones re-forming in diverticula. At present, correction of urethral strictures, diverticulectomy and adequate therapy to eradicate the infection are followed by extremely satisfactory end results.

URETHRAL CALCULI (FEMALE)

The occurrence of urethral calculi in the woman is infrequent when compared to that in the man. This may be attributed to two factors: (1) the short urethra in the woman which permits passage of the calculus, and (2) the infrequency of vesical calculi in women. Calculi in the female urethra are usually associated with a urethral diverticulum or urethrocele. In 1939, Gaston and Ferrucci collected thirty-three cases of calculi in urethral diverticula, and added one case. In 1943, Higgins and Roen reported a case, and I have operated upon eight additional patients since that time.

The urethral diverticulum is a pouch formed by dilatation of a portion of the urethrovaginal septum and it communicates with the urethral canal. The pouch may have a wide opening into the urethra, or the opening may be narrow or tubular. If the mouth of the diverticulum is wide, it is doubtful whether calculus formation can occur, for stone formation in a diverticulum is probably due to urinary stasis, stagnation with infection, which allows the precipitation of urinary salts to occur. Therefore, theoretically, the presence of a calculus in a diverticulum would presuppose a narrow opening between the urethra and the diverticulum. Such was the finding in our cases (Fig. 379).

Symptoms and Diagnosis. Symptoms of urethral diverticulum, with or without calculus, are those of infection of the lower urinary tract, including frequency, dysuria, nocturia, pyuria and, in rare instances, hematuria. Pain during coitus is a prominent symptom. Occasional discharge of pus may occur; this gives the patient temporary relief. Vaginal examination discloses a hard mass in the anterior vaginal wall.

Treatment. The treatment of a urethrocele or diverticulum containing a calculus is surgical, with excision of the sac containing the calculus. The surgical technique varies according to the personal preference of the operating surgeon. In our series, the postoperative convalescence has been uncomplicated.

PREPUTIAL CALCULI

From the standpoint of etiology, three types of preputial calculi may be observed: (1) calculi arising from inspissated smegma becoming impregnated with lime salts; these are soft in consistency, brown in color and may be single or multiple; (2) calculi, forming in stagnant urine retained in the sac in the presence of phimosis, which may be multiple or single, round or faceted, and composed of ammonium-magnesium phosphate and calcium phosphate; (3) calculi that have been expelled from the bladder into the urethra and have gained entrance into the preputial sac *via* the urethral meatus or by ulceration through the fossa navicularis. They are greyish and usually made up of phosphates.

Preputial calculi usually form when phimosis is present, and in this country are rare (Fig. 766). Thompson reported 116 cases from the Canton Hospital. The condition is rarely observed in childhood, but is primarily a disease of adult life. There may be no symptoms referable to the calculus, though the patient may be aware of the presence of a lump for a considerable period. The usual symptoms are those of balanoposthitis. A discharge from the small opening in the foreskin, edema, and in late stages, ulceration may be present. Carcinoma may also coexist when the calculus has been present for a long time.

The diagnosis is established by palpation of the stone.

When an acute infection is present, a dorsal slit should be performed to establish drainage. If such an infection is not present, the treatment consists of circumcision.

REFERENCES

ALBRIGHT, F., BAIRD, P. C., COPE, O. and BLOOMBERG, E.: Studies on the physiology of the parathyroid glands; renal complications of hyperparathyroidism. Am. J. M. Sc., *187:* 49–65, 1934.

ALBRIGHT, F. and BLOOMBERG, E.: Hyperparathyroidism and renal disease; with note as to the formation of calcium casts in this disease. J. Urol., *34:*1–7, 1935.

ALBRIGHT, F. and REIFENSTEIN, E. C., JR.: Parathyroid Glands and Metabolic Bone Disease. Baltimore, Williams and Wilkins Co., 1948.

ALBRIGHT, F., SUBY, H. and SULKOWITCH, H. W.: Cited by Albright and Reifenstein.

ALBRIGHT, F., SULKOWITCH, H. W. and CHUTE, R.: Non-surgical aspects of the kidney stone problem. J.A.M.A., *113:*2049–2053, 1939.

ALBRIGHT, F., et al.: Metabolic studies and therapy in a case of nephrocalcinosis with rickets and dwarfism. Bull. Johns Hopkins Hosp., *66:*7–33, 1940.

ANDERSON, W. A. D.: Renal calcification in infancy and childhood. J. Pediat., *14:*375–381, 1939.

ASSENDELFT, E.: Bericht über 630 stationär behandelte Steinkranke. Arch. f. klin. Chir., *60:*669–686, 1900.

BARNEY, J. D.: Observations on the treatment of vesical calculi. Boston M. & S. J., *81:* 462–464, 1919.

BARNEY, J. D.: Recurrent renal calculi. Surg., Gynec. & Obst., *35:*743–748, 1922.

BARNEY, J. D. and MINTZ, E. R.: Some newer concepts of urinary stone formation. J.A.M.A., *103:*741–743, 1934.

BEARD, D. E. and GOODYEAR, W. E.: Hyperparathyroidism and urolithiasis. J. Urol., *65:* 638–642, 1950.

BOSHAMER, K.: Blasensteine in Südchina. Ztschr. f. Urol., *30:*18–19, 1936.

BRAASCH, W. F.: Cited by Bumpus and Scholl.

BRAASCH, W. F.: Clinical data on nephrolithiasis. Surg., Gynec. & Obst., *24:*8–14, 1917.

BRAASCH, W. F.: Clinical data in cases of renal lithiasis. J. Iowa M. Soc., *16:*33–35, 1926.

BRAASCH, W. F. and FOULDS, G. S.: Postoperative results in nephrolithiasis. J. Urol., *11:*525–537, 1924.

BRAASCH, W. F. and MOORE, A. B.: Stones in the ureter. J.A.M.A., *65:*1234–1237, 1915.

BROWN, R. K. L. and EARLAM, M. S. S.: Relation of prolonged immobilization and urinary tract infection to renal calculus formation. Australian & New Zealand J. Surg., *3:*157–171, 1933.

BROWN and VINEBERG: Cited by Albright and Reifenstein.

BUGBEE, H. G.: Recurring pyelonephritis as an etiological factor in nephrolithiasis. Tr. Am. A. Genito-Urin. Surg., *25:*121–131, 1932.

BUMPUS, H. C., JR. and SCHOLL, A. J.: Ureteral stones. S. Clin. N. America, *5:*813–827, 1925.

BUMPUS, H. C., JR. and THOMPSON, G. J.: Stones in the ureter. Surg., Gynec. & Obst., *50:*106–109, 1930.

BUTLER, A. M., WILSON, J. L. and FARBER, S.: Dehydration and acidosis with calcification at renal tubules. J. Pediat., *8:*489–499, 1936.

BUTT, A. J., HAUSER, E. A., SEIFTER, J. and PERRY, J. G.: Prevention and treatment by increasing protective urinary colloids with hyaluronidase (in press).

CABOT, H.: Cited by Scholl, A. J.: Some common sources of error in the diagnosis of renal and ureteral calculi. Am. J. Urol., *8:*1–8, 1912.

CABOT, H. and CRABTREE, E. G.: Frequency of recurrence of stone in the kidney after operation. Surg., Gynec. & Obst., *21:*223–225, December, 1915.

CAHILL, G. F.: Cited by Lowsley and Kirwin, p. 1490.

CARP, I. J.: Ureteral calculus; analysis of 100 cases. Urol. & Cutan. Rev., *41:*587–589, 1937.

CAULK, J.: Litholapaxy; method of preference for removal of vesical calculi. Ann. Surg., *93:*891–898, 1931.

CIVIALE: Cited by Joly.

COPPRIDGE, W. M.: Clinical management of ureteral stones. South. M. J., *33:*18–21, 1940.

COUNCILL, W. A.: The treatment of ureteral calculi; report of 504 cases in which Councill stone extractor and dilator was used. J. Urol., *53:*534–538, 1945.

CRENSHAW, J.: Vesical calculi. Coll. Papers Mayo Clin., *13:*346–357, 1921.

DAVALOS, A.: Rarity of stones in the urinary tract in the wet tropics. J. Urol., *54:*182–184, 1945.

DENOS and MINET: Cited by Joly.

DOMANSKI, T. J.: Renal calculi; a new method of qualitative analysis. J. Urol., *37:*399–406, 1937.

DORRONSORO, B. and FERNANDEZ, O.: Reaction of nopic acid. An. Soc. Espan. Fis. Quim., *11:*411, 1913.

DOURMASHKIN, R. L.: Cystoscopic treatment of stones in the ureter with special reference to large calculi, based on a study of 1550 cases. J. Urol., *54:*245–283, 1945.

ENGEL, W. J.: Management of stone in the ureter. S. Clin. N. America, *19:*1275–1284, 1939.

ENGEL, W. J.: Nephrocalcinosis. J.A.M.A., *145:*288–294, 1951.

ENGLISCH, J.: Über eingelagerte und eingesackte Steine der Harnröhre. Arch. f. klin. Chir., *72:*487, 1904.

FEDEROFF: Cited by Joly, p. 728.

FISKE, C. H. and SUBBAROW, Y.: The colorimetric determination of phosphorus. J. Biol. Chem., *66:*375–400, 1925.

FLOCKS, R. H.: Cited by Lowsley and Kirwin.

FLOCKS, R. H.: Prophylaxis and medical management of calcium urolithiasis; role of quantity and precipitability of urinary calcium. J. Urol., *44:*183–190, 1940.

FLOCKS, R. H.: Studies on the nature of urinary calcium; its role in calcium urolithiasis. J. Urol., *64:*633–637, 1950.

FUJIMAKI, Y.: Formation of urinary and bile duct calculi in animals fed on experimental rations; note on treatment. Japan M. World, *6:*29–35, 1926.

GAHAGAN, H. Q. and REED, W. K.: Squamous cell carcinoma of the renal pelvis; review of the literature. J. Urol., *62:*139–151, 1949.

GASTON, E. A. and FERRUCCI, J.: Calculous formation in urethral diverticulum in woman; report of a case. New England J. Med., *221:*379–383, 1939.

GENTILE, A.: True prostatic calculus. J. Urol., *57:*746–754, 1947.

GERAGHTY, J. T. and HINMAN, F.: Ureteral calculus; special means of diagnosis and newer methods of intravesical treatment. Surg., Gynec. & Obst., *20:*515–522, 1915.

GILBERT, J. B. and MCMILLAN, S. F.: Cancer of the kidney; squamous-cell carcinoma of renal pelvis with special reference to etiology. Ann. Surg., *100:*429–444, 1934.

GUERSEL, A. E.: Une étude sur les lithiases urinaires en Turque. J. d'urol., *42:*447–466, 1936.

GUTZEIT, G.: Sur une méthode d'analyse qualitative rapide. Helv. Chim. Acta, *12:*713–740, 1929.

HAGER, B. H., and MAGATH, T. B.: The etiology of incrusted cystitis with alkaline urine. J.A.M.A., *85:*1352–1355, 1925.

HAMMARSTEN, O.: Lehrbuch der physiologischen Chemie. Wiesbaden, J. F. Bergmann, 1896, p. 837.

HARRINGTON, H. L.: Clinical study of 480 cases of urinary lithiasis. J. Urol., *44:*507–519, 1940.

HARRISON, J. H., BOTSFORD, T. W. and PIERCE, F. R.: The management of urolithiasis in the Army General Hospital. J. Urol., *53:*282–294, 1945.

HAWK, P. B. and BERGEIM, O.: Practical Physiological Chemistry. Philadelphia, Blakiston's Son & Co., 1931, Chapter 34.

HEATH, P. M.: Large ureteral calculus. Brit. J. Surg., *10:*153–155, 1922.

HERBST, R. H.: Recurrent renal calculus; its causes and prevention. Am. J. Surg., *12:*58–62, 1931.

HERMAN, L.: The Practice of Urology. Philadelphia, W. B. Saunders Co., 1938, p. 798.

HIGGINS, C. C.: Prevention of recurrent renal calculi. Surg., Gynec. & Obst., *63:*23–34, 1936 a.

HIGGINS, C. C.: Urinary lithiasis; experimental production and solution with clinical application and end-results. J. Urol., *36:*168–177, 1936 b.

HIGGINS, C. C.: Factors which influence the formation of urinary calculi; clinical application to prevention of recurrent renal calculi. New York State M. J., *36:*1620–1628, 1936 c.

HIGGINS, C. C.: Dietary regimen in the treatment of renal calculi. J. Lancet, *58:*9–12, 1938 a.

HIGGINS, C. C.: Recurrent renal lithiasis; review of 100 cases. J. Urol., *40:*184–192, 1938 b.

HIGGINS, C. C.: Squamous cell carcinoma of the kidney pelvis. Arch. Surg., *38:*224–244, 1939 a.

HIGGINS, C. C.: Urinary lithiasis; collective review. Internat. Abstr. Surg., *68:*392–405, 1939; in Surg., Gynec. & Obst., 1939 b.

HIGGINS, C. C.: Surgical removal of renal calculi. S. Clin. North America, *19:*1285–1294, 1939 c.

HIGGINS, C. C.: Factors in recurrence of renal calculi. J.A.M.A., *113:*1460–1465, 1939 d.

HIGGINS, C. C.: Ureteral calculi; review of 350 cases. New York State J. Med., *39:*2085–2093, 1939 e.

HIGGINS, C. C.: Ureteral calculi; review of 350 cases. Nebraska M. J., *27:*301–308, 1942.

HIGGINS, C. C.: Renal Lithiasis. Springfield, Ill., Charles C Thomas, 1943.

HIGGINS, C. C.: Etiology and management of renal lithiasis. J. Urol., *62:*403–409, 1949.

HIGGINS, C. C. and MENDENHALL, E. E.: Factors associated with recurrent formation of renal lithiasis, with report of new method for qualitative analysis of urinary calculi. J. Urol., *42:*436–450, 1939.

HIGGINS, C. C. and RAMBOUSEK, E. S.: Diverticula of the urethra in women; review of 12 cases. J. Urol., *53:*732–739, 1945.

HIGGINS, C. C. and ROEN, P. R.: Report of a case of calculus-containing urethral diverticulum in a woman. J. Urol., *49:*715–719, 1943.

HIGGINS, C. C. and WARDEN, J. G.: Modern concepts of ureteral calculi. Ann. Surg., *127:*257–268, 1948.

HINMAN, F.: Principles and Practice of Urology. Philadelphia, W. B. Saunders Co., 1935.

HOLMES, R. J. and COPLAN, M. M.: Study of geographic incidence of urolithiasis with consideration of etiological factors. J. Urol., *23:*477–489, 1930.

HUGGINS, C. and BEAR, R. S.: Course of prostatic ducts and anatomy; chemical and x-ray diffraction analysis of prostatic calculi. J. Urol., *51:*37–47, 1944.

HUNNER, G. L.: Ureteral stricture; report of unusual case illustrating influence on formation of urinary calculi and on recurring calculi. J.A.M.A., *82:*509–516, 1924.

JEANBRAU: Cited by Joly, p. 799.

JENSEN, A. T.: On concrements from the urinary tract. Acta chir. Scandinav., *84:*207–223, 1940.

JENSEN, A. T.: On concrements of the urinary tract. Acta chir. Scandinav., *85:*473–486, 1941.

JOLY, J. S.: Stone and Calculous Disease of the Urinary Organs. St. Louis, C. V. Mosby Co., 1931.

KEYSER, L. D.: The etiology of urinary lithiasis; an experimental study. Arch. Surg., *6:* 525–553, 1923.

KEYSER, L. D.: The relationship of urinary infection to recurrent calculi. J. Urol., *31:*219–238, 1934.

KEYSER, L. D., SCHERER, P. C. and CLAFFEY, L. W.: Studies in the dissolution of urinary calculi; experimental and clinical study. J. Urol., *59:*826–841, 1948.

KIMBROUGH, J. C. and DENSLOW, J. C.: Urinary tract calculi in recumbent patients. J. Urol., *61:*837–845, 1949.

KRETSCHMER, H. L.: Xanthin calculi, report of a case and review of the literature. J. Urol., *38:*183–193, 1937.

KRETSCHMER, H. L.: Stone in the ureter; clinical data based on 500 cases. Surg., Gynec. & Obst., *74:*1065–1077, 1942.

KUTZMANN, A. A.: Replacement lipomatosis of the kidney. Surg., Gynec. & Obst., *52:* 690–701, 1931.

LEADBETTER, W. F. and ENGSTER, H. C.: Problem of renal lithiasis in convalescent patients. J. Urol., *53:*269–281, 1945.

LETT, H.: On urinary calculus with special reference to stone in the bladder. Brit. J. Urol., *8:*205–232, 1936.

LICHTWITZ, L.: The formation of concretions. Colloid Chemistry. Vol. V, Jerome Alexander, ed., New York, Reinhold Publishing Co., 1944.

LIGHTWOOD, R.: Calcium infarction of kidneys in infants. Arch. Dis. Child., *10:*205–206, 1935.

LOWER, W. E. and BELCHER, G.: Massive lipoma of kidney with report of case. Surg., Gynec. & Obst., *45:*1–6, 1927.

LOWSLEY, O. S. and KIRWIN, T. J.: Clinical Urology. Vol. 2, Baltimore, Williams and Wilkins Co., 1940.

MCCARRISON, R.: Causation of stone in India. Brit. M. J., *1:*1009–1015, 1931.

MCLEAN, F. C. and HASTINGS, A. B.: Clinical estimation and significance of calcium ion concentration in the blood. Am. J. M. Sc., *189:*602–612, 1935.

MATHE, C. P.: Diagnosis and present day treatment of ureteral stone. J. Urol., *28:*133–155, 1932.

MATHEWS, A. P.: Physiological Chemistry. New York, Wm. Wood & Co., ed. 5, 1930.

MENDEL, L. B.: Urinary calculi. J.A.M.A., *69:*32, 1917.

MORRIS: Cited by Keyes, E. L.: Urology. New York, D. Appleton & Co., 1920, p. 385.

NAKANO, H.: Beiträge zur Kenntnis der in den Harnsteinen enthaltenen Substanzen. J. Biochem. Tokyo, *2:*437–441, 1923.

NEVILLE, D. W.: Constitutional factor in oxaluria. Urol. & Cutan. Rev., *39:*32–33, 1935.

NICHOLS, B. H. and LOWER, W. E.: Roentgenographic Studies of the Urinary System. St. Louis, C. V. Mosby Co., 1933.

NOBLE: Cited by Addison, O. L.: Urology in children. Proc. Roy. Soc. Med., London, *29:*1295–1306, 1936.

OPPENHEIMER, G. D.: Nephrectomy versus conservative operation in unilateral calculous disease of the upper urinary tract. Surg., Gynec. & Obst., *65:*829–836, 1937.

ORD, W. M. and SHATTOCK, S. G.: On microscopic structure of urinary calculi of oxalate of lime. Tr. Path. Soc., London, *46:*91–132, 1895.

OSBORNE, T. B., MENDEL, L. B. and FERRY: Incidence of phosphatic urinary calculi in rats fed on experimental rations. J.A.M.A., *69:*32–33, 1917.

PEARLMAN, C. K.: Xanthine urinary calculus. J. Urol., *64:*799–900, 1950.

PETERSON, H. O. and HOLMES, G. W.: Roentgen analysis of 100 cases of ureteral calculi. Am. J. Roentgenol., *37:*479–483, 1937.

PRATHER, G. C.: Spinal cord injuries; calculi of the urinary tract. J. Urol., *57:*1097–1104, 1947.

PRIEN, E. L. and FRONDEL, C.: Studies in urolithiasis; composition of urinary calculi. J. Urol., *57:*949–991, 1947.

QUINBY, W. C.: End results of operations for lithiasis. Tr. Am. A. Genito-Urin. Surg., *26:*285–286, 1933.

RAINES, S. L.: Personal communication.

RANDALL, A.: Giant vesical calculus. J. Urol., *5*:119, 1921.
RANDALL, A.: in Discussion of Higgins, C. C.: Further observations on the experimental production of urinary calculi. Tr. Am. A. Genito-Urin. Surg., *28*:157–170, 1935.
RANDALL, A.: Initiating lesions of renal calculus. Surg., Gynec. & Obst., *64*:201–208, 1927.
RANDALL, A., CAMPBELL, E. W. and BEESON, H. C.: A simple method of chemical analysis of urinary calculi with a report of recent series. Urol. & Cutan. Rev., *38*:29–32, 1934.
RAVICH, A.: A critical study of ureteral calculi based on a series of 758 private cases. J. Urol., *29*:171–185, 1933.
RIBA, L. W.: Urologic complications in cases of transverse myelitis. Transverse Myelitis Conference, Armed Service Forces, Ninth Service Command, June 24–25, 1945, pp. 4–5.
RIEGEL, C., ROYSTER, H. P., GISLASON, G. J. and HUGHES, P. B.: Chemical studies in hyperparathyroidism and urolithiasis. J. Urol., *57*:192–195, 1947.
ROSENOW, E. C. and MEISSER, J. G.: Nephritis and urinary calculi following the experimental production of chronic foci of infection. Coll. Papers Mayo Clin., *13*:253–256, 1921.
ROTH, L. J. and DAVIDSON, H. B.: Fibrous and fatty replacement of renal parenchyma. J.A.M.A., *111*:233–239, 1938.
ROVSING, T.: Kidney calculi. Ztschr. f. urol. Chir., *12*:358–384, 1923.
RUSCHE, C. F. and BACON, S. K.: Injury of ureter due to cystoscopic intraureteral instrumentation; report of 16 cases. J. Urol., *44*:777–793, 1940.
SANGREE, H. K.: Management and prevention of renal and ureteral calculi. J. Urol., *59*: 842–845, 1948.
SCHADE, H.: Die physikalische Chemie in der inneren Medizin. Ed. 3, Steinkoff, Dresden, 1923, p. 352.
SCHOLL, A. J.: Stones in the kidney and ureter, in Cabot, B.: Modern Urology, Philadelphia, Lea and Febiger, 1936, pp. 598–678.
SEEGER, S. J., and KEARNS, W. M.: Cystinuric lithiasis. J.A.M.A., *85*:4–7, 1925.
SHAW, E. C.: A study of the curve of elimination of phenolsulfonphthalein by normal and diseased kidneys. J. Urol., *13*:575–591, 1925.
SHORR, E.: The possible usefulness of estrogens and aluminum hydroxide gels in the management of renal stone. J. Urol., *53*:507–520, 1945.
SIMRIL, W. A. and ROSE, D. K.: Replacement lipomatosis and its simulation of renal tumors. J. Urol., *63*:588–590, 1950.
SUBY, H. I. and ALBRIGHT, F.: Dissolution of phosphatic urinary calculi by the retrograde introduction of a citrate solution containing magnesium. New England J. Med., *228*:81–91, 1943.
TENNANT, C. E.: Ureteral stone of unusual size. J.A.M.A., *82*:1122–1123, 1924.
THOMPSON, G. J. and KIBLER, J. M.: Treatment of ureteral calculus with particular reference to the urethral manipulation. J.A.M.A., *114*:6–12, 1940.
THOMPSON, J. C.: Urinary calculi at the Canton Hospital. Surg., Gynec. & Obst., *32*:44–55, 1921.
TWINEM, F. P.: A study of recurrence following operations for nephrolithiasis. J. Urol., *37*:259–267, 1937.
TWINEM, F. P.: Cited by Lowsley and Kirwin, Vol. 2, p. 1025.
VICKERY, E. P.: Urologist's letters, p. 83, 1936.
WHITE, H. P. W.: Calculous anuria. Lancet, *1*:918–919, 1929.
WHITE, J. L.: Stones in the prostate and seminal vesicles. Texas State J. Med., *23*:581–583, 1928.
WISHARD, W. N., JR.: Stone in the lower third of the ureter. J. Urol., *50*:775–783, 1943.
YOUNG, H.: Urinary lithiasis, in Annals of Roentgenology. New York, Hoeber, 1928, v. 7, pp. 302–413.

CHAPTER 2

Foreign Bodies in the Urinary Tract

DALTON K. ROSE, M.D.

INTRODUCTION

Foreign bodies from the animal, vegetable and mineral kingdom are found in the genitourinary tract. They may be introduced through the mouth, skin, urethra, rectum or vagina. Of abnormal psyche, most frequently sex difficulties (auto-eroticism) account for nearly all of those foreign bodies introduced through the urethra; a few instances are the results of transurethral surgical procedures. War, fights, surgery and accidents account for those introduced by way of the skin; relatively few swallowed sharp foreign bodies reach the genitourinary tract. Packs, drains and surgical instruments left in the vagina or the abdomen may migrate to the bladder and it may become of great medicolegal as well as clinical importance. Malingering is an infrequent incentive for introduction of foreign bodies into the urethra or bladder, and when it does occur in addition to the desire to arouse sympathy (often in one chronically ill) we find an abnormal psyche.

Obstruction to the flow of urine from the kidney pelvis to the urethral meatus by the foreign body itself may or may not be associated with the eventual urinary infection we expect to find in these cases. Inflammatory masses associated with foreign bodies may be contiguous to some part of the urinary tract and directly or indirectly interfere with renal function, inducing infection and interfering with the normal flow of urine from kidney to bladder, or from bladder to urethral meatus.

A foreign body in the urinary tract occasionally migrates from an unusual distance, passing vulnerable structures to emerge in the urinary tract where it may reside; it often closes off its pathway as it migrates and, therefore, we may not find an expected extravasation of urine. Rarely, a stone may migrate from the bladder to the alimentary tract. The place of residence of a foreign body often is transitory; a foreign body may pass down the ureter to the bladder or regurgitation of a foreign body from the bladder to the kidney pelvis may occur.

DIAGNOSTIC AIDS

Locating a foreign body in or near a part of the genitourinary tract is usually quite exact. An analysis of the patient's psyche and history; examination of the urine for blood, pus and bacteria; x-ray studies, particularly an intravenous pyeloureterogram with its associated nephrogram and cystogram; a cystogram by catheter bladder filling, noting ureteral reflux, will contribute the necessary information in a large majority of cases. Cystoscopic and urethroscopic examination and, when necessary, ureteral catheterization with retrograde pyelogram assist not only in locating and identifying the foreign body but will properly evaluate associated damage

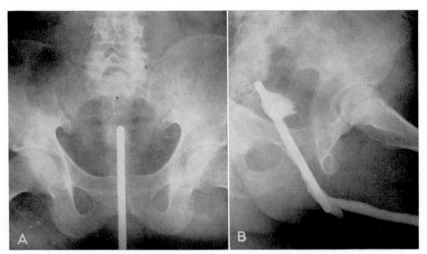

Fig. 380.   *A*, anterior-posterior view of steel rod introduced into bladder by a man in senility.

B, lateral view, supplemented with urethrogram by Dr. Wm. B. Wall, Jr., Barnes Hospital.

The steel bar was removed with a Lowsley cystoscopic rongeur with McCarthy for-oblique telescope.

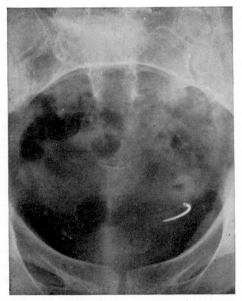

Fig. 381.   Plain film. Foreign body: surgical needle in pelvis. (Braasch and Emmett.)

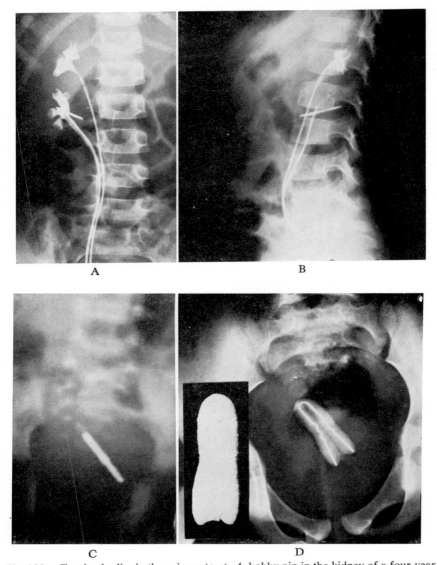

A   B

C   D

Fig. 382. Foreign bodies in the urinary tract. *A,* bobby pin in the kidney of a four-year-old girl examined because of persistent hematuria. *B,* lateral view. Nephrotomy removal of the friable rusted pin. It is assumed the object was swallowed, perforated the bowel (duodenum?) and lodged in the kidney. (Courtesy Dr. O. A. Nelson.) *C,* brass connecting unit and tip of an 8 F. Philips' follower catheter lost in the bladder of a three-day-old male. This child, born in chronic complete retention and unable to void or to be catheterized, was brought eight hours after birth to the Editor's office for examination. This disclosed complete obstruction of the deep bulbous urethra. This membrane was broken down with a miniature sound following which a new and never previously used 8 F. Philips' catheter with a short filiform screw tip was passed to the bladder and tied indwelling. The child was returned to his suburban hospital nursery with instructions for removal of the catheter in two days. Upon removing the catheter, the screw connecting segment and short filiform tip remained in the bladder. Cystoscopic attempts to remove this were fruitless. The infant was carefully observed and after three months spontaneously passed the foreign body. To my knowledge this is the earliest incidence of foreign body in the bladder. *D,* hairpin heavily encrusted with phosphatic crystals in the bladder of a three-year-old girl examined because of "chronic pyelitis." Suprapubic removal. Upon confronting the child with the surgical findings, she admitted having introduced the hairpin herself and obviously as a masturbatory act. Insert: removed specimen. (Campbell.)

that has been done to any part of the urinary tract. Laminagram, arteriography, perineal insufflation and gastrointestinal visualization may be helpful, and occasionally are essential for foreign body localization.

Harry S. Crossen of the School of Medicine and David F. Crossen, School of Law, Washington University, published a most comprehensive and authoritative book "Foreign Bodies Left in the Abdomen" (1940). I have drawn freely upon their excellent work; advice is given that smaller gauze sponges be made visible in open surgery by using an attached metal ring or wire or by impregnating the gauze with an x-ray opaque chemical such as

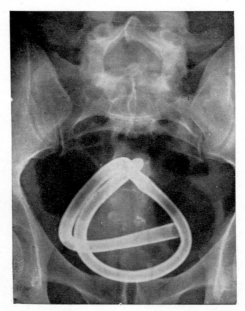

Fig. 383.   Plain film. Urethral catheter coiled in bladder. (Braasch and Emmett.)

lead tannate, zinc wolframmate, or tin phosphate silicate. For greater security Crossen and Crossen advise a continuous sponge in abdominal and vaginal surgery (Fig. 380).

Schachner (1901) stated "It is a surgical axiom that so long as surgery continues as an art just so long will foreign substances continue to be unintentionally left in the abdominal cavity (Fig. 381). These foreign bodies continuously find their way out by eventually forcing an entrance through the least resisting surface, which is usually some portion of the intestinal tract, or as it has occurred into the urinary tract."

Urologists may be confronted with foreign bodies left behind after surgery or treatment and ranging from drains to broken electric light bulbs or instruments (Fig. 382). Crossen and Scott (1939) present interesting findings in this connection in an experimental work, "The Lost Drain and Its Experimental Identification." They found that red rubber tubing gave the most distinct shadow, while black rubber gave the least distinct shadow. Red tubing contains antimony sulfide which gives the red color and also aids in x-ray visibility. Amber rubber tubing had no more x-ray visibility than black tubing (Fig. 383). He also found that a foreign body gave a more distinct shadow when it was near the x-ray film. Laminagraphy, therefore, should be helpful.

The incrustation of foreign bodies with urinary salts and notably with calcium, given sufficient time, occurred to some degree in nearly every instance. Highly polished metal or smooth glass incrusted slowly until rusting of the metal or minute roughing of the glass occurred. The broken surface or irregularities of even polished glass will in time incrust to some extent. Bullets incrust though much slower than gauze, silk, rubber, wood, bone or catheters. Incrustation materially aids in x-ray localization of foreign bodies that are not in themselves radiopaque.

LEGAL ASPECTS REGARDING FOREIGN BODIES

The urologist may leave a sponge in the abdomen during kidney, ureter or bladder surgery; all varieties of packs, instruments and catheters have been left in the prostatic cavity after open prostatectomy, as well as in the respective channels after urethral, bladder and ureteral instrumentation. What is the responsibility of the surgeon in such instances? Crossen (1940) states that "The plaintiff has the burden of proof. This means that the patient must show by a preponderance of confident evidence that the foreign body was permitted to remain in the patient through *negligence* of the physician, and that the patient suffered an injury as a result thereof . . . since the plaintiff patient is not versed in medical practice, and frequently is in no position during the operation to observe what takes place, he is often ignorant of what specific negligence on the part of the defendant caused his injury. To correct this the Courts have (a) applied the doctrine of res ipsa loquitur (the thing speaks for itself), or (b) held that the leaving of the sponge constitutes negligence per se." Crossen quotes Black's Law Dictionary, Ed. 2, p. 1539: res ipsa loquitur as "rebuttal presumption that defendant was negligent, which arises upon proof that instrumentality causing injury was in defendant's exclusive control, and that the accident was one which does not happen in absence of negligence." It is further stated "The defendant may overcome the presumption of negligence arising under the doctrine of res ipsa loquitur, or negligence per se, by producing competent evidence showing that he in fact exercised due care during the operation."

FOREIGN BODIES IN GENITOURINARY TRACT

Foreign Bodies in the Urethra and the Bladder. The method of introduction of a foreign body, portal of entrance, and its final place of residence have associated importance.

Articles and materials introduced into the bladder by youths and by intoxicated adults, by malingerers, the insane, masturbators and sex perverts are legion (Figs. 383–388). "Urological Oddities," edited and published by Dakin in 1948, lists a surprising assortment. A complete listing would be nigh impossible as any solid material small enough to pass through the urethral meatus may be "lost" in the bladder; however, an incomplete list of such objects is presented. Undoubtedly the oftimes frantic efforts to regain the object as it escapes into the meatus serves only to push it farther along the urethra, or into the bladder (Figs. 382–388). Both male and female masturbators introduce the most bizarre objects into the urinary tract, though the male is the more frequent offender in this regard. He

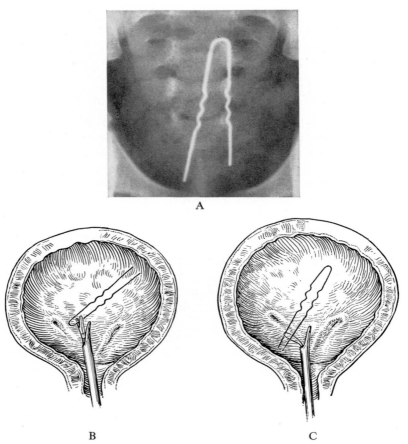

A

B   C

Fig. 384. Vesical foreign body. *A,* hairpin which was introduced into the bladder for masturbatory purposes by a six-year-old girl. *B,* cystoscopic removal of hairpin using Campbell 17 F. miniature cysto-urethroscope and grasping forceps. *C,* removal of hairpin by employing small wire loop.

passes into the urethra worms, larvae, small snakes, wasps, wire (Fig. 386), waxed thread, long strips of rubber, newspaper rolled into tight cylinders, gum, paraffin, even the tail-bone of a squirrel, and all types of round objects: stones, shot and so forth. Other objects cited by Dakin as having been introduced into the bladder through the urethra include pieces of vegetables, stalks of plants, cuticle pushers, nail files, tightly rolled condoms, electric light bulb (5½ by 2½ inches), rubber bands, leather-boot lace, eyebrow tweezers, safety pins, bobby pins, small bits of tightly rolled cloth, thermom-

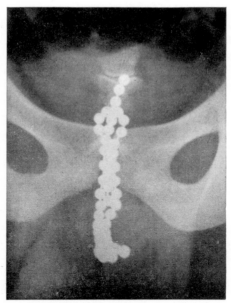

Fig. 385.   Plain film. Foreign body. String of beads in posterior urethra and bladder of man. (Courtesy of Dr. J. M. Pace.)

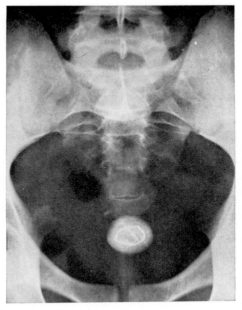

Fig. 386.   Plain film. Stone in bladder, nucleus of which was a copper wire. (Braasch and Emmett.)

eters, highball muddlers, watch chains, tooth-brush handles, handles of safety razors, pencils, penholders, meat skewers, hog's penis, medicine dropper, rubber ballons, crayon, candles, bamboo, contraception diaphragm, tallow, gravy that hardened in the bladder after cooling, and fish-line leaders. Sharp objects introduced through the urethral meatus may eventually protrude through the penis or perineum (Campbell, 1951). Objects such as tooth-picks and blades of grass may pass through the bladder and on to the kidney pelvis. Occasionally in females the urethral meatus is confused with the cervix uteri, and the urethra is plugged with gum to prevent conception; attempts to produce abortion again mistaking the urethral meatus for the cervix accounts for some of the pins, nails, glass tubes, slippery-elm sticks and so forth that we find in the bladder. Powell (1952) removed from the ureteral orifice of a four-and-a-half-month old female a hair from a cat (microscopic confirmation) to which the infant was exposed in the home.

Brewer and Marcus (1948) state that 566 foreign bodies in the bladder have been reported from 1880 to 1946. By no means are all of these patients insane or psychotic; they may be intoxicated or their sex life may be in the process of first exploration. Occasionally an individual entirely misdirected, with a chronic cystitis or urethritis will introduce objects in a clinically unsound effort to relieve the urethral or bladder irritation, though frequently in these cases sex aberration is also present and auto-eroticism is fundamental.

Foreign Bodies in the Bladder Introduced with Surgical Treatment. Catheters have been lost in the bladder and removed with bent wires and button hooks long before our modern cystoscopes and urethroscopes were conceived. It is interesting that the Journal of the American Medical Association, volume 1, 1883, reports three instances of stiff catheters broken off in the bladder and one of a soft rubber catheter lost in the bladder. At that time screw tipped obturators passed through catheters as well as bent wire, hooks, and loops recovered the lost catheters. The soft rubber catheter was just gaining wide acceptance (1883) over the more rigid catheter which evidently broke all too frequently.

Foreign Bodies within the Kidney Pelvis and Ureter Introduced Through the Urethra. Rusche and Bacon state that "Ureteral trauma occurs most commonly in the course of surgical procedures on the internal genitalia of the female, next as a result of cystoscopic intra-ureteral instrumentation, external violence, and finally as the result of foreign bodies."

Many ureteral instruments have contributed to our list of ureteral foreign bodies; broken ureteral catheters, metallic tips from instruments used to dislodge and remove ureteral stones; bougie tips from ureteral dilators. In one case a tip of a ureteral stone extractor basket became unscrewed; the empty shaft was reintroduced and the wire (basket) tip was screwed again onto the shaft, and the entire instrument was safely withdrawn. A wire ureteral basket has been used to trap and withdraw a broken end of a metal spiral instrument; in other instances open surgery has been necessary to remove the foreign object.

In one patient at nephrectomy Hale* had difficulty cutting across a ureter. It was soon discovered that a ureteral catheter had been "lost" some fourteen years previously and accounted for the renal destruction now requiring nephrectomy; the calcium accumulation on the catheter resisted the surgeon's knife.

Kretschmer (1916) clinically demonstrated the ureteral regurgitation of foreign objects, and stated, "It is rather striking, therefore, to see the frequency with which it was possible to demonstrate regurgitation of fluid into the ureter in children. As far as I know, this is the first time that regurgitation of fluid into the ureter has been demonstrated in children with normal bladders. In these cases examinations were carried out under anesthesia . . . the regurgitation was unilateral." He found that in one adult in whom the regurgitation occurred the bladder was perfectly normal; in another patient regurgitation occurred on one side during straining and there was no regurgitation when there was no straining. Kretschmer found an increased frequency of regurgitation in adults with a diseased bladder. From this work we can postulate that a contracted, irritable, inflamed bladder in trying to expel a foreign body would furnish the physical situation for unilateral and probably at times bilateral ureteral regurgitation.

Waring and Drane (1932) report the case of a thirty-seven year old male who presented himself with physical signs of so-called acute right pyelitis. He had had an attack of hematuria fourteen months previously and there had been a mild attack of cystitis recently. The patient confessed that he had introduced grass and straw into his urethra and that on one occasion seed-bearing grass had slipped into his bladder. A calcified foreign body 2.5 by 0.2 cm. was removed from the right renal pelvis, and examination disclosed it to be a portion of seed-bearing grass with calcific and phosphatic incrustation. These authors reviewed the works of Graves and Davidoff, Gruber, and Kirwin, and together with their own observations concluded that "During urination and bladder contraction, the end of the foreign body happened to be introduced into the ureter, and the sagittal arrangement of the seed on the stem caused it to work its way during muscular movements and peristalsis up the ureter" (cf. Fig. 382).

Reporting upon their experimental surgery in dogs, they deduced that as regards the transport of sagittate (arrowhead-shaped) grass seed: "The ureteral orifices could not be located, so the right ureter was severed at the bladder. No peristalsis was detected in the ureter, and very little urine was excreted. A portion of the seed-bearing grass sagittations pointing upward when placed in this ureter remained stationary as long as the ureter was not disturbed. However, the amount of manipulation which occurred in searching for the left ureter caused the grass to disappear and ascend 2 cm. up the (cut right) ureter." Waring and Drane found the reports of two urologists who cited cases suggestively similar. Braasch recorded a calculus formed about a hairpin in the ureter and which was removed; the hairpin had been introduced into the bladder. Barney reported a calculus which partially surrounded a toothpick and which was removed from a kidney pelvis by

* Quoted by Dakin (1948).

one of his colleagues. Waring and Drane concluded that the toothpick had been swallowed and found its way through the bowel to the kidney. A similar duodenal pelvic migration of a bobby pin was observed by Nelson (Fig. 382, *A, B*).

Small stones, a glass straw, toothpicks, and plugs for ureteral catheters have been reported gaining access to the kidney pelvis with the help of ureteral retrograde peristalsis. Also a ureteral orifice, abnormally large through disease or when congenitally wide open at all times, may allow free interchange of urine, stones and small foreign bodies between the bladder, ureter and kidney pelvis.

Foreign Bodies of the Urinary Tract in Orthopedic Surgery. Branham and Richey (1947) report the use of a Kirchner threaded wire together with two similar wires to pin a fracture of the neck of the left femur; one of the three threaded Kirchner wires passed below the fractured neck of femur. Two months after this operation the patient presented herself with pyuria, hematuria, chills and fever. Over the left greater trochanter there was a soft tissue tumor mass with two draining sinuses. A cystoscopic examination revealed the bladder mucosa to be markedly inflamed and an object thought to be the tip of a Kirchner wire was found penetrating the left lateral wall of the urinary bladder. By an extraperitoneal approach through an incision above the left inguinal ligament the wire was located and removed; three-quarters of an inch of its point was within the bladder. The other wires were removed through a separate incision over the greater trochanter and the patient made an uneventful recovery. McCrea (1945), cited by Branham and Richey, referred to a similar case in which the prostate gland had been pierced by a large screw which had been driven through the left acetabulum in an effort to pin a fractured hip.

Grant (1936) reported a case of intracapsular fracture of the left femur in a woman. Two days after the injury the left trochanter was explored by an orthopedist; the capsule was severed and under direct vision a beef-bone peg was inserted through the trochanter and into the head of the femur holding the two in apposition and without perforation of the acetabulum. One week later an abscess about the wound opened; after treating the patient at home for four months the orthopedic surgeon sought a urologic consultation. Cystoscopic examination disclosed a large irregular fungating mass lying in the center of the bladder. A roentgenogram revealed an unusual picture which was explained at operation; the point of the bone peg was found to be just entering the bladder and on the left side a sinus extended from the bladder to the head of the femur; no effort was made to excise the sinus which was simply curetted and the bladder was closed about a Pezzar catheter. The patient made an uneventful recovery. Six months had elapsed from the time of insertion of the bone peg until its removal.

Subsequently the orthopedic surgeon was sued for malpractice. The patient admitted that "The fortuitous lodging of the bone peg in the bladder was not due to any fault of the (orthopedic surgeon) defendant," but "claimed that he was negligent in failing to discover sooner that the peg had migrated." The defendant surgeon stated that there was "no case on record where any (bone peg) had ever worked inward, they all migrated out, and so felt that he was justified in not moving the patient and jeopardizing the union." The Court concluded that "The plaintiff had failed to prove that the defendant had left undone something that he should have done, or that he had done something that he should not have done." Accordingly, the Court affirmed the judgment for the (surgeon) defendant (Meador vs. Arnold).

Floyd and Pitman (1941) reported the case of a patient aged twenty-six years who stated that at the age of twelve he had an acute osteomyelitis involving the right hip joint. On several occasions a urinary odor was detected on the dressing. He suffered "cystitis," difficulty in voiding, and an ankylosed right hip. Radiography disclosed in the bladder area a shadow shaped like the head of a femur and absence of the head of the right femur from its normal position. At cystostomy the bladder was found intact but to have been pulled over and fixed to the right pelvis. The specimen removed was "the head of the right femur detached at the epiphysial line, and appears to be the head of a femur of a twelve year old person." The authors felt this case of interest because the bone had migrated from one part of the body to another leaving no trace of its migration other than cicatricial tissue, and because so little change had taken place in the bone itself.

Rubber tubing used in tuberculous hip operations has migrated to the bladder entering through its dome which was much more unusual than similar migration of sharp foreign bodies. Fractured pelves account for the occasional migration of bone splinters into the bladder.

Foreign Bodies in the Bladder Migrating from the Abdominal Cavity. Sponges, drainage tubes, surgical instruments, sutures and needles used in abdominal surgery may migrate through the bladder wall though a great number of such foreign bodies either become encysted or migrate into the bowel. Bladder sutures frequently incrust to form stones.

When sponges and needles, notably after pelvic surgery, migrate into the bladder cavity they usually become incrusted with urinary salts, yet instances have been cited in which the cystoscopist could recognize shreds of sponge extending through the bladder wall. Upchurch and Upchurch (1933) reported fabric shreds in calcified masses removed with an operating cystoscope, later to find more gauze extruding through the bladder wall. These repetitive piecemeal extraction procedures were continued until cystostomy was demanded and revealed a large extracystic mass of gauze contiguous to the bladder wall; in all, 102 procedures (transurethral and/or open operation) were carried out before the last shred of migrating gauze was removed (cf. Fig. 380).

An abdominal pregnancy was complicated by a urethral obstruction due to four small fetal bones; at operation an egg-sized mass, attached to the bladder wall, was found beneath the broad ligament. Dermoid cysts containing hair, teeth and bones have by propulsion by adjacent viscera migrated into the bladder.

Foreign Bodies in the Bladder Migrating from the Gastrointestinal Tract. There are not a great many instances of foreign bodies migrating from the alimentary tract to the bladder. The largest object known to thus migrate is the thigh bone of a rabbit that eroded slowly through the bladder wall and without leakage of urine. Even in severely infected cases the pathways that are formed by migrating foreign bodies to and through the bladder wall leak very infrequently except when the bladder has been incised.

A swallowed needle has penetrated the intestines in such a manner that it scratched the peritoneum over the bladder causing the same frequency of urination we should expect had the needle passed into the bladder cavity. A pin located in the appendix penetrated both the enteric and the bladder wall; the point of the pin became incrusted. The pin and appendix were removed at one operation.

Baron and Lipshutz (1947) reported the passage of a fiber bristle of a whisk broom from the bowel to the bladder. The patient swallowed the 12 cm. bristle while asleep, it having been in use as an applicator for a cotton pledget to stop bleeding from a tooth socket; twenty-six days later he had frequent bloody urination but two cystoscopic examinations failed to reveal the source of hematuria. Culture of the urine disclosed a B. coli infection, yet two weeks after the onset of the cystitis the point of a black bristle was cystoscopically observed to project ½ inch through the right dome of the bladder. Two days later using a Young's cystoscopic flexible biopsy forceps, the fiber bristle which measured 10 cm. long was removed from the bladder and the following day another piece of bristle 2 cm. long was spontaneously voided by the patient. This interesting case demonstrates how a foreign body may ulcerate through the wall of the bowel and into the urinary bladder without causing peritonitis. A barium enema just previously had revealed a hypertonic spastic colon. Prophylactically sulfadiazine had been given. The temperature of the patient did not exceed 100° F.

The possible wandering of soft gauze sponges is well illustrated in the case presented by Furniss (1913) who made the diagnosis before operation. A forty-three year old woman had a Dührssen interposition operation for prolapse and soon after the operation there was profuse discharge from the wound. Five months later cystoscopy showed bullous edema in the region of the right ureteral orifice and a later cystoscopic examination revealed a bit of gauze sticking from the middle of the edematous area. The next day she was unable to urinate; the following day a small probang sponge was removed from her bladder through a #12 Kelly speculum. The cystitis cleared rapidly. Three months later the patient again called and said that for two weeks she had had a profuse watery vaginal discharge. Upon examination with the patient in the knee-chest posture and the perineum retracted with Sims speculum, a bit of gauze was seen protruding from a small opening in the anterior vaginal wall. By constant traction another small probang sponge was removed; after this the patient recovered completely. The notable features of this case were (1) the complete closure of the wound in the presence of a foreign body, (2) the appearance of one sponge in the bladder many months after the operation, and (3) the other sponge in the vagina subsequent to this.

Foreign bodies may enter the urinary tract by way of the rectum, by forceful introduction, war, accident, or migration after rectal surgery.

Foreign Bodies in the Bladder Migrating from the Vaginal Tract. Occasionally sharp instruments used to produce abortion may pierce the bladder or enter the peritoneal cavity. These objects are seldom lost in the bladder except when the unhappy female confuses the urethra with the cervix.

When gauze sponges or packs are lost in the bladder in pelvic surgery through vaginal excision and when the bladder is incised, persistent leakage of urine and infection soon require surgical exploration. However, when the bladder wall is not incised and sponges are left in the pelvis leakage of urine is infrequent even when they migrate through the bladder wall there to be found later as thickly incrusted foreign bodies. Shivers (quoted by Dakin) reported that a gauze sponge overlooked during a salpingectomy sloughed into the bowel and then into the bladder. It was removed cystoscopically; catheter drainage was employed for two weeks. At first fecal material passed through the catheter, but the patient was discharged cured.

Foreign Bodies in the Bladder Entering by Way of the Skin. Bullets, fragments of shell, sharp objects penetrating the skin occasionally pass directly into the bladder or migrate into it with or without extravasation of urine. Hoover (quoted by Dakin) cites the instance of a 22 caliber bullet voided twenty minutes after a boy was shot in the buttocks. Indwelling catheterization promptly established prevented extravasation of urine. A large percentage of gunshot wounds of the bladder are complicated by injuries to adjacent organs and frequently extravasation of urine occurs. When the bony pelvis is fractured spicules of pubic or iliac bones may complicate the injury (cf. Section IX, Chapter 4).

Foreign Bodies in the Bladder Migrating from the Scrotum and the Urethra. Kretschmer (1909) has emphasized the extreme ease with which foreign bodies, especially sponges, gauze pads, artery forceps and so forth are left in the operative wound as proved by the large number of cases that have been reported in the literature but that foreign bodies left in an extraperitoneal wound have not been so carefully studied. He reported the removal of a gauze sponge from the scrotum two and a half years after an operation for double inguinal hernia and thought it unusual because of (1) the long time during which the sponge remained in such a relatively superficial part of the body without producing any symptoms, and (2) the rare occurrence of this condition and the ease with which the sponge was removed this being accomplished without the patient's knowledge. Kretschmer also cited a case reported by Louis E. Schmidt of Chicago in which a sponge previously left in the suprapubic space, upon cystoscopic examination showed long incrustations of lime salts lying in the bladder wall and hanging free in its cavity. A previous cystoscopic examination had disclosed long incrustations of lime salt swinging to and fro in the bladder fluid which led to the diagnosis of incrusted silk sutures in the bladder wall. After suprapubic removal of the sponge the patient made an uneventful recovery.

Symptoms caused by a foreign body within the urinary tract vary with the infection it may invite, the urethral or ureteral irritation and/or obstruction it may cause and when the bladder cavity is invaded, by the summating effort of the kidney, ureter, or bladder to expel the object. In normal bladders these painful, forceful voiding contractions often are stimulated and intensified by an associated and severe cystitis. Even when acute symptoms are present the patient may wilfully obscure the diagnosis until the urologist actually locates

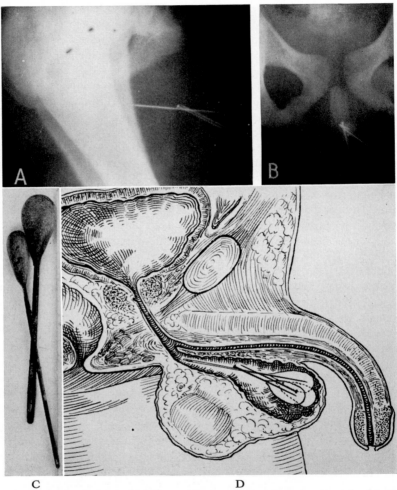

C   D

Fig. 387.   Foreign bodies in the urethra. *A,* two pins and a darning needle introduced into the urethra by an eight-year-old boy; lateral urogram. *B,* anterior posterior urogram. *C,* eighteen months previously these two darning needles, phosphatic encrusted at one end also had been removed from this boy's urethra by the Editor. Three weeks before this removal, these needles had been introduced into the urethra for masturbation, became covered with phosphatic deposits which formed stones and subsequent periurethral abscess. The patient was admitted to a hospital for contagious diseases and treated for a week for gonorrhea despite negative microscopy. X-rays revealed the needles which were removed by perineal section. *D,* schema of surgical findings in *A.* The needle and pins became phosphatic encrusted at one end, perforated the bulbous urethra to form a large pus-filled urethral diverticulum in the midline between the testicles, externally giving the appearance of a third testicle. Treatment: excision of the diverticulum with removal of the foreign bodies and urethral suture. (Essex County Isolation Hospital.)

and identifies the foreign body either in the kidney, ureter, bladder, urethra or genitalia. A foreign body in the urethra may provoke urethral discharge simulating that of gonorrhea and is occasionally so misdiagnosed (Fig. 387). By engendering periurethral abscess and secondary urethral diverticulum the resulting chronic pyuria too often causes the diagnosis of "chronic pyelitis" to be made (Fig. 387).

Genitalia. Nuts of large bolts or knot-holes in boards used by erotic youths in simulated intercourse may so constrict the penis that edema of the organ distal to the encircling object makes it impossible for the patient to remove the foreign body. In these instances mechanics have cut off the steel nuts and carpenters have first sawed off the board and then sawed open the knot-hole, as in May's case cited in Dakin.

Sharp objects introduced into the urethra may penetrate the prostate. A metal catheter guide pierced a large median lobe; it was removed cystoscopically. Once this accident reported by Fitzgerald (Dakin, 1948) occurred after the patient had been catheterizing himself for twelve years. Similar and/or comparable conditions engendered by foreign bodies are considered in Section IX, Chapter 4.

A celluloid ball recorded by Abeshouse (Dakin, 1948) was successfully used for thirty-four years as a prosthesis to replace a testicle removed by orchiectomy. Paraffin injected into the scrotum to simulate chronic tuberculous epididymitis for the purpose of avoiding compulsory military service in Russia is reported by Movitt. Not infrequently needles are driven into the testes by aged and/or psychotic individuals.

Foreign Bodies Reaching the Kidney by Way of the Alimentary Tract. Examples of foreign bodies reaching the kidney from the alimentary tract may be of soft material, gauze, rubber and so forth but usually they are rigid, bone, metal or wood; most often the foreign body ultimately reaches the perirenal fat rather than the interior of the renal pelvis. Many types of gauze and rubber drain have been left behind to complicate vesical and renal function. Mackby (1948) reported a case almost identical with that recorded by McEnery and Fox who described a two-year-old boy subject to persistent pyuria and intermittent fever. X-ray studies revealed a bobby pin in the second portion of the duodenum extending into the kidney pelvis. The pin was removed by open surgery. In neither case did the history suggest foreign body. Nelson's case is shown in Figure 394.

Foreign bodies penetrating the skin and migrating to or about a kidney or ureter are infrequent, and are predominantly projectiles. Bullets are found in kidney pelves; Fagerstrom (Dakin, 1948) recorded a .32 caliber revolver bullet that passed through the kidney near the point of entry, traversed the spinal cord, and spent itself exactly at the center of the pelvis of the opposite kidney. At autopsy the bullet was found to have started its passage down the ureter nose-first toward the bladder. In other instances bullets have been carried for years in a kidney pelvis; when removed eventually they were found to be heavily incrusted with urinary salts. Sponges, needles, pins introduced by abdominal surgery have encysted in or located near the ureter to influence drainage by juxtaposition.

Wilhelmi (1940) observed that an exhaustive search of the literature covering the past twenty-four years reveals surprisingly few cases of foreign bodies in the kidney. Eight cases were discovered, the foreign bodies being hairpins, rubber drains, broken needle, grass, straw, bullet, toothpick and a darning needle. In Wilhelmi's case the darning needle probably entered the skin at the groin during a fistic encounter; at operation a 1¾ inch needle was found, ¾ inch penetrated the kidney substance—not the kidney pelvis —and 1 inch remained in the perirenal fat. Upon removal at open surgery the needle was found to be incrusted with urinary salts. The incrustations were removed with a solution of phosphoric acid (1 to 2 per cent), after which the point of the needle was found to be sharp and the eyelet intact although there were several rust spots near the point.

TREATMENT

Conservative. Psychotic males may be helped in controlling their auto-eroticism by curing, if possible, their genitourinary infection and maintaining the patient in reduced sex stimulation with graded and interrupted doses of stilbestrol.

In the female, mentally near normal, who persists in passing small foreign bodies through her urethra, any medical or surgical intervention directed toward relieving her of the bladder, urethral or gynecologic irritations is indicated. These patients often confuse urinary and sex irritation.

Instrumental. Before the cystoscope was developed as a catheter, forceps, and scissors carrying instrument, it was used to locate and sound the bladder stone or foreign body. At that early period long-shafted narrow forceps were passed alongside this instrument to remove small foreign bodies. Even at that time the female urethra was digitally dilated to two fingers breadth and most foreign bodies in the bladder were readily removed with forceps, but the male urethra, often infected, constricted or blocked by a large prostate, presented surgical difficulties and cystostomy became necessary.

The Stern-McCarthy resectoscope, using the loop to lead the object into the sheath, or the Ellik evacuator operating through the 28 F. Stern-McCarthy resectoscope, is excellent for washing out small objects, as recently reported by Schloss and Solomkin (1950).

For selectivity in choosing the part of the object to be grasped, the flexible-stem cystoscopic forceps made by the American Cystoscope Makers, Inc., or a Huffman (1946) hook for looped structures (made by C. R. Bard, Inc.) introduced through a 24 F. Brown-Buerger operating cystoscope is generally satisfactory. With the forceps one may grasp the head of a pin. Many other instruments such as the Kirwin cystoscopic rongeur are available and will firmly grasp the object especially after some of the incrustations have been removed. Employment of the miniature cystourethroscope to remove a hairpin from the bladder of a child is shown in Figure 389.

Cotton pledgets, bits of wood applicators, broken small electric light bulbs from urethroscopes in particular are occasionally lost but can usually be quickly recovered by flushing the bladder or by grasping with cupped biopsy forceps passed through an operating cystoscope (Fig. 388).

Solvents. Paraffin and most other candles are soluble in heavy mineral oil. Wax, chewing gum, and paraffin are soluble in benzine or xylol. Consequently urologists have successfully used mineral oil to reduce the size of small (birthday) candles and have then had the patients void the remainder. Benzine or xylol is irritating to the vesical mucous membrane and requires twenty to thirty minutes to dissolve a fair-sized ball of chewing gum or

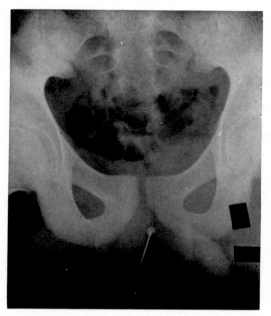

Fig. 388. Plain film. Foreign body: hatpin in bulbomembranous urethra in the male (Braasch and Emmett.)

wax. Here a general anesthetic is necessary, and the solvent solution must be changed two to four times.

Joelson (1950) recently advised that wax foreign bodies can be readily removed from the bladder with a McCarthy resectoscope if the bladder is distended with air instead of with water. With water filling the tendency of the wax or gum to float to the vesical dome makes it practically inaccessible to the ordinary cystoscopic instruments. Joelson considers the various recommended solvent mixtures to be quite satisfactory in most instances despite the severe and disturbing irritation of the vesical mucosa they may cause. In his hands the entire procedure is carried out through the McCarthy resectoscope under anesthesia. The water inflow stopcock is attached to its usual connection on the sheath of the instrument because occasional irrigation of the bladder may be necessary to remove pus and mucus which may be present, or the small amount of blood which may gather on the floor of the bladder during the procedure. The tube of a sterilized sphygmomanometer

bulb or, better still, a double bulb of a cautery set is attached to the outflow
cock which is mounted on the working element of the instrument. An
assistant keeps the bladder partially distended with air by pressing the
bulb whenever requested to do so by the operator. This method has
worked very satisfactorily with wax foreign bodies, and could probably be
used for other types of foreign bodies which float.

Lins (1945) synthetized a somewhat irritating solution to dissolve phosphate stones based on the brew of the Amazon buitach apple. The Indians
of the Amazon basin employ a native remedy to dissolve the skeleton of a
small fish which invades the urethra and bladder of river bathers. The fish

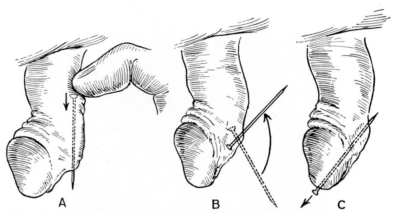

Fig. 389.   Urethral foreign body. Simple method of removing a pin from the anterior
urethra, especially when its point has perforated the canal. When there has been no perforation of the urethra, endoscopic removal is preferred. (Campbell, Clinical Pediatric
Urology.)

clings to the urethral and vesical mucosa, sets up inflammation and, unless
destroyed or removed, feeds on the flesh of its victim. A singular urinophilous instinct incites it to enter the excretory openings of the human body,
and it forces its way with great violence. The fish Candiru (*Vandellia
Cirrhosa*) is not quite 3 inches long and between 3 and 4 mm. in caliber.
Bathers usually protect themselves by wearing a small coconut-shell sheath
over their genitalia. A brew made of buitach apple of the Amazon region,
drunk very hot, will dissolve the skeleton of this fish clinging to the mucous
membrane of the native's bladder.

Suby and Albright's (1940) solution "G" for phosphatic deposits is also
somewhat irritating and has been improved in this regard with solution "M."
The formulas and use of these solutions are given in Section VIII, Chapter 1.
Gehres (1951) and, working entirely independently, Abeshouse and Weinberg (1951) presented a new solvent for calculi or incrustations.

Surgical. Foreign bodies in the urethra frequently can be removed with
forceps directly or through a urethroscope (Figs. 388, 389); a simple method
of removing pins is shown in Figure 389. In the male urethrostomy with
retention catheter may be necessary. Urinary obstruction by objects within
the urethra or by compression of the entire penis and urethra often leads

to heroic measures on the part of the patient, for removal of the object. They have incised their own urethras. In other instances, foreign bodies have eroded through the urethra and skin.

Cystotomy for removal of a foreign body in the bladder or deep urethra presents no special problem. Complications such as prostatic enlargement, urethral strictures, diverticula, masses contiguous to the bladder wall, and pyelonephritis should receive individual urologic diagnostic investigation and treatment. Antibiotic therapy today offers patients with foreign bodies in the urinary tract great advantage over their more unfortunate ancestors afflicted in a similar manner, many of whom the complicating urinary infection killed.

A scout or plain urogram may show a metallic object surrounded by dense incrustations (Figs. 380–387). Litholapaxy or dissolution of some of the phosphatic stone can be carried out in such instances with removal of the foreign body. Yet cystotomy is generally preferable and particularly if other pathologic conditions are present.

Lithotrites broken and/or locked in the bladder present a serious problem. It has been necessary at times to open the bladder, saw through the shaft of the instrument, and remove the shaft and jaws through the cystotomy wound.

Nicely (1946) is of the opinion that patients suffering gunshot wounds of the bladder operated upon a reasonable length of time following the injury, have a relatively good chance for recovery. Suprapubic cystotomy (including search for possible foreign body, bullet or shattered bone, and their removal) should be performed early and all wounds sutured.

Robinson et al. (1946) studied seventy-five gunshot or shell fragment wounds of the kidney which were suffered at the battle front during World War II. Sixteen had nephrectomy as the initial operation after injury, and eight required nephrectomy after evacuation to the rear. The remaining fifty-one had conservative surgery. These observers concluded that surgical intervention is indicated only when there is uncontrollable hemorrhage, evidence of increasing urinary extravasation, massive destruction or extensive infarction of the kidney. Operative treatment usually can be conservative, with removal of the foreign body, suture and packing of the kidney, and perirenal drainage.

REFERENCES

ABESHOUSE, B. S. and WEINBERG, TOBIAS: An experimental study of a new solvent action of versene on urinary calculi. J. Urol., *65:*316, 1951.

BARON, S. and LIPSHUTZ, H.: Unusual foreign body ulcerating into bladder from bowel. J. Urol., *58:*112–113, 1947.

BRANHAM, D. W. and RICHEY, H. M.: Kirchner wire removed from bladder. J. Urol., *57:* 869, 1947.

BREWER, A. C. and MARCUS, R.: Foreign body in the urinary bladder: an unusual case. Brit. J. Surg., *35:*324, 1948.

CAMPBELL, MEREDITH F.: Clinical Pediatric Urology. Philadelphia, W. B. Saunders Co., 1951.

CAULK, J. R.: Brooks Textbook of Surgical Nursing. 2nd ed. The C. V. Mosby Co., 1940.

CROSSEN, H. S. and CROSSEN, DAVID F.: Foreign bodies left in the abdomen. St. Louis, C. V. Mosby Co., 1940.

CROSSEN, H. S. and SCOTT, W. G.: The lost drain and its roentgen ray identification. J. Mo. State Med. Assoc., *36:*202, 1939.

DAKIN, WIRT B.: Urological Oddities. 1948.

FLOYD, E. and PITTMAN, JAMES L.: Transmigration of the head of the femur into the urinary bladder. Urol. & Cut. Rev., *45:*303–304, 1941.

FURNISS, H. D.: One gauze sponge removed from bladder, another from vagina, months after a Duehrssen operation for prolapse. J.A.M.A., *60:*1879, 1913.

GEHRES, R. F. and RAYMOND, S.: A new chemical approach to the dissolution of urinary calculi. J. Urol., *65:*474, 1951.

GRANT, O.: An unusual foreign body (bone peg) in the bladder. J.A.M.A., *107:*1632–33, 1936.

HUFFMAN, L. F.: A hook for removing foreign bodies from the bladder. J. Urol., *56:*57–58, 1946.

JOELSON, J. J.: Instrumental removal of wax foreign bodies from the bladder. J. Urol., *64:* 572, 1950.

KRETSCHMER, H. L.: Removal of a gauze sponge from the scrotum two and one half years after an operation for double inguinal hernia. Ann. Surg., *49:*814–819, 1909.

KRETSCHMER, H. L.: Cystography, its value in bladder surgery. Surg., Gynec. & Obst., *23:* 707–717, 1916.

LINS, E. E.: The solution of incrustations in the urinary bladder by a new method. J. Urol., *53:*702–709, 1945.

MACKBY, M. J.: Foreign body in second portion of the duodenum, perforation pelvis of right kidney. J. Mt. Sinai Hospital, *14:*929–930, 1948.

McCRAE, L. E.: Clinical Cystoscopy. Vol. 1, p. 345, Philadelphia, F. A. Davis Co., 1945.

MEADOR, vs. ARNOLD (Kentucky) 945 2nd, 626. Malpractice Fracture of Hip, Migration of Bone Peg Into Bladder. J.A.M.A., *108:*1997, 1937.

NICELY, E. PARK, MAJOR, MC: Gunshot wounds of the urinary bladder. J. Urol., *56:*59–67, 1946.

ROBINSON, J. N., CULP, SUBY, REISSER and MULLENIX: Injuries to the genito-urinary tract in the European theatre. J. Urol., *56:*498–507, 1946.

RUSCHE, C. R. and BACON, S. K.: Injuries of the ureter due to surgery, intraureteral instrumentation, external violence, and foreign bodies. See Chapter 2, this Section.

SCHANER, AUGUST: Foreign bodies accidentally left in the abdominal cavity. Ann. Surgery., *34:*498–523, 1901.

SCHLOSS, W. A. and SOLOMKIN, MARK: Removal of thermometer with Stern-McCarthy resectoscope. J.A.M.A., *143:*804–805, 1950.

SUBY, H. I. and ALBRIGHT, F.: Dissolution of phosphatic calculi by the retrograde introduction of a citrate solution containing magnesium. New England J. Med., *228:*81–91, 1940.

UPCHURCH, W. A. and UPCHURCH, W. E.: Unusual foreign body in bladder (gauze). Urol. & Cut. Rev., *37:*234, 1933.

WARING, T. P. and DRANE, R.: An ascending foreign body in the kidney pelvis. Am. J. Roentgenol., *28:*34–36, 1932.

WILHELMI, OTTO J.: Foreign body in the kidney. J. Urol., *43:*1, 1940.

INDEX TO
VOLUMES ONE, TWO AND THREE

(*Vol. One:* pp. 1 to 862. — *Vol. Two:* pp. 863 to 1665. — *Vol. Three:* pp. 1667 to 2356.)

1

Efferent nerves, function, 1257
Ejaculatory ducts, 34
    injury, epididymitis and, 950
    sealing of, sterility and, 444
Electrocardiogram, changes in potassium
        deficiency, 1710
    preoperative, 1703
Electrocautery, 1771
    of urethral caruncle, 1396
    of urethral mucosa in prolapse, 1396
Electrocoagulation of bladder tumor, 1077,
        2058
    of Skene's glands, 1581
Electroexcision of bladder papillomatosis,
        1074
    of bladder tumors, infiltrating, 1077
        noninfiltrating, 1073
Electroincision in bladder tumors, infil-
        trating, technique, 1077
Electrolyte balance, management, in renal
        insufficiency, 57
    in uremia, 2177
    metabolism, effect of cortisone and
        ACTH on, 1683
Electrourethrotomy in urethral stricture,
        2114
Elephantiasis in children, 1558
    nostra, 677
    of scrotum, 576, 677
    treatment, 579
Ellik evacuating syringe, 2024
Elliott machine, use of, in prostatitis, 640
Elliptical transplant, Nesbit, 1885
Embolism, arterial, 1752
    in hypertensive heart disease, treatment,
        2209
    postoperative, in suprapubic prostatec-
        tomy, prevention, 1952
Embryology
    of adrenals, 2285
    of bladder, 369
    of clitoris, 394
    of kidney, 233
    of labia majora, 394
    of male reproductive tract, 458
    of penis, 394
    of scrotum, 394
    of ureter, 307
    of urethra, 390
    of urogenital tract, 227–491
Embryonal sarcoma, 979
Embryonic cancer of kidney, 978
Emetine in amebiasis, 590
Emphysema of scrotum, 723
Empyema, postoperative, 1739
Encephalopathy, hypertensive, 2199
    symptoms, 2199
    in glomerulonephritis, acute, 2175
Encopresis, enuresis and, 1640
Endocrines
    control of water and salt, preoperative,
        1711

Endocrines (*continued*)
    prostatic hyperplasia and, 1107
        studies on, 1108, 1109
    therapy, effect on prostatic cancer, 1157
        metastases and, 1158
        of bladder tumors, 1089
Endocrinology in urology, 1667–1699
Endometriosis of bladder, 1062
    of kidney, 970
    of ureter, 1038
Endopelvic fascia, 34
Endoscopy in intersex diagnosis, 2108
Endothelioma of penis, 1179
    in children, 1627
Enuresis, 1634–1647
    cystometry in, 1642
    cysto-urethrography in, 1642
    diagnosis, 1641
    diurna, 1640
    etiology, 1635
    heredity, 1636
    incidence, 1635
    masturbation and, 1638
    neuromuscular vesical dysfunction and,
        1640
    nocturna, 1640
    obstruction and, 1640, 1647
    physiotherapy in, 1646
    prognosis, 1641
    prophylaxis, 1653
    psychiatric considerations, 1637
    psychotherapy in, 1639
    symptoms, 1640
    treatment, 1643
        behavior training, 1643, 1644
        drug therapy, 1643, 1645
        incontinence clamps, 1645
        urologic, 1646
    urethroscopy in, 1642
    urologic disease and, 1639
Environment, intersexuality and, 2103
Enzymes in prostatic fluid, 117
Eosinopenia in adrenal hemorrhage, 2303
    in Cushing's syndrome, 2313
Ephedrine, 1268
    in enuresis, 1646
Epidermophyton floccosum, 679
Epididymectomy, 2143
    complications, 949
    in epididymitis, 1566
        nonspecific, 695
        tuberculous, 701, 1576
    in tuberculosis, genital, 659
    prognosis after, 660
Epididymis, 31
    aberrant wolffian duct remnants in, 480
    amebiasis in, 590
    appendix, 32
    carcinoma of, 1245
    cysts of, 1248
    filariasis of, 573
    function, 739

Evisceration, postoperative, 1736
Examination
  cystoscopic, 167
    equipment for, 169
  history, 144
  instrumental, in children, 1461–1480
  physical, 153
    in children, 1438
  rectal, 155, 161
    in children, 1440
  urologic, 143–185. See also *Urologic examination.*
Examining table for cystoscopy in children, 1468
Excretory urography. See *Urography, excretory.*
Exercises for strengthening sphincter mechanism, 1424
Expandex in shock, 1732
Experimental data on cord bladder, 1286
  production of hypertension, 2185
  studies on temperature and scrotal function, 131
  on urinary tract absorption, 90
Exstrophy of bladder, 377
Extrarenal pelves, 294
Extravasation, urinary. See *Urinary extravasation.*
Extremities, examination of, 156
  lower, elastic bandaging, prophylactic, 1750

F

Facial contour, effect of cortisone and ACTH on, 1681
Facies, 154
Family history, 144
Fantus' test for urinary chlorides, 1705, 1708
Fascia, Buck's, 27
  Colles', 23
  endopelvic, 34
  Gerota's, 2
  lumbar, 10
  lumbodorsal, 10
  of Denonvilliers, 20, 34
  of Zuckerkandl, 2
  perirenal, 11
  rectovesical, 20
  renal, 2
  Scarpa's, 23
  transversalis, 16
  vesicopelvic, 20
Fat, perirenal, invasion of, 1528
Fatigue in hypertensive disease, 2197
Fecal impaction, postoperative, 1744
  masses vs. nephroma, 987
Female
  adrenal mixed syndrome in, 2326
  adrenogenital syndrome in, differential diagnosis, 2320
  bladder catheterization, technique, 1416

Female (*continued*)
  congenital urologic malformations in, 1388
  cystectomy in, 1913
  epispadias in, 418
  genitalia, schistosomiasis of, 569
  hypospadias in, 427
  prostate, 111
  pseudohermaphroditism, 1687, 2318
    treatment, 2321
  traumatic injuries of urinary tract, 1414–1420
  Trichomonas urethritis, in, 586
  ureteral obstruction in, 1399
  urinary infections in, 1403–1414
  urinary obstruction in, 1397
  urogenital tract, malformations of, 485
  urological symptoms in, interpretation, 1385, 1387
    renal, 1385
  urology in, 1385–1429
Feminization in males, 2331
Fertility. See also *Infertility.*
  following operations for cryptorchidism, 478
  history taking, 740
  methods of evaluating, 740
  reduced, treatment, methods of, 757
    surgical, 763
Fetal lobulation, 266
Fever
  evaluation, 152
  in children, 1436
  in glomerulonephritis, 2171
  in hypernephroma, 974
  in nephroma, 984
  in perinephritis, 515
  in pyelitis of pregnancy, 1405
  in renal adenocarcinoma, 977
  in renal infarction, 1522
  in renal tuberculosis, 541
  in urinary infections, 1409
  induced, in hypertension treatment, 2204
  postoperative, 1739, 1750
    list of possible causes, 1740
  with kidney tumors, 956
Fibrin calculi, 774
Fibrinogenase in prostatic fluid, 117
Fibrinolysin in prostatic fluid, 117
Fibroma of spermatic cord, 1235
  of testicular tunics, 1247
  of tunica albuginea, 1248
Filariasis, 570
  chylocele in, 722
  genital, 571
  of spermatic cord, 702
  symptoms, 572
  pathology, 571
Finney type of pyloroplasty, 1811
Fistula
  due to irradiation, 1419
  of bladder, 1922

Tunica vaginalis, in children, 1627
  sarcoma of, 1247
  tumors of, classification, 1246
    malignant, 1247
Tunics, infections of, 705
  proliferous periorchitis of, 706
Turner's syndrome in male, 1592

U

Ulcer, chancroid, treatment, 671
  Hunner's elusive, 172
Ulceration of external meatus, 1543
  of penis, 610
Ulcus molle phagedenicum, 670
Umbilicus, infection, 1534
  pain at, in horseshoe kidney, 272
Undecylenic acid, 679, 680
Urachus, 369
  cysts, 388, 1931
    differential diagnosis, 389
  patent, 389
    treatment, 1931
  tumors of, 1062
Urate calculi, 773
  test for, 795
Urea as diuretic, 2176
  clearance test, 46
    in glomerulonephritis, acute, 2171
  excretion, 43
  in blood, normal, 43
  in tubular reabsorption, 38
  nitrogen, blood, in childhood, 2225
    excretion, 43
    normal value, 43
Urea-splitting organisms, calculi formation
  and, 770
Urecholine, 1282, 1745
  for bladder tonicity, 2016
Uremia, 152
  benzodioxane test in, 2341
  definition, 2196
  in childhood, 1437, 1493
  in hypertensive disease, treatment, 2207
  in nephritis, chronic, 2176
  postoperative, 1732
  preoperative, care in, 1722
  symptoms, 152, 1734, 2196
  with valvular urethral obstruction, 439
Ureter
  agenesis, bilateral, 309
    unilateral, 309
  anastomosis, end-in-end, 1865
    end-to-end, 1865
  anatomy, 11
  anomalies, 308
    classification, 308
    of number, 309
    of form, 340
    of origin and termination, 314
  aplasia, 340
  areas of constriction, 12
  arteries of, 14

Ureter (*continued*)
  atony, primary, 359
  blind ending, 336
  blood supply of, 14, 17
  bud, 234
  calculi, 813. See also *Calculi, ureteral.*
    in childhood, 1611
      treatment, 1616
        surgical, 1616
    manipulation in, 819–821
      contraindications, 822
    pain in, 148
  catheterization, 176
    in childhood, 1470–1480
      reactions, 1480
      retrograde pyelography, 1472
      technique, 1470
    in kidney injuries, 877
  catheters, 165, 1462
    passage of, in children, 1599
    sterilization of, 169
  circumcaval, 1860
  colic, 1609
  congenital high insertion of, 336
  course of, 13
  cyst, intravesical, 324
  deligation, 1856
  dilatation of, 1361
    due to stricture, 343
    in pregnancy, 1404
      causes, 1405
    nonobstructive, 1362
    obstructive, 1361
      treatment, 1364
  dilation of stricture, 349
    caution in, 353
  diverticulum of, 363
  double, 309
  drainage, methods, 1406
  dynamic sections of, 65
  dynamics of, roentgenocinematography
    of, 66
  ectopic, 314
    diagnosis, 321
    etiology, 315
    pathology, 319
    symptoms, 320
    treatment, 322
  embryology, 234, 307
  empyema of, 1850
  endometriosis of, 1038
  exposure, 1843
    transvaginal, 1847
  fission of, 310, 311
  foreign bodies in, 850
  herniation of, 339
  in vesical reduplication, 372
  incisions, 15, 1843
  infection of, in children, 1529
  injuries of, 885–908, 1417
    anuria in, 1418
    calculus and, 896